Nutrition & Wellness for Life

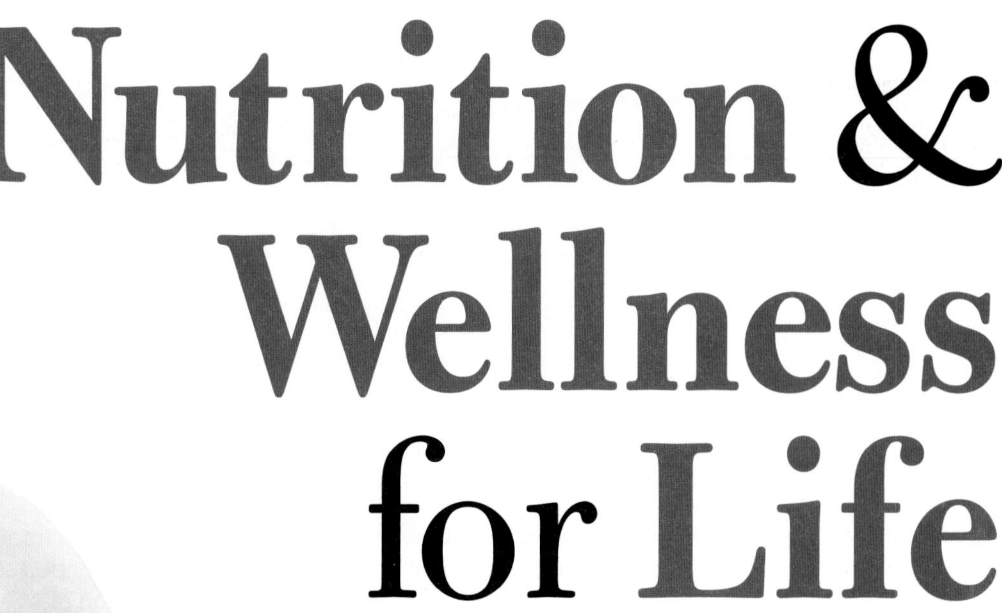

FIFTH EDITION

by
Dorothy F. West, PhD, CNWE
Food and Nutrition Author and Educator
Lansing, Michigan

Contributing Authors

Cindi Calhoun, MPH
Food and Nutrition Educator
Palisades Charter High School
Playa Vista, California

Jessica Peconi-Cook, MSS
Executive Director
Pennsylvania State Association for Health, Physical Education, Recreation, and Dance (PSAHPERD)
Pittsburgh, Pennsylvania

Publisher
The Goodheart-Willcox Company, Inc.
Tinley Park, Illinois
www.g-w.com

Previously published as *Nutrition, Food, and Fitness*
Formerly published as *Nutrition and Fitness: Lifestyle Choices for Wellness*
Previous editions copyright 2012, 2010, 2008, 2006, 2004, 2000

Manufactured in the United States of America.

ISBN 978-1-63563-076-3

1 2 3 4 5 6 7 8 9 – 19 – 23 22 21 20 19 18

Cover image: Olef/Shutterstock.com

Feature images—Case Study: gagarych/Shutterstock.com; Community Connections: irfan firdaus/Shutterstock.com; Extend Your Knowledge: Nizwa Design/Shutterstock.com; Featured Career: dizain/Shutterstock.com; Food and the Environment: Nizwa Design/Shutterstock.com; Recipe File: vickyphoto/Shutterstock.com; Wellness Tip: Tefi/Shutterstock.com

Features

Infographics

What's Your Nutrition and Wellness IQ?

UNIT 3 Managing Your Nutrition

UNIT 4 Serving Up Nutrition

Contents

Brief Contents

Reviewers

Goodheart-Willcox Publisher would like to thank the following teachers who reviewed selected chapters and contributed valuable input into the development of ***Nutrition & Wellness for Life.***

Donna Bixby-Stephens
Southwest High School
San Antonio, Texas

Cindi Calhoun
Palisades Charter High School
Playa Vista, California

Elizabeth Christensen
Osbourn Park High School
Woodbridge, Virginia

Alyssa Foote
Benjamin Logan High School
Arlington, Ohio

Karen Gay
General William J. Palmer High School
Colorado Springs, Colorado

Cheryl Landers
Grandview High School
La Tour, Missouri

Precision Exams Certification

Nutrition & Wellness for Life explores the knowledge and skills needed for successful careers in Food and Nutrition. Goodheart-Willcox is pleased to partner with Precision Exams by correlating *Nutrition & Wellness for Life* to Precision Exams' Food and Nutrition II Standards. Precision Exams' Standards and Career Skill Exams were created in concert with industry and subject matter experts to match real-world job skills and marketplace demands. Students who pass both the written and performance portions of the exam can earn a Career Skills Certification™. To see how *Nutrition & Wellness for Life* correlates to the Precision Exams Standards, please see the *Nutrition & Wellness for Life* correlations at www.g-w.com/nutrition-wellness-for-life-2019 and click on the Correlations tab. For more information on Precision Exams, please consult the accompanying *Nutrition & Wellness for Life Instructor's Resources* or go to www.precisionexams.com.

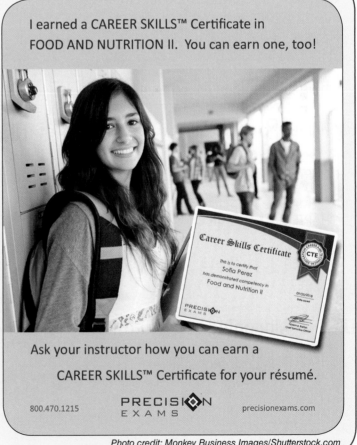

Photo credit: Monkey Business Images/Shutterstock.com

About the Authors

Dorothy West earned a bachelor's degree in dietetics and a master's degree in teacher education with an emphasis on family and consumer sciences from Pennsylvania State University. Dorothy received her doctorate in teacher education with an emphasis on home economics secondary education and family resource management from Michigan State University. She remained on the faculty there for over thirty years instructing both undergraduate and graduate courses in family and consumer sciences. She has developed and taught courses on curriculum, evaluation, and strategies for teaching nutrition at the secondary level. Dorothy played an active role in writing nutrition curriculum for the Michigan State Department of Education.

Dorothy has taught in the Netherlands, Okinawa, and England. She served as chairperson of the Social Sciences Department at the LCC International University in Lithuania and taught foods courses at Kodaikanal International School in India. She played a role in the development of the International Baccalaureate (IB) middle school food technology curriculum materials. During her career, Dorothy has been active in membership and leadership roles with the Michigan Association of Family and Consumer Sciences (MAFCS) and American Association of Family and Consumer Sciences (AAFCS). In 2017, she earned the Certified Nutrition and Wellness Educator (CNWE) credential.

Cindi Calhoun attended University of California, Los Angeles where she earned a bachelor's degree in anthropology and a master of public health with a focus on epidemiology to study health curriculum to reduce high risk behaviors in elementary and middle school students. She currently teaches classes in food preparation and nutrition principles at Palisades Charter High School.

Jessica Peconi-Cook authored the *Movement Connection* features found in each chapter. Jessica earned her bachelor of science degree in health and physical education from Slippery Rock University and a master of science in sport science from Indiana University of Pennsylvania. She taught physical education at Mt. Lebanon School District and now serves as Executive Director for the Pennsylvania State Association for Health, Physical Education, Recreation, and Dance.

Introduction

Nutrition & Wellness for Life stresses the importance of a nutritious eating plan and daily physical activity throughout the life span. The text will help you understand how decisions you make today affect your state of wellness at various stages of the life cycle.

The body's need for various nutrients may be greater at certain stages of the life cycle. This text helps you understand the sources and functions of the nutrients your body requires for a lifetime of optimal health. You will learn how to achieve healthy weight and body composition by balancing energy. The text also discusses the health consequences of unhealthy eating and exercise patterns.

Nutrition & Wellness for Life explores strategies for staying physically active through the life span. It covers the special needs of the competitive athlete. The text also discusses the relationship between social and mental health and your nutrition and activity. You will learn to recognize sources of stress and healthy strategies for reducing their impact on your total wellness.

Healthy eating requires planning and preparation. The text discusses safe food handling as well as planning, shopping for, and preparing healthy meals.

RECIPE FILE

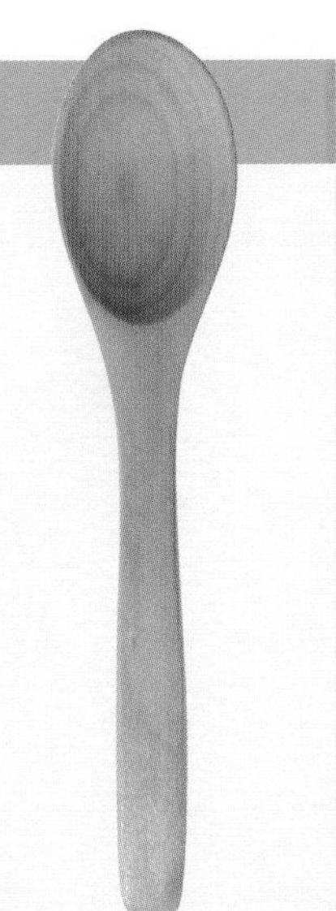

THE MOVEMENT CONNECTION

WELLNESS TIP

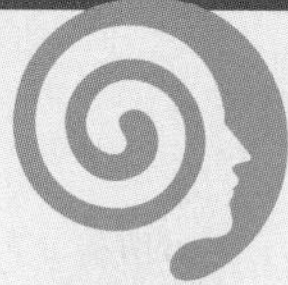

EXTEND YOUR KNOWLEDGE

FOOD AND THE ENVIRONMENT

COMMUNITY CONNECTIONS

CASE STUDY

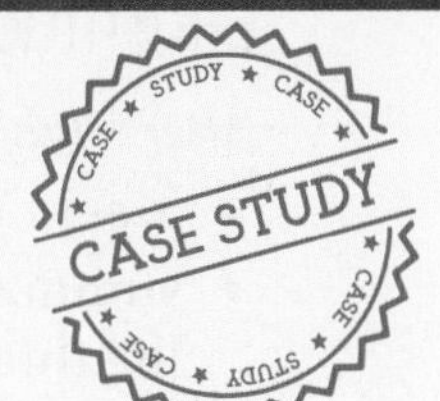

FEATURED CAREER

Making Wellness a Lifestyle

Learning Outcomes

After studying this chapter, you will be able to

- **assess** your location on the wellness continuum;
- **summarize** how physical, mental, and social aspects of wellness affect quality of life throughout the life span;
- **recall** factors that contribute to disease;
- **distinguish** those factors that affect wellness over which you have control;
- **judge** how your lifestyle choices affect your health now and in the future;
- **implement** a behavior-change contract to improve your health;
- **evaluate** the importance of nutrition and wellness research for changing wellness behaviors; and
- **understand** why use of the scientific process is important when conducting nutrition research.

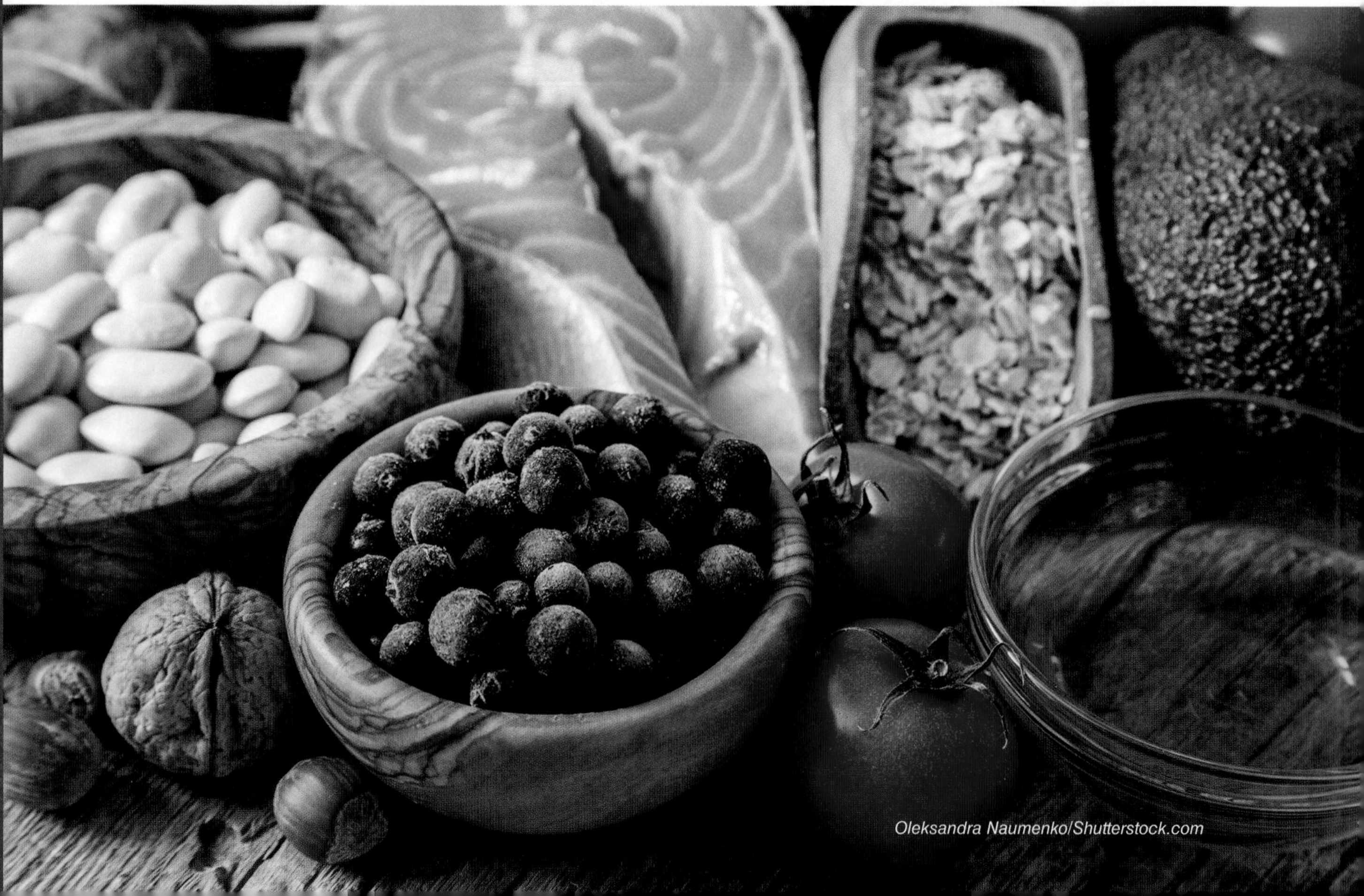

Oleksandra Naumenko/Shutterstock.com

Content Terms 

diagnosis
eating pattern
environmental quality
holistic medicine
hypothesis
life expectancy
mental health
nutrient
nutrition
optimum health
peer pressure
physical health
premature death
quality of life
risk factor
scientific method
social health
theory
wellness

Academic Terms 

chronic
diminished
endeavor
impair
induce

What's Your Nutrition and Wellness IQ?

Take this quiz to examine how much you already know about the relationship of lifestyle choices to wellness outcomes. If you cannot answer a question, pay extra attention to that topic as you study this chapter.

- Identify each statement as *True*, *False*, or *It Depends*. *It Depends* means in some cases the statement is true; in some cases it could be false.
- Revise false statements to make them true.
- Explain the circumstances in which each *It Depends* statement is true and when it is false.

Nutrition and Wellness IQ 

	Statement			
1.	Social health, mental health, and physical health are equally important for lifelong personal wellness outcomes.	True	False	It Depends
2.	Most people find themselves at one end of the wellness continuum or the other.	True	False	It Depends
3.	Genetics is the biggest factor for determining life expectancy.	True	False	It Depends
4.	Many chronic diseases can be prevented.	True	False	It Depends
5.	Eating patterns, activity levels, and tobacco usage are directly related to wellness outcomes.	True	False	It Depends
6.	Peer pressure has little to do with wellness.	True	False	It Depends
7.	The scientific methods used in nutrition research always start with stating a hypothesis.	True	False	It Depends
8.	Obesity is directly related to increased medical costs both for the individual and for society.	True	False	It Depends

While studying this chapter, look for the activity icon  **to**

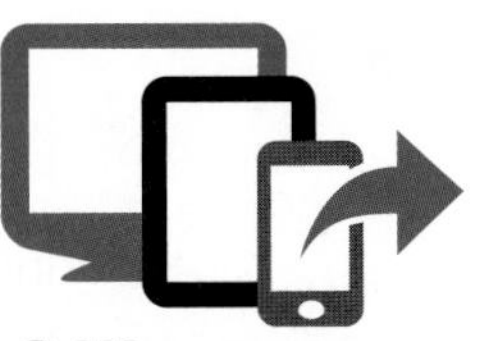

- **build** vocabulary with e-flash cards and interactive games;
- **assess** what you learn by completing self-assessment quizzes and completing review questions; and
- **expand** knowledge with interactive activities and activities that extend learning.

www.g-wlearning.com/foodsandnutrition/

You make choices every day that affect how you feel, think, and act. You decide what you will eat and when you will sleep. You choose how physically active you will be, too. Your actions affect who you are now and the person you will become. You are responsible for making decisions that benefit your health.

How healthy will you be 10 years from now? You could be healthier and in better physical shape than you are now! Choosing behaviors that promote health can have lifelong benefits. You can take steps to feel just as fit at age 50 as you do at age 15.

What Is Wellness?

Wellness is the state of being in good health. Your level of wellness contributes to your quality of life. ***Quality of life*** refers to a person's satisfaction with his or her looks, lifestyle, and responses to daily events. When people are in good health, they have a desire to stay fit and live a healthful lifestyle. They are energetic and have an enthusiastic outlook. They are able to successfully meet the challenges of each day. When people are not in good health, life's events can become harder to manage. This causes a decrease in quality of life. Most people want to improve their state of wellness and live a fulfilling life. Making choices that promote wellness is a way to improve your quality of life.

You can use a continuum to determine your personal state of wellness. Premature death is at one end of the continuum and optimum health is at the other. ***Premature death*** is death that occurs earlier than expected due to lifestyle behaviors that lead to a fatal accident or the development of an avoidable disease. The Centers for Disease Control and Prevention (CDC) reports that nearly 20 to 40 percent of premature deaths could be prevented. ***Optimum health*** is a state of wellness characterized by peak physical, mental, and social well-being (**Figure 1.1**).

Your health status determines your place along the wellness continuum. Being free from illness and having much energy indicate that you have a high level of physical wellness. If you are able to cope with life's challenges and maintain stable relationships, you exhibit mental and social wellness, too. This means you probably fall near the optimum health end of the continuum. A short-term decline in any of these areas may temporarily move you toward the other end of the continuum; however, the key is your overall state of health most of the time. This is your wellness point.

Figure 1.1
Evaluate your physical, mental, and social health to determine where you fall along the wellness continuum.

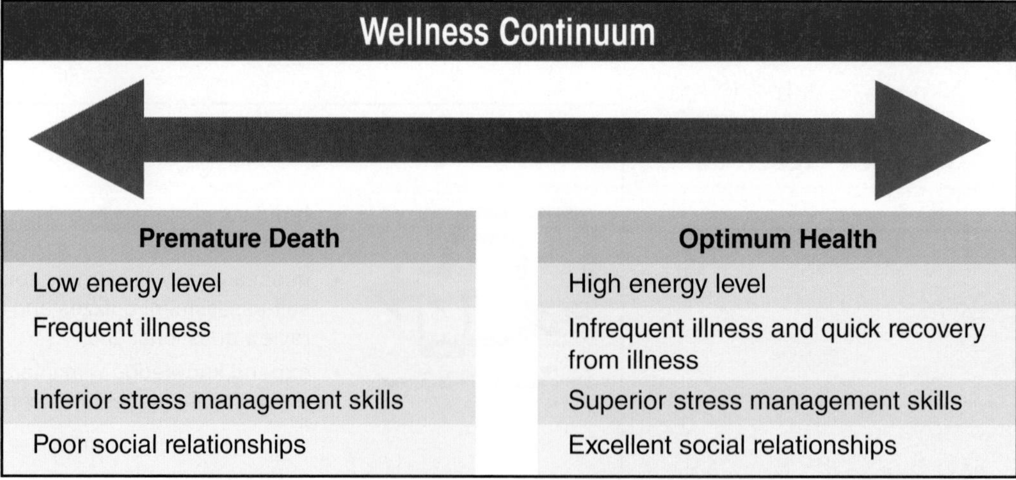

Premature Death	Optimum Health
Low energy level	High energy level
Frequent illness	Infrequent illness and quick recovery from illness
Inferior stress management skills	Superior stress management skills
Poor social relationships	Excellent social relationships

If you are already at optimum health, you will want to find out how to maintain this state of wellness. If you are not at optimum health, you can learn how to change your lifestyle to move toward that goal. The key to achieving wellness is accepting responsibility for your health. No one can force you to change. Moving toward optimum health happens when you want change to occur.

Once you begin taking steps to improve your health, you will start to notice the benefits. You might feel stronger and more alert. Maybe you will find it easier to cope with the daily problems of life. Perhaps you will feel more confident about your performance at home, school, work, and play. You may begin to experience better relationships with family members and friends. You may notice additional benefits of wellness in the future. Having optimum health will help you face the challenges of parenthood, career changes, and other aspects of active adult living.

Aspects of Wellness

Wellness means much more than being free from illness. It is more than eating healthful foods and being physically fit. Three major components—physical, mental, and social health—contribute to your state of wellness. Each component affects the others and your overall sense of wellness. Together, they influence how you look, feel, and act.

Physical Health

Physical health refers to the fitness of your body. It is achieved when numerous body parts work in harmony.

A number of factors can harm your physical health. For instance, getting insufficient rest can reduce your energy for exercising and doing chores. Eating too much or too fast may upset your stomach. Lack of physical activity, poor sanitation, and reckless actions can also keep your body below peak performance level. Too much stress can negatively impact your physical health. *Stress* is the inner agitation you feel in response to change. Tobacco, alcohol, and other drugs can harm physical health, too. Choosing lifestyle behaviors that avoid these factors will help you stay in good physical health (**Figure 1.2**).

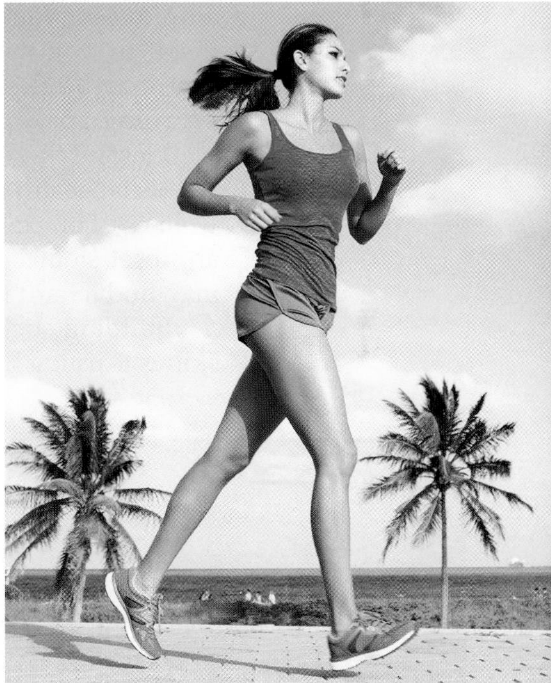

Matthew Ennis/Shutterstock.com

Figure 1.2 Getting regular exercise is an important requirement for maintaining good physical health. *What are other lifestyle behaviors that promote physical health?*

Healthcare professionals use medicine, physical therapy, diet, and surgery to care for the physical health of their patients. They stay informed on research about alternative treatments, such as the use of herbs and nutrient supplements. As healthcare costs rise, people are becoming more interested in learning how to prevent disease. Doctors often suggest that patients combine medical care with lifestyle changes. You will read more about making lifestyle changes later in this chapter.

Mental Health

Have you ever felt stressed, depressed, and emotionally exhausted? These feelings may be related to your current state of mental health. ***Mental health*** has to do with the way you feel about yourself, your life, and the people around you. People with good mental health generally like themselves for who they are.

They express positive attitudes and work to keep all social, physical, spiritual, and emotional aspects of their life in balance. They tend to act according to a set of socially acceptable values. They may also hold beliefs that help them see their relationship to a larger universe. When problems arise, people who are mentally healthy seek ways to resolve them.

Irrational fears, anxiety, and depression may be signs of a mental health problem (**Figure 1.3**). If you are concerned about your mental health, you should talk to a trusted adult. Share concerns and problems with parents, teachers, counselors, or clergypersons. These people may be able to help you better understand who you are and what you want to become. Building effective communication and problem-solving skills can help you improve your mental health.

Social Health

Social health describes the way you get along with other people. Friends and family members enrich your life. Social health can be negatively affected when disagreements occur and problems arise. Learning to resolve conflicts with others is an important skill that can help you achieve and maintain good social health.

Social health is related to an understanding and acceptance of roles. People have different role expectations for sons, daughters, husbands, wives, mothers, fathers, girlfriends, boyfriends, teachers, students, employers, and employees. You may want to analyze your roles for possible conflicts. For instance, you may be expected to be a follower in your role as an employee. You may be expected to be a leader, however, in your role as team captain. Learning appropriate ways to act in each role can contribute to your social wellness.

Social health affects a person's outlook on life and his or her personal state of wellness. For example, a teen on a first date might become so nervous that he gets an upset stomach. A student who worries about being accepted among friends may find it hard to fall asleep at night.

Building social skills allows you to improve your social health. One such skill is learning how to use good communication to resolve conflicts with others.

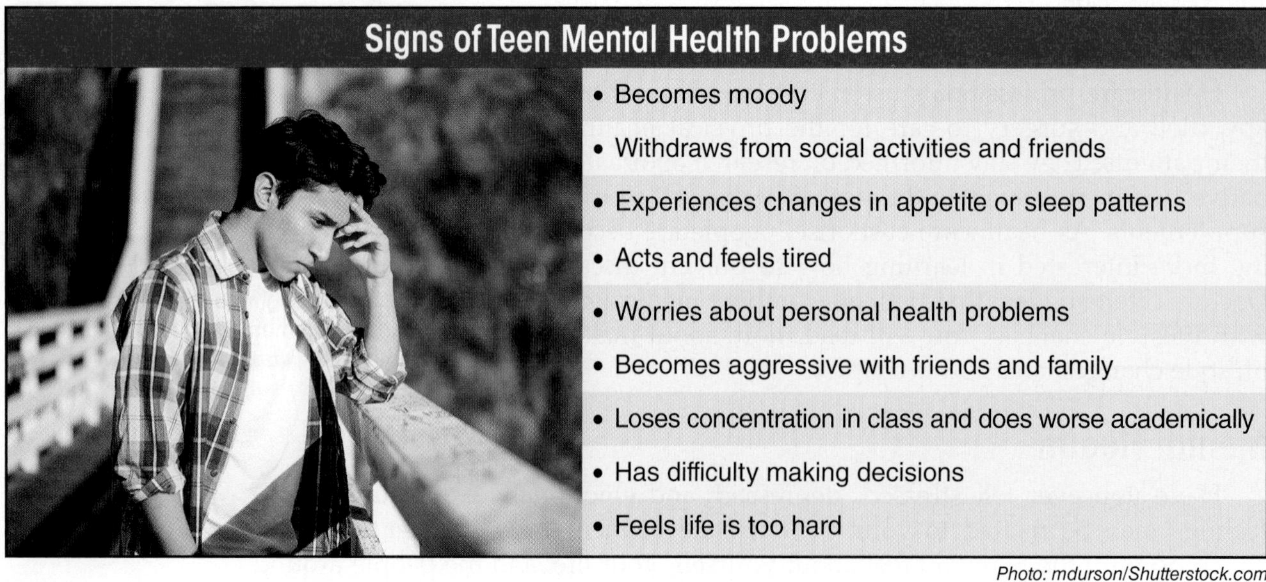

Signs of Teen Mental Health Problems
• Becomes moody
• Withdraws from social activities and friends
• Experiences changes in appetite or sleep patterns
• Acts and feels tired
• Worries about personal health problems
• Becomes aggressive with friends and family
• Loses concentration in class and does worse academically
• Has difficulty making decisions
• Feels life is too hard

Photo: mdurson/Shutterstock.com

Figure 1.3 A teen who is exhibiting these warning signs may need help.

THE MOVEMENT CONNECTION

Begin with Posture

Why

Chances are good that you are sitting as you read this. Most of us sit when we read, study, and attend class. Too much sitting can lead to tight hamstrings, hip flexors, shoulders, chest, and neck. The activity bursts in *The Movement Connection* features found throughout this text will help combat the negative impacts of too much sitting. These activities are designed to help re-energize your brain so you can focus and learn.

As explained in this chapter, wellness is a combination of good mental, physical, and social health. These components of wellness range on a continuum from premature death to optimal health. Oftentimes we put more emphasis on one area of wellness than the others. It is important to remember, it is about balance! Wellness is best achieved when we give equal attention to all three.

Good posture is fundamental to wellness. By standing with good posture, we decrease unnecessary stress on joints, ligaments, and bones that might otherwise occur as we begin to move.

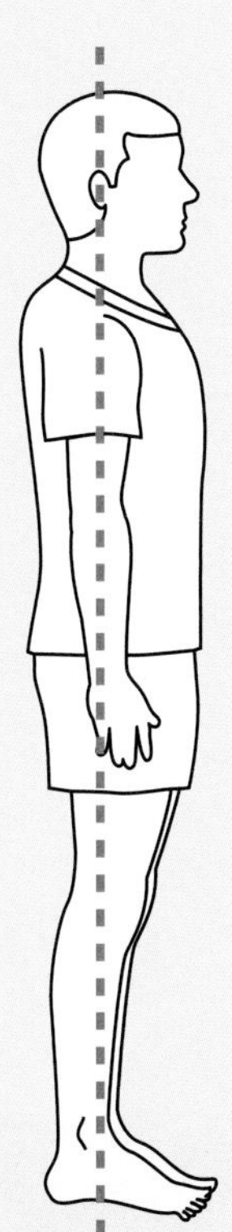

Apply

Assume a standing position with weight evenly distributed in both feet. Stand so your hips are stacked over your feet, your shoulders are over your hips, and your neck is straight with your head facing forward (your chin should be parallel to the ground).

Tighten your stomach muscles as if to squeeze your belly button toward your spine. This movement engages your core muscles.

Standing with good posture, slowly breathe in for 5 seconds and out for 6 seconds. Repeat three times. Slow, deliberate breathing can lower heart rate and calm the mind, helping you to relax.

Standing after a long period of sitting allows blood to flow and the brain to feel more alert.

Seeking and lending support to people who need your help is another important social skill. Building a positive self-image will also help you improve your relationships. Developing these skills will help you reach optimum social health. Reaching this optimum level means you can work, play, and interact with others cooperatively. Optimum social health contributes to your states of physical and mental health, too.

Learning how people develop physically, mentally, and socially can positively affect your sense of wellness. This knowledge may give you some sense of reassurance as you continue to develop and mature over your life span.

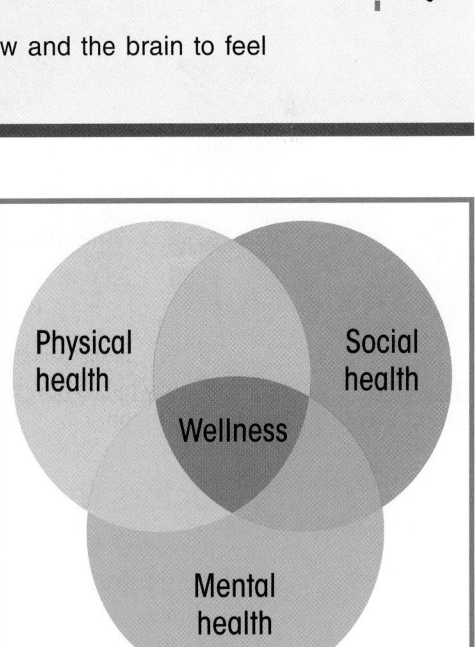

Figure 1.4 Physical, mental, and social health all contribute to a total sense of wellness. *Which component do you feel you could improve?*

Holistic Approach to Wellness

Holistic medicine is an approach to healthcare that focuses on all aspects of patient care—physical, mental, and social. It evolved because many medical doctors saw links among physical, mental, and social health (**Figure 1.4**).

Treatment programs and medicine may not be enough to cure a physical illness. The effect of physical treatment can depend on mental and social health. Low self-esteem or loneliness can reduce a person's desire to get better. These factors can **impair** (damage) the body's immune system and delay the healing process.

The trend is for healthcare professionals to work in teams to treat illness. This provides greater insight for understanding the various components of how best to help a patient. Specialists, consultants, and mental health professionals work with each other to understand the various aspects of treatment to improve patient health.

As an individual, your holistic approach to wellness must be well rounded. You need to be aware of your physical, mental, and social health needs. You must manage time, money, and other resources to address your needs in all of these areas. If you spend all of your time working out, you may end up neglecting relationships. This would cause your social health to suffer at the expense of your physical health. If you spend all of your money going out with friends, you may feel anxious because you cannot repay the money you borrowed from your parents to buy new sports equipment. Your state of mental health may be reduced in favor of your social health.

Taking a holistic approach to wellness means making choices that fit together to promote all facets of health.

Factors That Affect Wellness

Why is it important to recognize the impact of health-related decisions made in the teen years? The reason is that your present actions and attitudes are shaping the person you will be in the future (**Figure 1.5**). Habits are hard to change once established. This is true for good habits as well as bad habits. Once you perform an unhealthful behavior, you are more likely to repeat it. Likewise, once you choose a healthful behavior, you can easily make it a regular part of your life.

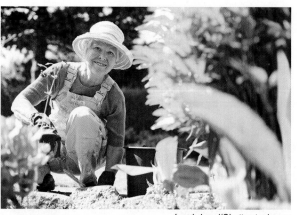

Jacob Lund/Shutterstock.com

Figure 1.5 Establishing healthy habits now will improve your quality of life in older adulthood.

Because you are responsible for making many decisions, you have much control over your personal state of wellness. You can engage in activities that lead to the decline of your health. You can also follow practices that help ensure good health.

Improving your odds for a long and healthful life requires an understanding of the consequences of poor choices. It also involves recognizing wise choices. Learning about exercise, healthcare, and which foods best nourish your body will aid you in making wise choices.

Factors That Contribute to Disease

A ***risk factor*** is a characteristic or behavior that influences a person's chance of being injured or getting a disease. Researchers identify risk factors by studying the traits and actions of large groups of people. Then the researchers determine what effects these traits and behaviors have on the people's health.

Certain lifestyle habits, environmental conditions, and healthcare limitations are known to be risk factors you can control. Hereditary factors affect your risk of disease, too. Genetic research continues to explore ways to help people avoid or delay the onset of inherited diseases. Heredity continues to be a factor that alerts people to their risk factors for specific diseases, however. Knowing your risk factors can encourage early prevention.

COMMUNITY CONNECTIONS

The Rewards of Volunteering

Do you believe people have a responsibility to help one another? If so, volunteering in your community is one way to make a difference in the lives of people who need help.

A *volunteer* is someone who chooses to act when a need is recognized and has no expectation of payment. When you volunteer, you have the opportunity to create positive change for others, as well as yourself. For instance, volunteering can provide you with hands-on learning experiences that may prepare you for a job. You may gain insight into how government funds finance agency work. Demonstrating dependability and responsibility is important for successful volunteering that potential employers will also value. These experiences can be used to build your résumé.

When volunteering, you will most likely meet and work with people from backgrounds that are different from your own. Working with diverse populations helps you develop and expand your cultural awareness. The hands-on experience gained and interpersonal skills learned during volunteering will give you an advantage when applying for jobs.

Volunteer experiences often provide opportunities for you to develop your teamwork and leadership skills. As you learn what is unique and special about your skills and talents, your confidence builds. This confidence is an important prerequisite for any career path you choose.

Many nonprofit organizations and agencies are very happy to have teens volunteer their services. Beyond gaining valuable job skills, teens report a growing sense of fulfillment, satisfaction, and "doing good" in the world. Volunteering can be as simple as collecting food to donate to a soup kitchen, or as involved as organizing a food drive for the local food bank.

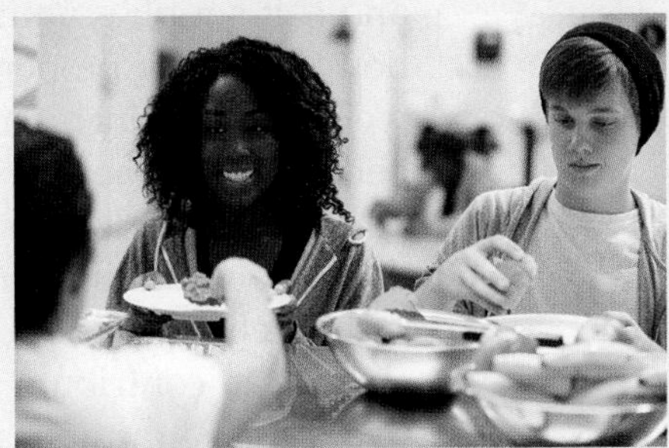

Monkey Business Images/Shutterstock.com

Volunteering in a community agency or organization can help you organize your thoughts about your career path. For instance, you may discover that you like helping people solve social or emotional problems. Or perhaps you will learn that you enjoy helping construct and reorganize the physical environment. These experiences allow you to explore what interests you the most.

Think Critically

1. In group discussion, identify which rewards and benefits of volunteering are of greatest importance for most teens. Explain why these rewards and benefits are important.
2. Provide examples of specific skills and abilities that a teen might have that could be applied to a volunteer situation. Then, list the skills you personally could bring to a volunteer position. Identify a volunteer experience that would be a good match for your interests and abilities. Research the steps required to participate in this experience.

Unhealthful Lifestyle Choices

Heart disease, cancer, **chronic** (recurring) lower respiratory diseases, unintentional injuries, and stroke are five major causes of death among adults in the United States. The Centers for Disease Control and Prevention (CDC) stresses the power of prevention through lifestyle choices across the life span. Many chronic diseases are preventable. Measures you can take to prevent these diseases are powerful wellness factors. Lifestyle choices account for more than half of the factors contributing to disease. One example of an important lifestyle choice is your decision about smoking. Smoking is a risk factor for cancer and heart disease. If you choose to smoke, you are at increased risk of getting these diseases.

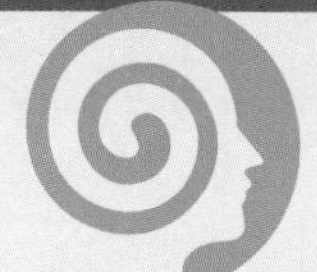

EXTEND YOUR KNOWLEDGE

Locate Community Wellness Resources

Complete an investigative inquiry about a health club, healthcare clinic, wellness center, or other community facility concerned with the health of citizens. Write a brief description stating who is encouraged to use this resource and how much it costs. Also, specify what services the center or agency provides and the expected benefits of participation.

Create a community wellness resource blog describing available activities, as well as locations where wellness activities occur. This may require a visit to the facilities to learn more about their goals, ease of use, requirements for membership, fee structure, and feedback from current users of the facility.

Write a description of each activity or facility, and include links to any online information you may find about wellness options in your community. Build your blog as you continue to gather new information. Consider how you will promote your blog to people in the community.

Other lifestyle choices include decisions about the foods you eat, seat belt use, texting while driving, alcohol consumption, use of drugs, stress management, and exercise. In these areas, you should avoid choices that increase your risk of disease and poor health outcomes.

Eating large amounts of fast foods that are high in saturated fats, added sugars, and salt supplies your body with many calories, but it provides little else that the body needs for proper growth and development. Excess calories contribute to overweight, which increases the risk for many diseases. Inappropriate and illegal driving behaviors all too often result in fatalities. Alcohol and drug misuse create health and social problems for the individual misusing these substances, their family, and their friends. Failing to manage your time can increase your stress level, which can negatively affect your health. Spending little time being active or participating in sports can contribute to weight problems and other health risks. Learning how to avoid unhealthful lifestyle choices is a powerful wellness life skill (**Figure 1.6**).

Poor Environmental Quality

Have you noticed that when your classroom is hot and stuffy, your concentration on learning decreases? While your health may not be in danger in this environment, your learning ability may be **diminished** (reduced). This is one example of how environmental factors affect quality of life.

Other, more serious environmental factors can cause significant illness or death. The National Cancer Institute at the National Institutes of Health reports that exposure to poor environmental quality may be responsible for as little as 4 percent or as much as 19 percent of all cancers. ***Environmental quality*** refers to the state of the physical world around you. It relates to the safety of the water you drink, the air you breathe, and the food you eat, as well as your exposure to the elements, such as the sun's ultraviolet rays.

Pollutants in the water and air, and contaminants in food decrease the quality of the environment. Consuming polluted water or contaminated food, or breathing polluted air can cause illness. In countries where food, water, and shelter are scarce or unsafe, the quality of life is greatly reduced because of poor environmental quality.

Some jobs require people to assume greater environmental health risks than others. You may want to think about the safety of various work environments as you evaluate career choices. Compare the job of an urban construction worker with that of a sales representative. What environmental risk factors can you identify in each job? Jobs that require the use of heavy equipment and exposure to dangerous conditions add risk to health and safety.

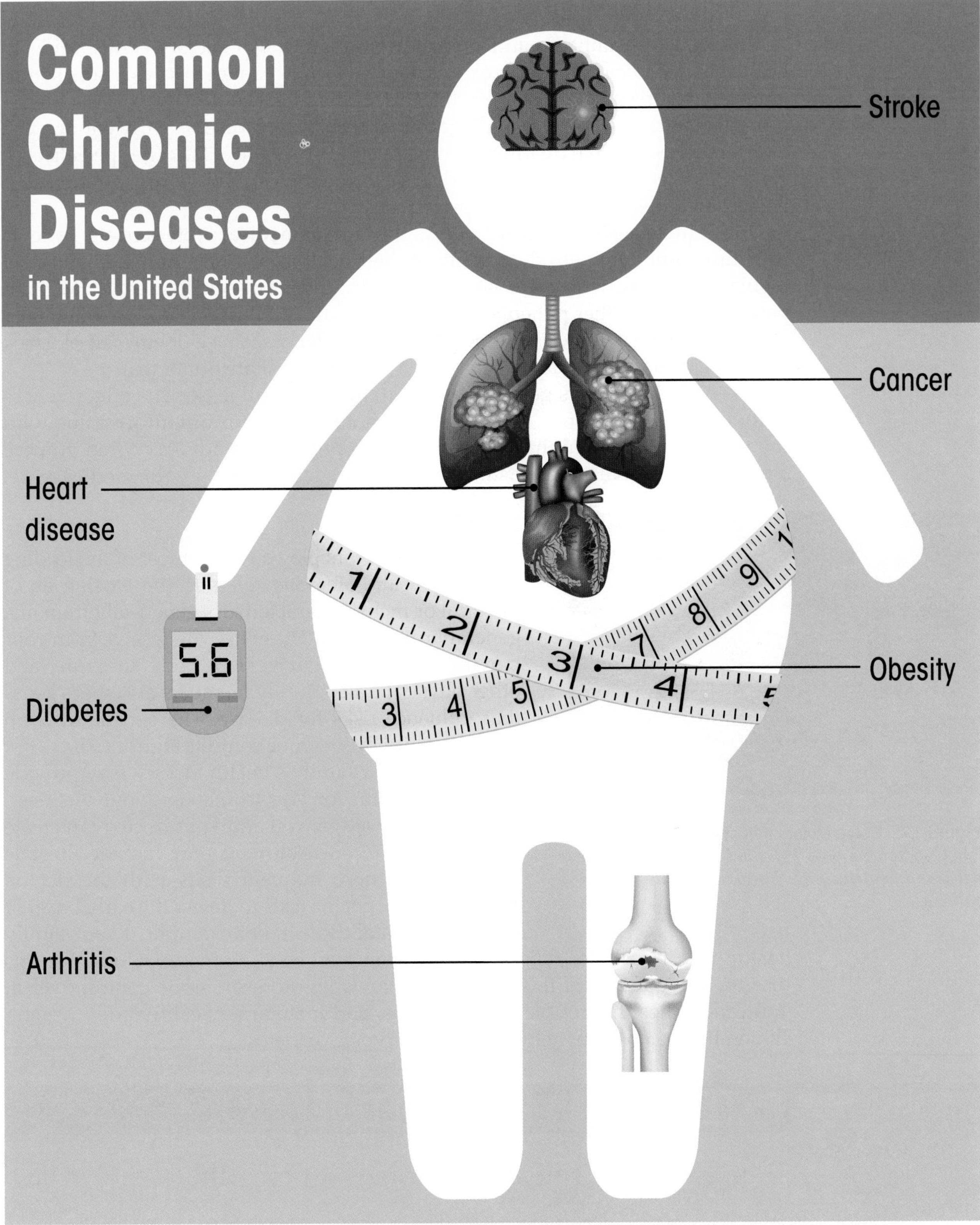

Body figure: vadim-design/Shutterstock.com; Top to bottom: ann131313/Shutterstock.com; BlueRingMedia/Shutterstock.com; Tefi/Shutterstock.com; Thana Thanawong/Shutterstock.com; wiki/Shutterstock.com; Designua/Shutterstock.com

Figure 1.6 The Centers for Disease Control and Prevention (CDC) estimates that changes in lifestyle, including elimination of poor diet, inactivity, and smoking, could prevent 80 percent of all heart disease, stroke, and type 2 diabetes, as well as more than 40 percent of cancers.

Inadequate Healthcare

Inadequate healthcare and medical errors are major factors contributing to health risk. Medicine is not an exact science. Doctors cannot always assess symptoms and test results to easily reach a correct diagnosis. A ***diagnosis*** is the identification of a disease. Failing to diagnose, or recognize, a disease early enough can interfere with effective treatment. Some healthcare facilities lack the specialists or equipment needed to treat certain diseases. Sometimes facilities are not managed well, or treatments are not given properly.

Inadequate healthcare is not always the fault of medical professionals. Patients sometimes interfere with the quality of their healthcare. Some patients fail to get regular checkups, which are needed to help physicians evaluate and maintain patients' health. Other patients do not seek medical care soon enough when they are experiencing symptoms. Some patients may delay seeing a doctor due to a lack of health insurance or inability to pay. Others may hesitate out of fear.

Even when patients go to a physician, they can still lessen the effectiveness of their care. For instance, patients might not share important information with the physician. They might fail to follow the physician's advice. When you are a patient, you have a responsibility to play an active role in your medical care.

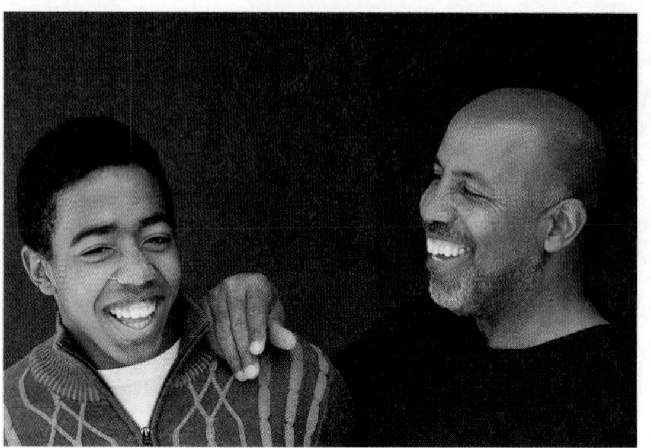

pixelheadphoto digitalskillet/Shutterstock.com

Figure 1.7 Some factors that affect health are inherited from parents. *Why is it important to be aware of health issues known to recur in your family?*

Heredity

Inherited factors play a role in most of the leading causes of death. Heredity refers to the passing on of physical or mental characteristics genetically from one generation to another. The genes you receive from your parents determine your gender, body structure, and other physical traits. Family members also share genes that influence risks for disease. The genetic makeup you inherit is beyond your control (**Figure 1.7**).

Tracing your family's health history may provide vital information for you to manage your wellness. With this knowledge, you and your doctor can create a plan to keep you healthy. It may include lifestyle changes and more frequent visits with the doctor. There may be specific tests to detect the early onset of a known familial disease. For example, if your family health history includes type 2 diabetes, you may be at an increased risk for this disease. Being aware of this risk factor allows you to exert some control over it. You can eat healthy, get plenty of exercise, and maintain a healthy body weight. Taking these steps may help you prevent type 2 diabetes.

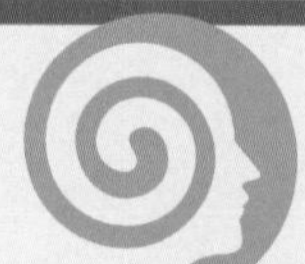

EXTEND YOUR KNOWLEDGE

The Effects of Lifestyle Choices on Health

Develop 10 interview questions about personal lifestyle choices. Include questions about topics such as foods typically eaten, number of meals eaten each day, daily activity level, quality of daily environment, availability of medical services, family health history, and other lifestyle choices that affect health and wellness.

Use your questions to interview an adult over age 70. Consider which factors contributed to this individual's long life and which may have reduced his or her quality of life.

You cannot change who your biological parents are. Likewise, you cannot change the genes you inherit from them. You can keep yourself in good physical condition, however. This helps you avert the influence of genetic risk factors. It also improves your body's ability to handle diseases if they do develop.

Health-Promoting Choices

Studies show that you have much control over the factors that influence your health. Healthcare experts have identified certain behaviors that make a difference in a person's quality of life and wellness level. By choosing these behaviors regularly, you can promote good health and perhaps lengthen your life.

Choose a Healthful Lifestyle

Because you can control your lifestyle choices, you can also control some of your risks for disease. Your eating pattern is a lifestyle factor that has a strong correlation with many diseases. An ***eating pattern*** is all of the foods and beverages you routinely consume over time, or your dietary intake. The terms *diet* or *dietary pattern* are often used interchangeably with the term *eating pattern*. In addition to decreasing your risk for disease, healthy eating patterns provide other benefits, such as

- increased energy level;
- improved performance at school or work;
- support for your body during physical and mental stress; and
- healthy skin, hair, weight, and overall appearance.

Choosing to become physically fit is also considered an important lifestyle choice. Researchers find that physically fit people often feel better about themselves and their relationships with others. Exercise is required for becoming physically fit. The benefits of becoming physically fit are clear—improved health and wellness, better weight management, reduced risks of certain diseases, and various mental and social health benefits.

The earlier you begin making healthful lifestyle choices, the more you decrease your risk of early disease.

Health experts recommend adopting the following practices into your lifestyle:

- Provide your body with fuel throughout the day by eating three or more regularly spaced meals, including breakfast (**Figure 1.8**).
- Supply your body with needed nutrients to support health, growth, and development.
- Sleep eight to nine hours each night.
- Maintain a healthy weight.
- Stay active. Accumulate at least 60 minutes of physical activity most days of the week.
- Do not use tobacco.
- Avoid drinking alcoholic beverages.
- Do not use street drugs.
- Carefully follow your physician's instructions when using prescription drugs.

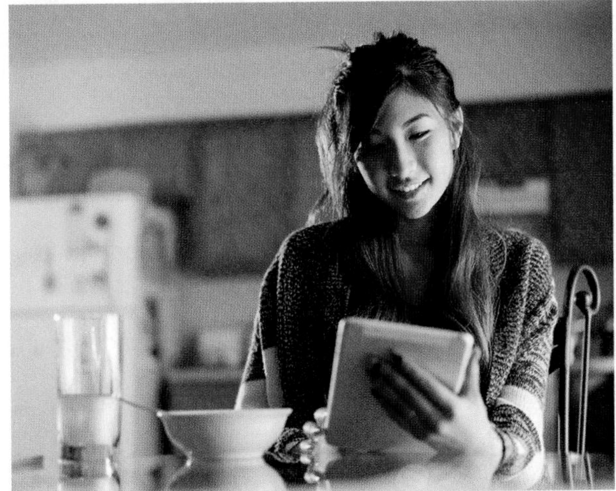

Joshua Resnick/Shutterstock.com

Figure 1.8 Establishing healthy eating patterns when you are young, such as eating breakfast, can reduce the risk of early disease.

Throughout this book, you will read about the impact of each of these practices on health. Although these behaviors may sound simple, many people fail to follow them. Instead, they develop poor health habits. This may occur for a number of reasons. Some people take good health for granted. Perhaps they feel they are strong enough to withstand the strain of poor health habits. Others do not notice the slow toll such habits take on their health. For instance, frequently eating high-calorie desserts and snack foods in place of fruits and vegetables deprives your body of needed nutrients. You may not notice, however, the gradual decrease in energy level and other health effects caused by this eating habit.

Another reason people form poor health habits is they fail to realize how addictive some behaviors can be. Perhaps you have heard someone say, "I can quit drinking alcohol whenever I want." This person may not realize how physically and emotionally dependent on alcohol he or she has become. Most people need the help of professional services to overcome addictions.

Resist Negative Peer Pressure

Peer pressure can play a role in the development of health habits. ***Peer pressure*** is the influence people in your age and social group have on your behavior. The desire to be accepted leads many teens to try activities their peers encourage. This can often be good, such as when friends invite one another to become involved with a sport. Peer pressure is negative, however, when it encourages people to pursue activities that can endanger their health. Teens who urge their friends to smoke cigarettes, drink alcohol, or drive recklessly are using negative peer pressure. Negative peer pressure may play a role in making accidents and suicide the leading causes of death among teens.

You can stand up against negative peer pressure and still come out a winner. Combating negative peer pressure requires self-confidence. You need to believe in your ability to evaluate the effect a choice will have on your health. You also need to be strong enough to say "no" to what you consider to be a poor choice. Be aware that people who have trouble resisting negative peer pressure may admire you for doing so (**Figure 1.9**).

Figure 1.9
Choose friends who share your values for health and wellness to avoid having to deal with negative influences.

Avoiding Negative Peer Pressure
• Role-play your response to a peer-pressure situation. Practice using firm, confident statements. Consider using humor, flattery, challenges, or topic changes to avoid undesirable situations.
• Talk to a trusted family member or friend about the situations and temptations with which you are struggling.
• Know what is important to you and what you hope to accomplish. This will help you build confidence to make positive choices.
• Demonstrate confidence in your decision and do not be embarrassed.
• Remember your personal goals and show respect for your personal limits to avoid being influenced negatively.
• Spend time with people who share your values for health and wellness. Avoid situations where peer pressure may tempt you to make harmful choices.
• Consider the consequences if you gave in to negative peer pressure.

CASE STUDY

A Healthier Lifestyle Choice

Raj is 16 years old. His 41-year-old father is currently receiving medical treatment for heart disease. Raj's father has smoked cigarettes since he was 14. Raj's 40-year-old mother is healthy, but she loves to cook the curried rice and chicken she enjoyed as a child. She loves making Indian desserts, too. She is now about 40 pounds (18.1 kg) overweight.

Raj has decided he wants his life to be different. He wants to be more physically active than his parents and is hoping to avoid health problems. His inherited factors place him at increased risk for acquiring heart disease.

Case Review

1. How do Raj's ideas about quality of life compare with those of his parents?
2. What lifestyle choices can Raj make now to reduce the risk for future heart and weight problems? Be specific with your suggestions.

Improve Your Environment

You can do your share to make your environment a healthful one. Carpool or take public transportation to avoid polluting the air with car exhaust. Use cleaning products that do not pollute water supplies with harmful chemical wastes. Handle food carefully to avoid contamination that can cause illness. These are just a few of the many steps you can take to improve the quality of your environment.

Besides these personal efforts, you can also work with others to improve the environmental quality of your area. Contact local industries about the efforts they are making to reduce their impact on the environment. Write to government officials if you have concerns about the quality of the air or water in your community. Talk with your employer about the benefits of creating a work environment that surpasses federal health and safety standards. These steps can help improve the health of many people.

Choose Quality Healthcare

Choosing quality healthcare will help you reduce health risks. The first step is to select a physician who has a reputation for providing quality care. Choose facilities that can meet your needs and are approved by your healthcare provider. See your doctor for regular checkups. Seek your doctor's advice when you first notice a health problem. Research has shown that early detection of health problems is the best way to prevent serious illness. When you visit your doctor, describe your symptoms completely and accurately. Ask questions to be sure you understand your symptoms and treatment (**Figure 1.10**).

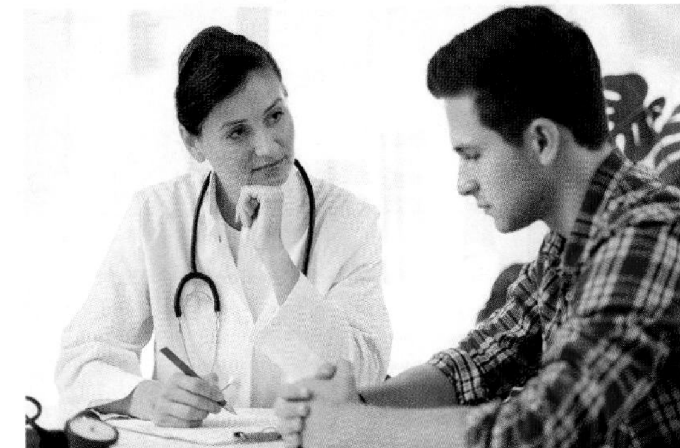

Alexander Raths/Shutterstock.com

Figure 1.10 Patients should feel free to ask their doctors questions.

Making a Change

Changing one behavior can affect all aspects of your health. Knowing this can increase your motivation to make positive changes. For instance, you may have heard that eating breakfast can help you concentrate better in school (mental health).

Assess Your Lifestyle Choices

Do you

- avoid the use of tobacco?
- avoid the use of alcohol and street drugs?
- regularly eat a nutritious diet, including breakfast?
- manage your weight?
- get daily physical activity to maintain fitness?
- manage stress effectively?
- get enough sleep?
- avoid taking unnecessary risks?
- carefully follow the instructions on medicine labels?
- wear protective clothing when participating in sports and fitness activities?
- avoid unsafe sexual practices?
- take appropriate safety precautions when using equipment and machinery?
- enthusiastically participate in school and community activities?

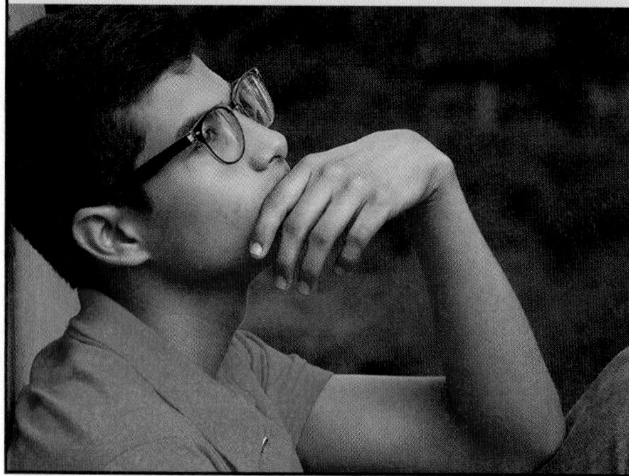

Photo: cheapbooks/Shutterstock.com

Figure 1.11 Ask yourself these questions. *Are you making lifestyle choices that promote good health?*

This may not be enough to encourage you to eat breakfast, however. Eating breakfast can also help you maintain a healthy weight (physical health). It can moderate mood swings and help you interact more positively with others, too (social health). Knowing these added benefits may be just the incentive you need to start eating breakfast.

Although you may be motivated to improve your health, you may not know how to start. Answering the questions in **Figure 1.11** can help you pinpoint areas in which you might improve.

Once you have identified an area you want to improve, set a goal for improvement. Setting and achieving goals is key to success in any **endeavor** (effort). To create effective goals, use the acronym **SMART** as a guide:

- **S**pecific—The goal should identify a specific action or event.
- **M**easurable—The goal and its benefits should be easily determined and assessed.
- **A**chievable—The goal should be attainable given the resources that are available.
- **R**ealistic—The goal should require you to stretch your limits but still allow the likelihood of success.
- **T**imely—The goal should state the specific time period in which it will be accomplished. Short-term goals may take days, weeks, or months, while long-term goals may take several years to achieve.

An example of a short-term SMART goal might be, "Complete research for my workplace wellness term paper by Friday afternoon. Prepare my bibliography to include a minimum of 10 research sites. Summarize the main points presented in each reference." Another practical SMART goal for teens may simply be stated as, "I will drink 8 glasses of water every 24 hours to stay hydrated."

If your SMART goal requires long-term planning to **induce** (cause) a personal behavior change, then you may want to craft a behavior-change contract to help you achieve your goal. Write your goal at the top of your document and create a chart below it. In the first column of the chart, list specific steps you will take to reach the goal. For instance, suppose your goal is to improve your eating pattern. You might list steps such as "Eat breakfast daily" and "Choose beverages with no added sugars, such as water, in place of sugary soft drinks." List the days of the week across the top of the chart. Each day you complete a listed step, give yourself a check. This allows you to see the progress you are making toward your goal.

WELLNESS TIP

Private Pep Talk

Manage your stress with a pep talk. Instead of thinking "I'll never be able to figure this out," say to yourself "I have the skills to solve this problem." In general, if you would not say a negative comment to someone else, do not say it to yourself.

It will take time for you to notice most physical, mental, and social health benefits of a lifestyle change. Follow the listed steps and maintain your chart for at least three weeks. After that time, evaluate the results of your efforts. Ask yourself what factors helped you complete steps you marked with a check. Then ask yourself what kept you from completing those steps left unchecked. For instance, you might notice that eating breakfast is easier on weekends because you have more time in the morning. You might find that limiting your soft drink consumption is harder on weekends, when you are socializing with friends.

Your evaluation will help you set new goals and plan steps for achieving them. Try to consistently reach your goal for a period of six weeks. After this time, you will have formed a new habit that will be an ongoing part of your wellness lifestyle. Achieving optimum health is a lifelong process of consciously evaluating daily lifestyle choices.

Seeing positive results in one lifestyle area can affect your desire to change other areas. For instance, if you improve your eating habits, you are likely to have more energy. This may increase your willingness to begin an exercise program or join a sports team.

Your confidence that good health practices will improve your state of wellness will help you follow such practices. Not all of your daily choices will be in the best interest of your health, however. Everyone skips a meal or overeats snack foods once in a while. Little harm is done unless you start making such choices on a regular basis.

The Science of Nutrition and Wellness

Clearly, nutrition has a big impact on wellness. ***Nutrition*** is the sum of the processes by which a person takes in and uses food substances. There has been widespread growth in the study of nutrition in recent years. Scientists once thought foods contained just a few nutrients. ***Nutrients*** are the basic components of food that nourish the body. Today, scientists know of over 45 nutrients needed by the body, which are supplied by foods (**Figure 1.12**).

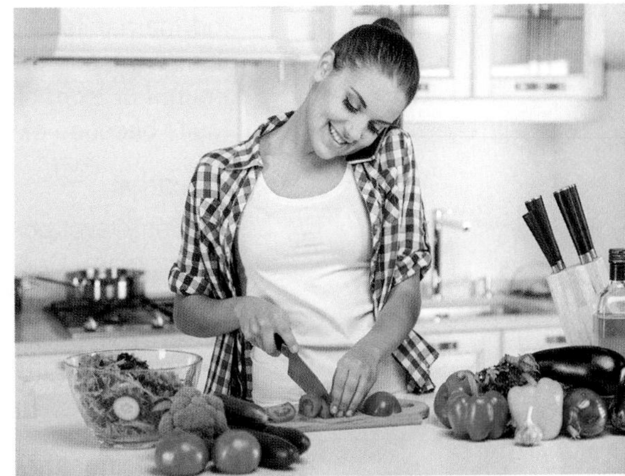

VGstockstudio/Shutterstock.com

Figure 1.12 Eating a variety of foods will help ensure your body is getting all of the nutrients needed for good health.

Growth in nutrition science is linked to growth in the field of epidemiology. *Epidemiology* is a branch of science that studies the incidence of disease in a population. After World War II, epidemiologists began exploring factors related to heart disease, cancer, and viral infections. One factor that interested them was diet. They conducted studies to learn how the eating patterns of large groups of people related to certain disease patterns.

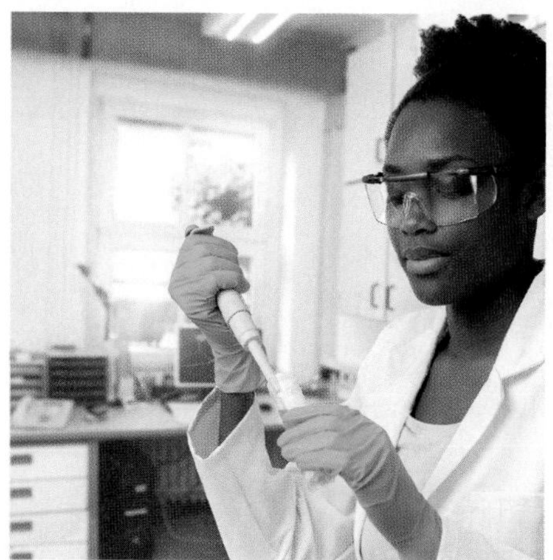

anyaivanova/Shutterstock.com

Figure 1.13 Scientists are discovering more about the connection between diet and health every day. ***What diet-related discoveries have you learned about recently?***

Sometimes nutrition studies involve comparing the effects of various food choices. For instance, researchers might want to compare the health of people who eat meat with the health of those who do not. They might compare the health effects of high-fiber diets with those of low-fiber diets. Researchers can also compare diet and lifestyle patterns among cultures.

What have researchers learned from their nutrition studies? They have learned that eating specific foods cannot cause or prevent certain diseases. They have found, however, that following certain eating patterns tends to increase or decrease a person's chances of developing illness. For instance, studies have shown that eating sugar does not cause diabetes. Nevertheless, eating a diet high in simple sugars can increase a person's risk of becoming overweight. This, in turn, can increase his or her risk of developing type 2 diabetes.

Nutrition scientists continue to research the roles food components play in the human body. They use research methods to discover answers to questions about the links between diet and health (**Figure 1.13**). As a student of nutrition, you will use tools similar to those used by scientists. Correct use of these tools will help you understand and apply information covered in this text.

In the future, you may find yourself eligible to participate in a medical or nutrition-based research project. *Clinical studies* use accepted research methods with human subjects. These studies often focus on new methods of screening, prevention, diagnosis, or treatment for the improvement of health. New therapy methods may be tested.

FEATURED CAREER

Health Educator

Health educators encourage healthy lifestyles and wellness. They work with people to encourage behaviors that can prevent diseases, injuries, and other health problems. They cover such health-related topics as proper nutrition, exercise and fitness, avoiding sexually transmitted infections (STIs), and the habits and behaviors necessary to avoid illness. Health educators must be able to assess the needs of a group and tailor their educational programs to that group. For example, programs for teens would vary greatly from programs for older adults because of the age and needs of each group.

Education

Entry-level positions generally require a bachelor's degree from a health education program. Courses in psychology, human development, and a foreign language are helpful. Experiences with internships or volunteer opportunities can make applicants more appealing to employers. A master's degree is generally required to work in public health, community health, school health, or health promotion.

Job Outlook

The demand will remain high. Due to the rising cost and complexity of healthcare, and the need for people to learn how to live healthy lives, career opportunities for health educators will continue to increase.

For example, a clinical study may focus on the role of exercise in preventing type 2 diabetes for people who have a family history of the disease. The study may be designed to learn more about how to treat the condition. Other studies focus on measuring safety factors and possible side effects of treatment. Clinical studies use scientific methods to gather and analyze data.

Using the Scientific Method to Study Nutrition and Wellness

Scientists and research dietitians use the scientific method when performing research. The ***scientific method*** is the process researchers use to answer a question. Once the question is determined, the researcher states the hypothesis. A ***hypothesis*** is a proposed answer to a scientific question, which can be tested and verified. An experiment is then devised to test the hypothesis to determine if it is true (**Figure 1.14**).

The following example illustrates the use of the scientific method. A researcher becomes aware of statistics showing that men tend to not live as long as women. This prompts her to raise the question: Why do males have a shorter life expectancy than females? The researcher begins observing males and females. Through these observations, she notes that men seem to exercise less than women. This causes her to form a hypothesis. The researcher's hypothesis states: Men do not live as long as women because men do not exercise as much as women. The researcher then compares the life spans of men and women who do the same amount of exercise.

Suppose the results revealed that men who exercise as much as women have the same life expectancy as women. This would indicate the hypothesis is true. Conversely, suppose the observations revealed that men who exercise as much as women still have a shorter life expectancy. This would indicate the hypothesis is false.

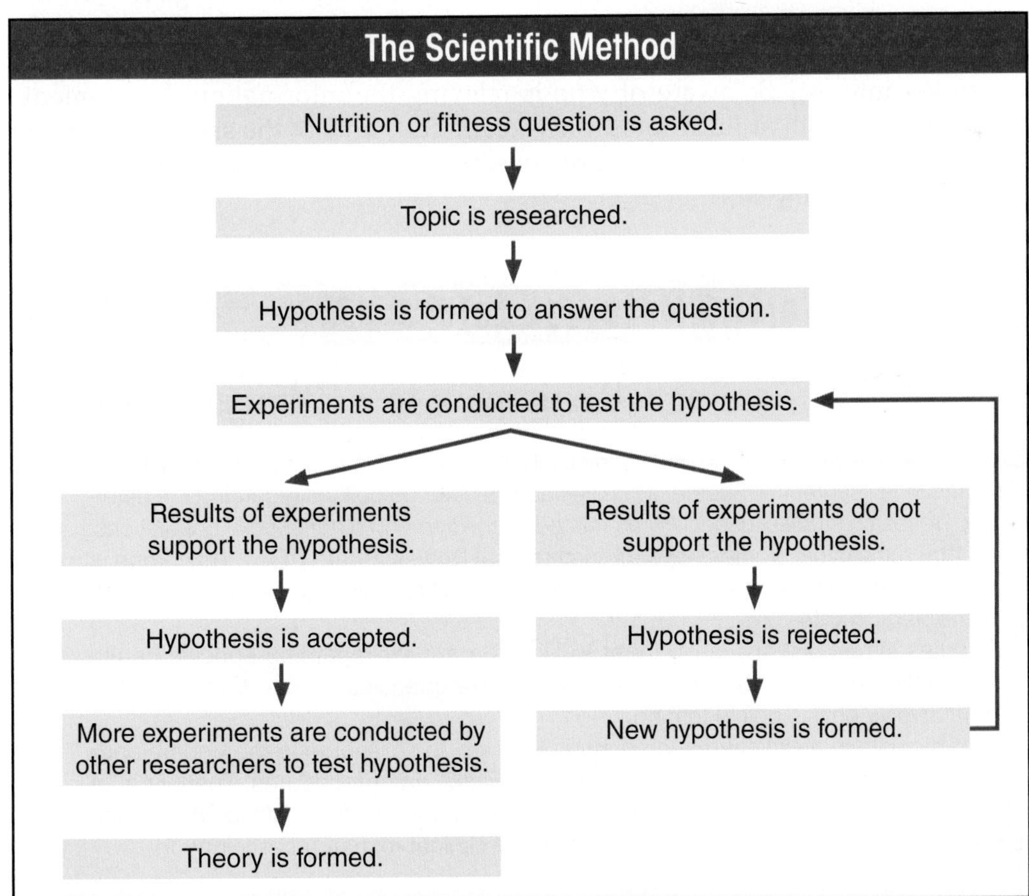

Figure 1.14 Using the scientific method, researchers are able to test and verify possible answers to their questions.

If other researchers conduct many experiments testing this hypothesis and reach the same conclusion, a theory forms. A ***theory*** is a principle that tries to explain something that happens in nature. Although it is based on evidence, a theory is not a fact. It still requires further testing.

There are still many unanswered questions about diet, disease, and health. Addressing the following questions helps researchers choose which food science, nutrition, and physical fitness topics to study:

- How is current technology affecting these areas?
- What gaps of knowledge currently exist related to the problems identified?
- How many people will be affected by learning about the information?
- Are resources available (money, time, staff, other resources) to do the research?
- How can current technology be used to advance research?
- Where will the study take place, and who will participate?
- Are the rights of people protected, and is the physical environment left unharmed?

Evaluating Research Reports

You can learn about some of the latest findings and recommendations for improving your wellness level. Television and radio newscasts often include brief reports about the results of health and nutrition studies. These studies are covered in greater detail in newspaper and magazine articles. Professional journals present technical information from the studies. Hundreds of health and nutrition websites provide a wealth of data.

As you evaluate information, identify important details to gain a clearer understanding of the content. For instance, identify the audience to which the report is directed. Is the information intended to update professionals or pique consumer interest? Be aware of who is relaying the information. Is it a media reporter or a health or nutrition professional? Take note of the size and length of the study. Did it involve eight people observed for three weeks or 8,000 people observed for three years?

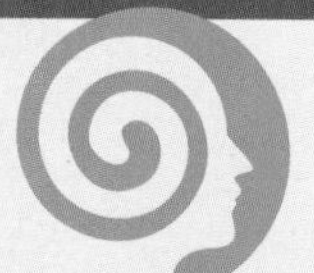

EXTEND YOUR KNOWLEDGE

Consider Becoming a Participant in a Clinical Study

Researchers look for people who qualify to participate in clinical studies. Usually, anyone who meets the specific criteria of the study can enroll. Federal agencies have stricter guidelines regarding the determination of eligibility for research studies, especially as related to children and other special populations.

Most institutions that run clinical studies have an Institutional Review Board (IRB). This group is given the responsibility for reviewing and approving a study. They will examine research procedures to ensure safety for the participants.

Some clinical studies simply ask the participant to fill out a survey regarding specific health problems, food consumption patterns, or exercise patterns. More intensive research may require more of your time and involve physiological testing.

Volunteering to participate in a clinical research study is a way to contribute to the understanding of human diseases and the development of new drugs, devices, and procedures. There is a lot to consider before making the decision to participate. Visit the National Institutes of Health website to learn more about personal and societal benefits and risks of clinical research participation.

Keep in mind that many experiments are conducted to prove or disprove a theory. Not all experiments will yield the same results. A single study is not a sufficient basis for recommending changes in behavior.

Evaluating Social Media Reports on Health and Wellness

Teens frequently look to social media and the Internet for answers to health-related questions such as the following:

- What are the healthiest food choices?
- How can I build stronger muscles or lose weight?
- Do some foods cause acne?

Not all websites and social media sites are reliable and accurate, however. Therefore, it is important to learn how to identify sources that can be trusted to provide accurate information.

In general, the most reliable information can be found on websites with the primary goal of educating the public rather than selling a product or a service. Web addresses that include a suffix such as *.gov*, *.edu*, or *.org* are considered more credible than others. These government agencies, educational institutions, or professional organizations share educational literature, post current research findings, and often provide healthcare guidance (**Figure 1.15**). Check with your school librarian if you are in doubt about the reliability of your media source.

Sources of Nutrition and Wellness Information	
Sources of Information	**URLs**
Academy of Nutrition and Dietetics	www.eatright.org
American Academy of Pediatrics	www.aap.org
American Cancer Society	www.cancer.org
American Diabetes Association	www.diabetes.org
American Heart Association	www.heart.org
American Red Cross	www.redcross.org
Centers for Disease Control and Prevention	www.cdc.gov
Institute of Medicine of the National Academies	www.nationalacademies.org/hmd/
Mayo Clinic	www.mayoclinic.org
MedlinePlus® (U.S. National Library of Medicine, National Institutes of Health)	www.medlineplus.gov
National Institute of Mental Health	www.nimh.nih.gov
National Institute on Drug Abuse	www.drugabuse.gov
Office of Disease Prevention and Health Promotion	www.healthfinder.gov
Office of the Surgeon General	www.surgeongeneral.gov
Tufts University Health & Nutrition Letter	www.nutritionletter.tufts.edu
United States Consumer Product Safety Commission	www.cpsc.gov
USDA MyPlate Food Guidance System	www.choosemyplate.gov
U.S. Food and Drug Administration	www.fda.gov
World Health Organization	www.who.int

Figure 1.15
Be sure to use reliable Internet sources of nutrition and wellness information when evaluating reports on health and wellness.

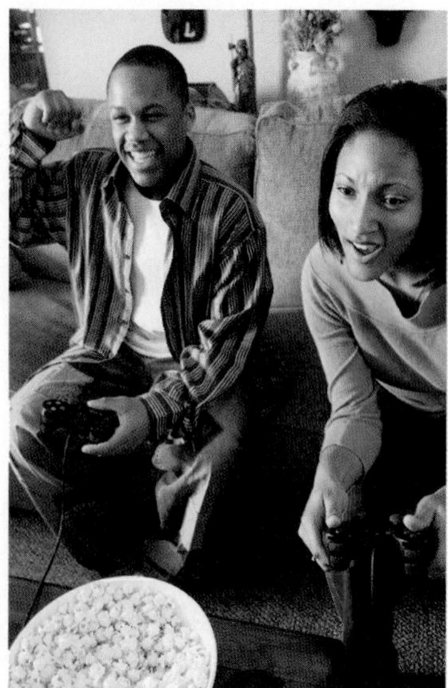

Blend Images/Shutterstock.com

Figure 1.16 Many people fail to balance sedentary work and leisure activities with physical activity. *How many minutes a day are you physically active?*

Healthful Living in the United States

Studies show that many people in the United States are not following the most healthful eating and physical activity patterns. Studies also show that nutritional problems tend to increase as income levels decrease. A number of health and fitness problems are affecting the nation's state of wellness:

- The percentage of overweight youth has more than doubled in the last 20 years. Now, 21 percent of youth ages 12 to 19 are obese. More than one-third of youth are overweight or obese.
- An estimated 69.2 percent of adults age 20 and older are overweight. Nearly 36 percent of adults are considered obese.
- Nearly one in four households struggles to afford needed food. Approximately one-third of the people in the United States have inadequate eating patterns.
- Popular lifestyles include less and less physical activity (**Figure 1.16**).
- Important nutrients are missing from the diets of some groups of people, such as teens and older adults.
- Saturated fat, sodium, added sugar, and calorie intake are higher than recommended for 64 percent of consumers.

These problems arise for several reasons. Some people do not have enough money to acquire adequate nutrition. Others lack the information, desire, or skills needed to select a nutritious diet. Some people may not know they need to make changes. Still others simply choose to ignore current nutrition recommendations.

One reason some people give for disregarding nutrition recommendations is that nutrition messages can appear unclear or contradictory. Findings from one study seem to dispute the findings from another study. One source says to eat more fiber. Another reference focuses on the importance of protein. Sports books say one thing, diet books say another, and advertisements say something else. Even government nutrition guidelines change periodically. What is a health-conscious person supposed to believe as he or she tries to make wise lifestyle choices?

Education can help you sort out conflicting messages. Learning the scientific method and studying the functions and food sources of nutrients will help you assess media reports. Asking questions will also help you evaluate nutrition information. Finding out who conducted a study and how it was conducted can help you decide whether the results are valid.

Past nutrition studies uncovered convincing information to support the need for improved eating habits. Researchers found that people who ate high-fat diets, especially the harmful fats, were more likely to have heart disease. Identifying this link helped researchers discover that eating a low-fat diet can reduce the risk of heart disease.

As people became more aware of these findings, they began to change their eating habits. Food manufacturers began to produce a wide selection of reduced-fat foods for consumers. For example, low-fat dairy products, nonfat muffins, and fat-free soups began to appear in supermarkets and restaurants. Consumers were buying and eating reduced-fat or nonfat products more than ever before. Despite this, population health issues related to overweight and obesity continued to increase. On average, consumers are now eating more total calories than in past decades, and they are more likely to be overweight. Consuming excess calories has kept the overall risk of weight-related diseases from decreasing.

More recently, there is new evidence suggesting a link between the consumption of added sugars and heart disease. As a result, the American Heart Association has revised its diet recommendations and now recommends individuals minimize their intake of beverages and foods containing added sugars.

One result of improved nutrition research, expanding food technology, and the increased availability of quality food is an increase in life expectancy in the United States over the last 100 years. ***Life expectancy*** is the average length of life of people living in the same environment. Life expectancy in the United States is about 78.8 years. With improved health, life expectancy tends to increase. Together, healthy people make a healthy nation. Following nutrition and physical activity guidelines will help you and your family maintain good health. In so doing, you contribute to the health of the nation.

RECIPE FILE

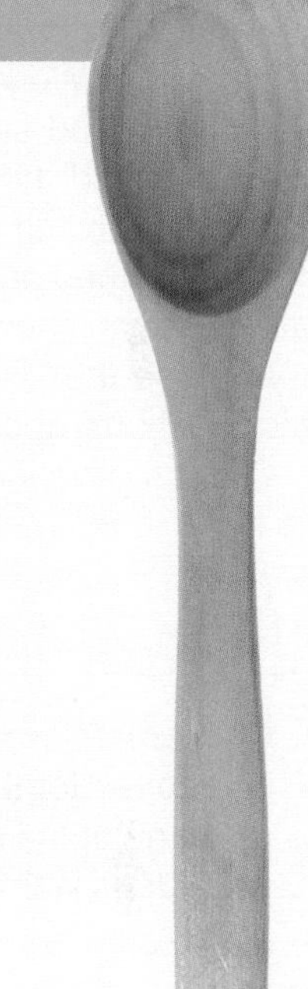

Vegetable Stir-Fry

6 SERVINGS

Ingredients

- 2 T. low-sodium soy sauce
- 2 t. toasted sesame oil
- ¾ c. broth, vegetable or chicken
- hot pepper sauce to taste (optional)
- 1½ T. cornstarch
- 2 T. avocado or peanut oil
- 2 cloves garlic, minced
- 2 t. ginger, minced
- ½ c. onion, chopped
- ¾ c. carrots, julienned
- 1 c. broccoli florets
- ¾ c. red bell pepper, sliced into ½-inch-wide strips
- ¾ c. yellow bell pepper, sliced into ½-inch-wide strips
- 1 jalapeño chile, julienned
- 1 c. purple cabbage, shredded
- ½ c. mushrooms, sliced
- ½ c. baby corn, cut into thirds
- 1 c. snow peas
- ½ c. green onion, chopped, green and white parts
- 3 c. cooked brown rice

Directions

1. Combine soy sauce, toasted sesame oil, broth, hot pepper sauce, and cornstarch. Set aside.
2. Heat wok over high heat.
3. When wok is hot, add oil to wok and swirl to coat the wok with oil.
4. Turn heat down to medium-high.
5. Add garlic and ginger and stir around for 30 seconds.
6. Add onions, carrots, and broccoli florets. Stir-fry for 2–3 minutes.
7. Add red and yellow bell peppers, and jalapeño. Stir-fry for 2–3 minutes more.
8. Add cabbage and sliced mushrooms. Stir-fry for 1–2 minutes.
9. Add baby corn and snow peas. Stir-fry for 1–2 minutes.
10. Pour soy sauce mixture over vegetables. Stir for one minute, or until thickened.
11. Serve over ½ cup brown rice and top with chopped green onion.

PER SERVING: 205 CALORIES, 6 G PROTEIN, 43 G CARBOHYDRATE, 8 G FAT, 6 G FIBER, 296 MG SODIUM.

Chapter 1 Review and Expand

Reading Summary

Wellness involves being in good physical, mental, and social health. People can define their personal states of wellness as points on a continuum between premature death and optimum health.

A number of factors can negatively affect wellness by contributing to disease. Most of these factors are unhealthful lifestyle choices, over which you have control. Poor environmental quality, inadequate healthcare, and heredity can also contribute to disease. You can counteract these factors by making health-promoting choices. Choose a healthful lifestyle and resist peer pressure to engage in unhealthful behaviors. Work to improve the quality of your environment and seek qualified healthcare services when you need them. You can set and work toward goals for improving behaviors that affect your health.

Nutrition and daily physical activity are two factors that have been shown to have a big impact on health. Experts use the scientific method to find answers to their questions about these factors. With education, skills, and motivation, people can eat better and exercise more to maintain better health.

Chapter Vocabulary

1. **Content Terms** In small groups, create categories for the following terms and classify as many of the terms as possible. Then, share your ideas with the rest of the class.

diagnosis	peer pressure
eating pattern	physical health
environmental quality	premature death
holistic medicine	quality of life
hypothesis	risk factor
life expectancy	scientific method
mental health	social health
nutrient	theory
nutrition	wellness
optimum health	

2. **Academic Terms** Write each of the following terms on a separate sheet of paper. For each term, quickly write a word you think relates to the term. In small groups, exchange papers. Have each person in the group explain a term on the list. Take turns until all terms have been explained.

chronic	impair
diminished	induce
endeavor	

Review Learning

3. Describe the characteristics of people functioning at the extreme points of the wellness continuum.
4. Provide an example of how physical, mental, and social health interrelate.
5. List common symptoms that may appear when a person has mental health problems.
6. What are two social skills that can help teens improve their social health?
7. Why is it important to choose health-promoting lifestyle patterns during the teen years? during the adult years?
8. In reducing the risk of disease, which risk factors are considered controllable and which are not?
9. Name the five major causes of death among adults in the United States.
10. List five lifestyle practices that health experts recommend people adopt.
11. Describe what is included in a behavior-change contract for achieving a goal for personal improvement.
12. Explain the difference between a hypothesis and a theory.
13. When evaluating research information, what details should you examine to ensure better and reliable understanding of the content?
14. What are two factors that have contributed to health and wellness problems in the United States?

Self-Assessment Quiz

Complete the self-assessment quiz online to help you practice and expand your knowledge and skills.

Critical Thinking

15. **Evaluate** If obesity is a national health problem in the United States, how does this affect the nation as a whole?
16. **Conclude** Think about where you currently fit along the wellness continuum. Draw conclusions about ways you can improve your physical, mental, and social health to achieve optimum wellness.

17. **Predict** If people in the United States continue along their current path of eating and fitness patterns, predict the effect of these behaviors on life expectancy for future generations.
18. **Evaluate** Draw a line representing the wellness continuum. Label one end "Premature Death" and the other end "Optimum Health." Place a star on the line to indicate where you place yourself on the wellness continuum. Write a brief explanation to support your assessment.
19. **Analyze** Interview a healthcare professional to learn more about the effects mental and social health can have on physical health. What are the implications of poor mental and/or social health on physical health?
20. **Identify** Working in small groups, identify five activities that are both fun and healthy. Then, brainstorm ways to motivate individuals to incorporate these activities into their daily life. Plan a blog for your class or school website to share your ideas about healthy, fun activities. Employ one or more of the motivational strategies your group generated. When writing your blog, consider the age of your audience and what would make them want to read it. Organize your content and give it an interesting title. Be sure to proofread your blog.
21. **Analyze** Use the Occupational Outlook Handbook website or other reputable resources to research the education requirements, work environment, pay, and job outlook for dietitians in the United States. Write a summary of your findings. Based on information you learned in this chapter and other sources, do you think the job outlook for this career is accurate? Provide evidence to support your opinion.

Core Skills

22. **Writing** Write and present a play on methods teens could use to avoid negative peer pressure.
23. **Technology Literacy** Create a list of websites that offer information on wellness. Rate each site for accuracy and usability of information and credibility of sources. Prepare a list of reliable sites and post it on your class or school website.
24. **Reading** Identify short stories about teens who made poor choices that had negative consequences in their lives. In each case, describe the choice that was made and the outcomes. Suggest ways to help change the situation so the outcomes are more positive.
25. **Writing** Research current legislation related to nutrition or wellness issues. Select one issue and write a brief summary to share with the class. Include your opinion of the legislation in the summary.
26. **Technology Literacy** Use infographic creation software to create an infographic about wellness.
27. **Science** Contact the state department of public health or a community hospital to obtain a health and wellness lifestyle questionnaire. Complete the questionnaire. Identify the top three lifestyle changes that would probably provide the greatest benefits to your health.
28. **Technology Literacy** Find a life expectancy calculator online to learn about which factors and lifestyle choices add years to life. Calculate your life expectancy and analyze the results. Identify your major health risk areas and suggest methods for changing risky behaviors into health-promoting behaviors.
29. **Math** In 2006, the share of young adults ages 18 to 24 who never smoked was 70.2 percent, according to the Centers for Disease Control and Prevention. In 1965, far fewer could make that claim—only 47.6 percent. Calculate the percentage increase in nonsmokers among members of this age group during that 41-year span.
30. **Speaking** Prepare and present a persuasive speech on the benefits of a healthful diet. Refer to evidence from the text as well as other research to present your case.
31. **Career Readiness Practice** Most employers value employees who can set and achieve reasonable, attainable goals. Think about your personal wellness goals and how they relate to you as a future employee. Create a **SMART** goal for changing one aspect of personal wellness. Determine how you will measure achievement of this goal and identify a deadline for meeting this goal.

Factors Affecting Food Habits

Learning Outcomes

After studying this chapter, you will be able to

- **explain** how culture influences people's eating patterns;
- **evaluate** the social influence of family and friends on people's eating patterns;
- **analyze** the effect of emotions on the way people eat;
- **relate** how agricultural resources, technology, economic factors, and politics affect the availability of food; and
- **analyze** the effects of global and local events and conditions on food choices and consumer practices.

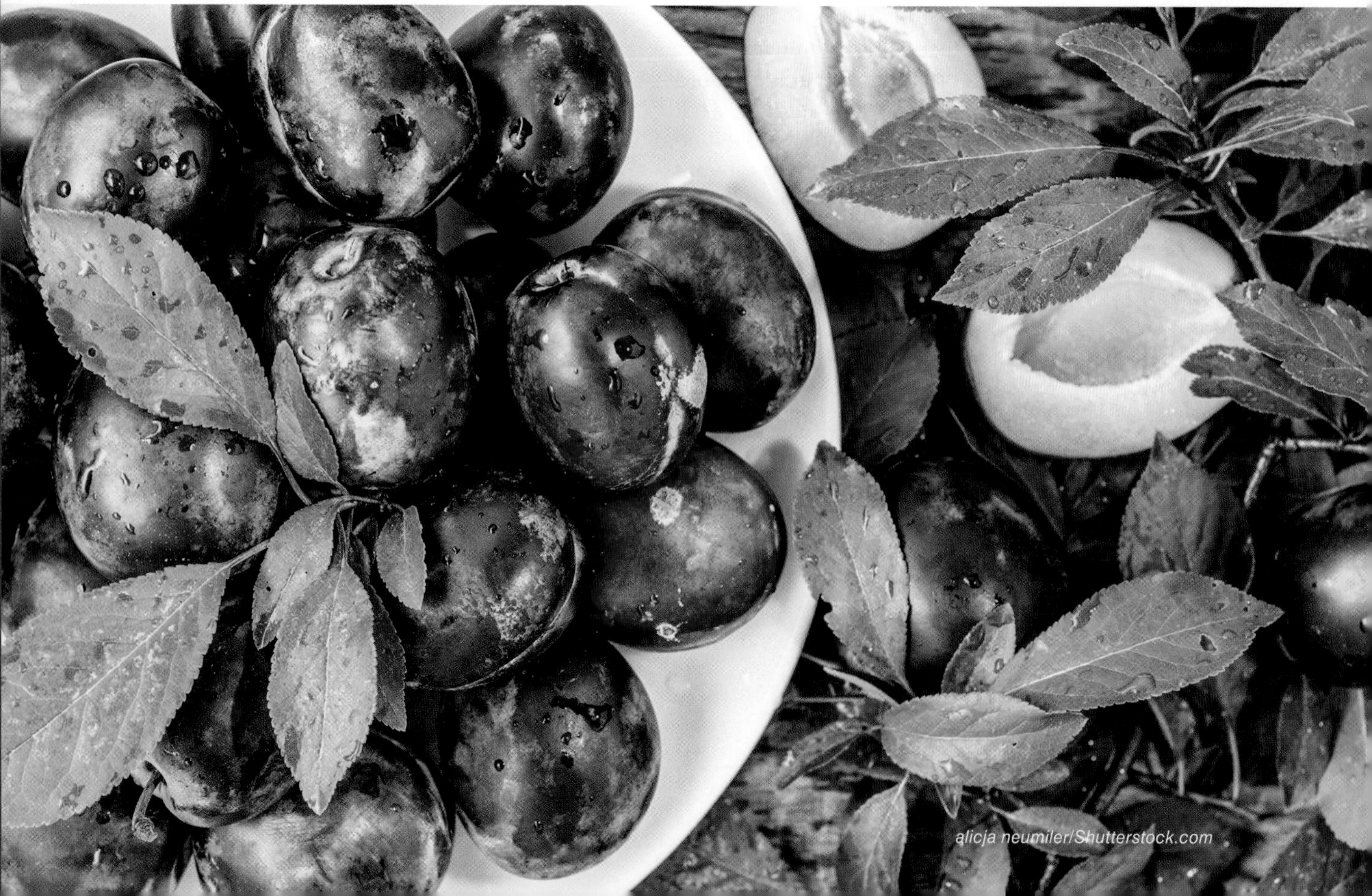

alicja neumiler/Shutterstock.com

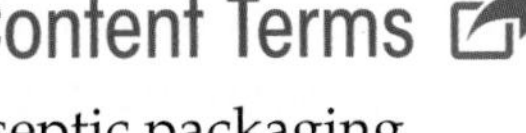

Content Terms

aseptic packaging
cultural heritage
culture
food biotechnology
food norm
food taboo
genetically modified (GM) food
kosher food
social media
staple food
technology
value

Academic Terms

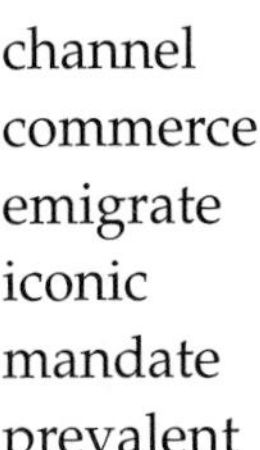

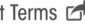

channel
commerce
emigrate
iconic
mandate
prevalent

What's Your Nutrition and Wellness IQ?

Take this quiz to examine how much you already know about the factors that affect your food habits. If you cannot answer a question, pay extra attention to that topic as you study this chapter.

- Identify each statement as *True*, *False*, or *It Depends*. *It Depends* means in some cases the statement is true; in some cases it could be false.
- Revise false statements to make them true.
- Explain the circumstances in which each *It Depends* statement is true and when it is false.

Nutrition and Wellness IQ

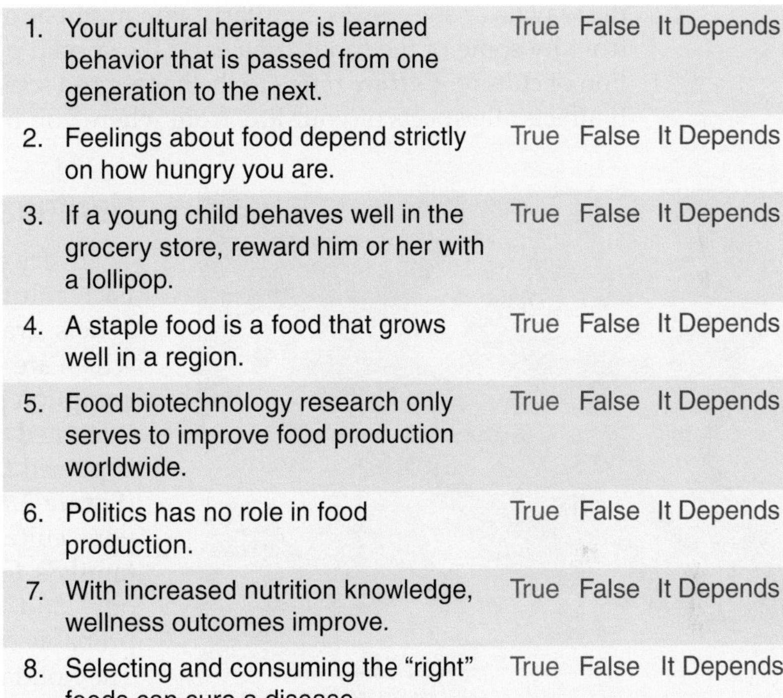

1.	Your cultural heritage is learned behavior that is passed from one generation to the next.	True	False	It Depends
2.	Feelings about food depend strictly on how hungry you are.	True	False	It Depends
3.	If a young child behaves well in the grocery store, reward him or her with a lollipop.	True	False	It Depends
4.	A staple food is a food that grows well in a region.	True	False	It Depends
5.	Food biotechnology research only serves to improve food production worldwide.	True	False	It Depends
6.	Politics has no role in food production.	True	False	It Depends
7.	With increased nutrition knowledge, wellness outcomes improve.	True	False	It Depends
8.	Selecting and consuming the "right" foods can cure a disease.	True	False	It Depends

While studying this chapter, look for the activity icon  **to**

- **build** vocabulary with e-flash cards and interactive games;
- **assess** what you learn by completing self-assessment quizzes and completing review questions; and
- **expand** knowledge with interactive activities and activities that extend learning.

www.g-wlearning.com/foodsandnutrition/

What people eat says a lot about them. Food tells a story about where people live, what they do, and what they consider important. Food reflects people's history and affects their future. In fact, one way to find out about a group of people is to study their daily food habits.

What factors affect people's food habits? When choosing food, you probably select food that tastes good. There are many other factors that affect people's daily food choices, however. Where you live and the people around you affect the foods you choose to eat. The resources available to you and your experiences with food are also likely to shape your food choices.

Cultural Influences on Food Habits

You may have had the experience of guessing where someone comes from by the way he or she speaks. Similarly, you might be able to guess where people come from by some of the foods they eat. Like speech patterns, food habits are a reflection of culture. ***Culture*** refers to the beliefs and social customs of a group of people. It affects all aspects of your life, from where you live to how you dress.

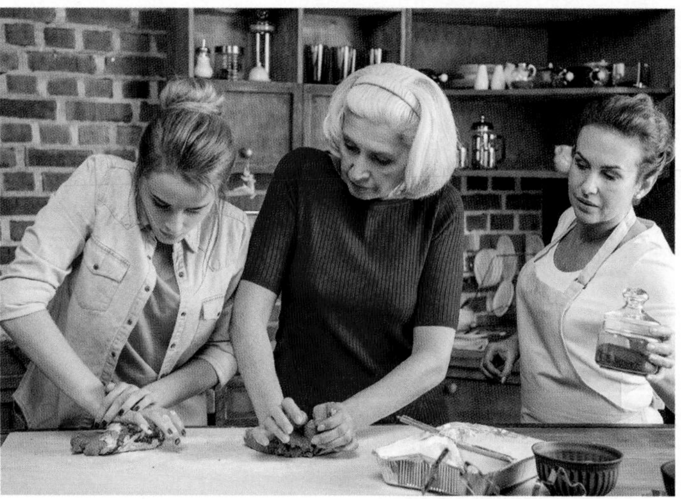

LightField Studios/Shutterstock.com

Figure 2.1 Recipes and food traditions are passed from one generation to the next. *What food traditions does your family keep?*

Heritage

Every culture has a unique way of life. Each culture's way of life is influenced by beliefs, traditions, and customs, some of which are related to food choices and consumption patterns. Your ***cultural heritage*** is learned behavior about a way of life that is passed from one generation to the next (**Figure 2.1**). Food is an important part of your cultural heritage. Think about your family's food choices, preparation methods, and eating patterns. These habits probably came from previous generations. The holidays you celebrate and the traditions or ceremonies you observe are also aspects of your cultural heritage.

When people **emigrate** (leave one's country to live elsewhere), they bring their food traditions with them. For example, an Asian family new to the United States will likely continue to make curry dishes and stir-fry meals using the recipes of their ancestors. Social groups form due to shared beliefs and values, and observing food traditions is one expression of those shared beliefs and values.

Foods that are typically identified with a particular region, race, or religion are frequently called *ethnic foods*. A collection of food preparations come to be associated with a particular region, race, or religion because they employ common ingredients and cooking methods of the region. The ingredients and cooking methods that form the basis for an ethnic food were influenced by both environmental and human factors. For instance, cooks in a landlocked region were less likely to use fish as an ingredient than cooks in coastal regions. A region with limited natural resources suitable for use as cooking fuel was likely to rely on cooking methods that required little fuel, such as stir-frying.

Historically, as merchants and explorers ventured farther around the world, they introduced ingredients of one culture to another culture. For example, spices were one of the earliest forms of **commerce** (business, trade). They were relatively easy to transport and highly prized. Availability of spices influenced the foods of a region.

These factors acted to shape the various foods of a region, race, or religion and continue to do so. With advances in transportation and technology, ingredients that were once difficult to obtain are now readily available. Recipes and preparation videos of **iconic** (important, recognizable) dishes of other cultures can be viewed on the Internet. Similar to culture, ethnic foods often change and evolve.

Food Norms and Traditions

Groups of people with different cultural heritages have different food norms and traditions. ***Food norms*** are typical standards and patterns related to food and eating behaviors. For example, a food norm common to the Pennsylvania Dutch heritage is to include both a sweet and a sour element in a meal. A typical meal might feature pickles or pepper cabbage as the sour element and a dessert as the sweet element.

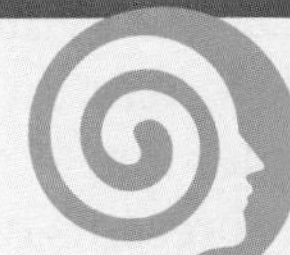

EXTEND YOUR KNOWLEDGE

What Can You Learn from Your Family Tree?

A family tree shows relationships among ancestors and descendants in one family. To learn about family history, you will need to do some detective work:

- Interview parents, aunts, uncles, and grandparents and record their stories.
- Ask questions about common health problems, favorite foods, and cultural history.
- Learn from which country and town your ancestors came.
- Ask what traditions they want to see passed on from this generation to the next.

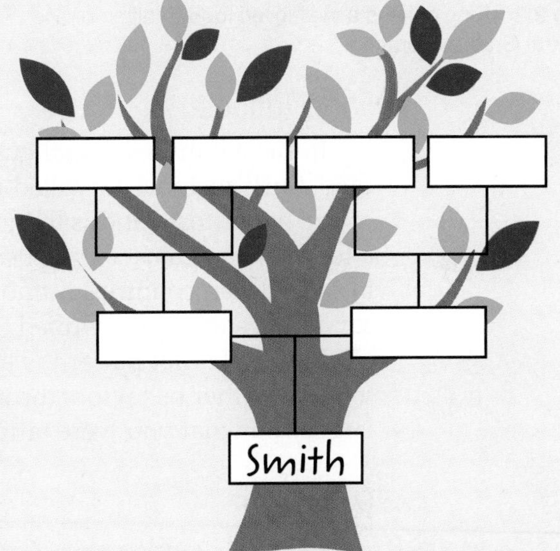

iris wright/Shutterstock.com

Obtain permission to gather more data from family photos, old family documents, or other papers found in special storage places.

Enter the information you find on a family tree chart. Many types of charts are available online. You can also draw your family tree, placing your name on the trunk of the tree and your parents' names on the lower branches. Include all of your grandparents, aunts, and uncles on higher branches. Go back in your history as far as possible. Family trees often include birth dates and places of birth. Age and cause of death can be noted for each person. You can add footnotes to your chart as you learn other stories of interest.

The tree will help you understand the source of your cultural values and traditions. Can you see a pattern in your preferences for certain foods on special occasions? Identify longevity patterns and potential inherited health issues in your family. How will this impact your lifestyle choices over your life span? In what ways will you alter your food and wellness behaviors?

A food norm for many Italian and French cooks is to shop for food every day to get the freshest fruits, vegetables, and meats for recipe ingredients. A food norm for the British is to serve tea with cookies or sandwiches as a light meal in the late afternoon. Adhering to food norms is a way to express deep-rooted, authentic ties to cultural identity and common heritage.

Many cultures have food traditions that include serving special foods on significant days to build positive emotions and connections to the cultures' roots. Holidays become more festive when traditional foods are served. Kwanzaa, for example, is a week-long celebration honoring people's African heritage. Traditional African dance, music, and food inspire participants to reconnect with their heritage. Such traditional foods as peanut soup, roasted chicken, and sweet potato pie can often be found on the family table.

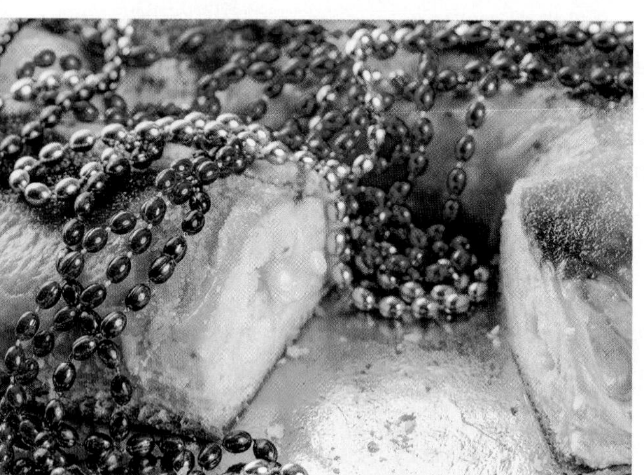

Arina P Habich/Shutterstock.com

Figure 2.2 King cake is a well-loved food tradition of the Mardi Gras celebration.

Mardi Gras, also known as *Carnival*, is celebrated in many countries around the world. Food celebrations occur on this day before a religious season begins. New Orleans Mardi Gras highlights the celebration with foods such as jambalaya, red beans and rice, and king cake (**Figure 2.2**). A Japanese food tradition is to eat black beans on New Year's Day to symbolize good health and fortune for the New Year. In the Jewish faith, it is common to serve apples and honey to celebrate the Jewish New Year. This represents hope that the coming year will be sweet. Think about your cultural heritage. What foods are part of your family's cultural traditions?

Food Taboos

In most cultures, social customs prohibit the use of certain edible resources as food. Such customs are called ***food taboos***. Many people in the United States enjoy eating beef. Most Hindus living in India and other parts of the world, however, have a food taboo against eating beef. Their culture considers cows to be sacred. People in some Asian countries cannot understand why people in the United States do not savor dog stew. In the United States, there is a food taboo against eating dog meat.

No single diet pattern is acceptable to all people. People learn feelings about food and other behaviors through cultural experiences. What tastes good depends largely on what you were taught to believe tastes good.

Religion

Religious beliefs have influenced people's food habits for centuries. Certain religious groups have rules regarding what members may or may not eat. For example, many Orthodox Jews follow dietary laws based on their interpretation of the Old Testament. These laws forbid the eating of pork and shellfish. They also specify that meat and dairy foods may not be stored, prepared, or eaten together. Foods prepared according to these laws are called ***kosher foods***.

Many other religions also have restrictions regarding food and drink. For instance, Muslims fast during the ninth month of their calendar year. Seventh-Day Adventists eat a vegetarian diet. They also abstain from drinking alcohol, tea, and coffee because of their effects on the body.

Some members of religious groups view food customs as strict commandments. Others observe the customs to help keep traditions alive for future generations.

CASE STUDY

Future Food Taboo?

In Japan, whale hunting is a tradition that dates back hundreds of years. Whale meat was once an important and common family food. Now, whale dishes are mostly found in restaurants, or the meat is canned and sold in supermarkets. Whale is not as popular as it once was, but it is still enjoyed by some people. The Japanese whaling ships catch primarily minke whales and lesser amounts of fin whales.

Environmental groups and others oppose the practice of killing whales. Their concerns focus on the harpooning methods used to kill whales and the threat to the number of minke whales in the sea.

Case Review

1. Do you think eating whale meat will become a food taboo? Why?
2. Name several common taboos that can be found in your family or community of friends. How do you think they became taboos? Will attitudes toward the taboos ever change? Why?

Growing Exposure and Access

In the United States, there is a growing interest in and taste for foods of other cultures. Specialty stores, farmers' markets, and supermarkets are carrying more and more of the ingredients needed to prepare the dishes of other cultures. Throughout this century, many more international visitors, immigrants, and refugees are likely to come to the United States. A growing number of people from the United States will travel internationally for business, study, and recreation. This is likely to expand the range of international food choices available to you.

A willingness to try the dishes of another culture will add variety to your palate and provide glimpses into the cultural heritage of others. It may inspire you to learn more about the influences that shaped the culture's cuisine (**Figure 2.3**).

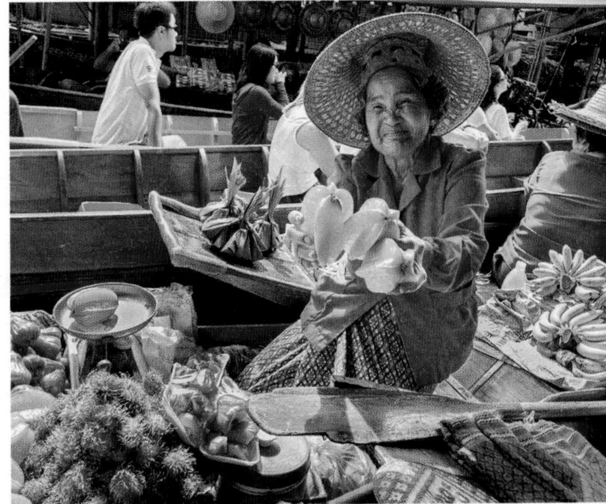

puwanai/Shutterstock.com

Figure 2.3 In many parts of the world, people settled next to rivers because much commerce occurred on and around the rivers. The floating markets in Thailand are a remnant of this past culture and are a popular tourist destination today.

Social Influences on Food Habits

Have you noticed that food seems to taste better when you share it with people you know and like? Food often plays a role in social relationships with family members and friends. These people, and other social factors, may influence the foods you choose to eat.

Family

The family is a major influence on the diets of young eaters. You no doubt formed many of your beliefs about food when you were much younger. By watching your family members, you learned about table manners and how to eat certain foods.

You learned about food traditions for holidays, birthdays, and other special occasions. You probably also adopted some of the food likes and dislikes of your family members.

Like culture, families change over time. Years ago, most households had two parents—a father who went off to work and a mother who stayed home. The mother was usually responsible for preparing food. Dinner was often served as soon as the father came home from work. Families have changed in many ways during the last century. The following changes have led to new trends in what, how, and when families eat:

- *More households are headed by working single parents.* A working single parent is likely to have a limited amount of time for meal preparation. Families today often rely on prepared foods to help save time. Meal preparation tasks may be shared among family members. The evening meal may be eaten later because preparation cannot begin until one or more family members arrive home.
- *Many dual-worker families have more income at their disposal.* Dual-worker families may be able to afford to buy more time-saving kitchen appliances and ready-made food products. They might have enough money to eat out more often. They might have sufficient means to hire someone to help with food preparation tasks, too. Dual-worker families have hectic schedules and eating times may vary from day-to-day. Family members sometimes find themselves eating meals on the run or preparing individual servings. Very few meals may be shared throughout the week.
- *The average family size is smaller.* Manufacturers are offering many food products in smaller portion sizes to better suit smaller households.
- *Family members are increasingly mobile.* Working family members may commute to their jobs. Children and teens are frequently involved in a variety of activities. Busy schedules often keep family members from eating meals together. Many family members are in the habit of serving themselves whenever they are hungry.

Values often influence family food habits. ***Values*** are beliefs and attitudes that are important to people. Traditions, such as making special foods and eating meals together, are important values in many families. Such traditions can bring family members closer emotionally and socially (**Figure 2.4**). This is probably why some families make a point to eat together at least once a day. Some may share these values but are unable to put them into practice for economic or other reasons.

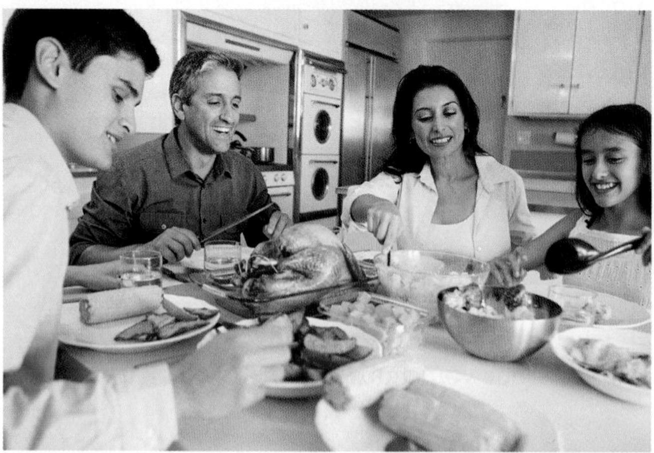

Monkey Business Images/Shutterstock.com

Figure 2.4 Teens who share family dinners three or more times per week are less likely to be overweight and take part in unhealthy behaviors. They are more likely to perform well in school and have better family relationships.

Friends

Your friends and peers play a major role in determining what, where, and when you eat. Have you noticed that your friends like many of the same foods you like? Specific favorites may vary from one region of the country to another, but some foods—such as pizza, tacos, hamburgers, and French fries—seem to be popular among teens everywhere.

WELLNESS TIP

Eating Out, Plan Ahead

To eat healthfully when eating out, plan ahead. Look at menus online and choose healthful foods from all food groups. Select foods that are baked, braised, broiled, grilled, steamed, or poached. For a lighter meal, order a child-size portion or an appetizer. Planning ahead and knowing what's available can help you stick to your healthy eating plan.

You are likely to see food anywhere people gather. Students eat lunch together in the school cafeteria. Fans eat hot dogs, popcorn, and nachos at sporting events. Friends enjoy sharing snacks and meals together at movie theaters, parties, church gatherings, and shopping malls.

Just as friends eat together almost anywhere, they also eat together almost anytime. Jogging partners may share breakfast after an early morning run. Neighbors may meet for midmorning coffee and rolls. Business associates often gather for lunch to discuss company decisions. A group of classmates may search the cupboards for an after-school snack. Couples and families enjoy sharing dinner in the evening at home and in restaurants. Teenagers may raid the refrigerator for a late-night study break.

When serving food to friends at a social event, people often choose foods that help create a festive mood. Certain foods add special meaning to social events. Thanksgiving turkey and wedding cake are popular examples.

When people serve food to friends, they want to serve foods their friends will like. Sometimes foods that people perceive as being popular are not the most healthful. For instance, adults may serve cake and cookies at a card party. Teens may serve chips and soft drinks to a group of friends. These foods are high in calories, saturated fat, and added sugar, and low in other nutrients.

You do not have to stop serving snack foods that are low in nutrients; however, you might want to offer your friends some healthful snacks, too. Fresh fruits or vegetables with an avocado or hummus dip make tasty, healthful alternatives to high-fat, high-calorie snacks (**Figure 2.5**).

Peers affect eating behaviors as well as food choices. Teens commonly worry about body weight, complexion problems, and the impressions they make on others. Some teens try new eating behaviors that are reported to address these problems. Dieting is one such behavior that is popular among teens.

When choosing eating behaviors, just as when choosing foods, you need to keep health in mind. For instance, choosing to follow an extreme diet to lose weight can be harmful. These diets often severely limit calories. Restricting calorie intake and failing to obtain essential nutrients during the teen years can inhibit growth.

Are your choices based on nutrition knowledge or the influence of your peers? Examine how much your friends influence your eating behaviors and food choices. Think about the extent to which they affect when, where, and what you eat. Ask yourself if you tend to eat after school or in the evenings because you are with your friends. Evaluate whether you order popcorn at the movies or hot dogs at a basketball game because your friends are doing so.

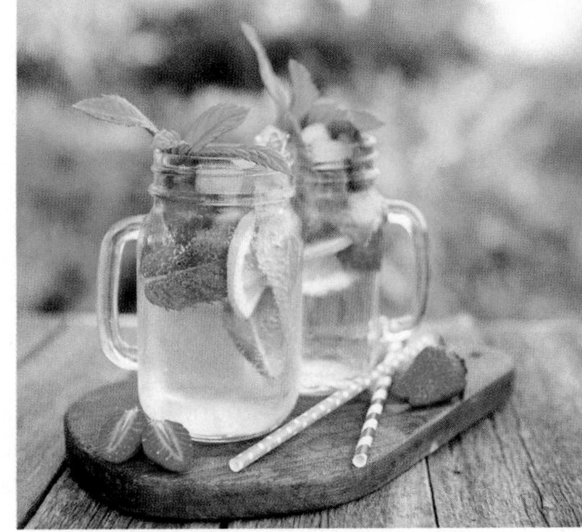

Ekaterina Iatcenko/Shutterstock.com

Figure 2.5 Nearly 50 percent of added sugars in the typical US teen's diet are from soft drinks, fruit drinks, and sport/energy drinks. Sparkling water with fruit is a delicious, healthier alternative.

Do you find yourself ordering a cheese and sausage pizza because that is what your friends like? Becoming aware of how others affect the quality of your diet can help you improve your overall health.

Prestige

Prestige is a person's reputation resulting from his or her achievement, rank, or other positive traits. Many people purchase or serve certain foods in an attempt to influence or impress others and gain prestige. For example, people may be willing to pay more for food that is considered fresh, wholesome, and healthful to impress others. They may serve more expensive bottles of water or other beverages to show they have the resources to buy such products. These people view shopping at pricey stores and at local markets that feature mostly organic foods as a way to display their success. Interestingly, healthful food purchases can be made in low-cost and high-cost supermarkets.

One specific food that is associated with prestige is caviar. Caviar is an expensive delicacy consisting of the unfertilized eggs (roe) of sturgeon fish. It is often served to impress others.

Media

The media is a strong social influence on food choices. Social media is used by millions of people worldwide. People may want to prepare foods in a way described in a newspaper or magazine, on social media, or on a television cooking channel.

THE MOVEMENT CONNECTION

Walk and Talk

Why

Taking a break from studies and homework to be mindful of eating whether you are alone or with family and friends can help you make healthy choices and relieve stress.

Apply

Food habits develop due to cultural, social, and emotional influences. Does your family have a favorite recipe they pass from one generation to the next? Or, is there a food that you identify with a particularly happy event in your life?

Walk around the classroom or hallway (with permission) and find three people with which to discuss this topic. After five minutes, gather by the whiteboard and remain standing. Take turns writing one similarity and one difference you discovered between the three people you spoke with and yourself. As a group, discuss the similarities and differences that exist within your class.

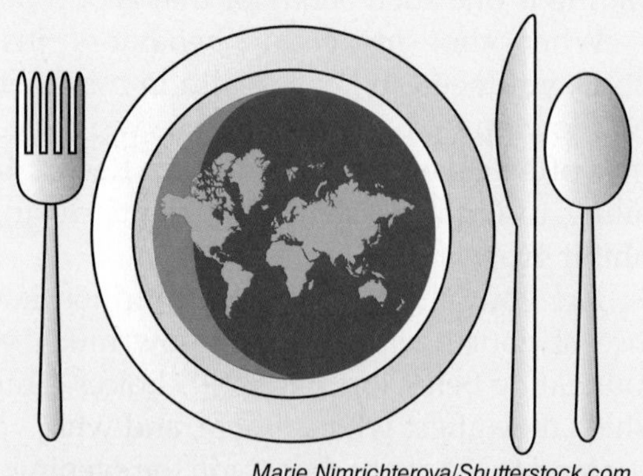

Marie Nimrichterova/Shutterstock.com

People frequently use social media to share photos of meals they ate at a restaurant or prepared themselves (**Figure 2.6**). ***Social media*** is defined as forms of electronic communication (such as websites) through which people create online communities to share information or ideas. People use these platforms to share brand name foods they recommend or foods they believe provide certain health benefits. Information shared on social media can affect the food choices of many who view this content.

The media is also a primary source for food advertisements. Television commercials have an especially strong impact on people's food choices. Commercials are designed to acquaint you with products. After you hear or see an ad over and over, you are more likely to buy the product.

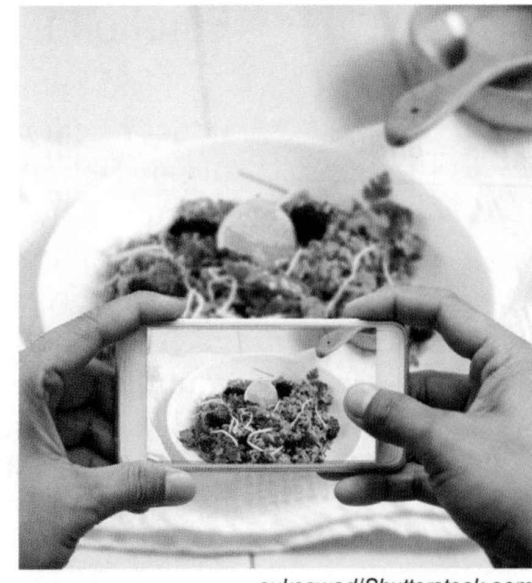

suksawad/Shutterstock.com

Figure 2.6 It is a common practice to take a photo of your meal and upload it to social media. *When you see photos of meals others have posted, how does this influence your food choices?*

Research shows that young people in the United States view an average of 40,000 commercials a year. Children become socialized to want the foods they see advertised. More than half of television commercials are for foods high in calories, sugar, fat, and salt. A daily eating pattern of such foods instead of fresh fruits, vegetables, and whole grains can harm children's health and development.

The impact of media on health and wellness across the life span continues to be researched.

Emotions Affect Food Habits

People use food to do more than satisfy physical hunger. Many people choose to eat or avoid certain foods for emotional reasons. For example, suppose you ate a hot dog for lunch and felt terribly sick later in the day. This may lead you to form a mental connection between hot dogs and illness. You may think, "Hot dogs make me sick, and I never want to eat one again!" Such an emotional response can outweigh hunger pangs and nutrition knowledge in its effect on your food habits (**Figure 2.7**).

Mental Connections with Foods and Eating Patterns

Food/Eating Pattern	Mental Connection
Luncheon salads	Femininity
Meat and potatoes	Masculinity
Carving meats	Strength, authority
Expensive foods	Status, elegance
Sharing food	Trust, friendship, hospitality
Giving food as a gift	Custom, affection
Snacking	Amusement, camaraderie
Family dining	Security
Formal dining	Tradition, ritual
Eating alone	Independence, loneliness, punishment
Refusal to eat	Sacrifice, retaliation
Overeating	Anxiety, greed, frustration, lack of self-control
Fad dieting	Insecurity, vanity, popularity

Figure 2.7 Emotional factors cause some people to form mental connections with certain foods and eating patterns. *What foods create emotional responses for you?*

Emotional Responses to Food

Food evokes many emotional responses. People develop most of their emotional reactions toward foods in early life. For some people, food creates feelings of satisfaction and happiness. For others, food produces feelings of frustration or disgust. Play a word association game with a friend to learn more about your emotional response to food. What feelings come to mind when you hear the words *chocolate*, *liver*, *spinach*, and *ice cream*?

You learn some emotional responses to food in the context of family, school, community, religion, and the media. In other words, your culture affects how you will react to the food presented to you.

Some emotional responses to food may be associated with gender. Research has shown that some people connect maleness with hardy foods, such as steak and potatoes. Similarly, some people link femininity with dainty foods, such as parfaits and quiches.

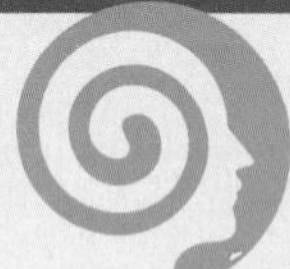

EXTEND YOUR KNOWLEDGE

Does Gender Affect Food Choices?

Do you make food choices because you are female or male? Probably. Your food choices may be affected by gender stereotyping. *Gender stereotyping* is an overgeneralization about characteristic differences between the genders. For example, research has shown that people often view light foods, such as salads and grilled foods, as feminine foods. Fried and high-fat foods, such as fried chicken or nachos and cheese, are viewed as masculine foods.

Advertisers try to target their ad promotions toward specific groups, knowing that food is viewed differently by males and females in this culture. Small containers of yogurt and prepared salads are marketed toward females. Commercials for "megaburgers" and French fries often employ muscular males to appeal to the male consumer. In general, there is a stereotype that women choose healthy foods more frequently than males. "Healthy" foods are frequently sold in smaller, more colorful packages that appeal to women.

Evidence that gender affects food choices is clearly reflected in the food and beverage packaging industry. Skinny bottles of beverages with a petite female on the label front are marketed to females. Oversized snack packages are marketed mostly to males. Packaging intended to appeal to males is often designed to look crisp, bold, or crinkly.

Evidence shows that targeting to a specific gender sells more products. Is it possible the food industry is encouraging stereotypes about gender food choices? As distinct gender roles disappear, is it possible that salads, yogurts, healthy grains, and fresh fruits and vegetables will be marketed to both males and females? In the same way? Will stereotyping of gender eating behaviors become more difficult to identify? What message does the packaging on the two bars shown in this feature communicate?

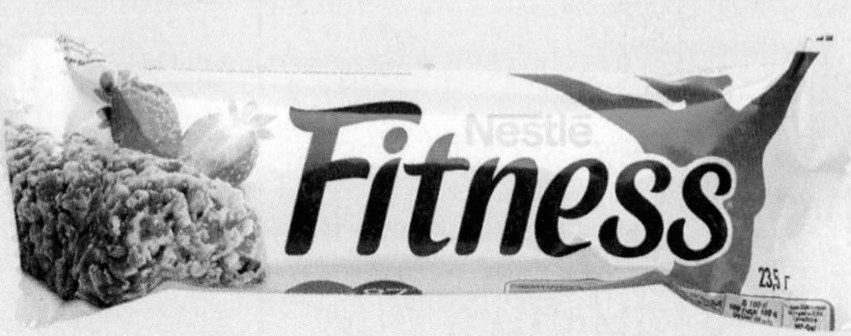

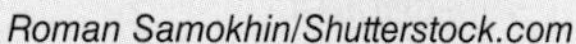
Roman Samokhin/Shutterstock.com

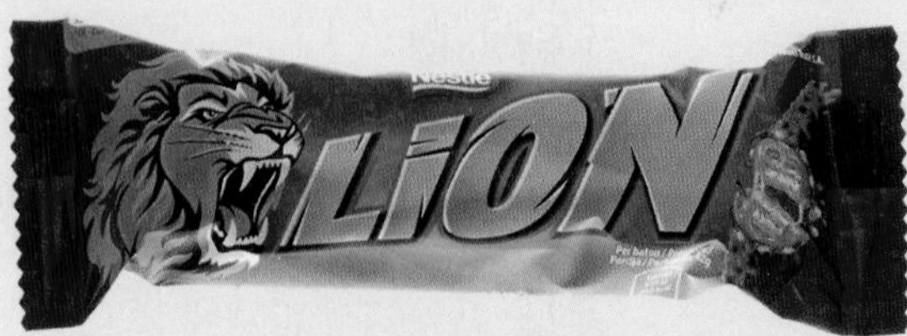

Toni Genes/Shutterstock.com

Using Food to Deal with Emotions

Food not only evokes emotions, it can also be used to express emotions. Many people offer food as a symbol of love and caring (**Figure 2.8**). People show concern by taking food to neighbors and friends who have an illness or a death in the family.

People often choose to eat certain foods to help meet emotional needs. For instance, a chocolate bar may cheer you up when you are depressed. Your grandmother's recipe for macaroni and cheese may comfort you when you are feeling lonely. A double scoop of ice cream might be just what you need to celebrate a good report card. Chicken noodle soup may nourish your emotions as well as your body when you have a cold.

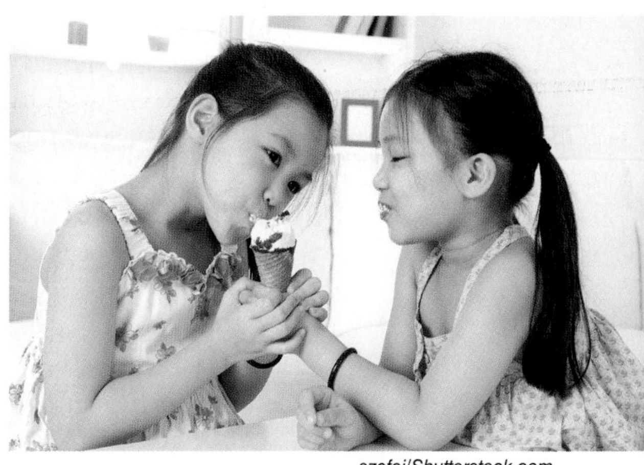

szefei/Shutterstock.com

Figure 2.8 Sharing food with others is a demonstration of love.

Frustration can lead some people to eat more or less food than their bodies need. Other people use food to help them deal with fears. Both types of people use the pleasure of eating to avoid thoughts that are annoying or scary. Have you ever found yourself wanting to snack heavily before a big event in your life? If so, you may have been associating food with emotional comfort.

Some feelings related to food can be harmful. Some teens and young adults, mainly girls, starve themselves to be very thin. This pattern of eating is grounded in emotions and requires the help of professional counselors. People must examine the way they use food to help put eating behaviors into a healthy perspective.

Food Used for Rewards or Punishment

Foods can be used to manipulate behaviors. For instance, parents may use food to change a child's behavior. If parents want to encourage a child to do something, they may give a special treat. Cookies, ice cream, and candy are popular rewards for good behavior.

People who have been rewarded with food as children may continue to reward themselves with food as adults. They may select food rewards even when they are not hungry. Following this learned pattern of behavior can lead to weight management problems.

CASE STUDY

CASE ★ STUDY ★ CASE
CASE STUDY
CASE ★ STUDY ★ CASE

Teaching Eating Behavior

Jenny is a hyperactive two-year-old child. When the family goes to a restaurant, Jenny can be very loud and has a hard time sitting still. Her parents give her lollipops to keep her quiet. At home, they tell her that if she eats her dinner, she can have a special treat of chocolate chip cookies.

Case Review

1. What is Jenny learning from these experiences?
2. How do you think the parents' behaviors will impact Jenny's life as an adult?

Sometimes parents take foods away from children as a punishment. For instance, a parent may withhold dessert when a child misbehaves at the dinner table. This can cause some children to develop negative emotions toward food and eating. Some children carry such negative associations into their adult years.

Individual Preferences Affect Food Habits

You choose to eat many foods simply because you like them. What causes you to like some foods more than others? Your emotions are one factor. You are likely to prefer foods that you associate with positive emotions, such as comfort and caring. However, you are apt to dislike foods that you associate with negative feelings, such as guilt and fear.

Your genes are partly responsible for your food preferences. You were born with personal preferences for certain tastes and smells. Everyone has taste buds that sense the tastes of sweet, salty, sour, bitter, and umami. Just how you perceive each of these tastes is part of your unique makeup. For instance, one person might wince in pain from the heat he or she feels when eating a jalapeño pepper. Another person may hardly notice the heat when eating one of these peppers.

This difference in taste perception is due to genetics. It helps explain why members of the same family, who have the same background, often prefer the same foods. If your taste preferences are different from other members of your family, you may have inherited a different set of genes.

Although genes play an important role in determining taste preferences, your experiences with food affect your preferences, too. Suppose someone offers you a choice between fried grasshoppers and a hamburger. If you have eaten hamburgers but never tried grasshoppers, you are more likely to choose the hamburger. Someone from China, where fried grasshoppers are a delicacy, might be more likely to choose the grasshoppers. People simply prefer what is familiar to them.

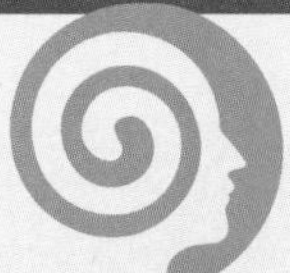

EXTEND YOUR KNOWLEDGE

Umami—A New Basic Taste?

Umami—the fifth basic taste—is somewhat new to Western culture, but it has been understood in Asian culture for centuries. Umami is a savory, meaty taste that results from glutamate. Glutamates occur naturally in some foods, such as mushrooms, aged cheeses, tomatoes, seafood, Chinese cabbage, and soy sauce. Monosodium glutamate (MSG) is a flavor additive that also produces umami taste. It is used to enhance the flavors of savory food by having an impact on the other ingredients in a dish.

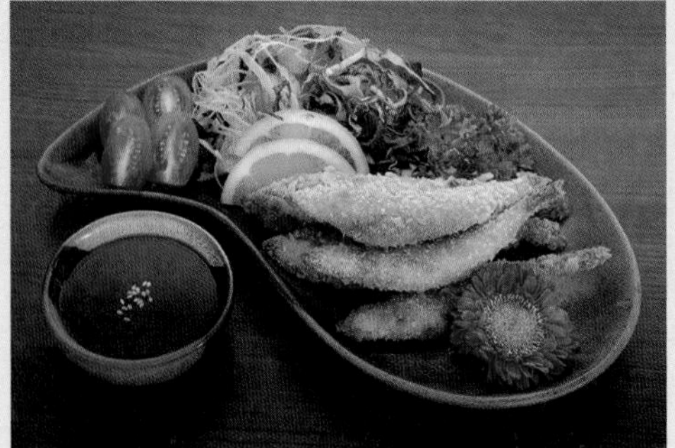

Thoyod Pisanu/Shutterstock.com

Next time you are eating your favorite stew, consider whether umami is a contributing factor in the flavor. Consider doing a taste comparison of a clear chicken broth with MSG and one without. How does the flavor differ? Use the Nutrition Facts panels to compare the sodium content of each product.

The Influences of Agriculture, Technology, Economics, and Politics

Sometimes you have control over what is available to eat and sometimes you do not. When you buy food, you have control over what is in your cupboards; however, you have little control over what foods are available in the supermarket. Factors that can affect what foods are sold in stores include agriculture, technology, economics, and politics.

Most people in the United States have many foods available to them. This is not the case for many people throughout the world. In poor countries, agriculture, technology, economics, and politics affect more than the variety of foods available. These factors can affect whether there is food available at all.

Agriculture and Land Use

Food production is plentiful when important resources are available to grow crops. These resources include

- fertile soil;
- adequate water supply;
- favorable climate;
- technical knowledge; and
- human energy.

The availability of these five resources differs greatly among regions throughout the world. Crops need fertile soil in which their roots can take hold. Fertile soil supplies the nutrients plants need to grow. In some regions, the soil quality is too poor to support crop growth.

Quality of soil varies from area to area in the United States and throughout the world. The typical diet of a region usually is based on the foods that grow well there. For example, soil quality in the Andes Mountains of South America is too poor to support many types of crops. Hardy crops such as potatoes grow well there, however, yielding large amounts in a small amount of acreage. Therefore, potatoes are a staple food in the countries through which the Andes extend, including Chile, Peru, and Bolivia (**Figure 2.9**). A ***staple food*** is a food that is eaten routinely and supplies a large portion of the calories people need to maintain health.

In Asia, rice grows well and is a staple food in the diet. Western Europe and the United States have conditions favorable for growing wheat. Bread made with wheat flour is a **prevalent** (main) part of the diets of these regions. Corn grows well in South American soil. Therefore, South American people eat many corn-based foods. Rye is a staple crop in Russia and northern Europe. This grain is used to make the hardy breads typical of this region.

Water availability affects food availability. Experts predict lack of fresh water will be one of the most serious concerns in this century.

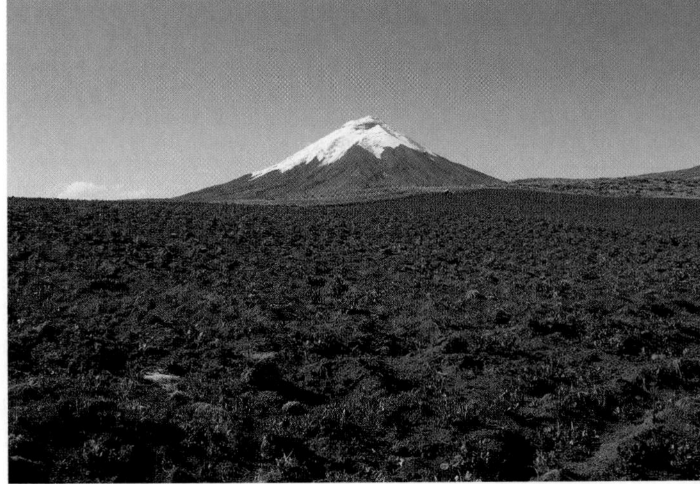

Ecuadorpostales/Shutterstock.com

Figure 2.9 Today, potatoes are still grown in the Andes Mountains but serve as a staple in the diets of many people around the world.

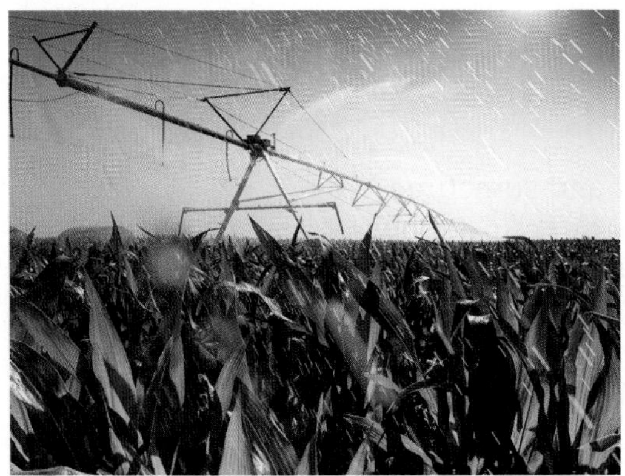

KSwinicki/Shutterstock.com

Figure 2.10 Agriculture is the largest user of freshwater on the planet. Water is pulled from rivers, lakes, and groundwater to irrigate fields. *What do you think is the second largest user of freshwater on the planet?*

Rainfall is not always plentiful enough to fill the rivers and streams. Watering crops to increase yields creates a heavy draw on underground water supplies. Thus, water resources are at risk of being depleted (**Figure 2.10**).

Climate refers to the average temperatures and rainfall in a region. Different crops grow best in different climates. For instance, citrus fruits require warm temperatures that last for an extended time. Apples, on the other hand, cannot withstand long periods of warm weather. That is why most oranges come from warm regions such as Florida, Israel, and Spain. Apples tend to grow well in cooler regions such as Washington, Oregon, and Russia. Wherever the weather can sustain plant life, people can raise some type of food.

Technical knowledge is specialized information. It helps farmers get the most from their land. Through experience and scientific study, farmers have learned ways to increase crop production. They have discovered what nutrients crops need to grow. This has helped them develop planting techniques and chemical fertilizers that replenish the soil with those nutrients. Farmers have determined how much water crops require, and have installed elaborate watering systems to provide it. They have identified what weeds and insects are damaging to plants. This has enabled them to take steps to control these pests.

Human energy is needed to plant seeds and harvest crops. In areas where the other four resources are readily available, a few people can produce an abundant food supply. When the other resources are scarce, however, many people may be needed to grow only small amounts of food. In the midwestern United States, the soil is fertile and an ample amount of rain falls each year. The climate is suitable for growing crops such as corn, wheat, and soybeans. Farmers in this area are able to take advantage of the latest information about the most productive farming methods. These factors allow a midwestern farmer to produce enough grain to feed thousands of people per year.

In contrast to the midwestern farmer, consider a farmer in a country such as Afghanistan. Much of the land is covered by mountains or desert, making it difficult to farm. Although some areas have fertile soil, rainfall is insufficient to support crop growth. Many farmers lack access to current technical knowledge.

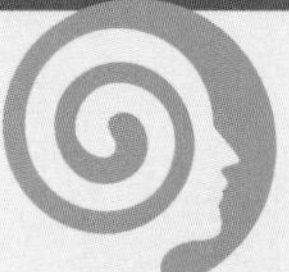

EXTEND YOUR KNOWLEDGE

Food and Agriculture Organization (FAO)

Many private and government agencies work to end global hunger. Some specialize in short-term crisis relief. Others work on long-term solutions, such as improving farming methods. The Food and Agriculture Organization (FAO) is an international organization that focuses on increasing crop yields in developing nations. FAO is also concerned with the fair distribution of food to rural people. FAO is part of the United Nations system. FAO offices are located worldwide.

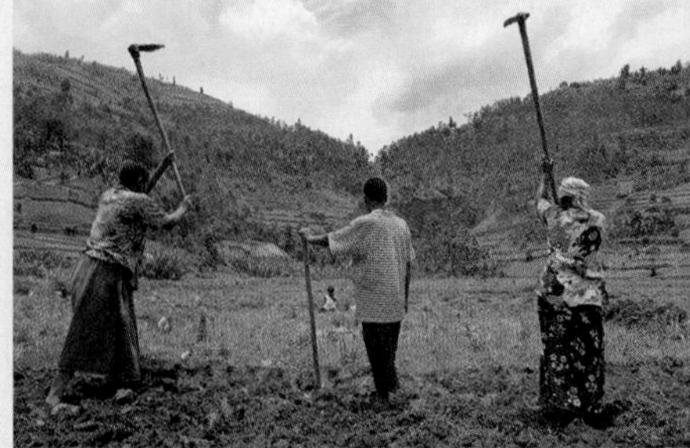

giulio napolitano/Shutterstock.com

They are also unable to obtain high-quality seeds, modern machinery, and chemicals to help stimulate plant growth and control insects. In Afghanistan, many farmers barely produce enough food to feed their families.

Technology

Shoppers in the United States often find Chilean kiwifruit and Mexican mangoes in the produce section of the supermarket. With the help of science and technology, as well as transportation resources, foods from many lands are as close as the local supermarket.

In the last 75 to 100 years, many changes in technology and agriculture have influenced how food gets from farm to table. ***Technology*** is the application of scientific knowledge for useful purposes to accomplish tasks or solve problems. Modern farming machinery, faster food-processing systems, and rapid transportation are all examples of technological advances. The invention of new foods and food-handling processes has increased the food supply (**Figure 2.11**).

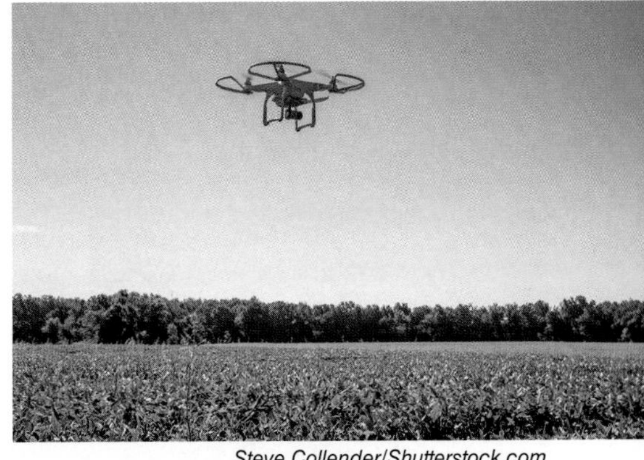

Steve Collender/Shutterstock.com

Figure 2.11 Farmers use drone technology for soil analysis, planting, spraying, monitoring, and irrigation.

Developing New Foods

New foods are being developed more rapidly with modern food biotechnology. ***Food biotechnology*** uses knowledge of plant or animal science and genetics to develop plants and animals with specific desirable traits while eliminating traits that are not wanted. Genes that carry the desirable trait are moved from one plant or animal to another. (Genes are units in every cell that control an organism's inherited traits.)

FEATURED CAREER

Food Technologist

Food technologists work in the food processing industry, in universities, and in government. They generally work in product development—applying the findings from food science research to improve the selection, preservation, processing, packaging, and distribution of food.

Education

Most jobs in this area require a bachelor's degree, but a master's or doctorate degree is usually a requirement for university research positions. Relevant coursework includes life and physical sciences, such as cell and molecular biology, microbiology, and inorganic and organic chemistry.

Job Outlook

The demand for new food products and safety measures will drive the job growth for food technologists. Food research is expected to increase because of heightened public awareness of diet, health, food safety, and *biosecurity*—preventing the introduction of infectious agents into herds of animals. Advances in biotechnology and nanotechnology should also spur demand, as food technologists apply these technologies to testing and monitoring food safety.

Food biotechnology uses a mix of traditional and modern breeding techniques to produce genetically modified foods. The World Health Organization defines ***genetically modified (GM) foods*** as "foods derived from organisms whose genetic material (DNA) has been modified in a way that does not occur naturally." Currently, most of the GM foods in the supermarket are plant-based foods. In the future, foods you buy may have clear labeling to indicate that genetically modified ingredients were used.

For centuries, farmers have worked to breed desirable qualities into plants and animals. Food biotechnology increases the speed and accuracy of this process. The new plants may be more resistant to factors such as disease, pests, or drought. By reducing or eliminating these factors, more food can be produced on less land using fewer chemicals and less water or other resources. Some food biotechnology focuses on enhancing the nutritional content of a food. For example, researchers have developed corn with higher concentrations of specific protein components and more healthful cooking oils.

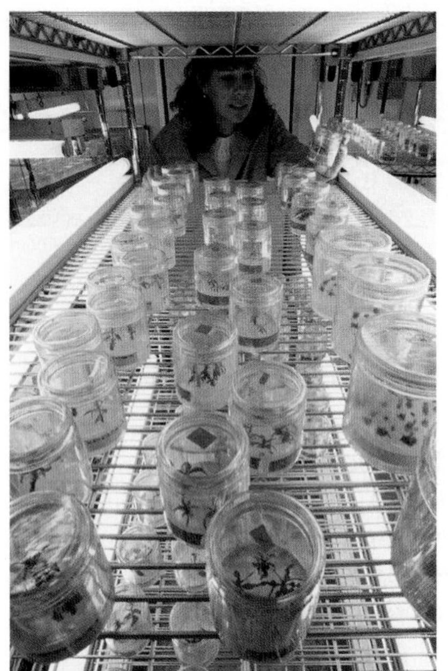

Scott Bauer/USDA

Figure 2.12 This USDA technician observes experimental peach and apple trees that are a product of food biotechnology.

The use of biotech foods has caused controversy in some groups and countries around the world. The safety of biotech foods concerns some consumers. Food biotechnology that is well regulated poses little threat to people or the environment. Agricultural scientists point out that biotech foods are just as safe as traditional foods. Developers must consult with the FDA before they can introduce a new biotech food. This process takes several years. It ensures these products pass the FDA's food safety assessment.

Many discoveries and advances in food biotechnology begin in USDA research centers. The USDA also oversees field trials and large-scale production of biotech plants and animals (**Figure 2.12**). The Environmental Protection Agency (EPA) regulates the pest-resistant properties of biotech crops. These many checkpoints assure consumers and product developers of the safety of food biotechnology.

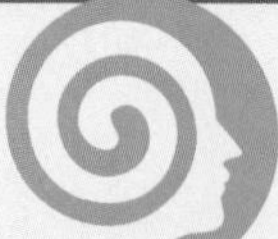

EXTEND YOUR KNOWLEDGE

Labeling Biotech Foods

Most genetically modified (GM) foods taste much like traditional foods. The FDA does not require special food labeling for GM foods at this time; however, labels are required for the following:

- food that causes an allergic reaction in some people
- food whose nutrient content is changed (for example, a bioengineered carrot with more vitamin A)
- food for which an issue exists regarding how the food is used or consequences of its use
- food that is new to the diet

New foods introduced to the public always require labeling. It does not matter whether the food is the result of biotechnology or traditional crossbreeding methods. Visit the FDA website to learn more about labeling of these foods. Next time you are in the supermarket, see if you can identify foods that are the result of biotechnology.

Social issues related to bioengineered foods center on how much the consumer has a right to know about food ingredients produced with genetically modified plants or animals. Federal laws will continue to be rewritten as consumers press for more information.

FOOD AND THE ENVIRONMENT

Nutrition from Edible Insects

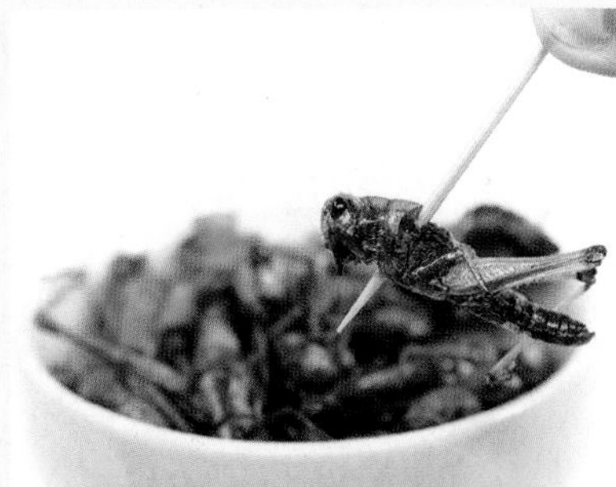
Napat/Shutterstock.com

A greater number of people in the United States and other Western countries are beginning to consider insects as a food option for human consumption. Part of the reason for this lies in the serious environmental challenges of global climate change and its effects on the ability to provide food for a growing world population. Another reason is that insects, such as beetles and grasshoppers, have an interesting taste that some people enjoy.

The Food and Agriculture Organization (FAO) reports that raising cattle, pigs, chickens, and other animals for meat production contributes to the production of greenhouse gases. Livestock feed production, food processing, and gas emissions from manure, along with transportation of animal products, are major sources of harmful environmental by-products. It takes a great deal more land and water to raise a cow or pig than it does to raise corn, beans, or potatoes, but all are good food sources of protein.

Why not consider farming insects—such as bees, ants, or beetles—as a food source for people? Insects can be fed on compost and require little space. Hunger remains a persistent global problem that affects over 900 million human beings worldwide. The production of insect food sources has few effects on the global climate, and they are safe to eat. Insects may soon be a common food option in the United States.

Most insects are a good source of protein. Their protein concentration can be equal to beef, but with less fat and fewer calories. Insects are also rich in other essential nutrients, including vitamin B_{12}, riboflavin, and vitamin A. Can you imagine an insect aisle at the supermarket? Mealworms, tiny crayfish, grasshoppers, and water bugs could be packaged attractively at the meat counter in the supermarket right next to ground beef and chicken legs. Or, imagine a fast-food restaurant that serves bug burgers!

Think Critically

1. What obstacles must be overcome for insects to become a viable food source in the United States?
2. Not all insects are edible. Consider when it might be unsafe to eat insects.
3. Why is it more common today to eat insects in some parts of the world than in other parts?
4. In what type of recipes or food dishes would you use insects as an ingredient?

Advances in Packaging

Improved food packaging is another way in which technology has affected the food supply. Researchers try to design packaging materials that will keep food safe without adding much to the cost of products. Plastic is one such material that is commonly used in food packaging. Plastics keep food fresh and protect food from contaminants in the air and on unclean surfaces. Another factor researchers must keep in mind when designing packaging is its impact on the environment. One option being studied is biodegradable packaging that will break down in landfills.

A packaging technology that preserves quality and extends the shelf life of food is called ***aseptic packaging***. This process involves packing sterile food into sterile containers. It is done in a sterile atmosphere. Bacteria cannot grow in aseptic packages. Therefore, food in aseptic packaging does not need to be refrigerated to remain wholesome. This means perishable foods can be safely stored in places where there is no refrigeration. These foods must be refrigerated once the package is opened.

Food products can now be safely and quickly transported all over the world. Staple foods can be stored for extended periods, and then used during times of food shortages. These foods can be shipped to areas where food production is low and people want to buy them.

The Economics of Food

Have you ever had to forego buying a candy bar because you had no money? This is a minor example of the fact that it takes money to buy food. It also takes money to buy the seeds to grow food.

Economics has much to do with the availability of food. If a country cannot afford agricultural supplies or other technological aids, such as tractors, its food production is limited. If farmers cannot buy fertilizer, crop yields decrease. Poverty is a close relative of hunger.

Poor countries lack the resources to build food-processing plants and store food safely. This can result in up to 40 percent of crops being lost to spoilage and contamination (**Figure 2.13**). Poor countries also lack the funds to import food from more productive countries. The nutritional status of the entire population can suffer when a country's economy cannot afford to produce adequate food.

In wealthy countries, food prices and availability are also affected by global events and situations. For example, when corn is used for the production of ethanol gas, less corn is available for consumption or distribution. The price of corn-based foods in stores increases. When drought affects rice-growing countries and production decreases, the price of rice in the local supermarket goes up, too. As you follow news events, you can identify ways global events directly affect the availability and cost of food in your local stores.

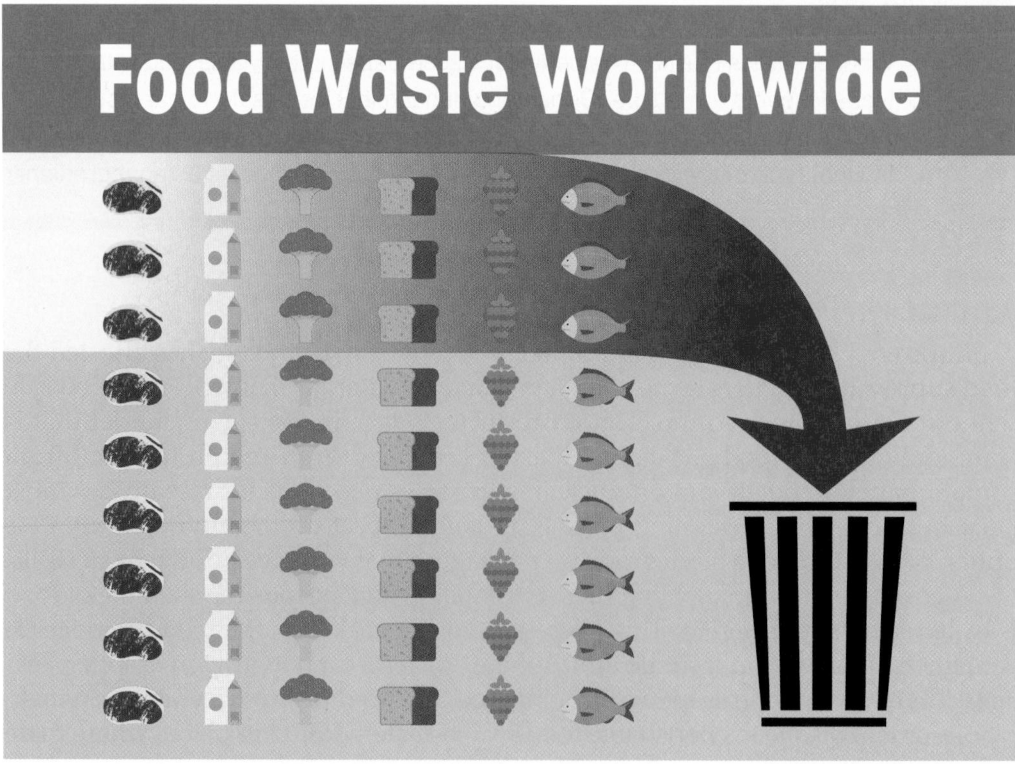

Red monkey/Shutterstock.com

Figure 2.13 Worldwide, nearly 900 million people are undernourished, while approximately one-third of the food produced is lost to spoilage or is thrown away. *Where do you see food being wasted?*

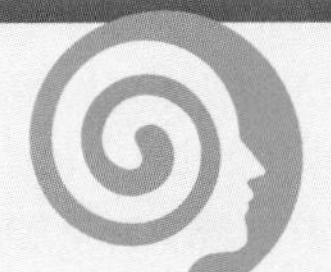

EXTEND YOUR KNOWLEDGE

The Power of Food

In many parts of the world, war and conflict create problems for farmers and affect food production. Fighting forces millions of people to flee their homes, leading to hunger. People without a home find themselves without the means to feed themselves. The recent conflict in Syria has caused many people to flee for safety and, subsequently, their food security was lost.

In war, food sometimes becomes a weapon. Soldiers will starve opponents into submission by seizing or destroying food and livestock, and by systematically wrecking local markets. Fields are often mined and water wells contaminated, forcing farmers to abandon their land. When war and strife end, hunger problems are reduced.

Research a country where there is strife, war, and hunger occurring today. Find current reports in the media to understand the role that food supply, political power, and upheaval play in creating the desperate hunger conditions in the country. Who do you think has the power to deny or permit the delivery of food to the hungry people? What political solutions are possible for reducing hunger at the local, national, and international levels?

The Politics of Food

The degree to which a country's economic resources are used to address food problems depends largely on politics. The people with political power make most of the decisions in some countries. Those who have political power may decide what lands will be used for food production. They might determine what crops will be grown. Sometimes the decision is made to raise crops that can be sold to other countries. Money from these crops often goes to the people in power rather than the farmers who grew the crops. While the politicians get rich, the farmers remain too poor to buy food. Land that could be used to raise nutritious food for hungry people is being used to grow the exported crops instead.

Some political decision makers invest a large percentage of a country's economic resources in military power. Sometimes leaders make these decisions to increase their personal power. Sometimes they feel compelled to **channel** (guide) resources to the military to protect their country from hostile neighbors. In any case, money spent on the military is not available to help develop a country's agricultural production. It cannot be used to buy food from other countries, either.

Political leaders may even decide how food will be distributed. Food needed by hungry people may be given to the military. People with higher status may receive more or better food than those who are poor (**Figure 2.14**).

Politics does not affect food only in other countries. The US government sets many policies that relate to the food supply. Some policies concern food products that are imported from other countries. Some of these policies are intended to ensure the wholesomeness of foods. Other policies are designed to protect the market for products produced in the United States. Still other policies are made to keep trade relations with other countries friendly.

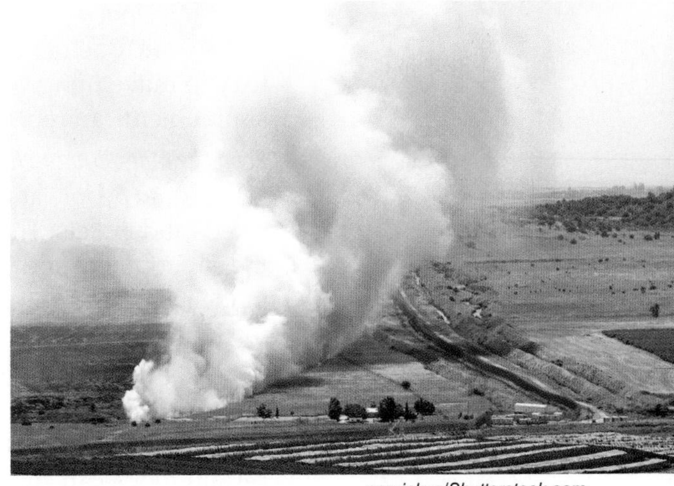

servickuz/Shutterstock.com

Figure 2.14 When politics result in war, food production declines due to a lack of access to seed, fertilizer, and feed, as well as destruction of land and equipment.

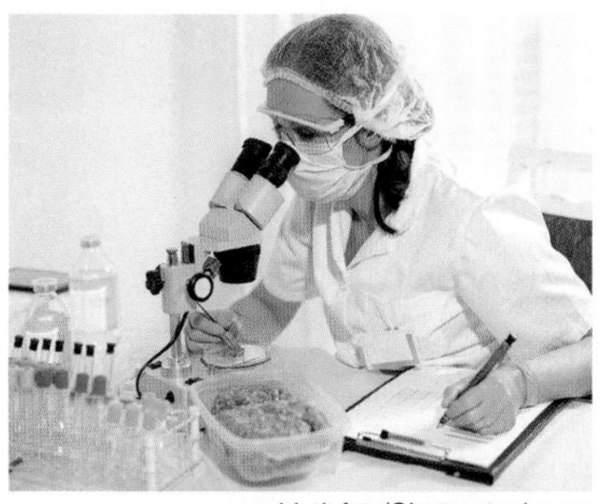

adriaticfoto/Shutterstock.com

Figure 2.15 Food processors conduct periodic analyses of samples to ensure foods meet product standards and maintain records for review by government investigators.

Many federal regulations **mandate** (direct) how food is to be produced and processed. The government requires that many foods, such as meat and poultry, be inspected to be sure they are wholesome. Guidelines state that manufacturers must pack foods in a sanitary setting (**Figure 2.15**). Laws require label information to be truthful. Federal acts designate what types of ingredients can be added to products, too. All of these factors affect the foods that are available to you in the marketplace.

Nutrition Knowledge Affects Food Habits

This chapter has addressed a number of factors that affect your food habits. As you have read, factors ranging from your culture to government policies have an impact on the foods you select. One other factor that influences your food habits is how much you know about nutrition.

To illustrate this point, answer the following question: Should you avoid vegetable oil because it is high in cholesterol? If you said yes, you would be agreeing with 68 percent of respondents to a nationwide survey. Unfortunately, you would be wrong. Vegetable oil, like all other foods from plant sources, contains no cholesterol. Therefore, you would be avoiding a food based on misinformation. This example should help you understand why correct information is so important. It can help you make knowledgeable decisions about food.

Fact or Fiction?

People have many beliefs about food and nutrition. The following are just a few examples reflecting a lack of knowledge that may lead people to make uninformed choices:

- *Certain foods have magical powers.* Eating fish will not make you a genius. Eating yogurt will not allow you to live to be over 100 years old. All nutritious foods have benefits for the body; however, you must eat a variety of foods. No single food provides all the nutrients you need.
- *Taking vitamin and mineral supplements eliminates the need to eat nutritious foods.* Some doctors suggest taking a multivitamin and mineral supplement to help make up for what is lacking in your eating pattern; however, no supplement can replace the nutrients supplied by nutritious foods.
- *Foods grown without chemical pesticides have greater nutritional value than other foods.* Some people are concerned about the effects of chemicals used to control weeds and insects. They worry about the impact these chemicals may have on the environment and the food chain. Farmers must use chemicals within safety guidelines set by government agencies, however. And most studies show that foods grown with and without chemical pesticides have similar nutritional value.
- *Certain foods can cure diseases.* Some people have heard an old story about British sailors. The story reports how the sailors stopped dying of scurvy when they started eating citrus fruits. Many people want to believe eating certain foods can similarly cure such diseases as arthritis and cancer. What these people may not understand is that scurvy is a nutrient-deficiency disease. A lack of vitamin C in the diet causes the disease. The vitamin C contained in the citrus fruit cured the sailors, not the fruit itself.

Some foods have been shown to be useful in preventing and treating certain diseases not caused by nutrient deficiencies. For instance, research has shown that regularly eating onions and garlic may help prevent some types of cancer. Diet is only one of several factors, however, that play a role in disease prevention and treatment.

Reliable Information

Where do you look for information about nutrition? Friends and relatives may offer advice, but they may lack knowledge. You can find an abundance of nutrition information through books, magazines, television, and the Internet. Be aware that details from these sources can be incomplete or inaccurate, however. For reliable information, look for materials reviewed by registered dietitians. These professionals have expert knowledge of nutrition.

Knowledge about your health is also important for making the best food choices. Certain illnesses, such as diabetes and hypertension, require a modified diet. A qualified physician must correctly diagnose illnesses. Then a registered dietitian can help people with illnesses plan diets that will meet their special needs.

RECIPE FILE

Spinach Omelet

1 SERVING

Ingredients

- 2 eggs
- 1 T. water or milk
- 1 t. butter or margarine (or cooking spray)
- ½ c. fresh spinach, chopped
- ¼ c. low-fat Monterey Jack cheese, grated
- scant pinch of nutmeg
- hot pepper sauce to taste (optional)

Directions

1. Break eggs into a large bowl and add water or milk.
2. Put butter or margarine into skillet, or if using cooking spray, coat the inside of the skillet well. Place skillet over medium heat.
3. Beat the eggs together with the water or milk with a whisk or fork.
4. Pour egg mixture into hot skillet. Mixture should set immediately around the edges.
5. With an inverted pancake turner, pull the cooked portion of the egg from the edge to the center of the pan, exposing the hot pan.
6. Tilt the pan so the uncooked egg can flow onto the exposed hot pan.
7. Continue until the egg is set and will not flow.
8. Place spinach on one half of the omelet and sprinkle with cheese. Place spinach/cheese filling on the left side if you are right-handed, or on the right side if you are left-handed. Sprinkle with nutmeg.
9. Slide a pancake turner around the edge of the omelet to loosen. If the edges do not stick to the pan, it will fold more easily.
10. With the pancake turner, fold the omelet in half.
11. Invert onto a plate. Sprinkle with hot pepper sauce if desired.
12. Serve immediately.

PER SERVING: 243 CALORIES, 21 G PROTEIN, 3 G CARBOHYDRATE, 16 G FAT, 0.5 G FIBER, 322 MG SODIUM.

Chapter 2 Review and Expand

Reading Summary

Many factors influence people's food habits. Food habits often reflect a person's culture. The culture's way of life is influenced by beliefs, traditions, and customs, some of which are related to food choices and consumption patterns. Religious beliefs also influence food habits.

People choose food for social reasons. Family members influence the food choices children make. Friends can also influence food habits, especially for teens. The media influences people's desire and willingness to eat certain foods, too.

Emotion is another factor that affects food habits. Some foods produce emotional responses in people. In the same way, some emotions cause people to desire certain foods. Some people use food to reward or punish themselves or others.

Agriculture, technology, economics, and politics affect what foods are sold in the supermarket. Foods that grow well in a region are likely to be widely available in that region. Technological advances have made it easier for foods from all over the world to reach local supermarkets. People with political power make decisions that affect the availability of food products among people in a country.

A final factor that affects food habits is nutrition knowledge. People are more likely to choose foods that are good for them when they understand their nutritional needs.

Chapter Vocabulary

1. **Content Terms** Working in small groups, locate a small image online that visually describes or explains each of the following terms. To create flash cards, write each term on a note card and paste the image that describes or explains the term on the opposite side.

aseptic packaging	genetically modified (GM) food
cultural heritage	kosher food
culture	social media
food biotechnology	staple food
food norm	technology
food taboo	value

2. **Academic Terms** Write each of the following terms on a separate sheet of paper. For each term, quickly write a word you think relates to the term. In small groups, exchange papers. Have each person in the group explain a term on the list. Take turns until all terms have been explained.

channel	iconic
commerce	mandate
emigrate	prevalent

Review Learning

3. Why does a collection of foods come to be associated with a particular region, race, or religion?
4. *True or false?* A social custom that prohibits eating dog meat is an example of a food norm.
5. What are four trends that have influenced family eating habits?
6. *True or false?* Some people shop at stores that feature mostly organic foods as a way to gain prestige.
7. What are two ways in which the media influences people's food choices and eating habits?
8. When do people develop most of their emotional reactions toward foods?
9. *True or false?* People who have been rewarded with food as children may continue to reward themselves with food as adults.
10. What factors most affect individuals' food preferences?
11. What five resources are needed to grow plentiful crops?
12. Name three technological advances that have improved the food supply in modern history.
13. How can lack of food processing plants and food storage facilities affect food availability in an economically disadvantaged country?
14. List three examples of lack of nutrition knowledge that may lead people to make misinformed food choices.

Self-Assessment Quiz

Complete the self-assessment quiz online to help you practice and expand your knowledge and skills.

Critical Thinking

15. **Cause and Effect** In your opinion, what is the cause-and-effect relationship between food advertisements in the media and increasing obesity levels among Americans of all ages? Cite evidence to support your opinion.
16. **Conclude** Biotechnology has the potential to impact the world food supply in regard to feeding hungry people. Research current areas of study in biotechnology related to food. Draw conclusions about whether these research areas are likely to impact the world food supply.
17. **Analyze** List several emotions you commonly experience, such as anger, love, and fear. Then list a food you associate with each emotion. Compare your list with other students' lists to decide if certain emotions make you think of the same foods.
18. **Examine** Use media sources, the Internet, or personal interviews to discover a belief about nutrition or a particular food that is based on misinformation. Research the topic to disprove the belief. Share your findings with the class.

Core Skills

19. **Speaking** Research the dietary laws of a cultural group in which you are interested. If possible, connect with a historian to learn where, why, and when the laws originated. Summarize your findings using presentation software.
20. **Math** Examine the food section of a local newspaper, magazine, or website. Select articles and advertisements that might influence readers' food choices and eating habits. Identify the group that is being targeted, for example, children, teens, and so on. Calculate the percentage of advertisements that is directed at each group.
21. **Technology Literacy** Look up the website of your state's department of agriculture to learn which fruits and vegetables are grown locally, as well as their growing seasons. Plan and write a two-day blog about locally grown foods that are available to purchase in your area.
22. **Science** Working in small groups, arrive at a consensus as to what aspect of food technology has had the greatest impact on food production in the past 50 years. Describe how the technology was developed and what impact it has had on the food industry. Use diagrams, drawings, or other visual support to share results with the class.
23. **Writing** Select a culture in a country other than the United States. Research the foods and preparation techniques associated with that culture. Write a paper describing the foods, equipment, and methods used in the dishes of that culture.
24. **History, Technology Literacy** Use time line creation software to prepare a food history time line showing the evolution of foods eaten and eating patterns from prehistoric times to current times. Include at least 20 significant points that represent changes in ways and foods people eat at that point in history. Share your time line in class.
25. **Speaking and Listening** Divide into groups of four or five students. Each group should choose one of the following influences on food availability: agriculture and land use, technology, economics, or politics. Using your textbook as a starting point, research your topic and prepare a report on how these factors affect availability of food. As a group, deliver your presentation to the rest of the class. Take notes while other students give their reports. Ask questions about any details that you would like clarified.
26. **Career Readiness Practice** The ability to gather and analyze information is an important skill in every workplace. Consider the following problem: As foodservice director for a multinational corporation, you have been informed that foods served in the company cafeterias are not meeting the cultural needs of all employees. Most offices in the United States have many employees from Asian and Middle Eastern cultures. You need to make changes in some types of foods served, but you need more information. Create a plan to gather and analyze needed information. List questions you need to ask and potential sources of reliable information.

Practicing Safe Food Habits

Learning Outcomes

After studying this chapter, you will be able to

- **identify** the common causes of food contamination;
- **practice** preventive measures to avoid foodborne illness when purchasing, storing, and preparing food;
- **identify** the population sectors that are most at risk for foodborne illness;
- **recognize** symptoms and treatment of foodborne illnesses; and
- **compare** the roles of food producers, food processors, government agencies, and consumers in protecting the safety of the food supply.

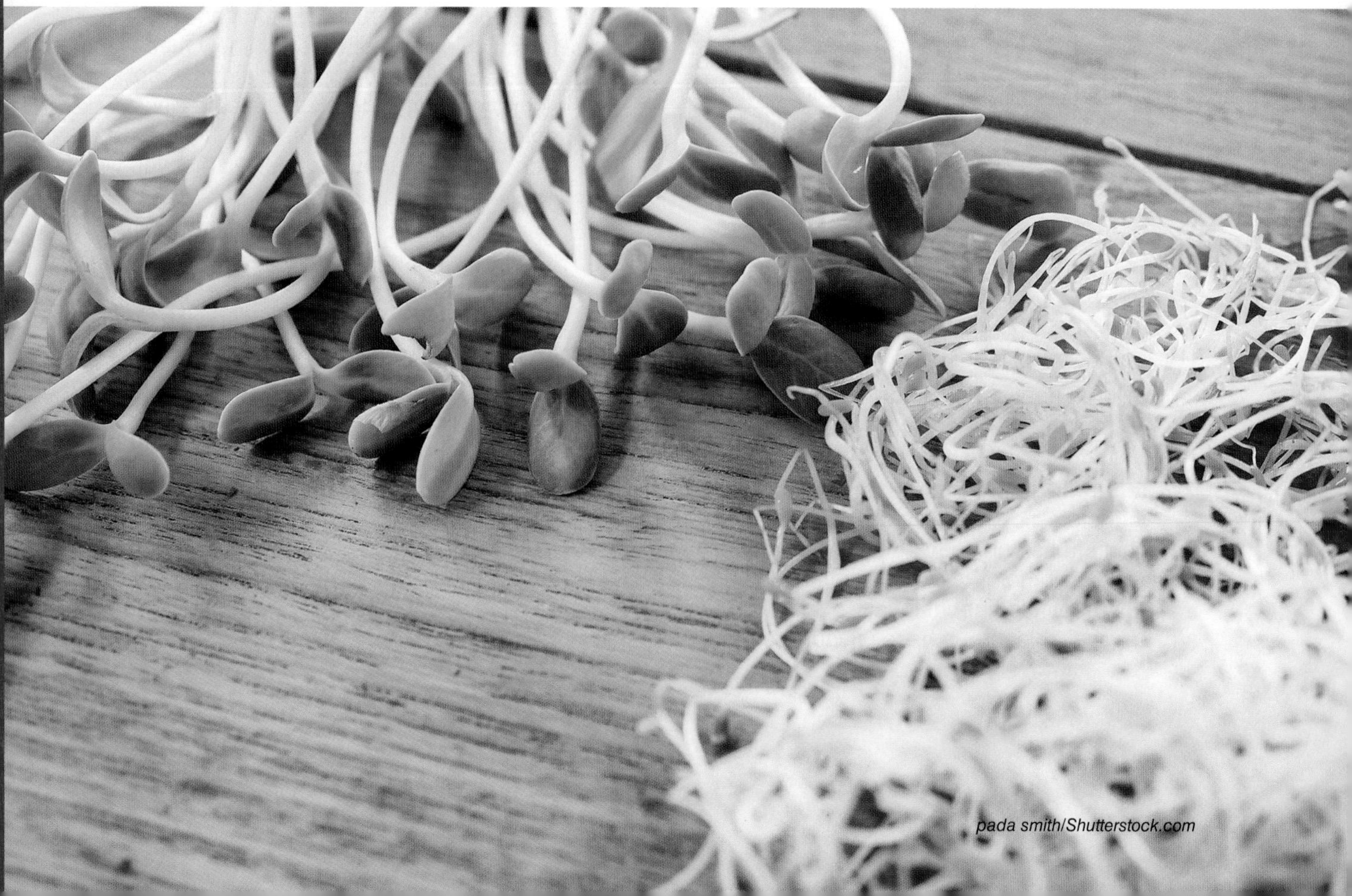

pada smith/Shutterstock.com

Content Terms

bacteria
contaminant
cross-contamination
environmental contaminant
foodborne illness
fungi
hazard analysis critical control point (HACCP) system
hygiene
microorganism
parasite
pathogen
pesticide residue
protozoa
sanitation
toxin
virus

Academic Terms

adhere to
ascertain
repel
reputable

What's Your Nutrition and Wellness IQ?

Take this quiz to examine how much you already know about the factors that keep your food safe. If you cannot answer a question, pay extra attention to that topic as you study this chapter.

- Identify each statement as *True*, *False*, or *It Depends*. *It Depends* means in some cases the statement is true; in some cases it could be false.
- Revise false statements to make them true.
- Explain the circumstances in which each *It Depends* statement is true and when it is false.

Nutrition and Wellness IQ

	Statement			
1.	Keeping foods safe to eat is solely the responsibility of the food producer.	True	False	It Depends
2.	The most common cause of food contamination is pathogens growing in the food.	True	False	It Depends
3.	When shopping for food, placing hot foods and cold foods next to each other in your cart or basket has no relationship to food safety.	True	False	It Depends
4.	While working in the kitchen making meals, washing hands once at the beginning of food preparation is adequate.	True	False	It Depends
5.	Babies are most at risk for foodborne illness.	True	False	It Depends
6.	All microorganisms in food are harmful to your health.	True	False	It Depends
7.	Symptoms of foodborne illness occur within an hour after eating tainted food.	True	False	It Depends
8.	Self-treatment for a foodborne illness requires drinking plenty of water and getting extra rest.	True	False	It Depends

While studying this chapter, look for the activity icon 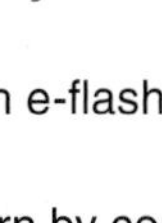 **to**

- **build** vocabulary with e-flash cards and interactive games;
- **assess** what you learn by completing self-assessment quizzes and completing review questions; and
- **expand** knowledge with interactive activities and activities that extend learning.

www.g-wlearning.com/foodsandnutrition/

Food safety is important to the health of the nation. People rely on a safe food supply to stay healthy and productive in their work. The national headlines are sometimes a reminder that the food supply could be safer, however. In the past, food producers and food handlers have distributed contaminated foods, and consumers have gotten sick. Consumers have handled and stored foods in a manner that causes them to spoil, also resulting in illness.

Foodborne illness, also called *food poisoning*, is a disease transmitted by food. In the United States, foodborne illness affects millions of people each year; however, many cases go unreported because people mistake their symptoms for stomach flu.

Foodborne illness can be avoided. This chapter will help you learn how organisms that cause foodborne illness get into food. It will also help you apply guidelines to prevent the spread of these organisms. You will read about steps to take if foodborne illness occurs. You will also study the agencies that are responsible for protecting the food supply.

Common Food Contaminants

Foodborne illness occurs when food is contaminated. A ***contaminant*** is an undesirable substance that is unintentionally introduced in food. The most common food contaminants are ***microorganisms***. These are living beings so small you can see them only under a microscope. ***Pathogens*** are microorganisms that cause foodborne illness. The types of pathogens that contaminate food are bacteria, parasites, viruses, and fungi. Although these organisms are tiny, the diseases they cause can have big impacts on people (**Figure 3.1**).

Major Pathogens That Cause Foodborne Illness (Bacteria, Parasites, Viruses)		
Pathogen	**Methods of Transmission**	**Symptoms and Potential Impact**
Anisakis simplex (parasite)	Raw and undercooked infected fish	Tingling in throat, coughing up worms
Campylobacter jejuni (bacterium)	Contaminated water Raw milk Raw or undercooked meat, poultry, or shellfish	Fever, headache, and muscle pain followed by diarrhea, abdominal pain, and nausea that appear 2 to 5 days after eating May spread to bloodstream and cause a serious life-threatening infection
Clostridium botulinum (bacterium)	Canned goods, improperly processed home-canned foods, luncheon meats	Bacteria produces toxin that causes double vision, inability to swallow, speech difficulty, and progressive paralysis of the respiratory system that can lead to death Symptoms begin 12 to 36 hours after toxin enters the body
Clostridium perfringens (bacterium)	Food left for long periods on steam tables or at room temperature Meats, meat products, and gravy	Intense stomach cramps and diarrhea begin 8 to 22 hours after eating Complications and/or death are rare

Continued

Figure 3.1 These pathogens can cause illnesses with symptoms of varying degrees.

Major Pathogens That Cause Foodborne Illness (Bacteria, Parasites, Viruses) *(Continued)*		
Pathogen	**Methods of Transmission**	**Symptoms and Potential Impact**
Escherichia coli O157:H7 (One of several strains of E. coli bacterium that can cause human illness)	Undercooked beef, especially hamburger Unpasteurized milk and juice Contaminated raw fruits and vegetables, and water Person-to-person	Severe diarrhea that is often bloody; stomach cramps and vomiting; little or no fever; can begin 1 to 8 days after eating Can cause acute kidney failure or even death, especially in the very young
Listeria monocytogenes (bacterium)	Contaminated hot dogs, luncheon meats, cold cuts, fermented or dry sausage, and other deli-style meat and poultry Soft cheeses and unpasteurized milk	Fever, chills, headache, stiff neck, backache; sometimes upset stomach, stomach pain, and diarrhea; may take up to 3 weeks to become ill At-risk patients (including pregnant women) should seek medical advice
Noroviruses (and other calciviruses)	Shellfish and foods or water contaminated by feces Ready-to-eat food touched by infected food workers; examples include salads, sandwiches, ice, cookies, and fruit	Nausea, vomiting, stomach pain, fever, muscle aches, and sometimes headache usually appear within 1 to 2 days Diarrhea is more prevalent in adults, and vomiting is more prevalent in children
Salmonella (over 2,300 types; bacterium)	Raw or undercooked eggs, poultry, and meat Raw milk or juice Cheese and seafood Contaminated fresh fruits and vegetables	Stomach pain, diarrhea, nausea, chills, fever, and headache usually appear 8 to 72 hours after eating A more severe illness may result if the infection spreads to the bloodstream
Staphylococcus aureus (bacterium)	Contaminated milk and cheeses Salty foods (such as ham), sliced meats Foods made by hand that require no cooking, such as puddings and sandwiches Infected food workers	Nausea, vomiting, stomach cramps, and diarrhea usually occur within 30 minutes to 6 hours after eating contaminated food
Toxoplasma gondii (parasite)	Accidental ingestion of soil contaminated with cat feces on fruits and vegetables; raw or undercooked meat	Flu-like illness usually appears 5 to 23 days after eating—may last months; those with a weakened immune system may develop more serious illness Can cause problems with pregnancy, including miscarriage
Vibrio vulnificus (bacterium)	Undercooked or raw seafood, such as fish and shellfish	Diarrhea, stomach pain, and vomiting may appear within 1 to 7 days after eating; may result in a blood infection; can result in death for those with a weakened immune system
Yersinia enterocolitica (bacterium)	Contaminated food-contact surfaces Raw milk, chitterlings (swine intestines), water, pork, other raw meats	Diarrhea, stomach pain, headache, fever, vomiting; can result in arthritis, meningitis, and inflammation of the skin for those with a weakened immune system

FEATURED CAREER

Food Inspector

Food inspectors work to ensure that your food will not make you sick. These workers monitor or audit quality standards for foods. Inspectors work to guarantee the quality of the goods their companies produce. Some jobs involve only a quick visual inspection; others require a longer, detailed one. Some companies have completely automated the inspection process with the help of advanced vision inspection systems and machinery installed at one or several points in the production process. Inspectors in these companies monitor the equipment, review output, and perform random product checks.

Education

Training requirements vary with the responsibilities of the inspector. For workers who perform simple "pass/fail" tests of products, a high school diploma and limited in-house training is generally sufficient. Training for new inspectors may cover the use of special meters, gauges, computers, and other instruments. There are some postsecondary training programs, but many employers prefer to train inspectors on the job. USDA food inspectors must have at least a bachelor's degree in food science.

Job Outlook

Employment is expected to decline slowly primarily because of the growing use of automated inspection.

Harmful Bacteria

Much foodborne illness in the United States is caused by harmful ***bacteria***. These single-celled microorganisms live in soil, water, and the bodies of plants and animals. Knowing how bacteria grow and multiply can help you prevent foodborne illnesses.

All foods contain bacteria, but not all bacteria are harmful. Certain types of bacteria are intentionally added to foods to produce desired effects. For instance, bacteria are used to make cultured milk products, such as buttermilk and yogurt (**Figure 3.2**).

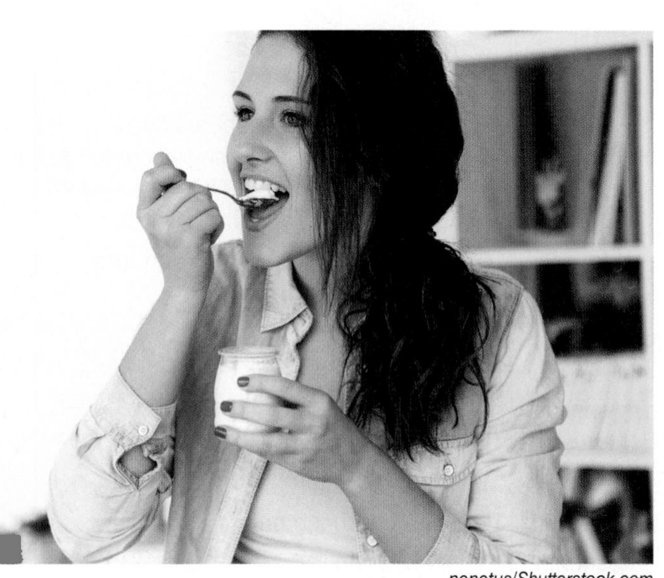

nenetus/Shutterstock.com

Figure 3.2 Helpful bacteria are behind the tangy taste and creamy texture of this yogurt. *What are some other foods that contain helpful bacteria?*

Bacteria can also cause foods to spoil; however, foods that contain illness-causing bacteria often look, smell, and taste wholesome. Spoilage and contamination are not the same. *Spoiled* food has lost its nutritional value and quality characteristics—such as flavor and texture—due to decay. *Contaminated* food has become unfit to eat due to the introduction of undesirable substances.

A number of bacteria are known to cause foodborne illness. Some bacteria cause sickness by irritating the lining of the intestines. Others produce ***toxins***, or poisons, that cause illness.

Other Harmful Organisms

Other organisms that can cause foodborne illness include parasites, viruses, and fungi. A ***parasite*** is an organism that lives off another organism, called a *host*. *Trichinella* is a parasite sometimes found in raw or undercooked pork. It can cause a disease called *trichinosis*. Improved feeding conditions of hogs have made trichinosis rare in the United States today. Pork should be cooked to an internal temperature of at least 145°F (63°C) and allowed to rest for three minutes before eating. Parasites that more commonly cause foodborne illness today are included in **Figure 3.1**.

Protozoa are single-celled organisms. Some types of protozoa are parasites that can cause foodborne illness. *Entamoeba histolytica* and *Giardia lamblia* are two such protozoa found in water polluted with animal or human feces. Safe drinking water is tested and treated to destroy these and other harmful microorganisms (**Figure 3.3**).

A ***virus*** is a disease-causing agent that must inhabit the living cell of another organism to grow or multiply. Viruses are the chief cause of foodborne illness. A few viruses, such as *hepatitis A* and *Norwalk virus*, can be transmitted in foods. These viruses are commonly spread through ready-to-eat foods prepared by infected food workers. People can also contract these viruses by eating raw or undercooked shellfish, such as oysters, clams, and mussels. Although most shellfish are safe, those taken from polluted waters may be contaminated.

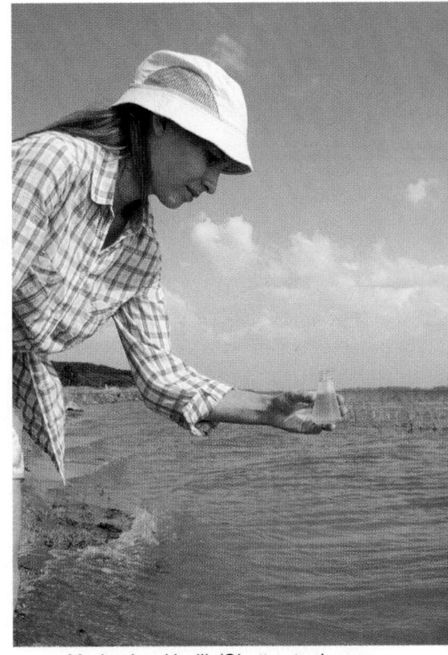

Merkushev Vasiliy/Shutterstock.com

Figure 3.3 Drinking water must be tested for the presence of certain harmful microorganisms before it can be declared safe.

Fungi are organisms that vary greatly in size and structure, and are classified as plants. Mold and yeast are two types of fungi. Molds are mainly associated with food spoilage, but they can cause illness. Molds often form on foods that have been stored for extended periods after opening. Some molds produce toxins.

EXTEND YOUR KNOWLEDGE

Nanotechnology and Food Safety

Nanotechnology is the understanding and control of extremely small matter that measures between 1 and 100 nanometers. A nanometer is one-billionth of a meter. One gold atom is approximately one-third nanometer in diameter.

Nanotechnology is a very new technology that many believe holds potential benefits for the food industry. Food packaging is one aspect of the food industry that might benefit from improved safety, quality, strength, and stability. Smart, or active, packaging is an example of nanotechnology's role in food quality and safety. For example, a nanolayer of aluminum is used to line many snack food packages.

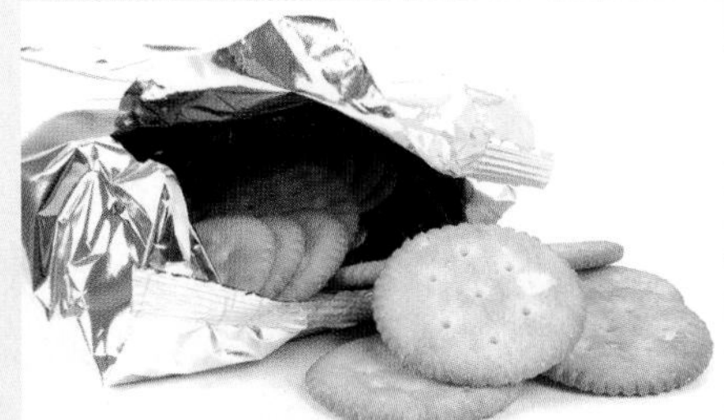

Graphic design/Shutterstock.com

In the future, nanosensors may be used in packaging to detect and signal the presence of contaminants such as chemicals, bacteria, viruses, toxins, or allergens in foods.

Some food safety experts have expressed caution regarding the use of nano-engineered materials. They question the potential health effects on people if the material is inhaled, ingested, or spread on the skin. The research data is not all collected as progress in nanotechnology continues.

Research further to learn about the potential challenges and concerns regarding nanotechnology and the food processing industry.

When mold forms on liquids or soft foods, such as jelly, soft cheese, or shredded cheese, you should discard the whole food. The mold cannot be safely removed.

With hard cheese, you can cut away the moldy part and eat the rest of the cheese. Keep the knife out of the mold itself so that it does not touch other parts of the cheese. Cut off at least one inch around and below the moldy spot. Discard the moldy portion.

Yeasts can spoil foods quickly. Discard food that smells or tastes like alcohol, which is an indication of yeast. Yeast can also cause discoloration or slime on foods.

Natural Toxins

Many plants produce substances to defend themselves against insects, birds, and animals. These substances are called *natural toxins*. Although many of these substances are not toxic to humans, others are toxic. For instance, eating some varieties of wild berries and mushrooms can cause illness. Avoid foods that do not come from **reputable** (trustworthy) food sellers.

Some types of fish, such as tuna and blue marlin, produce a natural toxin called *scombroid toxin* when they begin to spoil. The cooking process does not destroy this toxin. People who eat fish containing this toxin may develop symptoms of foodborne illness immediately. These symptoms last less than 24 hours.

Chemicals

Foodborne illness can also be caused by chemicals that come in contact with the food supply. Some chemicals are purposely used to produce and process foods. Such chemicals include pesticides and food additives. A *pesticide* is a substance used to **repel** (keep away) or destroy insects, weeds, or fungi that affect plant crops. Pesticides are also used to protect foods during transportation. Food additives are chemicals added to food during processing.

Pesticide residues are chemical pesticide particles that remain on or in food after it is prepared for consumption. Some consumers are concerned about the potential effects of long-term exposure to these residues. Farmers must follow strict guidelines when applying pesticides (**Figure 3.4**). They must keep residues within legal limits. State and federal agencies set these limits to protect public health. Government agencies also check the food supply to be sure foods are safe.

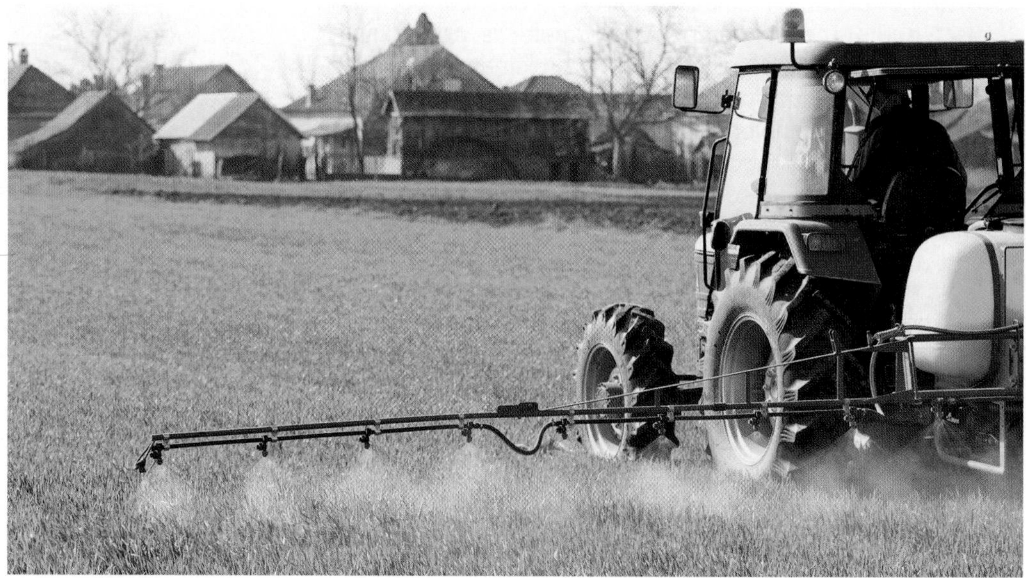

Figure 3.4
Strict guidelines govern farmers' use of pesticides on their crops. These guidelines are in place for our safety.

oticki/Shutterstock.com

Some chemicals unintentionally come in contact with the food supply. ***Environmental contaminants*** are substances released into the air or water by industrial plants. These substances eventually make their way into foods. They can build up in the body over time until they reach toxic levels.

Environmental contaminants can accumulate in fish that live in waters polluted by industrial wastes. The larger the fish, the more time it had to store toxins. Eating lean fish may help you avoid chemical toxins, which tend to be stored in fishes' fatty tissues. Become informed about fish advisories for the bodies of water being fished when eating fish caught by yourself or others. If the waters being fished are not monitored for contamination, you should eat fish from these sources no more than once a week. This helps you avoid the potential buildup of toxins, just in case contamination exists.

Helpful Microorganisms

Some microorganisms produce positive effects on food taste and texture. For instance, special molds are used to age some cheeses. Lactic acid bacteria are used to give yogurt its tangy taste and thick, creamy texture. One type of yeast is used as a leavening agent. A *leavening agent* is a substance used to produce a gas that causes batter or dough to rise (**Figure 3.5**).

How Does Yeast Make Bread Rise?

1. Liquid ingredients used to make bread dough are heated to a temperature that helps activate the yeast.
2. Bread is kneaded, or folded and pushed with the hands. This action helps develop an elastic protein in the dough called *gluten*.

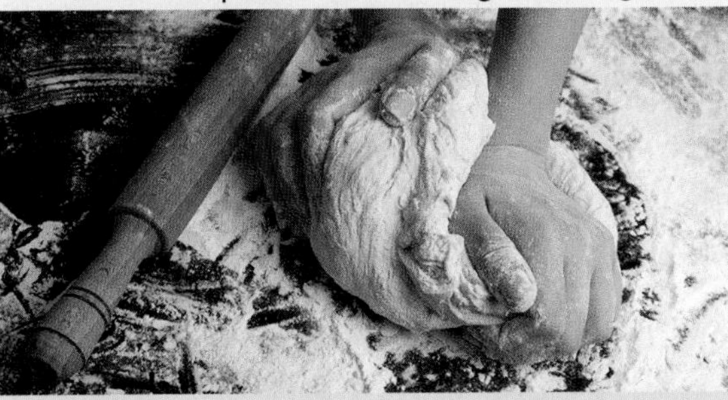

3. After being kneaded, the dough is allowed to rise in a warm environment, which promotes a process called *fermentation*. During this process, the yeast causes a chemical reaction that produces carbon dioxide gas.
4. After time, the carbon dioxide causes the dough to rise.
5. Physical changes to the size and shape of the dough result in a high-quality bread product that is flavorful and light in texture.

Photo: Africa Studio/Shutterstock.com

Figure 3.5 Yeast is a helpful microorganism that is used as a leavening agent to make bread rise.

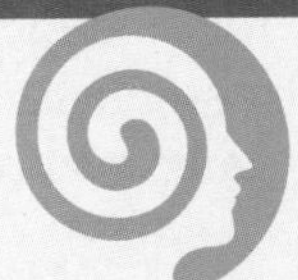

EXTEND YOUR KNOWLEDGE

Reduce Your Exposure to BPA

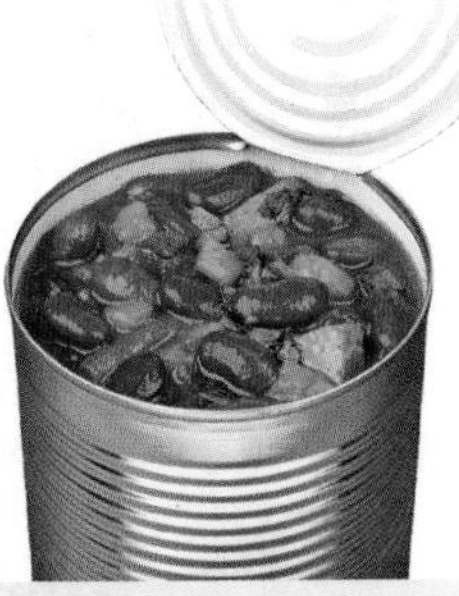

Pixelspieler/Shutterstock.com

Bisphenol A (BPA) is a chemical resin that is used as a coating on food and beverage containers. During storage and use, some BPA can seep into foods and beverages. The Food and Drug Administration (FDA) continues to support research on the long-term use of BPA, the health effects it may have on the brain, as well as the potential health outcomes for fetuses, infants, and children.

The FDA now reports that BPA is safe if consumed at very low levels. If you choose to reduce your exposure to BPA, you can take the following steps:

- Use containers marked "BPA free" (containers with recycle codes 3 and 7 may have BPA present).
- Reduce use of canned food containers lined with BPA resins.
- Avoid microwaving food in plastic containers and washing plastics in hot dishwashers to avoid leaching of BPA.
- Store and cook foods in glass, porcelain, or stainless steel containers instead of plastic.

Decide how important it is for you to take steps to reduce your BPA exposure. What can manufacturers do to reduce consumers' concerns about BPA? Continue to follow the research on the consequences of BPA exposure and report results to the class.

Outwitting the Food Contaminators

Most foodborne illness is due to improper food handling. You need to use care when buying, storing, and preparing food. You must correct conditions that allow bacteria to spread and multiply. This will help you protect yourself and your family from foodborne illnesses.

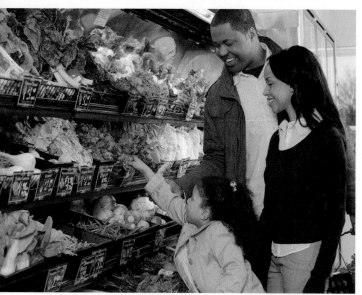

XiXinXing/Shutterstock.com

Figure 3.6 General cleanliness can indicate that a store practices safe food-handling techniques.

Shopping with Safety in Mind

Fortunately, the food supply in the United States is one of the safest in the world; however, you still need to be on guard for possible sources of contamination. Bringing safe foods into your home is your first step toward outwitting the food contaminators. Begin by shopping at stores known for food safety and sanitation.

Sanitation is the practice of clean food-handling habits to help prevent disease. Check to see if store refrigerators, shelves, and floors are clean (**Figure 3.6**). Poor sanitation in these areas may indicate low standards for food handling overall.

Bacteria grow most rapidly in the temperature range between 41°F and 135°F (5°C–57°C). This temperature range is called the *danger zone* because bacteria thrive in this range. The number of bacteria present in food can double in as little as 20 minutes spent in these temperatures. This is why time and temperature are two important factors to monitor for keeping food safe.

Food service professionals use thermometers to ensure that the foods they prepare spend as little time as possible in the danger zone. The USDA suggests that consumers **adhere to** (observe) a more conservative temperature danger zone of 40°F–140°F (4°C–60°C).

Transport food carefully when shopping. Place cold foods in refrigeration soon after purchase, and do not keep them out of refrigeration longer than two hours. If the outside temperature is 90°F (32°C) or higher, food should be refrigerated within one hour. Keep frozen items separated from warmer items when placing them in the cart or basket. Maintain frozen food quality by transporting items in coolers or thermal bags.

Protecting yourself and others from foodborne illness begins with following a few simple tips when selecting and transporting food purchases (**Figure 3.7**).

Storing Foods Safely

When you arrive home after shopping, put away your perishable foods first. The temperature in the refrigerator should be 40°F (4°C) or lower. The freezer should be 0°F (–18°C) or lower. These cold temperatures do not kill bacteria, but they do slow bacterial growth. Consider keeping refrigerator/freezer thermometers in your refrigerator and freezer. This can help you make sure your appliances are maintaining the correct temperatures.

Tips for Buying Safe Foods

- Select foods that appear fresh and wholesome.
- Check dates on packages. Choose the freshest foods with the latest use-by date.
- Do not buy food in cans that are swollen, rusted, or deeply dented.
- Check packages for leaking, which could be a source of contamination.
- Buy from stores that practice safe food handling.
- Research door-to-door food companies for safety and reliability before buying their food products.
- Ensure that labels on meat and poultry products display the USDA inspection stamp.
- Select meats, fish, and poultry that smell fresh and have good color. Avoid any that smell of ammonia.
- Place meats, poultry, and fish in separate plastic bags to avoid cross-contamination.
- Shop for refrigerated and frozen foods last to avoid prolonged time at room temperature.
- Avoid frozen products that are covered with a heavy layer of frost or have indications of thawing and refreezing.
- Take food home promptly and store it properly.

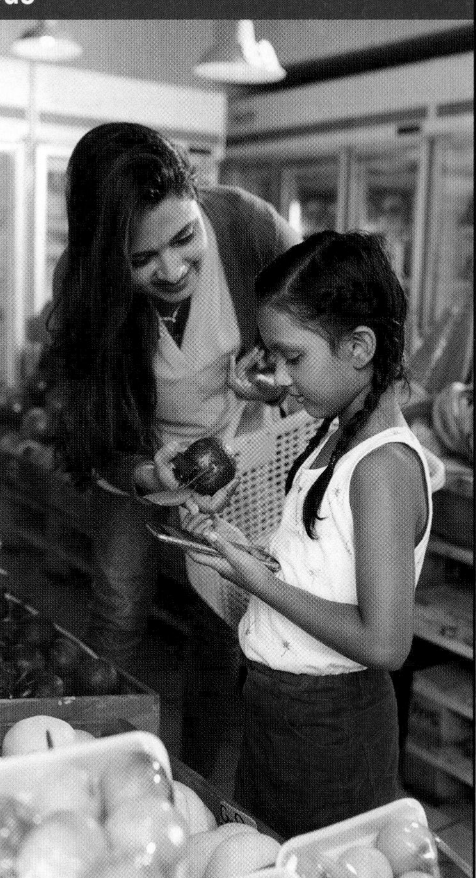

Photo: Dragon Images/Shutterstock.com

Figure 3.7 Following these tips can help you avoid foodborne illness.

Store eggs in the cartons in which you purchased them (**Figure 3.8**). These cartons help reduce the evaporation of moisture from the egg through the porous eggshell. Place eggs on an interior shelf of the refrigerator. The refrigerator door is not as cold as the interior.

Wrap or cover all foods for refrigerator or freezer storage. This keeps bacteria from settling on foods. It also prevents foods from dripping onto one another. Plastic or glass lids are good covers because they can be reused. Plastic wrap and aluminum foil also make fine food covers; however, they cannot be reused because they cannot be easily sanitized.

The sooner foods are chilled, the less time bacteria will have to grow to unsafe numbers. Store foods in shallow containers to promote quick cooling. Arrange foods in the refrigerator in a manner that allows air to circulate freely around the containers.

Put calendar dates on leftovers. This will help you remember how soon you must use the food (**Figure 3.9** on the next page).

Store foods that do not need refrigeration—such as dried beans, pasta, and canned goods—in a cool, dry place. Store foods away from cleaning supplies, which are likely to be toxic. Also, avoid storing foods in damp areas, such as under the sink. Dampness encourages bacterial growth. Check to be sure boxes and bottles are tightly closed, and plastic bags are completely sealed.

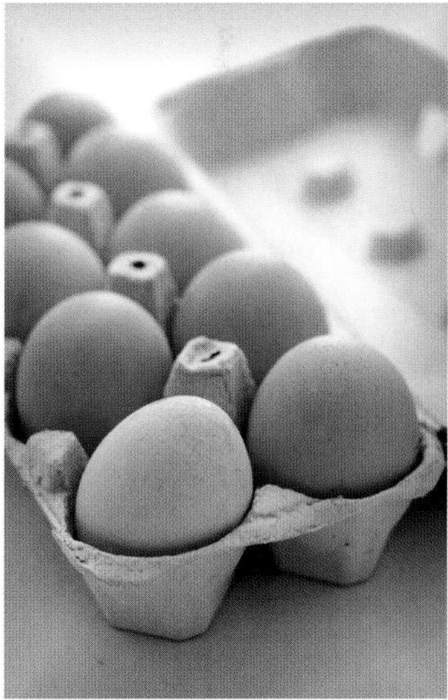

Gayvoronskaya_Yana/Shutterstock.com

Figure 3.8 The best way to store eggs is in the carton in which they came. *What are some other guidelines for refrigerator and freezer storage?*

Cold Storage Chart		
Product	**Refrigerator (40°F, 4°C)**	**Freezer (0°F, –18°C)**
Eggs		
Fresh in shell	3 weeks	Do not freeze
Hard cooked	1 week	Do not freeze well
Salads		
Egg, chicken, ham, tuna, and macaroni salads	3 to 5 days	Do not freeze well
Hot Dogs		
Opened package	1 week	1 to 2 months
Unopened package	2 weeks	1 to 2 months
Luncheon Meat		
Opened package or deli meat	3 to 5 days	1 to 2 months
Unopened package	2 weeks	1 to 2 months
Bacon and Sausage		
Bacon	7 days	1 month
Sausage, raw (chicken, turkey, pork, beef)	1 to 2 days	1 to 2 months
Hamburger and Other Ground Meats		
Hamburger, ground beef, turkey, veal, pork, lamb, and mixtures	1 to 2 days	3 to 4 months
Fresh Beef, Veal, Lamb, and Pork		
Steaks	3 to 5 days	6 to 12 months
Chops	3 to 5 days	4 to 6 months
Roasts	3 to 5 days	4 to 12 months
Fresh Poultry		
Chicken or turkey, whole	1 to 2 days	1 year
Chicken or turkey, pieces	1 to 2 days	9 months
Soups and Stews		
Vegetable or meat added	3 to 4 days	2 to 3 months
Leftovers		
Cooked meat or poultry	3 to 4 days	2 to 6 months
Chicken nuggets or patties	3 to 4 days	1 to 3 months
Pizza	3 to 4 days	1 to 2 months

Source: USDA Kitchen Companion: Your Safe Food Handbook

Figure 3.9 Knowing how long foods can be safely stored in the refrigerator or freezer is important for maintaining food safety.

Practicing Kitchen Cleanliness

Many people are unaware of basic safe food-handling techniques. When working with food, one of the most important points to remember is to use good personal hygiene. ***Hygiene*** refers to practices that promote good health. It involves making a conscious effort to keep dirt and germs from getting into food.

Handwashing

Always wash your hands with soap and warm running water for 20 seconds before beginning to work with food (**Figure 3.10**). Try singing "Happy Birthday" twice while you wash your hands to be sure you are spending a full 20 seconds washing. You need this much time to get hands thoroughly clean. Be sure to clean under your nails and around cuticles, too. Use paper towels or clean cloth towels to dry hands.

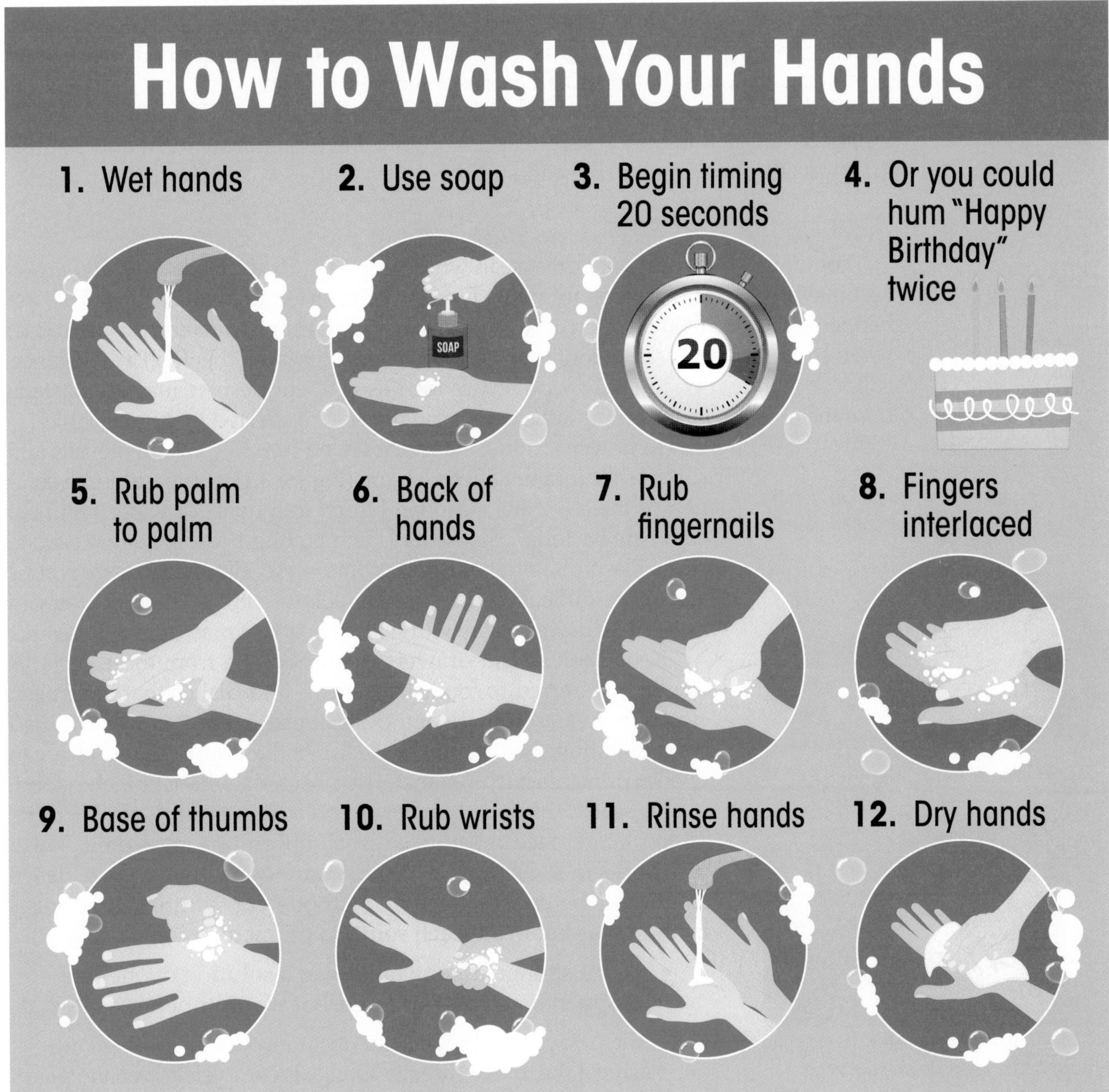
How to Wash Your Hands
1. Wet hands
2. Use soap
SOAP
3. Begin timing 20 seconds
20
4. Or you could hum "Happy Birthday" twice
5. Rub palm to palm
6. Back of hands
7. Rub fingernails
8. Fingers interlaced
9. Base of thumbs
10. Rub wrists
11. Rinse hands
12. Dry hands

Hands: Pro_Vector/Shutterstock.com; Stopwatch: Aleksandr Bryliaev/Shutterstock.com; Cake: vannilasky/Shutterstock.com

Figure 3.10 Washing your hands is the simplest and most important step you can take in practicing safe food-handling techniques.

If you have any kind of cut or infection on your hands, wear gloves when preparing foods. Bacteria grow in open wounds and may contaminate the food you are preparing. Change gloves whenever you move from one task to another, or when the gloves become contaminated. For example, if you answer the phone with your glove on, you must get a new glove before returning to food preparation.

Be sure to wash your hands when moving from one food preparation task to the next. Rewash your hands every time you touch another object, such as a pet, money, the refrigerator door, or unwashed utensils. Wash your hands after coughing, sneezing, touching your hair, and using the bathroom, too.

Wear clean clothes or a clean apron when working with food. If you have long hair, pull it back to keep loose strands from falling into food.

Washing Foods

Before preparing or eating fresh fruits and vegetables, wash them under cold water to remove dirt and other residue. Scrub root vegetables, like beets, yams, yucca, and potatoes, with a brush. Do not use soaps or detergents to wash food products, as these substances can be absorbed by the food.

Washing raw poultry, beef, pork, lamb, or veal before cooking is not recommended. This action may result in spreading the bacteria in raw meat and poultry juices to other foods, utensils, and surfaces.

Cleaning the Work Area

You must keep your work area clean when preparing foods. ***Cross-contamination*** occurs when harmful bacteria from one food are transferred to another food. This can happen when one food drips on or touches another. Cross-contamination can also occur when an object that touches a contaminated food later touches another food. For instance, suppose a knife used to cut raw poultry is then used to cut fresh vegetables. Bacteria from the poultry can get on the knife, and it can then be transferred to the vegetables.

To prevent cross-contamination, be sure to wash all utensils and surfaces thoroughly after each use (**Figure 3.11**). Using a bleach solution of three-fourths teaspoon bleach to a quart of water will help eliminate bacteria. Choose tools and cutting boards that are easy to clean. Plastic materials are good choices. Wooden surfaces are porous and more difficult to keep clean. Allow cutting boards to air-dry rather than drying them with cloth towels that may transmit bacteria.

Keep shelves and drawers clean. Bacteria from these surfaces can be transferred to foods by utensils and dishes that have been stored there. Carefully cleaning appliances is another way to avoid contamination. For example, cleaning the cutting edge of a can opener prevents it from transferring bacteria when it touches food.

Damp cloths and sponges are breeding grounds for bacteria. Therefore, replace or sanitize dishcloths and sponges daily. Wash dishcloths in the hot cycle of the washing machine or in a bleach solution. The most effective methods for sanitizing sponges include soaking in a bleach solution or microwaving.

- Soak a sponge for one minute in a solution of one-half teaspoon bleach per one quart of warm (not hot) water.
- Microwave a wet sponge for one minute on high. To guard against fire, make sure the sponge is completely wet and place it in a microwave-safe dish. Use caution when removing the sponge from the microwave as it may still be very hot.

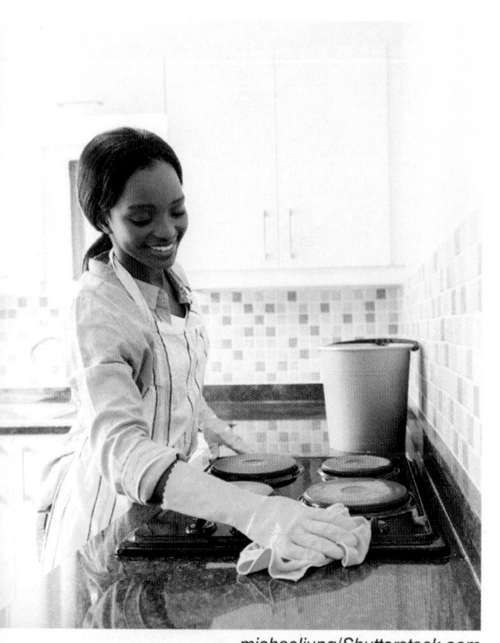

michaeljung/Shutterstock.com

Figure 3.11 Utensils and surfaces used in the kitchen must be thoroughly washed after use. This will help prevent cross-contamination of harmful bacteria.

Preparing Foods Safely

Following safety guidelines when preparing and serving food is another major part of food safety. The time food spends in the temperature danger zone is also important during food preparation and serving.

Thawing

Never thaw frozen meat at room temperature. Bacteria present in the portions of the meat that reach room temperature will reproduce rapidly. The safest way to thaw all foods is to defrost them in the refrigerator. Another acceptable thawing technique is to place foods under cold running water. You can also use a microwave oven for quick, safe defrosting just before cooking. Follow the directions of the microwave manufacturer.

Cooking

Do not eat or taste raw or partially cooked meat or poultry. Cook foods to the appropriate minimum internal temperatures required for safety (**Figure 3.12**). Appearance alone is not a good indication of doneness, so you should use a thermometer to check the internal temperature of food. When checking the temperature of meat, insert the tip of the thermometer into the thickest part of the meat, avoiding fat and bone.

Eggs may be contaminated with salmonella bacteria. Therefore, avoid eating raw or undercooked eggs. Cooking eggs until the whites are completely set and the yolks are solid helps destroy salmonella bacteria.

Serving

Do not place cooked meat on the same plate that held uncooked meat. Bacteria from the uncooked meat can remain on the plate and contaminate the cooked meat. Brush sauces only on cooked surfaces of meat and poultry. This prevents bacteria on the surface of raw meat and poultry from getting on the basting brush and contaminating the sauce. If you want to use a marinade as a sauce for cooked meat, reserve a portion before adding raw meat.

When serving foods, hold foods at room temperature for no more than two hours. This will help limit bacterial growth. If possible, it is best to hold cold foods at or below 40°F (4°C) and hot foods above 140°F (60°C) during serving times. Refrigerate leftover foods as soon as possible.

Using a Microwave Oven

When cooking foods in a microwave oven, be sure to follow instructions on product labels. Keep in mind that microwave ovens vary in power and operating efficiency. Also, remember that microwave ovens often do not cook foods evenly. Some parts of a food may not reach a high enough temperature to destroy harmful microorganisms.

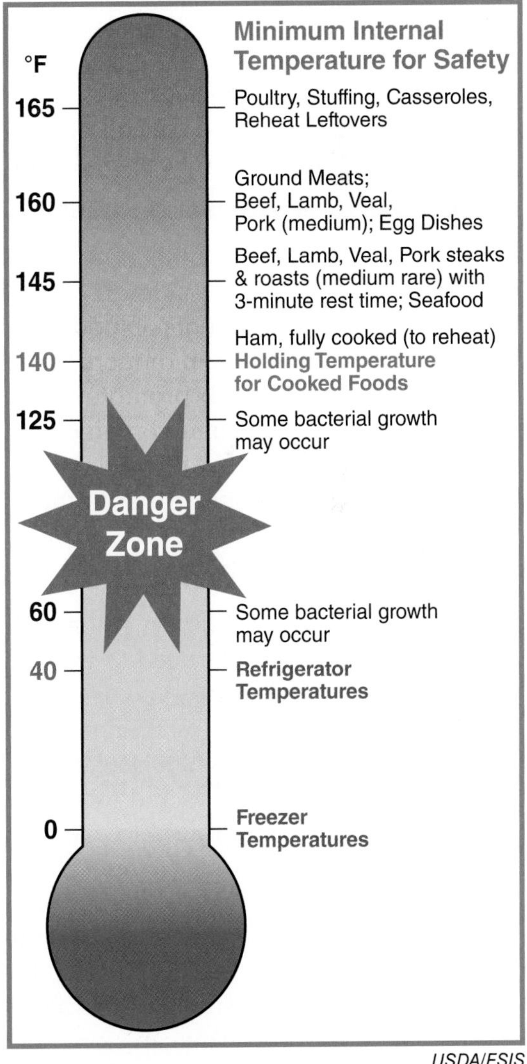

USDA/FSIS

Figure 3.12 Use a thermometer to ensure that meat has been cooked to the appropriate temperature. *To what temperature should ground beef be cooked?*

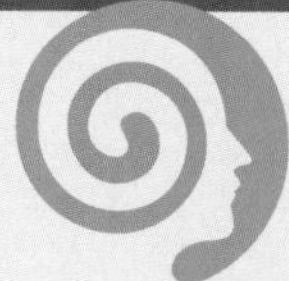

EXTEND YOUR KNOWLEDGE

Food Safety During an Emergency

Emergencies such as power outages, flooding, or fire can place your food supply at risk. The United States Department of Agriculture's Food Safety and Inspection Service asks that you plan ahead for such emergencies. For example, you are urged to keep an appliance thermometer in the refrigerator and freezer. Keep a freezer full of items to maintain coldness longer. Have large insulated coolers available with ice packs to put into them, if needed. Know where to buy dry ice or block ice if needed.

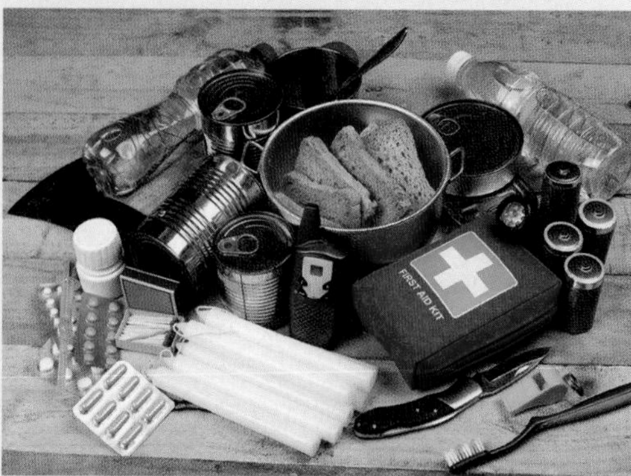

Alex Kosev/Shutterstock.com

You can take small steps toward emergency preparedness. Each month take one action that makes you more prepared. Prioritize your needs and keep the most important supplies on hand.

Select one emergency situation that could happen in your community and prepare a set of guidelines for maintaining a safe supply of food and water throughout the emergency. Refer to the food safety guidelines on the Department of Homeland Security's Ready America website. Share your guidelines with your family and work together to ensure readiness.

Incidents of food poisoning have occurred because people were not cooking frozen chicken dinners to recommended temperatures.

To promote uniform cooking in a microwave oven, arrange foods evenly in covered containers. Stir or rotate foods several times during the cooking period. (Many microwave ovens come with turntables for this purpose.) Use a temperature probe or thermometer to make sure food has reached a safe internal temperature.

Packing Food to Go

Some members of your family may pack lunches to take to work or school. You might need to transport a casserole to a relative's home for a holiday celebration. Perhaps you are going on a picnic with some friends. Whatever the situation, you need to take special steps to keep food safe when transporting it.

When packing food to go, place all perishable items in an insulated bag or cooler. Cold foods should be frozen or well chilled before packing. For instance, you might freeze sandwiches for lunches the night before. This ensures they will stay cold longer the next day. (Freezing sandwiches with mayonnaise or fresh lettuce on them is not a good idea. Mayonnaise tends to separate and lettuce wilts during freezer storage.) Use ice packs to keep cold foods cold and safe for several hours. Try to keep foods out of direct sunlight and avoid storage in a hot car. If possible, refrigerate packed food until you are ready to eat it.

You can store hot food in a wide-mouth thermal container to keep it at a safe temperature for several hours. Rinse the container with hot water before adding the food. Food should be hot to the touch at serving time. Throw away any uneaten perishable food.

When Foodborne Illness Happens

Foodborne illnesses can affect people differently. A contaminated food eaten by two people may cause different symptoms in each person. One person may become sick and the other may not. Genetic makeup may play a role in the way your body reacts to certain contaminants. Your age and state of health may also affect how you will react to foodborne contaminants.

Who Is Most at Risk?

Foodborne illness can be more serious for some groups of people than others. Infants, young children, pregnant women, older adults, substance abusers, and people with immune disorders are at the greatest risk. The immune systems of infants and children are not mature enough to fight a virus or buildup of harmful bacteria easily. A given amount of toxin poses more danger to their small bodies than to the larger bodies of adults. Pregnant women need to avoid any type of illness due to potential danger to their fetuses. Older people have lost some of their ability to fight off dangerous bacteria because immune systems weaken as people age (**Figure 3.13**). In addition, stomach acid decreases with age. Stomach acid plays an important role in reducing the number of bacteria in our intestinal tracts.

Contaminants from foods place added stress on the bodies of people who are already in poor health. People who are HIV positive or have AIDS are at a greater risk for problems from foodborne illness. People who have cancer, diabetes, or liver disease are also in more danger when foodborne illness occurs.

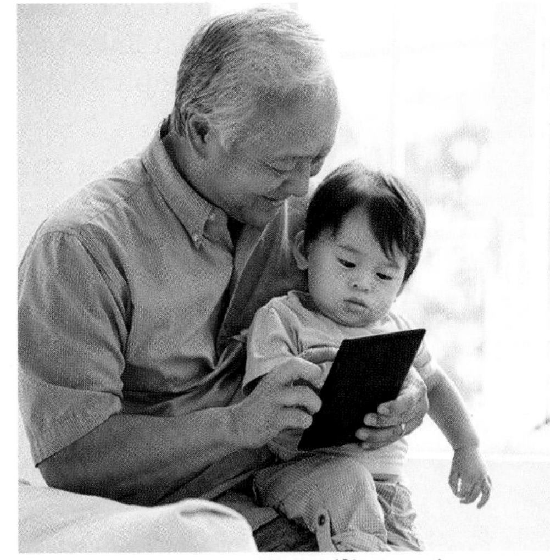

Monkey Business Images/Shutterstock.com

Figure 3.13 Older adults and infants are two groups of people for whom foodborne illnesses can cause serious complications. *What other groups are at risk for foodborne illness complications?*

WELLNESS TIP

Avoid Consuming Pesticide Residues

To limit potential exposure to pesticide residues, use the following tips:

- Thoroughly wash and dry fruits and vegetables with clear water. Do not use soaps and detergents to wash food—these products leave residues, too!
- Remove the outer leaves of vegetables such as cabbage and lettuce.
- Eat a moderate, nutritious diet with plenty of variety to reduce the risk of toxicity from any one food source.
- Trim fat from meat and poultry. Discard the fats and oils from broth and pan drippings since some residues from animal feed concentrate in the fatty tissue.
- Eat kidneys, liver, and other organ meats sparingly. Chemical residues from animal feeds may also be stored in these organs.
- Buy USDA-certified organic produce to avoid foods exposed to pesticides. Certified organic foods are pesticide free when they meet the standards of the National Organic Certification Program.

Recognizing the Symptoms

Foodborne illnesses produce an array of symptoms that range in severity. The most common symptoms are vomiting, stomach cramps, and diarrhea. The type and amount of bacteria in a food affects how sick a person becomes. The symptoms of most foodborne illnesses appear within a day or two after eating tainted food; however, some illnesses take up to 30 days to develop.

The symptoms of most foodborne illnesses last only a few days, but a small percentage of cases can lead to other conditions. For instance, foodborne illnesses have been linked to spontaneous abortions (miscarriages), kidney failure, and arthritis. Complications caused by foodborne illnesses result in thousands of deaths each year.

Treating the Symptoms

Prevention is the best approach to foodborne illness. Do not eat any food you suspect might be contaminated. If in doubt about a food, throw it out! Dispose of it safely away from other humans and animals.

THE MOVEMENT CONNECTION

Jump on Safety

Why

Most likely, you are preparing and packing the food for your school lunch. You do not want to gamble with food safety; therefore, it is important to learn and take preventive steps to avoid foodborne illness.

Don't gamble on whether the food you pack in the morning will still be safe to eat at lunch. Use freezer packs to help food stay cold and prevent the growth of potentially harmful bacteria.

You shouldn't gamble with your health either. Physical activity—even something as simple as jumping in place—will benefit your health and very possibly your academic performance!

Apply

First, find a partner and a location in the classroom where you have clear space around you. Partners should stand a few paces apart and turn to face each other. Now you are ready to play the "Rock, Paper, Scissors" game.

To start the game, make a fist with one hand. As you recite "rock, paper, scissors," jump once on every word. For example,

- "Rock" (Both partners jump.)
- "Paper" (Both partners jump.)
- "Scissors" (Both partners jump.)

On the fourth jump, simultaneously recite, "shoot" and reveal the hand signal you wish to play—either *rock*, *paper*, or *scissors*. To decide the winner, remember that rock "crushes" scissors, paper "covers" rock, and scissors "cut" paper. The player with the "stronger" hand signal is the winner of that round.

Play for the best of three rounds.

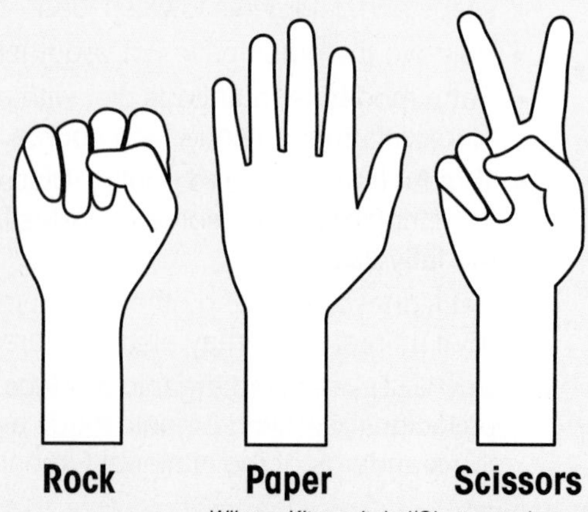

Wikrom Kitsamritchai/Shutterstock.com

If foodborne illness does occur, you may be able to provide treatment at home. Self-treatment is appropriate when symptoms are mild and the person affected is not in a high-risk group. Replace the fluids lost through diarrhea and vomiting by drinking plenty of water. This will help prevent dehydration. Get a lot of rest. If symptoms continue for more than two or three days, call a physician.

If symptoms are severe, you should not wait to call a doctor. Severe symptoms include a high fever (101.5°F), blood in your stools, and dehydration (noticed by dizziness while standing). Diarrhea or vomiting that lasts more than a few hours are also severe symptoms. You should also seek immediate medical advice when someone in a high-risk group presents symptoms of foodborne illness. Infants, young children, pregnant women, older adults, and chronically ill people need prompt medical care. If symptoms include double vision, inability to swallow, or difficulty speaking, you should go directly to a hospital. These symptoms suggest botulism, which is a type of foodborne illness that can be fatal without immediate treatment.

Reporting Foodborne Illness

Determining the source of foodborne illness can be hard. Symptoms may not appear until a day or two after eating contaminated food. If you suspect the contaminated food came from a public source, however, you should call your local health department. If you ate the food at a restaurant or large gathering, such as a party, you should file a report. You should also report commercial products suspected of causing illness, such as canned goods, prepared salads, or precooked meats. Be prepared to provide required information when you phone in your report to the local health department (**Figure 3.14**).

Information to Report When Foodborne Illness Is Suspected

- Your name, address, and phone number
- Description of what happened: where the food was purchased, how many people ate the food, when the food was eaten
- If food is a commercial product, the manufacturer's name and address listed on the container

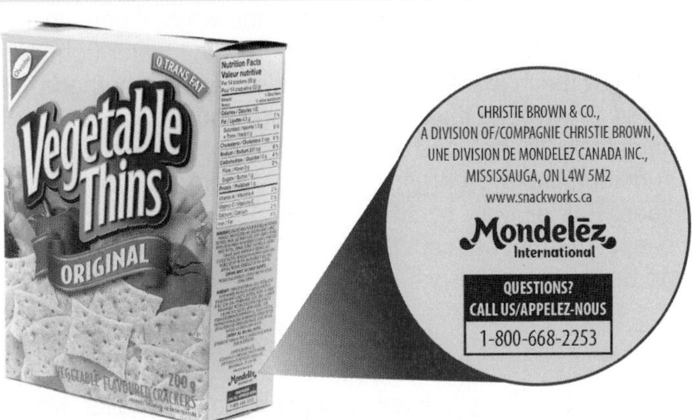

- On meat and poultry products, the USDA inspection stamp number for the identification of the processing plant or establishment number
- Lot or batch number, which will indicate on what day and during which factory shift the item was produced

Photo: Christopher Gardiner/Shutterstock.com

Figure 3.14
If foodborne illness is suspected and a number of people may be affected, health officials may request the information presented here.

If you still have some of the suspected food, wrap it in a plastic bag. Clearly mark the bag to warn people not to eat the food. Store the bag in the refrigerator. Health officials may want to examine the food to **ascertain** (to find out) if a *product recall* is necessary. This means removing the product from stores and warehouses and announcing a consumer alert to the public.

People and Public Food Safety

The food supply chain includes food producers, food processors and distributors, government agencies, and consumers. A weak link at any point in the chain may mean the difference between safety and illness. Poorly maintained farms and unclean processing plants can introduce microorganisms into the food supply. A careless inspection or improper handling at home can also allow tainted food to reach the dining table. Everyone in the chain has a role to play in keeping food safe.

FOOD AND THE ENVIRONMENT

Pesticides and Food: A Question of Sustainability

Pesticides are chemicals that can be applied to fruits and vegetables to control pests, such as insects, rodents, weeds, bacteria, mold, and fungus. *Herbicides* are used to kill plants, primarily weeds. Such chemicals improve product quality and increase both yield and income for the farmer.

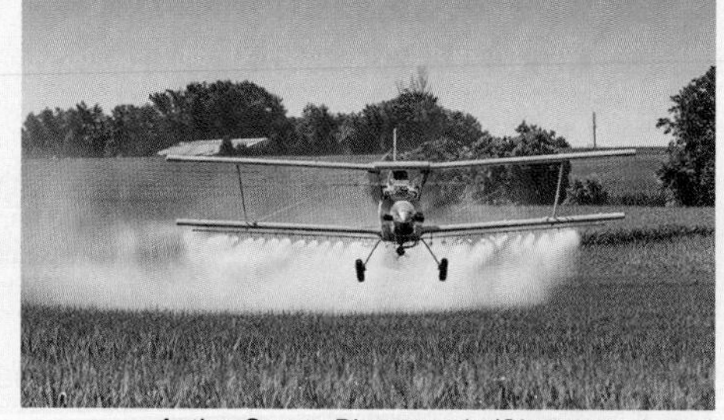

Action Sports Photography/Shutterstock.com

Problems can arise from the use of these chemicals, however. One problem is the danger to the farmer and the workers in the fields. They risk exposure to the chemicals by spray drift, which may be inhaled and/or deposited on the skin. Exposure to the chemicals may cause chronic diseases. Multiple applications of these chemicals are often made during a growing season, further increasing exposure.

Chemicals applied to crops may also contaminate the soil and the water it contains. Over time, this may be harmful to humans who eat the food grown there and drink the water from the *aquifers*, or underground water storehouses. How much exposure to pesticides is safe for humans? Does even low exposure create health problems for a young child? Farmers are required to use good management practices regarding which chemicals can be used and when they are applied relative to harvest.

Currently, much emphasis is being placed on organic farming—production of food without the use of toxic or synthetic pesticides. Rather than synthetic pesticides, organic farmers are using natural pesticides such as oils, soaps, or other safe solutions. For food crop producers, soil sustainability and food safety continue to be challenges.

Think Critically

1. If the use of all pesticides was prohibited and the food supply became smaller, how might food prices and consumer behavior be affected?
2. Organically grown foods are usually more expensive and may not be blemish free. Prepare an argument to support your views on buying organic versus conventionally grown foods.
3. What information about pesticides do you think should be required on food labels? Create a sample label for a box of strawberries found in the local supermarket that illustrates this.

A hazard analysis critical control point (HACCP) system is used to protect the wholesomeness of the food supply. A ***hazard analysis critical control point (HACCP) system*** identifies the steps at which a food product is at risk of biological, chemical, or physical contamination as it moves through an operation. Once the steps are identified, a plan is created to minimize or eliminate the risk. A seven-step process is used to develop a HACCP plan (**Figure 3.15**). Various links in the food supply chain use HACCP plans.

Food Producers

Farmers who raise plants and animals for food have a duty to use chemicals carefully. They must use pesticides according to label directions. They might also explore alternatives to chemical pesticides as part of a crop management system. Farmers need to follow regulations when treating animals with medications. They must also be sure medications have cleared the animal's system before selling the animal for meat.

Food Processors and Distributors

From the farm to the grocery store, the responsibility for safe foods lies with food processors and distributors. Reputable companies know safe food is good business. To compete in the food industry, they must provide wholesome foods. Processors should not accept farm products they suspect of being tainted. They need to keep their facilities clean. Distributors are responsible for keeping food at safe temperatures during shipping.

To ensure food safety, some processing companies set guidelines for handling food that exceed government standards. They may have their own inspectors in addition to government inspectors. These steps help guarantee the quality of products placed on grocery store shelves.

People who handle foods at supermarkets and restaurants also have a duty to protect public health. They must follow proper procedures to keep food wholesome.

Government Agencies

A number of federal and state agencies look after the food supply. Each agency plays a role in maintaining food safety.

Developing a HACCP Plan
1. Analyze how foods move through the operation.
2. Identify the points (critical control points) in the process at which risks to the food can be reduced or avoided.
3. Establish the limits that must be met at each step to achieve safety.
4. Establish a procedure to monitor the limits at each step.
5. Identify a corrective action to take when limits are not met.
6. Evaluate the plan regularly to make sure it works.
7. Establish a system for record keeping and documentation.

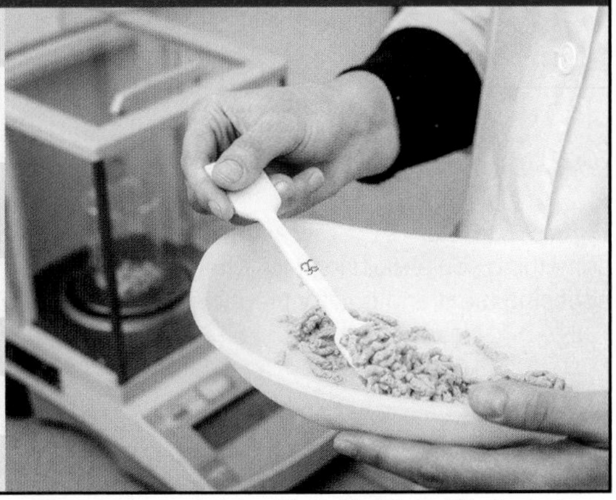

Photo: Mark Agnor/Shutterstock.com

Figure 3.15 HACCP plans are used to minimize risks as food moves through the supply chain.

CASE STUDY

Contaminated Peanut Butter

Blaine is listening to the news and hears a story about peanut butter being linked to incidents of foodborne illness across the country. ACME Peanut Butter Company sells peanut butter to food manufacturers. The news report states that this company is responsible for a nationwide salmonella outbreak. Five hundred cases of illness due to salmonella have been reported. This company ships peanut butter to many manufacturers who make products with peanut butter, such as cookies, crackers, and ice cream.

Blaine is interested in learning more about the outbreak and decides to research further online. He finds out the company had received multiple citations for food safety violations from inspectors in recent years. A company manager was quoted anonymously as "having concerns about the safety of the peanut butter, but was afraid to say anything for fear of losing his job." The more Blaine reads about the situation, the angrier he gets.

Case Review

1. Which link(s) in the food supply chain failed to protect the consumers in this situation? Explain.
2. What factors might contribute to another possible episode of food contamination in some other part of the food supply chain?

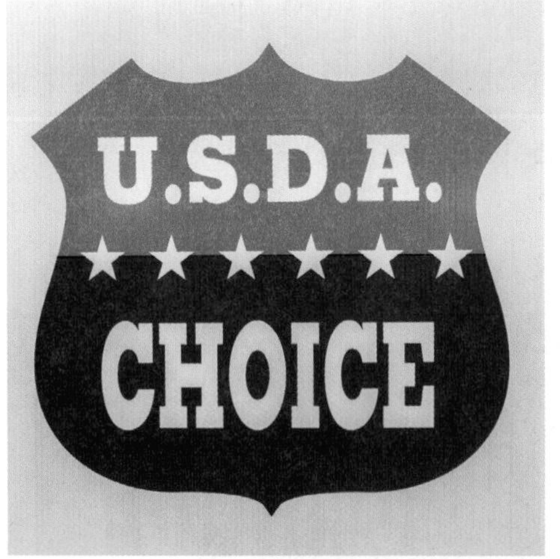

Ken Wolter/Shutterstock.com

Figure 3.16 USDA certification is something you should look for when choosing meat and poultry products.

US Department of Agriculture (USDA) and Food Safety and Inspection Service (FSIS)

The USDA and FSIS work together to monitor the safety and quality of poultry, egg, and meat products. USDA inspectors place a stamp of approval on food products that meet their standards for wholesomeness. They also inspect food handlers to ensure that they are practicing good sanitation.

Food processors may choose to have USDA inspectors judge the quality of their products. A grade shield stamped on products indicates their level of quality (**Figure 3.16**). Imported meat, poultry, and egg products must be produced under standards equivalent to US standards.

The USDA and FSIS also make an effort to educate the public. They developed a safe food-handling label to help consumers prepare and store foods with safety in mind. The USDA also maintains the Meat and Poultry Hotline to answer consumers' food safety questions. The government's food safety website also provides answers to many food safety questions.

US Food and Drug Administration (FDA)

The FDA is in charge of ensuring the safety of all foods sold other than the meat, poultry, and egg products regulated by FSIS. The FDA monitors pesticide residues left on farm products. FDA inspectors check farms, food-processing plants, and imported food products. They also oversee recalls of unsafe foods.

National Oceanic and Atmospheric Administration (NOAA)

NOAA's seafood inspection services help to ensure high-quality seafood. Inspectors travel to fishing vessels, seafood processors, and cold storage facilities around the world. The FDA runs a required fish inspection program for all seafood processors and retailers both domestic and international (**Figure 3.17**). The Fish Watch website also provides much information about seafood safety.

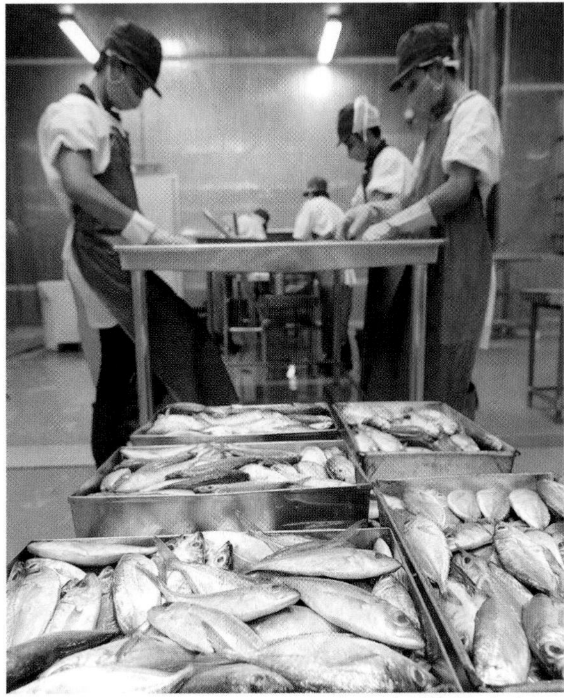

Jordan Lye/Shutterstock.com

Figure 3.17 As with other foods, fish must be inspected for safety. *What kinds of food safety problems are related to fish?*

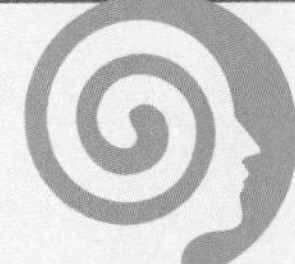

EXTEND YOUR KNOWLEDGE

Protecting the Food Supply

The United States has one of the safest food supplies in the world. Still, consumers want to be assured their food system is protected from contaminants. News reports and data collected by the government indicate that too many foodborne illnesses still sicken people.

In 2011, the Food Safety Modernization Act (FSMA) was passed. This act empowers the Food and Drug Administration (FDA) to regulate the way foods are grown, harvested, and processed. These food safety controls extend to producers, processors, and importers of food products.

Specifically, the law added five key changes to help regulate the protection of the food supply. The law provides the FDA with the authority and the mandate to

- require preventive controls across the food supply to stop or limit food safety problems from occurring;
- implement new inspection techniques that focus on risk;
- apply enhanced means to ensure that imported foods are safe for consumers;
- issue mandatory recalls; and
- strengthen partnerships among food safety agencies at all levels—federal, state, local, territorial, tribal, and foreign.

Form an opinion about government controls protecting food safety. Should there be more controls and inspections, or is government interfering with food production too much? If you were a farmer or a food producer, would you feel differently?

US Environmental Protection Agency (EPA)

The EPA plays a role in food safety by regulating pesticides. The EPA evaluates the safety of new pesticides and publishes directions for their safe use. It sets limits for pesticide residues and prosecutes growers who exceed these limits. The EPA also sets standards for water quality.

Federal Trade Commission (FTC)

The FTC's Bureau of Consumer Protection regulates food advertisements. Advertising claims must be truthful. They cannot mislead consumers about the contents or nutritional value of a product. The FTC handles complaints about a company, organization, or business practice.

State and Local Agencies

Federal agencies cannot keep the food supply safe without support. State and local government agencies help ensure the safety of food produced in their regions. State departments of agriculture set standards and inspect farms. Local health departments check food handling in grocery stores. They also inspect food-service operations, such as schools, nursing homes, and restaurants.

Food Consumers

As a consumer, you are the last link in the food supply chain. The responsibility for choosing wholesome food and handling it properly ultimately lies with you. You must select foods carefully to minimize food-related risks. You must practice safe food-handling techniques to prevent foodborne illnesses (**Figure 3.18**). If illness occurs, you need to report it to the appropriate agencies.

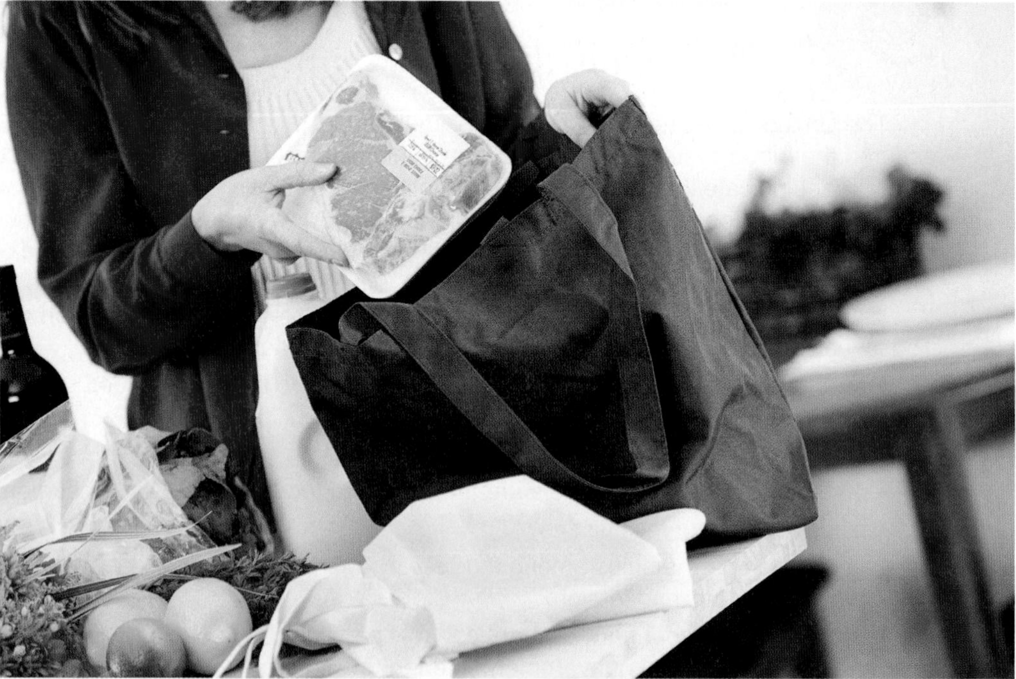

Figure 3.18 Putting perishable groceries such as meat into the refrigerator immediately when returning home from shopping helps prevent spoiling.

Sean Locke Photography/Shutterstock.com

RECIPE FILE

Roasted Vegetables with Chicken

6 SERVINGS

Ingredients

- 12 oz. boneless, skinless chicken breast, cut into 1-inch cubes
- 1 T. balsamic vinegar
- ½ t. garlic powder
- ½ lb. asparagus
- 1 yellow squash
- 1 zucchini
- 1 yellow potato
- 1 purple potato
- 1 red bell pepper
- 1 red onion
- 1 T. olive oil
- ½ t. dried thyme
- ½ t. garlic powder
- ½ t. pepper
- ¼ t. salt
- red pepper flakes, to taste (optional)
- cooking spray as needed
- ¼ c. grated Parmesan cheese

Directions

1. Preheat oven to 400°F (204°C).
2. In small bowl, mix together chicken cubes, balsamic vinegar, and garlic powder. Set aside.
3. Break off tough bottom ends of asparagus and throw away. Cut remaining spears into 2-inch pieces.
4. Cut yellow squash and zucchini into fourths, lengthwise. Then cut each fourth into 1-inch chunks.
5. Slice potatoes into fourths, lengthwise. Then slice each fourth into ¼-inch slices.
6. Slice red bell pepper into ½-inch strips. Then cut each strip in half.
7. Cut onion into 1-inch chunks.
8. Place all vegetables in a large bowl and drizzle with olive oil.
9. Sprinkle thyme, garlic powder, red pepper flakes (if desired), salt, and pepper over vegetables.
10. Toss until all vegetables are coated well with olive oil and herbs.
11. Line jelly roll pan with foil and spray well with cooking spray.
12. Spread vegetables out onto prepared pan in a single layer.
13. Roast in oven for 15 minutes.
14. Place chicken evenly around the pan and roast for 15 minutes more or until chicken reaches 165°F (74°C). Vegetables should begin to brown and chicken should be cooked through with no pink inside.
15. Remove from oven and sprinkle with Parmesan cheese.

PER SERVING: 181 CALORIES, 22 G PROTEIN, 13 G CARBOHYDRATE, 4 G FAT, 4 G FIBER, 114 MG SODIUM.

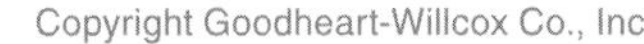

Chapter 3 Review and Expand

Reading Summary

Many foodborne illnesses are caused by harmful bacteria. Parasites, viruses, and fungi in foods can cause illness, too. Natural toxins and chemicals can also contaminate foods.

Steps to prevent foodborne illness include selecting only foods that appear wholesome, storing foods at safe temperatures, and using safe food-handling practices. You must take special precautions to keep food at safe temperatures when packing to eat away from home.

Knowing which populations are most at risk for foodborne illness and recognizing the symptoms will help you know how to react appropriately. Although mild symptoms may be treated at home, severe symptoms and people in high-risk groups require treatment from a physician.

Many people play a role in helping keep the food supply safe. Food producers, processors, and distributors each have a duty to maintain the wholesomeness of food before it reaches consumers. Government agencies set and enforce guidelines for food safety. Ultimately, consumers are responsible for practicing safe food handling.

Chapter Vocabulary

1. **Content Terms** In teams, play *picture charades* to identify each of the following terms. Write the terms on separate slips of paper and put the slips into a basket. Choose a team member to be the *sketcher*. The sketcher pulls a term from the basket and creates quick drawings or graphics to represent the term until the team guesses the term. Take turns being the sketcher until the team identifies all terms.

   bacteria
   contaminant
   cross-contamination
   environmental contaminant
   foodborne illness
   fungi
   hazard analysis critical control point (HACCP) system
   hygiene
   microorganism
   parasite
   pathogen
   pesticide residue
   protozoa
   sanitation
   toxin
   virus

2. **Academic Terms** For each of the following terms, identify a word or group of words describing a quality of the term—an *attribute*. Pair up with a classmate and discuss your list of attributes. Then, discuss your list of attributes with the whole class to increase understanding.

   adhere to
   ascertain
   repel
   reputable

Review Learning

3. Describe the differences between bacteria that are harmful and those that are helpful.
4. What causes food to spoil?
5. How are foodborne illnesses caused by viruses commonly spread?
6. What are three steps a person can take to limit his or her intake of pesticide residue?
7. Why is the temperature range from 40°F (4°C) to 140°F (60°C) called the *danger zone*?
8. When should you wash your hands during food preparation?
9. List three ways to thaw foods safely.
10. What six groups of people are most at risk when foodborne illness occurs?
11. What are the most common symptoms of foodborne illness?
12. Describe the treatment of mild symptoms of foodborne illness for someone who is not in a high-risk group.
13. What is the role of food distributors in keeping food safe?
14. How does the government help ensure a safe food supply for consumers?

Self-Assessment Quiz

Complete the self-assessment quiz online to help you practice and expand your knowledge and skills.

Critical Thinking

15. **Identify Evidence** Read an article about a recent recall on a food product. Follow the chain of evidence in the article. Who identified the problem? What was the source of the problem? When and where did the problem initially occur? How was the problem resolved?
16. **Draw Conclusions** Suppose you and a friend went out for dinner. Your friend had a chicken sandwich and green salad, and you had a well-done burger and fries. Two days later, your friend has a fever, severe headache, abdominal pain, and diarrhea, but you are fine. What conclusions can you draw about your friend's symptoms?
17. **Apply** Research to learn the factors a health inspector evaluates when he or she is inspecting a food service facility. Use these points to create an inspection form to inspect your home or school kitchen. Identify any food safety issues and recommend appropriate corrections on the form.
18. **Analyze** Select two websites that serve as food safety resources for consumers. Write a one-page review comparing their ease of use and quality of information.

Core Skills

19. **Technology Literacy** Research sources such as Food Poisoning: Medline Plus Medical Encyclopedia to find food safety information. Use infographic creation software to prepare an infographic that highlights potential sources of food poisoning, such as eating food prepared with unwashed hands or eating undercooked eggs and meat. Be sure to identify your target audience and tailor your infographic to that audience.
20. **Science** Traveler's diarrhea (TD) is the most common illness affecting international travelers. Research the symptoms, causes, and preventive measures for TD. Prepare an electronic presentation to share your findings with the social sciences classes or a geography club.
21. **Speaking** Much of the food we eat comes from the global marketplace. Select any food product produced in another country and investigate the inspection standards used in that country to keep foods safe for export. Give a presentation in class sharing your opinion about the safety of the global food supply based on your findings. Be sure to cite your sources.
22. **Technology Literacy** Select one section from this chapter on keeping foods safe and summarize the content in the form of a tweet (140 characters or less). Write your summary as if you are posting it to Twitter.
23. **Math** Lena took a piece of leftover chicken from the refrigerator, but before she could eat, her sister called needing a ride. Lena left the chicken on the counter and went to pick up her sister. She returned home two hours and forty minutes later. Knowing that bacteria can double in 20 minutes spent in the "danger zone," she wondered if the chicken was still safe to eat. If there were 12 bacteria on the chicken when Lena removed it from the refrigerator, how many bacteria are on the chicken now?
24. **Science** Select one of the pathogens studied in this chapter and draw a large picture of the specific microorganism present in the pathogen. Complete a Webquest to locate sample pictures of your organism. Name the organism, where it can be found, how it grows, and the dangers it poses to consumers. Display pictures in the science laboratory.
25. **Career Readiness Practice** Presume you work as waitstaff at a very busy, trendy restaurant. One of your customers has complained that he ordered his steak to be cooked to medium doneness, but the steak he received is well done. You return the steak to the kitchen and pick up an appropriately cooked one for your customer. As you turn to go to the dining area, you notice the chef replating the well-done steak for another customer. Health department code states that once food has been served to someone, it cannot be served to someone else. What is the ethical way to handle this situation?

CHAPTER 4 Nutrients and You

Learning Outcomes

After studying this chapter, you will be able to

- **identify** the six basic nutrient groups required for a lifetime of wellness;
- **distinguish** the functions of the major parts of the digestive system;
- **summarize** the processes of absorption and metabolism;
- **analyze** how lifestyle behaviors and food patterns can affect digestion and absorption processes; and
- **recognize** the characteristics associated with common digestive disorders.

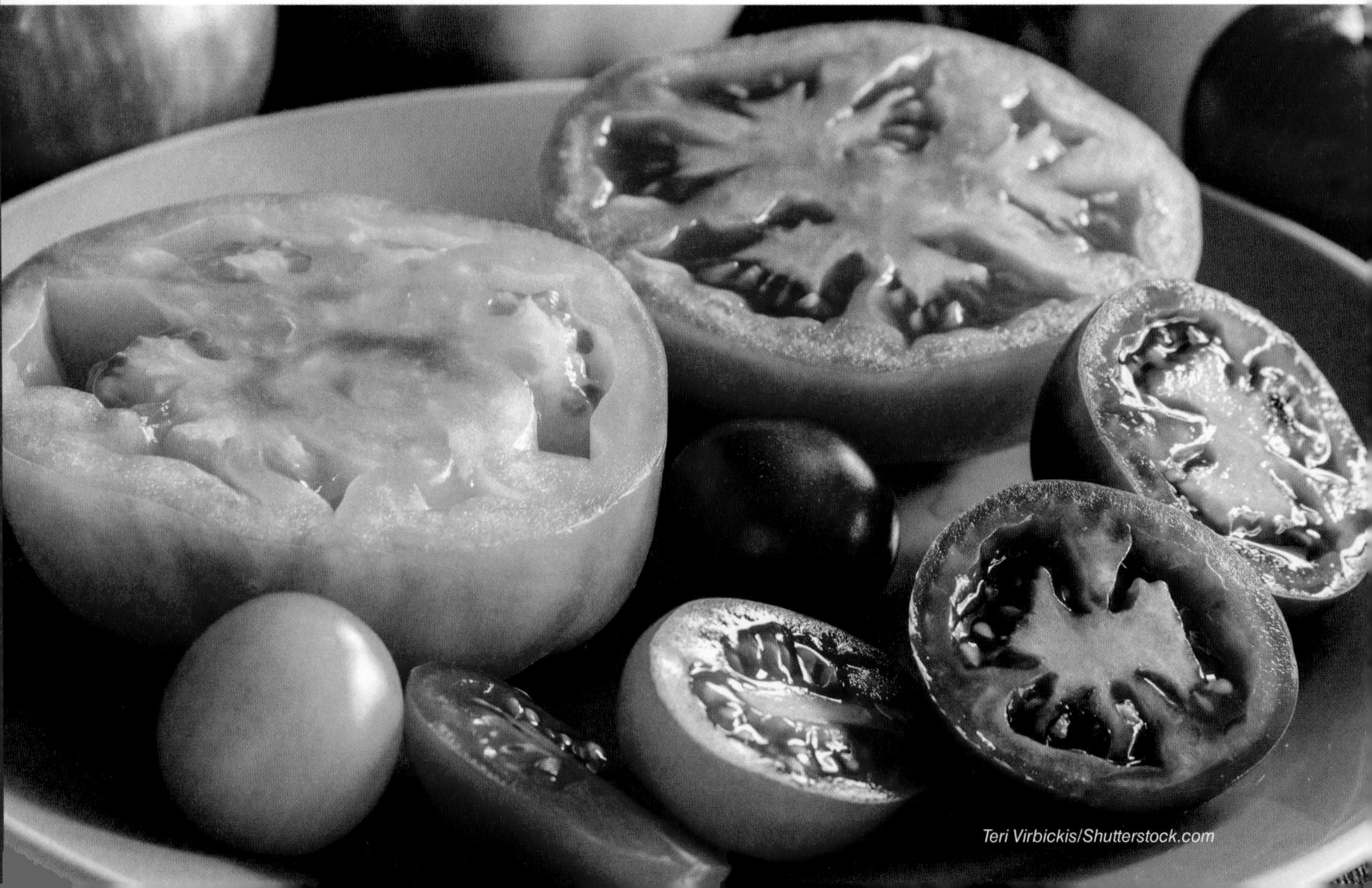

Teri Virbickis/Shutterstock.com

Content Terms 

absorption
ATP (adenosine triphosphate)
bile
chyme
constipation
diarrhea
digestion
diverticulosis
enzyme
feces
food allergy
food intolerance
gallstones
gastric juices
gastrointestinal (GI) tract
heartburn
indigestion
kilocalorie
macronutrient
mastication
metabolism
micronutrient
peristalsis
ulcer
villi

Academic Terms

disperse
erratic
neutralize
secrete
sloughed

What's Your Nutrition and Wellness IQ?

Take this quiz to examine how much you already know about nutrients and you. If you cannot answer a question, pay extra attention to that topic as you study this chapter.

- Identify each statement as *True*, *False*, or *It Depends*. *It Depends* means in some cases the statement is true; in some cases it could be false.
- Revise false statements to make them true.
- Explain the circumstances in which each *It Depends* statement is true and when it is false.

Nutrition and Wellness IQ

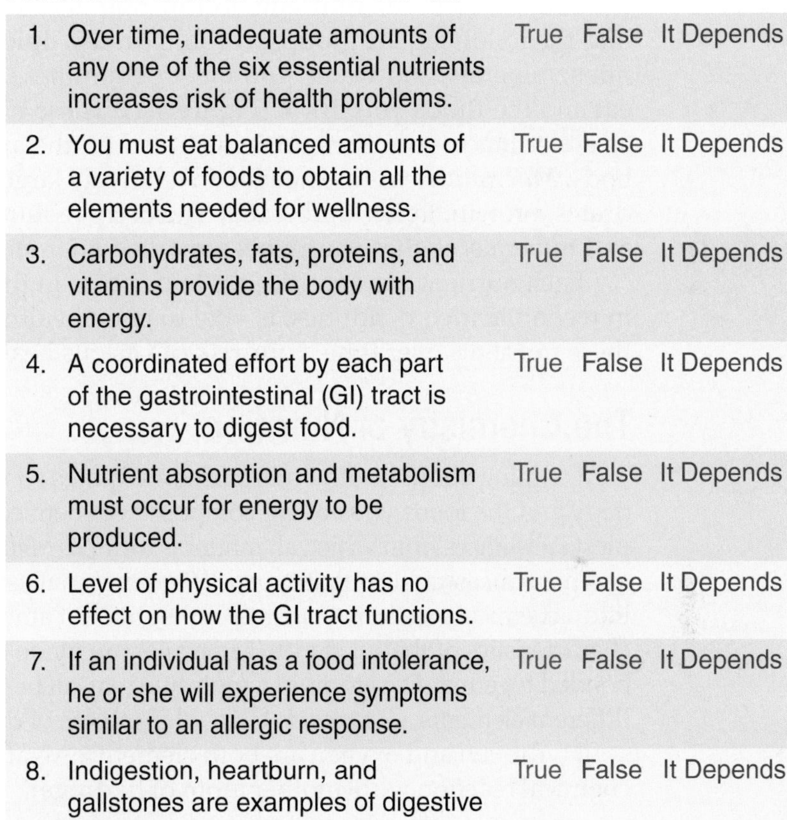

1. Over time, inadequate amounts of any one of the six essential nutrients increases risk of health problems.	True	False	It Depends
2. You must eat balanced amounts of a variety of foods to obtain all the elements needed for wellness.	True	False	It Depends
3. Carbohydrates, fats, proteins, and vitamins provide the body with energy.	True	False	It Depends
4. A coordinated effort by each part of the gastrointestinal (GI) tract is necessary to digest food.	True	False	It Depends
5. Nutrient absorption and metabolism must occur for energy to be produced.	True	False	It Depends
6. Level of physical activity has no effect on how the GI tract functions.	True	False	It Depends
7. If an individual has a food intolerance, he or she will experience symptoms similar to an allergic response.	True	False	It Depends
8. Indigestion, heartburn, and gallstones are examples of digestive disorders.	True	False	It Depends

While studying this chapter, look for the activity icon to

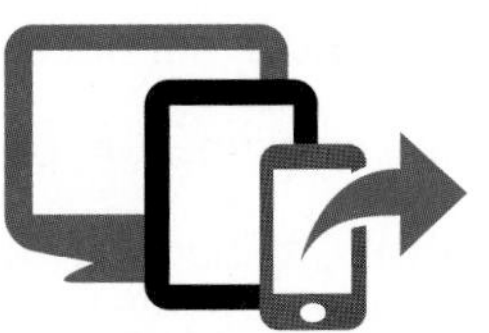

- **build** vocabulary with e-flash cards and interactive games;
- **assess** what you learn by completing self-assessment quizzes and completing review questions; and
- **expand** knowledge with interactive activities and activities that extend learning.

www.g-wlearning.com/foodsandnutrition/

The phrase "You are what you eat" is a true statement. Food is your body's fuel. When you eat, your body breaks down food and the nutrients it contains into simpler elements. Energy is released and nutrients are used to help build, repair, and maintain body cells. Then your body discards the by-products of this process as waste. This chapter will help you picture the process of how your body uses food from beginning to end.

Food, Nutrients, and Energy

Food plays more roles than simply satisfying hunger. The food you eat becomes part of you. Nutrients from food are your body's source of fuel and building materials.

The Six Nutrient Groups

Your body needs nutrients to function and thrive. The nutrients are divided into the following six groups: carbohydrates, lipids (fats and oils), proteins, vitamins, minerals, and water. You must obtain these substances from the foods you eat and the fluids you drink (**Figure 4.1**). These nutrients are further categorized as either macro- or micronutrients based on the amounts required by the human body. ***Macronutrients*** are needed in relatively large amounts and include carbohydrates, protein, lipids, and water. The body requires smaller amounts of vitamins and minerals, so these nutrients are called ***micronutrients***.

Each nutrient has specific jobs to perform in the body. Each of these nutrients, in recommended quantities, is vital to good health. Without adequate amounts of these nutrients over time, your risk of various health problems will increase.

The Chemistry of Nutrition

Learning about health and nutrition requires some knowledge of chemistry. Your body and the foods you eat are composed of chemical elements. *Elements* are the simplest substances from which all matter is formed. *Matter* is anything that takes up space and has a measurable quantity. An *atom* is the smallest part of an element that can enter into a chemical reaction. A *molecule* is the smallest amount of a substance that has all the characteristics of the substance. Molecules are made up of two or more atoms that are bonded together. The atoms in a molecule may all be the same element, or they may be different elements. *Compounds* form when atoms of different elements bond together.

Hydrogen and oxygen are both elements. An atom of hydrogen can enter into a chemical reaction with another atom of hydrogen. These two atoms can be bonded

Figure 4.1
Nutrients are obtained from a wide variety of sources.

Sources of the Six Nutrient Groups

Nutrient Group	Sources*
Carbohydrates	Pasta, corn, potatoes, bread, tortilla, rice
Lipids (fats and oils)	Butter, nuts, canola oil, salad dressing
Proteins	Beef, chicken, fish, pinto beans, quinoa
Vitamins	Carrots, spinach, avocados, liver, eggs, cabbage
Minerals	Milk, almonds, bananas, beef, black beans, shrimp
Water	Water, celery, apples

*List is not all-inclusive

together to form a hydrogen molecule. Two atoms of hydrogen can also bond to an atom of oxygen. The resulting substance would be a molecule of water. Water is a compound because this molecule is made up of two different elements.

Five of the basic nutrient groups—carbohydrates, lipids, proteins, vitamins, and water—are compounds. (The lipids group is made up largely of fats and oils, and the terms *lipids*, *fats*, and *oils* are often used interchangeably.) Minerals—the sixth basic nutrient group—are elements. There are at least 25 chemical elements involved in health and nutrition, including oxygen, hydrogen, carbon, nitrogen, sulfur, and cobalt.

It may be difficult to think of food as a list of chemicals. You do not need to carry out laboratory experiments to understand nutrition; however, having some chemistry background will help you grasp how nutrients interact in your body.

The Functions of Nutrients

Essential nutrients found in food

- build and repair body tissues;
- regulate all body processes; and
- provide energy.

When your body is performing all these functions in harmony, your potential for optimum wellness increases.

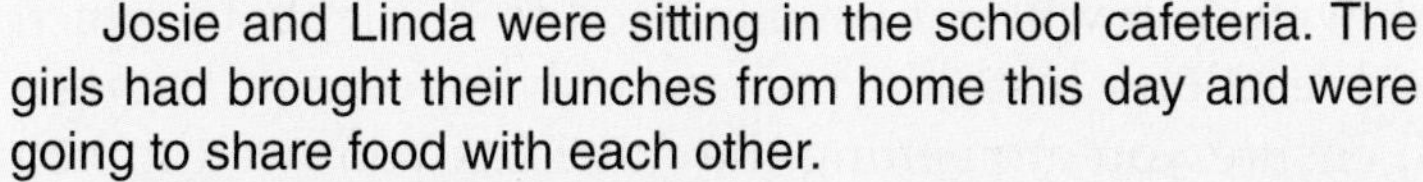

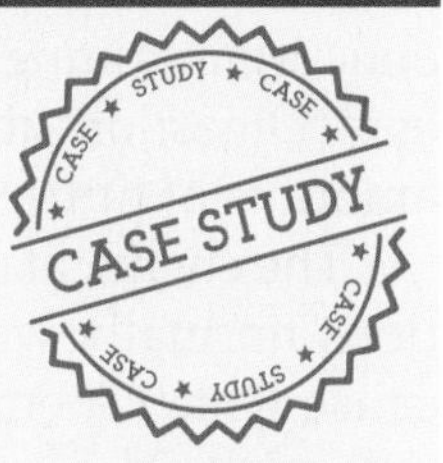

Chemistry of the Lunch Table

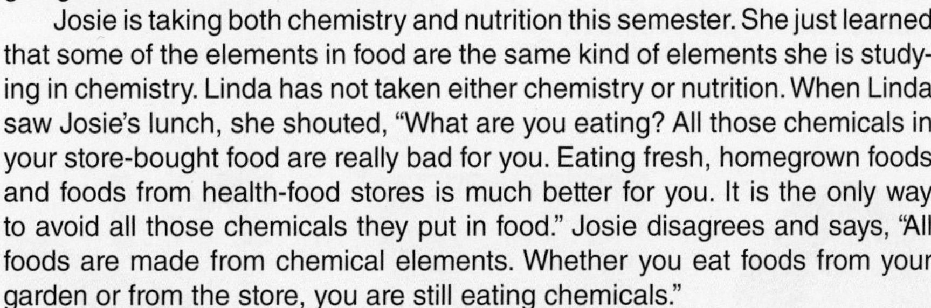

Josie and Linda were sitting in the school cafeteria. The girls had brought their lunches from home this day and were going to share food with each other.

Josie is taking both chemistry and nutrition this semester. She just learned that some of the elements in food are the same kind of elements she is studying in chemistry. Linda has not taken either chemistry or nutrition. When Linda saw Josie's lunch, she shouted, "What are you eating? All those chemicals in your store-bought food are really bad for you. Eating fresh, homegrown foods and foods from health-food stores is much better for you. It is the only way to avoid all those chemicals they put in food." Josie disagrees and says, "All foods are made from chemical elements. Whether you eat foods from your garden or from the store, you are still eating chemicals."

Josie knows that the chemicals added to the store-bought snacks in her lunch are not naturally occurring. She learned in class that these chemicals added to foods are not harmful for most people when eaten in moderation. However, she also knows that she wants to add more fresh fruits and vegetables to her lunch to include more naturally occurring chemicals in her diet.

Still, Josie cannot resist teasing Linda and states, "Did you know that *you* are made up mostly of chemical elements, too?" Linda looks confused.

Case Review

1. Why do you think Linda believes only store-bought foods are composed of chemical elements?
2. Do you agree or disagree that naturally occurring chemicals are better for you than chemicals added by the food manufacturers? Why?

Build and Repair Body Tissues

Your body is made up of billions of cells. From before you are born until you die, cells divide. Each time a cell divides, it produces two new cells. These new cells account for your growth. New cells are also used to repair damaged body tissues and to replace old cells. All cells are formed with materials that come from food. Therefore, your body needs adequate amounts of nutrients to help make new cells.

Nutrient needs during periods of rapid growth are greater than at any other time. Such periods include the prenatal period, infancy, and adolescence (**Figure 4.2**). Lacking adequate nutrition during periods of growth may affect a person's physical size, strength, and health. Learning abilities and behavior patterns could also be affected.

Every cell in your body contains genes. *Genes* carry hereditary information you received from your parents. Height, gender, skin color, and other details that are yours alone are on a genetic blueprint. Good nutrition is necessary, however, if you are to reach your full genetic potential. In other words, if your parents are tall, they may have passed along genes allowing you to become tall, too. Your body needs nutrients to grow, however. If your diet does not provide these nutrients, you will not grow to your full height potential.

Regulate Body Processes

A second function of nutrients is to keep body processes running smoothly. For instance, the circulation of body fluids requires a balance of essential nutrients. Maintaining the correct acid-base level in the blood is a function of nutrients. Digestion, absorption, and metabolism are also processes that rely on proper amounts of nutrients.

The chemical reactions that control body processes are complex, but these reactions normally work well. You will not usually need to think about which foods cause which chemical reactions. Instead, you need only to focus on eating a nutritious diet. This will ensure you are getting the nutrients you need to help your organs and tissues work properly.

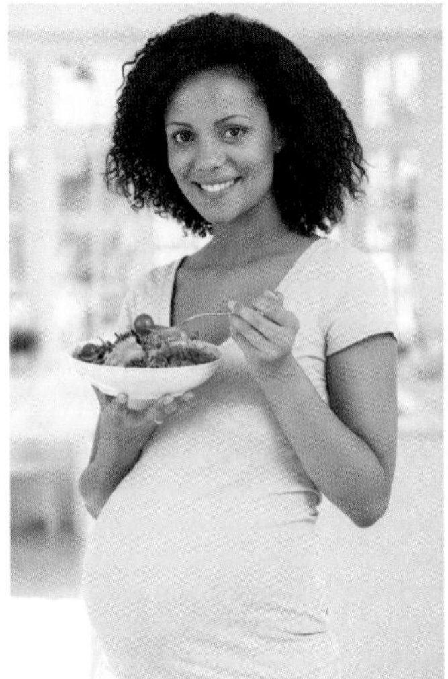
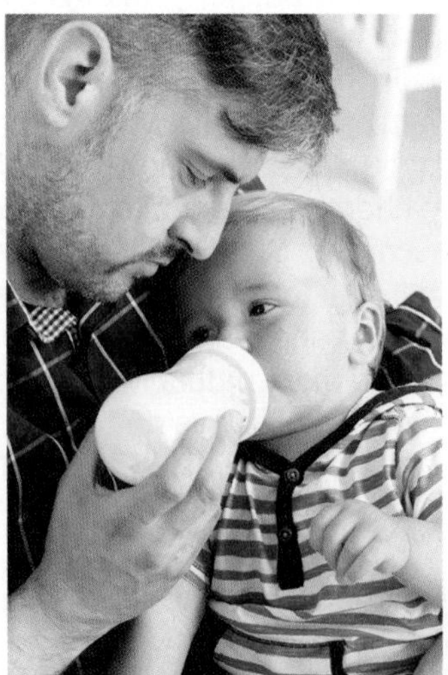
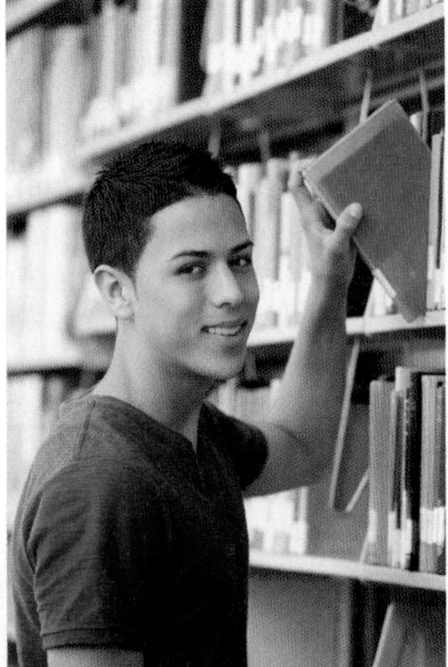

Monkey Business Images/Shutterstock.com; Photographee.eu/Shutterstock.com; Monkey Business Images/Shutterstock.com

Figure 4.2 Pregnant women, infants, and teenagers all have relatively greater nutrient needs than other life-cycle stages. *Why do you think nutrient needs are greater during these stages?*

Provide Energy

A third key function of nutrients is to provide energy. Food is to your body what gasoline is to a car. It is a source of energy for performance. The quality of the food you eat affects how well your body will run.

Energy is necessary for all life processes to occur (**Figure 4.3**). Your body needs energy to breathe, pump blood, move muscles, and provide heat. You need energy every minute of every day. If you go without food too long, your body will not have the energy needed to operate vital organs. The more active you are, the more energy you need to meet the physical demands placed on your body.

Chemical reactions that take place in your cells release energy from the nutrients you get from food. Carbohydrates and fats are the two main nutrients used for energy. Proteins may also be used, but the body prefers to save proteins for other vital functions. Vitamins, minerals, and water do not provide energy.

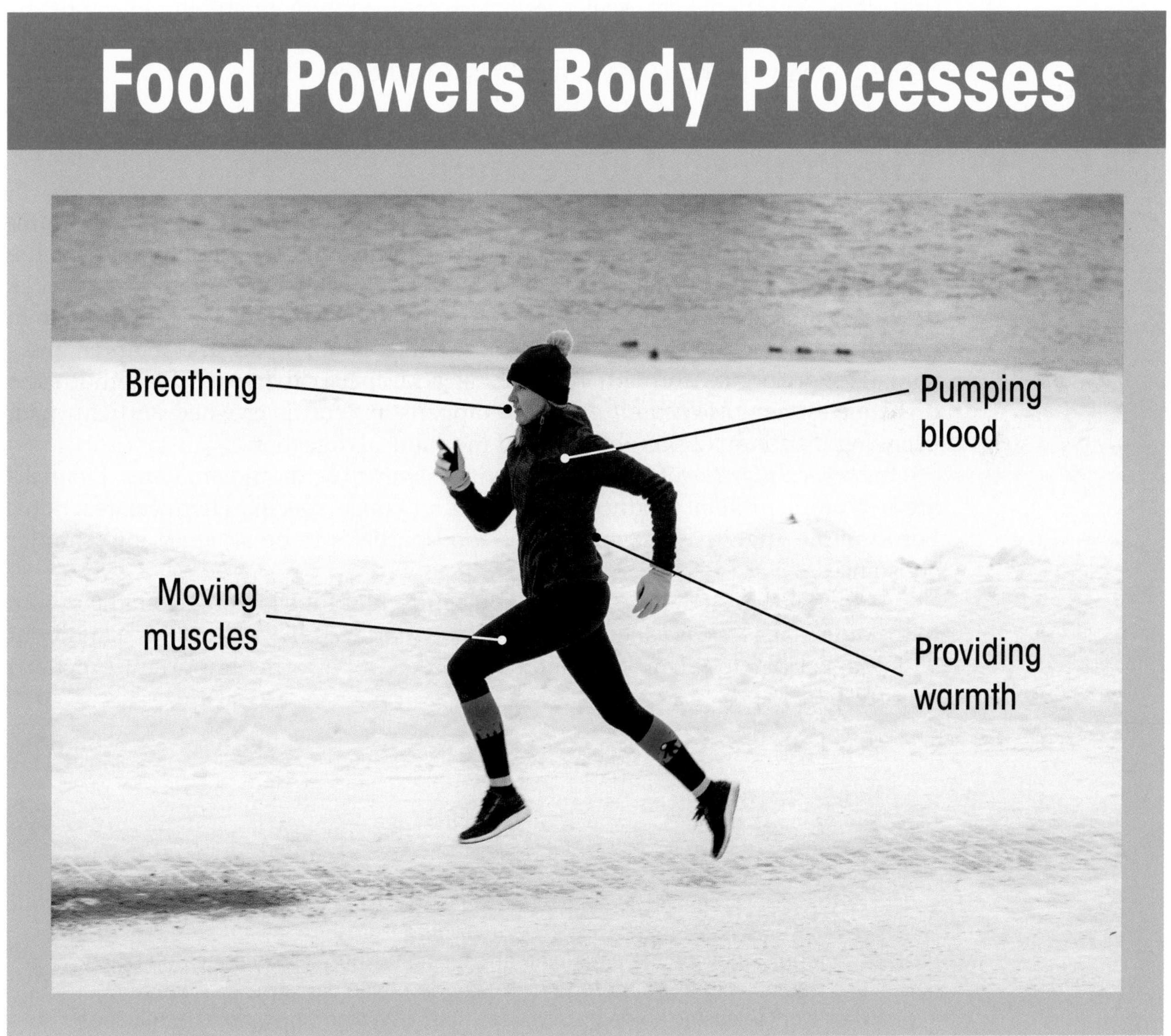

Pavel Korotkov/Shutterstock.com

Figure 4.3 Energy that you receive from food powers many different processes throughout your body. It allows you to perform daily activities.

The body needs these nutrients, however, to help regulate the release of energy from carbohydrates, fats, and proteins. If just one nutrient is missing from the diet, energy release will be hampered.

The Energy Value of Food

The energy value of food is measured in units called ***kilocalories***. A kilocalorie is the amount of heat needed to raise one kilogram of water one degree Celsius. More commonly, the term *calorie* is used instead of kilocalorie on food labels and other sources of nutrition information. In this book, the term *calorie* will be used when discussing the energy value of food.

As mentioned earlier, only certain nutrients provide energy. Each gram of carbohydrate in a food product supplies the body with 4 calories of energy. Fats provide 9 calories per gram. Proteins yield 4 calories per gram. Water, vitamins, and minerals do not yield energy. Therefore, they have no calorie content. The more calories in a food, the more energy it will provide.

Alcohol provides 7 calories per gram consumed. Nonetheless, alcohol is not considered a nutrient because it does not promote growth, maintain cells, or repair tissues. Alcohol is a drug. If consumed in excess, its harmful effects outweigh any positive energy contributions it might make to the diet.

The Process of Digestion

Digestion begins when you ingest food, but what happens to the food after you put it in your mouth? A detailed answer to this question would describe the complex process of digestion. ***Digestion*** is the process by which your body breaks down food, and the nutrients in food, into simpler substances. The blood can then carry these simple substances to cells for use in growth, repair, and maintenance.

Digestion occurs through mechanical and chemical means throughout the digestive system. *Mechanical digestion* happens as food is crushed and churned. Chewing food is an observable form of mechanical digestion.

In *chemical digestion*, food is mixed with powerful acids and enzymes. ***Enzymes*** are a type of protein produced by cells that cause specific chemical reactions. For example, digestive enzymes cause food particles to break apart into simpler substances.

As food is digested, it passes through a muscular tube leading from the mouth to the anus. This tube is called the ***gastrointestinal (GI) tract***. The GI tract is about 25 to 30 feet (7.6 to 9.1 m) in length. Each section performs important functions (**Figure 4.4**).

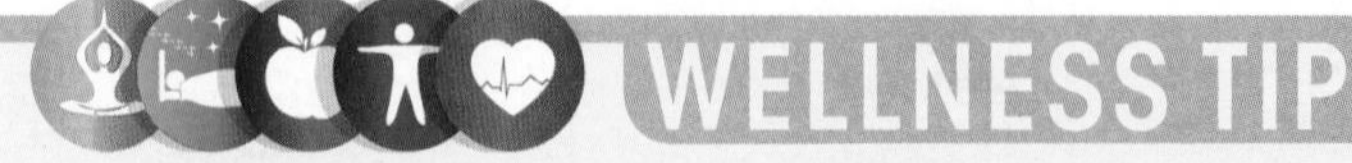

Chew on This!

What's the key to maintaining and losing weight? Chewing! Good digestion begins with chewing food well. As you chew, digestive enzymes begin their work releasing nutrients in your system. Chewing slowly not only releases nutrients, but also takes more time and can help you eat less. This strategy can help you to manage your weight.

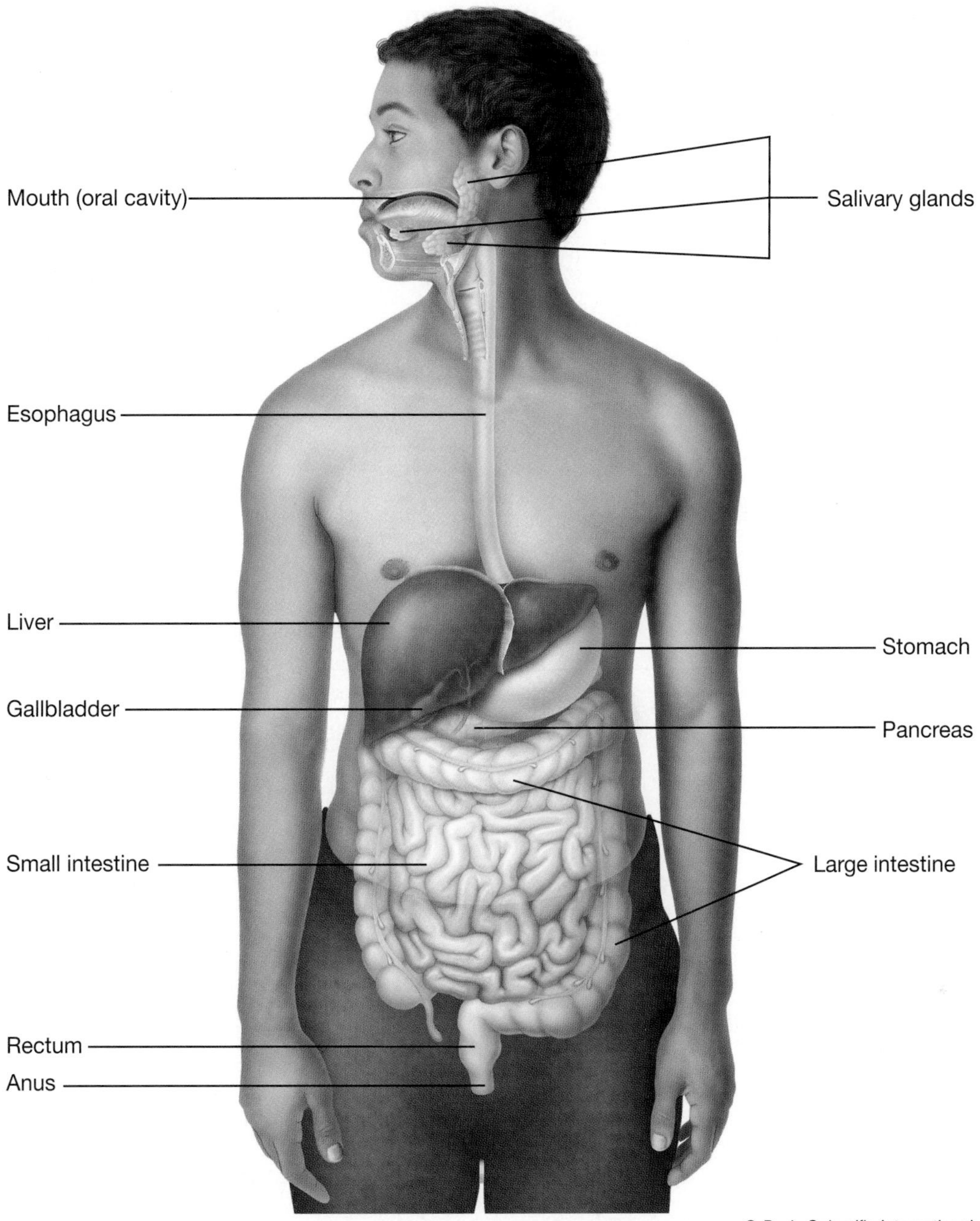

© Body Scientific International

Figure 4.4 The digestive system includes the gastrointestinal tract as well as some additional organs that are essential to digestion and absorption.

In the Mouth

Food enters the GI tract through the mouth. ***Mastication***, or chewing, is the first step in the digestive process. The teeth and tongue work together to move food and crush it into smaller pieces. This process prepares food for swallowing. Chewing your food well aids digestion because the body can break down small food particles faster than large particles.

There are about 10,000 taste buds on and around the tongue. These taste buds sense the flavors of food. This taste sensation, along with good food odors and the thought of food, trigger salivary glands in your mouth. These glands produce and **secrete** (release) a solution called *saliva*. Saliva is a mixture of about 99 percent water plus a few chemicals. One of these chemicals is an enzyme called *salivary amylase*. This enzyme, found only in the mouth, helps chemically break down (digest) the starches in foods.

Saliva plays other important roles in the digestive process besides the breakdown of starches. Without saliva, your mouth is dry and food seems to have little taste. Saliva moistens, softens, and dissolves food. It also helps cleanse the teeth and **neutralize** (counterbalance) mouth acids (**Figure 4.5**).

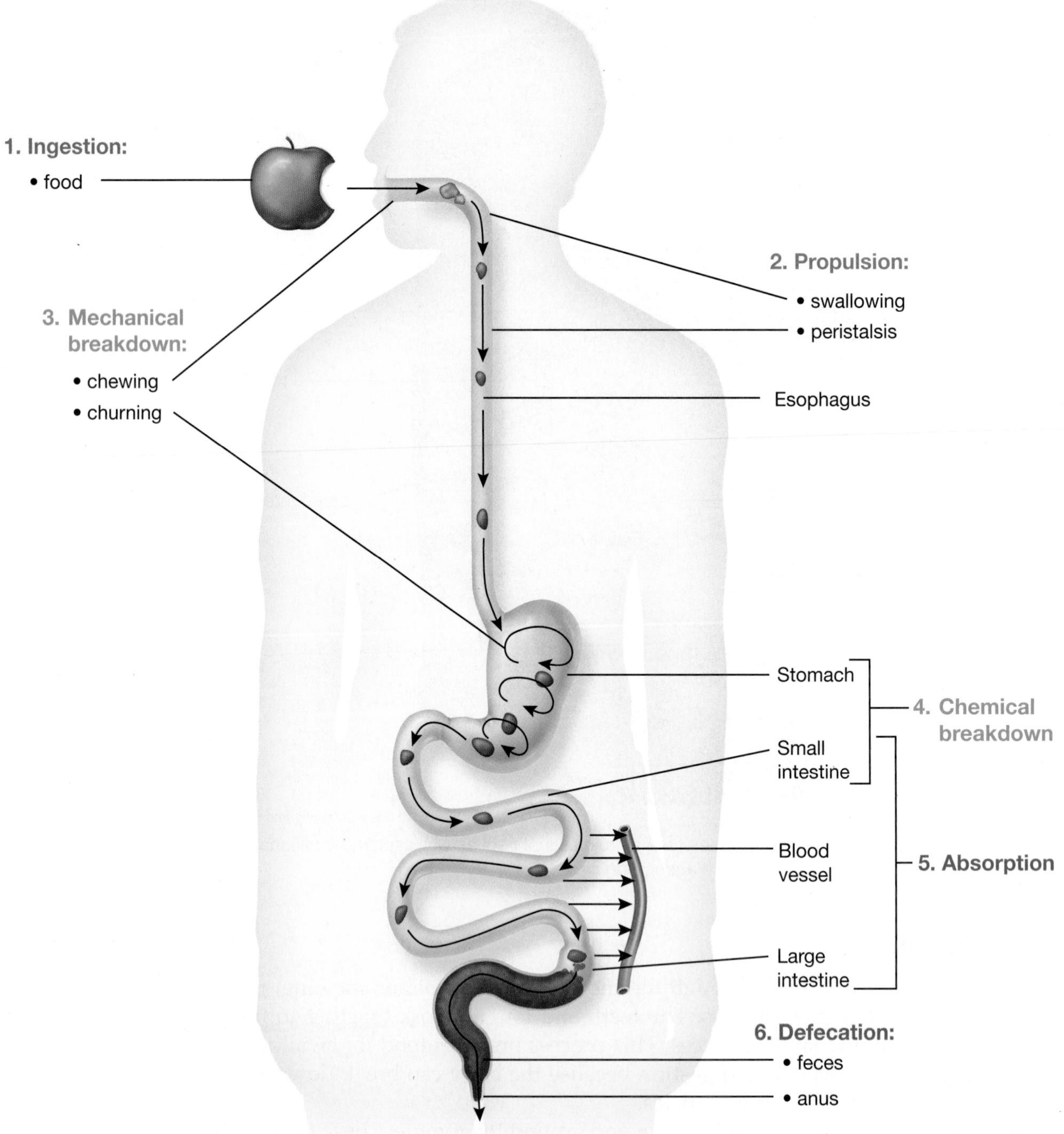

Figure 4.5 As food travels through your body, it undergoes several processes. These processes help break food down into nutrients for the body.

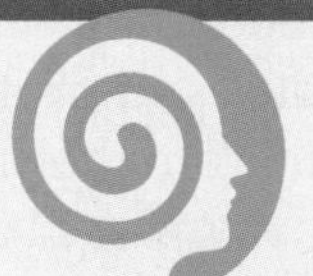

EXTEND YOUR KNOWLEDGE

What Affects the Sense of Taste?

Use print or reliable Internet sources to learn more about factors that affect taste. If something smells good, do you think it tastes better? Why? How does the sense of taste develop? What flavors and tastes are recognized first as a child? Research to learn which medicines older people take can affect taste. How do certain illnesses, food colors, or serving utensils affect taste? How does age affect a person's sense of taste?

In the Esophagus

As you chew, the muscles of your mouth and tongue form the food into a small ball. Your tongue moves this ball of food to the back of your mouth and you swallow it. As you swallow, food passes from the mouth to the stomach through the esophagus. The *esophagus* is a tube about 10 inches long. It connects the mouth to the stomach.

Another tube, called the *trachea*, is in the throat. It is frequently called the *windpipe*. When you swallow food, a flap of skin called the *epiglottis* closes to keep food from entering the trachea. Breathing automatically stops when you swallow food to help prevent choking.

A series of squeezing actions by the muscles in the esophagus, known as ***peristalsis***, helps move food through the tube. Peristalsis is involuntary. It happens automatically when food is present. You cannot feel or control the muscles as they move the food toward the stomach. Peristaltic action occurs throughout the esophagus and intestine to help mechanically move and churn food. Swallowing and peristalsis occur during the propulsion stage of digestion.

In the Stomach

When you eat, the stomach produces gastric juices to prepare for digesting the oncoming food (**Figure 4.6**). The term *gastric* means "stomach." ***Gastric juices*** contain hydrochloric acid, digestive enzymes, and mucus. The mixture of gastric juices and chewed and swallowed food combine in the stomach. This mixture is called ***chyme***.

The acid in the stomach is almost as strong as acid found in a car battery. The stomach wall has a thick lining called the *mucosa*. The mucosa secretes mucus. *Mucus* is a thick fluid that helps soften and lubricate food. It also helps protect the stomach from its strong acidic juices.

Protein digestion begins in the stomach. *Pepsin*, a major gastric enzyme, begins the chemical breakdown of protein in the stomach.

When empty, a stomach has a volume of about one-eighth cup. The inner wall of the stomach has folds, or *rugae* (ROO-gee), which allow the stomach to expand as a food is consumed. In fact, most people can hold one to two quarts of food in their stomachs when the rugae are fully extended.

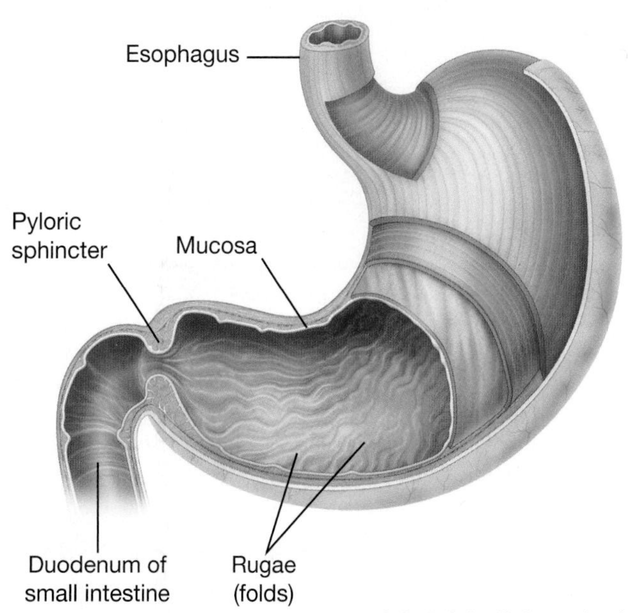

© Body Scientific International

Figure 4.6 The stomach is a hollow organ that holds and digests the food that you swallow.

Food generally remains in the stomach two to three hours, depending on the type of food. Liquids leave the stomach before solids. Carbohydrates and proteins digest faster than fats. Fatty foods stay in the stomach the longest. From the stomach, chyme moves to the small intestine.

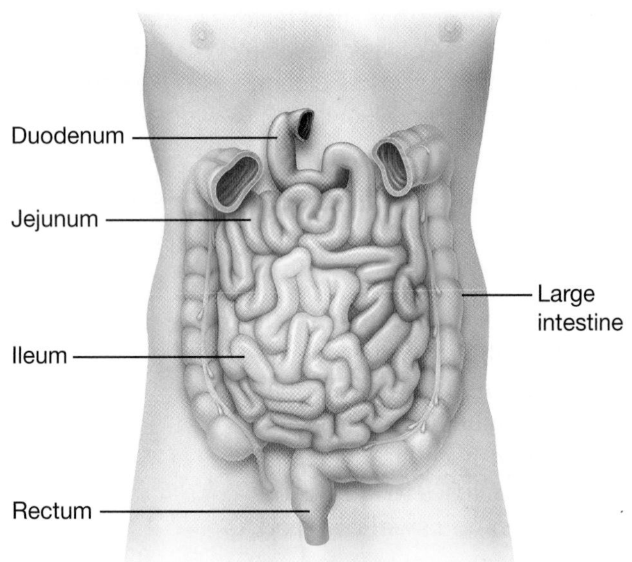

Figure 4.7 After it leaves the stomach, food travels through the three segments of the small intestine. *Which section of the small intestine is the longest?*

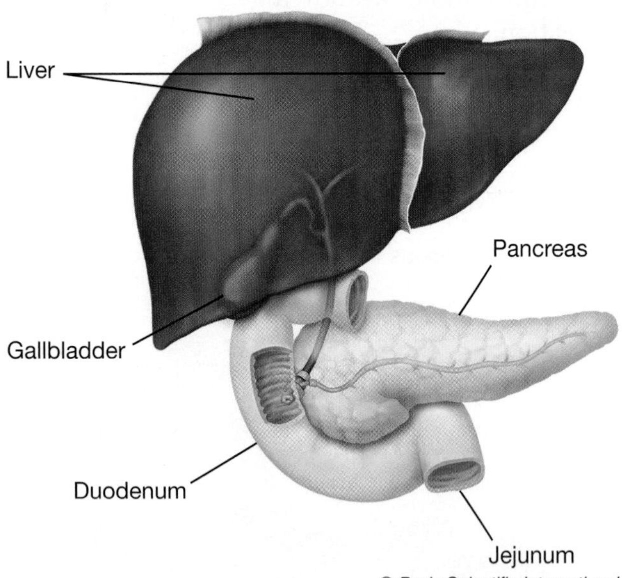

Figure 4.8 Bile from the liver is secreted into the duodenum of the small intestine. Bile helps enzymes break down fats in the foods you eat.

In the Small Intestine

About 95 percent of digestion occurs in the small intestine. The small intestine is coiled in the abdomen in circular folds (**Figure 4.7**). It has three sections: the duodenum, the jejunum, and the ileum. The *duodenum* is the first section and is about 12 inches (30.5 cm) long. The *jejunum* is the middle section and is about 4 feet (1.2 m) long. The *ileum* is the last section and is 5 feet (10.5 m) in length. When stretched, the small intestine measures about 20 feet (6.1 m) in length and 1 inch (2.5 cm) in diameter.

It takes about 5 to 14 hours for food to travel from the mouth through the small intestine. During this time, strong muscular contractions constantly mix and churn food, aiding in mechanical digestion. Peristalsis moves food through the small intestine.

The small intestine needs a less acidic environment than the stomach to perform its work. The *pancreas*, an elongated gland behind the stomach, helps create the correct environment. The pancreas secretes *bicarbonate*, which neutralizes hydrochloric acid that has come from the stomach with the partially digested food.

The pancreas also produces digestive enzymes that aid in the chemical digestion that takes place in the small intestine. These enzymes break down proteins, fats, and carbohydrates into their most basic parts so your body can use them. *Amino acids* are the most basic parts of proteins. *Monosaccharides* are the most basic parts of carbohydrates. *Fatty acids*, *glycerol*, and *monoglycerides* are the most basic parts of fats. *Proteases* break down proteins into amino acids. *Lipases* are fat-digesting enzymes, which break down fats and oils into fatty acids, glycerol, and monoglycerides. *Saccharidases* break carbohydrates into monosaccharides (simple sugars).

The liver is also involved in the chemical digestion that happens in the small intestine. The *liver* is a large gland that sits above the stomach (**Figure 4.8**). It produces a digestive juice called ***bile***, which aids fat digestion. Bile helps **disperse** (distribute) fat in the water-based digestive fluids. This gives enzymes in the fluids access to the fat so they can break it down. The *gallbladder* is the muscular sac in which bile is stored until it is needed for digestive purposes. Bile is secreted into the first part of the small intestine.

In the Large Intestine

The small intestine is connected to the large intestine, which is sometimes called the *colon*. The large intestine measures about 3½ feet (1.1 m) in your body, or 5 to 6 feet (1.5 to 1.8 m) when stretched. Very little digestion occurs in the large intestine. The main job of the large intestine is to reabsorb water. (Chyme is liquid when it enters the large intestine.)

Chyme usually stays in the colon for about one to three days before elimination. During this time, water is absorbed through the walls of the colon. Useful bacteria in the colon work on fiber. They also help manufacture small amounts of some vitamins.

THE MOVEMENT CONNECTION

Nutrient Squats

Why

Squats are a great way to build muscle and even work on flexibility and range of motion in hips and legs.

Apply

We now know that only certain nutrients provide energy. Carbohydrates and proteins yield 4 calories per gram, while fats provide 9 calories per gram. Water, vitamins, and minerals do not provide energy.

Working with a partner, cut or carefully rip a sheet of paper into 6 roughly equal pieces. On each card, write *carbohydrate*, *protein*, *fat*, *water*, *vitamin*, and *mineral* as well as the number of calories per gram provided by each nutrient. Shuffle the cards and lay them face down on the desk. Take turns flipping a card over. Read the card to determine the number of calories supplied by that nutrient. Then, you perform that number of chair squats using the correct form described below.

Chair Squat

- Starting on the edge of the chair in a seated position, place your legs in front of you so feet are planted firmly on the ground. Your knees should be at 90-degree angles.
- Keeping your torso and shoulders upright, rise to a standing position pushing equally through both heels until you are upright with an erect spine, and your head, hips, and feet are stacked on top of each other.
- When lowering back down to the seated position, send your hips back slightly before you bend your knees. This will ensure your knees remain stacked over your ankles.

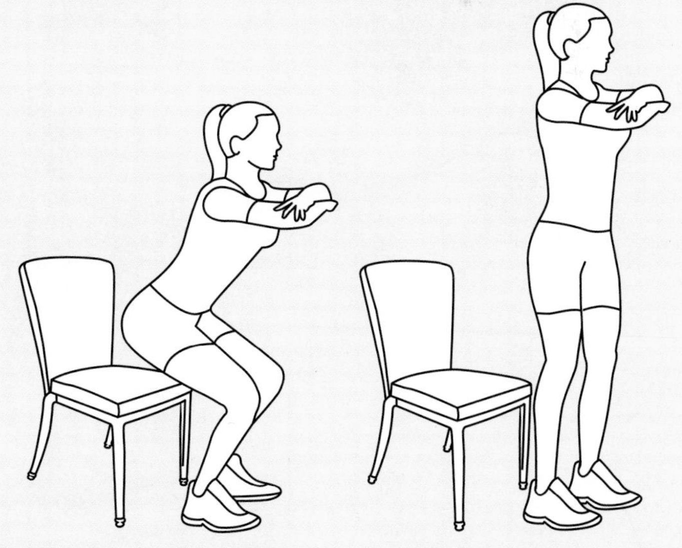

Modifications

- To make this move more difficult, barely touch the top of your chair in the lowest portion of the "squat."
- To ease up on the intensity, take a brief moment to rest as you reach the chair before standing, or do fewer repetitions!

Feces are solid wastes that result from digestion. These wastes include mucus, bile pigments, fiber, cells that have been **sloughed** (shed) from the lining of the large intestine, and water. The end of the large intestine is called the *rectum*. Feces collect here until they are ready to pass from the body through the *anus*.

Absorption of Nutrients

After being digested in the small intestine, the nutrients in food are ready for absorption. ***Absorption*** is the passage of nutrients from the digestive tract into the circulatory or lymphatic system. Most nutrients pass through the walls of the small intestine. Alcohol and a few other drugs can be absorbed in the stomach, however. Alcohol can be absorbed in the mouth, too.

The inside surface area of the small intestine is about 600 times larger than that of a smooth tube. This is because the wall of the small intestine is pleated with thousands of folds. The folds are covered with villi. ***Villi*** are tiny, fingerlike projections that give the lining of the small intestine a velvetlike texture. Each cell of every villus is covered with *microvilli*, which are like microscopic hairs that help catch nutrient particles (**Figure 4.9**).

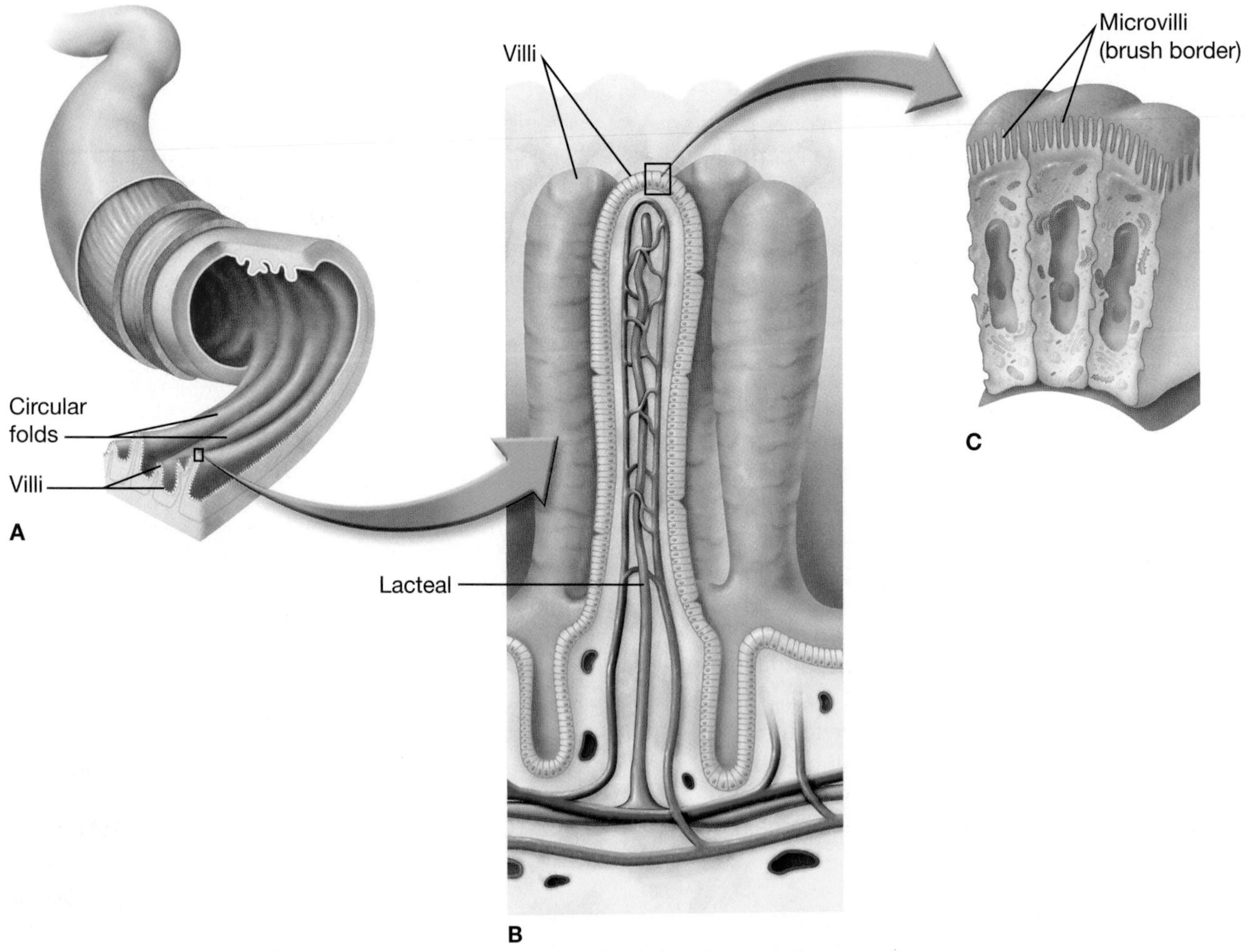

Figure 4.9 The wall of the small intestine. A—The lining of the small intestine contains circular folds. B—The surfaces of the folds are covered with villi. C—The cells of each villus are covered with microvilli.

Some nutrients dissolve in water and are called *water-soluble nutrients*. These nutrients include amino acids from proteins, monosaccharides from carbohydrates, minerals, most vitamins, and water. Tiny blood vessels in the villi, called *capillaries*, absorb water-soluble nutrients into the bloodstream. Then these nutrients are carried to the liver through the portal vein.

Some nutrients can dissolve in fat. They are called *fat-soluble nutrients*. These nutrients include a few vitamins as well as fatty acids, glycerol, and monoglycerides from fats. Lymph vessels in the villi, called *lacteals*, absorb fat-soluble nutrients into the lymphatic system. These nutrients then make their way to the bloodstream.

The large intestine finishes the job of absorption. Small amounts of water and some minerals are absorbed in the large intestine. Bacteria, plant fibers, and sloughed off cells from the lining of the large intestine make up the remaining waste material.

Metabolism

Once nutrients are digested and absorbed, the circulatory system takes over. The circulatory system carries nutrients and oxygen to individual cells. ***Metabolism*** is all the chemical changes that occur as cells produce energy and materials needed to sustain life.

During metabolism, cells make some compounds. They use some of these compounds for energy and store others for later use. For example, cells can make new proteins to be used for growth. The body will shed worn cells and replace them with new cells.

Through metabolism, cells convert some nutrients into energy. The body stores this energy as ***ATP (adenosine triphosphate)***. ATP is the source of immediate energy found in muscle tissue. When the body needs energy, chemical reactions break down ATP to release energy. Every cell makes ATP to help meet all your energy needs.

The body must discard waste products that result from cell metabolism. Waste products leave the body through the kidneys, lungs, and skin. The *kidneys* are part of the urinary system. They act like a filter to remove wastes and excess water from the blood and form *urine*, a liquid waste material. The urine collects in the *bladder* until it is excreted. Drinking six to eight glasses of water daily helps keep waste products flushed out of your system.

Breath from your lungs and perspiration through your skin also excrete waste products from cell metabolism. The harder and faster you breathe, as when exercising, the more moisture and carbon dioxide you lose (**Figure 4.10**).

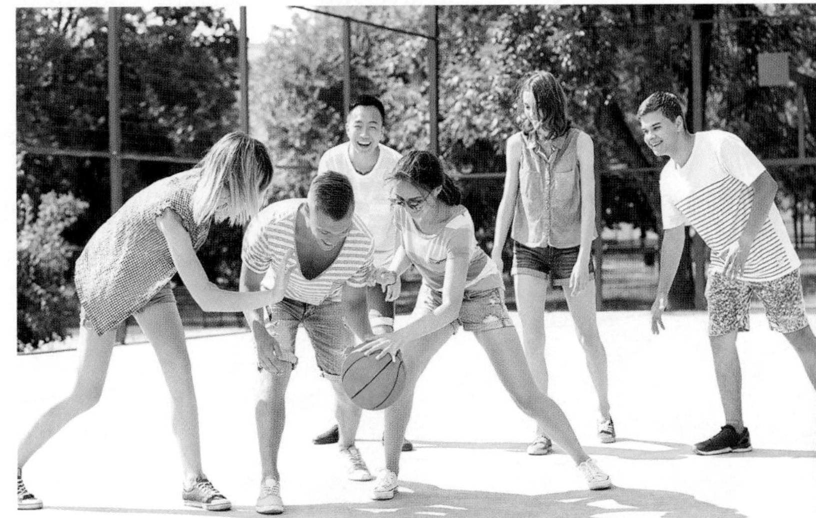

Africa Studio/Shutterstock.com

Figure 4.10 Waste products created through cell metabolism, such as carbon dioxide and perspiration (sweat), are excreted more during exercise.

FEATURED CAREER

Clinical Dietitian

Clinical dietitians provide nutritional services to patients in hospitals, skilled nursing facilities, and other institutions. They assess patients' nutritional needs, develop and implement nutrition programs, and evaluate and report the results. Clinical dietitians also confer with doctors and other healthcare professionals to coordinate medical and nutritional needs. Some specialize in weight management or in the care of diabetic or critically ill patients. In addition, clinical dietitians may manage the food service department in nursing care facilities, small hospitals, or correctional facilities.

Education

Clinical dietitians need at least a bachelor's degree. Licensure, certification, or registration can vary by state. After graduation, dietitians typically have supervised training for several weeks, in the form of an internship. Some schools offer this training as part of their undergraduate work.

Job Outlook

High employment growth is projected. Food and nutrition are seen more and more as a part of preventative healthcare for nutrition-related illnesses (like diabetes or kidney disease) and as having a major role in promoting health and wellness. Applicants with specialized training, advanced degrees, or certifications beyond their particular state's minimum requirements should have the best job opportunities.

Factors Affecting Digestion and Absorption

Have you ever been nervous or worried and felt food sitting in your stomach like a rock? The GI system usually works as it should, but sometimes people have problems. Factors that affect this complex system include your eating habits and emotions. Food sensitivities and physical activity can affect digestion, too. Healthy lifestyle choices can help you avoid many GI problems.

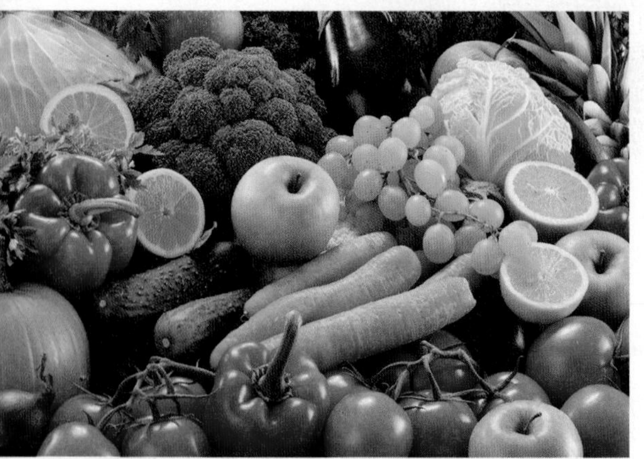

monticello/Shutterstock.com

Figure 4.11 Foods like fruits, vegetables, and whole-grain products like certain breads can provide fiber. *Why is fiber important for health?*

Eating Habits

The foods you choose to eat and the manner in which you eat them can affect digestion. If you eat too little food or your diet lacks variety, you may be missing important nutrients. The lack of a single nutrient can affect how your body will digest and absorb other nutrients. To ensure normal digestion, choose a nutritious diet that includes a wide range of foods.

Be sure to include fresh fruits and vegetables, and whole-grain products in your varied diet (**Figure 4.11**). These plant foods are high in an indigestible material called *fiber*. Fiber helps strengthen intestinal muscles the way weight training helps strengthen arm and leg muscles. Fiber forms a mass in the digestive tract that creates resistance against which the muscles of the intestine can push.

Eating too much food too quickly places stress on the mechanical and chemical reactions needed for normal digestion. To avoid such stress, take time to enjoy your food instead of rushing through a meal. Also, be aware of the size of your portions. Eat moderate amounts of food rather than stuff yourself.

The makeup of a meal affects how long it will take your body to digest. Foods high in fat take longer to digest than foods high in carbohydrates or protein. In the stomach, fats separate from the watery part of the chyme and float to the top. They are the last food component to leave the stomach. A steak dinner, including baked potato with sour cream, oily salad dressing, and chocolate cream pie, is high in fat. This meal will take longer to digest than a high-carbohydrate meal, such as spaghetti, bread, and fruit salad. Because fats take longer to digest, you will feel full longer after eating the high-fat meal.

You should be aware of the wholesomeness of the foods you choose. Spoiled and contaminated foods are unsafe and can cause intestinal problems. Symptoms of these problems often include nausea, stomach cramps, and other intestinal disturbances. Illnesses caused by some contaminated foods can even lead to death.

Emotions

Emotions such as fear, anger, and tension can lead to digestive difficulties. You can avoid most of these problems by making a few lifestyle changes. Making a point of reducing stress and tension while eating will aid digestion. Try to enjoy food in a peaceful, quiet, cheerful atmosphere (**Figure 4.12**). Avoid arguments at mealtime. Also, chew foods slowly and thoroughly to ease swallowing. Taking these steps will help promote normal digestion.

Food Allergies and Intolerances

A ***food allergy*** is a reaction of your body's immune system to certain proteins found in foods. Allergic reactions to food occur in a small percent of the population.

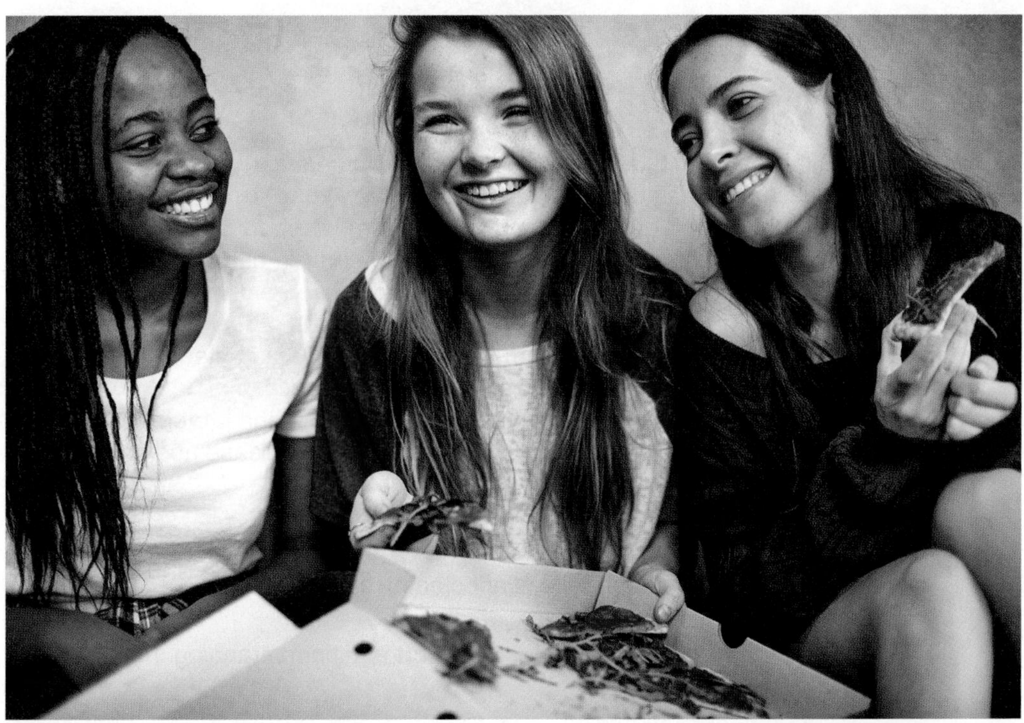

Rawpixel.com/Shutterstock.com

Figure 4.12
Mealtime should be free from stress and tension.

They occur more often during infancy and young adulthood. Reactions occur after a certain food is eaten and the immune system responds. The *immune system* is the body's defense system. The tonsils, thyroid, lymph glands, spleen, and white blood cells make up this system. The immune system protects the body against disease and foreign materials. It produces proteins called *antibodies*. Antibodies combat foreign materials that get into your bloodstream.

The protein that stimulates the immune system to produce antibodies is called an *allergen*. When an allergen enters the body, the release of antibodies leads to allergy symptoms. Vomiting, stomach pain, and intestinal distress are common symptoms of a food allergy. Some people experience skin rashes, swelling, and breathing problems, however.

Experts cannot predict who will develop allergies or how allergies will affect people. Heredity seems to play a role in the development of some allergies. Very small amounts of an allergen may be a problem for one person. Another person may be able to tolerate much more of the same substance. Allergic reactions can change over a life span. As some children get older, their allergies go away. Conversely, other people develop new allergies as adults.

Which foods can cause allergies? Most people are allergic to only one or two foods. The foods most often identified with allergic reactions are tree nuts, peanuts, eggs, milk, soybeans, wheat, fish, and shellfish. People who are allergic to such foods must avoid or limit eating them. If milder reactions occur, after consuming a food, you may be sensitive to the food but not experience a full allergic reaction. People with food allergies must carefully read labels to be sure prepared foods do not contain allergens.

A ***food intolerance*** also causes an unpleasant reaction to food. Unlike a food allergy, a food intolerance does not cause an immune system response. Food intolerances often cause little or no discomfort when the offending food is consumed in small quantities. In contrast, allergic responses may occur from exposure to very small amounts of an allergen. Food intolerances are caused by deficiencies or

CASE STUDY

CASE STUDY ★ CASE STUDY ★ CASE STUDY ★

Adjusting to Food Intolerance

Tom, Sara, Katie, and Josh decided to go for burgers and drinks at a fast-food restaurant after school. They wanted to get a head start on their group science project. Tom watched as Josh pushed the hamburger bun from his plate and ate only the tomato, lettuce, pickle, and meat. Tom asked Josh, "Why don't you eat the bun? Are you on a diet or something?"

Josh said, "No, I am a celiac." Tom wondered if it was a contagious disease. Katie chimed in to ask, "What is that? It sounds weird!"

"I know what it is," said Sara, "He has an intolerance to the protein found in wheat and some other grains. My cousin has the same disease and she is on a gluten-free diet. It is not contagious, it is genetic!"

Case Review

1. How do you suppose Josh's life is affected by having a food intolerance?
2. How could Josh's friends show their support and understanding the next time they go out to eat?

reactions in the digestive tract. Intolerance can be experienced through a reaction to certain food colors, sulfates in food, or food contaminants from unhealthy bacteria. For example, some people lack the necessary enzyme in their digestive tract to digest milk properly. Some symptoms can be similar to an allergic response and may include elevated blood pressure, sweating, and headache. Treatment focuses on eliminating or reducing the amounts of the offending foods from the diet.

Physical Activity

Physical activity can improve health in many ways. It can aid digestion and metabolism. Physical activity stimulates a healthy appetite and strengthens the muscles of internal organs. It helps move food through the GI tract. It also helps reduce stress and adds to your total sense of well-being. For a healthy digestive system, include some physical activity in your lifestyle (**Figure 4.13**).

Digestive Disorders

Most people experience digestive disorders from time to time. Consumers spend many dollars on medications to relieve these problems. Most of these medications are not needed. The digestive system normally functions better without drugs. To help avoid problems, focus on eating a nutritious diet. Be sure to include a variety of high-fiber fruits, vegetables, and whole-grain products. Drinking plenty of water can also help resolve many digestive difficulties.

Long-term illnesses, including ulcers and gallstones, can have serious effects on digestion. They can alter the kinds and amounts of nutrients that reach the cells. Such illnesses require medical supervision.

Diarrhea

Diarrhea is frequent expulsion of watery feces. Food sensitivity, harmful bacteria, and stress are just a few of the factors that can cause diarrhea. Diarrhea causes food to move through the digestive system too quickly for nutrients to be fully absorbed. In addition, diarrhea can lead to a loss of body fluids. Drinking plenty of water will help restore fluid losses when diarrhea occurs. Prolonged diarrhea may be a sign of other health problems and indicates a need to see a doctor.

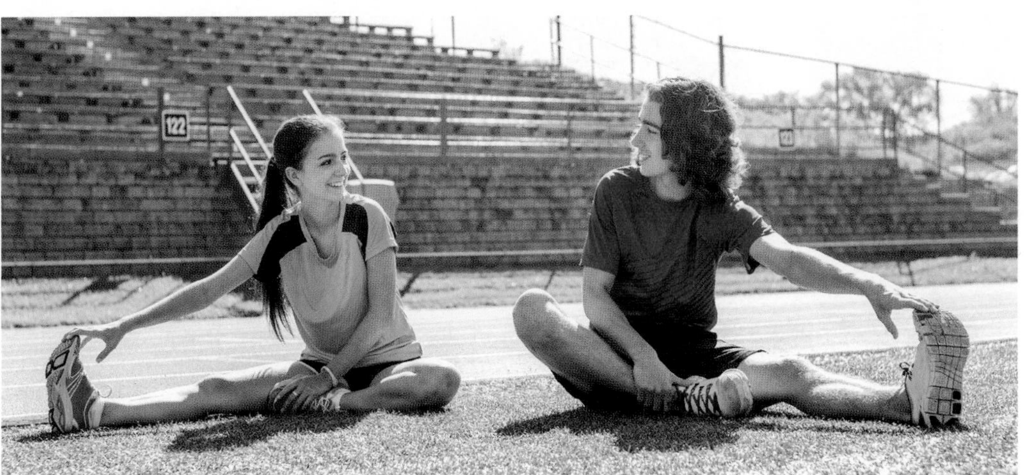

Lopolo/Shutterstock.com

Figure 4.13
Physical activity stimulates a healthy appetite, aids digestion, and offers many other health benefits.

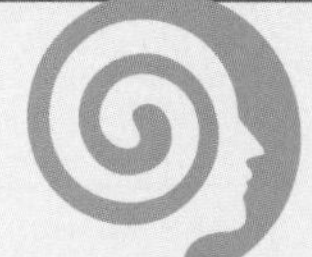

EXTEND YOUR KNOWLEDGE

What Is Crohn's Disease?

Crohn's disease is a chronic inflammatory disease of the gastrointestinal tract that belongs to a group of illnesses called inflammatory bowel disease (IBD). Nutritional complications are common with this disease since it affects the intestines. According to the National Institute of Allergy and Infectious Diseases, about one in 500 people suffer from IBD. Conduct research to learn about the occurrence, symptoms, and treatment of Crohn's disease. Is Crohn's disease hereditary? Is it more common in one gender than another? Which age groups are most affected? Which segments of the population are most affected? How is Crohn's disease treated? Is there a cure?

Constipation

Constipation occurs when chyme moves very slowly through the large intestine. When this happens, too much water is reabsorbed from the chyme. This causes the feces to become hard, making bowel movements painful. Straining during elimination can lead to the added problem of hemorrhoids. Hemorrhoids are swollen veins in the rectum.

Constipation can result from **erratic** (irregular) eating habits, low fiber intake, and lack of physical activity. Drinking too little water and failing to respond to a bowel movement urge can also add to this problem.

Many people use laxatives when they are constipated. The body can start to depend on the use of laxatives, however. This can cause constipation to worsen. A better approach to treating and preventing constipation is to choose a diet high in fiber, get regular physical activity, and drink plenty of water (**Figure 4.14**).

Indigestion

Indigestion is abdominal discomfort that begins soon after eating and relates to difficulty digesting food. Indigestion may be caused by stress, eating too much or too fast, or eating particular foods. Symptoms of indigestion may include gas, stomach cramps, and nausea.

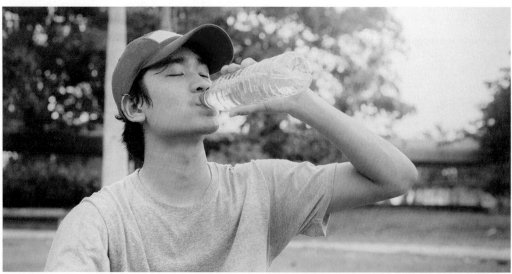

Figure 4.14 Among other health benefits, drinking enough water can help you avoid constipation.

socrates471/Shutterstock.com

People often take antacids for indigestion. *Antacids* are medications that neutralize stomach acids. Taking too many antacids, however, can alter the acidity levels of the stomach and interfere with nutrient absorption rates. Frequent use of antacids can also cause constipation. Instead of taking antacids, try to modify your diet. Avoid eating too much of one food or too many calories at one meal. Avoid eating foods that seem to upset your stomach. Also, eat in a relaxed atmosphere to help reduce stress.

Heartburn

Heartburn is a burning pain in the middle of the chest, but it has nothing to do with the heart. Stomach acid flowing back into the esophagus causes heartburn. This condition is known as *reflux*.

Many people have heartburn after a meal now and then. Antacids can help relieve occasional discomfort. You should see a doctor, however, if you have ongoing or recurrent heartburn. This may be a sign of a more serious condition called *gastroesophageal reflux disease (GERD)*. This disease is common among older adults. If left untreated, it can cause damage to the esophagus and other complications.

You can sometimes prevent heartburn symptoms by changing dietary behaviors. You may need to avoid certain foods and drinks that make your symptoms worse. Often symptoms can be reduced by decreasing fatty or spicy foods, or by eating small, frequent meals instead of very large meals. Refraining from eating several hours before bedtime is often helpful.

Ulcer

An ***ulcer*** is an open sore in the lining of the stomach or small intestine. This disease is caused by a bacterium. The ulcerated area becomes inflamed, and the person who has the ulcer experiences a burning pain.

Some people get ulcers more quickly than others do. People may have a hereditary tendency for the disease. Those who are under stress or use alcohol or aspirin excessively may also be at greater risk (**Figure 4.15**). You can avoid factors that contribute to ulcers by making healthful lifestyle choices.

Depending on the cause of the ulcer, various treatments may be used. Usually doctors prescribe antibiotic therapy to kill the bacterium often present in ulcer patients. Other treatments can be used to reduce stomach acid. Treatment of acid blockers can help reduce the amount of acid produced and released in the digestive tract. Reducing the level of acid in your digestive system also helps the healing process. Over-the-counter antacids and acid blockers may relieve some or all of the pain, but the relief is always short-lived. You will need medical help if the problem persists and you want a cure.

Doctors also encourage ulcer patients to eat a nutritious diet. They recommend increasing physical activity and decreasing stress levels. They tell patients getting enough sleep

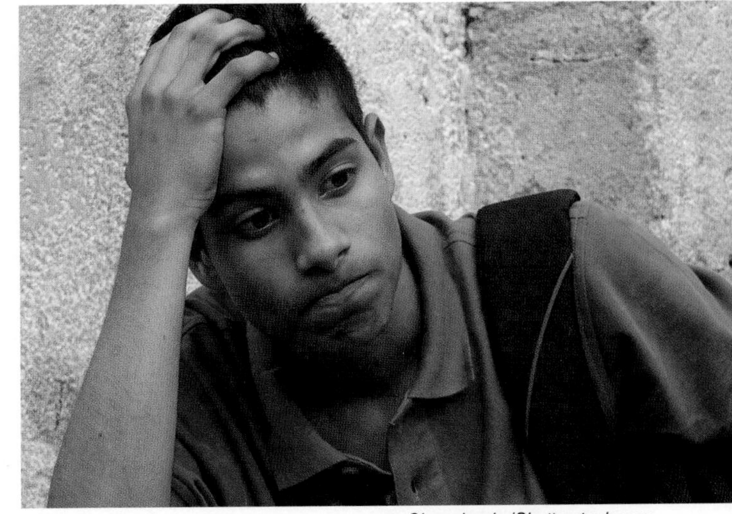

Cheapbooks/Shutterstock.com

Figure 4.15 Stress can increase your risk of developing an ulcer. *How could you reduce the stress you experience each day?*

is important. Avoiding caffeine and alcohol in your diet may help to reduce irritation. If you do have caffeine, combine it with a meal or snack. Eliminate foods that may cause added ulcer discomfort, such as chocolate, certain herbs, and spicy foods. Small meals throughout the day work better than one big meal. Tobacco is to be avoided.

Gallstones

Gallstones are small crystals that form from bile in the gallbladder. Bile, which is produced by the liver to help digest fat, is stored in the gallbladder. When food is present in the small intestine, the gallbladder contracts to release bile. When gallstones are blocking the duct between the gallbladder and the small intestine, this contraction causes severe pain. The presence of gallstones may slow fat digestion. This can cause fluids to pool and back up into the liver.

The treatment of gallstones often requires medical supervision. A physician may recommend a diet low in fats. In severe cases, the doctor may remove the gallbladder.

FOOD AND THE ENVIRONMENT

Air Pollution and the Impact on Food Digestion

Air pollution is known to harm the lungs causing respiratory diseases. But does air pollution also relate to diseases of the gut (stomach) or bowel? Currently, the relationship between air pollution and diseases of the bowel, such as Crohn's disease, is at the forefront of research. Not all evidence is clear, but people with a genetic history of a gastrointestinal (GI) tract disease who are also exposed to high levels of air pollution for longer periods of time, show higher incidences of stomach pains and bowel distress.

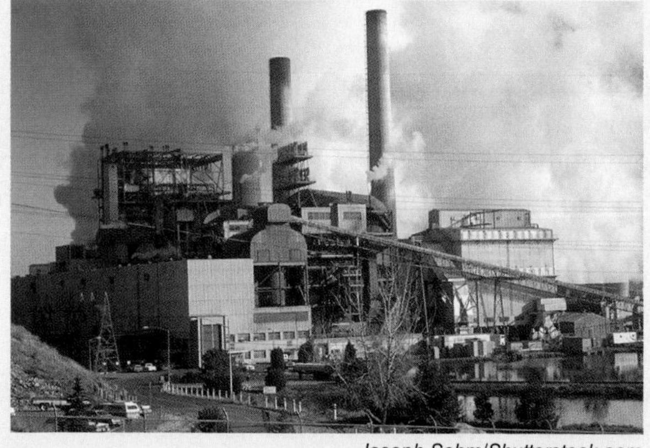

Joseph Sohm/Shutterstock.com

The research focuses on how pollution particles in the air from traffic emissions, other fossil fuel burning, noxious gases, and cigarette smoke enters the body and affects the functions of the GI tract. The complex relationship of pollutants to the work of the immune system, bacteria growth patterns, and the formation of inflammation causing disease is being researched. Understanding how pollution contributes to intestinal disease will help identify ways to reduce exposures to dangerous pollutants found in the air.

Think Critically

1. If you had a GI tract disease, what could you do to avoid exposure to pollutants in the air?
2. What options are available to community officials to keep the common airspace pure and pollutant free?

Diverticulosis

Diverticulosis is a disorder in which many abnormal pouches form in the intestinal wall. When these pouches become inflamed, the condition is called *diverticulitis*.

Diverticulosis can occur when intestinal muscles become weak, such as when the diet is too low in fiber. A high-fat diet and an inactive lifestyle can also increase the risk of getting this disease. The best prevention method is to eat a high-fiber diet, which will help keep intestinal muscles toned.

RECIPE FILE

Vegetable Quesadilla

6 SERVINGS

Ingredients

- 1⅛ t. vegetable oil
- ½ c. green bell pepper, small dice
- ½ c. yellow bell pepper, small dice
- 1 jalapeño chile, julienned
- ½ c. onion, small dice
- ½ c. tomato, chopped
- 2 T. fresh cilantro, chopped
- ¼ t. salt
- ¼ t. ground black pepper
- ¼ t. cumin
- ¼ t. dried oregano
- ¼ t. chili powder
- 6 each whole-grain tortillas (6-inch diameter)
- 1½ c. low-fat cheddar or Monterey Jack cheese, shredded

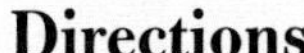

Directions

Prepare Filling

1. Heat 1 teaspoon of oil in a skillet over medium heat.
2. Sauté bell peppers, jalapeño, and onions over medium heat until soft, about 3–5 minutes.
3. Add tomatoes and cook until heated through, about 1 minute.
4. Stir in cilantro, salt, pepper, cumin, oregano, and chili powder.
5. Set aside.

Prepare Quesadilla

6. Place a couple drops of vegetable oil in a skillet. Use a paper towel to coat skillet with oil.
7. Place skillet over medium heat.
8. Place tortilla in skillet. Spread one-sixth of vegetable mixture and ¼ cup of cheese over one-half of the tortilla.
9. Fold tortilla in half and brown one side, then flip to brown the other side.
10. Remove from skillet and serve.
11. Repeat for remaining quesadillas.

PER SERVING: 159 CALORIES, 12 G PROTEIN, 29 G CARBOHYDRATE, 6 G FAT, 3 G FIBER, 481 MG SODIUM.

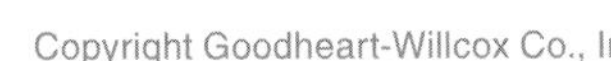

Chapter 4 Review and Expand

Reading Summary

Your body needs six types of nutrients—carbohydrates, lipids, proteins, vitamins, minerals, and water. These nutrients, like your body, are made up of chemical elements. Your body uses them to build and repair tissues and control body processes. Carbohydrates, fats, and proteins are also used to provide energy.

Digestion occurs in the gastrointestinal (GI) tract. Throughout the GI tract, crushing and churning help digest food mechanically. Enzymes and other fluids help digest food chemically.

After digestion, your bloodstream is able to absorb nutrients and carry them to your cells. Most absorption takes place in the small intestine.

Several factors can affect digestion and absorption. These include eating habits, emotions, food allergies and intolerances, and physical activity.

The digestive system is complex. You can prevent most digestive problems by forming healthful lifestyle habits that aid digestion.

Chapter Vocabulary

1. **Content Terms** On a separate sheet of paper, list words that relate to each of the following terms. Then, work with a partner to explain how these words are related.

   absorption
   ATP (adenosine triphosphate)
   bile
   chyme
   constipation
   diarrhea
   digestion
   diverticulosis
   enzyme
   feces
   food allergy
   food intolerance
   gallstones
   gastric juices
   gastrointestinal (GI) tract
   heartburn
   indigestion
   kilocalorie
   macronutrient
   mastication
   metabolism
   micronutrient
   peristalsis
   ulcer
   villi

2. **Academic Terms** Individually or with a partner, create a T-chart on a sheet of paper and list each of the following terms in the left column. In the right column, list an *antonym* (a word of opposite meaning) for each term in the left column.

   disperse
   erratic
   neutralize
   secrete
   sloughed

Review Learning

3. List the six nutrient groups and summarize the three main functions of nutrients in your body.
4. How is the energy value of food measured?
5. What is the difference between mechanical digestion and chemical digestion?
6. Why is saliva important in the digestive process?
7. How does the epiglottis help prevent you from choking on food while eating?
8. What is the function of mucus secreted in the stomach?
9. Describe the function of three digestive enzymes that help break down foods in the small intestine.
10. What is the main job of the large intestine?
11. What are the water-soluble and fat-soluble nutrients and how are they absorbed?
12. How does metabolism provide for the body's energy needs?
13. How can eating food too quickly or when you are stressed affect your digestion and absorption?
14. Describe the body's response when a food to which you are allergic is consumed.
15. Describe two digestive disorders and recommended treatment for each.
16. What is the difference between diverticulosis and diverticulitis?

Self-Assessment Quiz

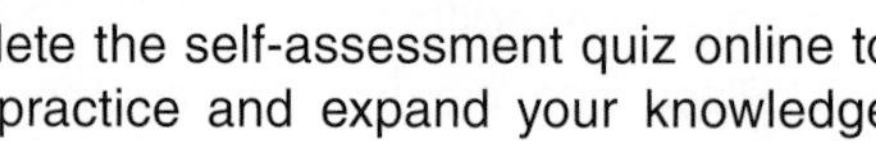

Complete the self-assessment quiz online to help you practice and expand your knowledge and skills.

Critical Thinking

17. **Compare** Compare positive and negative behaviors that impact digestion. For each negative behavior, identify a change for improving digestion.
18. **Conclude** How might long-term use of acid-reducing medicines impact health? Make a list of your conclusions.

19. **Evaluate** Visit the website of a store that sells medications for digestive disorders. List the various disorders and identify the names of drugs available to "treat" each one. Which disorder seems to offer the greatest variety of drug choices? Talk to the pharmacist to learn why so many choices are available. Report your findings in class.
20. **Analyze** Find a nutrition-related article using a reliable online newspaper service. Print out the article. Highlight three important facts you learned about how your body uses nutrients.
21. **Evaluate** Evaluate the credibility of an Internet site reporting on causes, prevention, and treatment of a particular digestive disease. Write a summary of your findings.
22. **Identify** Take an online tour of the human body and its systems. Create a list of the systems in the human body. Investigate how the various body systems relate to each other. Organize your findings in a chart and note an interesting fact that you learned about each system. Present your facts in class.

Core Skills

23. **Technology Literacy** Prepare a digital collage illustrating healthful lifestyle choices that can help people avoid problems with digestion and absorption.
24. **Science** Research how a cow's digestive system works. Compare the cow's digestive system to the human digestive system. How are they different? similar?
25. **Speaking** Human digestion has been studied throughout history, and understanding about digestion and digestive organs has evolved. Select a time period and learn about the accepted beliefs, myths, and traditions of that time regarding human digestion. Use presentation software to present your findings in a manner and style appropriate to your audience.
26. **Technology Literacy** Research the digestion and absorption process for alcohol. Prepare an electronic presentation on how alcohol is digested, absorbed, and metabolized in the body. Include in your report the effects of alcohol on the liver, kidneys, and other organs.
27. **Math** If a food supplies 260 calories from carbohydrate, 45 calories from fat, and 24 calories from protein, how many grams of carbohydrates, fat, and protein does this food contain?
28. **Listening** Peanut allergies are one of the most common types of food allergies for children. Interview a teacher of young children or the school foodservice manager to learn what the school does to promote a safe, allergen-free environment. What process is used by the school to learn if students have food allergies or intolerances? Share findings with the class.
29. **Speech** In small groups, debate the topic "You are what you eat." Identify factors that support the expression referring to the facts of digestion. Identify factors that may interfere with the process of digestion.
30. **Writing** Research and write a paper on the changes that occur in the digestive system as people age. Compare the GI tract characteristics of a young person with that of a person in his or her later years. Gather information from a variety of authoritative print and digital sources. Integrate information into your paper selectively to communicate your ideas effectively. Provide citations for your sources.
31. **Science** Create a diagram of the digestive system. On your diagram, identify where each nutrient found in a BLT sandwich (bacon, lettuce, tomato, mayonnaise, whole-wheat bread) would be absorbed.
32. **Math** Robert consumes a snack that contains 46 grams of carbohydrates, 9 grams of fat, and 2 grams of protein. Calculate how many calories are in Robert's snack.
33. **Career Readiness Practice** Presume you are the human resources director for a small manufacturing company. Recent research shows that employees who have good eating habits and total wellness have a positive impact on productivity. You are forming a workplace "Wellness Council." Meet with your council members (two or more classmates) and brainstorm a list of possible ideas for encouraging healthful eating and wellness behaviors among employees. Then narrow the list down to the three best options. List the steps you would take to implement one of these options.

Nutrition Guidelines

Learning Outcomes

After studying this chapter, you will be able to

- **differentiate** among the six types of Dietary Reference Intakes (DRIs);
- **summarize** the eating pattern advice offered in the *Dietary Guidelines for Americans 2015–2020;*
- **apply** the MyPlate food guidance system to make healthy eating choices;
- **identify** the equivalent amounts commonly used to estimate portion size in each of the five food groups;
- **use** information on food labels to make healthful food choices; and
- **identify** how to analyze and improve your eating patterns by using a variety of dietary planning tools.

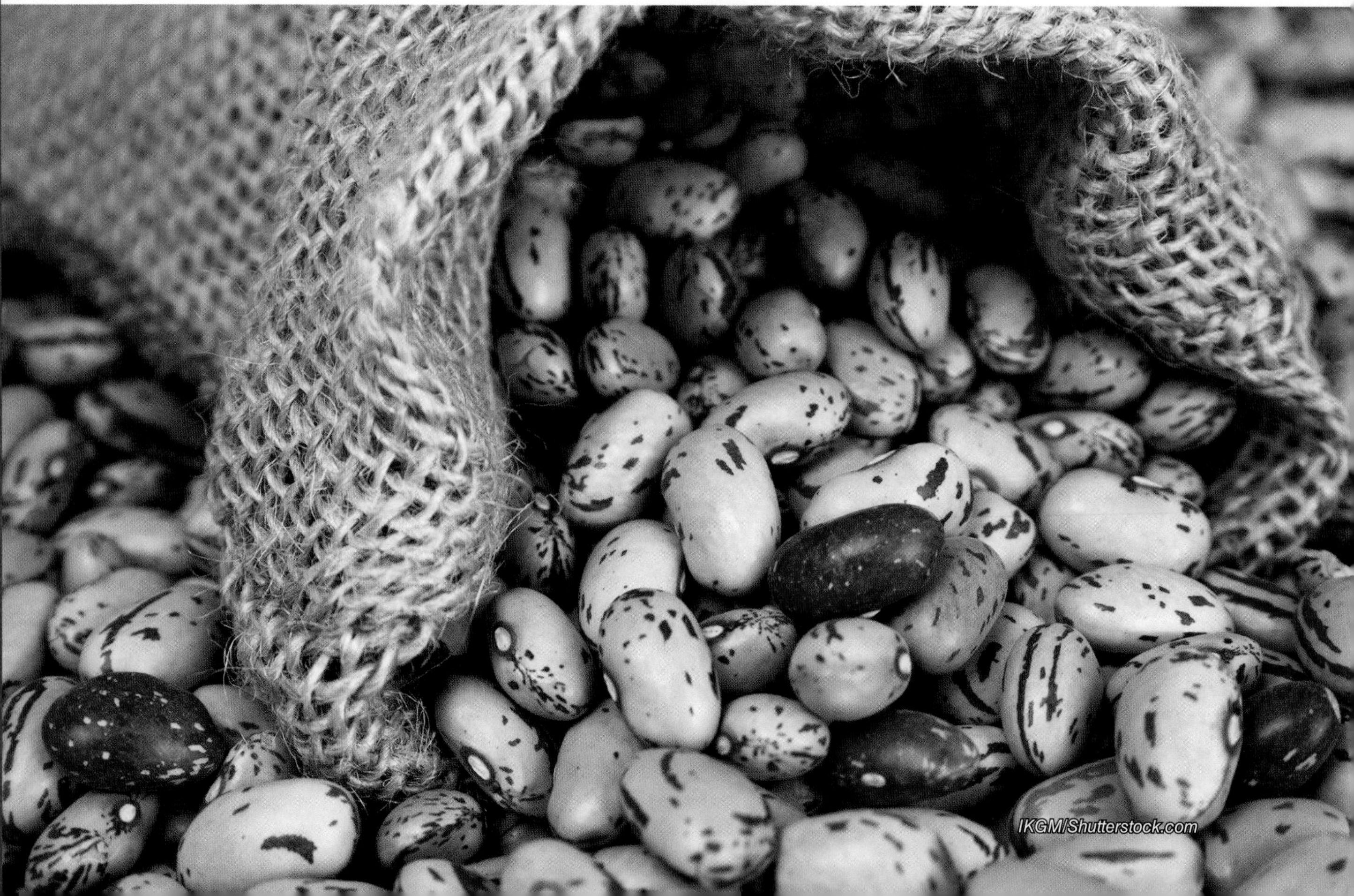

IKGM/Shutterstock.com

Content Terms

Acceptable Macronutrient Distribution Ranges (AMDR)
Adequate Intake (AI)
Daily Values (DV)
Dietary Guidelines for Americans
Dietary Reference Intakes (DRI)
Estimated Average Requirement (EAR)
Estimated Energy Requirement (EER)
food journal
MyPlate
nutrient dense
Physical Activity Guidelines for Americans
Recommended Dietary Allowance (RDA)
Tolerable Upper Intake Level (UL)

Academic Terms

adept
amended
comprise
undermine

What's Your Nutrition and Wellness IQ?

Take this quiz to examine how much you already know about nutrition guidelines. If you cannot answer a question, pay extra attention to that topic as you study this chapter.

- Identify each statement as *True*, *False*, or *It Depends*. *It Depends* means in some cases the statement is true; in some cases it could be false.
- Revise false statements to make them true.
- Explain the circumstances in which each *It Depends* statement is true and when it is false.

Nutrition and Wellness IQ

	Statement			
1.	The Recommended Dietary Allowance (RDA) and Dietary Reference Intakes (DRIs) are tools used for planning and evaluating diets for healthy individuals.	True	False	It Depends
2.	The *Dietary Guidelines for Americans* advises individuals what to eat every day.	True	False	It Depends
3.	MyPlate Daily Checklist creates a healthy eating plan based on age, sex, height, and weight.	True	False	It Depends
4.	Portion size and serving size are always consistent amounts.	True	False	It Depends
5.	If a nutrition label indicates the product provides 20% of your Daily Value for fiber, then you have met your fiber needs for the day.	True	False	It Depends
6.	If the first ingredient listed on a food product is sucrose (sugar), then this ingredient is the largest by volume.	True	False	It Depends
7.	Keeping a food journal means you are eating the proper foods for healthy growth.	True	False	It Depends

While studying this chapter, look for the activity icon to

- **build** vocabulary with e-flash cards and interactive games;
- **assess** what you learn by completing self-assessment quizzes and completing review questions; and
- **expand** knowledge with interactive activities and activities that extend learning.

www.g-wlearning.com/foodsandnutrition/

Many resources are designed to promote wellness across the life span. This chapter introduces some common references and guidelines available to health professionals and consumers. You will read about guidelines for making health-promoting dietary plans. You will then evaluate your eating pattern and practice applying the guidelines to your food choices.

Tools for Planning Healthy Eating

Health experts are challenged to inform people about how to meet their nutritional needs. Many boards, councils, and committees work to develop tools to aid consumers in selecting a healthy diet. These tools continue to be revised as new information is discovered. Some of these tools are intended for use by public policy makers or by health professionals as they work with clients. Other tools discussed in this chapter are intended for use by consumers to aid them in planning for healthy eating.

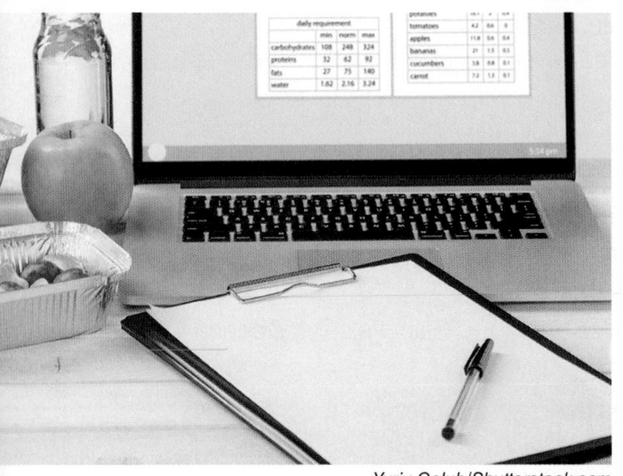

Yuriy Golub/Shutterstock.com

Figure 5.1 Dietitians and nutrition educators use the Dietary Reference Intakes for dietary planning and assessment.

Dietary Reference Intakes

In the 1990s, the Food and Nutrition Board of the National Academy of Sciences and Health Canada began to develop new dietary standards for Americans and Canadians. In 2005, the final set of Dietary Reference Intakes (DRIs) was released. The ***Dietary Reference Intakes (DRI)*** are reference values for nutrients and food components that can be used to plan and assess diets for healthy people (**Figure 5.1**). The purpose of the DRIs is to promote health, and to prevent chronic disease and the effects of excessive or deficient nutrient intakes.

Types of DRI

The DRIs include six types of nutrient reference standards—Estimated Average Requirement (EAR), Recommended Dietary Allowance (RDA), Adequate Intake (AI), Tolerable Upper Intake Level (UL), Estimated Energy Requirement (EER), and Acceptable Macronutrient Distribution Ranges (AMDR).

The ***Estimated Average Requirement (EAR)*** is a nutrient recommendation estimated to meet the needs of 50 percent of the people in a defined group. If a group of people consumes a nutrient at this level, half of them would be deficient. This standard is based on scientific evidence and is used for calculating the Recommended Dietary Allowance.

The ***Recommended Dietary Allowance (RDA)*** is the average daily intake of a nutrient required to meet the needs of most (97 to 98 percent) healthy individuals. RDAs are based on EARs. The RDA can be used as a goal for typical daily intake for individuals in a particular life stage and sex group.

Adequate Intake (AI) is a reference value that is used when there is insufficient scientific evidence to determine an EAR for a nutrient. Since an EAR cannot be established, an RDA cannot be determined either. Instead, the intake recommendation is based on estimates and observations of people who appear to be healthy and well nourished. As more research becomes available, AIs for some nutrients may be replaced by EARs and RDAs. AIs are used for all nutrients for infants.

The ***Tolerable Upper Intake Level (UL)*** is the maximum level of ongoing daily intake for a nutrient that is unlikely to cause harm to most people in a defined group. Daily intake of a nutrient above its UL could be harmful. ULs are not recommended levels of intake. Not enough information is available to set ULs for all nutrients.

When evaluating the macronutrients in a diet, two additional DRIs are used: Estimated Energy Requirement (EER) and Acceptable Macronutrient Distribution Ranges (AMDR). ***Estimated Energy Requirement (EER)*** is an estimate of the calories a healthy person needs based on height, weight, age, sex, and physical activity level.

The ***Acceptable Macronutrient Distribution Ranges (AMDR)*** are ranges of recommended dietary intake for a particular macronutrient energy source that are intended to help people achieve a balanced, healthy diet. Macronutrients are the energy nutrients, and they include carbohydrates, fats, and proteins. The AMDR is associated with reduced risk of chronic disease. Consuming amounts of certain macronutrients outside of the recommended ranges increases the risk of chronic disease.

Intended Use

DRIs are primarily intended for use by health professionals, policy makers, and scientists. These standards are used for planning and evaluating the diets of groups of people. For example, DRI values are used by scientists and nutritionists who work in research areas, such as sports medicine, or academic settings. Scientists analyze diets to determine the levels of nutrients being supplied. If the diet is not supplying enough of a nutrient, a disease state can result. Too much of some nutrients may be toxic.

FEATURED CAREER

Dietetic Technician

Dietetic technicians assist dietitians in evaluating, organizing, and conducting nutrition services and programs for schools, hospitals, and industry. Under the supervision of dietitians, dietetic technicians gather and evaluate diet histories, assist in planning patient meals, conduct foodservice operations, and maintain records.

Education

Students wanting to become dietetic technicians should graduate from high school with a well-rounded program. High school business courses may prove helpful. Dietetic technicians must complete a two-year associate's degree program that is accepted by the Academy of Nutrition and Dietetics. They must then meet other state requirements.

Job Outlook

Employment opportunities for dietetic technicians are expected to grow faster than average. This is largely due to the emphasis that the medical community is placing on disease prevention through improved dietary habits. The aging population will also increase demand for dietetic technicians because they will need balanced meals and nutritional counseling.

DRIs can be used by nutritionists to develop menus that meet nutritional requirements for specific groups, such as the elderly, a prison population, or the military (**Figure 5.2**). DRIs also serve as a foundation for other nutrition-related guidance for Americans.

Dietary Guidelines for Americans

The *Dietary Guidelines for Americans* is published by the United States Departments of Health and Human Services and Agriculture. The ***Dietary Guidelines for Americans*** provides information and advice that promotes health through improved nutrition and physical activity. Revised every five years, the *Guidelines*

- reflects current science on diet and health;
- provides guidance for healthy food and beverage choices for individuals two years of age and older;
- aids policy makers in designing and implementing nutrition-related initiatives;
- provides direction for relevant organizations and industries; and
- functions as the basis for nutrition education programs, federal nutrition assistance programs such as school meals and Meals on Wheels, and dietary advice provided by health professionals.

Poor dietary patterns, physical inactivity, and overweight and obesity continue to be issues that **undermine** (weaken) the health of Americans. These issues increase an individual's risk for a variety of chronic diseases. The *2015–2020 Dietary Guidelines* focuses on overall eating and physical activity patterns, as well as their relationship to health and risk of disease.

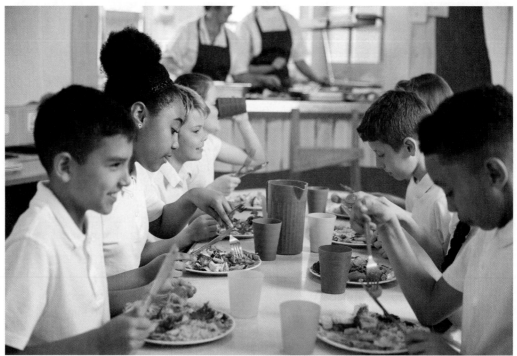

Monkey Business Images/Shutterstock.com

Figure 5.2
Dietary reference standards are used by government agencies that design, operate, and evaluate food and nutrition assistance programs such as the school lunch program.

EXTEND YOUR KNOWLEDGE

Nutrition Evidence Library (NEL)

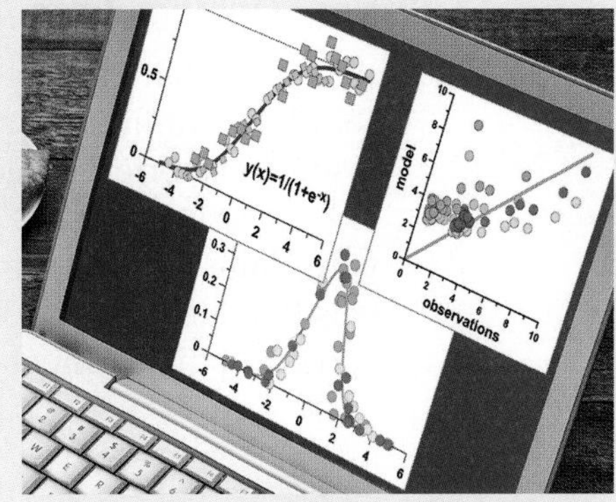

marekuliasz/Shutterstock.com

The first step in revising the *Dietary Guidelines* involves a committee reviewing and analyzing current scientific information on diet and health. The committee prepares a report summarizing its findings, which serves as a major resource for creating the *Guidelines*. The committee used the USDA's Nutrition Evidence Library (NEL) for its work on the *2015–2020 Dietary Guidelines*. The NEL is a government resource that evaluates, synthesizes, and grades food and nutrition-related research.

To facilitate its review of the scientific information, the committee submitted specific questions to the NEL. The NEL then found studies related to the question. The evidence from all the relevant studies was integrated. From this collection, a conclusion statement was formed and graded.

Locate the Nutrition Evidence Library online and learn what questions the committee submitted for its work on the *2015–2020 Dietary Guidelines*. Select a question of particular interest to you. Find the summary of evidence for that question, the conclusion statement, and how it was graded.

The goal of the *Guidelines* is for Americans to meet the nutrient levels established in the DRIs by consuming a variety of foods. Five basic themes summarize the message of the *2015–2020 Dietary Guidelines*:

- Follow a healthy eating pattern across the life span.
- Focus on variety, nutrient density, and amount.
- Limit calories from added sugars and saturated fats and reduce sodium intake.
- Shift to healthier food and beverage choices.
- Support healthy eating patterns for all.

Follow a Healthy Eating Pattern Across the Life Span

All foods you eat are important. Balance the amount and types of food you eat with physical activity to maintain a healthy body weight, support your nutrient needs, and reduce your risks for chronic diseases. Preventing unhealthy weight gain as a young person is often easier to accomplish than trying to lose excess weight later in life.

Focus on Variety, Nutrient Density, and Amount

Choose nutrient-dense foods more often. ***Nutrient-dense*** foods and beverages provide vitamins, minerals, and other substances that contribute to adequate nutrition or may have positive health effects. Nutrient-dense foods contain little or no solid fats, added sugars, refined starches, and sodium. These foods are proportionately higher in nutrient content relative to the number of calories per serving. In addition, it is important to vary the nutrient-dense foods you choose. Be sure to include foods from each of the food groups and in the recommended amounts.

People sometimes use terms such as *health food* or *junk food* to describe a food's quality. As you begin to analyze foods, you will find there is no such thing as a perfect food. Likewise, few foods supply absolutely no nutrients. Therefore, *health food* and *junk food* are less useful than the terms *high nutrient density* and *low nutrient density*.

Limit Calories from Added Sugars and Saturated Fats and Reduce Sodium

Foods that are high in solid fats and/or added sugars, also referred to as *SoFAS*, should be limited or avoided. An eating pattern that includes excess SoFAS may result in calorie imbalance, weight gain, and other negative health consequences. The *Dietary Guidelines for Americans* recommends that no more than 10 percent of your daily calories come from added sugars. Salty snacks and processed food products that are high in sodium **comprise** (make up) a significant portion of many teen and adult diets. Choose these foods less often to achieve a healthier eating pattern.

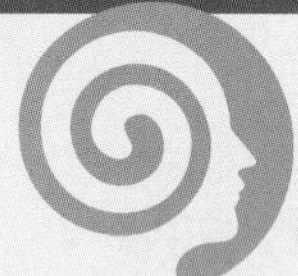

EXTEND YOUR KNOWLEDGE

Choose Nutrient-Dense Foods

Individuals must consume a limited number of calories if they want to avoid unhealthy weight gain. Therefore, you should choose foods that supply the nutrients you need for health, but which contain few additional calories from unnecessary solid fats and added sugars. In other words—choose nutrient-dense foods and beverages.

Unfortunately, many Americans choose foods that are not nutrient dense. You do not have to give up your favorite foods, just choose the more nutrient-dense form of your favorite food. Which food would you choose?

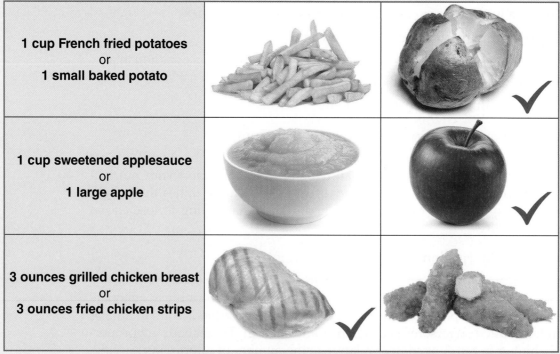

1 cup French fried potatoes or **1 small baked potato**		✓
1 cup sweetened applesauce or **1 large apple**		✓
3 ounces grilled chicken breast or **3 ounces fried chicken strips**	✓	

Top row: nito/Shutterstock.com; Joe Gough/Shutterstock.com; Middle row: Moving Moment/Shutterstock.com; Tim UR/Shutterstock.com; Bottom row: amenic181/Shutterstock.com; koss13/Shutterstock.com; Check mark: Fine Art/Shutterstock.com

Shift to Healthier Food and Beverage Choices

Most Americans exceed the recommendations for consumption of added sugars, saturated fats, and sodium. Adopting a healthier eating pattern is easier when small, incremental changes are made over a period of time. Consider each food and beverage choice an opportunity to improve your eating pattern.

Support Healthy Eating Patterns for All

Shifting to healthy eating behaviors requires the support of home, school, work, communities, healthcare providers, and everyone who cares about the health of the nation. By implementing changes to improve eating behaviors in all of these settings, efforts are more effective.

Physical activity is important not only for calorie balance, but also for prevention of many chronic diseases. The *2015–2020 Dietary Guidelines* addresses the importance of physical activity in health and encourages Americans to meet the *Physical Activity Guidelines for Americans*. The ***Physical Activity Guidelines for Americans*** is a set of recommendations that specify amounts and types of exercise that individuals at different life-cycle stages need each day. Just as healthy eating patterns must be supported at home, school, work, and across the community, so too must physical activity.

MyPlate

The United States Department of Agriculture (USDA) offers a food guidance system called ***MyPlate*** that is based on the *Dietary Guidelines for Americans*. The website ChooseMyPlate.gov offers tools and resources that help individuals make changes to their eating habits that are consistent with the *Dietary Guidelines*. The MyPlate icon is a simple, visual message to help Americans build a healthy plate at mealtime.

MyPlate divides foods into five main food groups—fruits, grains, vegetables, protein foods, and dairy. Foods from each of these categories are required for a healthy eating pattern. The plate is split into four sections to represent fruits, grains, vegetables, and protein. The sections differ in size based on the recommended portion of your meal each food should be. The circle next to the plate represents the dairy group. The MyPlate image communicates the message that half of your meal plate should be fruits and vegetables. Oils are not a food group and are not included on the MyPlate image (**Figure 5.3**).

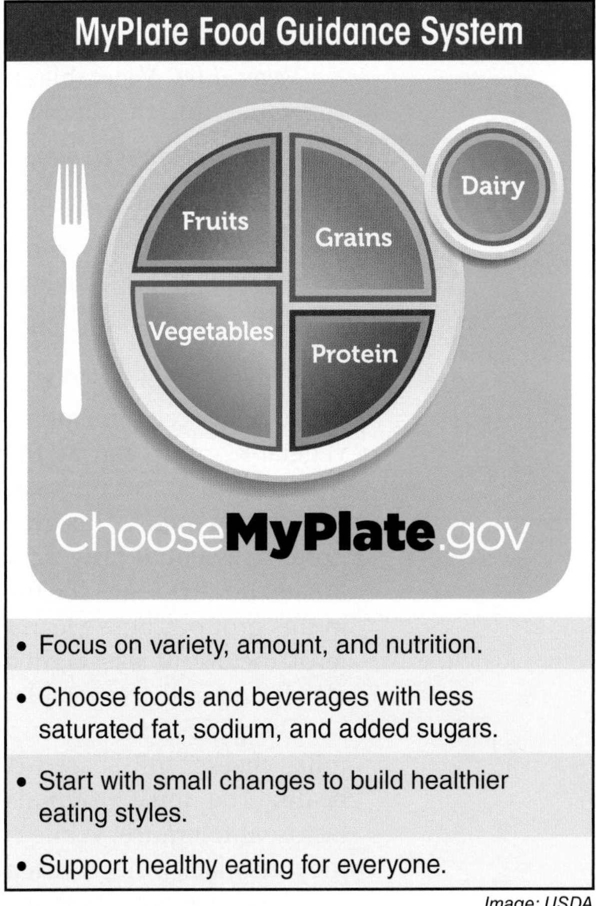

Image: USDA

Figure 5.3 The MyPlate food guidance system was created to help consumers implement the recommendations from the *Dietary Guidelines*.

MyPlate Food Groups

The MyPlate food guidance system emphasizes eating a variety of foods from each of the food groups. It helps you identify which foods are in each group, what amounts you should eat, and how to make a healthy selection.

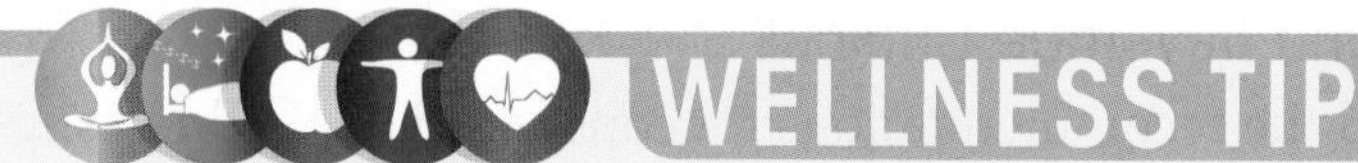

Healthy Eating for Life

The *Dietary Guidelines for Americans* helps people examine eating behaviors with a lifestyle perspective. One day's meals are not nearly as important as the total picture. Work toward improving your eating patterns over the long haul to build a healthful lifestyle.

Fruits. This group is rich in nutrients and fiber. Examples of fruits include bananas, oranges, peaches, blueberries, and kiwifruit. Fruits may be fresh, frozen, puréed, canned, or dried. Select whole fruit more often than fruit juice. Whole fruit contains fiber and is more nutrient dense than juice.

Grains. The grains group includes foods made from wheat, rice, oats, cornmeal, barley, and other grains. Grains can be either whole or refined. Whole grains include the entire grain kernel, whereas refined grains are milled to remove the bran and germ.

Guidelines from MyPlate recommend that half of the grains you eat should be whole grains. Examples of whole grains include whole-wheat flour, bulgur, oatmeal, brown rice, and whole cornmeal. Refined grains include white bread, white rice, and other white flour products often used in pastas and crackers. Grains are a source of fiber, some B vitamins, and some minerals.

Vegetables. Vegetables provide a variety of nutrients and fiber. MyPlate divides vegetables into the following five subgroups:

- *dark green vegetables*, such as broccoli, spinach, and kale
- *red and orange vegetables*, such as carrots, red peppers, tomatoes, and sweet potatoes
- *beans and peas*, such as kidney beans, soybeans, and lentils
- *starchy vegetables*, such as green peas, corn, and potatoes
- *other vegetables*, such as celery, onions, and zucchini

MyPlate recommends an amount from each group weekly. Foods from the vegetable group can be fresh, frozen, dehydrated, or canned. They may be raw, cooked, whole, cut up, mashed, or juiced.

Protein foods. This group supplies a variety of nutrients to the diet, including protein, essential fatty acids, B vitamins, iron, zinc, magnesium, and vitamin E. Meats, poultry, eggs, beans and peas, nuts and seeds, and seafood are all found in this group. Choose lean meats and poultry to reduce saturated fats and cholesterol. Include at least eight ounces of cooked seafood per week. Beans and peas are also found in the vegetable group.

Dairy. The dairy group includes foods high in protein and calcium, such as milk, cheese, milk-based desserts, and yogurt. These foods help improve bone health. The dairy group also includes calcium-fortified soy milk for people with lactose intolerance. While calcium-fortified foods and beverages provide calcium, they may lack other nutrients supplied by foods in this group.

Oils. Oils are fats that are liquid at room temperature and are obtained from a variety of plants and fish. Oils are not a food group, but some are needed in the diet to provide essential nutrients. For this reason, there is an allowance for oils in your daily food plan. Only small amounts of oils are recommended because they are high in calories and can easily cause an imbalance between calories consumed and daily activity level. Foods that are rich in oils, such as soft margarines, mayonnaise, and salad dressings, are counted in this allowance for oils.

Fats that are solid at room temperature are *not* included in the allowance for oils. Common solid fats include butter, beef fat, chicken fat, pork fat, stick margarine, and shortening. The fat in milk is also considered solid fat because milk fat, or *butterfat*, is solid at room temperature. Solid fats are not essential for good health and are considered empty calories. *Empty calories* such as those from foods high in solid fats and added sugars (SoFAS) provide few or no nutrients. Empty calories should be limited to avoid exceeding your recommended calorie intake.

A Personalized Food Plan

ChooseMyPlate.gov offers a number of interactive tools to help individuals plan and assess their daily food and activity choices. One of these tools is the "MyPlate Daily Checklist," which helps you create a personalized food plan based on your age, sex, height, weight, and activity level. After you enter this data, the plan selects the food intake pattern that is right for you. Many teens require 2,000 calories each day (**Figure 5.4**).

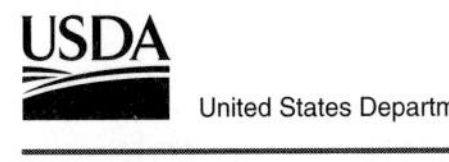

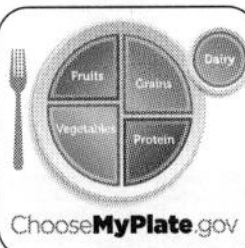

MyPlate Daily Checklist

Find your Healthy Eating Style

Everything you eat and drink matters. Find your healthy eating style that reflect your preferences, culture, traditions, and budget—and maintain it for a lifetime! The right mix can help you be healthier now and into the future. The key is choosing a variety of foods and beverages from each food group—*and making sure that each choice is limited in saturated fat, sodium, and added sugars.* Start with small changes—**"MyWins"**—to make healthier choices you can enjoy.

Food Group Amounts for 2,000 Calories a Day

Fruits	Vegetables	Grains	Protein	Dairy
2 cups	**2 1/2 cups**	**6 ounces**	**5 1/2 ounces**	**3 cups**
Focus on whole fruits	Vary your veggies	Make half your grains whole grains	Vary your protein routine	Move to low-fat or fat-free milk or yogurt
Focus on whole fruits that are fresh, frozen, canned, or dried.	Choose a variety of colorful fresh, frozen, and canned vegetables—make sure to include dark green, red, and orange choices.	Find whole-grain foods by reading the Nutrition Facts label and ingredients list.	Mix up your protein foods to include seafood, beans and peas, unsalted nuts and seeds, soy products, eggs, and lean meats and poultry.	Choose fat-free milk, yogurt, and soy beverages (soy milk) to cut back on your saturated fat.

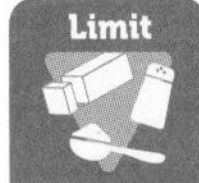

Drink and eat less sodium, saturated fat, and added sugars. Limit:

- Sodium to **2,300 milligrams** a day.
- Saturated fat to **22 grams** a day.
- Added sugars to **50 grams** a day.

Be active your way: Children 6 to 17 years old should move **60 minutes** every day. Adults should be physically active at least **2 1/2 hours** per week.

Use SuperTracker to create a personal plan based on your age, sex, height, weight, and physical activity level.

SuperTracker.usda.gov

USDA

Figure 5.4 Your MyPlate Daily Checklist shows how much you should eat from each food group to stay within your calorie allowance. ***How many ounces of whole grains does this Checklist recommend?***

Additionally, the plan makes recommendations for physical activity to help people balance food intake and to promote healthy weight. Your level of physical activity influences the amount of food you should consume.

MyPlate also has tools for children, women who are pregnant or breast-feeding, and individuals who speak Spanish. You will want to access the other tools on ChooseMyPlate.gov as you read this textbook.

Measuring Food Amounts

You must know how to measure the various amounts of foods your MyPlate Daily Checklist recommends. Because people often have very different ideas about the size of a serving, MyPlate uses volume and weight measures to describe the amounts of food you should eat. MyPlate lists amounts of foods using measures such as cups, teaspoons, tablespoons, ounces, or their equivalents. For example, 32 seedless grapes are equivalent to one cup of fruit, or one cup-equivalent.

The amount of food that is served at restaurants or that you serve yourself at home may be larger than the amounts suggested on your MyPlate Daily Checklist. Frequently eating more calories than you need to balance your activity level can cause you to gain weight. Therefore, it is important to be aware of the amounts your Daily Checklist recommends, and then read the labels on food products to learn how many cup- or ounce-equivalents the package contains.

The serving sizes used on food labels are the amounts that people typically consume, not *recommended* amounts. Therefore, you need to determine how the serving size on the label fits into your Daily Checklist. **Figure 5.5** lists some common foods from each of the food groups and describes how to measure amounts of each. (ChooseMyPlate.gov provides more extensive lists of food amounts.)

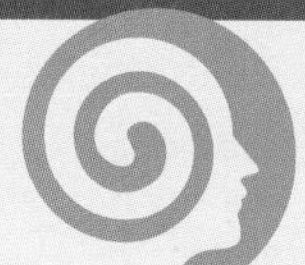

EXTEND YOUR KNOWLEDGE

Mediterranean-Style Eating Pattern

The Healthy Mediterranean-Style Eating Pattern is similar to the US (*MyPlate*) Healthy Eating Pattern. Both of these eating patterns are recommended in the *Dietary Guidelines*. How do these eating patterns compare?

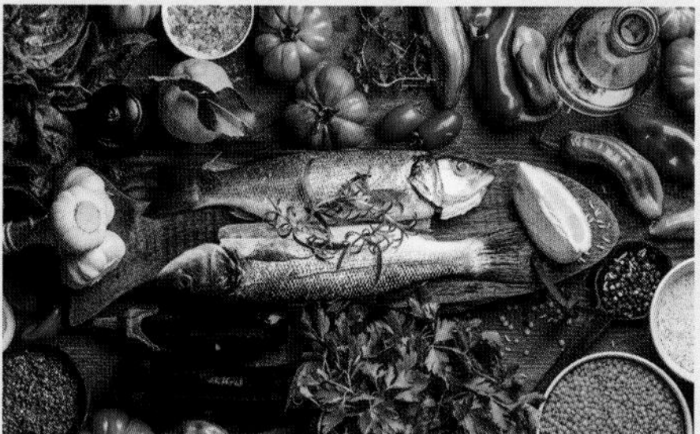

Foxys Forest Manufacture/Shutterstock.com

The Mediterranean-style eating pattern is based on typical foods, beverages, and recipes of Mediterranean-style cooking. It includes more fruits and seafood, and less dairy than the US Healthy Eating Pattern. It focuses on fresh, unprocessed foods, whole grains, and plant-based foods. Butter is often replaced with olive or canola oil. Herbs and spices are used instead of salt.

For someone who consumes 2,000 calories per day, a Mediterranean-style eating pattern includes

- 2½ cup-equivalents of vegetables;
- 2½ cup-equivalents of fruit;
- 6 ounce-equivalents of grains;
- 2 cup-equivalents of dairy; and
- 6½ ounce-equivalents of protein foods, including fatty fish, beans, nuts, seeds, poultry, and eggs in moderation, and little red meat.

Socializing at mealtime and engaging in physical activity are a large part of the Mediterranean culture. Evidence has been gathered over time that this diet pattern has the health benefit of heart disease prevention.

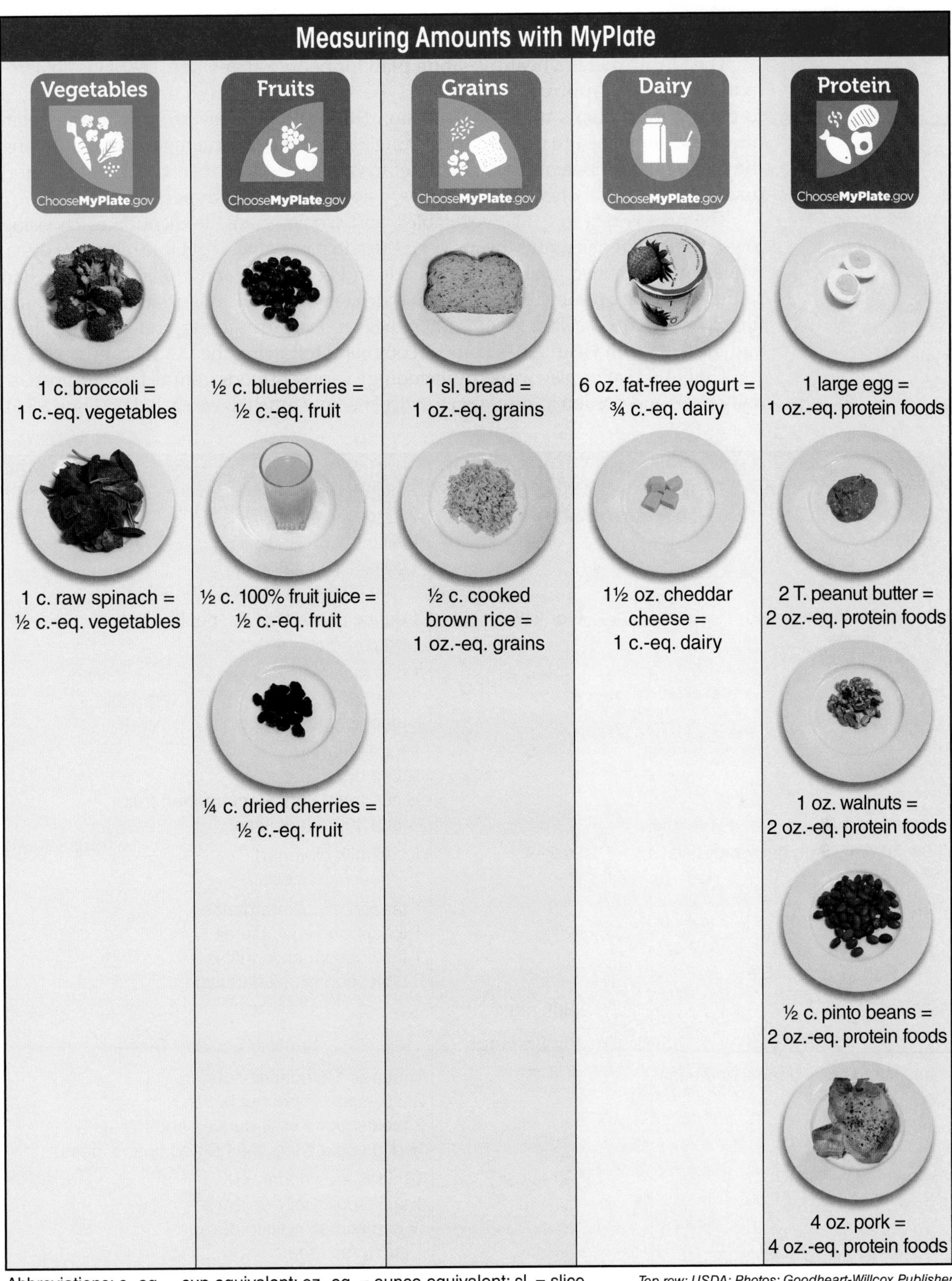

Measuring Amounts with MyPlate
Vegetables
ChooseMyPlate.gov
Fruits
ChooseMyPlate.gov
Grains
ChooseMyPlate.gov
Dairy
ChooseMyPlate.gov
Protein
ChooseMyPlate.gov
1 c. broccoli = 1 c.-eq. vegetables
1 c. raw spinach = ½ c.-eq. vegetables
½ c. blueberries = ½ c.-eq. fruit
½ c. 100% fruit juice = ½ c.-eq. fruit
¼ c. dried cherries = ½ c.-eq. fruit
1 sl. bread = 1 oz.-eq. grains
½ c. cooked brown rice = 1 oz.-eq. grains
6 oz. fat-free yogurt = ¾ c.-eq. dairy
1½ oz. cheddar cheese = 1 c.-eq. dairy
1 large egg = 1 oz.-eq. protein foods
2 T. peanut butter = 2 oz.-eq. protein foods
1 oz. walnuts = 2 oz.-eq. protein foods
½ c. pinto beans = 2 oz.-eq. protein foods
4 oz. pork = 4 oz.-eq. protein foods

Abbreviations: c.-eq. = cup equivalent; oz.-eq. = ounce equivalent; sl. = slice

Top row: USDA; Photos: Goodheart-Willcox Publisher

Figure 5.5 Amounts of foods within the same food group that count as an ounce- or cup-equivalent can differ significantly because some foods are more concentrated sources of nutrients and other foods contain more air or water. *Can you identify two foods from the same food group that require different amounts to equal a ½ cup-equivalent?*

DASH Diet

The DASH diet is a healthy eating plan for people at any age. DASH is an acronym for **D**ietary **A**pproaches to **S**top **H**ypertension. Although originally intended to benefit individuals with hypertension (high blood pressure), this eating plan offers additional health benefits, including healthy weight management. Following the recommendations of the DASH diet may reduce risk for certain cancers, heart disease, stroke, diabetes, kidney stones, osteoporosis, and hypertension.

The plan is rich in fruits, vegetables, and whole grains. It encourages choosing low-fat or nonfat dairy, nuts, beans, seeds, poultry, fish, and vegetable oils more often, while limiting refined grains, sugary foods and beverages, and foods that are high in saturated fat. As a result, this eating plan is rich in potassium, magnesium, calcium, and fiber. The *Dietary Guidelines for Americans*; the National Heart, Lung, and Blood Institute; and the American Heart Association recommend following the DASH eating plan.

The DASH eating plan works by including a variety of foods from all food groups. Use daily totals and portion information to calculate how much to eat each day (**Figure 5.6**).

DASH Eating Plan Goals*

Food Group	Daily Servings	Sample Serving Sizes
Grains	6–8	1 slice bread 1 ounce dry cereal ½ cup cooked rice, pasta, or cereal
Meats, poultry, and fish	6 or fewer	1 ounce cooked meats, poultry, or fish 1 egg
Vegetables	4–5	1 cup raw leafy vegetable ½ cup cut-up raw or cooked vegetable ½ cup vegetable juice
Fruit	4–5	1 medium fruit ¼ cup dried fruit ½ cup fresh, frozen, or canned fruit ½ cup 100% fruit juice
Low-fat or fat-free dairy products	2–3	1 cup milk or yogurt 1½ ounces cheese
Fats and oils	2–3	1 teaspoon soft margarine 1 teaspoon vegetable oil 1 tablespoon mayonnaise 2 tablespoons salad dressing
Sodium	2,300 mg**	
Food Group	**Weekly Servings**	**Sample Serving Sizes**
Nuts, seeds, dry beans, and peas	4–5	¼ cup or 1½ ounces nuts 2 tablespoons peanut butter 2 tablespoons or ½ ounce seeds ½ cup cooked legumes (dried beans, peas)
Sweets	5 or fewer	1 tablespoon sugar 1 tablespoon jelly or jam ½ cup sorbet, gelatin dessert 1 cup lemonade

*Based on a 2,000-calorie diet

Source: National Heart, Lung, and Blood Institute

**1,500 milligrams (mg) sodium lowers blood pressure even further than 2,300 mg sodium daily.

Figure 5.6 The DASH Diet has been called a "diet for all diseases" because it emphasizes food choices that provide many health benefits.

FOOD AND THE ENVIRONMENT

What Is Your Dietary "Food Print"?

A dietary "food print" is the impact of per-person food choices on agricultural land use. Environmentalists believe there is a need to think about how food choices affect land use and how many people can be fed per acre. Meeting food needs for an entire population depends on not only effective agricultural yield and production, but also people's choice of foods to consume. Agricultural scientists want to know which dietary patterns can feed the most people with the land available. This is called *carrying capacity*. The way land is used has important ecological consequences!

As you might expect, *omnivores*, or people who eat both meats and plant-based foods, require about eight times more land use than people who eat only plant-based foods and dairy. A vegetarian dietary pattern can feed the most people from the cultivatable land that is available. The conclusion remains that as meat consumption is reduced, the amount of land needed for crops to feed livestock is also reduced.

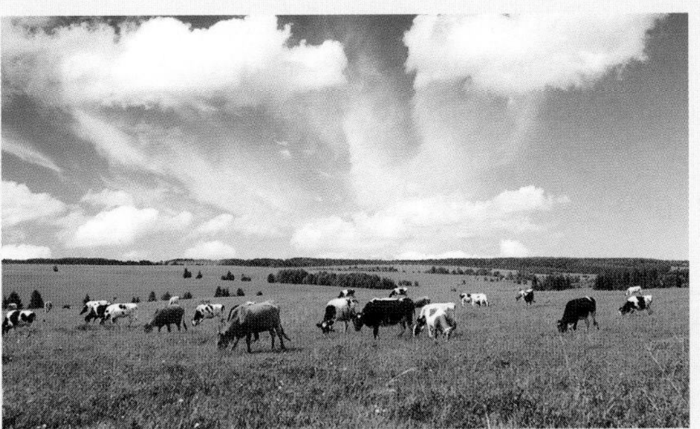

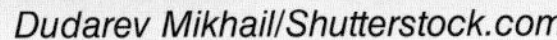

Dudarev Mikhail/Shutterstock.com

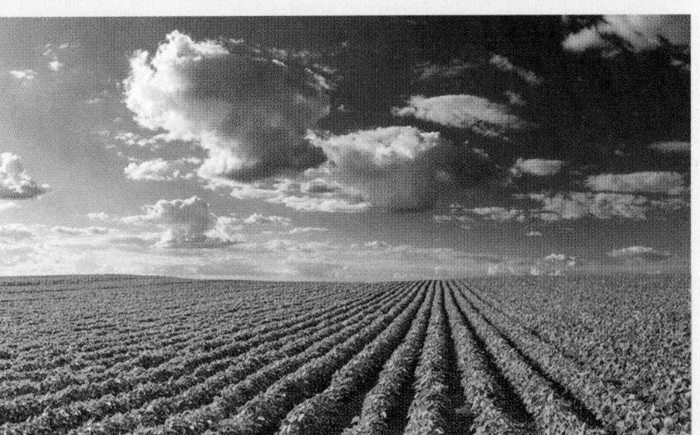

Rasica/Shutterstock.com

Think Critically

1. Should our personal food preferences be viewed as more important than the "food prints" we may leave behind?
2. How important is the need to have equitable distribution of food to all people?
3. What is the relationship between choice of food intake and other environmental concerns, such as water and air quality?

Food Lists

Another tool that can be used to plan a healthy meal or follow a special diet is the *Choose Your Foods: Food Lists system*. The Food Lists system (previously called the *Exchange Lists for Meal Planning*) classifies foods of similar nutrient and caloric content into groups.

The Food Lists were developed by the American Dietetic Association (now the Academy of Nutrition and Dietetics) and the American Diabetes Association. The lists can be used to balance the amounts of carbohydrate, protein, fat, and calories eaten each day. The system was originally used to help individuals with diabetes manage their food plans and stabilize their blood sugar. The Food Lists can also be used successfully for weight management.

To successfully use the Food Lists, you must first know what your particular dietary requirements are, as well as the number of calories you need each day. A doctor or dietitian will often explain how many choices from each list are needed to meet daily requirements.

With practice, this system can be used to plan a meal pattern that fits your individual dietary needs. Once you are familiar with the Food Lists, managing and balancing food intake become simple to master. See the *Food Lists Appendix E*.

Food Labels

Reading food labels can help you plan and manage your daily food choices. Food labels display a range of information from nutrient content to the manufacturer's address.

Nutrition Labeling

The 1990 Nutrition Labeling and Education Act (NLEA) requires most foods to include nutrition labeling. This regulation resulted in development of the Nutrition Facts label for use on food packaging. In 2016, the regulation was **amended** (revised) and the label was updated to reflect new scientific information. Changes also made the label easier for consumers to read (**Figure 5.7**).

In June 2017, the FDA extended the compliance date for the Nutrition Facts label to a future date; however, some manufacturers chose to proceed on their original schedule with implementation of the new label.

The information listed on a food's Nutrition Facts label can help you understand how the food will contribute to your daily eating pattern. Serving size and calories are the two most important elements in making healthier food choices.

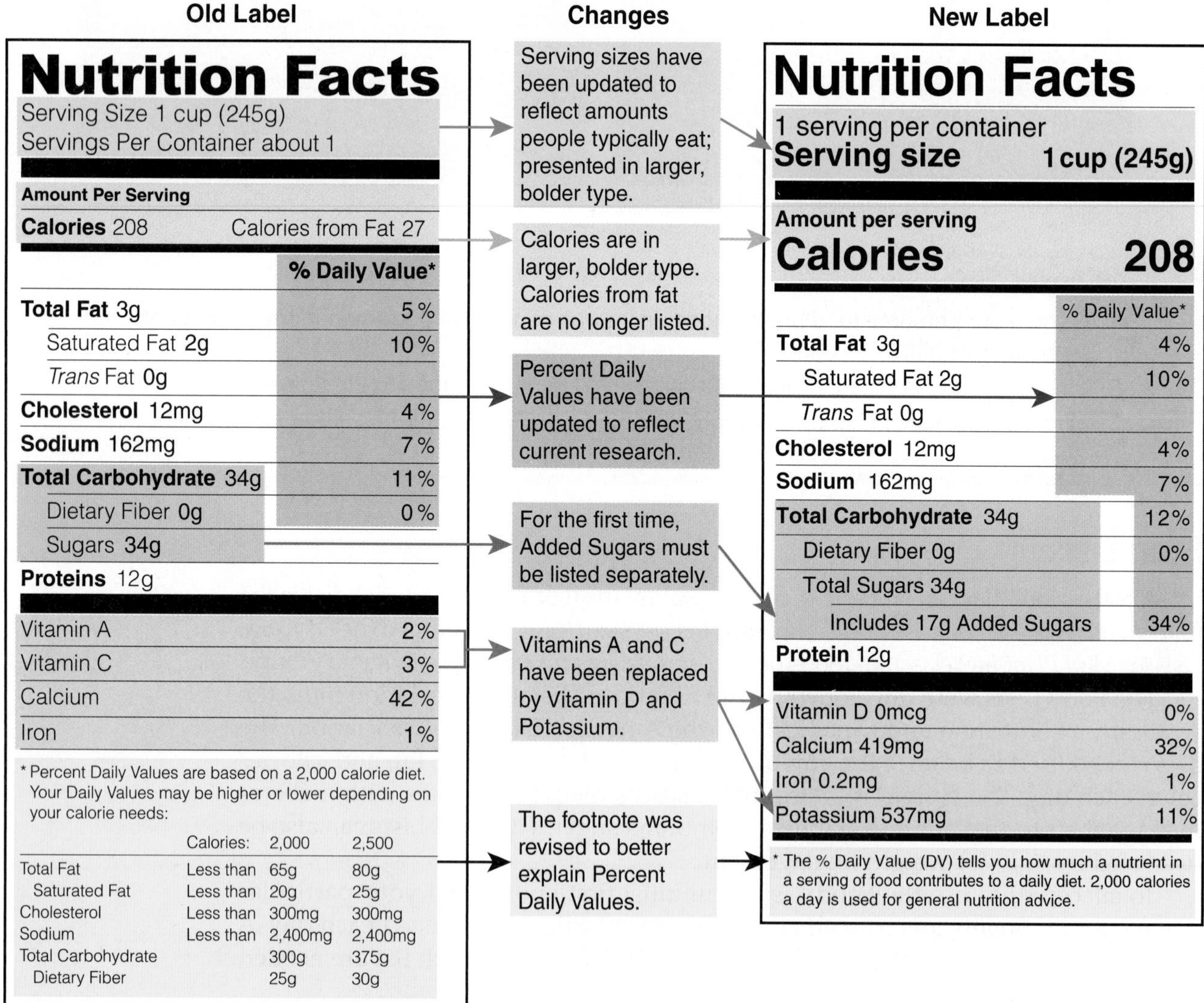

Figure 5.7 The Nutrition Facts label was revised to reflect current scientific research. There will be a period of transition during which you may see both labels in use.

With this information from the Nutrition Facts label, you can quickly compare two similar products and choose the healthier one for you. The label can also help you meet special dietary needs. For instance, information on the label can help you select foods that are lower in sodium or higher in fiber.

In addition to serving size and calories, the new label lists amounts of fats (saturated and *trans*), cholesterol, sodium, carbohydrate, fiber, sugars, added sugars, protein, vitamin D, calcium, iron, and potassium. Some of these nutrients should be limited in the diet, while others should be consumed in sufficient quantities (**Figure 5.8**).

Percent Daily Value

The Percent Daily Values (%DV) shown on the Nutrition Facts label are useful for evaluating food choices. ***Daily Values (DV)*** are recommended nutrient intakes developed to represent the needs of a typical individual. The Daily Values are based on individuals who require 2,000 calories to meet their daily energy needs. If you need more or fewer than 2,000 calories daily, you will need to adjust your Daily Values accordingly.

The Percent Daily Value is the portion of the daily requirement for a nutrient that is provided by one serving of the food. For example, if a cereal label states that it supplies five percent Daily Value for added sugars, this means one serving of the cereal supplies five percent of the added sugar that a person on a 2,000-calorie diet is allowed for one day. For a person who requires 1,800 calories per day to meet her energy needs, however, this cereal would supply a greater Percent Daily Value for added sugar.

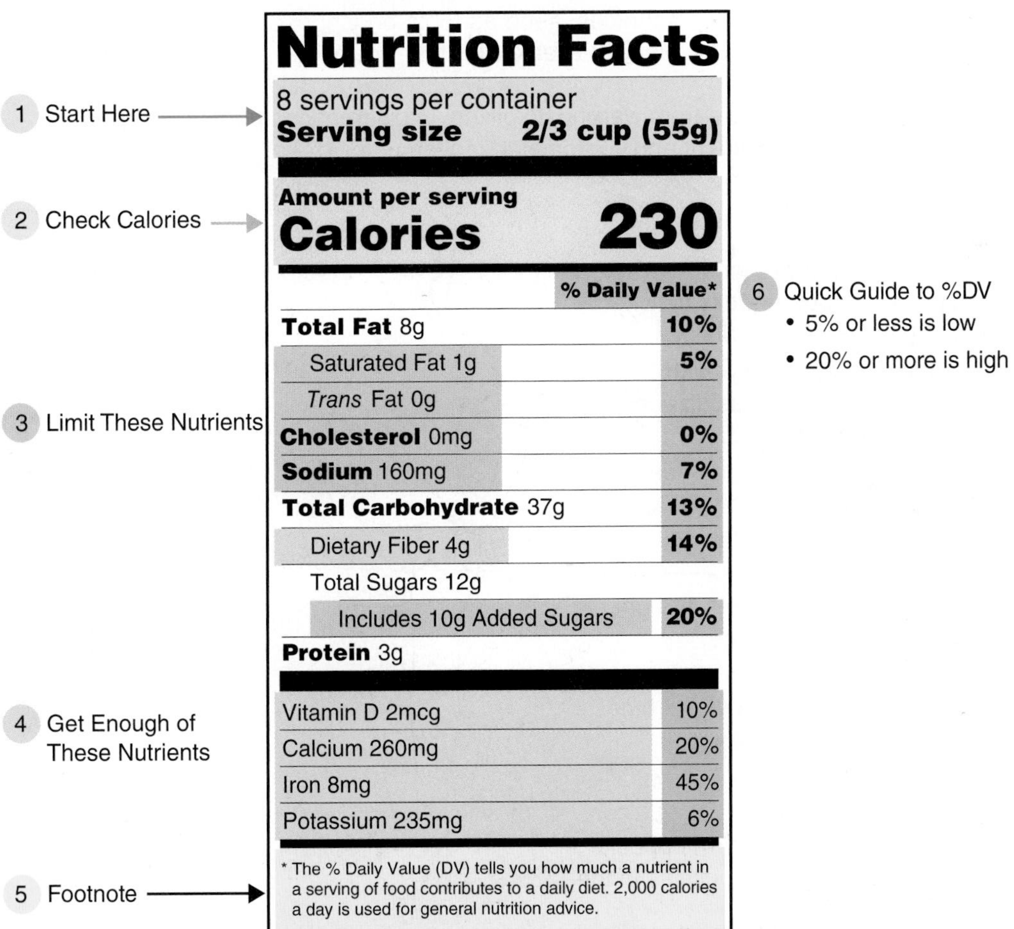

1 Start Here
2 Check Calories
3 Limit These Nutrients
4 Get Enough of These Nutrients
5 Footnote
6 Quick Guide to %DV
• 5% or less is low
• 20% or more is high
Nutrition Facts
8 servings per container
Serving size 2/3 cup (55g)
Amount per serving
Calories 230
% Daily Value*
Total Fat 8g 10%
Saturated Fat 1g 5%
Trans Fat 0g
Cholesterol 0mg 0%
Sodium 160mg 7%
Total Carbohydrate 37g 13%
Dietary Fiber 4g 14%
Total Sugars 12g
Includes 10g Added Sugars 20%
Protein 3g
Vitamin D 2mcg 10%
Calcium 260mg 20%
Iron 8mg 45%
Potassium 235mg 6%
* The % Daily Value (DV) tells you how much a nutrient in a serving of food contributes to a daily diet. 2,000 calories a day is used for general nutrition advice.

Figure 5.8 The Nutrition Facts label can help consumers make healthy food choices. *Is the %DV for saturated fat in this food low or high?*

This is because the amount of added sugar in the cereal remains constant, but the person requires fewer daily calories. For a person who requires 2,500 calories per day, the cereal would supply a smaller Percent Daily Value for added sugar.

The Percent Daily Values serve as general guidelines. They can help you understand how a food serving fits into your daily nutrient needs. A high Percent Daily Value (20 percent or more) for a given nutrient means a food provides a lot of that nutrient. A low percentage (5 percent or less) means the food provides a small amount of the nutrient.

Learn to use the information listed on the Nutrition Facts label on a regular basis. Ask yourself what combination of foods in how many serving sizes will best meet your nutritional needs for the day. You can also compare food products by using the Percent Daily Values to find food products with the greatest nutrient value.

THE MOVEMENT CONNECTION

It's About Balance

Why

This chapter provides you with the content to analyze your current eating patterns using a variety of different tools.

Many resources exist to help guide food choices, such as tools on ChooseMyPlate.gov that help you balance your caloric intake. This activity break will help you work on your *physical* balance!

Balance is a part of everything we do—from walking, to biking, to different components of sport. Good balance can lead to posture alignment and coordinated movements.

Apply

- Select a location at least an arm's length away from the nearest person to perform this activity. Keep a chair nearby if needed for stability.
- Select a location near a chair or desk with sufficient space around you. Stand using correct posture with your core engaged.
- Balance on one foot as you lift the other foot off the ground about 6 inches by raising your knee slightly toward your chest. Your leg should form a 45-degree angle.
- Keep your spine in line, with shoulders straight and your abdominal muscles engaged.
- Rotate the ankle on the raised foot in a clockwise circle 5 times and then counterclockwise 5 times. Repeat with the other ankle.

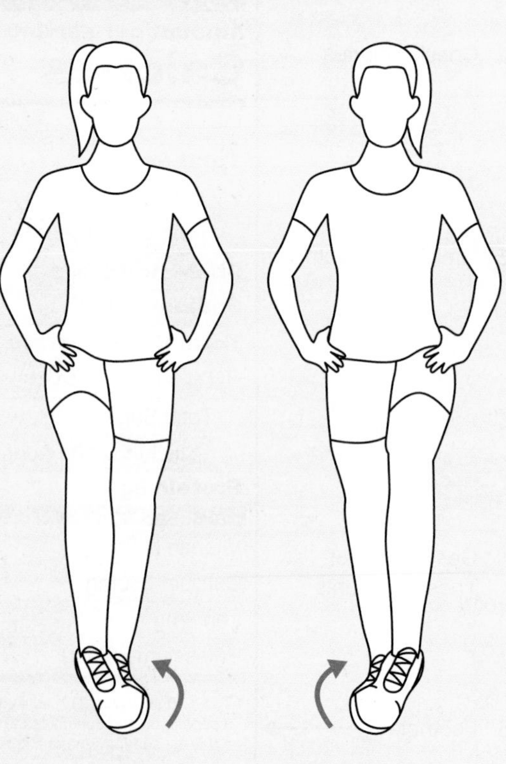

Modification

- For more of a challenge, add in the arm opposite from the lifted leg and complete wrist circles in the opposite direction from your ankle!

Product Claims

You may be swayed by words used on food packaging to make products sound healthful. Manufacturers use claims on their labels to convince you to buy their products. In addition to regulating nutrition labeling, the FDA requires any food labels that make product claims to meet specific criteria. There are four types of claims that may be used on food labels—nutrient content claims, health claims, qualified health claims, and structure/function claims.

- **Nutrient Content Claims.** A nutrient content claim either directly states or implies a level of nutrient in a food. For example, a cereal label that reads "Low-fat granola" is stating that the cereal contains a low level of the nutrient fat. Labels may use terms that can be confusing. For instance, light whipped topping sounds more healthful than regular whipped topping. You need to know what the term *light* means before you can decide if eating light foods will improve the quality of your diet. Products must meet specific definitions for manufacturers to use terms, such as *light*, *low sodium*, and *fat free* on labels (**Figure 5.9**).

Nutrient Content Claims

Claim	Definition (per serving)
Calorie free	Fewer than 5 calories
Low calorie	40 calories or fewer
Reduced or fewer calories	At least 25% fewer calories
Light or lite	One-third fewer calories or 50% less fat
Sugar free	Fewer than 0.5 grams sugars
Reduced sugar or less sugar	At least 25% less sugars
No added sugar	No sugars added during processing or packing, including ingredients that contain sugars, such as juice or dry fruit
Fat free	Fewer than 0.5 grams fat
Low fat	3 grams or fewer of fat
Reduced or less fat	At least 25% less fat
Saturated fat free	Fewer than 0.5 grams saturated fat and less than 0.5 grams *trans* fatty acids
Low saturated fat	1 gram or less saturated fat and 15% or less calories from saturated fat
Reduced/less saturated fat	At least 25% less saturated fat
Cholesterol free	Fewer than 2 milligrams cholesterol and 2 grams or fewer saturated fat
Low cholesterol	20 milligrams or fewer cholesterol and 2 grams or fewer saturated fat
Reduced or less cholesterol	At least 25% less cholesterol and 2 grams or fewer saturated fat
Sodium free	Fewer than 5 milligrams sodium
Very low sodium	35 milligrams or fewer of sodium
Low sodium	140 milligrams or fewer of sodium
Reduced or less sodium	At least 25% less sodium
Light in sodium	At least 50% less sodium

Figure 5.9 Food that includes a nutrient content claim on its label must meet the FDA's requirements for that claim.

- **Health Claims.** Besides claims about nutrient content, manufacturers may put certain health claims on product labels. These claims are based on research showing solid evidence of links between foods or nutrients and diseases. For instance, a yogurt container might include a claim about the link between calcium and a reduced risk of osteoporosis. The most frequently made health claims are related to heart disease. Claims cannot state that a certain food prevents or causes a disease, only that it may reduce risk for the disease. In some instances, the claim may need to include the amount of the beneficial food or nutrient that is supplied by the product. Health claims must be reviewed and evaluated by the FDA before they can be used on labels. The FDA approves a health claim only if it finds "significant scientific agreement (SSA)" to support the claim.
- **Qualified Health Claims.** Similar to health claims, qualified health claims suggest a link between a food or nutrient and its ability to reduce risk for a disease or health condition. Qualified health claims do not require scientific support as strong as a health claim requires, but these claims include a disclaimer to that effect. The following statement is an example of a qualified health claim that includes the disclaimer in the second sentence: "Green tea may reduce the risk of breast or prostate cancer. The FDA has concluded that there is very little scientific evidence for this claim." Truthful dietary guidance statements that are not deceptive do not require review and approval from the FDA before being used on a label. If the FDA decides the statement is misleading, however, its use may be disallowed (**Figure 5.10**).
- **Structure/Function Claims.** A fourth type of claim found on food labels is a structure/function claim. A structure/function claim describes the effect that a food or nutrient has on the structure or function of the body. This type of claim differs from health and qualified health claims because it does not reference a disease or health condition. An example of a structure/function claim is "Calcium (the nutrient) builds strong bones (the body structure)."

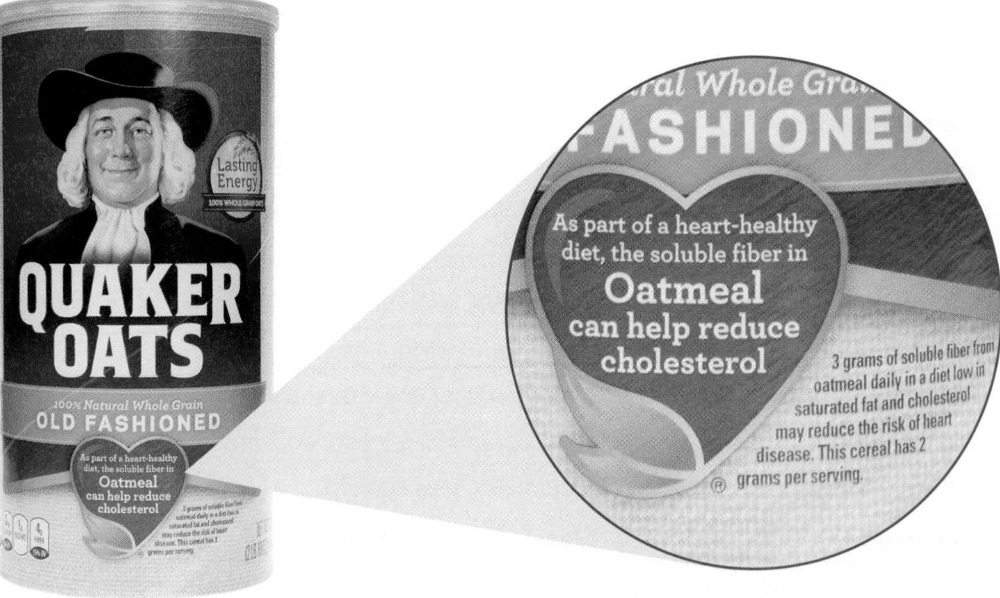

Figure 5.10 Food manufacturers include claims on their food labels to market their products. *What type of claim is on this oatmeal package?*

Sheila Fitzgerald/Shutterstock.com

A healthy food does not necessarily have a health claim. Some companies may choose to not use health claims. Minimally processed foods and whole foods, such as fruits and vegetables, may not display a product claim. These foods continue to be very healthful food choices.

Ingredient Labeling

Federal law requires manufacturers to list product ingredients in descending order by weight. Flavorings, color additives, and some spices must be listed by their common names.

A complete list of ingredients helps consumers know what is in the foods they buy. People are interested in this information for various reasons. They may want to buy the canned beef stew that contains more beef than any other ingredient. Others want to avoid certain ingredients for religious or cultural reasons. For instance, a vegetarian would want to know that a can of vegetable soup contains beef broth.

Some consumers want to avoid substances to which they may be allergic or sensitive. Eight foods or food groups are responsible for 90 percent of food allergies. The eight major food allergens include milk, eggs, fish, crustacean shellfish, tree nuts, wheat, peanuts, and soybeans. Food manufacturers are required by law to list ingredients found in their products that are major food allergens (**Figure 5.11**). Some states require that foods containing genetically modified organisms (GMOs) or genetically engineered foods in their ingredients be identified on the label.

Product Dating

The USDA estimates that 30 percent of food is lost or wasted every day. Oftentimes wholesome food is discarded because consumers are confused by product dating on packages.

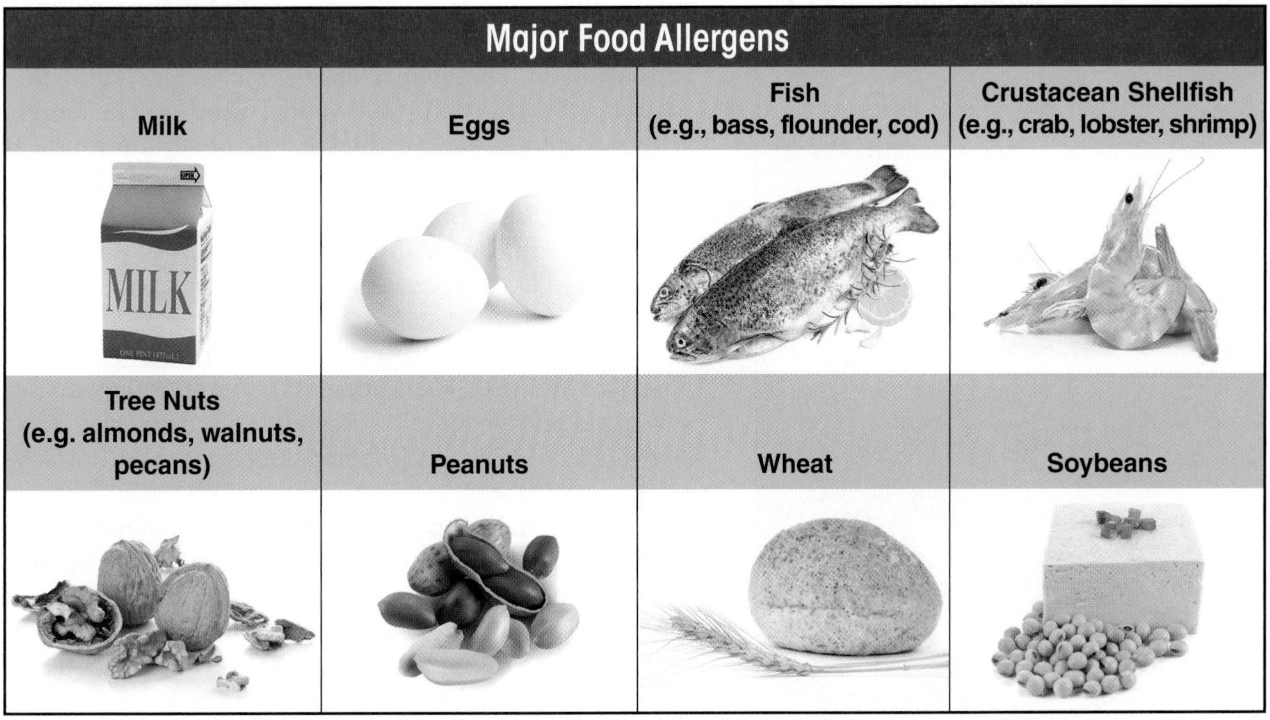

Major Food Allergens

Milk	Eggs	Fish (e.g., bass, flounder, cod)	Crustacean Shellfish (e.g., crab, lobster, shrimp)
Tree Nuts (e.g. almonds, walnuts, pecans)	Peanuts	Wheat	Soybeans

Top row: Hurst Photo/Shutterstock.com; Dancestrokes/Shutterstock.com; Creative Family/Shutterstock.com; nito/Shutterstock.com; Bottom row: Vitalina Rybakova/Shutterstock.com; kaband/Shutterstock.com; schankz/Shutterstock.com; NIPAPORN PANYACHAROEN/Shutterstock.com

Figure 5.11 Food manufacturers are required to list any ingredient that is one of the eight major food allergens on the label.

Although product dating on food packages is not required by law, except for infant formula, most manufacturers voluntarily provide dating on their products anyway. The dating is intended to inform you about when the food is of best quality. With the exception of infant formula, these dates are not an indication of the food's safety. You should not buy or use infant formula after its "Use-By" date.

In the past, product dating has used phrases such as "Best if Used By/Before," "Sell-By," or "Use-By." To reduce confusion and food waste, the USDA recommends that food manufacturers use only the "Best if Used By" phrase. This date indicates when the food product will be of best flavor and quality. This date *does not* convey when a food must be purchased by or when a food is no longer safe to consume.

If foods have been stored properly, they should still be wholesome after their "Best if Used By" dates. Food products are safe to consume past the date on the label; however, you should always evaluate the quality of the food product before consuming it. If the food has developed an off odor, flavor, or texture, you should discard it.

If you plan to store foods for an extended time and want to achieve maximum keeping quality, avoid buying products with expiration dates that have passed. Rotate items in kitchen storage to use products with older product dating first.

Other Basic Food Label Information

Federal laws require certain information to appear on the label of every processed or packaged food product. This information includes the name and form of the food, such as French cut green beans. The label must also state the amount of food in the package in both US and metric units of measure. The name and address of the manufacturer, packer, or distributor must also be listed.

Foods Covered by Country-of-Origin Labeling Law

- Muscle cuts of chicken, goat, and lamb
- Ground chicken, goat, and lamb
- Fish and shellfish (wild and farm raised)
- Fresh and frozen fruits and vegetables
- Peanuts
- Pecans and macadamia nuts
- Ginseng

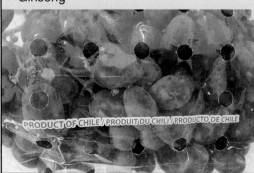

Photo: Goodheart-Willcox Publisher

Figure 5.12 Certain foods must display country-of-origin labeling.

Country-of-Origin Labeling (COOL)

Much of the food supply in the United States comes from other countries. Grapes and blueberries may come from Chile, avocados from Mexico, and apples from Canada. The *country-of-origin labeling (COOL)* law requires that full-line food stores provide consumers with information about the sources of certain foods at the point of purchase. Not all foods are covered by this law (**Figure 5.12**). Processed foods such as canned tuna, roasted peanuts, or fruit medley are examples of foods not covered by COOL. Beef and pork are also excluded from the law.

Businesses such as butchers and fish markets do not have to provide COOL information because they do not sell fruits and vegetables. Restaurants, cafeterias, food stands, salad bars, and delicatessens are also not covered by this law.

The COOL information may appear on a food label, sign, twist tie, band, or other display, but it must be easy to read. The label must list the country (or countries) where the food was grown, or born, raised, and slaughtered. In some cases, an animal may have been born and raised in Canada, but slaughtered in the United States. The label for this food would include both Canada and the United States.

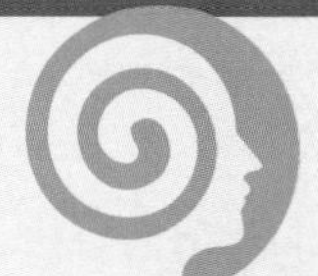

EXTEND YOUR KNOWLEDGE

Modified Food Labels

You will find modified nutrition labels on some foods. For example, the Nutrition Labeling and Education Act (NLEA) includes the use of dual column labels. These labels list the "per serving" and "per package" calorie and nutrition information. For instance, you may notice two columns of nutrient amounts on boxed mixes for products like muffins and pudding. Manufacturers must list nutrient amounts per serving of the products as packaged. However, manufacturers may also list nutrition information for the products as prepared.

You may find a simplified label on products like candy, which do not provide significant amounts of some nutrients. In addition, smaller food items, such as canned tuna, may include simpler labels that fit more easily on their packages. Fresh fruits, vegetables, meats, poultry, and fish may not have labels. However, most stores have posters, notebooks, or pamphlets with nutrition information about these foods. The produce department should offer information about the most popular raw fruits and vegetables. The fish department should provide nutrition details about the fish most commonly sold raw. The meat department should have nutrient data on the best-selling cuts of raw meat and poultry.

Vegetables

Nutrition Facts

Raw, edible weight portion. Percent Daily Values (%DV) are based on a 2,000 calorie diet.

Vegetables Serving Size (gram weight/ounce weight)	Calories	Calories from Fat	Total Fat		Sodium		Potassium		Total Carbohydrate		Dietary Fiber		Sugars	Protein	Vitamin A	Vitamin C	Calcium	Iron
			g	%DV	mg	%DV	mg	%DV	g	%DV	g	%DV	g	g	%DV	%DV	%DV	%DV
Asparagus 5 spears (93 g/3.3 oz)	20	0	0	0	0	0	230	7	4	1	2	8	2g	2g	10%	15%	2%	2%
Bell Pepper 1 medium (148 g/5.3 oz)	25	0	0	0	40	2	220	6	6	2	2	8	4g	1g	4%	190%	2%	4%
Broccoli 1 medium stalk (148 g/5.3 oz)	45	0	0.5	1	80	3	460	13	8	3	3	12	2g	4g	6%	220%	6%	6%
Carrot 1 carrot, 7" long, 1 1/4" diameter (78 g/2.8 oz)	30	0	0	0	60	3	250	7	7	2	2	8	5g	1g	110%	10%	2%	2%
Cauliflower 1/6 medium head (99 g/3.5 oz)	25	0	0	0	30	1	270	8	5	2	2	8	2g	2g	0%	100%	2%	2%
Celery 2 medium stalks (110 g/3.9 oz)	15	0	0	0	115	5	260	7	4	1	2	8	2g	0g	10%	15%	4%	2%
Cucumber 1/3 medium (99 g/3.5 oz)	10	0	0	0	0	0	140	4	2	1	1	4	1g	1g	4%	10%	2%	2%
Green (Snap) Beans 3/4 cup cut (83 g/3.0 oz)	20	0	0	0	0	0	200	6	5	2	3	12	2g	1g	4%	10%	4%	2%
Green Cabbage 1/12 medium head (84 g/3.0 oz)	25	0	0	0	20	1	190	5	5	2	2	8	3g	1g	0%	70%	4%	2%
Green Onion 1/4 cup chopped (25 g/0.9 oz)	10	0	0	0	10	0	70	2	2	1	1	4	1g	0g	2%	8%	2%	2%
Iceberg Lettuce 1/6 medium head (89 g/3.2 oz)	10	0	0	0	10	0	125	4	2	1	1	4	2g	1g	6%	6%	2%	2%
Leaf Lettuce 1 1/2 cups shredded (85 g/3.0 oz)	15	0	0	0	35	1	170	5	2	1	1	4	1g	1g	130%	6%	2%	4%
Mushrooms 5 medium (84 g/3.0 oz)	20	0	0	0	15	0	300	9	3	1	1	4	0g	3g	0%	2%	0%	2%
Onion 1 medium (148 g/5.3 oz)	45	0	0	0	5	0	190	5	11	4	3	12	9g	1g	0%	20%	4%	4%
Potato 1 medium (148 g/5.3 oz)	110	0	0	0	0	0	620	18	26	9	2	8	1g	3g	0%	45%	2%	6%
Radishes 7 radishes (85 g/3.0 oz)	10	0	0	0	55	2	190	5	3	1	1	4	2g	0g	0%	30%	2%	2%
Summer Squash 1/2 medium (98 g/3.5 oz)	20	0	0	0	0	0	260	7	4	1	2	8	2g	1g	6%	30%	2%	2%
Sweet Corn kernels from 1 medium ear (90 g/3.2 oz)	90	20	2.5	4	0	0	250	7	18	6	2	8	5g	4g	2%	10%	0%	2%
Sweet Potato 1 medium, 5" long, 2"diameter (130 g/4.6 oz)	100	0	0	0	70	3	440	13	23	8	4	16	7g	2g	120%	30%	4%	4%
Tomato 1 medium (148 g/5.3 oz)	25	0	0	0	20	1	340	10	5	2	1	4	3g	1g	20%	40%	2%	4%

Most vegetables provide negligible amounts of saturated fat, *trans* fat, and cholesterol.

U.S. Food and Drug Administration (January 1, 2008)

USDA

Using Food Recommendations and Guidelines

You now know about a variety of tools for healthy eating. The next step is to learn how to use them to improve your eating pattern.

Keep a Food Journal

Before you can determine whether you are getting enough nutrients, you need to know which foods you are eating. One way to be aware of what you eat is to keep a food journal. A ***food journal*** is a record of the kinds and amounts of foods and beverages consumed for a given time. Food journals are sometimes called *food logs* or *food diaries*. The record includes all snacks and foods eaten throughout the day. It also includes condiments, such as catsup, pickles, salad dressings, syrups, and jellies.

You need a complete journal if you want a true analysis of your diet. You will find it easy to forget what you ate if you wait too long to record information. Keeping a notepad and pencil handy will help you remember to record each food item you eat. Alternatively, you may choose to use a food journal app on your smartphone or computer.

CASE STUDY

Change for the Better

Kiara enrolled in a physical conditioning class for her physical education elective this semester. However, she is finding that she tires easily, is weaker than her peers, and has little stamina. One day, the class instructor discussed the importance of nutrition for optimal health and performance. Kiara isn't sure how good or bad her eating habits are, but she is sure she could do better. Kiara is determined to improve her overall health—she just doesn't know where to start.

Case Review

1. What steps can Kiara take to achieve her goal of improving her overall health?
2. What resources might be helpful to Kiara during this process?
3. Do you think Kiara will succeed? Why?

For your diet analysis to be valid, you need to become **adept** (skilled) at estimating food amounts. Look at measuring utensils to help you become familiar with what amounts such as one tablespoon and one cup look like. Find out how many ounces your cups, bowls, and glasses hold. Consider using your hand as a reference for judging food amounts (**Figure 5.13**). This will help you correctly record the amounts of foods you consume.

Record what you eat for several days. This will give you a more accurate picture of your eating habits than a one-day record. You will also get a better account if you record your food consumption on typical days. Avoid keeping a record on birthdays, holidays, and other days when you are likely to follow different eating patterns.

Analyze Your Diet

Use the information recorded in your food journal to determine whether you are meeting your daily nutrient needs. A number of software programs are available to help you quickly analyze your diet on a computer. Most of these programs include a database of *food composition tables*. These tables are reference guides listing the nutritive values of many foods in common serving sizes.

USDA Food Composition Database

The US Department of Agriculture provides a national nutrient database for consumers to use. Name brand packaged foods and prepared foods sold in restaurants and supermarkets are included in the database. You can reference this database, enter data about the foods you ate into analysis software, and the program will generate a report showing the calorie and nutrient values of those foods. You can print a detailed analysis of how your daily nutrient values compare to the RDAs and AIs. This comparison will show you which nutrient needs you have and have not met.

Food Tracker

You can also use the "Food Tracker" tool on the SuperTracker website to analyze your diet. Does your food journal show you are getting the recommended daily amounts from each food group? The different groups are good sources of different nutrients.

Serving-Size Comparison Chart

Food	Symbol	Comparison	Serving Size
Dairy: Milk, Yogurt, Cheese			
Cheese (string cheese)		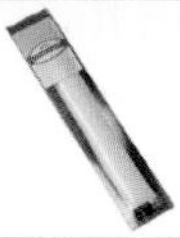 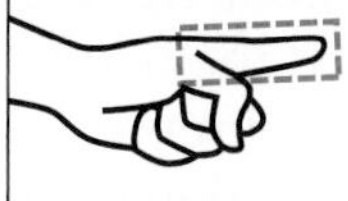 Pointer finger	1½ ounces
Milk and yogurt (glass of milk)		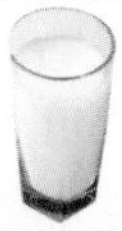 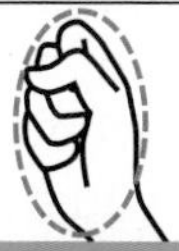 One fist	1 cup
Vegetables			
Cooked carrots		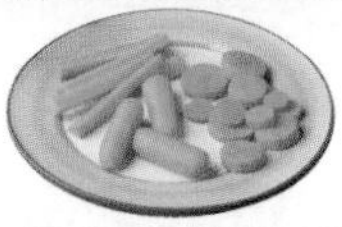 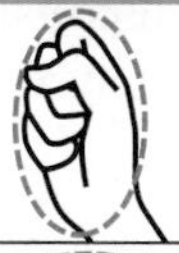 One fist	1 cup
Salad (bowl of salad)		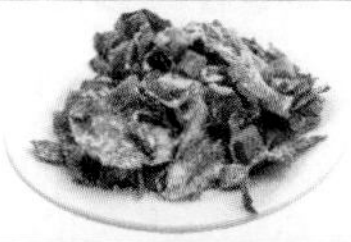 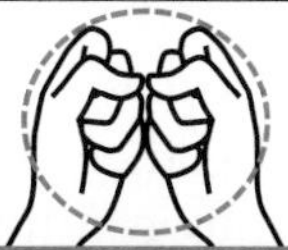 Two fists	2 cups
Fruits			
Apple		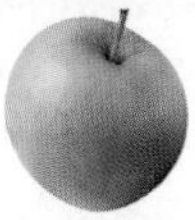 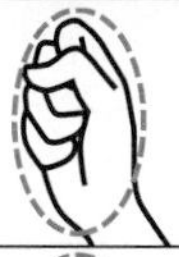 One fist	1 medium
Canned peaches		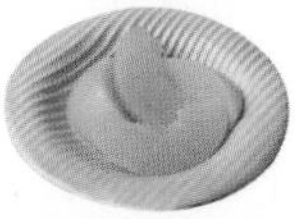 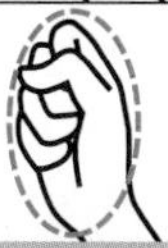 One fist	1 cup
Grains: Breads, Cereals, Pasta			
Dry cereal (bowl of cereal)		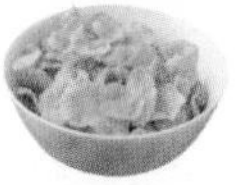 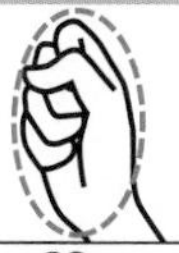 One fist	1 cup
Noodles, rice, oatmeal (bowl of noodles)		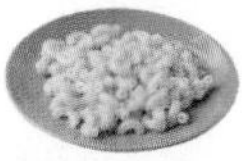 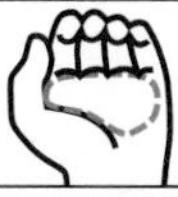 Handful	½ cup
Slice of whole-wheat bread		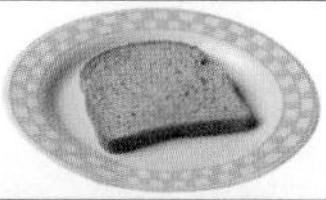 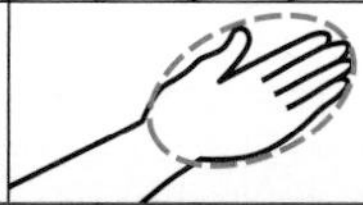 Flat hand	1 slice
Protein: Meat, Beans, Nuts			
Chicken, beef, fish, pork (chicken breast)		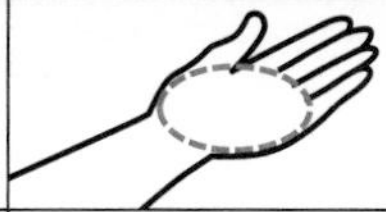 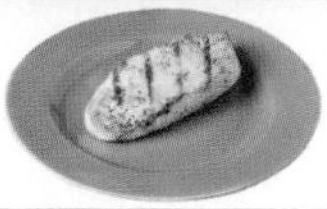 Palm	3 ounces
Peanut butter (spoon of peanut butter)		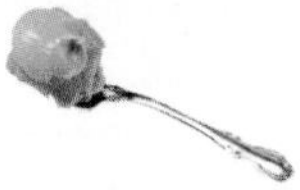 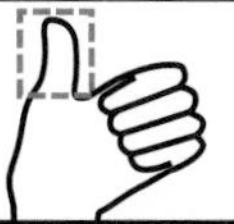 Thumb	1 tablespoon

Reprinted with the permission of Dairy Council of California, 2016

Figure 5.13 Learning to estimate food amounts accurately will help you avoid consuming too many calories. *How could you estimate 1 tablespoon of peanut butter using your hand as a reference?*

Eating the recommended amounts from each group every day will help you get all the nutrients you need (**Figure 5.14**).

Calculate Manually

If you do not have access to diet analysis software, you can analyze your diet yourself. Make a chart with columns for the foods you ate, the calories you consumed, and all of the major nutrients. List the foods recorded in your food journal in the first column. Look up each food in the USDA's Nutritive Value of Foods (see Appendix D). Record the calories and amounts of nutrients supplied by each food in the appropriate columns of your chart.

After you have filled in the information for each food, total the amounts in the nutrient columns. Compare these totals to the RDAs and AIs.

As you complete your chart, remember to think about amounts. Compare the amount of each food you consumed to the amount listed in the USDA's table. If your amount differs, you will have to adjust the nutrient amounts you list in your chart. For instance, the amount listed in the USDA's table for milk is 1 cup. If you drank 1½ cups, you will have to multiply the quantity of each nutrient listed for milk by 1½.

Plan Menus Using MyPlate Daily Checklist

Your diet analysis may show you are eating too much from some of the food groups and not enough from others. Planning a daily menu using "MyPlate Daily Checklist" at ChooseMyPlate.gov can help you correct such problems. Following the pattern planned for your age, sex, and physical activity level will help you get the balance of nutrients you need. The Checklist guides you in selecting foods low in saturated fats, sodium, and added sugars, and rich in fiber and nutrients as needed for good health.

You can create a more personalized daily food plan using MyPlan on the SuperTracker website. There is a "My Recipe" option on SuperTracker, which allows you to upload and analyze your favorite recipes for use when planning your menu.

Eating right may be easier and tastier than you think. ChooseMyPlate.gov is flexible enough for anyone to use. It can suit different family lifestyles, cultural backgrounds, and religious beliefs. It can accommodate all of your favorite foods.

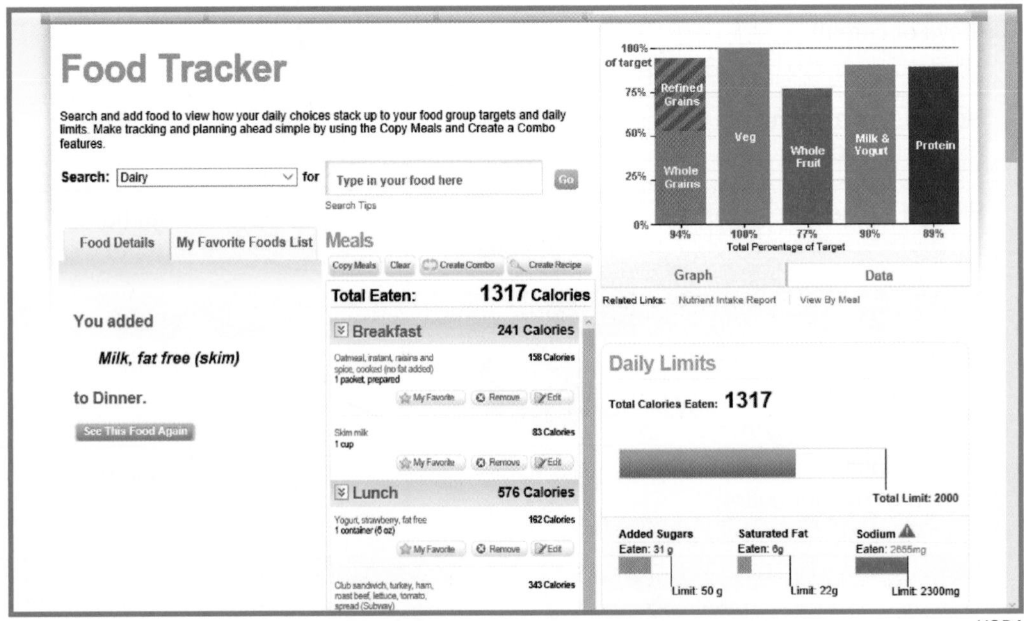

Figure 5.14 The Food Tracker on the SuperTracker website is useful for analyzing your diet.

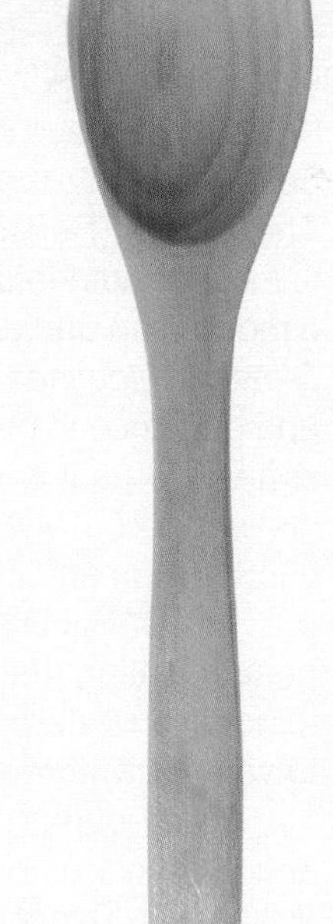

RECIPE FILE

Buffalo Chicken Tacos

6 TACOS

Ingredients

Filling

- 1 lb. chicken breast, cut into small pieces
- ¼ c. flour
- ½ t. black pepper
- ¼ t. salt
- 2 T. hot sauce
- 1½ T. olive oil
- ½ green bell pepper, chopped
- ½ red bell pepper, chopped
- ½ yellow bell pepper, chopped
- 2 garlic cloves, minced
- 6 each corn tortillas (6-inch diameter)

Toppings

- ½ avocado, sliced
- ½ c. mozzarella cheese, shredded
- 2½ c. cabbage, shredded
- ½ c. low-fat ranch dressing
- 6 green onions, chopped, green and white parts

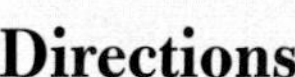

Directions

Prepare Filling

1. In large bowl, combine flour, pepper, and salt.
2. Add chicken pieces, toss to coat, and remove chicken from bowl. Discard flour that remains in the bowl.
3. Heat 1 tablespoon olive oil in large skillet over medium heat until a drop of water sizzles in the pan.
4. Place floured chicken in skillet. Brown chicken on all sides. Then sauté until chicken reaches 165°F (74°C), and is no longer pink inside and the juices run clear.
5. Remove chicken from the pan and place in a medium bowl.
6. Toss chicken with hot sauce and set aside.
7. Wipe out the skillet with a paper towel and add remaining ½ tablespoon olive oil.
8. Add peppers and sauté for 4–5 minutes over medium heat.
9. Add garlic and sauté for 1 minute more.

Prepare Tortillas

10. Use one of the following methods to warm the tortillas:

    Oven Method—Preheat oven to 350°F (177°C). Wrap 6 tortillas in aluminum foil. Place pouch directly on oven rack and heat for 15 minutes, or until heated through.

    Microwave Method—Place 6 tortillas on a microwave safe plate. Cover with a damp paper towel. Microwave in 30-second intervals until tortillas are heated through.

    Stovetop Method—Place one tortilla at a time in a clean, dry skillet over medium heat. Heat for 30 seconds, turn, and heat for 30 seconds more. Tortillas can also be heated directly over the burner on a gas stovetop.

Serve Tacos

11. Place warmed tortilla on plate.
12. Top tortilla with chicken, peppers, and toppings of your choice.

PER SERVING: 204 CALORIES, 20 G PROTEIN, 18 G CARBOHYDRATE, 7 G FAT, 4 G FIBER, 324 MG SODIUM.

Chapter 5 Review and Expand

Reading Summary

Experts have developed a number of tools to help people evaluate their diets and make wise food choices. The Dietary Reference Intakes (DRIs) are reference values for nutrients and food components that can be used to plan and assess diets for healthy people. The *Dietary Guidelines for Americans* provides information and guidance to promote healthy eating across the life span. The goal is to help reduce the risks of chronic diseases. The MyPlate food guidance system can be used to plan and implement a healthy diet.

The DASH Diet and Food Lists system are other healthy eating plans. Food labels display information to help you determine how a food product contributes to your daily nutrient needs.

A food journal can be used to keep track of the kinds and amounts of foods and beverages consumed on a daily basis. This information can be analyzed to determine if an individual's daily nutrient needs are being met. Use the recommendations and tools from the ChooseMyPlate and SuperTracker websites to plan balanced menus and track progress toward meeting nutrient needs.

Chapter Vocabulary

1. **Content Terms** On a separate sheet of paper, list words that are related to each of the following terms. Then, working with a partner, explain how these words are related.

   - Acceptable Macronutrient Distribution Ranges (AMDR)
   - Adequate Intake (AI)
   - Daily Values (DV)
   - *Dietary Guidelines for Americans*
   - Dietary Reference Intakes (DRI)
   - Estimated Average Requirement (EAR)
   - Estimated Energy Requirement (EER)
   - food journal
   - MyPlate
   - nutrient dense
   - *Physical Activity Guidelines for Americans*
   - Recommended Dietary Allowance (RDA)
   - Tolerable Upper Intake Level (UL)

2. **Academic Terms** Write each of the following terms on a separate sheet of paper. For each term, quickly write a word you think relates to the term. In small groups, exchange papers. Have each person in the group explain a term on the list. Take turns until all terms have been explained.

   - adept
   - amended
   - comprise
   - undermine

Review Learning

3. *True or false?* Dietary Reference Intakes are used to plan and assess diets for individuals who have a chronic disease.
4. What are the five basic themes of the *2015–2020 Dietary Guidelines for Americans*?
5. Why does the *2015–2020 Dietary Guidelines* address the topic of physical activity?
6. What message does the MyPlate image communicate?
7. How do you create a personalized food plan using MyPlate?
8. *True or false?* MyPlate uses volume and weight measures rather than number of servings to calculate the amounts of food recommended for an individual.
9. How does the Food Lists system organize foods into Food Lists?
10. List six foods the DASH diet suggests you choose more often.
11. Percent Daily Values used as references on food labels are based on a ______-calorie diet.
12. *True or false?* Food must be discarded after the "Best if Used By" date on the package.
13. Give two tips for keeping a food journal that will increase the validity of a diet analysis.

Self-Assessment Quiz 

Complete the self-assessment quiz online to help you practice and expand your knowledge and skills.

Critical Thinking

14. **Evaluate** What evidence can you give to support the theory that many people lack understanding about portion size? How can using the various healthy eating tools discussed in this chapter increase understanding of how much to eat each day?
15. **Apply** Use the *Food Lists Appendix E* to estimate the nutrient and calorie content of your breakfast.
16. **Analyze** Develop a survey to assess people's adherence to the *Dietary Guidelines for Americans*. Use your survey to interview three people in different age groups. Analyze the results to identify any patterns. Share your findings in class.

17. **Evaluate** Prepare a plate using foods and amounts you typically eat for a meal at home. Take a photo of the plate. Then, compare the amounts and types of foods on your plate with your recommendations from the MyPlate food guidance system. Prepare a brief summary of your findings to submit with your photo.
18. **Compare** Read the Nutrition Facts panel from your favorite cereal. Find a similar cereal that is healthier by comparing the Nutrition Facts panel from your favorite cereal with other cereals' Nutrition Facts panels. Using one serving size of each cereal, which nutrients add greater nutrient density value to the food?
19. **Create** View videos from the *MyPlate, MyWins Video Series* on ChooseMyPlate.gov. Then produce your own video illustrating how you put MyPlate guidance into practice.

Core Skills

20. **History** Research the history of the *Dietary Guidelines for Americans*, and then write a paper about what you learned. Discuss why the *Dietary Guidelines* was developed, who the intended audience is, and how it has evolved. Gather information from a variety of authoritative print and digital sources. Selectively integrate information into your paper to communicate your ideas in the most effective way. Provide citations for your sources.
21. **Research and Listening** Research current legislation and regulations related to nutrition and wellness issues. Select one that interests you and prepare to lead a group discussion in class. Prompt others to participate by posing thought-provoking questions. Reiterate group members' ideas or conclusions to encourage involvement and ensure understanding.
22. **Speaking** Create a one-minute media message promoting healthy food choices that could be broadcast over the school's public announcement system. Take your audience into consideration as you formulate your message. Practice delivering the nutrition message with enthusiasm.
23. **Writing** Imagine you are a member of the committee charged with preparing the next edition of the *Dietary Guidelines for Americans*. Identify a nutrition topic you believe should be addressed and formulate a question as if you were submitting it to the Nutrition Evidence Library (NEL). Be sure to use exact language and vocabulary that is appropriate to the field of nutrition and the expertise of the readers.
24. **Math** A meal plan based on the Food Lists provides for the following food choices: 2 starches, 1 fruit, 2 lean proteins, 1 nonstarchy vegetable, 1 fat-free milk, 1 fat. Calculate the total grams of carbohydrate, protein, and fat in this meal plan, as well as the calories provided by this meal.
25. **Listening** Find a podcast or video of an individual speaking on a nutrition topic. Evaluate the speaker's point of view, reasoning, and use of evidence. Identify any misleading content or unclear evidence. Be sure to determine the speaker's credentials and his or her authority on this topic. Write a brief analysis and share with the class.
26. **Math** Use *Appendix C Dietary Reference Intakes* to calculate the range of Recommended Dietary Allowance for iron for individuals six months of age and older. (*Hint:* range is the difference between the lowest and highest values in a set of numbers.) Include values for women who are pregnant or lactating in your calculation.
27. **Math** Jenna's food plan calls for 2,000 calories per day. Her goal is to select nutrient-dense foods as often as possible. One morning, she began reading the Nutrition Facts panel for the whole-grain bread she was toasting for breakfast. She discovered that each slice contains 3 grams of dietary fiber. She knows her Daily Value for dietary fiber is 28 grams. If Jenna has 2 slices of toast, what Percent Daily Value of fiber has she consumed?
28. **Career Readiness Practice** As a new employee, you are taking on the challenge of keeping your mind and body healthy. Part of this challenge includes taking the initiative to maintain a healthy body weight. Use the "MyPlate Daily Checklist" to plan healthful meals, and use the "Food Tracker" to keep track of your food consumption and fitness activities. Continue to use these tools found on ChooseMyPlate.gov for one month or more. After a couple of months, write a summary indicating how healthful eating and adequate physical activity have helped you maintain a healthy body weight. What would you tell other "employees" about the benefits of using these tools?

CHAPTER 6

Carbohydrates

Learning Outcomes

After studying this chapter, you will be able to

- **identify** the three types of carbohydrates and their food sources;
- **list** the major functions of carbohydrates;
- **interpret** how the body uses carbohydrates for energy production;
- **state** the relationship between adequate fiber in the diet and a healthy digestive system;
- **judge** the value and limitations of using the glycemic index; and
- **evaluate** the role of carbohydrates in a variety of health issues.

Victority/Shutterstock.com

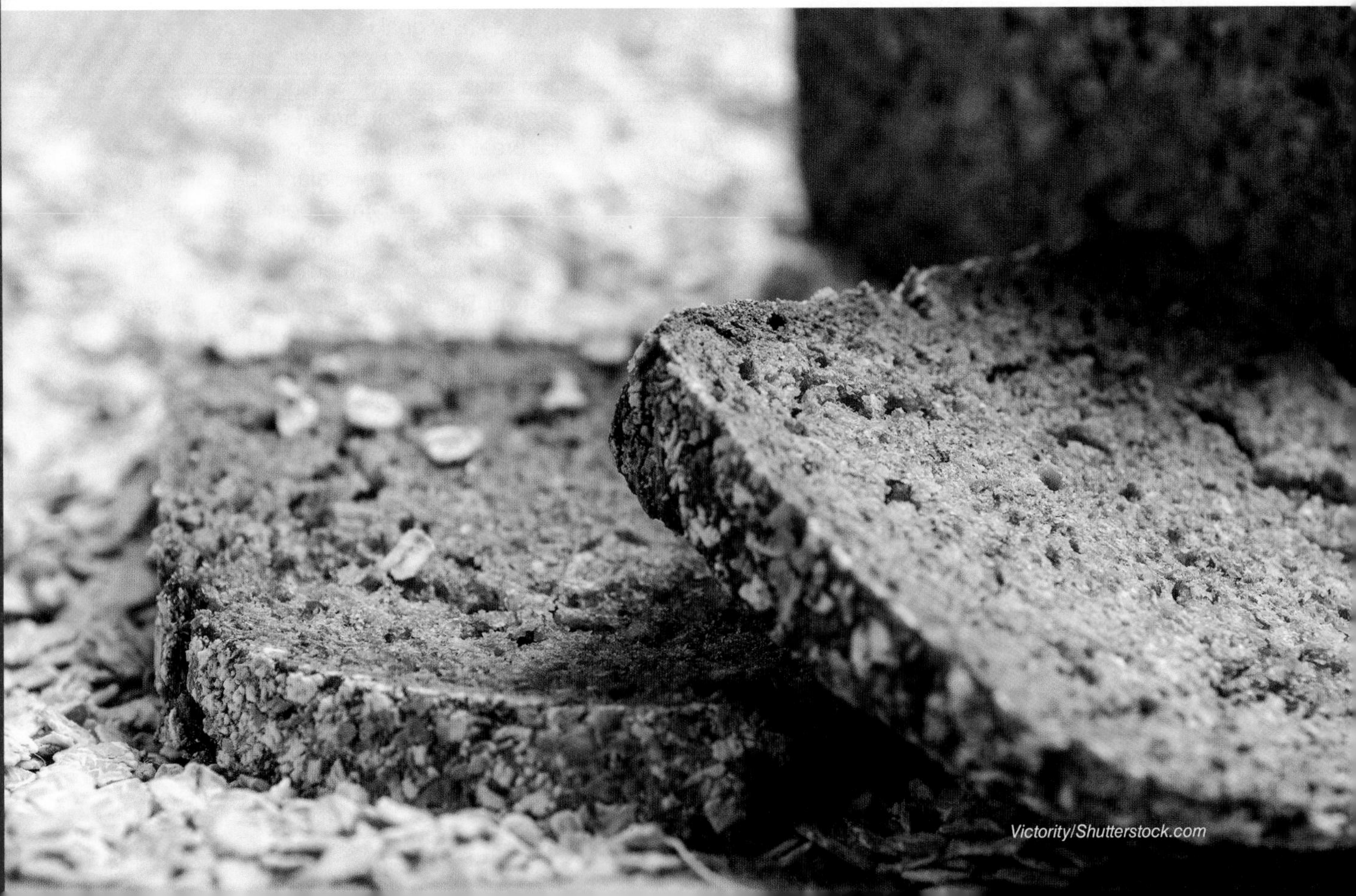

Content Terms 

carbohydrates
complex carbohydrate
dental caries
diabetes mellitus
dietary fiber
disaccharide
functional fiber
functional food
glucose
glycemic index (GI)
glycogen
hormone
hypoglycemia
insulin
lactose intolerance
monosaccharide
polysaccharide
simple carbohydrate
starch
sugars
supplement
total fiber

Academic Terms 

addiction
erode
replenish
satiety

What's Your Nutrition and Wellness IQ?

Take this quiz to examine how much you already know about carbohydrates. If you cannot answer a question, pay extra attention to that topic as you study this chapter.

- Identify each statement as *True*, *False*, or *It Depends*. *It Depends* means in some cases the statement is true; in some cases it could be false.
- Revise false statements to make them true.
- Explain the circumstances in which each *It Depends* statement is true and when it is false.

Nutrition and Wellness IQ 

	Statement			
1.	Carbohydrates supply most of the energy you need to do daily activities.	True	False	It Depends
2.	All carbohydrates contain about the same amount of fiber.	True	False	It Depends
3.	A physically active person draws on the glucose in the cells for energy production.	True	False	It Depends
4.	Inadequate insulin production results in too much glucose in the blood.	True	False	It Depends
5.	Dietary fiber is an important carbohydrate associated with aiding the work of the digestive system.	True	False	It Depends
6.	Added sugars in foods have contributed to rising obesity rates among children and teens.	True	False	It Depends
7.	Referring to the glycemic index is an accurate way to predict how long it will take food to turn into glucose in your body.	True	False	It Depends
8.	Research shows some people are addicted to sugar.	True	False	It Depends

While studying this chapter, look for the activity icon  **to**

- **build** vocabulary with e-flash cards and interactive games;
- **assess** what you learn by completing self-assessment quizzes and completing review questions; and
- **expand** knowledge with interactive activities and activities that extend learning.

www.g-wlearning.com/foodsandnutrition/

What comes to mind when you hear the word *carbohydrates*? If you are thinking about bread, crackers, muffins, rice, and spaghetti, you are correct. You might also wonder if these foods promote health or if they are fattening. Read this chapter to learn which carbohydrate choices have the most health-promoting benefits, and which carbohydrates you may want to limit as part of your lifelong eating pattern.

Types of Carbohydrates

Carbohydrates are one of the six essential nutrients and are a major source of energy for your body. They are the sugars, starches, and fibers in your daily food plan. Except for the natural sugar in milk, nearly all carbohydrates come from plant sources. Carbohydrates should make up the majority of your diet.

Carbohydrates are categorized as either simple or complex. ***Simple carbohydrates*** include the naturally occurring sugars in fruits, vegetables, and milk. Added sugars such as table sugar or honey are also considered simple carbohydrates. ***Complex carbohydrates*** include starch and fiber. Rich sources of starch include potatoes, rice, corn, and wheat. Fiber is found in foods derived from plants, often from the part of the plant that plays a role in its structure.

Both simple and complex carbohydrates are made of three common chemical elements—carbon, hydrogen, and oxygen. These elements are bonded together to form *saccharides*, or sugar units. The elements can be combined in several ways. The arrangement of the elements determines the type of sugar unit. Sugar units may be linked in various arrangements to form different types of carbohydrates (**Figure 6.1**).

The distinction between simple and complex carbohydrates is important when making food choices. Choosing more food sources of complex carbohydrates and fewer sources of simple carbohydrates has health and nutrition benefits. You will read about these benefits later in the chapter.

Monosaccharides

Monosaccharides are carbohydrates composed of single sugar units. (The prefix *mono-* means "one.") These are the smallest carbohydrate molecules. The three monosaccharides are glucose, fructose, and galactose. ***Glucose*** is sometimes called *blood sugar* because it circulates in the bloodstream. It supplies energy to the body's cells and—except in the case of starvation—is the only fuel used by the brain. Fructose has the sweetest taste of all sugars. It occurs naturally in fruits and honey. Galactose does not occur alone as a monosaccharide in foods. Instead, it is found bonded to glucose. Together, these two monosaccharides form the sugar in milk.

Disaccharides

The ***disaccharides*** are made up of two sugar units. (The prefix *di-* means "two.") The body splits disaccharides into monosaccharides during digestion. The disaccharides are sucrose, maltose, and lactose. All of the mono- and disaccharides are collectively referred to as ***sugars***.

Sucrose is the sugar you use in recipes or add to foods at the table. One glucose molecule and one fructose molecule bond together to form sucrose. Many foods contain sucrose. Beet sugar, cane sugar, molasses, and maple syrup are concentrated sources of sucrose.

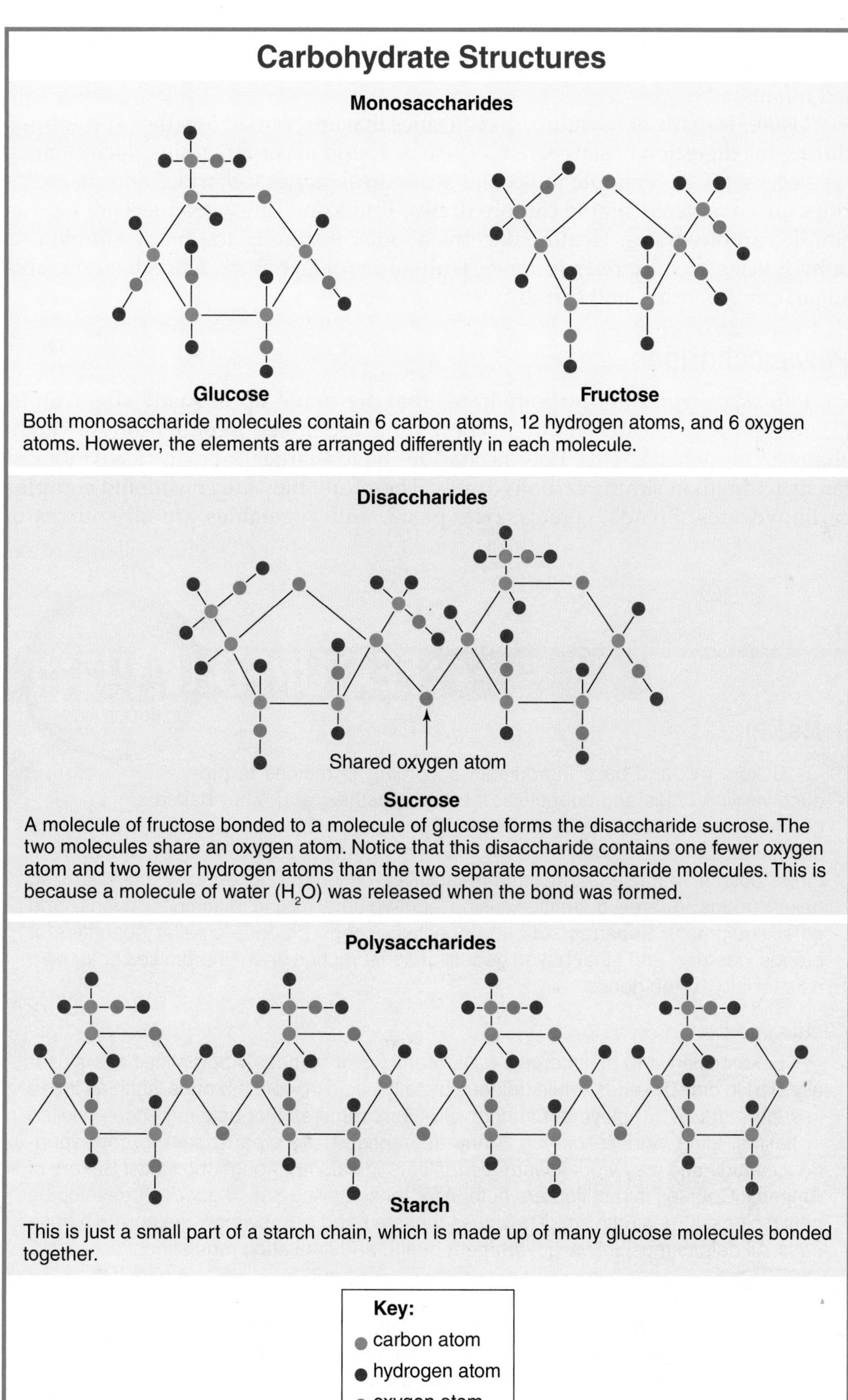

Carbohydrate Structures
Monosaccharides
Glucose
Fructose
Both monosaccharide molecules contain 6 carbon atoms, 12 hydrogen atoms, and 6 oxygen atoms. However, the elements are arranged differently in each molecule.
Disaccharides
Shared oxygen atom
Sucrose
A molecule of fructose bonded to a molecule of glucose forms the disaccharide sucrose. The two molecules share an oxygen atom. Notice that this disaccharide contains one fewer oxygen atom and two fewer hydrogen atoms than the two separate monosaccharide molecules. This is because a molecule of water (H2O) was released when the bond was formed.
Polysaccharides
Starch
This is just a small part of a starch chain, which is made up of many glucose molecules bonded together.
Key:
carbon atom
hydrogen atom
oxygen atom

Goodheart-Willcox Publisher

Figure 6.1 Carbohydrates are comprised of carbon, hydrogen, and oxygen, but differ in how these elements are arranged.

Lactose is found in milk. It is made of one glucose molecule and one galactose molecule that are bonded together. Lactose serves as a source of energy for breast-fed infants.

Maltose is made of two glucose molecules that are bonded together. It is formed during the digestion of starch. It may also be found in certain grains, such as malt.

Because of their simple molecular structures, monosaccharides and disaccharides are considered simple carbohydrates. Fruits and dairy products are high in simple carbohydrates. Health concerns about consuming too many simple carbohydrates generally refer to foods with added sugar. Such foods include table sugar, candy, syrups, and soft drinks.

Polysaccharides

Polysaccharides are carbohydrates that are made up of many sugar units. (The prefix *poly-* means "many.") These units are linked in either long, straight chains or branched chains. Polysaccharides have a larger, more intricate molecular structure than simple carbohydrates. Therefore, they are considered complex carbohydrates. Breads, cereals, rice, pasta, and vegetables are all sources of

FEATURED CAREER

Baker

Bakers mix and bake ingredients according to recipes to produce varying types and quantities of bread, pastries, and other baked goods. Bakers are commonly employed in commercial bakeries that distribute breads and pastries through established wholesale and retail outlets, mail order, or manufacturers' outlets. In these manufacturing facilities, bakers produce mostly standardized baked goods in large quantities, using high-volume mixing machines, ovens, and other equipment. Supermarkets and specialty shops produce smaller quantities of breads, pastries, and other baked goods for consumption on their premises or for sale as specialty baked goods.

Education

Bakers often start their careers as apprentices or trainees. Apprentice bakers usually start in craft bakeries, while trainees usually begin in store bakeries, such as those in supermarkets. Employment in both situations requires that bakers become skilled in baking, icing, and decorating. Many apprentice bakers participate in correspondence study and may work toward a certificate in baking through the Retail Bakers of America. Courses in nutrition are helpful for those selling baked goods or developing new recipes. If running a small business, bakers need to know how to operate a business. All bakers must follow government health and sanitation regulations.

Job Outlook

Highly skilled bakers should remain in demand because of growing interest in specialty products and the time it takes to learn to make these products. Opportunities for bakers in food manufacturing, however, are projected to decline in response to a rise in automated machines for mass-producing baked goods.

complex carbohydrates. Like the disaccharides, the polysaccharides must be broken down during digestion. Starches and most fibers are polysaccharides (**Figure 6.2**).

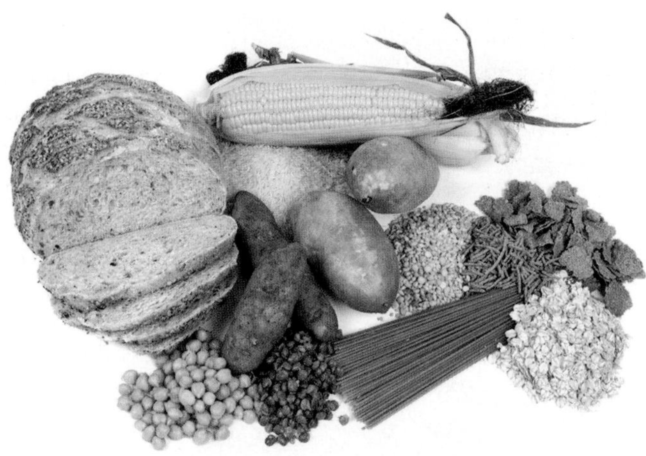

Robyn Mackenzie/Shutterstock.com

Figure 6.2 Starches and fibers found in these foods are polysaccharides. This means they are made up of many linked sugar units.

Starch

Starch is a polysaccharide that is the stored form of energy in plants. Starch is made of many glucose molecules that are bonded together. Grain products, such as breads and cereals, and starchy vegetables, such as corn, potatoes, and legumes, are high in starch.

Fiber

The carbohydrates and lignins found in plants, which cannot be digested by human enzymes are referred to as ***dietary fiber***. (*Lignins* are not carbohydrates, but act as the binder in cell walls.) ***Functional fibers*** are isolated, nondigestible carbohydrates that have been proven to have beneficial effects on human health. These functional fibers may be either extracted from plants or created in a laboratory. For example, *resistant starch* is produced when cereals and grains are processed and baked. It is considered a functional fiber when it is extracted from the original food source and added to another food to enhance that food's health benefits. ***Total fiber*** is the sum of dietary and functional fibers in a food.

When food ingredients, such as fiber, are added to foods to provide health benefits beyond basic nutrition, the foods are called ***functional foods***. These foods are promoted in the media to improve health. The added ingredient means the food is more than simply a source of nutrients, but also has the potential for preventing disease or promoting health.

Human digestive enzymes cannot digest fiber, but bacteria in the large intestine can break down some fibers. Because most fibers pass through the digestive system unchanged, these carbohydrates provide almost no energy (calories). Read food labels to find various terms for fiber, such as *cellulose*, *gum*, *beta glucan*, *psyllium*, and *pectin*.

Functions of Carbohydrates

Carbohydrates provide essential nutrients for healthy eating. They are found in fruits, vegetables, grains, and dairy food groups. To avoid or severely restrict carbohydrates in your diet can lead to health problems. Carbohydrates serve the following four key functions in the body:

- provide energy
- spare proteins
- assist in the breakdown of fats
- provide bulk in the diet

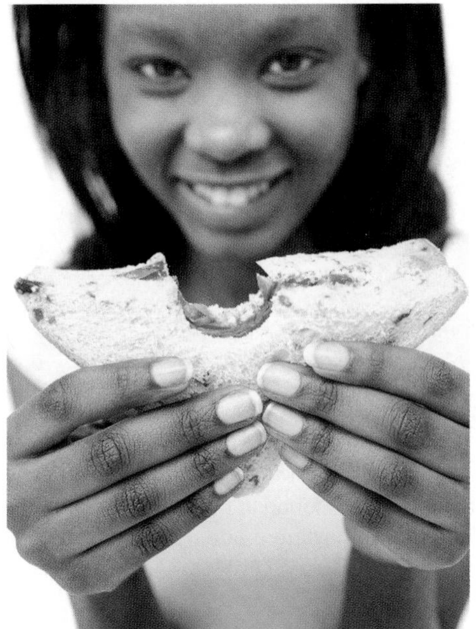

wavebreakmedia/Shutterstock.com

Figure 6.3 The meat in this sandwich provides you with protein, while its bread and vegetables provide carbohydrates. *How does obtaining an adequate amount of carbohydrates affect the proteins in your body?*

Provide Energy

Meeting the energy needs of all of your cells as they work to sustain life is your body's main goal. Carbohydrates provide four calories of energy per gram. Carbohydrates are the preferred source of energy because your body can use and store them so efficiently. Every time you are physically active, your body draws on its carbohydrate stores for energy. When the stored form of carbohydrates becomes depleted, you feel signs of fatigue. If you do not consume enough carbohydrates, your body begins to draw mainly on proteins for fuel needs. A small amount of fat can also be converted into energy during long periods of physical activity.

Spare Proteins

If necessary, your body can use proteins as an energy source, but it is not ideal. Your body is less efficient in using proteins for energy than it is in using carbohydrates. More importantly, if proteins are being used for energy, your body cannot use them to build and maintain cell structures. By eating adequate amounts of carbohydrates, you spare the proteins (**Figure 6.3**). That means you allow the proteins to be used for their more vital roles.

FOOD AND THE ENVIRONMENT

Climate-Friendly Food Production

The Worldwatch Institute reports that agricultural production is a major cause of climate change. Farming practices are estimated to be responsible for 25 to 35 percent of global greenhouse gas emission, which contributes to global warming.

What can be done to encourage farmers to reduce their contributions to the rising temperatures of the Earth's oceans and atmosphere? Worldwatch educates farmers about the need to use manure instead of chemical fertilizers, to plant more trees on farms to reduce soil erosion, and to help remove more carbon dioxide from the air.

Worldwatch also promotes growing food in urban areas to reduce transportation costs and fuel emissions. It encourages the use of responsible irrigation methods that conserve water.

If climate conditions continue to change for farmers, technology may have to look for solutions to help them adapt. Review the ongoing Worldwatch global projects to learn more about ways to support climate-friendly food production.

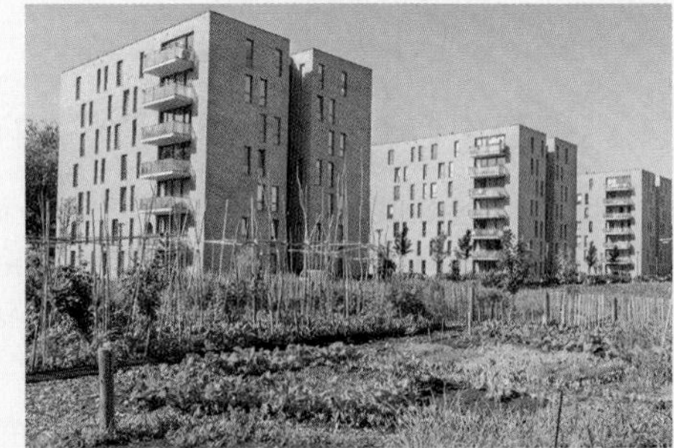

HildaWeges Photography/Shutterstock.com

Think Critically

1. Explain why consumers should be concerned about farming practices.
2. Predict how future technology will help farmers feed a growing population.

Break Down Fats

If the diet is too low in carbohydrates, the body cannot completely break down fats. When fats are not broken down completely, compounds called *ketone bodies* are formed. These compounds then collect in the bloodstream, causing the blood to become more acidic than normal. This acidity can damage cells and organs. This condition is called *ketosis*. The breath of a person in ketosis has the characteristic smell of nail polish remover. He or she also feels nauseous and weak. If the ketosis continues, the person can fall into a coma and die.

Provide Bulk in the Diet

One other important function of carbohydrates is to add bulk to the diet. Fiber is the carbohydrate responsible for this task (**Figure 6.4**). It helps promote normal digestion and elimination of body wastes.

Like the muscles in your arms and legs, the muscles in your digestive tract need a healthy workout. Fiber is the solid material that provides this workout, helping intestinal muscles retain their tone.

Fiber acts like a sponge. It absorbs water, which softens stools and helps prevent constipation. Softer stools are easier to pass, reducing the likelihood of *hemorrhoids*, or swollen veins in the rectum. Some fibers form gels that add bulk to stools. This helps relieve diarrhea.

Bulk in the diet has added benefits for people who are trying to lose weight. As fiber swells, the volume helps you feel full. Fiber also slows the rate at which the stomach empties. Fibrous food sources are usually lower in calories than foods that are high in fat.

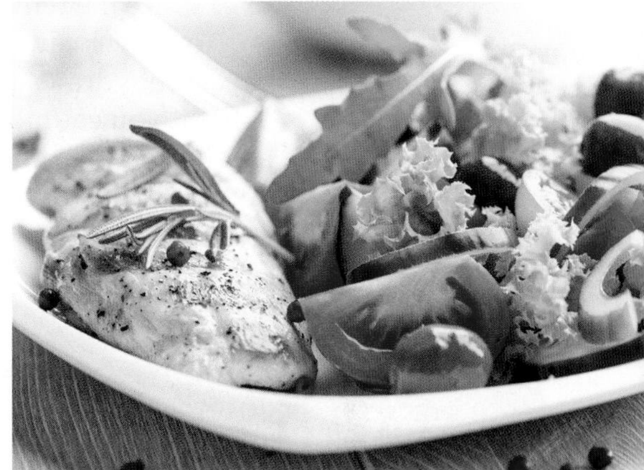

Barbara Dudzinska/Shutterstock.com

Figure 6.4 The vegetables in this meal provide fiber that is important for maintaining digestive health. They are also low in calories and fat.

How Your Body Uses Carbohydrates

Eating carbohydrates, regardless of their source, sets off a complex chain of events in your body. The way your body uses carbohydrates is explained here in simplified terms.

Energy Source

All carbohydrates must be in the form of glucose for your cells to use them as an energy source. To achieve this, your digestive system first breaks down poly- and disaccharides from foods into monosaccharides. The monosaccharides are small enough to move across the intestinal wall and into the blood. They travel via the blood to the liver. Any fructose and galactose in the blood is converted into glucose in the liver.

When the amount of glucose in the blood increases (this happens after you eat), a hormone called *insulin* is released from the pancreas. ***Hormones*** are chemicals produced in the body and released into the bloodstream to regulate specific body processes. ***Insulin*** helps the body lower blood glucose back to a normal level. Insulin does this by triggering body cells to burn glucose for energy. It also causes muscles and the liver to store glucose. In healthy bodies, blood glucose is carefully managed. If carbohydrates are not broken down, then the body begins to break down protein and fats for energy. When blood glucose levels become too high, cells can be damaged. Diabetes—the disease related to insulin use and production—is described in a later section.

Energy Storage

If your cells do not have immediate energy needs, the excess glucose from the bloodstream is stored (**Figure 6.5**). The cells convert the glucose into glycogen. ***Glycogen*** is the body's stored form of glucose. Two-thirds of your body's glycogen is stored in your muscles for use as an energy source during muscular activity. Your liver stores the remaining one-third of the glycogen for use by the rest of your body.

Your liver can store only a limited amount of glycogen. Therefore, you need to eat carbohydrates throughout the day to **replenish** (restore) your glycogen stores. What if you eat more carbohydrates than your body can immediately use or store as glycogen? In this case, your liver converts the excess carbohydrates into fat. An unlimited amount of fat can be stored in the fatty tissues of your body. Unlike glycogen stores, fat stores cannot be converted back into glucose.

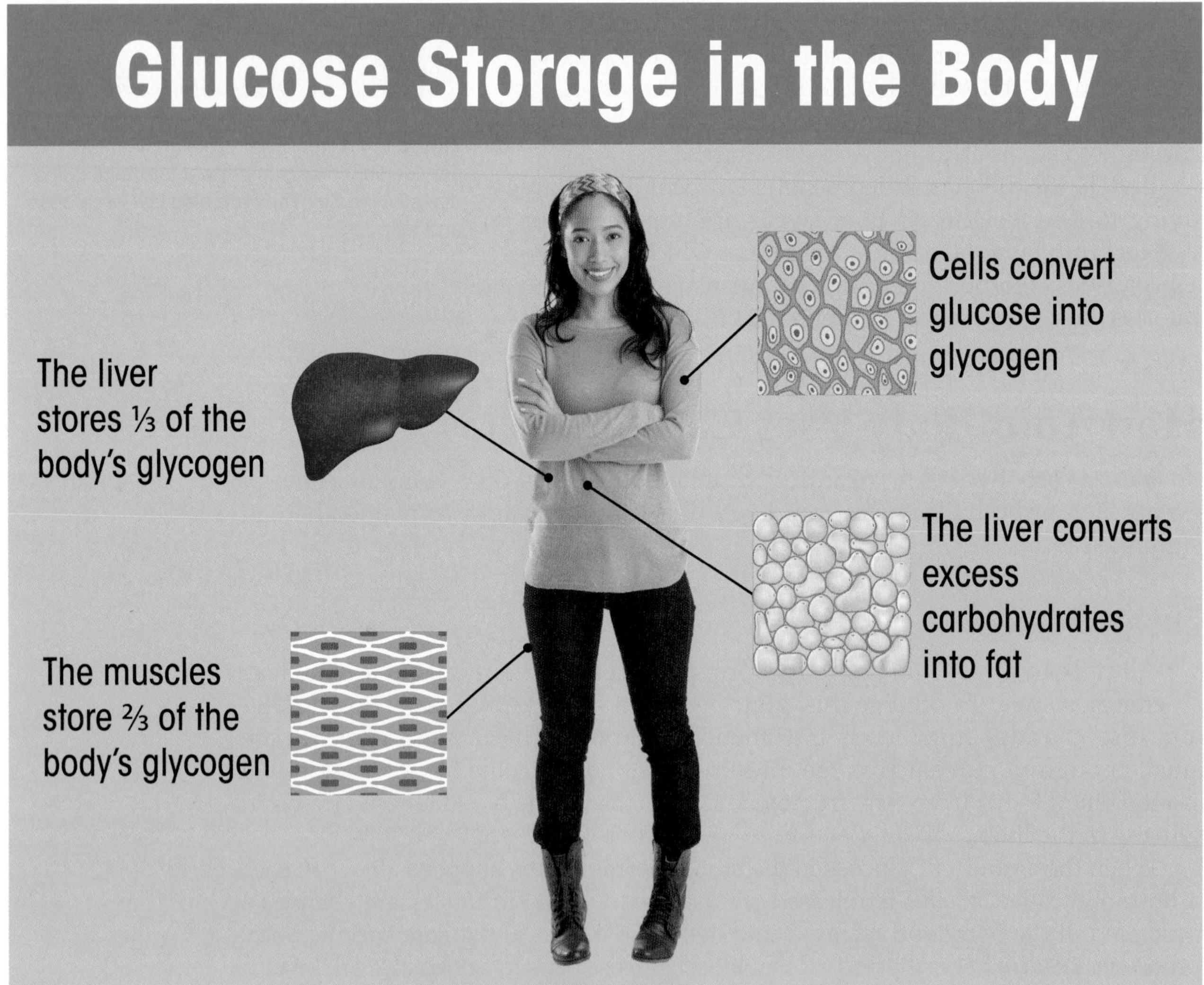
Glucose Storage in the Body
Cells convert glucose into glycogen
The liver stores ⅓ of the body's glycogen
The liver converts excess carbohydrates into fat
The muscles store ⅔ of the body's glycogen

Clockwise, from the top: tmcphotos/Shutterstock.com; Marochkina Anastasiia/Shutterstock.com; WhiteDragon/Shutterstock.com; Designua/Shutterstock.com; Exclusivelly/Shutterstock.com

Figure 6.5 The storage of glucose in the body.

THE MOVEMENT CONNECTION

Fueling Activity

Why

We learned in this chapter that "carbs" are the body's preferred fuel. Carbohydrates produce energy, spare proteins, breakdown fats, and provide bulk.

The human body requires energy for exercise and physical activity, as well as to perform daily activities. Higher intensity activities will require more energy from sources like a balanced diet and adequate sleep.

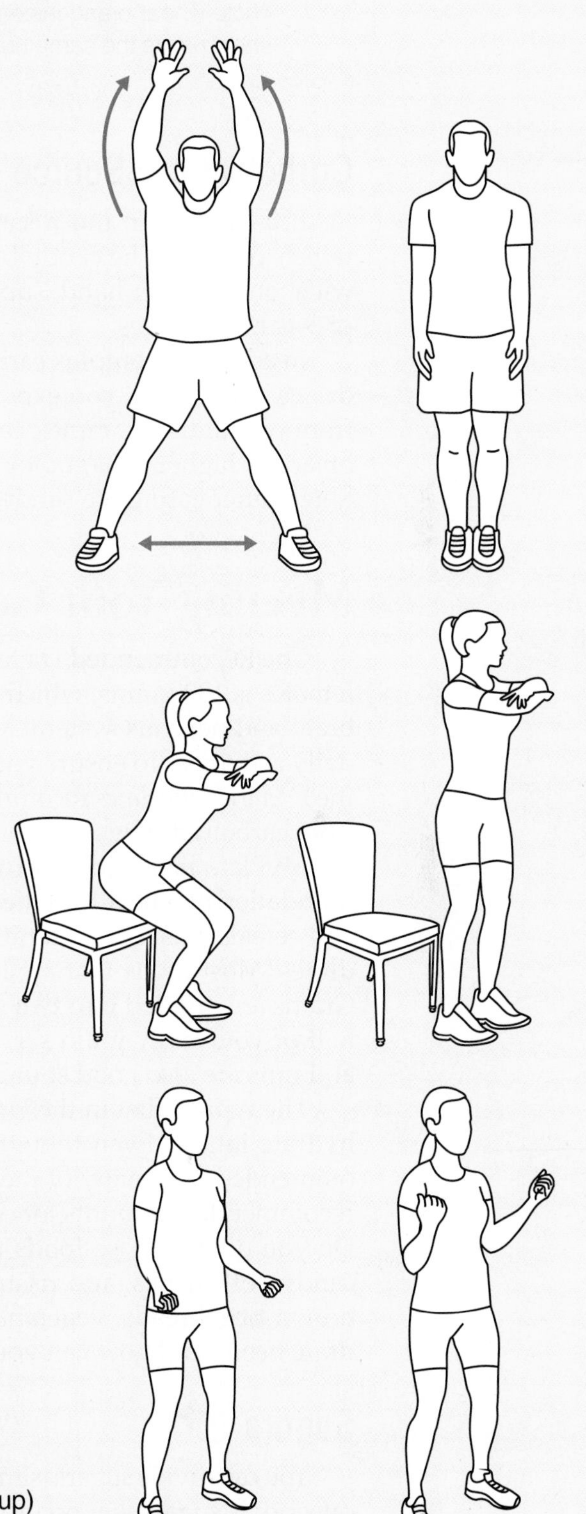

Apply

For this exercise, you will need a partner. One partner will call out a function of carbohydrates. The other partner will perform the activity listed with that function as follows:

Produce energy–perform 3 jumping jacks
Spare proteins–rest
Breakdown fats–perform 3 chair squats
Provide bulk–perform 3 air bicep curls

Jumping Jacks

- Simultaneously jump up and open legs to a wide stance while clapping your hands together overhead.
- Return arms to sides and feet together. If injury or attire prevent you from jumping safely, only perform the arm movements.

Rest

- Stand for 5 seconds.

Chair Squats

- See *The Movement Connection* in Chapter 4.
- Ensure proper form to avoid injury.

Air Bicep Curls

- Stand with good posture and arms at side.
- Rotate arms slightly so that palms are facing forward and then make loose fists with both hands.
- Bend at the elbows and slowly raise your fists to shoulders. Arms should raise slowly (2 seconds up) and lower slowly (2 seconds down).

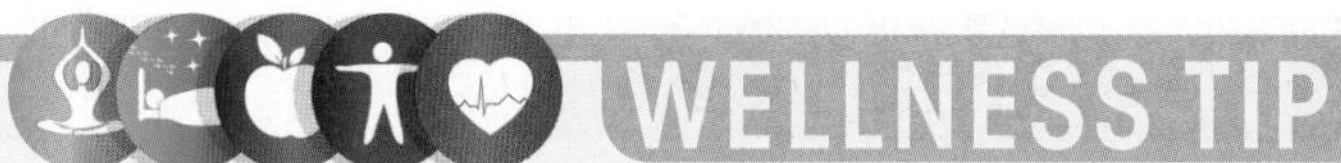

Choose White Whole Wheat

If you find the flavor and texture of whole-wheat bread unappealing, try white whole-wheat bread instead. Made from an albino variety of wheat, white whole wheat packs the same nutritional benefits and fiber as its red wheat counterpart.

Carbohydrate Source Matters

If a candy bar and a sandwich both end up as glucose, why does it matter which you eat? The candy bar provides little more than added sugars. The sandwich, on the other hand, supplies vitamins, minerals, and protein, as well as complex carbohydrates.

In addition, complex carbohydrates take longer to digest than simple carbohydrates. As a result, you experience greater **satiety** (feeling of fullness after eating) from consuming complex carbohydrates. The sandwich, made with whole-grain bread, is higher in complex carbohydrates. Therefore, you are likely to feel full longer after eating the sandwich than after eating the candy bar.

Meeting Your Carbohydrate Needs

The Recommended Dietary Allowance (RDA) for carbohydrates for males and females is 130 grams, which is the amount required to meet glucose needs for the brain and nervous system. More carbohydrates are needed to provide energy for daily activities. To ensure you are providing your body with the nutrients it needs, the *Dietary Guidelines* recommends that 45 to 65 percent of your total calories come from carbohydrates.

MyPlate lists and describes a variety of carbohydrate foods to make up the foundation of a healthful diet. Many popular foods, including whole-grain breads and cereals, pasta, nonfat milk, fruits, and vegetables, are rich sources of carbohydrates. Most foods that are high in carbohydrates are found in the grains group. Grains are divided into two subgroups—whole grains and refined grains. At least half of your daily grain servings should be whole grains. Legumes, peas, beans, and nuts are also good sources of carbohydrates.

The typical diet in the United States fails to meet recommendations for carbohydrate intake. Even though most Americans eat more carbohydrates than recommended, too many of these are simple carbohydrates. Many diets fall short of recommended amounts for complex carbohydrates. How does your diet compare? Do you often choose foods that are high in simple sugars, such as milk shakes, candy, soft drinks, and pastries? Do you choose complex carbohydrates such as brown rice, breads, vegetables, and legumes less often? What are your carbohydrate needs and how can you choose foods to meet them?

Sugars

You can divide sugars (simple carbohydrates) in foods into two categories. The first category is sugars that occur naturally in foods. These sugars include lactose in milk and fructose in fruits. Naturally occurring sugars are generally accompanied by other nutrients in foods. Therefore, they do not cause great concern among nutrition experts.

Sources of Added Sugar

The second category, added sugars, includes sugars and syrups that are added to foods and beverages during either processing or preparation. They come from such sources as sugarcane, sugar beets, and corn. Sugars are added to foods for reasons other than just sweetening. They may also be added to foods to increase bulk or aid in browning.

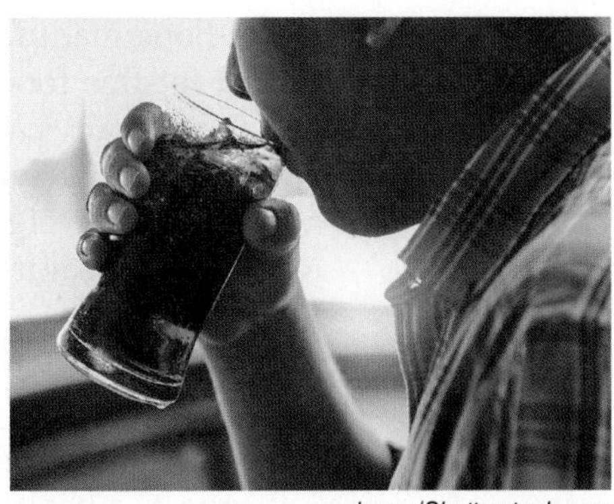

nednapa/Shutterstock.com

Figure 6.6 Intake of sugar-sweetened beverages should be limited. Added sugars in these beverages provide calories but no nutrients.

Sugar-sweetened beverages, such as soft drinks, fruit drinks, sweet teas, coffee drinks, sports drinks, and energy drinks, are the main source of added sugar in teen diets (**Figure 6.6**). Many other foods high in added sugar, such as candy, cakes, cookies, and donuts, are also high in fat. Eating too many of these foods can mean too many calories and not enough nutrients. This can lead to overweight and malnutrition.

Many processed foods, such as ketchup and ready-to-eat cereals, are also high in added sugars. Although sugar is an excellent source of simple carbohydrates, it contributes no other nutrients to foods. In other words, sugars increase the calories a food provides without increasing the nutrients it provides. Added sugars reduce the nutrient density of processed foods.

Food manufacturers often use *high-fructose corn syrup (HFCS)* to add sweetness to foods. HFCS is made by converting about half of the glucose found in cornstarch into fructose. The resulting product is sweeter than sucrose. HFCS is produced and sold to food manufacturers for its enhanced sweetening power. It is used in sports drinks, high-energy food bars, and other popular snack foods.

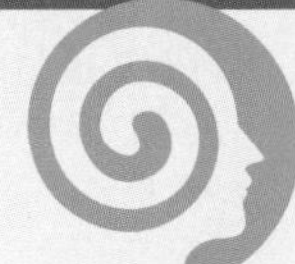

EXTEND YOUR KNOWLEDGE

Nonnutritive Sweeteners

Many people turn to low-calorie sweeteners to satisfy their sweet tooth while limiting calories. These low-calorie sweeteners contribute no or very few calories to foods and beverages, but provide more than 100 times the sweetening power of sugar. A number of low-calorie sweeteners have been approved for use in foods and drinks including

- Acesulfame potassium (known as acesulfame K or Ace-K)
- Advantame
- Aspartame
- Luo han guo (monk fruit extract)
- Neotame
- Saccharine
- Rebaudioside A (Reb-A) stevia
- Sucralose

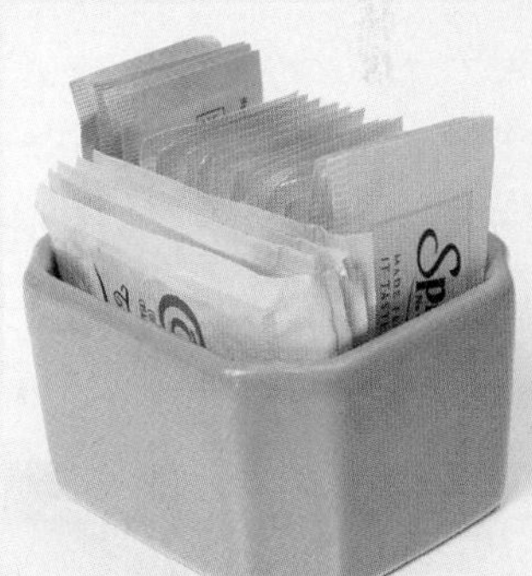

PeterG/Shutterstock.com

Saccharin, Ace-K, sucralose, and Reb-A stevia can be substituted for sugar in baking. Refer to each product's package for directions on substitution amounts when replacing sugar in a recipe. Substitution equivalents vary depending on the product being used and its form (granular, liquid, or other). Neotame is stable when heated, but is not sold to consumers in packet or bulk form and does not include cooking instructions.

Another group of reduced-calorie sweeteners called *polyols* or *sugar alcohols* are most often used in desserts, candy, and chewing gum.

Search the Internet or study food labels at the supermarket to learn the brand names of the low-calorie sweeteners.

Food manufacturers often replace fat with added sugar to produce reduced-fat and fat-free food products. Although these products are lower in fat, they often have as many calories as regular products. Some consumers mistakenly think they can eat more when they choose reduced-fat snacks. These consumers may end up gaining weight rather than losing it. You can read food labels to determine the number of calories per serving and the total calorie content.

Added Sugar Recommendation

Results of a nationwide survey reveal that Americans consume more than 13 percent of their total calories per day from added sugars. The *Dietary Guidelines* suggests a healthy eating pattern should limit added sugars to 10 percent of total calories. For a person following a 2,000-calorie food plan, the daily limit for added sugars would be about 200 calories per day.

How much sugar can you consume for 200 calories? Since one teaspoon of sugar contains approximately 16 calories, that means approximately 12 teaspoons of sugar will yield 200 calories.

200 calories ÷ 16 calories/teaspoon sugar = 12½ teaspoons

Just one 12-ounce orange soda contains slightly more than 11 teaspoons of sugar! With just this one beverage, you will have nearly reached the recommended limit of added sugars in your daily diet (**Figure 6.7**).

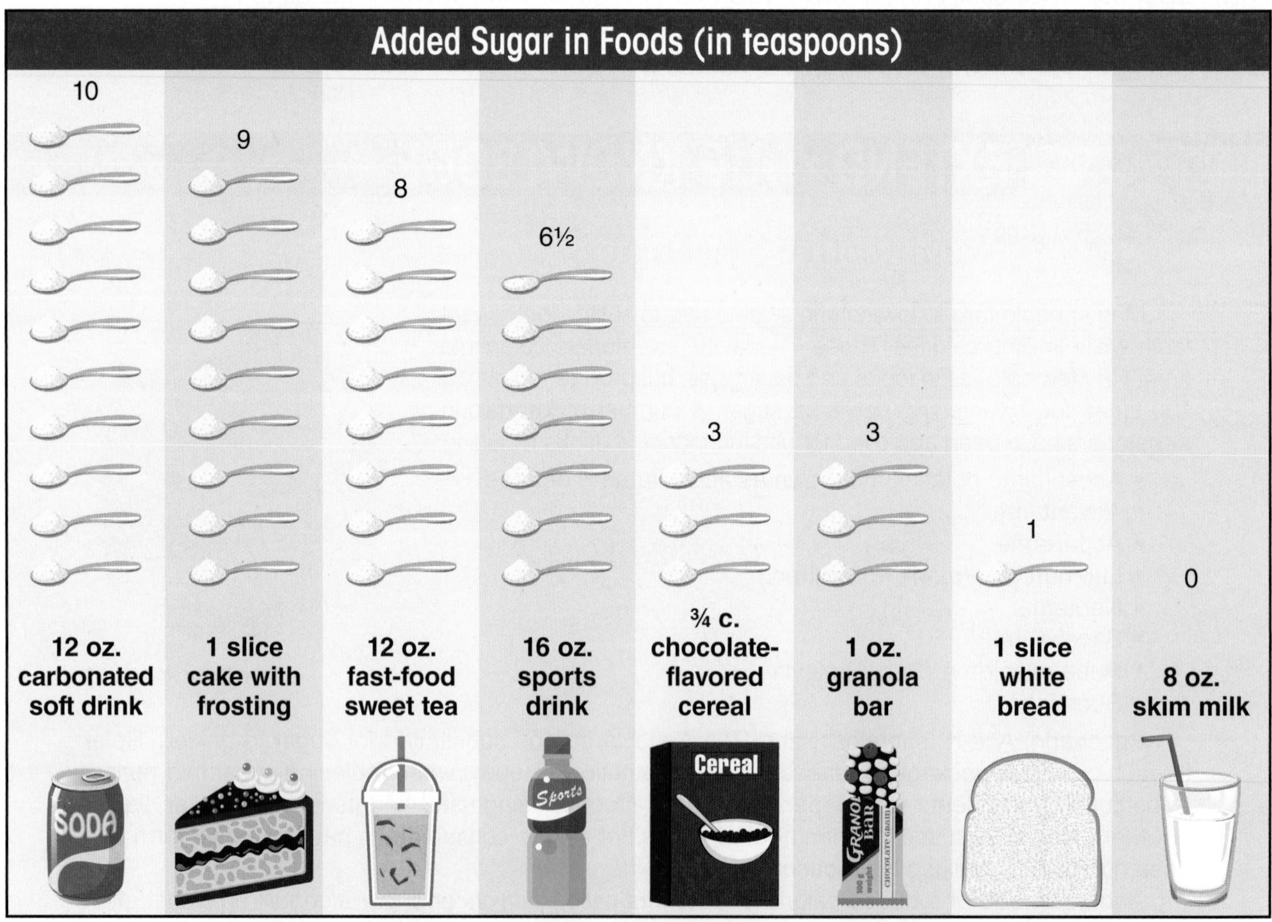

L to r: Altagracia Art/Shutterstock.com; Wor Sang Jun/Shutterstock.com; Suriyub/Shutterstock.com; Natykach Nataliia/Shutterstock.com; Banana Walking/Shutterstock.com; vectorisland/Shutterstock.com; Rinat Sultanov/Shutterstock.com; Tribalium/Shutterstock.com; nicemonkey/Shutterstock.com; MicroOne/Shutterstock.com; moremari/Shutterstock.com; Zeki Michael/Shutterstock.com; (spoons) Vasilyeva Larisa/Shutterstock.com

Figure 6.7 The number of teaspoons of added sugar in your favorite foods may surprise you.

The American Heart Association (AHA) recommends lower limits for added sugars. They suggest that women limit their added sugar intake to about 6 teaspoons per day and men limit theirs to about 9 teaspoons per day. The AHA reported findings that too much added sugar in the diet increases the risks of cardiovascular disease and contributes to the obesity epidemic.

The *Dietary Guidelines for Americans* recommends that calories from solid fats and added sugars combined should account for no more than 5 to 15 percent of total daily calories.

Starches

Starches are the body's preferred source of fuel. Your body can burn them efficiently for energy, and they have greater satiety value than simple sugars. Many starchy foods are also excellent sources of vitamins, minerals, and fiber.

Nutrition experts agree that your carbohydrate intake should primarily consist of fruits, vegetables, whole-grain breads and cereals, and beans. Following MyPlate helps you achieve this goal. The grain group is an excellent source of foods high in starch. Foods in the vegetable group and legumes from the protein foods group are also high in starch.

Fiber

The recommended intakes for fiber are

- 38 grams per day for males ages 14 through 50;
- 26 grams per day for 14- to 18-year-old females; and
- 25 grams per day for women ages 19 through 50.

These recommendations are based on intakes that have been shown to help protect against heart disease. Most people must at least double their current fiber intakes to meet these recommendations.

You can begin increasing your fiber intake by choosing whole-grain products in place of refined-grain products whenever possible. Whole-grain products contain all three edible parts of the grain kernel—bran, germ, and endosperm (**Figure 6.8**).

- *Bran* is the outer layer of the grain, which is a good source of fiber.
- *Germ* is the nutrient-rich part of the kernel.
- *Endosperm* is the largest part of the kernel and contains mostly starch.

Processing that produces refined-grain products also removes the bran, germ, and most of the fiber from grain. White flour and white rice are examples of refined-grain products.

Some people use fiber supplements to add fiber to their diets. A ***supplement*** is a concentrated source of a nutrient, usually in pill, liquid, or powder form. Supplements do not offer the range of nutritional benefits provided by food sources of nutrients.

For most people, fiber supplements are unnecessary. Meeting your fiber needs is easy if you eat the recommended amounts from MyPlate. An average serving of most whole-grain breads and cereals, vegetables, or fruits provides three grams of fiber. Dry beans provide up to eight grams per serving. Other high-fiber foods include cooked lentils, peas, and nuts.

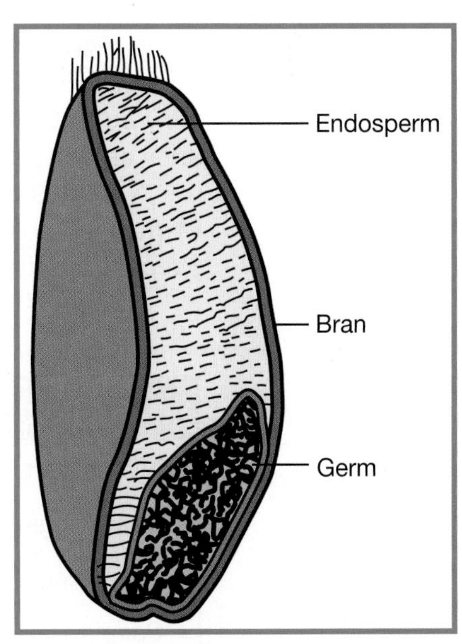

Goodheart-Willcox Publisher

Figure 6.8 Refined grains have had the germ and the fiber-rich bran layer removed. Choose whole-grain bread and cereal products for the nutrients contained in all three parts of the kernel.

As you change your eating habits, increase your intake of dietary fiber slowly. This helps your body adjust. A sudden large increase of dietary fiber may cause digestive discomfort. Be sure to drink plenty of water as you increase your fiber intake.

Using Food Labels to Meet Your Carbohydrate Needs

Reading food labels can help you meet your carbohydrate needs. The Nutrition Facts panel on a food label lists the amount of carbohydrates a food product contains. The amount labeled "Total Carbohydrate" includes all of the starches, fiber, and sugars present in the food product. Subtotals are listed under Total Carbohydrates to identify the amounts of Dietary Fiber, Total Sugars, and Added Sugars in the product. The amount listed for "Total Sugars" includes naturally occurring sugars—such as those found in milk or fruit—as well as any added sugars.

You can identify the sources of added sugar in a food product by reading the ingredient list (**Figure 6.9**). Reading the ingredient list can also help you increase your intake of whole grains. When selecting carbohydrate foods, look for the word "whole" in the first ingredient listed. For example, choose breads that list whole-wheat flour as the first ingredient rather than simply wheat flour or enriched flour. Other whole-grain ingredients include whole-grain cornmeal, brown rice, wheat berries, whole-grain rye, oats, and buckwheat.

The Glycemic Index (GI)

The term *glycemic index* is frequently used by people on special diets or people trying to lose weight when they make carbohydrate choices. The ***glycemic index (GI)*** is a measure of the speed at which various carbohydrates are digested into glucose, absorbed, and enter the bloodstream. Pure glucose raises blood glucose levels more quickly than any other carbohydrate. Foods with a high GI score produce a quick, steep increase in blood glucose, often followed by a rapid drop in blood glucose levels. Foods with a lower GI score result in slower, less dramatic increases in blood glucose levels. Dramatic swings in blood glucose are not healthy. The glycemic index may be a helpful tool for individuals trying to prevent or manage chronic illnesses such as heart disease and diabetes.

A food is assigned a GI score based on how it compares to an equal amount of pure glucose (GI = 100). Assigning GI scores to foods is not a precise science. Preparation methods, food combinations, and individual differences in metabolisms

Figure 6.9
Read the ingredient lists on food labels to learn what added sugars the food contains.

Identifying Added Sugars on the Label		
• Agave syrup	• Fructose	• Maltose
• Brown sugar	• Fruit juice concentrate	• Malt syrup
• Cane juice	• Glucose	• Molasses
• Cane syrup	• High-fructose corn syrup	• Raw sugar
• Corn sweetener	• Honey	• Sucrose
• Corn syrup	• Invert sugar	• Syrup
• Dextrose	• Lactose	• White granulated sugar

affect GI measurements. A person can have different GI scores for the same food eaten at different times of the day. Carbohydrates consumed with fat, protein, or fiber are digested and absorbed more slowly. Therefore, a plain slice of white bread has a much higher GI score than a slice of white bread with peanut butter (**Figure 6.10**).

Using the glycemic index can be a valuable strategy when combined with other tools that help you select healthful whole-grain foods, legumes, and nuts along with a varied selection of other fruits and vegetables. These foods are absorbed slowly and provide more stable levels of blood glucose levels. The complex carbohydrates take longer to digest than simple carbohydrates, and their satiety value is greater. The greater satiety value provided by complex carbohydrates helps people who are trying to reduce their calorie intake eat less (**Figure 6.11**).

Categorizing Foods by Glycemic Index

- **Low glycemic index** (GI of 55 or less): Most fruits and vegetables, beans, legumes, dairy products, and nuts
- **Moderate glycemic index** (GI 56 to 69): White and sweet potatoes, corn, brown rice, couscous, rolled oats
- **High glycemic index** (GI of 70 or higher): Potatoes, rice, white bread, rice cakes, most crackers, bagels, cakes, candy, doughnuts, croissants, waffles, most packaged breakfast cereals

Figure 6.10 Glycemic index scores are measured using glucose as a reference.

Health Questions Related to Carbohydrates

As you read about the importance of carbohydrates in your diet, you may find yourself thinking of specific questions. Many teens and their parents want to know the answers to these frequently asked questions.

Are Starchy Foods Fattening?

Some people believe eating foods high in starch causes weight gain. Starchy foods are rich in carbohydrates. At four calories per gram, carbohydrates have the same amount of calories per gram as protein and less than half the calories per gram of fat.

Some people may think starchy foods are fattening because of the way these foods are served. Pasta is often served with cream sauce, rice with gravy, and baked potatoes with sour cream. Such high-fat toppings can send the total calories in carbohydrate dishes soaring.

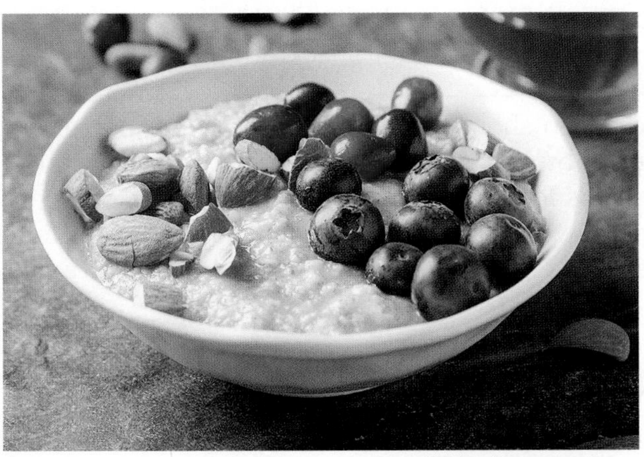

A Gaus Nataliya/Shutterstock.com

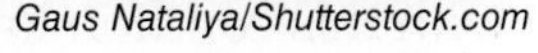

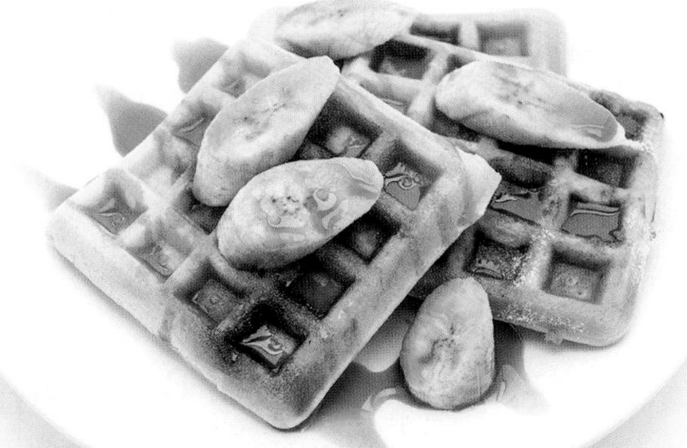

B topnatthapon/Shutterstock.com

Figure 6.11 A complex carbohydrate like whole-grain oatmeal will likely make you feel full longer. *Which of these breakfasts do you think has a lower glycemic index?*

Consider the example of a slice of bread, which has about 12 grams of carbohydrates and 65 calories. Spreading one teaspoon of butter on the bread adds 4 grams of fat and 36 more calories. If you are trying to reduce calorie intake, limit the use of high-fat toppings. Also, remember the recommended portion size and serving size of the carbohydrate foods you are consuming. For example, eating three pieces of plain bread provides more calories than eating one piece of bread with one tablespoon of butter.

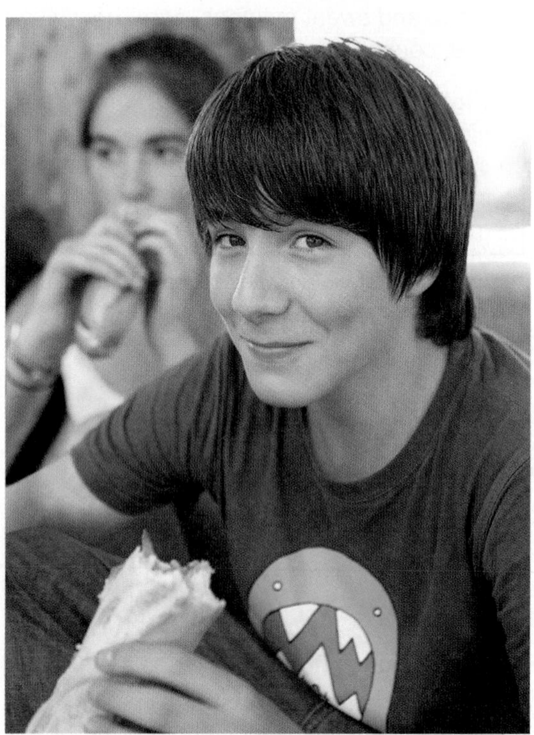

Phovoir/Shutterstock.com

Figure 6.12 This teen is eating a sandwich for lunch. The bread in the sandwich is a source of carbohydrates. ***How does the risk of cavities from eating this bread now differ from eating bread for a snack?***

Is Sugar a Hazard to Your Teeth?

There is a clear connection between sweets and ***dental caries*** (tooth decay). People who eat too much sugar throughout the day are likely to have a higher incidence of tooth decay than people who eat less sugar. Sugar is not the only culprit, however. Starches can promote tooth decay, too.

Bacteria that live in the mouth feed on the carbohydrates in food particles. The bacteria form a sticky substance called *plaque* that clings to teeth. As the bacteria grow, they produce acid that eats away the protective tooth enamel, forming pits in the teeth. In time, these pits can deepen into cavities.

The risk of dental caries depends on two main factors—the type of food and when you eat it (**Figure 6.12**). Sticky carbohydrate foods, such as raisins, cookies, crackers, and caramels, tend to cling to teeth. They are more harmful than foods that are quickly swallowed and removed from contact with the teeth. Likewise, sugars and starches eaten between meals tend to be more harmful to tooth enamel than carbohydrates consumed at meals. Food particles from between-meal snacks tend to remain in the mouth—and in contact with teeth—for longer periods. When carbohydrates are eaten in a meal, beverages and other foods from the meal help remove food particles from the mouth.

Avoiding sticky, carbohydrate-rich foods between meals is good advice for keeping teeth healthy. If you do eat sticky foods, drink plenty of water to wash your teeth. If brushing and flossing your teeth after snacking is possible, this is even better.

People who care for young children should know tooth damage can begin in early infancy. Regularly allowing a baby to sleep with a bottle in his or her mouth can destroy the baby's teeth. The acids formed by constant contact of bacteria with sugars in the milk will **erode** (wear away) the baby's tooth enamel. After feeding, caregivers should gently clean the baby's gums and teeth by wiping them with a soft, clean cloth.

Does Sugar Cause Hyperactivity?

Hyperactivity is a condition in which a person seems to be in constant motion and is easily distracted. Children with this condition may disrupt their classmates and have trouble concentrating on their schoolwork. Many teachers and parents observe that children are more active after parties and other events at which sweets are served. This has led some people to believe sugar causes hyperactivity.

Although researchers have conducted many studies, they have found no proof that consuming sugars causes behavior changes in most people. It is true that eating sugars gives children the energy needed to fuel activity; however, children at a party may exhibit rowdy behavior simply because they are excited (**Figure 6.13**). After all, eating and playing with friends are fun social activities. Caregivers may find that leading children in less-active games at the end of a party helps reduce post-party excitement.

Caregivers should also keep in mind that children who eat large amounts of sweets may be missing some important nutrients in their diets. If you know a child who has trouble concentrating, look at his or her total diet. Eating a well-balanced diet that replaces sweets with nutritious snacks can help improve performance.

Is Sugar Addictive?

Some people seem to crave sweets all the time. There are those who believe this type of craving qualifies as an **addiction** (dependence).

Experiments have shown that if animals do not have a nutritious diet, they will eat excessive amounts of sugar. When the animals are allowed to eat a variety of foods, they seem to be less dependent on sugar. This indicates the animals did not truly need the sugar. Therefore, *addiction* is not the best word to use to explain the animals' excessive consumption of sugar.

Research has shown that people are born with a preference for sweet-tasting foods. Researchers now seem to think the need for sugar is more psychological than physiological. In other words, people seem to eat sweets because they enjoy them, not because they are addicted to them.

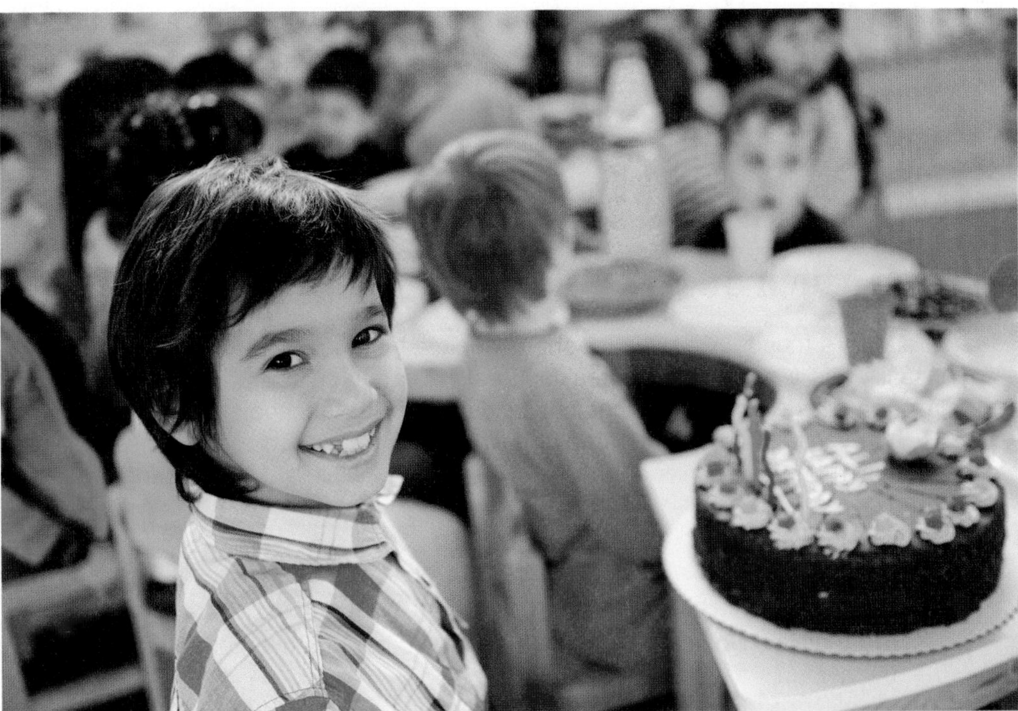

ESB Professional/Shutterstock.com

Figure 6.13
Excitable behavior is more likely to be caused by the party itself and not the cake being served there.

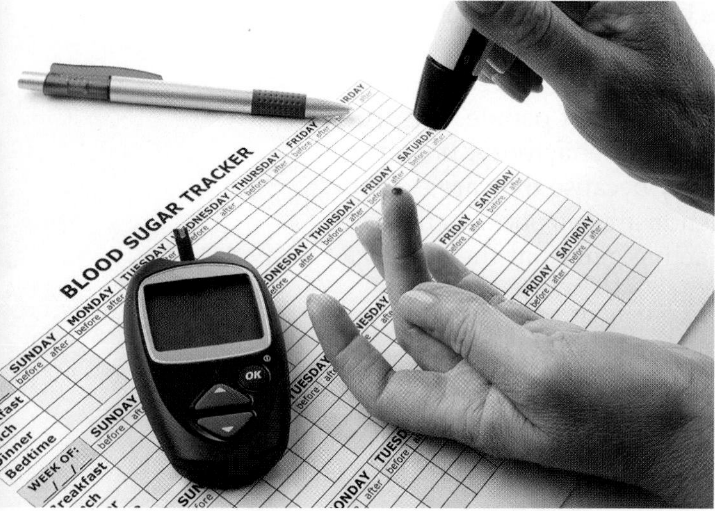

Zaretska Olga/Shutterstock.com

Figure 6.14 People with type 1 diabetes must check their blood glucose level regularly throughout the day.

Does Eating Too Much Sugar Cause Diabetes?

Diabetes mellitus, or *diabetes*, is characterized by a lack of or an inability to use the hormone insulin. Sugars and starches in the foods you eat are converted into glucose, which then enters the bloodstream. Insulin regulates the blood glucose level by stimulating cells to pull glucose from the bloodstream. When the body does not make enough insulin, or it fails to use insulin correctly, glucose builds up in the bloodstream.

There are two main types of diabetes. In *type 1 diabetes*, the pancreas is unable to make insulin. This type occurs most often in children and young adults, so it is also known as *juvenile-onset diabetes*. People with type 1 diabetes must take daily injections of insulin to maintain normal blood glucose levels (**Figure 6.14**). This type represents 5 to 10 percent of all diagnosed cases.

In *type 2 diabetes*, body cells do not respond well to the insulin the pancreas makes. This type of diabetes is much more common and represents about 90 to 95 percent of all diagnosed cases. Sometimes called *adult-onset diabetes*, this type usually occurs in adults over age 40. As rates of overweight and obesity increase, however, so does the incidence of type 2 diabetes. People who are overweight and eat diets high in refined carbohydrates and low in fiber are at greater risk of developing this type of diabetes. People in the later stages of this disease may require insulin injections. In the earlier stages, however, type 2 diabetes can often be controlled with diet and physical activity.

CASE STUDY

Too Much Sugar?

Mary's friends often tell her she is addicted to sugar. She usually has a soft drink for breakfast, eats a candy bar for a mid-morning snack, and brings cupcakes for lunch at school. In the evening, her parents always have ice cream or cookies for dessert. She often has soft drinks and more sweet snacks while studying during the evening.

Case Review

1. Why do you think Mary is or is not addicted to sugar?
2. What advice would you give to Mary to help her improve her eating behaviors?

Both types of diabetes tend to run in families. Symptoms of both types include excessive hunger and thirst accompanied by weakness, irritability, and nausea. Changes in eyesight; slow healing of cuts; drowsiness; and numbness in the legs, feet, or fingers are symptoms, too.

In both types of diabetes, the blood glucose level rises too high. Although eating sugar increases the blood glucose level, it does not cause diabetes to develop. However, diabetics need to regulate their sugar intake by following a diet plan prescribed by a physician or registered dietitian.

What Is Hypoglycemia?

Hypoglycemia refers to a low blood glucose level. In this condition, an overproduction of insulin causes blood sugar to drop sharply two to four hours after eating a meal. The central nervous system depends on a constant supply of glucose from the blood. Low blood sugar causes physical symptoms of sweating, shaking, headaches, hunger, and anxiety.

A medical test is required to diagnose true hypoglycemia. This condition is rare and may point to a more severe health problem. Many people who believe they have hypoglycemia may just be reacting to stress.

The dietary advice for people with hypoglycemia is sensible for all people. That is, avoid eating large amounts of sugar all at once. Also, eat nutritious meals at regular intervals.

What Is Lactose Intolerance?

Lactose intolerance is an inability to digest lactose, the main carbohydrate in milk. This condition is caused by a lack of the digestive enzyme *lactase*, which is needed to break down lactose (**Figure 6.15**). People who are lactose intolerant may experience gas, cramping, nausea, and diarrhea when they consume dairy products.

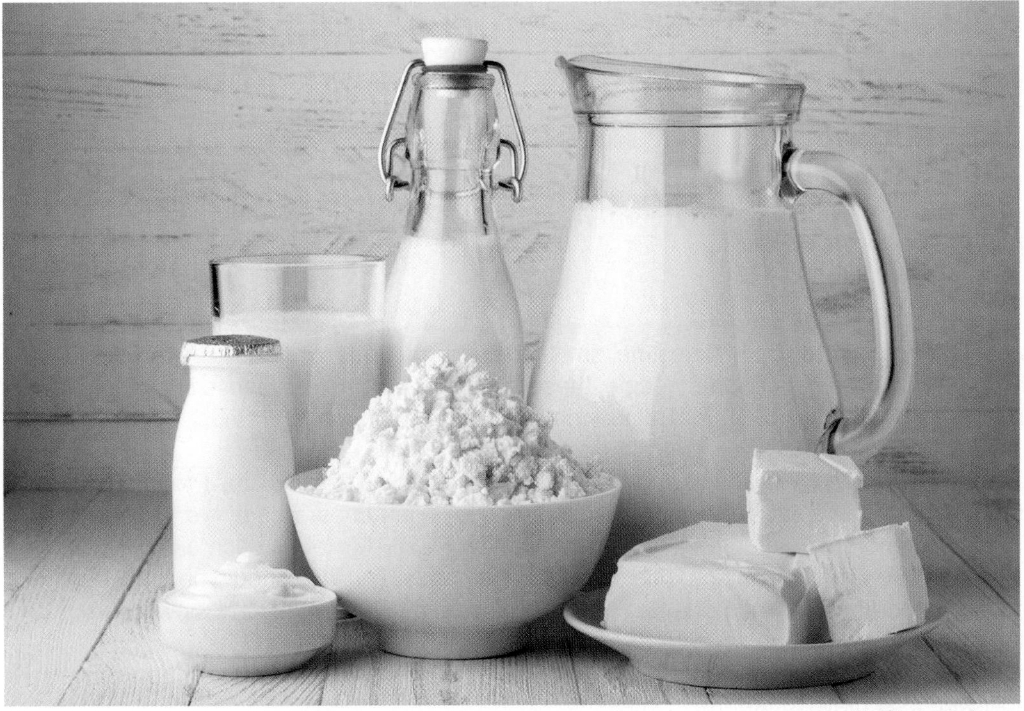

nevodka/Shutterstock.com

Figure 6.15 Someone who is lactose intolerant may be able to digest cheese more easily than milk.

Lactose intolerance is common throughout the world. It occurs more often among nonwhite populations and tends to develop as people age.

Milk and other dairy products are the chief sources of calcium and vitamin D in the diet. These nutrients help build strong bones and teeth. They are especially important for children and pregnant women.

People who are unable to drink milk must meet their calcium needs through other sources. Some people can tolerate small amounts of milk if they consume it with a meal. They may also be able to consume cultured milk products such as yogurt, cheese, and buttermilk. Lactose in these products is changed into lactic acid or broken down into glucose and galactose during the culturing process. Another option is to take lactase pills or add lactase drops to dairy foods to ease digestion.

Soy milk is a lactose-free beverage alternative. This nondairy beverage is made from soybeans. Calcium-fortified soy milk can meet calcium needs without producing unpleasant digestive issues.

Does Dietary Fiber Prevent Disease?

Fiber has been shown to have many benefits besides providing bulk in the diet. Current interest in fiber stems from observations made by British scientists around 1923. They noted that African populations had lower rates of certain gastrointestinal (GI) tract diseases, such as colon cancer, compared to Western industrialized populations. This led the scientists to study the differences in the eating patterns of the two populations. They found that people in Western countries had rather low fiber intakes. In contrast, people in the African nations tended to have high fiber intakes. The scientists hypothesized the difference in the disease rate could be related to the difference in fiber consumption.

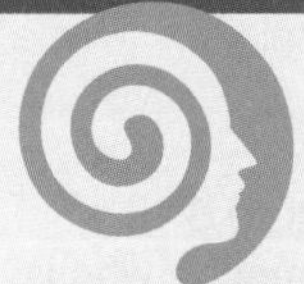

EXTEND YOUR KNOWLEDGE

What Are FODMAPs?

FODMAP is an acronym that describes types of carbohydrates that cause digestive issues for some individuals.

Fermentable
Oligosaccharides
Disaccharides
Monosaccharides
And
Polyols

FODMAPs are poorly absorbed in the intestine, small in size, and fermented easily by the bacteria found in the digestive system. For some people, these sugars and fibers can cause symptoms similar to irritable bowel syndrome (IBS), including stomach bloating, stomach cramps, diarrhea, and nausea.

To alleviate these symptoms, individuals may be instructed to follow the FODMAP diet. This diet restricts high-FODMAP foods such as onions, pears, cow's milk, legumes, wheat, rye, cashew, and some artificial sweeteners. The diet replaces these with low-FODMAP foods such as carrots, bananas, soy milk, meat, poultry, fish, quinoa, rice cakes, and almonds. This diet should be followed for a limited time and under the guidance of a healthcare professional. Then foods are slowly reintroduced to determine which foods are causing distress.

Research other foods that are considered either high- or low-FODMAP foods. Learn how this diet should be followed to achieve long-term success.

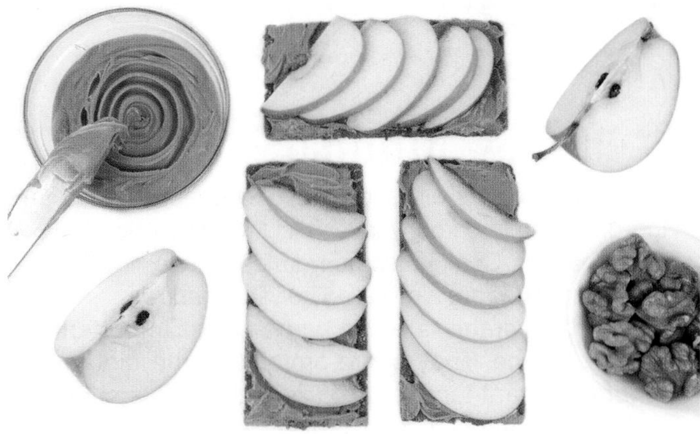

Kitamin/Shutterstock.com

Figure 6.16 To obtain the recommended amount of fiber each day, try substituting these tasty snacks for snacks that contain added sugars. *Can you think of other high-fiber snacks?*

Numerous studies have been conducted to find out more about the role fiber plays in promoting wellness. Research results indicate that including plenty of fiber in a low-fat diet appears to have many health benefits. For example, dietary fiber along with adequate fluids can help prevent *appendicitis*, or inflammation of the appendix. It may lower the risk of heart disease. Dietary fiber may reduce the risk of colon cancer. It also helps control blood glucose levels.

Fibers vary in their composition and in the jobs they perform in the GI tract. Eating a variety of fruits, vegetables, and whole grains gives you the full range of benefits from dietary fiber. Foods such as raisins, nuts, oranges, apples, carrot sticks, and seeds are high in fiber and make great snacks (**Figure 6.16**). These foods also provide health-promoting nutrients, including starch, protein, vitamins, minerals, and other important compounds.

RECIPE FILE

Chicken Minestrone Soup

6 SERVINGS

Ingredients

- 1 can (28 oz.) low-sodium crushed tomatoes in juice, undrained
- 4 c. low-sodium chicken broth
- 1 lb. boneless, skinless chicken thighs, cut into 1-inch chunks
- 1 medium red potato, diced
- ½ c. onion, chopped
- ½ c. carrots, chopped
- ½ c. celery, chopped
- ¼ t. ground pepper
- 1 can (14 oz.) cannellini beans, drained and rinsed
- 1 medium zucchini, diced
- ¼ c. prepared basil pesto

Directions

1. Mix all ingredients except cannellini beans, zucchini, and pesto, in a large pot over high heat.
2. Once ingredients reach boiling, reduce heat to a simmer.
3. Cover and simmer for 30–45 minutes, or until chicken is cooked through and vegetables are tender.
4. Stir in cannellini beans, zucchini, and pesto.
5. Continue simmering until zucchini is tender-crisp.
6. Ladle into bowls and top each with 2 teaspoons pesto.

PER SERVING: 369 CALORIES, 30 G PROTEIN, 40 G CARBOHYDRATE, 10 G FAT, 9 G FIBER, 389 MG SODIUM.

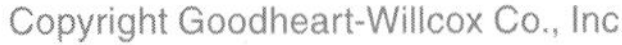

Chapter 6 Review and Expand

Reading Summary

Carbohydrates are sugars, starches, and fibers in the diet. Simple carbohydrates include the mono- and disaccharides. Complex carbohydrates include starches and fibers. They are also called *polysaccharides*.

Carbohydrates are the body's most important energy source. They spare proteins in the diet for other important functions. Carbohydrates also help with fat metabolism and provide bulk in the diet as fiber.

During digestion, carbohydrates are broken down and converted into glucose with the help of the liver. The bloodstream delivers glucose to cells, where it is used for energy or converted into glycogen for storage. Insulin from the pancreas helps regulate this process. Excess carbohydrates are converted into fat.

Carbohydrates should make up a large portion of your diet. About 45 to 65 percent of your daily calories should come from carbohydrates. The *2015–2020 Dietary Guidelines for Americans* recommends reducing added sugar consumption and increasing dietary fiber intake. Reading food labels can help you meet these dietary goals.

Chapter Vocabulary

1. **Content Terms** In teams, create categories for the following terms and classify as many of the terms as possible. Then, share your ideas with the remainder of the class.

carbohydrates	hormone
complex carbohydrate	hypoglycemia
dental caries	insulin
diabetes mellitus	lactose intolerance
dietary fiber	monosaccharide
disaccharide	polysaccharide
functional fiber	simple carbohydrate
functional food	starch
glucose	sugars
glycemic index (GI)	supplement
glycogen	total fiber

2. **Academic Terms** For each of the following terms, identify a word or group of words describing a quality of the term—an *attribute*. Pair up with a classmate and discuss your list of attributes. Then, discuss your list of attributes with the whole class to increase understanding.

addiction	replenish
erode	satiety

Review Learning

3. Identify the monosaccharide units that make up each of the three disaccharides.
4. List ten food sources of carbohydrates.
5. How do simple carbohydrates differ from complex carbohydrates?
6. If the diet does not provide enough carbohydrates, how does the body meet its needs for energy?
7. What are two benefits of including fiber in the diet for people who are trying to lose weight?
8. *True or false*? A person is likely to feel full longer after eating popcorn than after eating cotton candy.
9. Where is the body's glycogen stored and how is it used?
10. Why do added sugars cause greater concern among nutrition experts than naturally occurring sugars?
11. How many calories from carbohydrates should a person on a 3,000-calorie eating plan consume? What is the preferred type of carbohydrate?
12. List three good food sources of dietary fiber.
13. What two factors affect the risk of dental caries?
14. Compare and contrast type 1 diabetes and type 2 diabetes.
15. What causes lactose intolerance?

Self-Assessment Quiz

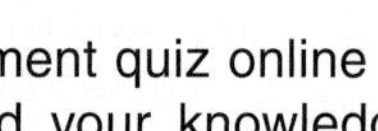

Complete the self-assessment quiz online to help you practice and expand your knowledge and skills.

Critical Thinking

16. **Analyze** What reasons can you identify for people choosing simple carbohydrates over complex carbohydrates? What factors may affect this behavior?
17. **Critique** Make a list of your favorite snack foods. Identify those that are high in added sugars. Then make a list of snack alternatives that are high in naturally occurring sugars and/or complex carbohydrates. Make sure half of your alternative snacks are whole grain. Share your lists with the class.
18. **Analyze** Analyze the labels of five cereal products. Make a chart and record the amount of total carbohydrate, dietary fiber, and sugars in each product. Also, list all types of added sugars included in each product. Rank the cereals based on their nutritional value. Present your rankings to the class.
19. **Analyze** Review one week of your school lunch menu. Evaluate the menu for the use of whole-grain products, fruits, vegetables, legumes, and other high-fiber foods. Prepare a brief summary of your findings.

Core Skills

20. **Research** Use the American Diabetic Association website and other useful sites to prepare an electronic presentation on healthful eating plans for a person with diabetes. Include a discussion of why and how carbohydrates are counted. Share your presentation with the class.
21. **Math** Select four bread products. Be sure to include a variety of products, such as whole-grain bread, plain bagel, rye bread, and so on. Use information from the Nutrition Facts panels to create a histogram comparing the grams of fiber found in each product.
22. **Writing and Technology Literacy** Write an entertaining and informative public service announcement (PSA) for television that encourages people to increase their fiber intake. Show pictures of foods high in fiber content. Describe the benefits of fiber.
23. **Writing** Research a grain that you have never eaten. Write a brief paper summarizing your findings.
24. **Speaking and Listening** Using digital media, prepare a presentation to inform your class about global sugar crops used to produce sweeteners. Include a map showing locations around the world where crops such as sugarcane, sugar beets, and corn are grown. Discuss the climate and topographies of the regions. Make the presentation interesting and appropriate to the audience.
25. **Science** Use credible resources to research the chemical makeup of the following sweeteners: honey, brown sugar, molasses, raw sugar, agave nectar, and high fructose corn syrup. Compare their chemical structures, their nutrient contents, and how they are digested by the human body. Prepare a summary of your findings.
26. **Math** Every morning, Tonya starts her day with a serving of cereal and half-cup of milk. According to their Nutrition Facts panels, these foods contain the following Total Carbohydrates: cereal—24 g, milk—6 g. Tonya follows an 1,800-calorie food plan. Her goal is to obtain 60% of her calories from carbohydrates. How many more grams does Tonya need to meet her daily goal?
27. **Listening** To find out more about the relationship between nutrition and dental health, interview a dentist. Identify and implement strategies you learn to keep your teeth healthy.
28. **Career Readiness Practice** The ability to teach skills to others is a transferrable skill that employers desire. Presume your new employer has noticed you have this ability. A group of employees has decided to form a team of runners to train for a fund-raising marathon next spring. Because you are a dedicated marathon runner and have knowledge about healthful eating, your employer has asked you to lead a lunchtime discussion group once a week. This week's topic is the importance of eating the right carbohydrates, especially when training for a marathon. What questions would you ask your coworkers about their past and current carbohydrate eating behaviors? What information would you want to teach them about carbohydrate choices?

Lipids: Fats and Oils

Learning Outcomes

After studying this chapter, you will be able to

- **compare and contrast** the three classes of lipids;
- **differentiate between** saturated and unsaturated fatty acids;
- **list** five functions of lipids in the body;
- **summarize** how the body digests, absorbs, and transports lipids;
- **recognize** food choices that contribute to an eating pattern with healthy fat content;
- **explain** the role fats play in your health; and
- **reflect** on controllable and uncontrollable heart-health risk factors.

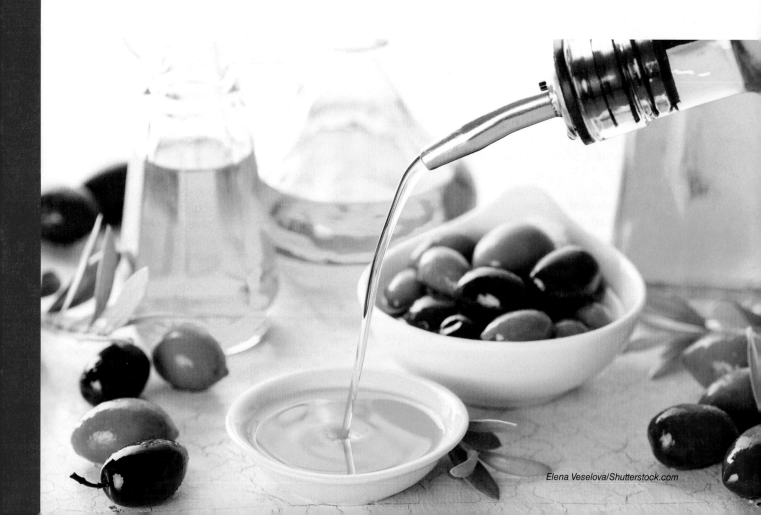

Elena Veselova/Shutterstock.com

Content Terms

adipose tissue
atherosclerosis
cancer
cardiovascular disease (CVD)
cholesterol
chylomicron
emulsifier
essential fatty acid
fatty acid
heart attack
high-density lipoprotein (HDL)
hydrogenation
hypertension
lecithin
lipid
lipoprotein
low-density lipoprotein (LDL)
monounsaturated fatty acid
omega-3 fatty acids
phospholipids
plaque
polyunsaturated fatty acid
rancid
saturated fatty acid
sterols
stroke
trans fatty acid
triglycerides
unsaturated fatty acid
very low-density lipoprotein (VLDL)

Academic Terms

abundant
extracted
ingrained
inherent
predominant
ruminant
synthesis

What's Your Nutrition and Wellness IQ?

Take this quiz to examine how much you already know about lipids. If you cannot answer a question, pay extra attention to that topic as you study this chapter.

- Identify each statement as *True*, *False*, or *It Depends*. *It Depends* means in some cases the statement is true; in some cases it could be false.
- Revise false statements to make them true.
- Explain the circumstances in which each *It Depends* statement is true and when it is false.

Nutrition and Wellness IQ

Statement			
1. The words *lipid* and *fat* have the same meaning.	True	False	It Depends
2. Following a fat-free diet is a healthy strategy for losing weight.	True	False	It Depends
3. The fat that is stored around the body's organs acts like a shock absorber.	True	False	It Depends
4. During digestion, fats are broken down into fatty acids and chylomicrons.	True	False	It Depends
5. Atherosclerosis is a preventable disease.	True	False	It Depends
6. Inactivity affects body weight, but has little to do with heart health issues.	True	False	It Depends
7. Fish are a good source of dietary fats.	True	False	It Depends
8. The *Dietary Guidelines* recommends that saturated fats account for less than 10 percent of your total daily calories.	True	False	It Depends

While studying this chapter, look for the activity icon to

- **build** vocabulary with e-flash cards and interactive games;
- **assess** what you learn by completing self-assessment quizzes and completing review questions; and
- **expand** knowledge with interactive activities and activities that extend learning.

www.g-wlearning.com/foodsandnutrition/

Historically, dietary fat has had a bad reputation, and there are some good reasons to be concerned about fat. Consuming too much of certain types of fats is linked to a variety of health problems; however, fats are not all bad. In fact, fats perform many important functions in the body. You need to eat foods containing some fat every day. The goal is to choose foods with the recommended amounts and types of fats for a healthful diet.

Types of Lipids

You are likely familiar with the word *fat*, but the word *lipid* may be new to you. ***Lipid*** is a broader term for a group of compounds that includes fats, oils, lecithin, and cholesterol. Lipids can be grouped into three main classes—triglycerides, phospholipids, and sterols.

As you read about lipids, remember that these compounds may come from the foods you eat or from sources within your body. For example, the butter you spread on bread is a *dietary* fat; whereas the extra cushion you may be carrying around your waist or in your thighs is an example of *body* fat.

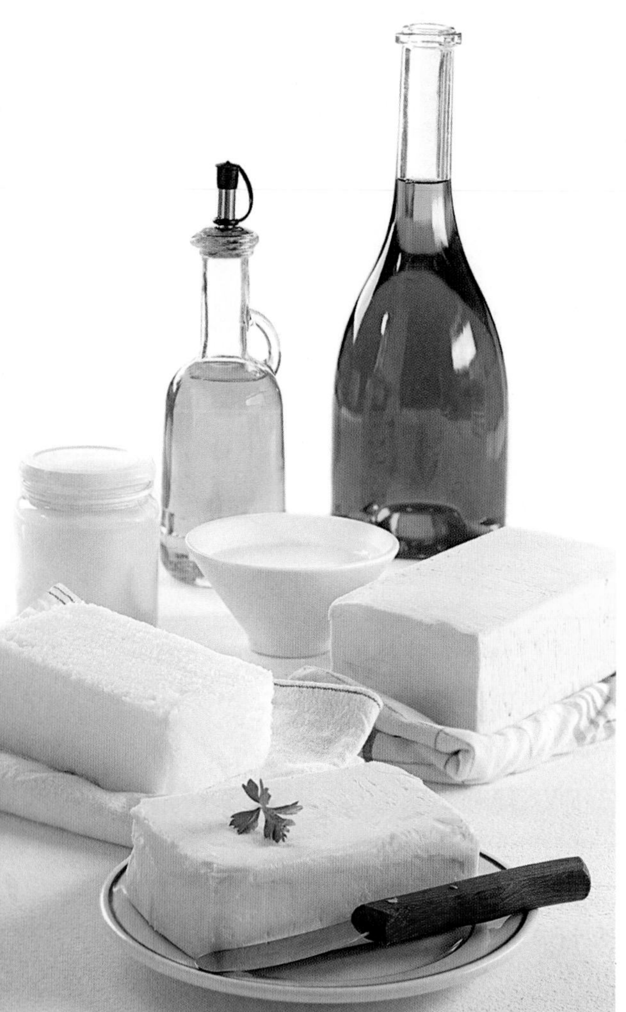

JPC-PROD/Shutterstock.com

Figure 7.1 The foods pictured here include a variety of fats and oils. *What differences in physical characteristics do you observe?*

Triglycerides

Triglycerides are the major type of fat found in foods and in the body. Food sources of triglycerides are referred to as *fats* and *oils*. These are a major source of energy for the body (**Figure 7.1**). The terms *triglycerides*, *fats*, and *oils* are often used interchangeably.

A triglyceride consists of three fatty acids attached to a glycerol molecule. *Glycerol* is an alcohol that has three carbon atoms. It is the backbone of the triglyceride molecule. A ***fatty acid*** is an organic compound made up of a chain of carbon atoms to which hydrogen atoms are attached. The last carbon atom at one end of the chain forms an *acid group* with two oxygen atoms and a hydrogen atom. Fatty acid chains vary in length. The fatty acids commonly found in foods have 16 to 18 carbon atoms.

Saturated and Unsaturated Fatty Acids

Fatty acids can be saturated or unsaturated. ***Saturated fatty acids*** have no double bonds in their chemical structure. They have a full load of hydrogen atoms. An ***unsaturated fatty acid*** has at least one double bond between two carbon atoms in each molecule. If a double bond is broken, two hydrogen atoms can be added to the molecule. The number of double bonds and hydrogen atoms in the fatty acid chain determine the degree of saturation. A ***monounsaturated fatty acid*** has only one double bond between carbon atoms. A ***polyunsaturated fatty acid*** has two or more double bonds (**Figure 7.2**).

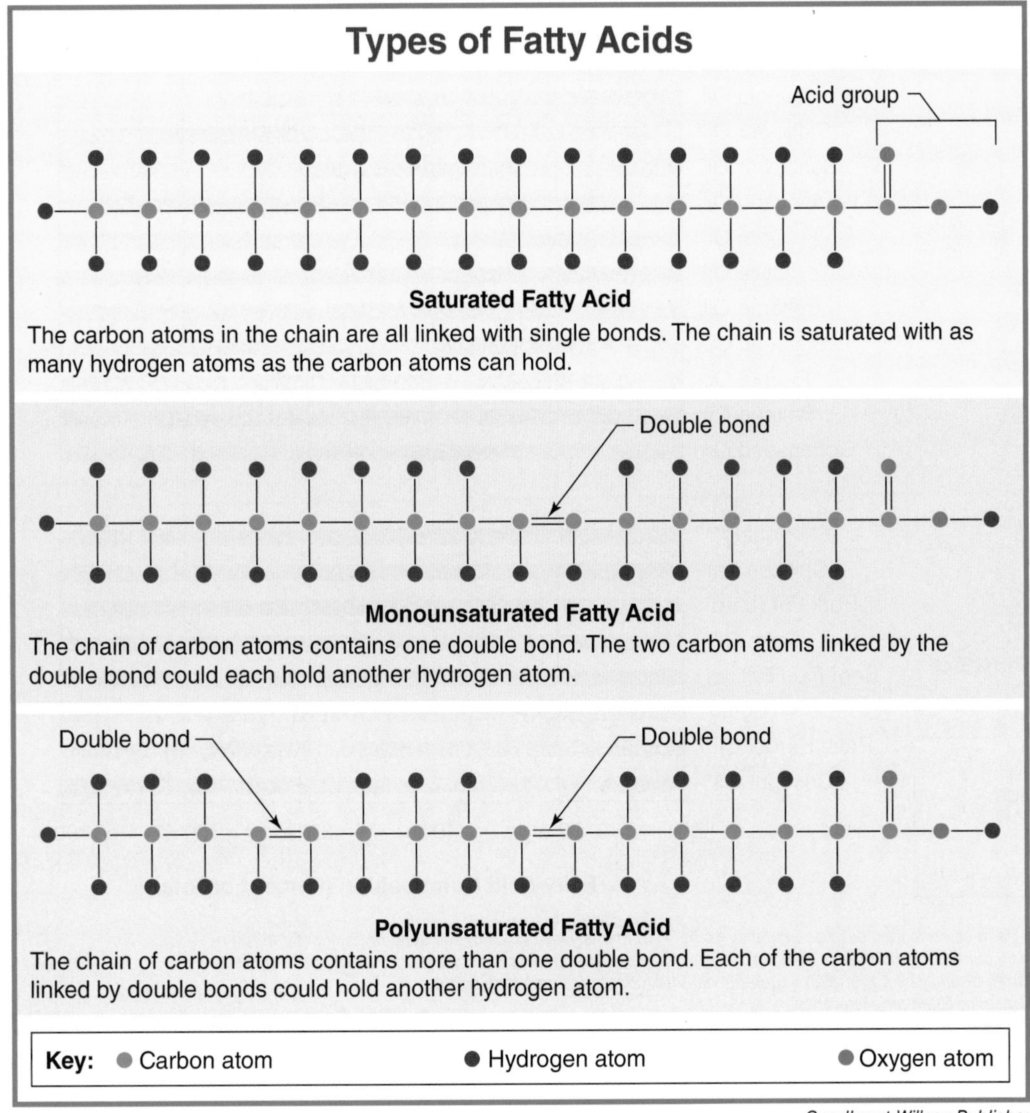

Types of Fatty Acids
Acid group
Saturated Fatty Acid
The carbon atoms in the chain are all linked with single bonds. The chain is saturated with as many hydrogen atoms as the carbon atoms can hold.
Double bond
Monounsaturated Fatty Acid
The chain of carbon atoms contains one double bond. The two carbon atoms linked by the double bond could each hold another hydrogen atom.
Double bond
Double bond
Polyunsaturated Fatty Acid
The chain of carbon atoms contains more than one double bond. Each of the carbon atoms linked by double bonds could hold another hydrogen atom.
Key: Carbon atom
Hydrogen atom
Oxygen atom

Goodheart-Willcox Publisher

Figure 7.2 The number of double bonds and hydrogen atoms present in a fatty acid determine whether it is saturated, monounsaturated, or polyunsaturated.

Nearly all fats and oils contain a mixture of the three types of fatty acids. For instance, corn oil is 13 percent saturated, 25 percent monounsaturated, and 62 percent polyunsaturated. The fats in meat and dairy products, including beef fat, lard, and butterfat, tend to be high in saturated fatty acids. Fats from plants are usually high in unsaturated fatty acids. Olive and peanut oils are high in monounsaturated fatty acids. Corn, safflower, and soybean oils are high in polyunsaturated fatty acids. The tropical oils, such as coconut and palm oils, are an exception to the rule about fats from plants. These oils are high in saturated fatty acids.

The **predominant** (main) type of fatty acid in a lipid determines whether a lipid is liquid or solid at room temperature. Lipids that are high in saturated fatty acids tend to be solid at room temperature. Lipids that are high in unsaturated fatty acids tend to be liquid at room temperature. Unsaturated fats have a lower melting point than more highly saturated fats. This is why chicken fat melts at a lower temperature than butterfat, which is more highly saturated (**Figure 7.3** on the next page).

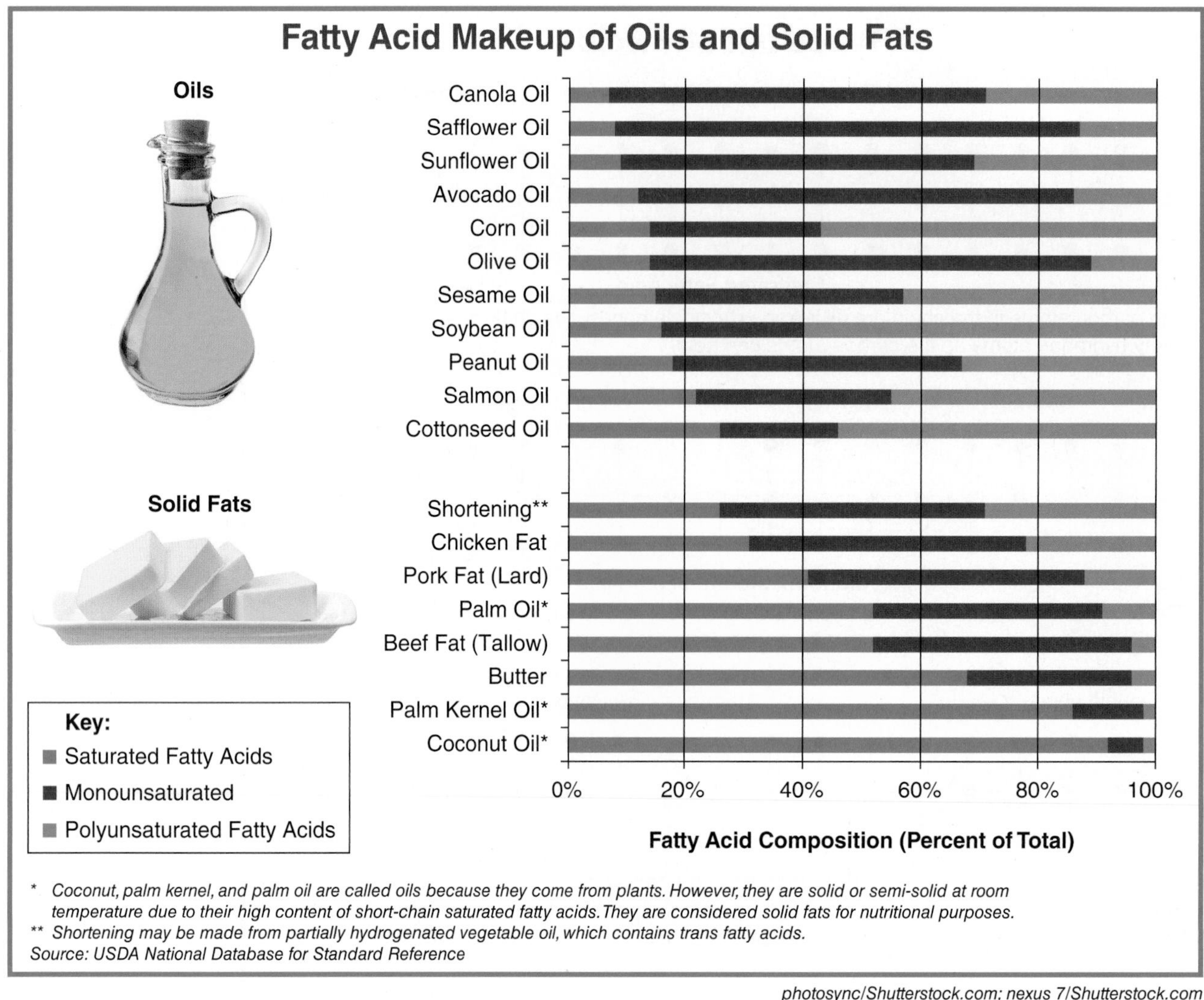

photosync/Shutterstock.com; nexus 7/Shutterstock.com

Figure 7.3 Fats and oils vary greatly in their fatty acid makeup. *Which of the products in this graph has the lowest saturated fatty acid content?*

Trans Fatty Acids

Unsaturated fatty acids can be hydrogenated. ***Hydrogenation*** is the process of breaking the double carbon bonds in an unsaturated fatty acid and adding hydrogen. This process converts liquid oils into solid fats. The resulting fatty acids are known as ***trans fatty acids***, also called *trans fats* or *partially hydrogenated vegetable oils*. *Trans* fats are naturally found in some food sources. The solid fats created through hydrogenation are considered artificial *trans* fats.

Besides changing the texture, the main reason for hydrogenating oils is to improve their keeping quality. Until recently, food manufacturers favored the use of artificial *trans* fats over unsaturated oils. The longer shelf life of *trans* fats saved the manufacturers money and improved consumer satisfaction. Oils turn rancid when exposed to air or stored for a long time. The term ***rancid*** describes a food oil in which the fatty acid molecules have combined with oxygen. This causes them to break down, and the oil spoils. Rancid oils have an unpleasant smell and taste.

Current research shows that *trans* fats act much like saturated fat in the body. Saturated fat contributes to heart disease, as do *trans* fats. *Trans* fats have been found to increase levels of fatty deposits on the walls of the arteries, which increases the chance for heart disease. *Trans* fats in the diet are also linked to high blood cholesterol levels.

Reducing saturated and *trans* fats in your diet helps reduce heart health risks. This is important because heart disease is a leading cause of illness and death worldwide.

In recent years, manufacturers and restaurants have been removing *trans* fats from food products in anticipation of the federal government's ban on the use of artificial *trans* fats in foods, effective June 2018. However, *trans* fats are **inherent** (belonging by nature) in some foods, such as beef, lamb, and butterfat (**Figure 7.4**). It is not yet understood whether these naturally occurring *trans* fats have the same negative health effects as artificial *trans* fats.

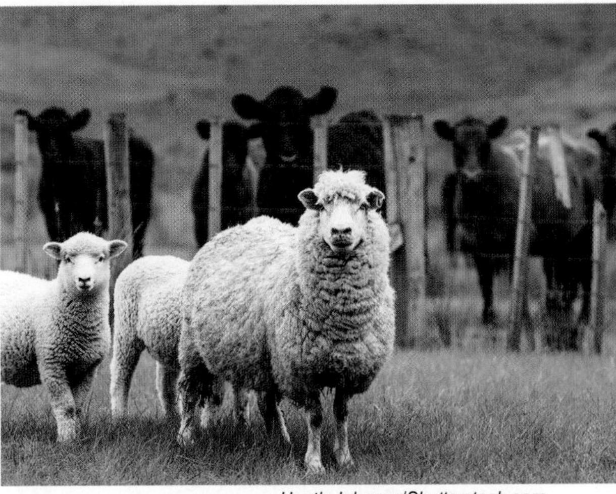

Heath Johnson/Shutterstock.com

Figure 7.4 Animals that chew cud, such as goats, cows, and sheep, are called *ruminants*. Foods from these animals are sources of naturally occurring *trans* fats.

The American Heart Association (AHA) recommends reducing the percentage of calories from *trans* fats in your diet. The *Dietary Guidelines* suggests limiting intake of *trans* fats to as low as possible by limiting foods that contain artificial *trans* fats. To limit your intake of *trans* fats, read the Nutrition Facts label on foods to determine the amount of *trans* fats they supply. The amount listed includes naturally occurring and artificial *trans* fats. Although they can no longer use artificial *trans* fats in foods, food manufacturers will still be able to petition the FDA for permission to use them as a food additive.

Phospholipids

Phospholipids are lipids that have a phosphorus-containing compound in their chemical structure. ***Lecithin*** is a phospholipid that is made by the liver, so it is not essential to the diet. Lecithin is also found in many foods of animal origin, including egg yolks.

Lecithin, like other phospholipids, is an emulsifier. An ***emulsifier*** is a substance that can mix with both water and fat. For example, egg yolk acts as an emulsifier in mayonnaise to prevent the oil and vinegar from separating. The lecithin in the egg yolk keeps the oil particles suspended in the watery vinegar. In the body, lecithin is part of cell membranes.

Sterols

Another class of lipids is called ***sterols***. Sterols have a molecular configuration that features complex ring structures. Vitamin D, some hormones, and cholesterol are examples of sterols. Sterols should not be confused with steroids. A steroid is a manufactured chemical substance that is a drug. Sterols are often associated with heart health.

Cholesterol is a white, waxy lipid found in every cell in the body. This fat-like substance performs essential functions in the body. For example, your body uses cholesterol to make sex hormones and bile acids. Cholesterol provides structure for all cell membranes. The human body makes cholesterol; therefore, it is not essential in the diet.

Cholesterol is found only in animal tissues. It is never present in plants. Therefore, plant foods such as peanut butter and corn oil margarine contain no cholesterol. All animal foods, including milk, cheese, hamburgers, eggs, and butter, contain cholesterol. It is **abundant** (plentiful) in egg yolks, organ meats (liver and kidney), crab, and lobster.

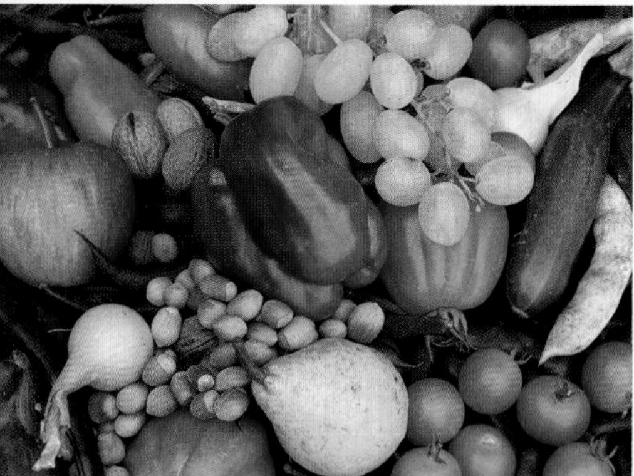

Corrado Baratta/Shutterstock.com

Figure 7.5 Phytosterols are naturally occurring in the cell membranes of these foods. *Are these foods also sources of cholesterol?*

Phytosterols are compounds from plants that are similar in structure to cholesterol. Phytosterols include plant sterols and stanols. Although plant sterols and stanols are different from animal cholesterol, they carry out similar cellular functions in plants. Stanols and sterols are essential components of plant membranes. Stanols and sterols can only be obtained through dietary sources. They are naturally present in small quantities in many fruits, vegetables, nuts, seeds, cereals, legumes, vegetable oils, and other plant sources (**Figure 7.5**).

Foods containing phytosterols may have health benefits. Including plant sterols and stanols in the diet may help lower LDL cholesterol levels and the risk for heart disease.

Functions of Lipids

Lipids serve many important functions in the body. Phospholipids and sterols are part of the structure of every cell. These substances are needed for the formation of healthy cell membranes. Phospholipids play an important role in transporting fats throughout the body. Cholesterol—the best-known sterol—is necessary for the **synthesis** (forming, building) of some hormones, vitamins, and other secretions.

Triglycerides are the most abundant type of lipids found in the body and in food. Triglycerides serve several important functions, including the following:

- providing energy
- storing energy
- insulating and protecting organs
- transporting fat-soluble substances
- providing pleasing flavor and texture

FEATURED CAREER

Research Dietitian

Research dietitians implement, collect, and enter food records. They also develop nutrition education materials. Research dietitians primarily work with dietary-related research in the clinical aspect of nutrition in disease, and with foodservice aspects in issues involving food. Many research dietitians work with the biochemical aspects of nutrient interaction in the body. Research dietitians normally work in a hospital or university research facility. Quality improvement in dietetics services is another area of research.

Education

Research dietitians often have a master's degree. They must have a strong background in health science, including anatomy, chemistry, biochemistry, biology, physiology, and nutrition.

Job Outlook

Employment in the dietetics field will experience average growth about as fast as other occupations. Population growth, aging, and emphasis on health education cause a steady expansion of the health services industry.

Providing Energy

Triglycerides provide a concentrated source of energy. All fats and oils provide 9 calories per gram. In comparison, proteins and carbohydrates provide only 4 calories per gram. This energy density is useful during life stages of accelerated growth. On the other hand, this concentrated source of energy can easily contribute to unhealthy weight gain.

Storing Energy

In excess, triglycerides are stored in the fat cells and in the liver. The body stores a large share of this excess energy in ***adipose tissue***. This stored energy is available for use during times when food is unavailable or insufficient. About half of this adipose tissue is just under your skin. It serves as an internal blanket that holds in body heat. The fat cells in adipose tissue can expand to hold an almost unlimited amount of fat. Overweight people have excess stores of fat in their adipose tissue.

Insulating and Protecting Organs

Body fat surrounds organs such as the heart and liver. This fat acts like a shock absorber. It helps protect internal organs from the bumps and bruises of body movement. In fact, fat plays an important role in the brain's function and health as well. The brain is nearly 60 percent fat!

Transporting Fat-Soluble Substances

Vitamins A, D, E, and K dissolve in fat. They are carried into your body along with the fat in foods. Lipids help move these vitamins around inside your body.

Providing Pleasing Flavor and Texture

Fats play a role in foods as well as in your body. Both naturally occurring and added fats affect the tastes, textures, and aromas of foods. Fats make meat moist and flavorful. They make biscuits tender and piecrusts flaky (**Figure 7.6**). Fats help fried foods become brown and crisp. Fats also disperse the compounds that allow you to smell bacon cooking.

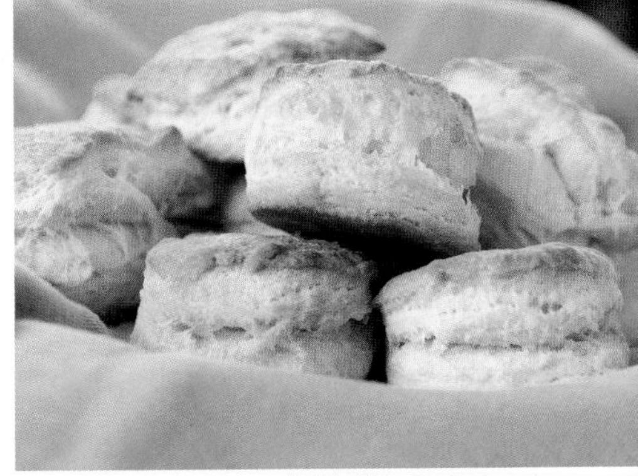

farbled/Shutterstock.com

Figure 7.6 Fats provide baked goods with a tender, flaky texture.

How Your Body Uses Lipids

You probably include sources of fat in your diet throughout the day. You may have an egg for breakfast, an avocado on your sandwich at lunch, and a pork chop for dinner. How does your body use the fat in these foods to perform vital functions?

Digestion and Absorption

After you chew it and swallow it, fat reaches the stomach along with carbohydrates, proteins, and other food elements. The fat—comprised largely of triglycerides— separates from the watery contents of the stomach and floats in a layer on top.

In the small intestine, fat mixes with bile, which acts as an emulsifier. Bile helps break fat into tiny droplets and keep it suspended in watery digestive fluid. Breaking fat into tiny droplets increases its surface area. This makes it easier for pancreatic enzymes to break the triglycerides down into glycerol, fatty acids, and monoglycerides. (A monoglyceride is one fatty acid attached to a glycerol molecule.) Bile's emulsifying effect improves absorption of the fat by the cells lining the intestine.

Transport in the Body

Once the glycerol, fatty acids, and monoglycerides pass through the intestinal walls, they must be transported in the bloodstream to tissues throughout the body. The smaller components resulting from fat digestion—glycerol and short-chain fatty acids—pass through the intestinal lining, directly into the bloodstream. In the intestinal cells, the larger, long-chain fatty acids rejoin with glycerol or monoglycerides. These fatty acids are then converted back into triglycerides. The newly formed triglycerides are clustered together. These clusters of triglycerides are thinly coated with cholesterol, phospholipids, and proteins to form ***chylomicrons***. The chylomicrons are absorbed into the lymphatic system and eventually move into the bloodstream.

Blood is mostly water and therefore does not mix well with fat. The protein and phospholipid exterior of a chylomicron enables the fat housed in the core of the chylomicron to travel in the water-based blood (**Figure 7.7**). This helps fat from your diet move efficiently through your blood vessels to the tissues where fatty acids can be absorbed for fuel or stored.

As the chylomicron travels through the bloodstream, it yields its triglycerides to the body's cells either to be used for energy or stored as fat. The enzymes on the lining of a blood vessel attack the chylomicron and remove a triglyceride. The enzymes proceed to break down the triglyceride into glycerol and fatty acids. These smaller components are able to pass into the cell. The cell can break the fatty acids down further to release energy for immediate needs. If the cells do not have immediate energy needs, they can rebuild the fatty acids into triglycerides. The cells then store these triglycerides for future energy needs.

Most cells can store only limited amounts of triglycerides; however, fat cells can hold an almost unlimited supply. Fat cells can break down stored triglycerides when they are needed. These cells send fatty acids through the bloodstream to other body cells that use the fatty acids for fuel.

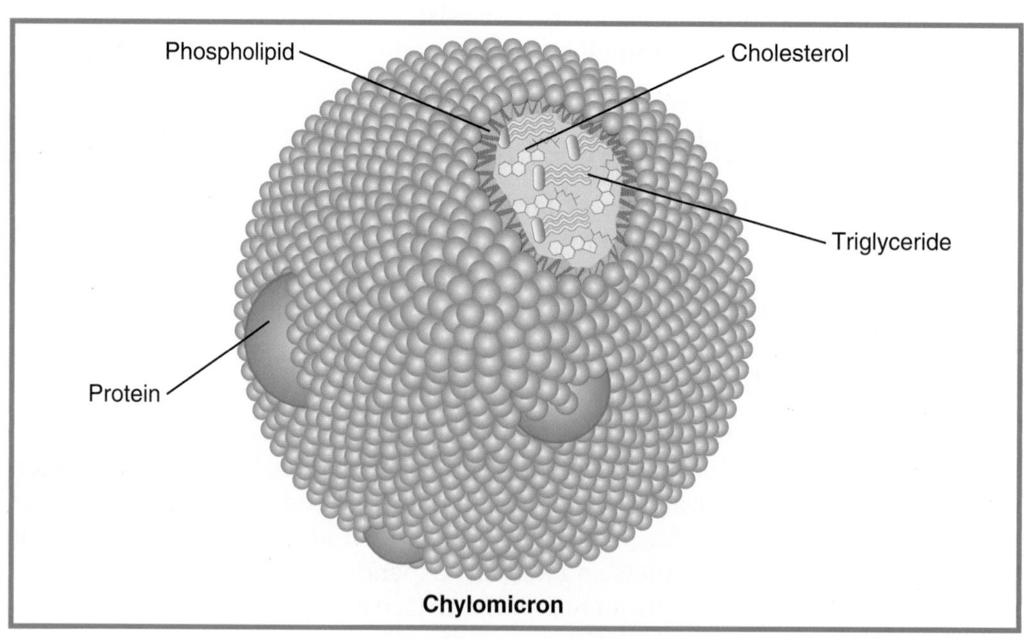

Figure 7.7 Water-loving proteins cover the outer surface of a chylomicron. This enables it to transport water-fearing lipids through the bloodstream, which is composed largely of water.

Goodheart-Willcox Publisher

EXTEND YOUR KNOWLEDGE

What's on Your Bread?

Compare several types of margarine, such as stick margarine, soft spreads, and reduced-calorie margarine. Compare their costs, tastes, and textures with traditional butter. Examine the Nutrition Facts panels on their labels for grams of saturated fat, as well as polyunsaturated and monounsaturated fats, if listed. Decide for whom and when you might use each product. Reflect on which brands you think would be most heart healthy. Explain your answer.

Chylomicrons are a type of lipoprotein. ***Lipoproteins*** consist of fats and proteins, and they help transport fats in the body. Chylomicrons are one of four types of lipoproteins found in the blood. ***Very low-density lipoproteins (VLDL)*** are a second type of lipoprotein. VLDLs carry triglycerides and cholesterol made by the liver to body cells. Once in the bloodstream, some of the triglycerides in VLDLs are broken down into glycerol and fatty acids and released. Losing triglycerides causes VLDLs to become denser, with a larger percentage of cholesterol.

At this point, VLDLs become ***low-density lipoproteins (LDL)***. LDLs are a type of lipoprotein that carries cholesterol through the bloodstream to body cells. A fourth type of lipoprotein is the ***high-density lipoproteins (HDL)***. HDLs pick up cholesterol from around the body and transfer it to other lipoproteins for transport back to the liver. The liver processes this returned cholesterol as a waste product for removal from the body. You will read more about LDL and HDL later in this chapter.

Meeting Your Lipid Needs

The *2015–2020 Dietary Guidelines* recommends that daily fat intake represent 25–35 percent of total daily calories, with most of this coming from unsaturated fats. To avoid calorie imbalance and unhealthy weight gain, unsaturated fats should replace existing saturated fats in the diet rather than add to them. The goal is for saturated fats to make up less than 10 percent of total daily calories (**Figure 7.8**).

How Much Fat Is Recommended?

If Your Daily Calorie Level Is:	Your Total Fat Intake Should Fall within this Range:		And Your Saturated Fat Should Not Exceed:
	25% of Total Daily Calories from Fat (grams)	35% of Total Daily Calories from Fat (grams)	10% of Total Daily Calories from Saturated Fat (grams)
1,800	50	70	20
2,000	56	78	22
2,200	61	86	24
2,400	67	93	27
2,800	78	109	31
3,000	83	117	33

Figure 7.8 Saturated fats should supply less than 10 percent of your daily calories. *For an individual who requires 2,400 calories per day, what is the maximum number of calories from saturated fats this person should consume?*

Unsaturated Fats

Oils are a source of unsaturated fats. They are composed of a high percentage of mono- and polyunsaturated fatty acids. Oils are an important part of a healthy eating pattern because the body needs a variety of fatty acids for normal growth and development.

In addition to being an essential component of a healthy eating pattern, oils are also a rich source of energy. Oils supply 9 calories per gram compared with the 4 calories per gram supplied by carbohydrates and protein. For this reason, you should limit the amount of oils in your eating pattern to ensure you maintain a healthy weight. Oils are also a major source of vitamin E.

Foods such as the oils **extracted** (separated) from plants are the most recognizable sources of oil in the diet. These include corn oil, olive oil, and soybean oil. These oils may be used as a heat transfer medium for cooking foods. Oils are also commonly used as recipe ingredients or as flavoring. Sources of oils also include whole foods such as nuts, seeds, seafood, avocados, and olives. These foods are naturally high in oil. Certain prepared foods, such as mayonnaise, some salad dressings, and margarine, are mainly oil.

Essential Fatty Acids

Your body can make most polyunsaturated fatty acids; however, your body cannot synthesize two specific polyunsaturated fatty acids—*linolenic acid* and *linoleic acid*. These are called ***essential fatty acids***, and you must obtain them from the foods you eat. If your diet is lacking in these nutrients, the skin, reproductive system, liver, and kidneys may all be affected. Most people include plenty of fats and oils in their diets, so essential fatty acid deficiencies are rare.

THE MOVEMENT CONNECTION

Elevate Your Heart Rate

Why

We learned about the hazards of physical inactivity in this chapter. Performing physical activity elevates your heart rate. Elevating heart rate for 30–60 minutes each day with physical activity along with a healthy diet can decrease risks of diabetes and excess weight.

Apply

Your heart rate is simple to measure:

- Sitting at your desk, place your index finger and middle finger along the side of your neck midway between your throat and your ear to find your pulse.
- Set a timer for 10 seconds and begin counting every time you feel a heartbeat. Record this number.
- Paying careful attention to items in the room and other students, complete 2 laps around the perimeter of the classroom.
- Find your pulse and measure it again. Did your heart rate increase?

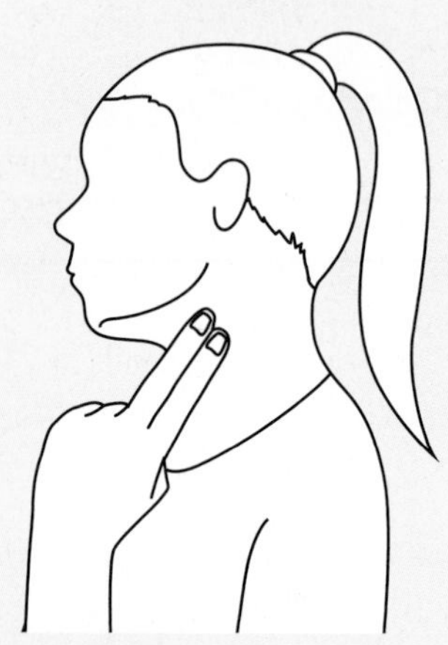

·ed and *Trans* Fats

ǥh in saturated fats and *trans* fats have been shown to disease. There is strong and consistent evidence that *ıns* fats with unsaturated fats can decrease the risk for

·ial *trans* fats were once widely used in foods such as es, and canned icings. They have since been removed e to public health concerns. In fact, artificial *trans* fats cognized as safe" for use in human food.

ed recommendations for total fat and saturated fat nsisting of a quarter-pound cheeseburger, French fries, h fat do you think is in this meal? The answer is about saturated—nearly the fat equivalent of half a stick of kfast consisted of a sausage-and-egg biscuit, and din- coleslaw, and ice cream. Add in a bag of chips and a ‹s between meals and the daily total is 147 grams of fat, ›eing saturated. Clearly, this is beyond the daily recom- ıd that these examples did not include any side dishes. he breakfast biscuit would add 8 more grams of fat.

snacks with care, however, a teen could occasionally ies in a nutritious diet. Food labels and nutrition infor- s describe the amount of calories and the grams of total ing of a food product. This information can be used to s.

hanges in daily food choices, you can lower your satu- y (**Figure 7.10**).

esterol

Guidelines no longer includes a Key Recommendation l. The decision to remove this recommendation was earch does not identify a clear relationship between ood cholesterol levels. However, the recommended lietary cholesterol because foods that are high in satu- o higher in dietary cholesterol. The *Dietary Guidelines* ·ated fats, so dietary cholesterol is limited by associa- *uidelines* suggests that foods higher in dietary choles- , such as eggs and shellfish, can be part of a healthy

WELLNESS TIP

ıy weight, try monitoring how much fat you eat. Start panel to identify the types and amount of fat in your k at the label ingredient list and note which items are t is one of the first ingredients listed, you may want to ative. For example, a container of low-fat macaroni and alories per serving than regular macaroni and cheese.

Some polyunsaturated fatty acids are called ***omeg*** location of the first double bond in their structure. between the third and fourth carbon atoms. Linolenic a that the body converts into other long-chain fatty acid ered to promote human health.

The other essential fatty acid, linoleic acid, is an *om* omega-6 fatty acids are far more prevalent in the US di fatty acids. Some estimates show that Americans con omega-6 fatty acids than omega-3 fatty acids. By contr prehistoric man's diet consisted of equal amounts of t cant imbalance of these fatty acids in modern eating pa negative impact on overall health. For this reason, hea include foods rich in omega-3 fatty acids.

Sources of Essential Fatty Acids

Certain fatty fish, such as mackerel, albacore tuna, sardines, salmon, halibut, and herring, are good sources of omega-3 fatty acids (**Figure 7.9**). Larger predatory fish, such as shark, swordfish, king mackerel, or tilefish, should be avoided due to high levels of toxins. Furthermore, children and pregnant women should limit certain fish, such as albacore tuna, to no more than one serving per week due to toxins.

Food manufacturers are now producing foods such as peanut butter, margarine, milk, and yogurt with added omega-3 fatty acids. However, the quality and quantity of omega-3 fatty acids in these foods are not equivalent to that of fish. Although foods such as walnuts, soybean oil, or canola oil are sources of omega-3 fatty acids, they also contain much larger amounts of omega-6 fatty acids. Therefore, consuming these foods could further disrupt the ratio of these nutrients in your diet.

Saturated Fats, *Trans* Fats, and Cholesterol

Saturated fats are easily identified because they are solid at room temperature, whereas unsaturated fats are liquid at room temperature. Saturated fats are found primarily in animal foods. The fat that gives a steak its flavor, the butter you spread on bread, and the drippings from bacon are all examples of saturated fats. Some tropical oils—coconut, palm, and palm kernel oils—are solid at room temperature because they contain large amounts of saturated fatty acids. For this reason, these oils are classified as saturated fats.

Trans fats can be solid or liquid at room temperature. *Trans* fats occur naturally in food from **ruminants** (animals that chew cud) such as cows, sheep, and goats. However, *trans* fats can also be manufactured.

Comparing Saturated Fat and Calories in Foods

Food	Amount	Saturated Fat (grams)	Calories
Added Fat			
Butter	1 T.	7.3	102
Olive oil	1 T.	1.9	119
Beverages			
Mocha caffe latte	15½ oz.	3.0	158
Nonfat milk	1 c.	0.1	83
2% milk	1 c.	3.1	122
Whole (3.25%) milk	1 c.	4.6	150
Breakfast			
Fast-food breakfast sandwich (sausage and egg)	1	9.9	452
Quick-service breakfast sandwich (egg white and avocado)	1	6	410
Fast-Food Sandwiches			
Crispy chicken filet	1	3.7	420
Double cheeseburger	1	10.8	437
Hamburger	1	3.3	251
Sandwich Toppers			
American cheese	½ oz.	4.0	70
Avocado	1 oz.	0.6	50
Snacks			
Almonds	1 oz.	1.2	170
French fries	1 small	1.6	229
Tortilla chips	1 oz.	0.8	135
Vegetables			
Pinto beans	1 c.	0.2	168
Refried beans	1 c.	2.7	231

Left to right: 1989studio/Shutterstock.com; Volosina/Shutterstock.com; Louella938/Shutterstock.com; Binh Thanh Bui/Shutterstock.com; Robyn Mackenzie/Shutterstock.com; Tiger Images/Shutterstock.com; Jiri Hera/Shutterstock.com; gresei/Shutterstock.com; johnfoto 18/Shutterstock.com

Figure 7.10 Small changes in food choices can greatly reduce your intake of saturated fats. *Which sandwich topper listed in this table is lower in saturated fats?*

People who have high blood cholesterol may want to increase their intake of plant foods. In fact, all people can benefit from a diet high in plant foods. Plant foods provide fiber and other heart-protective substances, such as plant sterols and stanols, that can help lower blood cholesterol.

For most people, dietary cholesterol does not affect blood cholesterol as much as total dietary fat does, especially saturated and *trans* fats.

Healthy Fat Choices

The American Heart Association (AHA) recommends the following steps to improve the fat content of your eating pattern:

- Eat a variety of fresh, frozen, and canned fruits and vegetables without high-calorie sauces or added salt.
- Select low- or fat-free dairy products.
- Eat a variety of fish at least twice a week, especially fish containing omega-3 fatty acids (for example, salmon, trout, and herring).
- Choose fish, skinless poultry, and plant-based proteins, and prepare them without added saturated and *trans* fats.
- If you choose to eat meat, choose lean cuts of meat and prepare them in healthy ways.
- Avoid foods containing partially hydrogenated vegetable oils.
- Limit saturated and *trans* fats and replace them with monounsaturated and polyunsaturated fats.

Avoid or limit fried foods, such as potato chips and fried chicken. Some people prefer the thick, rich flavor of whole milk to nonfat milk. These people may find it easier to switch to reduced-fat (2%) milk for a while before trying nonfat milk.

A significant percentage of the fat in many people's diets comes from meat products. You can reduce the amount of fat you get from meats by choosing lean cuts. Trim all visible fat before cooking (**Figure 7.11**). Use low-fat cooking methods, such as roasting, broiling, and grilling. Limit portion size to 3 ounces (85 g) of cooked meat, which is about the size of your palm.

Making Dietary Changes

Old eating habits are not easy to change. As a teen, your habits are less **ingrained** (firmly fixed). You are young and your body is strong. You are in a good position to make a fresh start. Forming a program of good nutrition will help you feel your physical and mental best.

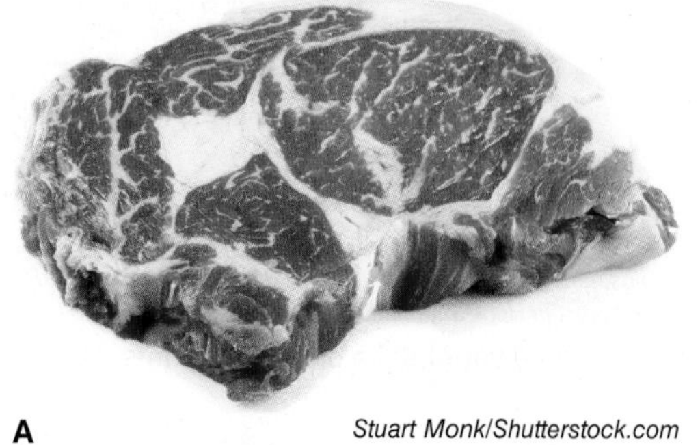

A Stuart Monk/Shutterstock.com

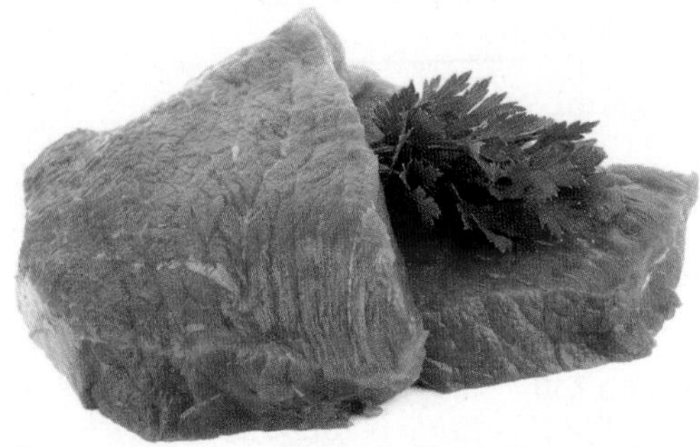

B Sergiy Kuzmin/Shutterstock.com

Figure 7.11 Some cuts of meat have fat around the edge as well as distributed throughout the muscle. ***Which of these cuts is the leaner choice?***

Most people in the United States need to reduce their consumption of saturated fats and *trans* fats to meet current recommendations. When making changes to your eating pattern, where do you start? First, assess your current eating pattern. Keep a food journal for a few days, recording everything you eat and drink. Use the information in your food journal to learn about the types and amounts of fats that you typically eat (**Figure 7.12**). Nutrition analysis software or a food composition table can help you.

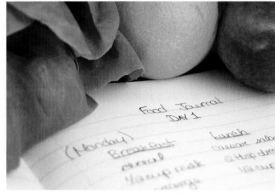

gvictoria/Shutterstock.com

Figure 7.12 A food journal is a useful tool when you are trying to improve your eating pattern.

Your analysis will help you identify the amounts of saturated and unsaturated fats you are consuming each day. Then you can calculate the percentage of calories in your eating pattern that come from total fat, as well as saturated, monounsaturated, and polyunsaturated fats.

The next step is to evaluate your current eating patterns and identify changes you can make to improve the fat content of your diet. Set realistic goals to make these changes gradually. Then make choices that support your goals. For instance, you might decide to eat French fries no more than once a week. Sticking with this decision might mean ordering a salad with oil and vinegar instead of fries at your next meal.

Support from your family can affect your ability to reach your goals. Talk to family members about your desire to make changes in your dietary behaviors. See if they might be willing to make changes as well. If not, ask for their respect and encouragement as you work to change your eating habits.

Look for the Hidden Fats

If you want to limit saturated and *trans* fats in your daily eating choices, you must be able to identify the sources of fat components in foods. Then you can replace the solid fats in your diet with more health-promoting unsaturated and polyunsaturated fats.

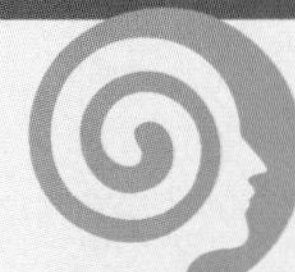

EXTEND YOUR KNOWLEDGE

What About Using Fat Replacers in Food?

Have you ever eaten a food that uses fat replacers? A *fat replacer* is an ingredient that is designed to replace some or all of the fat typically found in a food product. Fat replacers were developed to have a flavor and texture similar to fats and oils, while providing less fat and fewer calories. For example, a tablespoon of regular mayonnaise provides 11 grams of fat and 100 calories. A tablespoon of fat-free mayonnaise made with a fat replacer provides no fat and only 10 calories.

There are three categories of fat replacers: carbohydrate-based, protein-based, and fat-based. Some carbohydrate-based fat replacers can be used only in foods that are not cooked for a long time. You may find them in foods such as salad dressings, cheese, sour cream, ice cream, sauces, gravies, and yogurts. Some foods containing fat replacers use added sugar to improve their flavor, and therefore are not much lower in calories than their high-fat counterparts. Some fat replacers have been found to cause diarrhea and stomach cramps and interfere with absorption of fat-soluble vitamins.

Research fat replacers and form an opinion about their health benefit.

Lipids can be deceiving—sometimes they are easy to see, but sometimes they are not. The *visible fats* are those that you can readily see. Butter, fat on meats, and salad oil are visible fats. It is easy to recognize that you should limit your intake of these foods because you can see the fat.

Many times you cannot see the fat but it is there. These are called *invisible fats*. Baked goods, snack foods, and processed meats and poultry are often sources of invisible fat. For instance, one hot dog has about 145 calories, and 117 of those calories are from fat. You are more likely to consume excess fat and calories when you cannot see the fat in foods (**Figure 7.13**).

Foods that are high in solid fats and added sugars are found in all of the food groups. Foods such as biscuits and muffins, which contain invisible fat, are found in the MyPlate grains group. Eat these types of foods sparingly because they add more unhealthy fat to your diet. A better choice would be nutrient-dense selections from the grains group, such as oatmeal or whole-wheat bread.

The other food groups can also contribute hidden fat to your diet. Vegetables served with butter and fruits topped with cream are sources of fat. Whole milk and yogurts are high in fat. Drinks such as cappuccinos and lattes contain fat. To reduce the fat content of these drinks, request that they be made with fat-free dairy products.

When you buy prepared food, read the Nutrition Facts panel on the product label. The label states Percent Daily Values and the grams from total fat and saturated fat.

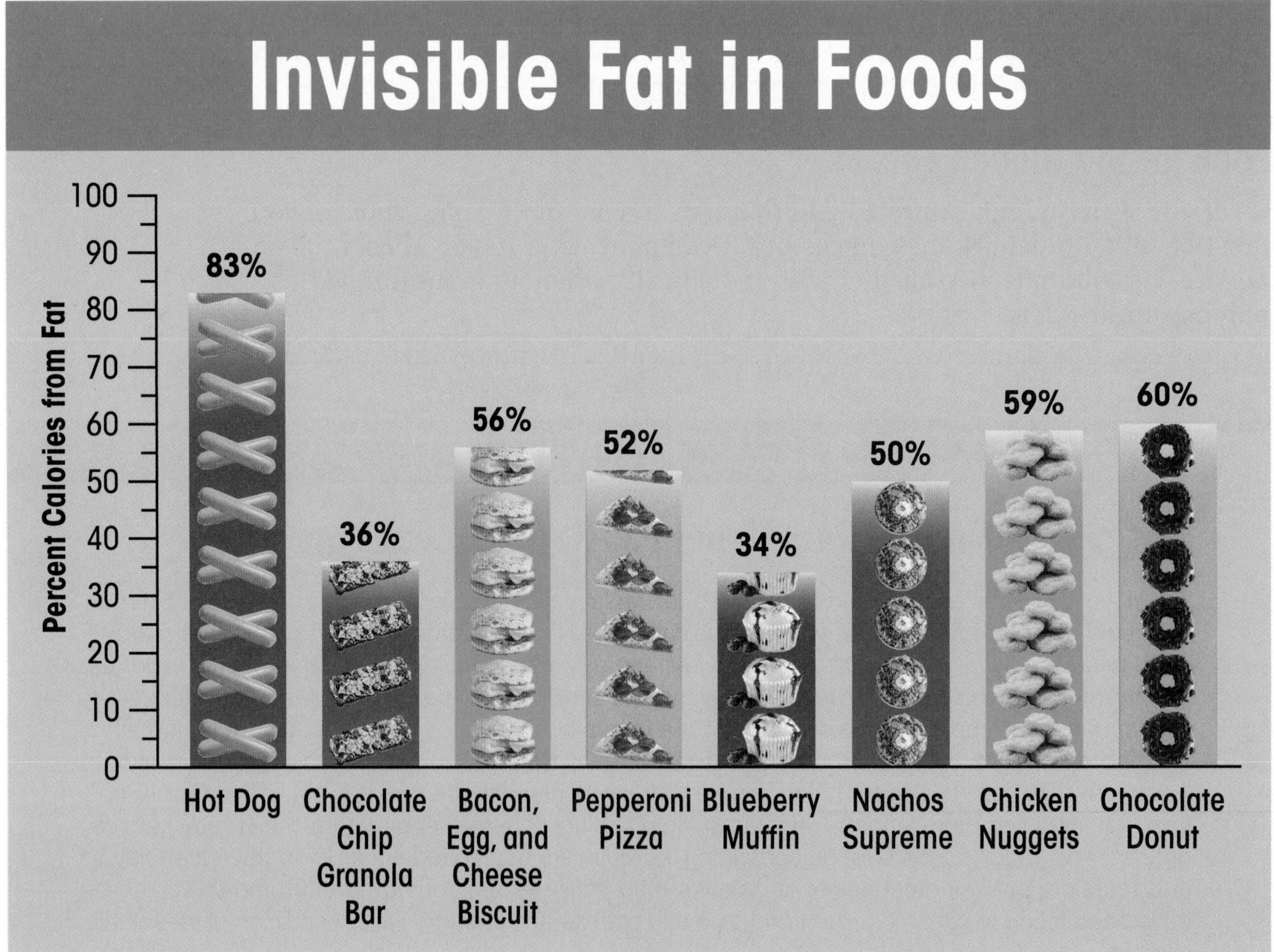

Olga Popova/Shutterstock.com; nito/Shutterstock.com; Andrea Skjold Mink/Shutterstock.com; Mike Flippo/Shutterstock.com; 5 second Studio/Shutterstock.com; LifetimeStock/Shutterstock.com; Rabits/Shutterstock.com; Nataliia K/Shutterstock.com

Figure 7.13 You may be eating far more fat than you realize because it is not visible in some foods.

COMMUNITY CONNECTIONS

Feeding the Hungry in Your Community

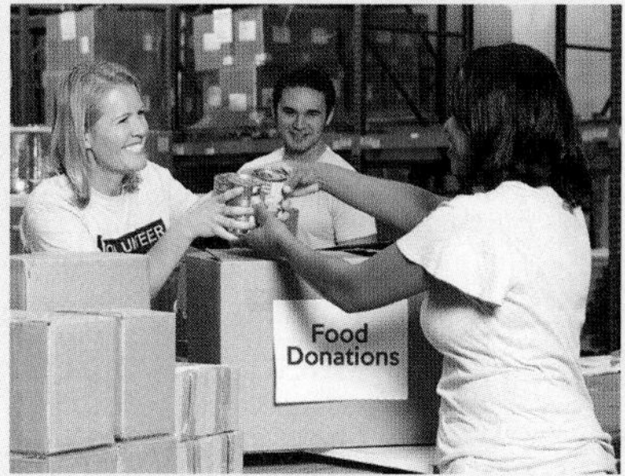

Monkey Business Images/Shutterstock.com

The USDA estimates that one in eight households is food insecure. *Food insecurity* means that a household has insufficient resources to provide food for all its members at some time during the year. People who worry where their next meal will come from have food insecurity. When food insecurity and hunger occur, people do not receive adequate nutrition to thrive and be healthy.

Hunger affects people of all ages living in many locations—children, teens, adults, older adults, city dwellers, and those living in rural areas. Hunger and food insecurity are the result of poverty. When people experience a loss of job, have a medical crisis, lose their homes, or experience other unexpected emergencies, food insecurity occurs. Many working families earn incomes below the poverty level. When an individual or a family has little or no money, choices must be made whether to spend money on food, medicine, or housing.

Fortunately, many community organizations exist to act as a safety net during times of need. For instance, food banks, church community meals, community garden projects, and Meals on Wheels are all examples of local programs working to feed the hungry. In the many thousands of food programs around the country, more than half of their services are provided by volunteers. However, many community-based programs are unable to meet the demand of hunger in America.

Understanding how and why hunger exists encourages many people to help. You can learn more about hunger in America at the Feeding America website. This may inspire you to volunteer your services with one of your local community food programs.

Think Critically

1. Imagine you are living at the poverty level. With limited money to feed your family, would you choose to buy food for the next day, pick up needed medicine, or pay the water bill that is overdue? What is the rationale for your decision?
2. Locate the places where you or your classmates could volunteer individually or as a group. Select one place to use as a class project.

Health Questions Related to Lipids

As you read about the importance of fat in your diet, you may find yourself thinking of specific questions. Many teens and their parents want to know the answers to these frequently asked questions.

Are Fats Bad for Heart Health?

Fats can be both good and bad for your heart—it depends on the type of fat. Current research suggests that replacing saturated fats with polyunsaturated fats may reduce the risk of heart disease, or cardiovascular disease. ***Cardiovascular disease (CVD)*** refers to disease of the heart and blood vessels, such as narrowed or blocked blood vessels. CVD is the leading cause of death in the United States.

Arteries are the blood vessels that carry oxygen and nutrients to body tissues. Fatty compounds made largely of cholesterol can attach to the inside walls of arteries, forming a buildup called ***plaque***. Plaque begins to form early in life in everyone's blood vessels.

As plaque increases, it hardens and narrows the arteries. This condition is called ***atherosclerosis***, the most common form of heart disease. The heart has to work harder to pump blood through narrowed arteries. This strains the heart and causes blood pressure to rise.

Blood clots are more likely to form at the sites of plaque buildup. Blood clots can become lodged in narrowed arteries and cut off the blood supply to tissues fed by the arteries. A buildup of plaque in the arteries feeding the heart muscle can lead to a ***heart attack***. A buildup of plaque in the arteries leading to the brain may result in a ***stroke***. These conditions can be life threatening. In both cases, cells are destroyed because the blocked arteries cannot supply enough nutrients or oxygen to the tissue (**Figure 7.14**).

Scientists have identified risk factors that contribute to CVD. The chances of developing CVD increase rapidly as more factors apply to you. You can reduce the risks of factors beyond your control by carefully managing the factors within your control.

The Uncontrollable Heart-Health Risk Factors

Unfortunately, you cannot control some factors that greatly affect your state of health. Risks for CVD are associated with certain age, gender, and ethnic groups. Certain inherited traits present risks, too. If any of these risks apply to you, getting regular medical checkups can help detect potential problems.

- **Age.** The risk of heart attack increases with age. Most heart attacks occur after the age of 65. Following healthy lifestyle behaviors when you are young can help prevent heart disease later in life.
- **Gender.** If you are male, you are at a greater risk of heart disease than females. Female hormones tend to protect against heart disease. However, hormonal changes that occur during menopause reduce this protective factor in older women. As a result, if other factors are equal, women older than 50 years of age have a risk for CVD equal to men.

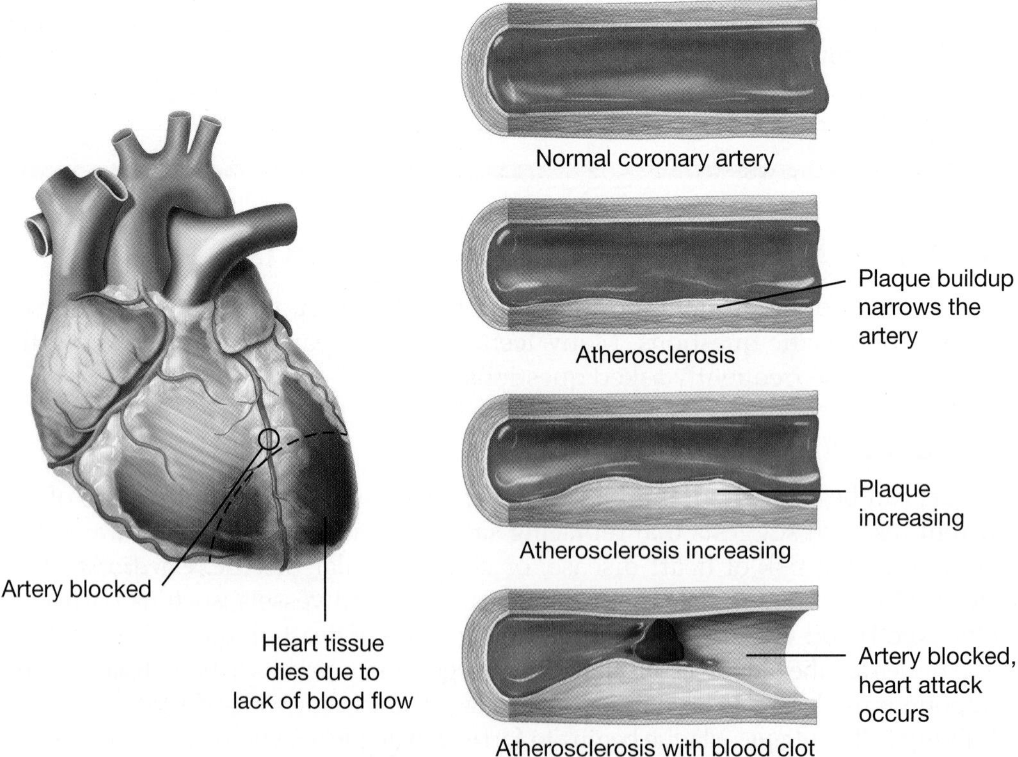

Figure 7.14 Plaque builds up on artery walls, causing cardiovascular disease.

- **Ethnicity.** Some groups of people with a specific ethnic heritage are at greater risk of heart disease than others. For instance, African Americans are twice as likely to have heart attacks as people with Northern European heritage. African Americans also have a higher incidence of high blood pressure. The reasons for this are unclear.
- **Family History.** If one or more of your blood relatives have had heart disease or stroke, your risk increases. Blood relatives include parents, grandparents, aunts, uncles, brothers, and sisters. Use a family health tree diagram to learn more about your family's incidences of heart disease (**Figure 7.15**).

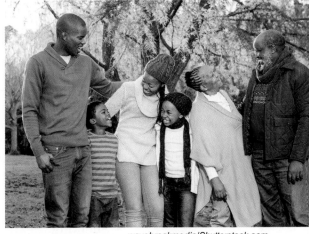

wavebreakmedia/Shutterstock.com

Figure 7.15 The health history of your relatives is a good predictor for your health.

The Controllable Heart-Health Risk Factors

Can your actions help prevent heart attacks? People who have survived heart attacks are the first to tell you that you can and should change your lifestyle behaviors. Many heart attack survivors are motivated to make drastic changes. They quit smoking. They start exercising more. They learn how to manage stress. They also lose weight and eat diets low in saturated fats and *trans* fatty acids.

The biggest risk factors for CVD are smoking, high blood pressure, and high blood cholesterol. Diabetes mellitus, inactivity, stress, and overweight are also risk factors. Through your lifestyle choices, you have some control over all of these risk factors. Changing lifestyle behaviors to control these factors could reduce CVD risk for up to 95 percent of the population.

CASE STUDY

Change of Heart

George is 14 years old. He is 5 feet 4 inches (162.6 cm) tall and weighs 210 pounds (95.3 kg). He knows he is overweight, but he had not given the problem much thought until recently. His 43-year-old uncle suffered a heart attack this year.

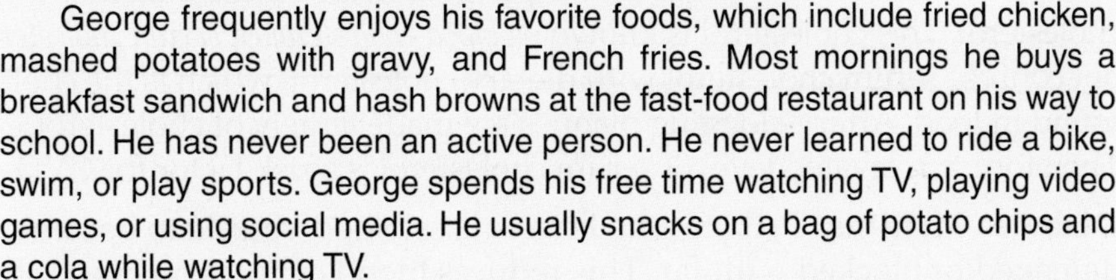

George frequently enjoys his favorite foods, which include fried chicken, mashed potatoes with gravy, and French fries. Most mornings he buys a breakfast sandwich and hash browns at the fast-food restaurant on his way to school. He has never been an active person. He never learned to ride a bike, swim, or play sports. George spends his free time watching TV, playing video games, or using social media. He usually snacks on a bag of potato chips and a cola while watching TV.

George worries that he might suffer an early heart attack like his uncle. He wants to make changes to improve his health but does not know how to begin.

Case Review

1. Which health risk factors are within George's control? Which are not?
2. What lifestyle changes should George make to reduce his risk for heart disease?

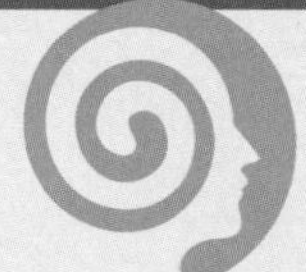

EXTEND YOUR KNOWLEDGE

Women and Heart Health

Recently, medical research has identified special concerns regarding women's heart health. This information has become known as more research focuses on women's health issues. Historically, heart health research has focused heavily on men.

Visit the National Heart, Lung, and Blood Institute's website and read "The Healthy Heart Handbook for Women" to learn about heart disease symptoms, the risks of heart attack, and treatment for women. Reflect on the differences between males and females regarding their health risks and healthcare needs.

- **Smoking.** Heart attacks that occur before age 55 can often be traced to cigarette smoking. Smokers have two to four times more risk of dying from a heart attack than nonsmokers.

  By quitting, people can undo most of the damage caused by smoking. The best advice is never to begin smoking.

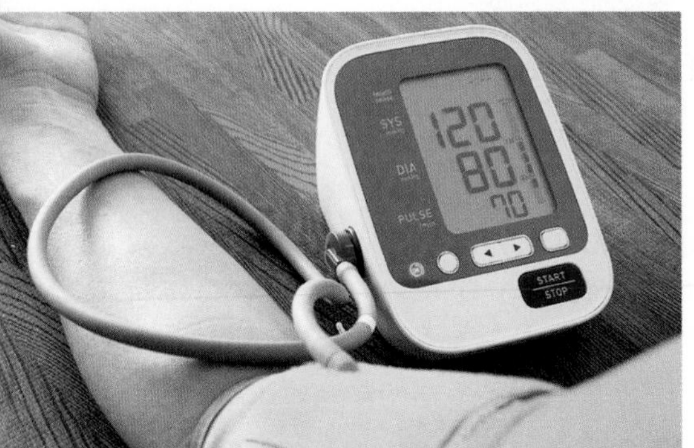

Seasontime/Shutterstock.com

Figure 7.16 A normal blood pressure reading is no higher than 120/80 mmHg.

- **High Blood Pressure.** Abnormally high blood pressure, or ***hypertension***, is a heart-health risk factor. It involves excess force on the walls of the arteries as blood is pumped from the heart. A normal blood pressure reading is no higher than 120/80 mmHg (**Figure 7.16**). The first number in this reading measures *systolic pressure*. This is the pressure on the arteries when the heart muscle contracts. The second number in a blood pressure reading measures *diastolic pressure*. This is the pressure on the arteries when the heart rests between beats. In adults, blood pressure higher than 140/90 mmHg is hypertension.

  High blood pressure places added stress on the heart. It contributes to CVD by damaging the walls of the arteries. The walls then accumulate plaque more easily.

  Doctors cannot cure high blood pressure. However, some people can control it through diet, exercise, and stress management. Doctors often prescribe medication for people who have trouble controlling their blood pressure.

- **High Blood Cholesterol.** Blood serum is the watery portion of blood in which blood cells and other materials are suspended. One of these materials is cholesterol. This cholesterol is known as *blood cholesterol* or *serum cholesterol*. Do not confuse serum cholesterol with dietary cholesterol, which is the cholesterol found in food. Artery-clogging plaques are made largely of cholesterol. Therefore, an elevated level of serum cholesterol is a risk factor for CVD.

- **Diabetes Mellitus.** Diabetes mellitus causes blood vessels to become damaged or blocked with fat. This reduces blood circulation even more than the effects of normal plaque buildups. Therefore, people with diabetes mellitus are at a higher risk of CVD.

  People with type 1 diabetes cannot view their disease as a controllable heart-health risk factor. They must take insulin injections to manage their condition. They cannot control it through lifestyle behaviors.

  However, about 80 percent of people who have diabetes mellitus have type 2. These people do have some control over this risk factor. Type 2 diabetes can often be managed through diet and physical activity.

- **Excess Weight.** Because fats are such a concentrated source of energy, calories from fat mount up surprisingly fast. For example, 2 tablespoons of chocolate hazelnut spread adds 108 calories to a slice of bread. The body can easily convert excess calories from fat into adipose tissue. Excess calories from carbohydrates and proteins are also stored as body fat.

  Every pound of stored body fat is equal to 3,500 calories of energy. One way your body can get energy needed between meals is to break down these fat stores. Many people regularly consume more calories than they need and are physically inactive. Therefore, their fat stores continue to build rather than being used for energy. These people become overweight.

  As fat stores in the body increase, the number of blood vessels must increase to nourish the added tissue. This creates more work for the heart, which increases blood pressure. High blood pressure stretches and injures blood vessels. Points of injury attract cholesterol, adding to plaque buildups. If blood pressure remains high, blood vessels begin to lose their elasticity. This makes it harder to control blood pressure.

  Statistically, overweight people have shorter life spans. Being overweight increases a person's risk of diabetes mellitus and high blood cholesterol, as well as high blood pressure. Each of these factors is also a risk factor for CVD. Therefore, an overweight person is more likely to have a combination of heart-health risk factors. Multiple risk factors place a person's heart health in greater danger than a single factor.

- **Physical Inactivity.** In the United States, only 30 percent of teen males and 13 percent of teen females meet the recommended guidelines for physical activity. Physical inactivity contributes to many people's excess weight problems. In addition, inactive people fail to give their heart the kind of regular workout it needs to remain healthy. People who spend most of their time sitting need to make a point of getting some exercise nearly every day. Exercise helps people manage weight, reduce stress, control cholesterol, and strengthen the heart muscle. Exercise improves the flexibility of your arteries. Muscles receive their blood supply more efficiently. All of these benefits have a positive impact on heart health (**Figure 7.17**).

  Strength training and lifting weights is important. When you contract your muscles, you begin to improve their ability to use glucose and respond with insulin more effectively. Keeping muscles strong protects against high blood pressure and can lower blood sugar.

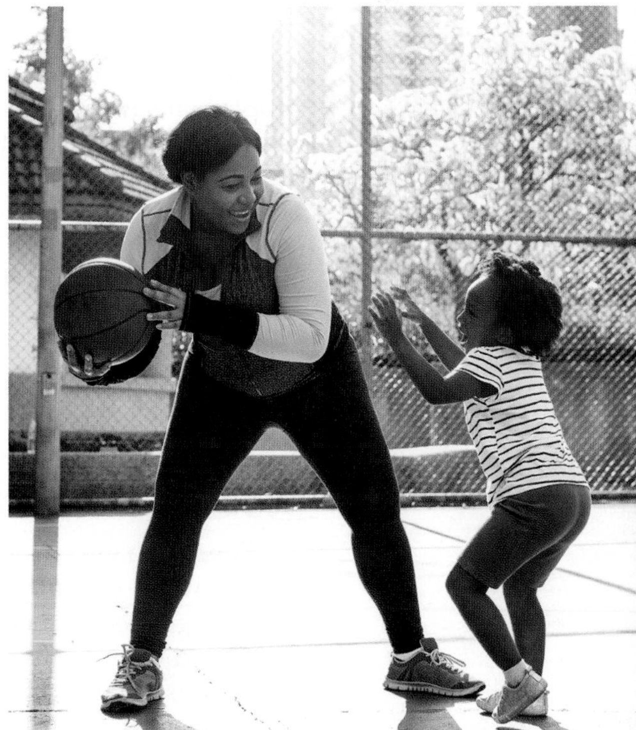

Rawpixel.com/Shutterstock.com

Figure 7.17 Physical activity does not have to be structured to be healthy.

- **Stress.** Research has linked stress and personality to a person's potential for developing heart disease. People who overreact to life's demands on a continual basis may suffer negative heart health. Those who are competitive, impatient, irritable, and easily angered may also be at greater risk.

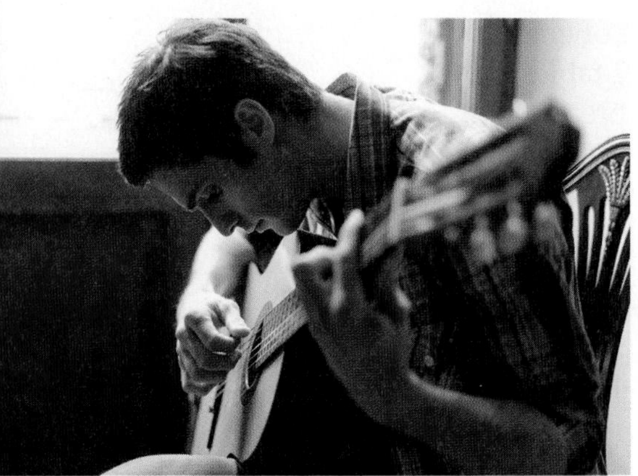

BlueSkyImage/Shutterstock.com

Figure 7.18 Hobbies such as playing a musical instrument can help alleviate stress. *What do you do to manage stress in your life?*

People can learn ways to reduce stress and work toward emotional balance. They can also acquire skills that will help them adapt to the stresses in life. For instance, eating right, establishing healthy eating behaviors, and getting enough rest and exercise can give people the strength they need to handle stress. Finding enjoyable hobbies can help them get their minds off stressful conditions (**Figure 7.18**). Setting priorities and using time effectively can keep some stressful situations from arising. Using these and other techniques can help people manage this heart-health risk factor.

Is Fish Oil Good for You?

Several years ago, the health community focused much attention on the effects of fish oils on heart health. This arose from the observation that the incidence of cardiovascular disease was low among native Alaskans. When analyzing the diet of this culture, researchers found that the Alaskans ate high-fat, high-cholesterol fish. This led the researchers to question why this high-fat diet did not cause the Alaskans to have clogged arteries.

The researchers discovered that fish oils are rich in omega-3 fatty acids. Further research found that omega-3 fatty acids lowered the risk of heart disease. This finding led people to ask if taking fish oil in pill form would improve their health.

The American Heart Association has found no conclusive evidence that fish oil pills lessen the risks of heart disease. In fact, including large amounts of fish oil supplements in the diet can cause health problems. Large amounts of fish oil have been found to thin the blood and may prevent clotting of the blood. Some fish oil, such as cod liver oil, contains large amounts of the fat-soluble vitamins A and D. Therefore, dose instructions should be followed.

Seafood, including fish and shellfish, contain high-quality protein, a variety of vitamins and minerals, and omega-3 fatty acids. You cannot get this range of nutrients from fish oil pills or foods fortified with omega-3 fatty acids, alone. The benefits of eating seafood include improving heart health and potentially helping to reduce the risk of obesity. Including fish in your diet at least once a week offers more benefits than taking fish oil supplements.

Does Fat Cause Cancer?

Cancer is a general term that refers to a number of diseases in which abnormal cells grow out of control. This is in sharp contrast to normal cell growth, which is highly regulated. Cancers can spread throughout the body. As a group, they are the second largest cause of death in the United States.

Scientists have spent years researching the causes and prevention of cancer. Much remains to be learned, but researchers have determined that many factors increase your chances of developing cancer. Diet is among these factors. The National Cancer Institute continues to support research to determine which foods and dietary components are associated with increasing or reducing cancer risk. Up to half of all cancer cases appear to be related to dietary habits and behaviors.

The American Institute for Cancer Research (AIRC) reports that lifestyle choices have a great impact on cancer development. Lifestyle choices are grouped as *cancer promoting* or *cancer protective*. For example, the AIRC suggests you should carefully choose the types and amounts of fat you eat. A diet that includes foods high in saturated fats may promote the development of colon, prostate, breast, and some other types of cancer (**Figure 7.19**). On the other hand, choosing a diet that includes monounsaturated fats and foods high in omega-3 fatty acids may protect against cancer. Eating excess amounts of any food results in weight gain, and excess weight increases cancer risk.

Adding a variety of fruits, vegetables, and whole grains to your daily eating plan is a cancer-protective lifestyle choice. These foods are often low in fat and contain fiber and certain chemicals that have anticancer effects. Maintaining a healthy weight and being physically active on a daily basis are cancer-protective choices as well. This lifestyle helps to prevent a high percentage of body fat, which increases the risks of some types of cancer.

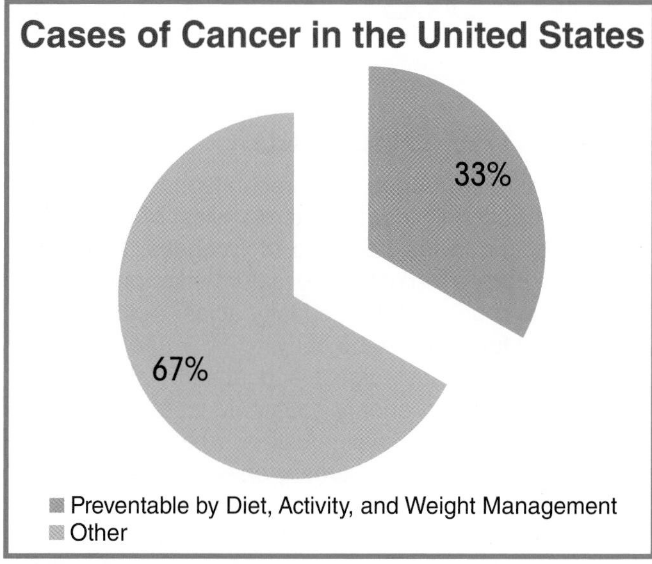

Figure 7.19 The American Institute for Cancer Research estimates that about one-third of common cancers could be prevented with diet, activity, and weight management. *Will this knowledge affect your food choices in the future?*

RECIPE FILE

Marinara Sauce

4 SERVINGS

Ingredients

- 1 T. olive oil
- ½ c. diced onions
- 2 cloves garlic, chopped
- crushed red pepper flakes, to taste (optional)
- 1½ c. canned crushed tomatoes
- 1½ c. canned tomato sauce
- 2 T. tomato paste
- ¼ t. dried basil leaves
- ¼ t. dried oregano leaves
- salt and pepper, to taste
- ½ t. balsamic vinegar
- ½ lb. spaghetti, cooked and drained

Directions

1. Heat the olive oil in a Dutch oven over medium-high heat.
2. Add the onions and cook until softened and translucent, about 8 minutes.
3. Add the garlic and crushed red pepper and cook, stirring, for 1 minute.
4. Add the crushed tomatoes, tomato sauce, tomato paste, basil, oregano, salt, and pepper.
5. Bring to a simmer over medium-high heat, stirring occasionally.
6. Simmer, partially covered, for an additional hour. Stir occasionally to prevent the sauce from sticking to the bottom of the pot.
7. After the sauce has been simmering for 40 minutes, prepare the spaghetti.
8. Bring a large pot of water to a boil and add pasta.
9. Cook until al dente as package directs, approximately 8 minutes for whole-grain spaghetti.
10. Drain pasta in colander.
11. Remove sauce from the heat and serve over cooked spaghetti.

PER SERVING: 270 CALORIES, 10 G PROTEIN, 52 G CARBOHYDRATE, 4 G FAT, 9 G FIBER, 31 MG SODIUM.

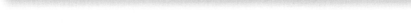

Chapter 7 Review and Expand

Reading Summary

Lipids are grouped into three categories—triglycerides, phospholipids, and sterols. Most of the lipids in foods and in the body are triglycerides. Triglycerides are composed of a mix of saturated, monounsaturated, and polyunsaturated fatty acids. Lipids serve important functions in the body.

The body must digest and absorb fats before using them as an energy source. Most fat digestion takes place in the small intestine, where bile keeps fats emulsified while pancreatic enzymes break down triglycerides. Because blood is mostly water, fats are clustered and covered in a thin coating of cholesterol, phospholipids, and proteins for transport in the bloodstream.

The *Dietary Guidelines* recommends that most of daily fat intake be from unsaturated fats. Two essential fatty acids—*linoleic acid* and *linolenic acid*—must be supplied by the diet. Saturated fats are found primarily in animal foods. *Trans* fats can be artificial or naturally occurring. Recommended eating patterns are low in dietary cholesterol because it is often present in foods that are high in saturated fats. Healthy eating patterns recommend limiting saturated fat.

Saturated and *trans* fats can form deposits in the arteries, which contribute to cardiovascular disease (CVD). A number of factors contribute to a person's risk of CVD. Some of these factors are uncontrollable and some are controllable.

Chapter Vocabulary

1. **Content Terms** Working in pairs, choose two words from the following list to compare. Create a Venn diagram to compare your words and identify differences. Write one term under the left circle and the other term under the right. Where the circles overlap, write three characteristics the terms have in common. For each term, write a difference of the term for each characteristic in its respective outer circle.

adipose tissue
atherosclerosis
cancer
cardiovascular disease (CVD)
cholesterol
chylomicron
emulsifier
essential fatty acid
fatty acid
heart attack
high-density lipoprotein (HDL)
hydrogenation
hypertension
lecithin
lipid
lipoprotein
low-density lipoprotein (LDL)
monounsaturated fatty acid
omega-3 fatty acids
phospholipids
plaque
polyunsaturated fatty acid
rancid
saturated fatty acid
sterols
stroke
trans fatty acid
triglycerides
unsaturated fatty acid
very low-density lipoprotein (VLDL)

2. **Academic Terms** Individually or with a partner, create a T-chart on a sheet of paper and list each of the following terms in the left column. In the right column, list an *antonym* (a word of opposite meaning) for each term in the left column.

abundant
extracted
ingrained
inherent
predominant
ruminant
synthesis

Review Learning

3. What are the three main classes of lipids?
4. List two food sources that are high in each of the three types of fatty acids.
5. How do saturated and *trans* fats contribute to heart disease?
6. What are five major functions of lipids in the body?
7. How do chylomicrons play a role in moving lipids in the body?
8. What percentage of total calories is recommended for daily fat intake?
9. What is a food source of omega-3 fatty acids?
10. How can you differentiate between saturated and unsaturated fats simply by observation?
11. List five choices for improving the fat content of your eating pattern.
12. List three examples of foods with invisible fat.
13. *True or false?* Changing lifestyle behaviors could reduce cardiovascular disease risk for up to 95 percent of the population.
14. List six controllable heart-health risk factors.
15. What effect does diet have on cancer development?

Content Terms 

acid-base balance
amino acid
antibody
buffer
complementary proteins
complete protein
deficiency disease
denaturation
essential amino acid
incomplete protein
kwashiorkor
legume
marasmus
nitrogen balance
nonessential amino acid
protein
protein-energy malnutrition (PEM)
vegetarianism

Academic Terms 

crucial
deficient
excreted
impede
vital

What's Your Nutrition and Wellness IQ?

Take this quiz to examine how much you already know about proteins. If you cannot answer a question; pay extra attention to that topic as you study this chapter.

- Identify each statement as *True*, *False*, or *It Depends*. *It Depends* means in some cases the statement is true; in some cases it could be false.
- Revise false statements to make them true.
- Explain the circumstances in which each *It Depends* statement is true and when it is false.

Nutrition and Wellness IQ 

1.	The molecular structure of protein includes nitrogen, but the structures of fats and carbohydrates do not.	True	False	It Depends
2.	The body can synthesize nonessential (dispensable) amino acids, but essential (indispensable) amino acids must be obtained from the foods you eat.	True	False	It Depends
3.	Adequate amounts of protein in each day's food plans are necessary for healthy growth and development.	True	False	It Depends
4.	Pinto beans are a complete protein and supply all the essential amino acids.	True	False	It Depends
5.	Males have greater protein requirements than females.	True	False	It Depends
6.	Most healthy, growing children are in negative nitrogen balance.	True	False	It Depends
7.	A diet excessively high in protein has few health consequences.	True	False	It Depends
8.	Most athletes need a protein supplement to build muscles and train successfully.	True	False	It Depends

While studying this chapter, look for the activity icon  **to**

- **build** vocabulary with e-flash cards and interactive games;
- **assess** what you learn by completing self-assessment quizzes and completing review questions; and
- **expand** knowledge with interactive activities and activities that extend learning.

www.g-wlearning.com/foodsandnutrition/

As a child, you probably heard people say, "You must eat your meat and drink your milk to get your protein." It is true that meat and milk are good protein sources; however, there are other foods that can supply your body with protein. People are often confused about how much and what type of protein they need.

This chapter will help you determine your protein needs and sources of protein in the diet. It will also help you understand the effects of too little and too much protein in eating patterns.

What Is Protein?

Protein is an energy-yielding macronutrient composed of carbon, hydrogen, oxygen, and nitrogen. The presence of nitrogen in the molecular structure makes this nutrient different from carbohydrates and fats.

Structure of Protein

Amino acids are the building blocks of protein molecules. Most proteins are made up of different patterns and combinations of 20 amino acids, which are linked in strands. An important part of the amino acid structure is the side chain. The side chains give each amino acid an identity and a unique chemical makeup. Most amino acids have the following basic chemical structure:

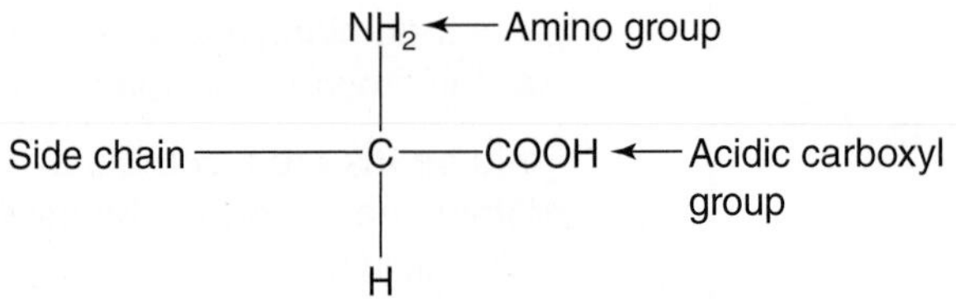

NH_2 ← Amino group

Side chain — C — COOH ← Acidic carboxyl group

H

Proteins make up a major part of the human body, second only to water. At least 30,000 types of protein function within the body. Each type performs a specific job. The number of amino acids and the order in which they are linked determine the type of protein.

Think of amino acids as letters in the alphabet. You can combine the different letters to make words. The words can contain any letters in any sequence. There is no limit to the number of letters in a word. That is why it is possible to have so many different words. In a similar way, amino acids are combined in different sequences to form different proteins. The amino acids can be arranged one after the other in a straight line, or they may be stacked up and branched like a tree. Each protein structure serves a specialized function. *DNA (deoxyribonucleic acid)* is found in the nucleus of every cell. It provides the instructions for how the amino acids will be linked to form the proteins in your body.

You need all the amino acids to make the proteins your body needs for good health. Your body can synthesize 11 of the amino acids from the other 9 amino acids. (The term *synthesize* describes when your body uses one or more compounds to make a new and different compound.) The 11 amino acids your body can make are called ***nonessential amino acids*** (also called *dispensable amino acids*). Your body is not able to make the remaining nine amino acids. These are called ***essential amino acids*** (also called *indispensable amino acids*). You must get essential amino acids from the foods you eat since your body cannot make them.

Certain health conditions interfere with the body's ability to make a nonessential amino acid from an essential amino acid. When this happens, a nonessential amino acid becomes a *conditionally essential amino acid* (sometimes called *conditionally indispensable amino acid*). Since the body is no longer able to create the amino acid, it must be obtained through a dietary source.

Changing Protein Structure

Heat, acids, bases, alcohol, agitation, and oxidation can cause the structure of a protein molecule to change. This is called ***denaturation***. When proteins are denatured, their shape changes and they take on new characteristics.

You can see the effects of denaturation when you cook an egg or marinate a roast—both of these are high-protein foods. Applying heat to an egg changes it from a runny fluid to a solid mass. Soaking a roast in an acidic marinade makes the meat more tender. The shapes of the protein molecules in these foods have changed.

Once proteins are denatured, they can never return to their original state. For example, a hard-boiled egg can never become liquid again (**Figure 8.1**).

Functions of Protein

Your cells can use amino acids from food proteins to build new proteins. Cells can also convert amino acids into other compounds, including other amino acids.

The proteins built by cells are custom designed to perform a wide variety of functions in the body. The following sections describe several key functions of proteins.

Build and Maintain Tissues

Protein is a necessary part of every cell. You need protein to form the structure of muscles, organs, skin, blood, hair, nails, and every other body part. As your body grows, it uses protein to help make new tissue. This is why it is important for you to get enough protein during your growth years, or you may not achieve your physical potential.

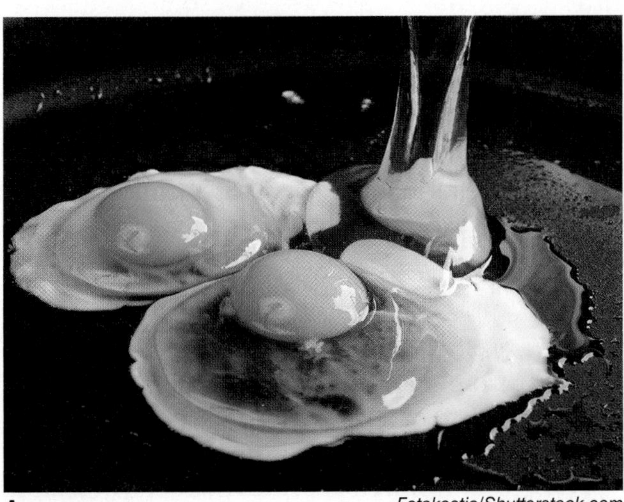

A Fotokostic/Shutterstock.com B Wow Pho/Shutterstock.com

Figure 8.1
A number of factors can denature protein. *Which factors caused the eggs in these photos to denature?*

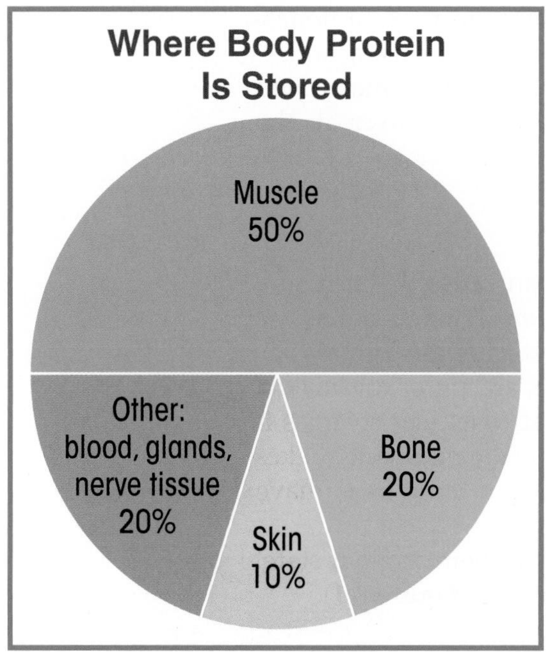

Goodheart-Willcox Publisher

Figure 8.2 Most body protein is stored in muscle tissue. Protein is also located in bone, skin, blood, and all other cell tissue.

Protein makes up about 18 to 20 percent of your body. Skeletal muscle accounts for more than half of body protein (**Figure 8.2**). About three percent of this protein is lost each day as cells wear out and are shed or **excreted** (eliminated). Each cell has a limited life span. To maintain tissue, your body constantly makes new cells to replace those that have died. Therefore, your body needs sufficient protein each day not only to build new tissue, but also to maintain existing tissue.

When you make nutritious eating choices and exercise regularly, your body uses proteins for normal growth and repair of tissue. Growth and repair are possible only when your eating choices provide the necessary mix of amino acids.

Make Important Compounds

Your body uses proteins to make a number of important compounds. These compounds include enzymes, which cause specific chemical reactions in the body. For instance, digestive enzymes cause the chemical breakdown of carbohydrates, fats, and proteins from foods. Proteins are also used to make some hormones. Hormones are chemicals released into the bloodstream to control specific body processes. For example, the hormone insulin helps regulate the level of glucose in the blood. Your body's immune system uses proteins to make antibodies. ***Antibodies*** are proteins that defend the body against infection and disease.

Regulate Mineral and Fluid Balance

Proteins help carry the minerals sodium and potassium from one side of cell walls to the other. These minerals and other proteins control the flow of water through cell membranes. A balance of fluid inside and outside the cells is **crucial** (important). This balance is needed for normal functioning of the heart, lungs, brain, and every other cell.

Maintain Acid-Base Balance

Ongoing processes in the body continually produce *acids* (compounds with low pH) and their counterparts, *bases* (compounds with high pH). Proteins help maintain the acid-base balance of the body. ***Acid-base balance*** refers to the maintenance of stable levels of acids and bases in body fluid. A life-threatening condition can result if the blood becomes too acidic or too basic. Proteins in the blood act as chemical buffers. A ***buffer*** is a compound that can counteract an excess of either acid or base in a fluid.

Carry Vital Substances

Proteins linked with fats form *lipoproteins*, the compounds used to carry fats in the bloodstream. Proteins also transport iron and other nutrients. Oxygen transport in the blood also depends on the presence of a protein. Each cell in the body has proteins that act as "cargo carriers." Protein carries chromosomes and other bundles of protein to other parts of cells. Health suffers if proteins are not available to carry these **vital** (needed) substances throughout the body.

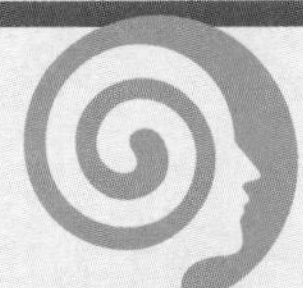

EXTEND YOUR KNOWLEDGE

pH Scale/Acid-Base Balance

The pH scale is used to measure the acidity (amount of acid) or alkalinity (amount of base) of a fluid. The pH scale uses a range of 0 to 14, with 0 being the most acidic measurement and 14 being the most basic measurement. A pH measurement of 7 is neutral. For example, battery acid has a pH of 0, water has a pH of 7, and concentrated lye has a pH of 14.

The ideal blood pH ranges from 7.35 to 7.45. Only seemingly slight moves in either direction of this range—above 8.0 or below 6.8—can result in deadly consequences within a few hours. A blood pH higher or lower than the ideal range can cause proteins to denature.

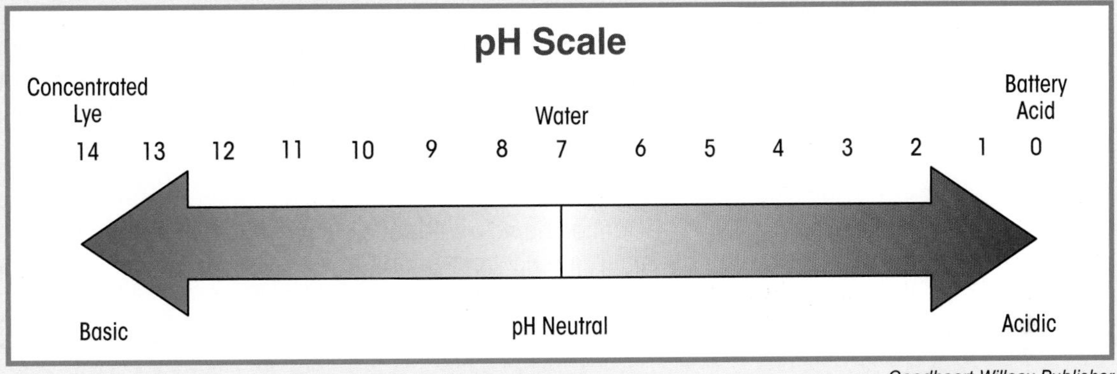

Goodheart-Willcox Publisher

Provide Energy

Only protein can perform the critical functions of cell growth and repair; however, the body's number one priority is to provide the cells with the energy they need to exist. Therefore, if carbohydrates and fats are lacking in the dietary patterns, the body can use protein as an energy source. Protein can be converted into glucose, which becomes the fuel used for energy. Protein yields 4 calories of energy per gram. Unfortunately, protein that is used for energy cannot be used for other purposes, such as building cells.

A shortage of dietary carbohydrates and fats is not the only condition that causes the body to burn protein for energy. The body also uses protein as an energy source when there is an excess of protein in the daily food plan. An excess of protein may also be stored as fat.

How Your Body Uses Protein

Your body must digest and absorb the food protein you eat so that it can make body protein. When you eat a food protein, stomach acids present in the stomach denature the protein. As the protein is denatured, it unfolds and becomes more accessible to enzymes. The enzymes in the stomach begin breaking down protein molecules into shorter strands of amino acids and single amino acids. The strands vary in length from two amino acids (called *dipeptides*), to three amino acids (called *tripeptides*), to some longer strands.

FEATURED CAREER

Food Scientist

Food scientists work to create food products that are healthy, safe, tasty, and easy to use. They find better ways to preserve, process, package, store, and deliver foods. Some food scientists discover new foods and analyze foods to see how much fat, sugar, or protein is in them. Others search for better food additives. Some food scientists work in the food processing industry, while others work in universities and government agencies.

Education

Most jobs require a bachelor's degree, but a master's or doctoral degree is usually required for research positions at universities. Students preparing to be food scientists take courses such as food chemistry, food analysis, food microbiology, food engineering, and food processing operations.

Job Outlook

Job growth in food science should be about as fast as the average for all occupations. This growth will stem primarily from efforts to increase the quantity and quality of food produced for a growing population.

The single amino acids, dipeptides, tripeptides, and longer strands move into the small intestine. In the small intestine, the cells lining the intestinal walls finish splitting the di- and tripeptides and absorb them along with the single amino acids. The amino acids are then released into the bloodstream. The blood carries these amino acids to body cells that need them. The cells use these single amino acids to assemble new proteins as needed.

If a cell is lacking a nonessential amino acid necessary for the construction of a new protein, it will make the needed nonessential amino acid and continue building the protein. If a cell is lacking an essential amino acid, however, construction of the new protein will cease. Imagine if the protein being constructed were an antibody. Now suppose the lack of this essential amino acid was a chronic condition in your diet. How might this affect your health?

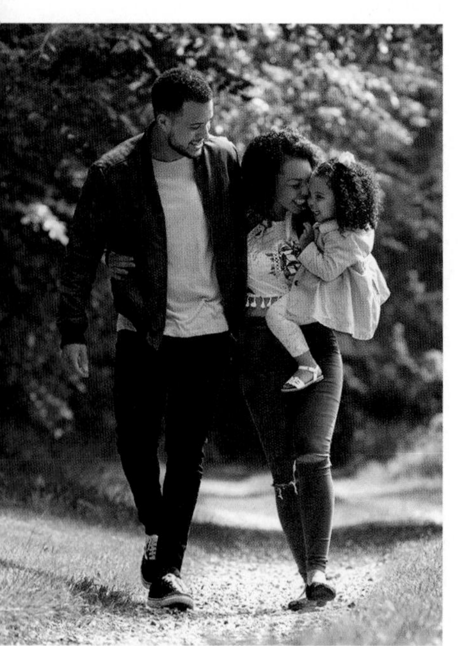

Monkey Business Images/Shutterstock.com

Figure 8.3 Each member of this family has different protein needs.

Meeting Your Protein Needs

Your body does not store protein. Therefore, you need protein every day. Your age, gender, and body size affect the amount of protein you need (**Figure 8.3**). It also depends on your state of health. If you are like most people in the United States, you need less protein than you are consuming.

As children and teens grow, their bodies are building new tissue as well as maintaining existing tissue. Therefore, children and teens have a higher proportional need for protein than people who are no longer growing. In other words, they need more protein per pound of body weight. Similarly, women who are pregnant need extra protein to support the growth of their babies. Women who are breast-feeding also need extra protein to produce milk.

Protein needs vary between males and females. The body needs protein to replace lean tissue (muscle) that wears out and is lost on a daily basis. Men generally have a higher percentage of lean tissue than women do. Therefore, teen and adult males usually require more protein than females of similar age and body size.

The more lean tissue a person has, the more protein is needed to maintain it. Therefore, a large, tall person has a slightly greater protein need than a small, short person.

Illness and injury increase the need for protein. When someone is sick, his or her immune system needs extra protein to build antibodies. When someone is injured, extra protein is needed to rebuild damaged tissue.

Protein Intake Recommendations

The Recommended Dietary Allowance (RDA) for protein is 52 grams per day for 14- to 18-year-old males. The RDA for females in the same age range is 46 grams of protein daily. RDAs for this age range are calculated based on 0.85 grams of protein per kilogram of body weight per day. (One kilogram is equivalent to 2.2 pounds. To convert pounds to kilograms, divide the number of pounds by 2.2.) After age 19, most individuals meet their protein needs with 0.8 grams of protein per kilogram of body weight per day. These are generous allowances that include a margin of safety. RDAs are intended for healthy individuals who eat adequate amounts of carbohydrates and fats. They are also based on the assumption that people are choosing high-quality sources of protein (**Figure 8.4**).

For individuals 4 to 18 years of age, the Acceptable Macronutrient Distribution Range (AMDR) for protein is 10 to 30 percent of calories. This represents a range of intakes to reduce the risk of chronic disease. For individuals 19 years of age and older, the range is 10 to no more than 35 percent. This means a physically active 18-year-old woman who needs 2,400 calories a day should include a minimum of 240 calories from protein daily.

By reading the Nutrition Facts panel on food products, you can estimate how much protein you consume each day. A daily food journal will also help you analyze what percentage of calories in your eating pattern is from protein. How does your daily intake of protein compare with your calculated RDA? Are you eating more or less than the RDA for protein?

Calculating Individual Protein Requirements
For 14- to 18-year-old males and females, use the following equation: 0.85 grams protein × kilograms of body weight = grams of protein per day
Sample calculation for a 150-pound, 16-year-old male: 150 pounds ÷ 2.2 kilograms/pound = 68.2 kilograms 0.85 grams protein × 68.2 kilograms = 58 grams of protein per day
For males and females 19 years of age or older, use the following equation: 0.85 grams protein × kilograms of body weight = grams of protein per day
Sample calculation for a 138-pound, 22-year-old female: 150 pounds ÷ 2.2 kilograms/pound = 62.7 kilograms 0.85 grams protein × 62.7 kilograms = 50 grams of protein per day

Figure 8.4
Protein needs can be calculated based on weight and age. *Why do you think the amount of protein needed per kilogram decreases after 18 years of age?*

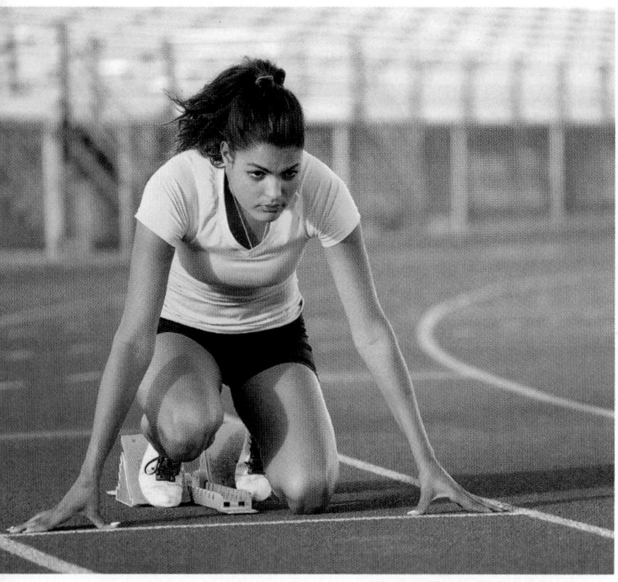

LifetimeStock/Shutterstock.com

Figure 8.5 RDAs are nutrition recommendations for *groups* of people, but an *individual's* requirement may be higher or lower than the RDA.

Factors Affecting Athletes' Protein Needs

Some athletes associate eating a solid piece of meat with building greater masses of body muscle. Serious athletes may wonder if they need more protein in their daily eating pattern than others who are less active. Many athletes—both competitive and casual—are able to meet their needs by consuming their RDA for protein (**Figure 8.5**). Protein and amino acid supplements or large servings of red meat are usually not necessary. Supplements may actually create greater health problems and **impede** (slow) performance gains.

Most athletes perform at their peak by consuming natural sources of protein from foods. Following the MyPlate plan allows adequate protein to meet the daily needs of most athletes.

Availability of Other Nutrients

Exercise involves a big increase in energy expenditure when compared to the resting state. The availability of energy from carbohydrates during exercise affects the body's protein needs. For this reason, an athlete needs to consume adequate carbohydrates and fats in his or her eating pattern so protein can be used to build and repair muscle rather than for energy. Other factors affect the body's protein needs during exercise. Such factors include the intensity, duration, and type of exercise, as well as the gender and age of the athlete.

Gender and Age

An athlete's gender and age may influence his or her protein needs. Some studies report that during distance running events, female athletes may use less protein as an energy source than males. Teens may need more protein since they are still growing. This additional protein is needed for both development and energy needs.

Type of Exercise

Most research on the impact of exercise intensity on protein needs focuses on sports involving strength training, or *resistance training*. Due to the high intensity of these activities, the athletes' protein needs are greater than the needs of athletes participating in low-intensity sports. For example, weight lifting requires high muscular intensity with few repetitions (low endurance) to build muscle. To support this muscle growth, weight lifters require sufficient amounts of amino acids from protein. Heavy resistance training coupled with adequate protein intake improves muscle mass.

When studying how duration of an activity influences protein needs, researchers focus on endurance sports such as long distance cycling, marathons, or triathlons. Distance runners are involved in high-endurance, low-intensity activity and may require protein in excess of the RDA. Since increasing muscle mass is not the goal of these endurance athletes, however, their protein needs are typically less than those of strength (high-intensity) athletes.

Meeting the Protein RDA

One of the simplest ways to meet protein needs is to follow the recommendations of MyPlate. The protein foods and dairy groups include the food sources richest in protein.

THE MOVEMENT CONNECTION

Shoulder Flexibility

Why

Proteins serve multiple functions and help provide growth and maintenance of body tissues. Just like proteins, our joints serve multiple functions. They help us perform work, bear weight, and move in certain directions. It is important to work on flexibility so we maintain the ability of our joints to move through their full range of motion.

This activity burst will focus on flexibility. It is important to note that stretching should never cause high levels of pain or discomfort. The phrase "no pain, no gain" does not apply here! Anytime you have questions about proper stretching techniques, ask your health and physical education teacher, athletic trainer, or other qualified exercise specialist.

Apply

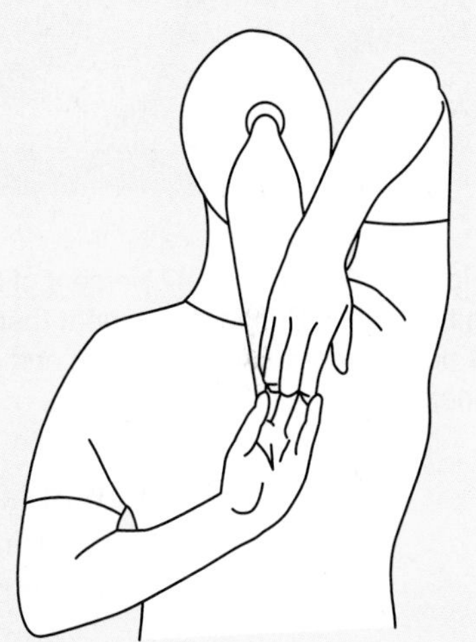

- Stand in front of your desk with good posture. Extend your right arm and raise it over your head, leaving your left arm hanging at your side.
- Bend your right arm at the elbow and reach behind your right shoulder and down your back. (Imagine you are trying to pull a zipper up on the back of your shirt.)
- At the same time, bend your left arm at the elbow and reach up behind your back toward your right hand.
- Try to touch the fingertips of your right hand to those of your left hand. Hold this reach for 5 seconds, then release.
- Repeat with the left arm raised over your head and your right arm at your side.

Did you notice a difference between your right and left side?

For most people, three cup-equivalents from the dairy group are recommended every day. One cup of yogurt, one and one-half ounces of cheese, or two ounces of processed cheese are equivalent to one cup of milk.

For most teens, five to six ounce-equivalents from the protein foods group are recommended daily. Each of the following count as one ounce-equivalent in the protein foods group:

- 1 ounce of meat, fish, or poultry
- ¼ cup of cooked dry beans or peas
- 1 egg
- ½ ounce of nuts or seeds
- 1 tablespoon of peanut butter

When choosing protein food sources, select a variety of foods and avoid consuming saturated fats to reduce certain health risks. Choose protein foods lower in saturated fats, such as fat-free milk, low-fat cheese, fish, nuts, seeds, and beans and peas. Select lean cuts of meat or trim visible fat from fattier cuts. Remove skin from poultry. Use low-fat cooking methods such as grilling, baking, braising, or poaching. Limit the use of high-fat cooking oils, sauces, and gravies with protein foods. Add flavors by using spices and herbs.

Food Sources of Protein

Most people meet their protein needs by eating both animal and plant food sources. Many factors influence which protein foods people choose. Availability, cost, health concerns, food preferences, religious beliefs, and environmental factors all affect people's food choices.

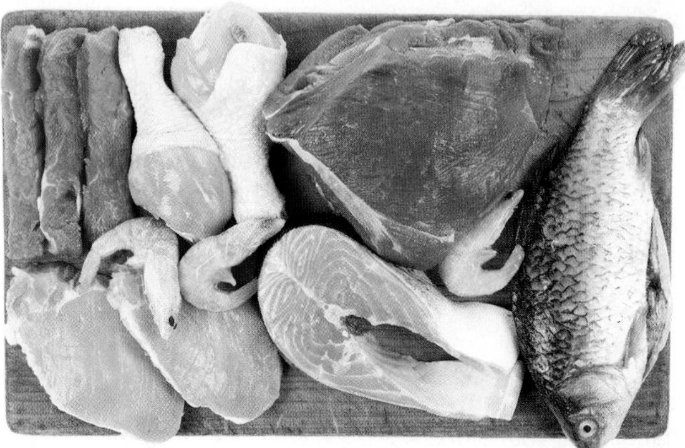

Africa Studio/Shutterstock.com

Figure 8.6 Roughly 47 percent of animal protein consumed in the United States is red meat (beef and pork), 46 percent is poultry (chicken and turkey), and only 7 percent is fish or seafood.

Animal Sources of Protein

Animal flesh is by far the largest source of protein in a meat-eating culture, such as the United States. Animal foods include beef, veal, pork, lamb, poultry, and fish. Other animal sources of protein include eggs, milk, yogurt, and cheese.

The USDA reports that US citizens eat an average of 200 pounds (90.7 kg) of meat, poultry, and seafood annually (**Figure 8.6**). Over the last 100 years, meat consumption has increased dramatically. The fast-food chains that serve hamburgers, chicken, and fish sandwiches provide much of the protein in teens' eating patterns.

Although meat is an excellent source of protein, some meat and dairy products are high in saturated fat. For instance, 57 percent of the calories in regular ground beef come from fat. Of the calories in whole milk, 48 percent come from fat. In contrast to many plant sources of protein, these foods provide no dietary fiber.

Animal sources of protein can be expensive. For example, one ounce (28 g) of a pork loin roast would provide about 8 grams of protein. One ounce (28 g) of sliced Swiss cheese would provide about 7 grams of protein. The cost of the pork roast is about 31 cents, and the cost of the cheese is about 46 cents. In contrast, a ½-cup serving of baked beans provides about 6 grams of protein and costs only about 9 cents. High costs often limit the amount of animal food sources low-income families can buy.

Plant Sources of Protein

A plentiful supply of protein is available from plant foods. Protein is found in grains, nuts, seeds, and legumes. ***Legumes*** are plants that have a special ability to capture nitrogen from the air and transfer it to their protein-rich seeds.

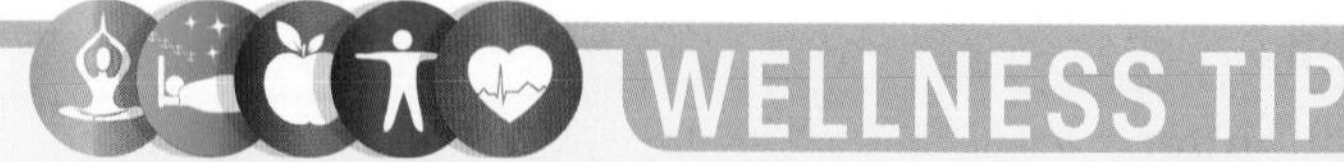

Consider Quinoa

Quinoa (KEEN-wah) is a grain that has been a staple for the people of the Andes Mountains for 5,000 years. Quinoa is considered a high-quality protein because it supplies all the essential amino acids. It is gluten free and a good source of iron and magnesium.

Examples of legumes that are harvested as dry products (also called *pulses*) include black-eyed peas, kidney beans, black beans, lentils, chickpeas, and lima beans. Pulses are rich in fiber and protein, and they contain no fat.

Soybeans and peanuts are also legumes. In contrast to pulses, soybeans and peanuts contain fat. Soybeans are an especially rich source of plant protein. These legumes can be processed and modified to form a variety of food products. For example, tofu is a curd product made from soybeans. It is used as a meat alternative in some dishes. Other pastes and meatlike products can also be made from soybeans (**Figure 8.7**).

Protein Quality

Protein quality differs in various food sources. The quality of the protein in meat, poultry, and fish is very high. Animal foods are sources of ***complete proteins***. This means all the essential amino acids humans need are present in these proteins. Eggs, milk, cheese, and yogurt are also excellent sources of high-quality protein.

The protein provided by plant sources is of lower quality than protein from animal sources. Plants furnish ***incomplete proteins***. These proteins are **deficient** (lacking) in one or more of the nonessential amino acids.

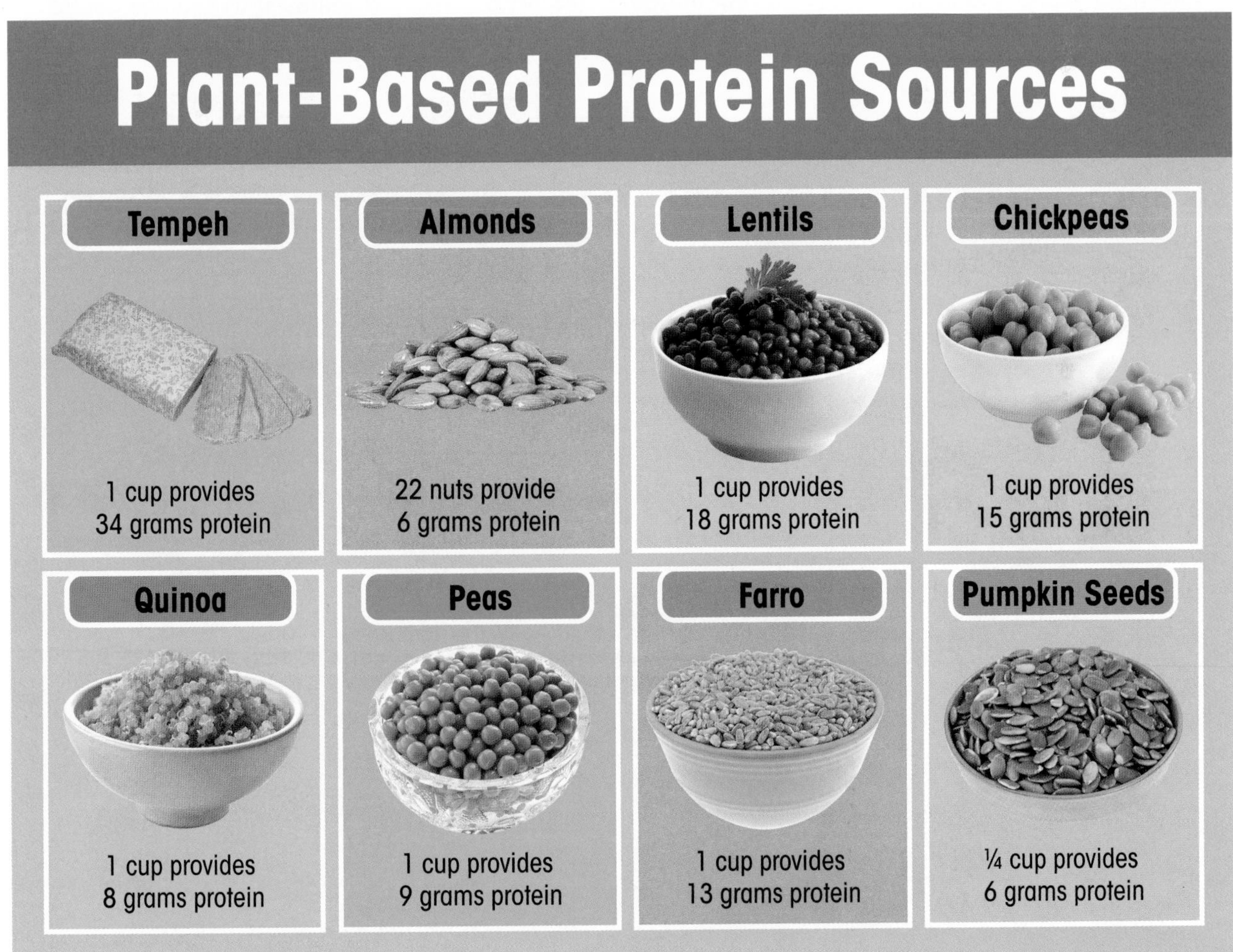

Top row: lavizzara/Shutterstock.com; ang intaravichian/Shutterstock.com; Moving Moment/Shutterstock.com; Moving Moment/Shutterstock.com; bottom row: MaraZe/Shutterstock.com; Scanrail1/Shutterstock.com; BW Folsom/Shutterstock.com; BW Folsom/Shutterstock.com

Figure 8.7 There are many options when choosing a plant-based protein. Some options, such as nuts and seeds, also supply a significant amount of fat and should be consumed in smaller portions.

Complementary Proteins

You can obtain the amino acid missing from an incomplete protein source by including another incomplete source in your eating pattern. When eaten within the same day, these two incomplete protein foods provide all the amino acids that a complete protein source provides. Two or more incomplete proteins that can be combined to provide all the essential amino acids are called ***complementary proteins***.

How do you know which plant foods complement each other? A general guideline is to combine grains, nuts, or seeds with legumes. For example, peanuts (legumes) and wheat (grain) are complementary proteins. Each of these is an incomplete source of protein. When peanut butter is combined with wheat bread, however, the sandwich becomes a source of complete protein (**Figure 8.8**).

People from all over the world combine complementary proteins. For example, Mexican cuisine often combines corn tortillas with refried beans (grain plus legumes). People in the Middle East combine sesame seeds and chickpeas (seeds plus legumes) to make a dip called *hummus*. How many combination foods and meals can you think of that contain complementary proteins?

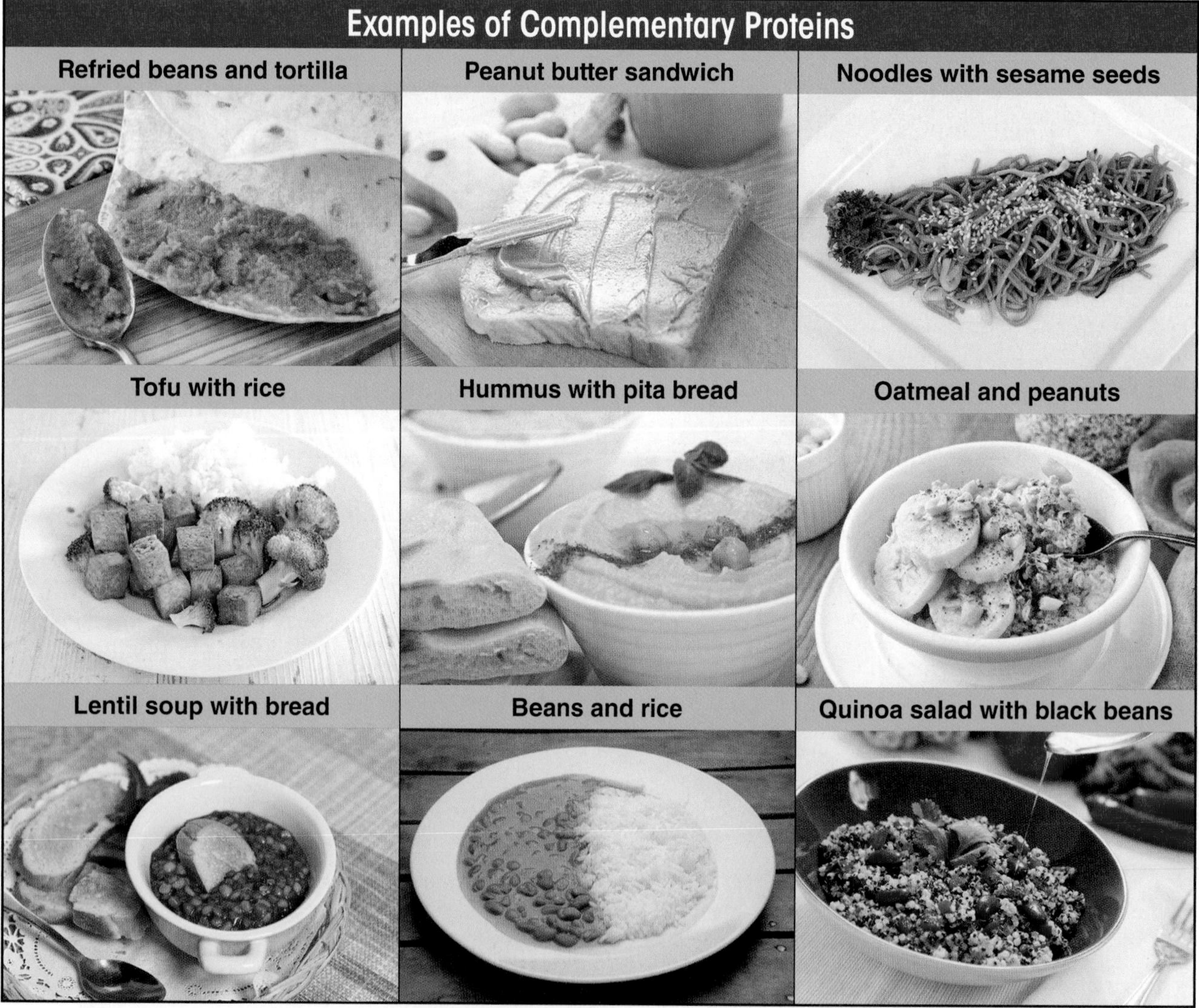
Examples of Complementary Proteins
Refried beans and tortilla
Peanut butter sandwich
Noodles with sesame seeds
Tofu with rice
Hummus with pita bread
Oatmeal and peanuts
Lentil soup with bread
Beans and rice
Quinoa salad with black beans

Top row: Natalia Wimberley/Shutterstock.com; Jiri Hera/Shutterstock.com; keko64/Shutterstock.com; middle row: margouillat photo/Shutterstock.com; TalyaAL/Shutterstock.com; Elena Larina/Shutterstock.com; bottom row: alisafarov/Shutterstock.com; Vanessa Volk/Shutterstock.com; zstock/Shutterstock.com

Figure 8.8 Many popular dishes feature complementary proteins. *Can you think of other examples of dishes with complementary proteins?*

Another way to improve the quality of incomplete protein foods is to combine them with complete protein foods. For instance, you might add a small amount of pork (complete protein) to a large amount of rice (incomplete protein). This improves the protein value of the rice.

Strict vegetarians must think carefully about using complementary proteins. High-quality protein is essential for normal growth and development in children and teens. Dietary patterns that focus on only one incomplete protein, such as rice, are harmful to long-term good health.

FOOD AND THE ENVIRONMENT

Sustainable Seafood

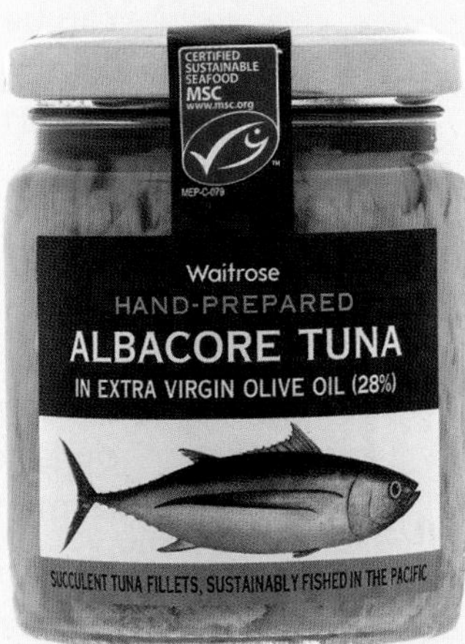

urbanbuzz/Shutterstock.com

Did you know the oceans cover over 70 percent of Earth's surface? Most people thought the oceans' resources were limitless, but this is no longer the belief.

Efficient fishing techniques and the growing consumer demand for fish have tested the limits of the oceans' resources. Now the challenge is how to keep the oceans free from pollution and unsustainable harvesting of fish.

There may not be enough fish to feed the world by 2050 unless there is a change in mindset to *sustainable seafood*. Sustainable seafood requires maintaining thriving, healthy oceans without reducing important marine species. The management of ocean resources is needed to supply the continuing needs for future generations of people.

The fishing industry is a segment of the economy dependent on the oceans' supplies of fish. In many areas, the world's fish stocks are unsustainably caught and marketed. In some cases the aquaculture (fish farming) industries are involved in unsustainable and unfair practices, including overfishing and destruction of other species caught or injured in nets.

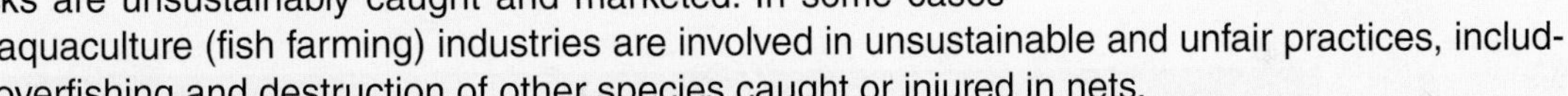

The growing consumer demand for types of seafood that take years to mature (for example, halibut, orange roughy, and Pacific Bluefin tuna) is cause for concern. A shift in eating patterns to smaller fish species found lower on the marine food chain (for example, bass, clams, oysters, and catfish) is necessary for sustainability. These species are more abundant and repopulate quickly. The food choices you make can contribute to restoration of the oceans.

Sustainable fisheries target plentiful species such as Atlantic spiny dogfish and mussels. Destructive fishing practices like bottom-trawling the ocean floor are avoided because of the potential danger to the coral reefs. Sustainable wild fisheries are managed well with accurate population monitoring and regulations that track seafood from the fishing boats to the retailer.

Before buying a fish product, look at the information on the seafood label or ask the retailer about sustainable practices used by the fishery. Responsible retailers care about the future of the oceans. More fish products have MSC-certified seafood (Marine Stewardship Council) labeling to indicate to consumers, retailers, and traders that they are helping to encourage and reward responsible fisheries.

Think Critically

1. What questions would you ask a grocery retailer to determine if the fish was produced using sustainable seafood practices?
2. Why should maintaining a sustainable seafood supply be a concern to individuals living in landlocked areas such as the Great Plains?

Vegetarian Diet

Vegetarianism is the practice of making eating choices consisting entirely or largely of plant foods. Forms of vegetarianism have existed since history began. Today, as in the past, many people choose to avoid eating foods from animal sources. Interest in vegetarianism, especially among young people, seems to be growing. This may explain the increasing popularity of vegetarian cookbooks and restaurants. The eating patterns of people who call themselves vegetarians vary greatly (**Figure 8.9**).

Ask a vegetarian why he or she prefers not to eat foods of animal origin. The answer may simply be that the person grew up in a vegetarian household. Other reasons may include the following:

- *Health reasons* are mentioned by people who want to avoid the saturated fat in meat. They may also want to avoid certain hormones and chemicals used in raising livestock. Some people are concerned about illnesses that can be transmitted by animal foods. These people may claim some animal foods give them digestive problems. They say they feel better when they eat primarily fruits, vegetables, and cereals.
- *Socioeconomic reasons* are given by people who believe eating animals is wasteful. About 90 percent of the soybeans, corn, oats, and barley grown in the United States is fed to livestock. These crops could feed many more people directly than can be fed by the animals that eat the crops.
- *Environmental reasons* are given by people who say animal grazing is hard on land. These people may also mention that meat processing uses a tremendous amount of water and energy.
- *Humanitarian reasons* are stated by people who believe sacrificing the life of an animal for food is wrong. Some oppose the conditions in which animals are raised and prepared for slaughter.

Figure 8.9 Vegetarians are identified by the degree to which they refrain from eating animal foods.

Types of Vegetarians
Vegans, or strict vegetarians, eat no foods from animal sources. Their diet is limited to foods from plant sources.
Fruitarians eat vegan diets based on fruits, nuts, and seeds. Vegetables, grains, beans, and animal products are excluded. (This diet is very restrictive and risk for malnourishment is high.)
Lacto-vegetarians eat animal protein in the form of milk, cheese, and other dairy products. They do not eat meat, fish, poultry, or eggs.
Ovo-vegetarians do not eat meat or dairy products, but do eat eggs. The prefix "ovo" comes from the Latin word for egg. Many people are ovo-vegetarians because they are lactose-intolerant.
Lacto-ovo vegetarians eat animal protein in the form of dairy products and eggs. However, they do not eat meats, fish, or poultry.
Pescetarians eat any combination of vegetables, fruits, nuts, beans, and fish or seafood, but reject animal or poultry food products.
Semivegetarians, also called *flexitarians*, eat mostly plant-based foods along with some dairy products, eggs, poultry, and seafood. They eat little or no red meat—beef, veal, pork, and lamb.

- *Religious reasons* for vegetarianism are cited by followers of many Eastern religions, such as Buddhists and Hindus. Seventh-Day Adventists and other Christian groups who express a compassion for animals also choose to be vegetarians.

In recent years, the health benefits of vegetarianism have received much attention. Most of the fats in plant foods are polyunsaturated. Plant foods contain no cholesterol, and they are generally high in fiber and low in saturated fat. These are positive factors in terms of heart health and cancer risk reduction.

Plant-based protein is not as easily digested as meat-based protein; however, the RDAs for protein are no different for vegetarians. Most people can easily meet their protein needs by eating a variety of whole grains, legumes, nuts, seeds, and vegetables in adequate amounts on a daily basis. The *Dietary Guidelines* includes a Healthy Vegetarian Eating Pattern (**Figure 8.10**).

Vegetarian Eating Pattern

Food Group	Calorie Level of Pattern				
	1,600	1,800	2,000	2,200	2,400
Vegetables	2 c.-eq.	2½ c.-eq.	2½ c.-eq.	3 c.-eq.	3 c.-eq.
Dark-green vegetables (c.-eq./week)	1½	1½	1½	2	2
Red and orange vegetables (c.-eq./week)	4	5½	5½	6	6
Legumes (beans and peas) (c.-eq./week)[a]	1	1½	1½	2	2
Starchy vegetables (c.-eq./week)	4	5	5	6	6
Other vegetables (c.-eq./week)	3½	4	4	5	5
Fruits	1½ c.-eq.	1½ c.-eq.	2 c.-eq.	2 c.-eq.	2 c.-eq.
Grains	5½ oz.-eq.	6½ oz.-eq.	6½ oz.-eq.	7½ oz.-eq.	8½ oz.-eq.
Whole grains (oz.-eq./day)	3	3½	3½	4	4½
Refined grains (oz.-eq./day)	2½	3	3	3½	4
Dairy	3 c.-eq.	3 c.-eq.	3 c.-eq.	3 c.-eq.	3 c.-eq.
Protein Foods	2½ oz.-eq.	3 oz.-eq.	3½ oz.-eq.	3½ oz.-eq.	4 oz.-eq.
Eggs (oz.-eq./week)	3	3	3	3	3
Legumes (beans and peas) (oz.-eq./week)[a]	4	6	6	6	8
Soy products (oz.-eq./week)	6	6	8	8	9
Nuts and seeds (oz.-eq./week)	5	6	7	7	8
Oils	22 g	24 g	27 g	29 g	31 g

c.-eq. = cup equivalent
oz.-eq. = ounce equivalent
[a]About half of total legumes are shown as vegetables, in cup-equivalents, and half as protein, in ounce-equivalents. Total legumes in the patterns, in cup-equivalents, is the amount in the vegetable group plus the amount in protein foods group, in ounce-equivalents, divided by four.
Source: *2015–2020 Dietary Guidelines for Americans*, Appendix 5

Figure 8.10 Although the Healthy Vegetarian Eating Pattern includes dairy and eggs, it can be used to follow a vegan diet by substituting fortified soy beverages or other plant-based products for dairy choices.

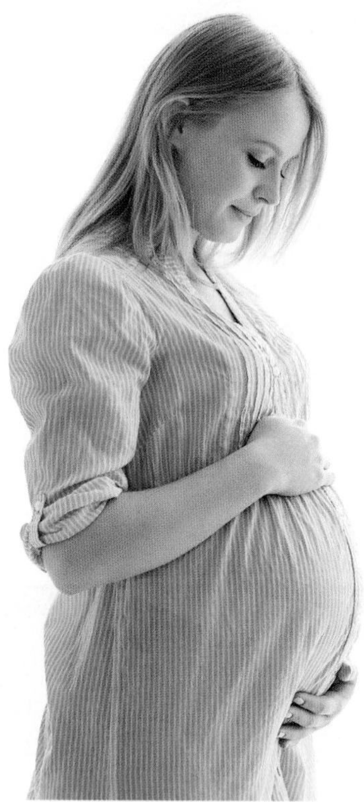

Africa Studio/Shutterstock.com

Figure 8.11 A pregnant woman is in positive nitrogen balance. *What are other situations in which a person might be experiencing positive nitrogen balance?*

Health Questions Related to Protein

As with all nutrients, you need to consume enough protein, but you should avoid getting too much. A lack of protein and a surplus of protein can both cause health problems.

Nitrogen balance is a comparison of the nitrogen a person consumes with the nitrogen he or she excretes. Protein is the only energy nutrient that provides nitrogen. Therefore, nitrogen balance is used to evaluate a person's protein status. Most healthy adults are in *nitrogen equilibrium*. This means they excrete the same amount of nitrogen they take in each day. A person who is building new tissue takes in more protein than he or she excretes. This person is said to be in *positive nitrogen balance*. A pregnant woman or a growing child would be in positive nitrogen balance. Someone whose tissues are deteriorating loses more nitrogen than he or she consumes. This person is said to be in *negative nitrogen balance*. A person whose body is wasting due to starvation would be in negative nitrogen balance (**Figure 8.11**).

Protein Deficiency

A deficiency is a shortage. In nutrition, the term *deficiency* refers to an amount of a nutrient that is less than what the body needs for optimum health. A ***deficiency disease*** is a sickness caused by the lack of an essential nutrient.

For a large portion of the US population, protein is easy to get in amounts that exceed daily recommendations. For people who are living in poverty, however, protein deficiency is common. This is especially true in countries where there is simply not enough food. If the only foods eaten are low in protein, a protein deficiency is likely to occur.

Protein-energy malnutrition (PEM) is a condition caused by a lack of calories and protein in a person's eating pattern. Symptoms of PEM include diarrhea and various nutrient deficiencies.

Kwashiorkor—a protein deficiency disease—is a form of PEM. This disease most frequently occurs in a child when the next sibling is born. The disease is common in poor countries where mothers stop breast-feeding an older child to begin breast-feeding a newborn. The weaned older child is no longer receiving protein-rich breast milk. He or she experiences an eating pattern that may provide sufficient calories but not enough protein.

A child with kwashiorkor does not reach his or her full growth potential. The child develops a bloated abdomen and has skinny arms and legs. Lack of protein also affects the body's fluid balance and immune system. Many children with kwashiorkor die of simple illnesses such as a fever or the common measles.

Another PEM disease is marasmus. ***Marasmus*** is a wasting disease caused by a lack of calories and protein. It most often affects infants. The muscles and tissues of these children begin to waste away. The children become thin, weak, and susceptible to infection and disease. In short, they are suffering from starvation.

Excess Protein

If you are like most people in the United States, you consume more than the RDA for protein. On average, women in the United States eat almost one and one-half times the RDA for protein. Men eat nearly twice the RDA for protein.

CASE STUDY

Building Muscle

Spence is 15 years old and wants to build up his muscles. He does not enjoy much physical activity, but he would like to change the way his body looks. All the guys his age seem to be taller and stronger than him. Spence decides to add more protein to his diet to build his muscles. His friends tell him about protein drinks and other protein food supplements that might help him out. Spence adds the following to his usual daily food plan: 2 whey protein shakes, 3 hard-boiled eggs, and 1 protein snack bar.

Case Review

1. What results do you think Spence will have with his new food plan?
2. What advice would you give Spence?

Some people take protein or amino acid supplements, thinking these products offer health benefits (**Figure 8.12**). Supplements are commonly available as protein powders, whey shakes, protein bars, and capsules. When milk is coagulated to make cheese, the liquid portion that remains is whey protein. This is used to make supplements that are marketed for muscle building or weight loss. Some people consume high-protein diets that consist largely of foods rich in protein, such as meats, poultry, fish, beans, nuts, cheese, and eggs. There is no evidence to show that excess protein contributes to bodybuilding or sports performance success. Using protein supplements is likely a waste of money. In fact, excess protein may hurt your body.

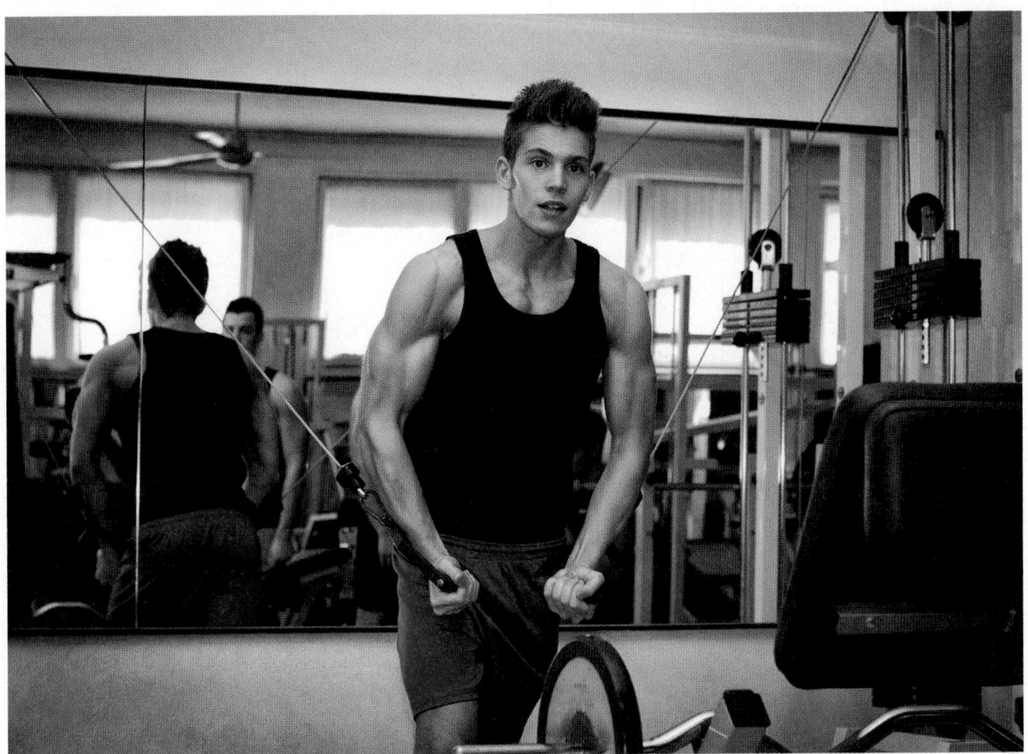

ArtOfPhotos/Shutterstock.com

Figure 8.12 Bodybuilders should be aware of the health risks of taking amino acid supplements and following a high-protein eating pattern.

People should consider the problems associated with high-protein eating patterns. Several health issues and serious complications have been linked to excess protein, including liver and kidney problems, decreased bone density, and excess body fat.

Liver and Kidney Problems

High-protein eating patterns produce an overabundance of nitrogen waste. The body must excrete this waste before it builds up to toxic levels. The liver turns nitrogen waste into urea. The kidneys are responsible for excreting urea in urine. Therefore, excess protein creates extra work for the liver and kidneys. Stress on these organs can be a problem and may cause them to age prematurely. Extra work for the kidneys is a special problem for diabetics, who may already have problems with kidney disease.

Excess Body Fat

Many common high-protein foods, such as whole milk, beef, and cheese, are also high-fat foods. Extra calories from fat can contribute to weight problems. Foods high in fat are also associated with heart-health and cancer risks (**Figure 8.13**).

The body cannot store excess amino acids as a protein source. However, it can store them as an energy source by converting them to body fat. Whether fat accompanies the protein in food or is manufactured from excess amino acids, the consequences are the same. Excess body fat is associated with a number of health problems.

Bone Health

When protein intake is very low, growth and development are impaired; however, calcium absorption may improve during periods of low protein intake. This could be a response to the body's increased need for bone density.

Comparing Protein Sources

Ground Beef Patty	White Beans
4 ounces	1 cup
330 calories	250 calories
16 grams protein	17 grams protein
13 grams saturated fat	less than 0.5 grams saturated fat
0 grams fiber	11 grams fiber

Photos: DronG/Shutterstock.com; onair/Shutterstock.com

Figure 8.13 Compare protein sources to determine which foods contribute more total nutrition.

At one time, high-protein diets were believed to contribute to decreased bone density based on observed increases in calcium excretion during periods of high protein intake. The assumption was that the calcium being excreted was being pulled from bone. More recent studies have shown slight increases in calcium absorption when dietary protein is increased up to 20 percent of total calories. It is possible that protein intakes at the high end of the recommended range produce moderate improvements in bone health when sufficient calcium, fruits, and vegetables are present in the diet.

The relationship between protein and calcium metabolism is complex, and there is currently no basis to recommend high protein intake above 10 to 35 percent of total daily calories for most healthy adults.

RECIPE FILE

Chicken Teriyaki

4 SERVINGS

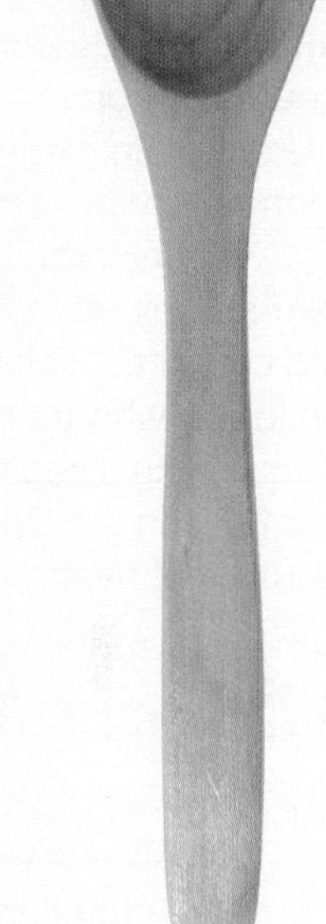

Ingredients

- 8 oz. chicken thighs
- 1 t. fresh ginger, grated
- ¼ t. salt
- 2 t. vegetable oil
- 1 T. honey
- 1 T. rice wine vinegar
- ½ t. sugar
- 2 T. low-sodium chicken broth
- 1 T. soy sauce

Directions

1. Rub ginger and salt into chicken and let sit for at least 30 minutes.
2. After marinating, dry chicken with paper towels to remove any ginger pulp.
3. Heat oil in pan over medium heat.
4. Sauté chicken pieces until golden brown on one side.
5. Turn the chicken and add 1 tablespoon of broth and quickly cover the pan.
6. Steam the chicken until just cooked through, about 5 minutes.
7. Prepare sauce by mixing 1 tablespoon each of: honey, vinegar, sugar, broth, and soy sauce.
8. Remove lid and drain any remaining liquid by tilting pan and spooning liquid out.
9. Use a paper towel to soak up any excess oil.
10. Turn heat up to high and add teriyaki sauce.
11. Let mixture boil, while turning chicken to coat evenly.
12. The chicken is done when it reaches 165°F (74°C) and most of the liquid has evaporated.
13. The sauce will form a thick glaze around the chicken.
14. To serve, slice chicken and pour remaining sauce over slices.

PER SERVING: 114 CALORIES, 12 G PROTEIN, 4 G CARBOHYDRATE, 4 G FAT, 0 G FIBER, 436 MG SODIUM.

Chapter 8 Review and Expand

Reading Summary

Protein is an energy nutrient that is constructed from a combination of amino acids. Proteins serve multiple functions in the body. They provide for growth and maintenance of body tissues. Proteins are used to make important compounds, and they regulate fluid and acid-base balance. They carry vital substances, and they provide energy under special conditions.

Protein needs depend on age, gender, body build, and state of health. RDA for protein can be met by following your MyPlate recommendations for food amounts from the dairy and protein foods groups. Most people in the United States consume more than the recommended amount of protein.

Proteins come from animal food sources, including meat, fish, poultry, milk, and eggs. They also come from plant sources, such as cereals, legumes, seeds, and nuts. Complete proteins provide all the essential amino acids; incomplete proteins do not. Incomplete sources of protein can be combined to make a complete protein. Vegetarian diets must incorporate complementary proteins to supply essential amino acids.

Kwashiorkor and marasmus are two types of protein-energy malnutrition that are common in developing countries. These diseases especially affect young children, who then become susceptible to other life-threatening diseases and infections. Excess protein is common in the United States and may contribute to a number of health conditions.

Chapter Vocabulary

1. **Content Terms** Work with a partner to write the definitions of the following terms based on your current understanding before reading the chapter. Then pair up with another pair to discuss your definitions and any discrepancies. Finally, discuss the definitions with the class and ask your instructor for necessary correction or clarification.

acid-base balance	incomplete protein
amino acid	kwashiorkor
antibody	legume
buffer	marasmus
complementary proteins	nitrogen balance
complete protein	nonessential amino acid
deficiency disease	protein
denaturation	protein-energy malnutrition (PEM)
essential amino acid	vegetarianism

2. **Academic Terms** On a separate sheet of paper, list words that relate to each of the following terms. Then, work with a partner to explain how these words are related.

crucial	impede
deficient	vital
excreted	

Review Learning

3. Compare the chemical structure of protein with that of carbohydrates and fats.
4. What is the difference between an essential and a nonessential amino acid?
5. What role do stomach acids play in protein digestion?
6. How does protein affect growth during the teen years?
7. How do carbohydrates and fats affect the body's use of protein?
8. Name three animal sources and three plant sources of protein.
9. Describe two reasons vegetarians might give for eating little or no food from animal sources.
10. How can vegans meet their needs for complete sources of protein?
11. About what percentage of daily calories should come from protein?
12. List six protein food choices that are low in saturated fats.
13. Compare the nitrogen balance status of a healthy teen with one who is undernourished.
14. A disease brought on by a protein deficiency is called ______.
15. What factors might influence an athlete's requirements for protein in his or her food plan?

Self-Assessment Quiz

Complete the self-assessment quiz online to help you practice and expand your knowledge and skills.

Critical Thinking

16. **Conclude** Research vegan eating patterns and lifestyles using print and Internet resources. Then interview two people who are vegan. Based on your findings, write a persuasive paper arguing for or against a vegan eating pattern.

17. **Analyze** Research three possible solutions to the problem of protein-energy malnutrition in developing countries. Write an opinion paper or give an oral report on the solution you think is most viable. Give reasons for your choice.
18. **Apply** Keep a food diary for three days. Use nutrition analysis software to compare your actual daily protein consumption with the RDA for protein.
19. **Evaluate** Learn how textured-vegetable protein is used to make meat substitutes. Research the comparative costs and nutritional value of these meat substitutes and the foods they are intended to replace. Sample a product made from textured-vegetable protein and evaluate its taste. Write a short summary to report your findings.
20. **Organize** Contact a local food bank to learn which foods are most needed. Identify nonperishable protein food items that could be donated. Organize a nonperishable food donation drive at your school.
21. **Analyze** Use the Internet to learn the various nutritional supplies the World Food Program distributes to people during emergencies or in refugee situations. Compare the calories and protein content of the various products to the RDA. Use spreadsheet software to create a bar chart to present your findings.
22. **Apply** Write a one-day menu to accommodate a vegetarian who eats no meat, fish, or poultry, but does eat dairy products and eggs. Be sure to include the use of complementary proteins. Draw arrows to the different foods to show where protein complements occur.
23. **Analyze** Collect food diaries from a vegetarian and a nonvegetarian friend. Complete a nutrition analysis to determine if protein needs are met in both cases. On the SuperTracker website, select the Other Tools tab, and click on "Food Tracker" to assess food intake.

Core Skills

24. **Science** Interview a biology teacher to learn how muscle develops. How does resistance training make muscle stronger? What other factors are important for muscle builders to consider?
25. **Math** In the United States, an individual's weight is typically stated in units called *pounds.* The scientific field commonly uses the metric system of measurement. The metric system measures weight in units called *kilograms (kg).* One kilogram is equivalent to 2.2 pounds. To convert pounds to kilograms, divide the number of pounds by 2.2. To convert kilograms to pounds, multiply the number of kilograms by 2.2.
    A. Convert 135 pounds to kilograms. (Round to one decimal place.)
    B. Convert 48 kilograms to pounds. (Round to one decimal place.)
26. **Science** Construct a model of a protein molecule using materials such as toothpicks, marshmallows, and other materials available in the classroom or at home.
27. **Speaking** Investigate a manufacturer's claims about their amino acid supplements. Determine whether the claims are valid. Compare the cost and nutritional value of these supplements to whole food protein sources. Consider any dangers posed by the use of these products. Create a video of yourself role-playing an investigative reporter presenting the findings.
28. **Math** Visit the local supermarket or go online and select three different sources of protein—one animal source, one fish source, and one plant source. Calculate the price per ounce, grams of protein per ounce, and the price per gram of protein for each. Rank the protein sources from highest to lowest price per gram of protein.
29. **Writing** Research and write an informative paper examining the health benefits and drawbacks of each type of protein source (meat, fish, plant-based). Organize your thoughts logically and provide a concluding section that summarizes your findings about the type(s) of protein necessary for a healthful diet. Cite your sources.
30. **Career Readiness Practice** Presume you are a department manager at a local social services agency. Your department works with people who have limited resources for food, including families with young children and older adults. For most clients, obtaining adequate daily protein is a financial problem. Develop a resource listing how much high-protein foods—both animal and plant protein sources—cost and where they can be purchased locally. Determine the relative costs by comparing cost per ounce for each food type. Provide tips to help your clients more accurately calculate and budget costs for serving high-quality protein foods to their families.

CHAPTER 9 Vitamins

Learning Outcomes

After studying this chapter, you will be able to

- **recall** the major roles of vitamins in the diet and their effect on health and wellness;
- **understand** the relationship of fat-soluble and water-soluble vitamins with their common dietary sources;
- **summarize** functions and sources of specific vitamins;
- **explain** common health problems of various vitamin deficiencies and excesses;
- **apply** dietary recommendations for meeting vitamin needs;
- **examine** the role phytochemicals and healthful microorganisms play in promoting good health;
- **evaluate** the use of vitamin supplements; and
- **compare** ways to select, cook, and store foods to maximize vitamin content.

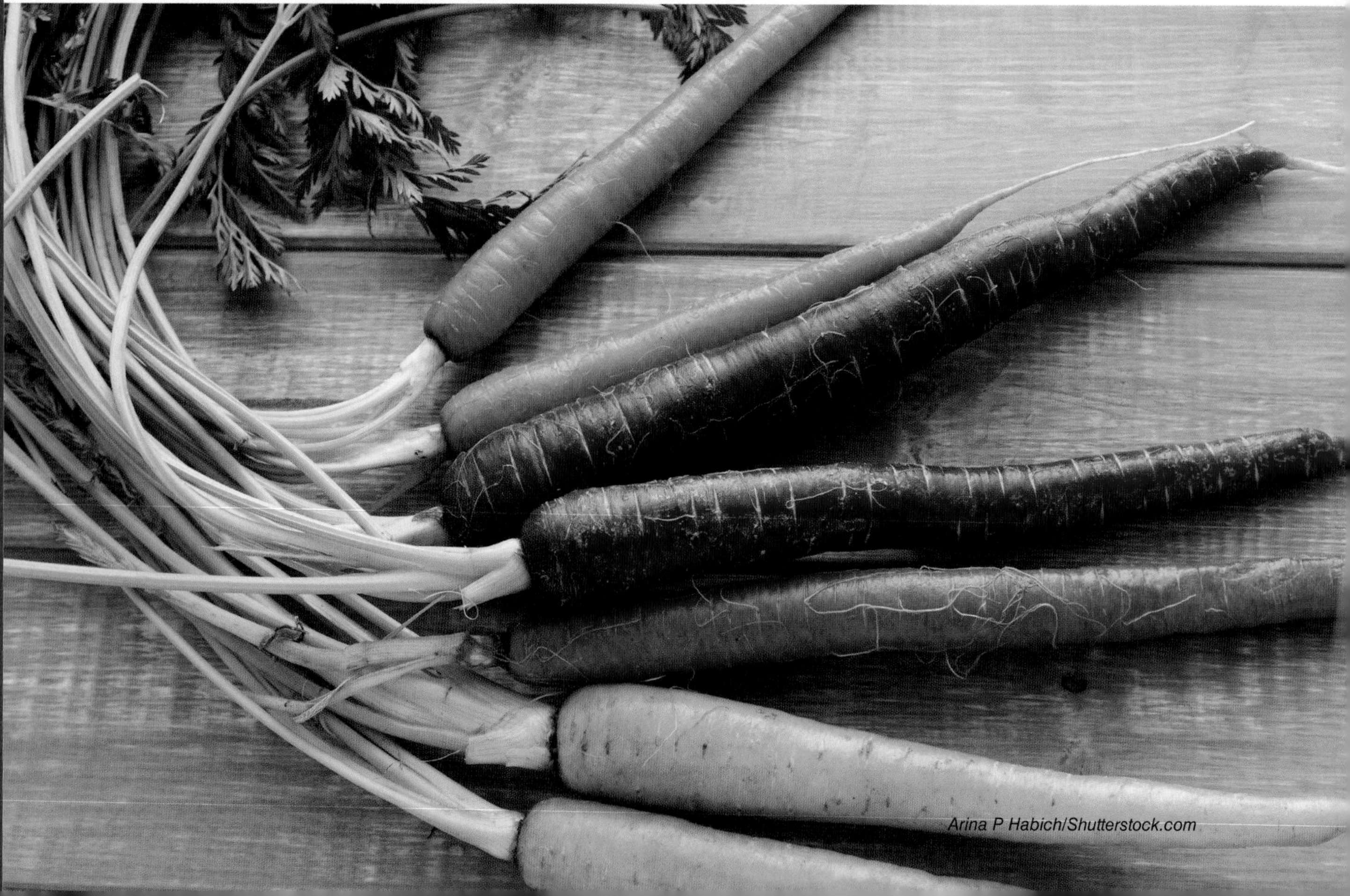

Arina P Habich/Shutterstock.com

Content Terms

antioxidant
beriberi
coagulation
coenzyme
collagen
enriched food
epithelial cells
erythrocyte hemolysis
fat-soluble vitamin
fortified food
free radical
night blindness
osteomalacia
pellagra
pernicious anemia
phytochemicals
placebo effect
prebiotics
probiotics
provitamin
rickets
scurvy
toxicity
vitamin
water-soluble vitamin

Academic Terms

apt
augment
conclusive
dilated
surplus
versatile

What's Your Nutrition and Wellness IQ?

Take this quiz to examine how much you already know about vitamins. If you cannot answer a question; pay extra attention to that topic as you study this chapter.

- Identify each statement as *True*, *False*, or *It Depends*. *It Depends* means in some cases the statement is true; in some cases it could be false.
- Revise false statements to make them true.
- Explain the circumstances in which each *It Depends* statement is true and when it is false.

Nutrition and Wellness IQ

Statement			
1. The main function of vitamins is to provide extra energy.	True	False	It Depends
2. Most water-soluble vitamins are found in fruits and vegetables.	True	False	It Depends
3. Pregnant women need to meet the RDA for folate to avoid potential health risks for their baby.	True	False	It Depends
4. The body can manufacture most vitamins from the food that is consumed.	True	False	It Depends
5. Vitamin D and calcium work together to form strong bones.	True	False	It Depends
6. Phytochemicals have an antioxidant effect and help with the prevention of certain chronic diseases.	True	False	It Depends
7. Using a vitamin C supplement is important to treat a cold.	True	False	It Depends
8. Soaking peeled potatoes in water for an extended period has no effect on vitamin content.	True	False	It Depends

While studying this chapter, look for the activity icon to

- **build** vocabulary with e-flash cards and interactive games;
- **assess** what you learn by completing self-assessment quizzes and completing review questions; and
- **expand** knowledge with interactive activities and activities that extend learning.

www.g-wlearning.com/foodsandnutrition/

Although nutrition research began in the nineteenth century, vitamins were not identified until the beginning of the twentieth century. Today, vitamins continue to be in the news. Scientists have learned much about vitamins. However, many questions concerning the roles of vitamins in the diet remain.

Will taking extra vitamin C prevent a cold? Should you take vitamin supplements rather than trying to get vitamins from food? Do fresh, raw vegetables supply more vitamins than canned or cooked vegetables? These are among the questions for which researchers have already found answers. You will learn about these and other topics related to vitamins as you study this chapter.

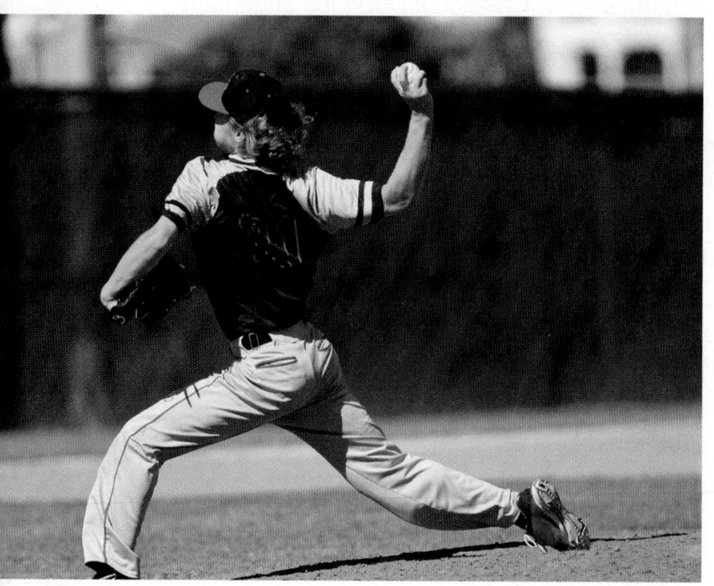

tammykayphoto/Shutterstock.com

Figure 9.1 Vitamins help the body release energy needed for physical activity.

What Are Vitamins?

A ***vitamin*** is an essential nutrient needed in very small amounts to regulate body processes. Vitamins are organic compounds because they contain carbon. Vitamins have no calorie value because they yield no energy; however, the body needs vitamins for the chemical reactions involved in releasing energy from other nutrients (**Figure 9.1**).

Vitamins in the foods you eat are essential for regulating body processes. Each vitamin has specific functions. As a nutrient group, vitamins assist with the following functions:

- nutrient metabolism
- energy production and release
- tissue maintenance
- normal digestion
- infection resistance

Vitamin Names

In 1912, Casimir Funk, a food science professor in Poland, coined the word *vitamine*. *Vita* means life; *amine* refers to a certain organic chemical structure that contains carbon and nitrogen. After years of research, scientists discovered that few vitamins had the amine structure in their chemical compounds. As a result, the final *e* was dropped.

Vitamins were named as they were discovered. The first vitamin discovered was named *vitamin A*. Logically, the next vitamin discovered was named *vitamin B*. However, scientists later discovered that vitamin B was several different vitamins. Additionally, some compounds originally thought to be vitamins turned out not to be. Therefore, the pattern to the naming of the vitamins became harder to recognize.

Today, there are 13 known vitamins. Some vitamins are most often referred to by a letter, such as vitamins A, C, D, E, and K. On the other hand, most of the B vitamins are better known by a name, such as riboflavin (B_2), thiamin (B_1), and niacin (B_3).

Most vitamins have several *active forms* that perform in the body. All of the active forms have similar molecular structures; however, not every form may be able to do every function associated with the vitamin. The different active forms are like different car models. Some models have navigation systems and some do not, but they can all provide transportation.

There are different names for each form of the same vitamin. For example, *pyridoxine*, *pyridoxal*, and *pyridoxamine* are all forms of vitamin B_6. You may have noticed some of these complex names on the ingredient lists of food labels (**Figure 9.2**).

The Chemistry of Vitamins

Unlike carbohydrates, fats, and proteins, the different vitamins do not share a typical molecular structure. Each vitamin is unique. Although all vitamins contain carbon, hydrogen, and oxygen, some also contain nitrogen, sulfur, or cobalt in their structures.

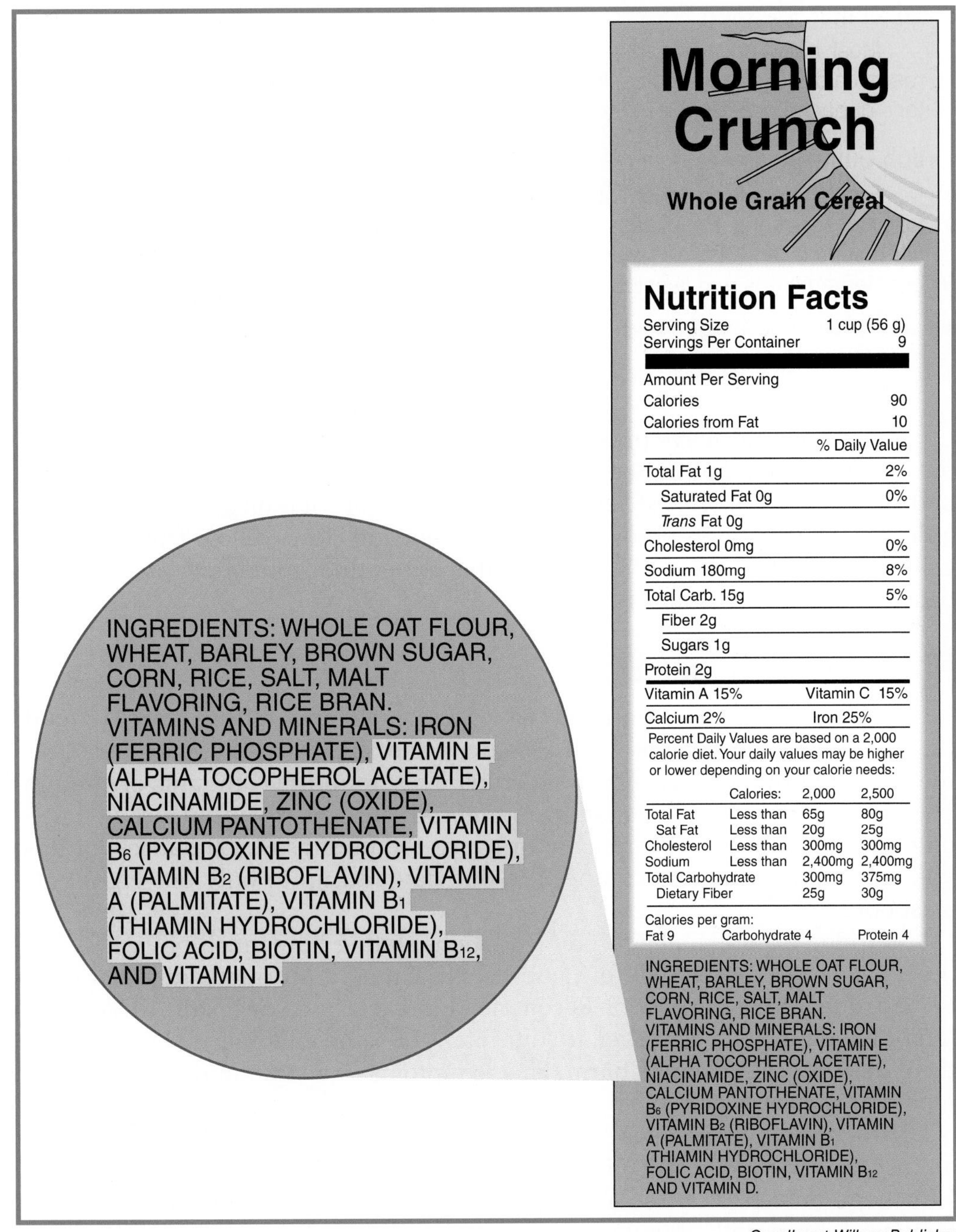

Morning Crunch
Whole Grain Cereal
Nutrition Facts
Serving Size 1 cup (56 g)
Servings Per Container 9
Amount Per Serving
Calories 90
Calories from Fat 10
% Daily Value
Total Fat 1g 2%
Saturated Fat 0g 0%
Trans Fat 0g
Cholesterol 0mg 0%
Sodium 180mg 8%
Total Carb. 15g 5%
Fiber 2g
Sugars 1g
Protein 2g
Vitamin A 15% Vitamin C 15%
Calcium 2% Iron 25%
Percent Daily Values are based on a 2,000 calorie diet. Your daily values may be higher or lower depending on your calorie needs:
Calories: 2,000 2,500
Total Fat Less than 65g 80g
Sat Fat Less than 20g 25g
Cholesterol Less than 300mg 300mg
Sodium Less than 2,400mg 2,400mg
Total Carbohydrate 300mg 375mg
Dietary Fiber 25g 30g
Calories per gram:
Fat 9 Carbohydrate 4 Protein 4
INGREDIENTS: WHOLE OAT FLOUR, WHEAT, BARLEY, BROWN SUGAR, CORN, RICE, SALT, MALT FLAVORING, RICE BRAN. VITAMINS AND MINERALS: IRON (FERRIC PHOSPHATE), VITAMIN E (ALPHA TOCOPHEROL ACETATE), NIACINAMIDE, ZINC (OXIDE), CALCIUM PANTOTHENATE, VITAMIN B6 (PYRIDOXINE HYDROCHLORIDE), VITAMIN B2 (RIBOFLAVIN), VITAMIN A (PALMITATE), VITAMIN B1 (THIAMIN HYDROCHLORIDE), FOLIC ACID, BIOTIN, VITAMIN B12 AND VITAMIN D.

Goodheart-Willcox Publisher

Figure 9.2 Ingredient lists on food labels often include the complex chemical names of added vitamins. *How might this affect the consumer's opinion about the food product?*

FEATURED CAREER

Biochemist

Biochemists study the chemical composition of living things. They analyze the complex chemical combinations and reactions involved in metabolism, reproduction, and growth. Many conduct further research to understand the effects of foods, drugs, serums, hormones, and other substances on tissues and vital processes of living organisms.

Education

Most biochemists need a Ph.D. (doctorate) in biology to work in independent research or development positions. Other positions are available to those with a master's or bachelor's degree in the field.

Job Outlook

Employment for biochemists is expected to increase about as fast as the average for all occupations. Population growth will fuel a need for more genetic and biomedical research, and there is also a quickly increasing demand for work in genetically engineered crops and livestock to combat rising food prices.

Several vitamins have provitamin forms. A ***provitamin*** is a compound that is not a vitamin, but that can be converted into the active form of a vitamin by the body. For example, *beta-carotene* is a provitamin for vitamin A. Beta-carotene is a deep-yellow compound found in dark green and deep yellow fruits and vegetables, including carrots. When you eat this compound, your body can change the beta-carotene into vitamin A.

How Much Is Needed?

Long ago, doctors wondered why just small amounts of specific foods improved health problems, such as scurvy and night blindness. They learned the answer with the discovery of vitamins. They found the amounts of vitamins you need for growth, maintenance, and reproduction were tiny. In fact, you need only about one ounce of vitamins for every 150 pounds (2,400 ounces) of food you eat. All the vitamins you need in one day add up to only one-eighth of a teaspoon.

Nutrition experts make recommendations stating how much of various vitamins people need each day for good health. Eating a nutritious diet that meets the Adequate Intakes (AIs) or Recommended Dietary Allowances (RDAs) is an important daily goal. However, if your intake of some vitamins is short now and then, there is no immediate harm. First symptoms of a vitamin deficiency take a month or so to appear in most people.

There are two main causes of vitamin deficiency diseases. The first cause is an insufficient amount of a vitamin in the diet. In cases of poverty, people may lack the resources to choose a variety of foods that can provide all the vitamins they need. Even with abundant food choices, some people simply fail to choose vitamin-rich food sources, and as a result, deficiencies can occur.

Getting enough vitamins in the daily food plan can be more of a challenge for people who have increased vitamin needs. Pregnant women have increased needs for a number of nutrients, including most vitamins. Infants and adolescents need extra nutrients to aid in the growth of body tissues (**Figure 9.3**). People who are sick or recovering from injuries also have greater vitamin needs. Lifestyle behaviors can also increase the need for certain vitamins. For instance, cigarette smokers need more vitamin C in their daily food plan than nonsmokers.

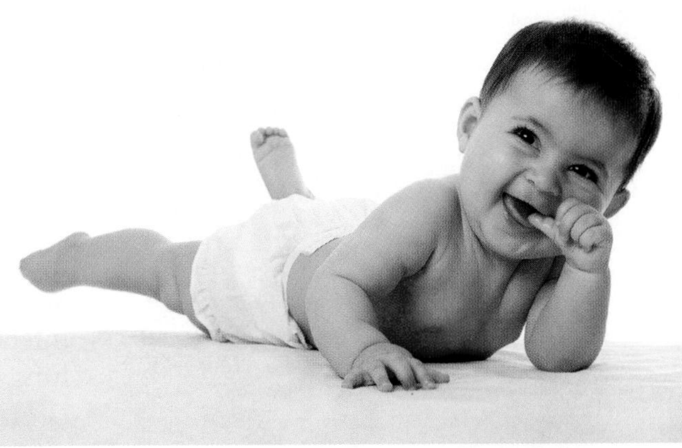

Paul Hakimata Photography/Shutterstock.com

Figure 9.3 Infants need relatively large amounts of vitamins to support their rapid growth.

The second cause of a vitamin deficiency disease is a failure of the body to absorb a vitamin. For instance, changes in the body that occur with age can affect a person's ability to absorb vitamin B_{12}. When food moves through the intestinal tract too quickly, vitamins do not have a chance to be absorbed adequately. Diarrhea or a very high-fiber diet may affect absorption in this way. Malabsorption of some nutrients can also be due to a lack of other nutrients.

Vitamin Classifications

All vitamins are grouped in two categories—fat-soluble or water-soluble. *Soluble* refers to a substance's ability to dissolve. Some vitamins dissolve in fats. The four ***fat-soluble vitamins*** are vitamins A, D, E, and K. Other vitamins dissolve in water. The nine ***water-soluble vitamins*** are the eight B-complex vitamins and vitamin C.

Your body stores excess fat-soluble vitamins when your intake exceeds your body's needs. For this reason, it is not crucial to consume the fat-soluble vitamins every day. On the other hand, megadoses of these vitamins can result in vitamin toxicity in the body. ***Toxicity*** means a level or degree that is poisonous. Simply eating vitamin-rich foods will not result in harmful levels of these nutrients in the body, but taking large quantities of vitamin supplements may.

Your body stores very little, if any, water-soluble vitamins. Excesses are normally excreted in the urine and may cause the urine to become more yellow. Consequently, water-soluble vitamins do not readily build up to toxic levels in the body. Without large stores of these vitamins, however, deficiency symptoms may not take long to develop. Therefore, you should consume sufficient water-soluble vitamins most days.

The Fat-Soluble Vitamins at Work

The fat-soluble vitamins, A, D, E, and K, are present in a wide range of foods in the diet. They are absorbed through the intestinal walls with fats from foods. Your body can usually draw on stored reserves of these vitamins when your intake is low.

Vitamin A

Vitamin A deficiency is the leading cause of preventable blindness in children living in Africa, Southeast Asia, and South America. According to the World Health Organization (WHO), vitamin A deficiency results in blindness in an estimated 250,000 to 500,000 children every year. Half of them die from severe infections within 12 months of losing their sight.

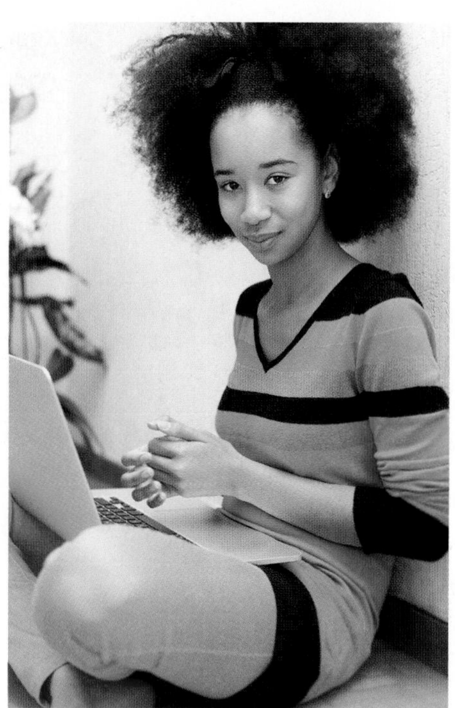

Samuel Borges Photography/Shutterstock.com

Figure 9.4 Vitamin A helps maintain healthy skin, hair, and eyes.

Functions of Vitamin A

Vitamin A is necessary for the formation of healthy epithelial tissue. The ***epithelial cells*** are the surface cells that line the outside of the body. Epithelial tissue also covers the retinas of the eyes and lines the passages of the lungs, intestines, and reproductive organs. Because of this function, vitamin A plays a role in keeping skin and hair healthy. Adequate amounts of vitamin A help keep the eyes moist and free from infections (**Figure 9.4**). Vitamin A also helps the linings of the lungs and intestines stay moist and resistant to disease.

Maintaining healthy eyesight is another main function of vitamin A. Without sufficient vitamin A, eyes cannot make the compounds needed to see well in dim light. As a result, the eyes adapt slowly to darkness and night vision becomes poor. This condition is called ***night blindness***.

Vitamin A is also crucial for the development of bone tissue. If bone formation is hampered, normal growth will not occur.

Meeting Vitamin A Needs

The RDA for vitamin A is 900 micrograms for males ages 14 years and older. The RDA is 700 micrograms for females over 14 years old. (Males need more of many nutrients to support their higher percentage of lean body tissue.)

Another unit of measure for vitamin A is the *retinol activity equivalent (RAE)*. This unit measures the strength of various vitamin A compounds and the ease with which the body can use them.

Vitamin A in foods exists in two basic forms—one from animal sources and the other from plant sources. Animal foods usually provide vitamin A as a *preformed* vitamin. This is an active form the body can use. Plant foods provide vitamin A as provitamin *carotenes*, including alpha- and beta-carotene. The body can convert these compounds into the more usable form of vitamin A. However, they are not in an active form your body can use when you consume them. Therefore, they have a lower RAE value than preformed vitamin A.

Liver, fish oils, egg yolks, and whole-fat dairy products are good sources of preformed vitamin A. Removing the fat from dairy products also removes the fat-soluble vitamin A. Therefore, reduced-fat dairy products are fortified with vitamin A. ***Fortified foods*** have one or more nutrients added during processing. Good sources of provitamin A carotenes include winter squash, carrots, broccoli, cantaloupe, and apricots.

Following the MyPlate guidelines for a healthy eating pattern is a sure way to get sufficient vitamin A for healthy growth and development.

Effects of Vitamin A Deficiencies and Excesses

People who drink little milk or eat few vegetables may show signs of vitamin A deficiency. Symptoms of the deficiency may include night blindness; dry, scaly skin; and fatigue.

Vitamin A deficiency is one of the major causes of blindness in the world. It is a serious problem in underdeveloped nations. Without adequate vitamin A, the membrane covering the eyes becomes dry and hard. Infection and blindness can develop. If detected early enough, vision problems caused by deficiency can be reversed with large doses of vitamin A.

While getting enough vitamin A is important, consuming too much can also cause health problems. The Tolerable Upper Intake Level (UL) is 2,800 micrograms for 14- to 18-year-olds. The body can store vitamin A to toxic levels. Symptoms of vitamin A toxicity include severe headaches, bone pain, dry skin, hair loss, vomiting, and liver damage. Toxicity poses a greater risk for children. Very high vitamin A intake is especially dangerous during pregnancy. Such intakes can cause babies to be born with disabilities.

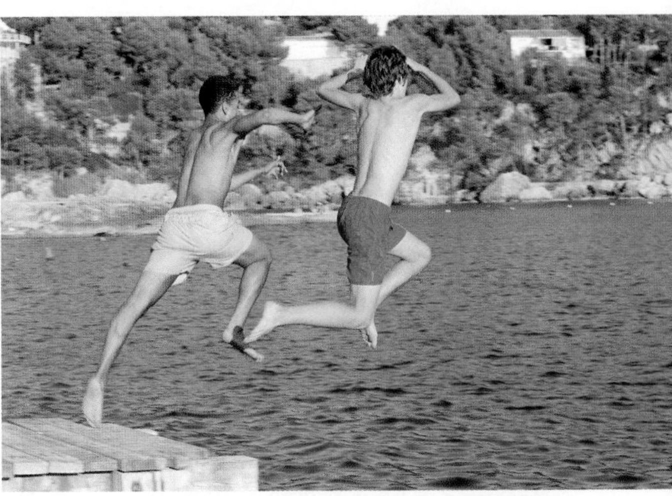

MANDY GODBEHEAR/Shutterstock.com

Figure 9.5 The body can make vitamin D with exposure to sunlight.

Vitamin D

Vitamin D is a unique fat-soluble vitamin. With direct sunlight exposure, your body can make most of the vitamin D it needs (**Figure 9.5**).

Functions of Vitamin D

An important function of vitamin D is to help regulate the levels of calcium in the bloodstream. Normal amounts of calcium in the blood are needed for healthy nerve function, bone growth and maintenance, and other functions. Vitamin D performs this function by triggering the release of calcium from the bones. Vitamin D also controls blood calcium levels by enhancing the absorption of calcium from the intestines. When blood calcium levels are low, vitamin D also reduces the amount of calcium the kidneys excrete.

Vitamin D plays a major role in bone health. Bone tissue is the chief user of blood calcium. This mineral makes bones rigid and strong. However, nerve, muscle, and other cells also require calcium drawn from the bloodstream to function properly. Therefore, vitamin D plays a role in maintaining all body tissues. More recently, vitamin D has been discovered to play a major role in regulating the cell cycle. It affects cell growth and *cell differentiation*. Cell differentiation is the process by which a cell changes from a generic cell to a more specialized cell such as a nerve cell or a bone cell.

Meeting Vitamin D Needs

A growing body of research indicates that both calcium and vitamin D deficiency is widespread throughout the world as well as in the United States, particularly in adults 70 and older. The RDA for vitamin D is 15 micrograms per day for all people through age 70. The RDA is higher for older adults. This is to help older adults avoid developing porous, fragile bones—a condition that is more common in later life.

Vitamin D occurs in 10 different forms. The two forms important to humans are the provitamins D_2 (ergocalciferol) and D_3 (cholecalciferol). The provitamin D_2 is found in plant foods. D_3 is found in animal foods, but is also made by the human body in the skin when exposed to sunlight. When sunlight shines on skin, a cholesterol-like compound in the skin forms the D_3 provitamin. The liver and kidneys then change the provitamin into the form of vitamin D best used by the body.

Spending too much time in the sun without protecting the skin increases the risk of skin cancer. Fortunately, the skin does not need prolonged sun exposure to make vitamin D. A light-skinned person can make enough vitamin D to meet the body's needs in 15 minutes of sun exposure. Dark-skinned people require a somewhat longer time to produce the same amount of vitamin D.

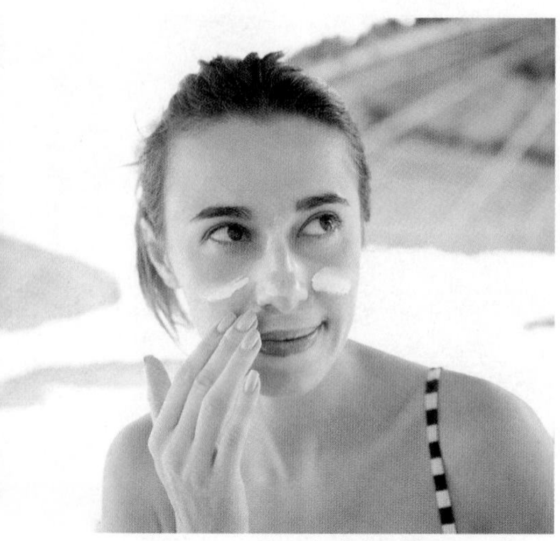

Tymonko Galyna/Shutterstock.com

Figure 9.6 Sunscreen inhibits vitamin D production. *What other factors inhibit vitamin D production?*

Anything that filters sunlight, including clouds, smog, window glass, sunscreen, and heavy clothing, inhibits vitamin D production (**Figure 9.6**). People living in the Northern Hemisphere can experience many days with little or no sunshine. Anyone who does not receive enough sunshine must get vitamin D from food sources.

Vitamin D occurs in a limited number of foods. Fish oil and fatty fish, such as salmon, lake trout, and tuna, are good food sources. Eggs, butter, and vitamin D-fortified milk and margarine are also good sources of vitamin D.

Effects of Vitamin D Deficiencies and Excesses

Rickets was once a common childhood disease. ***Rickets*** is a deficiency disease in children caused by lack of vitamin D. Without adequate vitamin D present, insufficient calcium is deposited in the bones. This causes the bones to be soft and misshapen. The leg bones may bow in or out. The chest bones may bulge outward. The disease is now rare in the United States. It may occur in countries where infants do not receive vitamin D supplements with breast milk or formula. Children who receive little exposure to sunlight, or who live in smog-filled urban areas, are at greater risk for vitamin D deficiency.

Osteomalacia is a vitamin D deficiency disease—similar to rickets— that afflicts adults. It can cause the leg and spine bones to soften and bend. Osteomalacia is different from *osteoporosis*, which is a bone condition related to calcium that affects older adults.

Too much vitamin D can be poisonous and toxicity occurs most quickly in children. Excessive sun exposure does not cause vitamin D toxicity. Obtaining too much vitamin D from food would be difficult. Therefore, toxic intakes are usually the result of consuming supplements in amounts greater than the UL. The UL for vitamin D is 100 micrograms per day for anyone over eight years old.

Excessive amounts of vitamin D cause too much calcium to be absorbed into the bloodstream. This **surplus** (excess) calcium is then deposited in the kidneys and other soft organs. This causes the organs to become hard and unable to perform their vital functions.

Vitamin E

Many dramatic claims are made about the benefits of vitamin E. It has been promoted as an aid for enhancing athletic performance and reducing the signs of aging; however, research does not provide strong evidence to support such claims.

Functions of Vitamin E

Vitamin E helps maintain healthy immune and nervous systems, but its main function is as an antioxidant. ***Antioxidants*** are substances that react with oxygen to protect other substances from the harmful effects of oxygen exposure. Vitamin C and provitamin A are also antioxidants. As an antioxidant, vitamin E ties up oxygen that could otherwise damage the membranes of white and red blood cells. It also protects the cells of the lungs.

In Earth's atmosphere, oxygen typically bonds with a second oxygen molecule to form a compound (O_2). When bound together, they are stable. On the other hand, a single oxygen molecule is highly reactive. This lone molecule wants to react with other compounds as quickly as possible. Such a highly reactive, unstable, single oxygen molecule is called a ***free radical***. Free radicals regularly form in the body due to ordinary cell processes and environmental conditions. These single oxygen molecules can generate a harmful chain reaction that can damage tissue.

Vitamin E and other antioxidants help deactivate or transform free radicals. In the absence of antioxidants such as vitamin E, tissue damage can occur (**Figure 9.7**).

Antioxidants

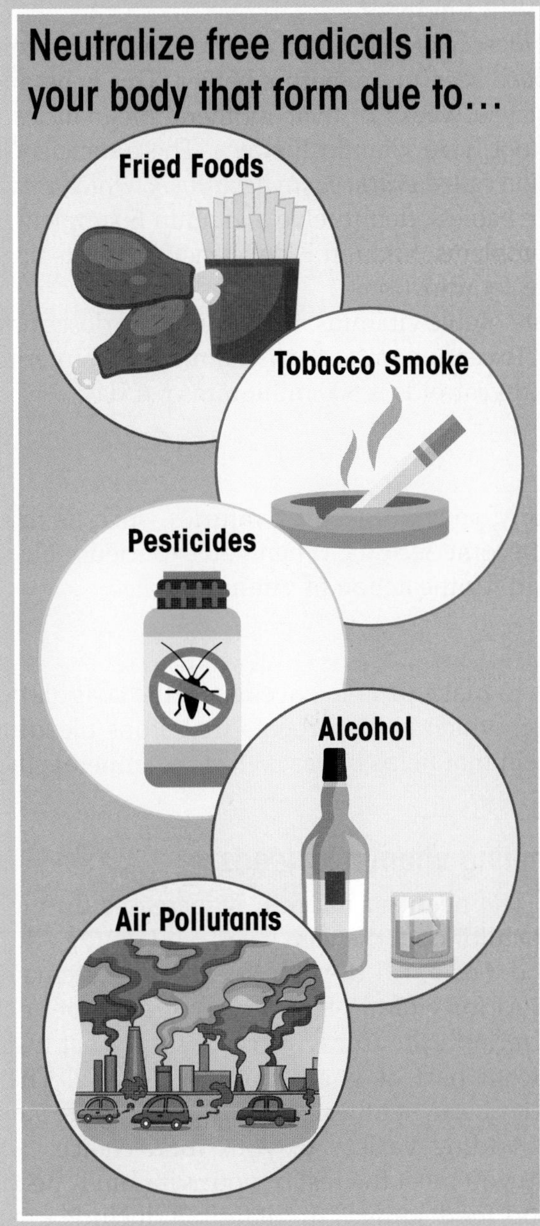

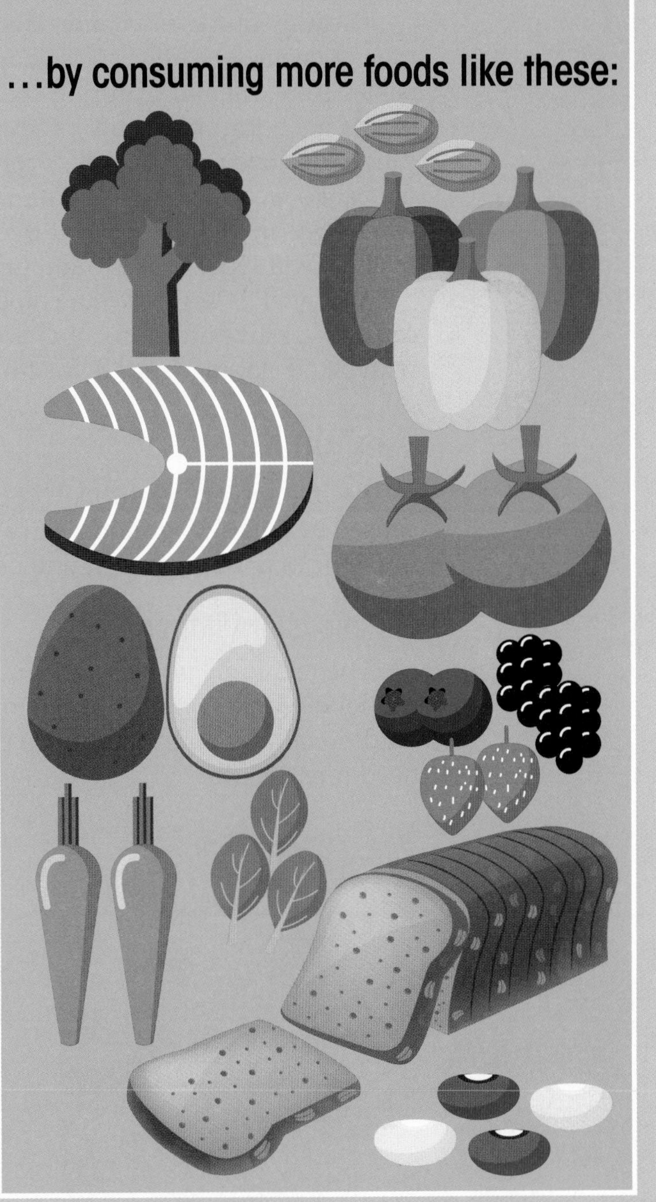

Left side, top to bottom: Voinau Pavel/Shutterstock.com; Voinau Pavel/Shutterstock.com; Macrovector/Shutterstock.com; MicroOne/Shutterstock.com; Alexander Ryabintsev/Shutterstock.com; Lorelyn Medina/Shutterstock.com; Right side, all except bread: KJNNT/Shutterstock.com; Bread: Netta07/Shutterstock.com

Figure 9.7 Vitamins E and C, and provitamin A are antioxidants that work to neutralize free radicals in your body before they can damage cell membranes, DNA (your genetic code), or enzymes.

Meeting Vitamin E Needs

The RDA for vitamin E is 15 milligrams per day for males and females over 14 years old. Research provides no strong support for consuming large amounts of vitamin E. There is also no support for taking vitamin E supplements instead of obtaining it from food sources.

Choosing a variety of foods across the food groups may provide many sources of vitamin E. The best food sources of Vitamin E are wheat germ, whole grain and fortified cereals, and nuts, particularly almonds. Peanut butter, broccoli, and spinach are also good sources.

High temperatures destroy vitamin E. Therefore, foods that are prepared or processed with high heat lose their vitamin E value.

Effects of Vitamin E Deficiencies and Excesses

Because sources of vitamin E are widespread in the diet, deficiencies are not common. Nonetheless, deficiencies have been seen in premature babies. This is because babies store vitamin E during the last few weeks of their mothers' pregnancies. If babies are born prematurely, they do not have vitamin E stores. These deficiencies cause red blood cells to break, a condition called ***erythrocyte hemolysis***, which makes the babies weak and listless. Premature babies often receive a vitamin E supplement when they are born to prevent these problems. Vitamin E deficiency in adults negatively affects speech, vision, and muscle coordination.

Vitamin E is less toxic than other fat-soluble vitamins. However, large doses have caused digestive problems and nausea. Excessive amounts of vitamin E may interfere with blood clotting. The UL for 14- to 18-year-olds is 800 milligrams per day.

Vitamin K

Facing surgery is difficult for many people. Bleeding injuries, such as those caused by cuts and wounds, can also become serious. When you experience bleeding injuries or surgery, you will be glad for the action of vitamin K.

Functions of Vitamin K

The main function of vitamin K is to make proteins needed in the coagulation of blood. ***Coagulation*** means clotting, which is the process that stops bleeding. Additionally, vitamin K makes a protein that helps bones collect the minerals they need for strength.

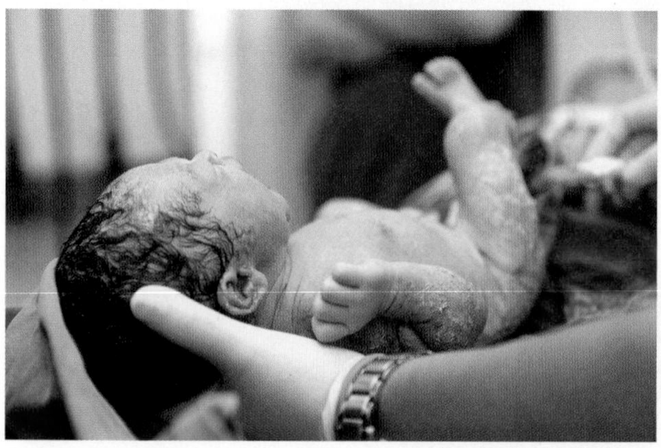

Naypong/Shutterstock.com

Figure 9.8 Newborns may lack vitamin K because they have not yet acquired the intestinal bacteria that produce the vitamin.

Meeting Vitamin K Needs

The need for vitamin K increases throughout childhood, the teen years, and young adulthood. For 14- to 18-year-old males and females, the AI for vitamin K is 75 micrograms per day. Bacteria in the intestinal tract help meet a significant part of your vitamin K needs. These bacteria can synthesize vitamin K (**Figure 9.8**).

Adding variety to your food choices will help you meet the rest of your vitamin K needs. Good food sources of vitamin K include green leafy vegetables, cabbage, and broccoli. Prunes, blueberries, blackberries, eggs, grain products, and nuts also supply small amounts of this vitamin.

Effects of Vitamin K Deficiencies and Excesses

There are few cases of vitamin K deficiency. However, a deficiency can occur among people who take antibiotics that kill intestinal bacteria. Newborns can also be at risk for vitamin K deficiency. This is because they do not yet have enough bacteria in their intestines to synthesize the vitamin. Newborns typically receive a vitamin K supplement. This helps meet their needs until bacteria in their intestines can begin producing enough vitamin K.

Although vitamin K can be toxic, toxicity is rare. A symptom of toxicity is *jaundice*, which is a yellow coloring of the skin. Vitamin K toxicity can cause brain damage. There is no UL established for vitamin K at this time (**Figure 9.9**).

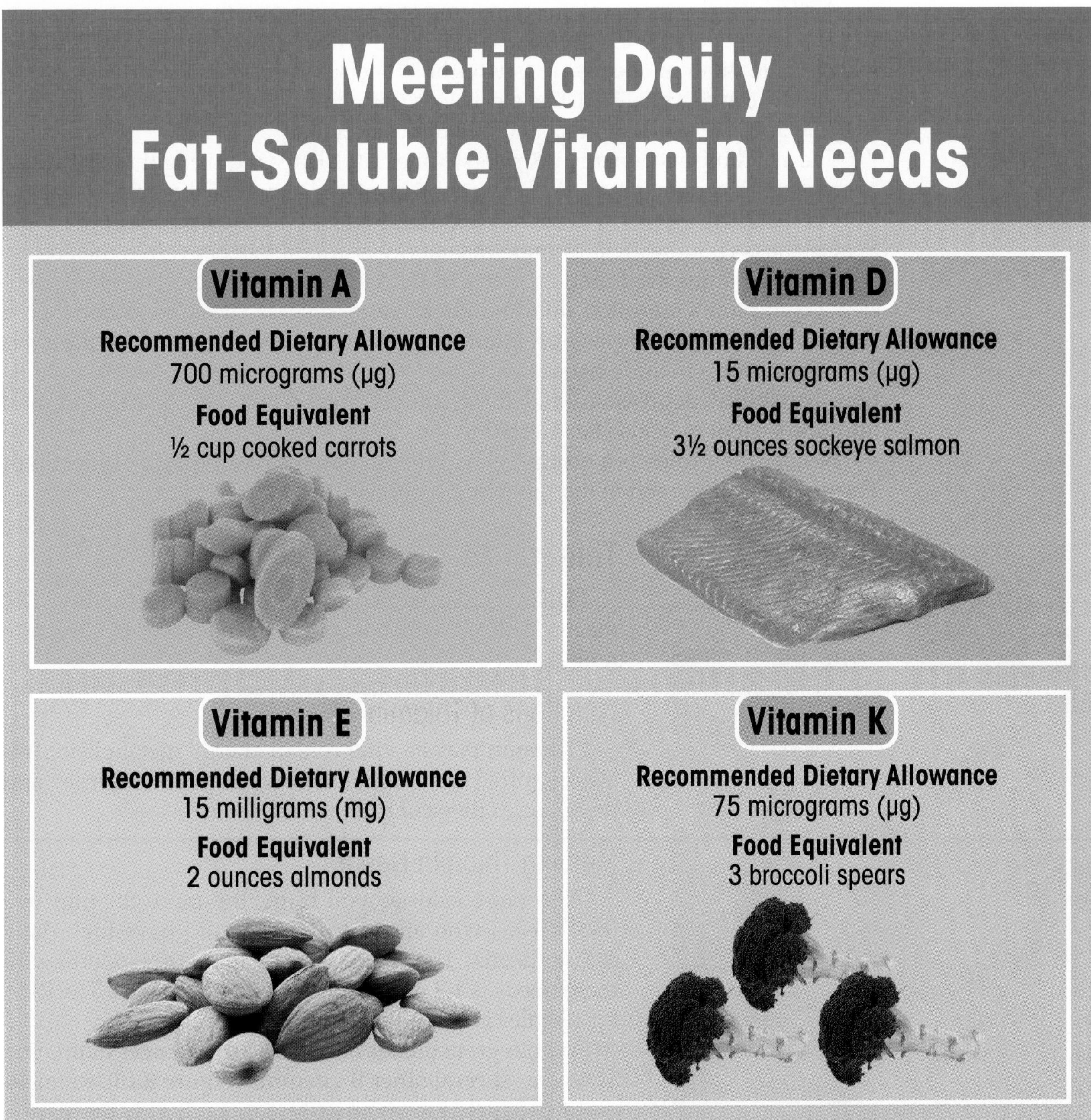

Top row, l to r: BW Folsom/Shutterstock.com; Edward Westmacott/Shutterstock.com; bottom row, l to r: Africa Studio/Shutterstock.com; Hank Shiffman/Shutterstock.com

Figure 9.9 Carrots, salmon, almonds, and broccoli are some examples of how to meet your Dietary Reference Intakes (RDAs and AIs) for fat-soluble vitamins.

The Water-Soluble Vitamins at Work

The water-soluble vitamins include all of the B vitamins and vitamin C. Lean tissues may store surpluses of these vitamins for short periods, but excesses are generally excreted in the urine. Therefore, the accepted recommendation is that you include them in your eating pattern most every day.

The Teamwork of B Vitamins

The B vitamins are thiamin (B_1), riboflavin (B_2), niacin (B_3), pantothenic acid (B_5), pyridoxine (B_6), biotin (B_7), folate (B_9), and cobalamin (B_{12}). These vitamins work as a team. They are all parts of coenzymes.

A ***coenzyme*** is a nonprotein compound that combines with an inactive enzyme to form an active enzyme system. Think of an inactive enzyme as a car without wheels. The vitamin coenzyme is like the wheels. When you put the wheels on the car, the car can move. Just as a car does not work without wheels, an inactive enzyme does not work without the vitamin coenzyme.

The metabolism of energy nutrients is one critical area requiring the joint action of enzymes and coenzymes. Without coenzymes, the enzymes that release energy from carbohydrates, fats, and proteins could not do their jobs. As parts of the coenzymes, the B vitamins help provide the energy needed by every cell in the body.

The B vitamins are found in many of the same food sources. Therefore, deficiency symptoms are often due to a shortage of several vitamins rather than a single vitamin. Deficiencies of B vitamins can cause a broad range of symptoms. These symptoms include nausea and loss of weight and appetite. Severe exhaustion, irritability, depression, and forgetfulness may occur. The heart, skin, and immune system may also be affected.

Besides their roles as a group, each of the B vitamins has individual functions. These will be discussed in the following sections.

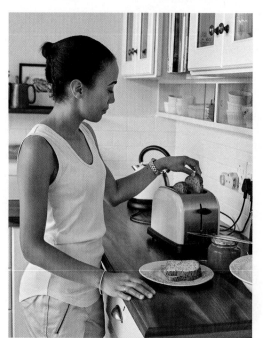

Daxiao Productions/Shutterstock.com

Figure 9.10 Whole-grain and enriched breads and cereals are good sources of several B vitamins.

Thiamin (B_1)

Thiamin was named for its molecular structure. *Thi-* means "sulfur," which is one of the elements in a thiamin molecule.

Functions of Thiamin

Thiamin plays a vital role in energy metabolism. It is also required for normal functioning of the nerves and the muscles they control.

Meeting Thiamin Needs

The more calories you burn, the more thiamin you need. Teens who are 14 to 18 years old have high daily calorie needs. The thiamin RDA that corresponds with these needs is 1.2 milligrams per day for males. The RDA for females is 1.0 milligrams per day.

Whole-grain breads and cereals are sources of thiamin as well as several other B vitamins (**Figure 9.10**). Refined-grain products are commonly enriched with these vitamins as well as iron. An ***enriched food*** has vitamins and minerals added to replace those lost during processing. Enriched foods can be important sources of nutrients.

Other foods that are good sources of thiamin include pork products, dried beans, nuts, seeds, and liver. Because the body does not store much thiamin, you need to consume thiamin-rich foods most days.

Effects of Thiamin Deficiencies and Excesses

Beriberi is the thiamin deficiency disease. *Beriberi* means "I can't, I can't." Without enough thiamin, the body "can't" perform the tasks required for everyday living. Symptoms include weakness, loss of appetite, and irritability. Poor arm and leg coordination and a nervous tingling throughout the body are also symptoms of thiamin deficiency. Some people develop edema and heart failure. *Edema* is an excess accumulation of fluid.

Alcoholism increases the risk of thiamin deficiency because alcohol diminishes the body's ability to absorb and use thiamin. A diet in which a large percentage of calories comes from alcohol also lacks calories from nutritious food sources. These two factors create serious health problems for alcoholics.

Symptoms of thiamin toxicity have not been identified. However, nutrition experts state there is no health benefit in consuming thiamin at levels higher than the RDA. The UL for thiamin has not been established.

Riboflavin (B_2)

The word riboflavin comes from the yellow color of this vitamin compound. *Flavus* means "yellow" in Latin.

Functions of Riboflavin

Riboflavin helps the body release energy from carbohydrates, fats, and proteins. You also need it to maintain healthy skin and normal eyesight.

Meeting Riboflavin Needs

Daily riboflavin needs for males 14 years and older is 1.3 milligrams per day. The RDA for 14- to 18-year-old females is 1.0 milligrams per day, but increases to 1.1 milligrams per day for females 19 years and older. Milk and milk products are excellent food sources for meeting these needs (**Figure 9.11**). Enriched and whole-grain cereals, meats, poultry, and fish are also good sources of riboflavin. Healthy people who eat a variety of nutrient dense foods generally get enough riboflavin.

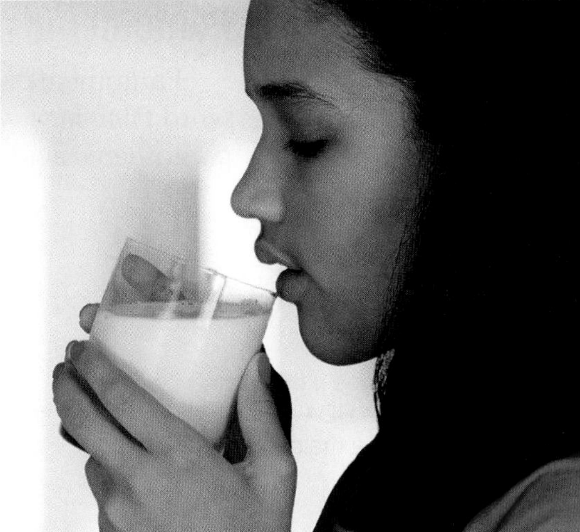

Rob Marmion/Shutterstock.com

Figure 9.11 Milk and other dairy products are good sources of riboflavin. *What are other sources of riboflavin?*

Effects of Riboflavin Deficiencies and Excesses

Many symptoms are associated with riboflavin deficiency. They include an inflamed tongue and cracked skin around the corners of the mouth. Various eye disorders and mental confusion are also symptoms.

Toxicity symptoms have not been reported. Established ULs have not been set. And, because it is a water-soluble vitamin, excess riboflavin is excreted in the urine.

Niacin (B_3)

There are several types of niacin. These include *nicotinic acid* and *nicotinamide.* All types of niacin are water-soluble.

Functions of Niacin

Like the other B vitamins, niacin is involved in energy metabolism. It also helps maintain healthy skin and a healthy nervous system. Niacin also promotes normal digestion.

Meeting Niacin Needs

Niacin in foods is available as a preformed vitamin. It is also available in a provitamin form—tryptophan—which is one of the amino acids in many protein foods.

The RDA for niacin is stated in terms of *niacin equivalents (NE)*. This unit accounts for both the provitamin and preformed forms of niacin. Males in the 14- to 18-year age range need the equivalent of 16 milligrams of niacin daily. Females in this age range need the equivalent of 14 milligrams.

Whole-grain and enriched breads and cereals, meat, poultry, and nuts are popular sources of niacin (**Figure 9.12**). Tryptophan is found in protein foods, such as meats and dairy products.

Effects of Niacin Deficiencies and Excesses

Pellagra is the niacin deficiency disease. The symptoms of pellagra are often known as the *four Ds*. These symptoms are diarrhea, dermatitis (dry, flaky skin), dementia (disorder of mental processes), and death. Early disease symptoms include poor appetite, weight loss, and weakness.

Niacin can be toxic when too much is consumed through supplements. Toxicity is characterized by **dilated** (enlarged) blood vessels near the surface of the skin. The resulting painful rash is sometimes called *niacin flush*. Nausea, dizziness, and low blood pressure are also symptoms of too much niacin. UL for 14- to 18-year-olds is 30 milligrams daily.

Pantothenic Acid (B_5)

Pantothenic acid is another B-complex vitamin. It gets its name from the Greek word *pantothen*, which means "from all sides." This name is **apt** (fitting) because pantothenic acid is found in all living tissues.

Figure 9.12
Three ounces of turkey supplies more than half the RDA of niacin for a male teenager.

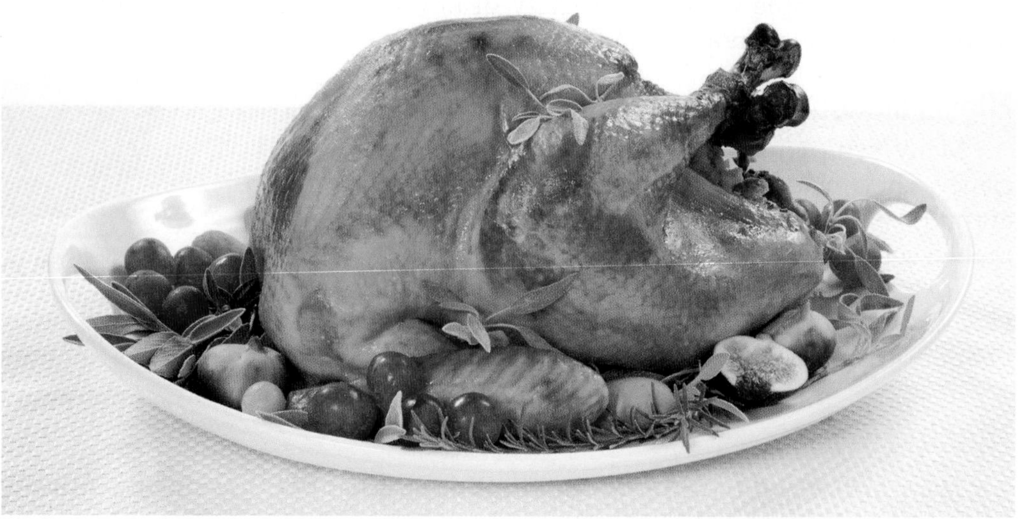

Bochkarev Photography/Shutterstock.com

Functions of Pantothenic Acid

Pantothenic acid promotes growth. It is part of a coenzyme that is critical to the metabolism of the energy nutrients. It is also involved in synthesizing a number of vital substances in the body.

Meeting Pantothenic Acid Needs

Studies on pantothenic acid have not produced enough **conclusive** (convincing) data to set an RDA. Therefore, an AI has been established as a guide for intake. For people ages 14 years and older, the AI for pantothenic acid is 5 milligrams per day.

Effects of Pantothenic Acid Deficiencies and Excesses

Pantothenic acid is found in many food sources. Therefore, deficiency symptoms are rarely a problem. Toxicity is also rare and no UL has been established for this vitamin.

THE MOVEMENT CONNECTION

Hamstring Stretch

Why

Just as vitamins help maintain healthy body tissues, daily stretching helps maintain pliable muscles and joints. Did you know that too much sitting negatively impacts your health, including flexibility levels?

Sitting shortens the muscles of our legs, hips, and back. If you sit too much, and do not get adequate amounts of stretching or physical activity, your range of motion is negatively impacted. So how can you combat this? Fortunately, there are simple stretches you can do to help combat the negative effects of sitting. When flexibility is increased, you will notice more comfort and ease of movement in your daily life.

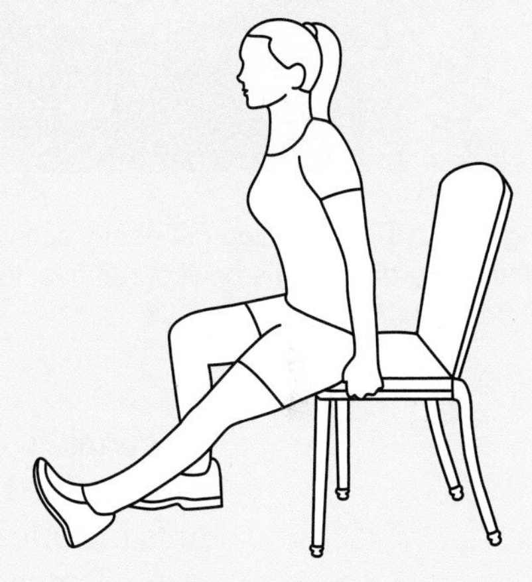

Apply

- Sitting at the edge of your chair, straighten one leg in front of the body with the heel on the floor. The other leg should remain bent with the foot flat on the floor.
- Good posture is key! Sit up straight and imagine squeezing your belly button to your spine before beginning the movement. This engages your core muscles and protects your lower back.
- Bring your torso toward your thigh without rounding your lower back. (Your back should remain straight at all times.)
- Hold this stretch for 30 seconds and repeat 3 times for each leg.

Modification

- This stretch can be performed while standing.

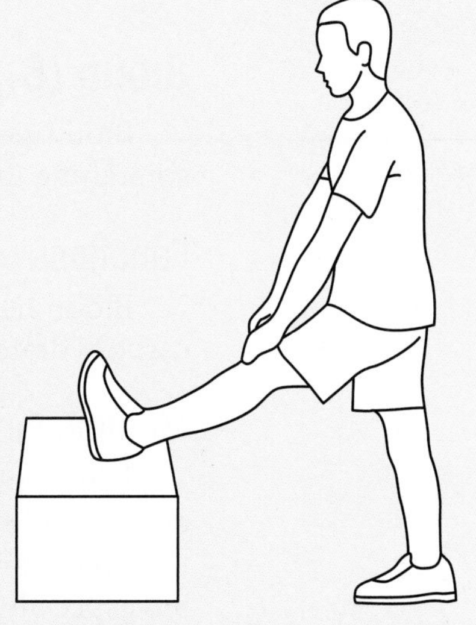

Pyridoxine (B_6)

Pyridoxine is instrumental in a wide variety of tasks in the body and is very **versatile** (capable of many uses). For example, this vitamin is thought to play a role in more than 100 enzyme reactions.

Functions of Vitamin B_6

In addition to playing a key role in synthesizing the nonessential (dispensable) amino acids, vitamin B_6 helps make the protein that allows red blood cells to carry oxygen. Pyridoxine helps regulate metabolism and affects the health of the immune and nervous systems. Additionally, it is needed for normal brain development and function.

Meeting Vitamin B_6 Needs

The RDA for vitamin B_6 for males ages 14 through 50 is 1.3 milligrams per day. Females ages 14 to 18 need 1.2 milligrams per day. Needs increase to 1.3 milligrams daily for adult females through age 50. Vitamin B_6 needs increase further for people of both sexes after age 50.

Vitamin B_6 is found in meats, fish, and poultry. Dairy products and some fruits and vegetables, such as bananas, cantaloupe, broccoli, and spinach, are also good sources (**Figure 9.13**).

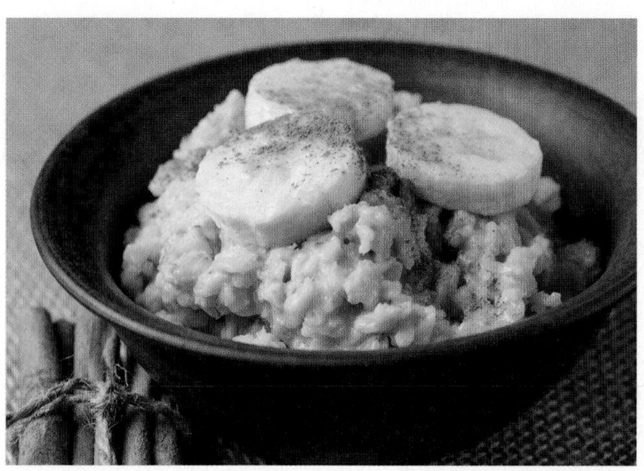

Julia Ardaran/Shutterstock.com

Figure 9.13 A teenage girl nearly satisfies her RDA for vitamin B_6 by eating a bowl of oatmeal topped with bananas at breakfast.

Effects of Vitamin B_6 Deficiencies and Excesses

Vitamin B_6 deficiencies are rare. Symptoms of deficiencies are related to poor amino acid and protein metabolism. Symptoms include skin disorders, fatigue, irritability, and convulsions.

People who have taken large doses of vitamin B_6 have reported symptoms of toxicity. The UL is set at 80 milligrams per day for 14- to 18-year-olds. These symptoms include walking difficulties and numbness in the hands and feet. Irreversible nerve damage can also result from excessive intakes of this vitamin.

Biotin (B_7)

Biotin gets its name from the Greek word for "sustenance," which means something that helps support life.

Functions of Biotin

Biotin helps activate several enzymes involved in the release of energy from carbohydrates, fats, and proteins. Biotin also helps the body make fat and glycogen.

Meeting Biotin Needs

Like pantothenic acid, there is no RDA for biotin. The AI for males and females ages 14 to 18 years is 25 micrograms per day.

Biotin is widespread in foods. Egg yolks, yeast, beans, nuts, cheese, and liver are especially good sources.

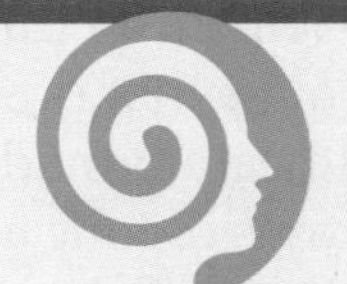

EXTEND YOUR KNOWLEDGE

Alcohol's Effect on Vitamins

How does excessive alcohol use affect nutrient absorption? When people consume large amounts of alcohol—especially in the case of people with alcohol addiction—appetite suppression often occurs. Poor eating habits and greater alcohol consumption tend to go hand-in-hand. In addition to taking in fewer nutrients, alcohol can interfere with the way the body absorbs nutrients, especially vitamins. For example, alcohol interferes with the way the body metabolizes and absorbs folate, vitamin A, and vitamin B_{12}.

Effects of Biotin Deficiencies and Excesses

Because biotin is widely available in foods, deficiencies among people who eat a variety of nutrient-dense foods are uncommon. A biotin deficiency produces similar symptoms of the circulatory and muscular systems as a thiamin deficiency. These symptoms include abnormal heart rhythms, pain, weakness, fatigue, and depression. Nausea, loss of appetite, hair loss, and dry, scaly skin are other symptoms.

Nutrition researchers have found no evidence of biotin toxicity. Although there may be no health risk, there are no advantages to biotin intakes above the recommended range.

Folate (B_9)

Folate, which was also called *folacin* in the past, is another B vitamin. The term *folate* is derived from the Latin word *folium*, which means "leaf." This is a logical name because leafy green vegetables are good sources of folate. *Folic acid* is a synthetic form of this vitamin found in nutrient supplements and fortified foods.

Functions of Folate

The main function of folate is to help synthesize DNA, the genetic material in every cell. Without folate, cells cannot divide to form new cells.

Another function of folate is especially important to any woman of childbearing age. Women who have inadequate folate intakes are more likely to give birth to babies with *neural tube damage*. Such damage affects the brain and spinal cord and can cause intellectual disabilities, paralysis, and premature death.

Meeting Folate Needs

The RDA for folate is 400 micrograms per day for everyone age 14 and over. Pregnancy increases folate needs. Pregnant women need 600 micrograms of folate daily.

Dark green, leafy vegetables are excellent sources of folate. Liver, legumes, oranges, cantaloupe, and broccoli are also good sources. In addition, most enriched breads, flours, and other grain products are fortified with folic acid.

Meeting daily folate recommendations is especially important for women of childbearing age. This is because neural tube damage occurs during the first weeks of pregnancy, before many women realize they are pregnant. Fully meeting folate requirements before becoming pregnant reduces a woman's risk of having a baby with neural tube damage.

Research confirms that folic acid from fortified foods and supplements reduces the risk of neural tube damage. Researchers do not know if the folate that occurs naturally in foods has the same preventive effect. Therefore, healthcare providers recommend all women of childbearing age consume 400 micrograms of folic acid daily from supplements or fortified foods. Eating a nutritious diet will provide additional folate from foods (**Figure 9.14**).

Effects of Folate Deficiencies and Excesses

You have already read about the increased risks of neural tube damage due to folate deficiency in pregnant women. Additional complications during pregnancy may include spontaneous miscarriage or the placenta separating from the uterus before delivery. Folate deficiencies affect other population groups as well.

Folate deficiencies are not uncommon. They usually result from low intakes of folate; however, several medications such as aspirin and oral contraceptives can interfere with the body's ability to use folate.

The first signs of a folate deficiency appear in the red blood cells. Without sufficient folate, the red blood cells are fragile and cannot mature and carry oxygen. With a reduced number of mature red blood cells, a person feels tired and weak. Other symptoms of a folate deficiency include diarrhea and increased risk of infection.

Little information is available about folate toxicity. However, large intakes of folic acid may conceal symptoms of a vitamin B_{12} deficiency. This reduces the likelihood the vitamin B_{12} deficiency would be diagnosed and treated. Irreparable nerve damage could result. The UL for 14- to 18-year-olds is 800 micrograms of folate per day.

Cobalamin (B_{12})

Vitamin B_{12} is a chemical compound that contains cobalt. That is why the vitamin is named *cobalamin*.

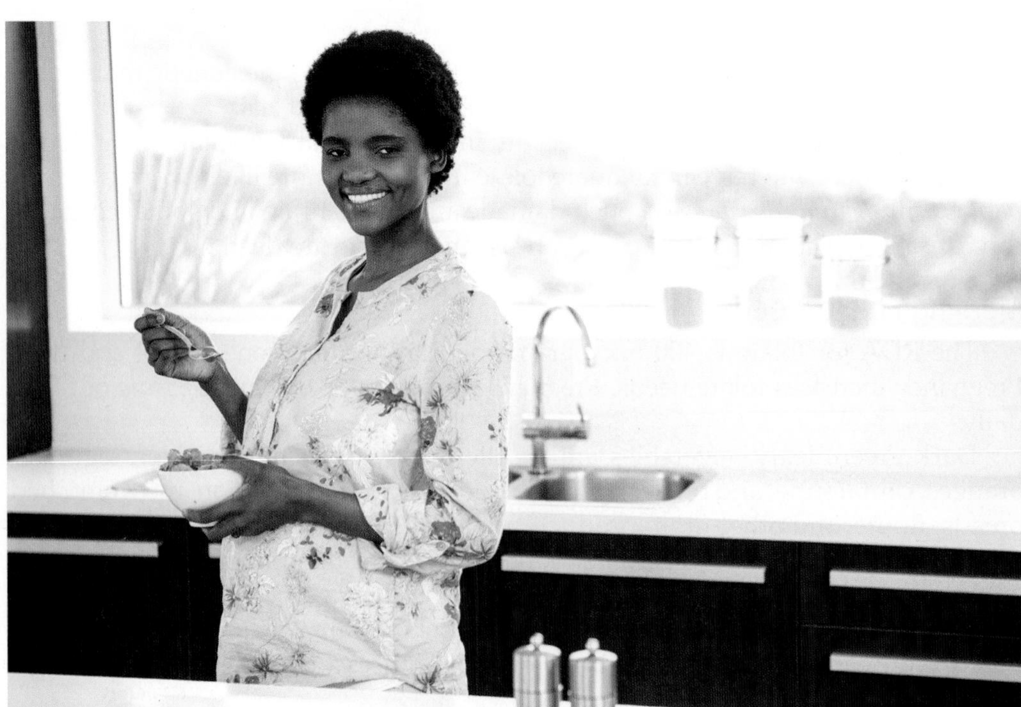

wavebreakmedia/Shutterstock.com

Figure 9.14 Women should be sure to meet their folate needs before and during pregnancy to help prevent neural tube damage in their babies.

Functions of Vitamin B_{12}

Vitamin B_{12} helps folate function. It is needed for growth, maintenance of healthy nerve tissue, and formation of normal red blood cells. It also is needed for the release of energy from fat.

Meeting Vitamin B_{12} Needs

The RDA for vitamin B_{12} for males and females ages 14 and over is 2.4 micrograms per day. People who eat foods from animal sources easily meet these needs. Meats, particularly in liver and muscle parts of meats, are good sources of vitamin B_{12}. Fowl, like chicken and turkey, and most varieties of fish are all good sources. Some breakfast cereals, soy products, and energy bars are fortified with vitamin B_{12}, but this vitamin does not naturally occur in foods from plant sources.

Effects of Vitamin B_{12} Deficiencies and Excesses

Pernicious anemia, the deficiency disease associated with vitamin B_{12}, is actually caused by an inability to absorb the vitamin. Impaired absorption is due to the lack of a compound made in the stomach. An injury or a rare genetic disorder can cause the stomach to stop producing this important compound. As people grow older, they may lose their ability to make this compound. Pernicious anemia prevents red blood cells from maturing and dividing properly. This causes a person to feel tired and weak.

Symptoms of pernicious anemia also include a red, painful tongue and a tingling or burning in the skin. Nerve damage can eventually lead to walking difficulties and paralysis. Nerve damage can also cause memory loss and mental slowness.

Fortunately, pernicious anemia can be treated. Periodic injections of vitamin B_{12} will allow red blood cells to mature normally. (The vitamin is injected because the body is unable to absorb it when taken by mouth due to the absence of the compound that facilitates absorption.) The injected vitamin B_{12} will help maintain the remaining insulation remaining around nerve cells; however, nerve damage that occurred before the deficiency was diagnosed usually cannot be reversed.

People who eat animal foods and can absorb vitamin B_{12} are unlikely to develop deficiencies. Vegans, who eat no animal products, must include alternative sources of vitamin B_{12} in their diets. Such sources might be vitamin supplements and fortified soy milk. Older adults are also at risk for developing pernicious anemia (**Figure 9.15**). Regular blood tests can help identify those people who need vitamin B_{12} injections.

The body can maintain long-term stores of vitamin B_{12}. Despite this, no toxicity symptoms are known and there is no reported UL.

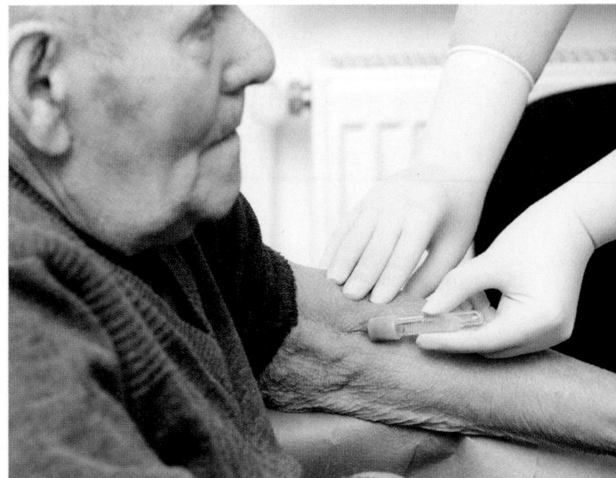

Barabasa/Shutterstock.com

Figure 9.15 Pernicious anemia is a disease that affects the elderly, but strict vegans are also at risk for developing this disease. *Why are strict vegans also at risk for pernicious anemia?*

Vitamin C

Vitamin C is also referred to as *ascorbic acid*. Long before this vitamin was identified, sailors who went on lengthy voyages often developed the deadly disease scurvy. In a search for a cure, a British doctor, James Lind, carried out the first nutrition experiment using human subjects. He added different substances to the diets of each of several groups of sailors with scurvy. Lind found those sailors who ate citrus fruits were cured.

Nutritionists now know it was the vitamin C in the citrus fruits that helped cure the disease. ***Scurvy*** has been correctly identified as a disease caused by vitamin C deficiency.

Functions of Vitamin C

Vitamin C performs a number of important functions in the body. It assists in the formation of collagen. ***Collagen*** is a protein substance in the connective tissue that holds cells together. Collagen is needed for healthy bones, cartilage, muscles, and blood vessels. Collagen helps wounds heal quickly. It also helps maintain capillaries and gums.

Vitamin C increases iron and calcium absorption. It plays a role in synthesizing thyroxine, the hormone that controls basal metabolic rate. Vitamin C is also vital to the body's immune system.

Vitamin C is an antioxidant that works with vitamin E to protect body cells from free radicals. Some experts believe this may allow vitamin C to help prevent some cell damage. This may include the cell damage that leads to the development of some cancers, cataracts, and heart disease.

Meeting Vitamin C Needs

The RDA for vitamin C for males ages 14 to 18 years old is 75 milligrams per day. After age 19, it increases to 90 milligrams per day. For females ages 14 to 18 years, the RDA is 65 milligrams per day. After age 19, it increases to 75 milligrams per day. The body does not store vitamin C, so a daily intake is necessary.

People exposed to tobacco smoke need extra vitamin C. The exposure to smoke results in increased free radicals in the body. More vitamin C is needed to function as an antioxidant and protect cells from the free radicals. Smokers and anyone exposed to smoke should include an extra 35 milligrams of vitamin C in their daily diets.

Vitamin C is found in many fruits and vegetables. Fruits rich in vitamin C include citrus fruits, kiwifruit, and strawberries (**Figure 9.16**). Good vegetable sources include red peppers, broccoli, cabbage, and potatoes.

Effects of Vitamin C Deficiencies and Excesses

Most people in the United States meet their daily needs for vitamin C through diet. However, low intakes of vitamin C are common among older adults. As a group, they tend to eat diets that contain fewer fruits and vegetables.

What happens if there is inadequate vitamin C in the diet? Scurvy is the most severe vitamin C deficiency disease. It rarely occurs in developed countries because the causes and cure of the disease are known. In poorer countries where diets are inadequate, however, scurvy is more common.

The symptoms of scurvy are many. They include tiredness, weakness, shortness of breath, aching bones and muscles, swollen and bleeding gums, and lack of appetite. Wounds heal slowly. The skin becomes rough and covered with tiny red spots. The marks are small patches of bleeding just under the skin that appear as capillaries break.

The UL for Vitamin C is 1,800 milligrams per day for 14- to 18-year-olds. Some extra vitamin C may not be harmful because most excess vitamin C is excreted. However, large doses of one to three grams (1,000 to 3,000 milligrams) have had reported side effects. People taking large doses have complained of nausea, diarrhea, and stomach cramps. Large doses may also reduce the ability of vitamin B_{12} to function.

Many people believe that taking extra vitamin C can prevent or cure the common cold. Current research does not support this claim. However, adequate amounts of vitamin C do help protect the body against infections.

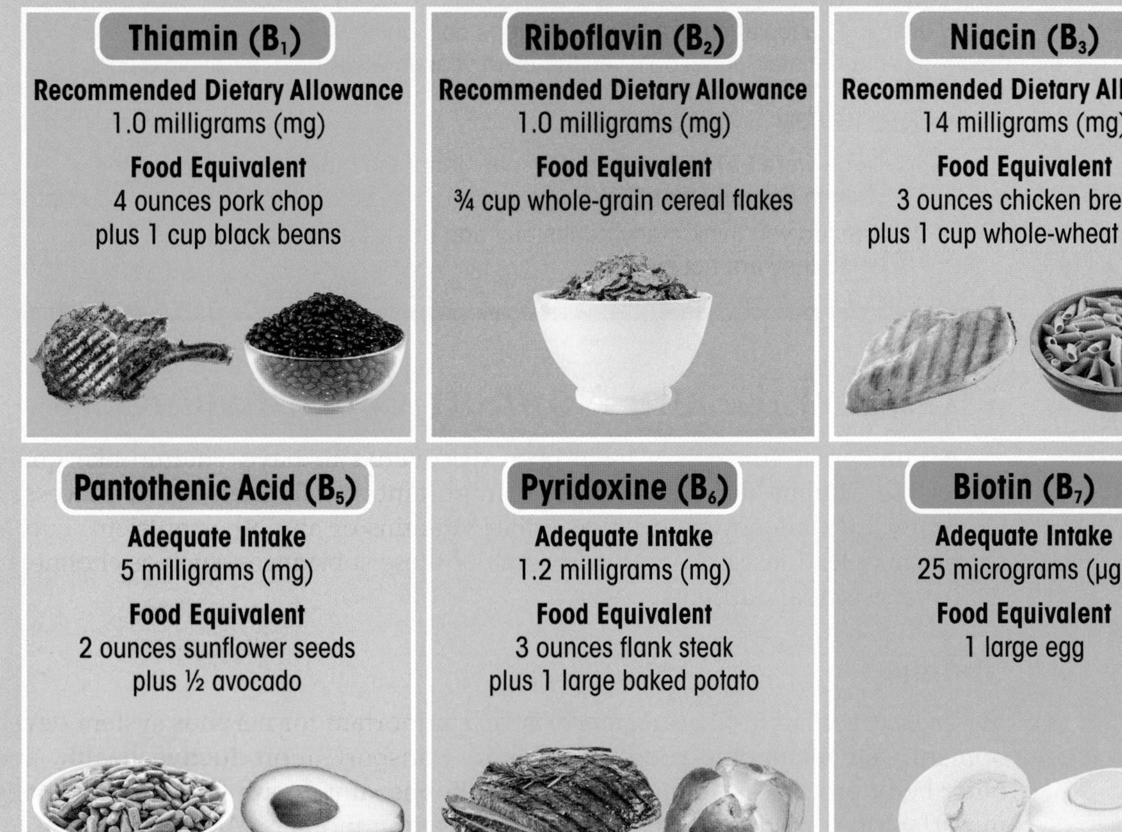

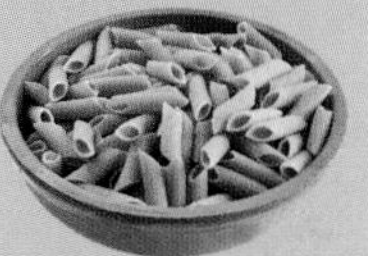

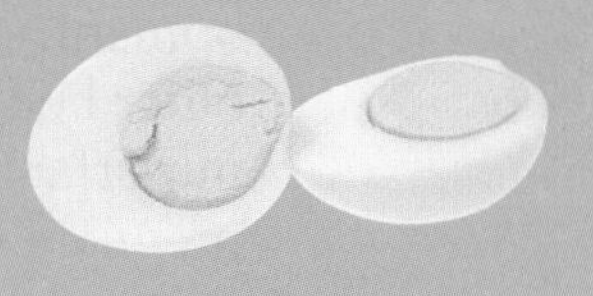

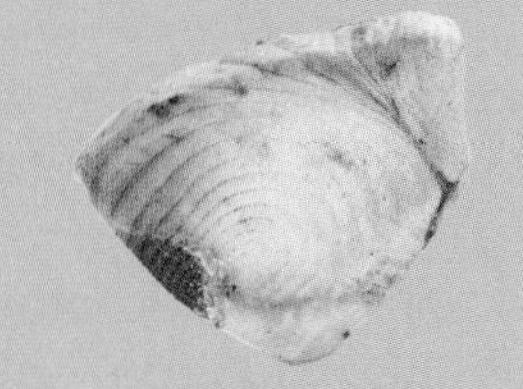

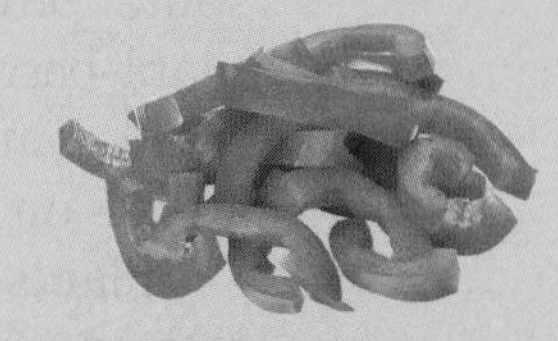

Top row, l to r: Robyn Mackenzie/Shutterstock.com; Da-ga/Shutterstock.com; Nils Z/Shutterstock.com; Tim UR/Shutterstock.com; Antonio Gravante/Shutterstock.com; 2nd row, l to r: MaraZe/Shutterstock.com; Olga Guchek/Shutterstock.com; stockcreations/Shutterstock.com; Joe Gough/Shutterstock.com; Richard Griffin/Shutterstock.com; 3rd row, l to r: Moving Moment/Shutterstock.com; Armas Vladimir/Shutterstock.com; ampFotoStudio/Shutterstock.com; Nattika/Shutterstock.com

Figure 9.16 Examples of how to meet your Dietary Reference Intakes (RDAs and AIs) for water-soluble vitamins.

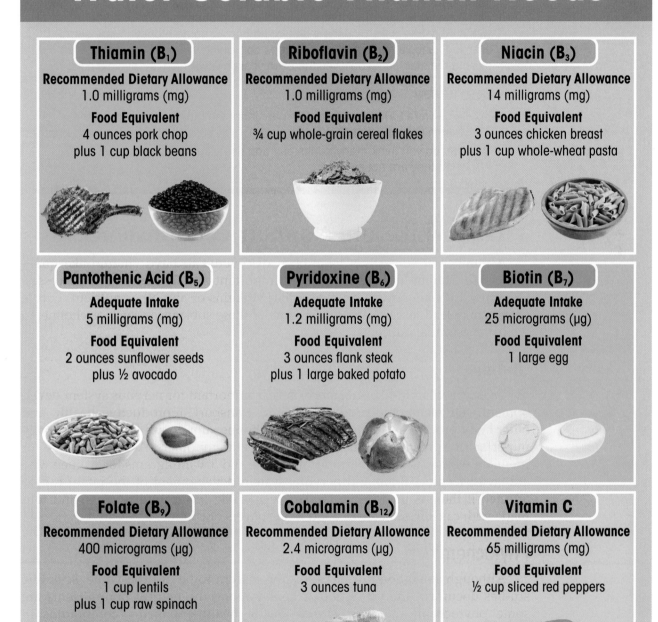

CASE STUDY

A Pill to Cure Janet's Cold?

Janet and LaTisha were at the mall shopping. Janet had just spent the last of her money in the food court on French fries and a soft drink. Janet has been feeling like she is coming down with a cold. She asks LaTisha if she could borrow some money to buy some vitamin C supplements and cough drops containing vitamin C at the nutrition store in the mall. Janet believes the extra vitamin C will help her avoid a cold.

Case Review

1. If you were LaTisha, would you loan Janet the money to purchase the vitamin C supplement? Why?
2. Why do you think many adults buy and use vitamin supplements, even when they are not sick?

Vitamin-Like and Nonnutrient Substances

A number of substances have been discovered to have vitamin-like qualities. These vitamin-like substances play important roles in many body processes. Currently, they are not regarded as either vitamins or any other nutrient. Future studies may lead researchers to add some of these substances, such as choline, to the list of essential nutrients.

Choline

Choline, a vitamin-like substance, is very important for nervous system development, cell membrane production, lipid transport, reproductive health, and other body processes. Adequate intake of choline, along with folate, is especially important for pregnant women and breast-feeding mothers. Adequate intake for pregnant women is 450 milligrams of choline and 550 milligrams for women who are breast-feeding. Brain and nervous system development of the infant can be affected if there is inadequate intake. Eggs, milk, meat, poultry, nuts, and tofu made with calcium sulfate are good food sources of choline.

Phytochemicals

Although some nonnutrient substances seem to be of little value, scientific studies document the benefits of others. Among the helpful nonnutrients are some phytochemicals. ***Phytochemicals*** are health-enhancing compounds in plant-based foods that are active in the body's cells. In comparison to nutrients, these compounds may not be essential for life, but are believed to have positive effects on health.

Plants make hundreds of phytochemicals to protect themselves against such factors as ultraviolet light, oxidation, and insects. Scientists have just begun to learn about the useful roles some of these compounds play in the human body.

One major group of dietary phytochemicals is *flavonoids*, also known as *polyphenols*. The flavonoids contribute a strong antioxidant effect. Green tea, extra virgin olive oil, and pomegranates are good sources of flavonoids.

COMMUNITY CONNECTIONS

International Volunteering

Sometimes the word "community" refers to more than just your local community; it can also mean the international, or global, community. Have you ever considered volunteering in the global community? Today, countries and peoples are more economically, socially, and politically interdependent than at any other time in history. As a result, it becomes apparent that in some parts of the world, people lack essential resources.

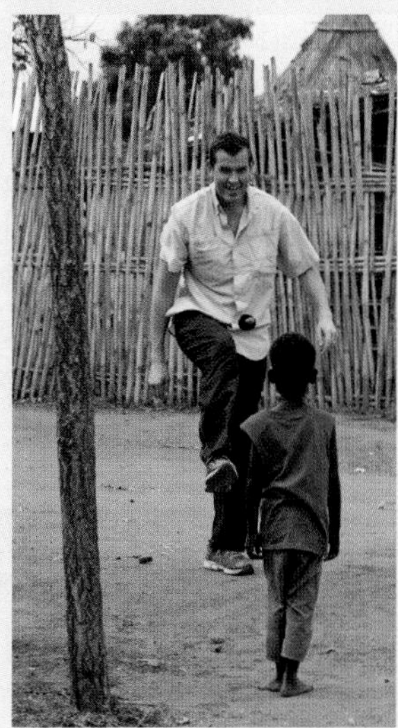
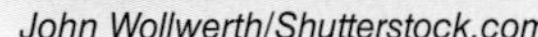
John Wollwerth/Shutterstock.com

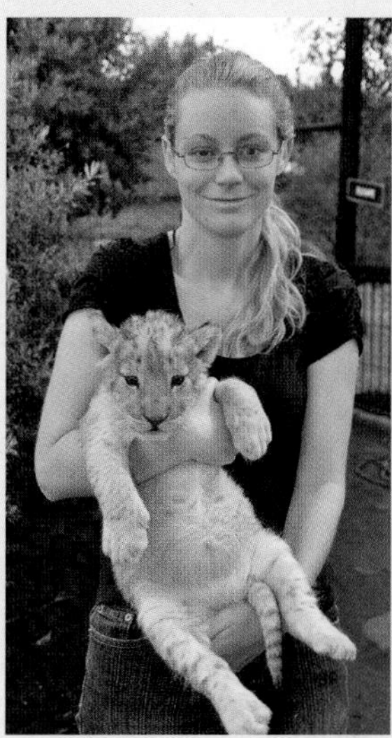
niall dunne/Shutterstock.com

Choosing to volunteer internationally to find solutions to problems of health, nutrition, or education can provide a vital service for others as well as a learning opportunity for you. While volunteering, you benefit by learning about a culture, language, and environment different from your own. And, you will likely make international friends that will last a lifetime.

Most programs require that volunteers are 16 years or older. Programs can vary in length from one week over winter break to an entire summer, or a gap year following graduation. You should research the requirements and guidelines for the program before making a commitment. A well-planned volunteer program will provide:

- a host leader to help you adjust to a new living and learning environment, including adjustments to language, social expectations, and cultural differences;
- clearly outlined volunteer responsibilities and limitations;
- safe, clean housing and living arrangements; and
- documented procedures for emergencies that might happen on-site or in your home country.

Costs of volunteer experiences can range greatly, so you will need to research the program's fees. For example, excluding travel costs, a typical assignment in an orphanage in India might cost $250 for one week and as much as $1,000 for eight weeks. Some students plan fund-raising projects to help support the costs of international volunteer work. Ethical volunteer programs are transparent about how program dollars are spent. Learn if the sponsoring organization provides detailed information about how program fees are spent. Look at a variety of programs to compare how fees are allocated to overhead costs and to the host country's program needs.

Think Critically

1. Evaluate several international volunteer programs that work with teens. Write a short summary comparing the programs.
2. What would an international volunteer experience offer you that a local volunteer experience could not?
3. Prepare a list of your skills, knowledge, and experiences. Analyze your list to determine a volunteer experience that is well-matched to your skills and experience.

Research has shown that flavonoids and other phytochemicals may help prevent heart disease and some forms of cancer. They achieve this preventive effect through various chemical reactions in the body. Phytochemicals prompt the body to make enzymes, bind harmful substances, and act as antioxidants.

Currently, there are no recommendations for intake of phytochemicals. More research is needed. Studies citing the value of certain phytochemicals have led many people who follow nutrition fads to buy phytochemical supplements. However, research has not proven these supplements to be safe and effective. The combinations of phytochemicals and nutrients found in foods cannot be duplicated in a supplement. Therefore, supplements cannot perform the same way foods can.

Eating a variety of plant foods in a rainbow of colors is the best way to include phytochemicals in your diet. Include a variety of fruits, vegetables, herbs, spices, legumes, and whole grains to maximize phytochemicals in your diet (**Figure 9.17**).

Phytochemicals		
Class	**Plant Source**	**Possible Health Benefits**
Carotenoids (such as beta-carotene, lycopene, lutein, zeaxanthin)	Red, orange, and green fruits and vegetables, including broccoli, carrots, cooked tomatoes, leafy greens, sweet potatoes, winter squash, apricots, cantaloupe, oranges, and watermelon	May inhibit cancer cell growth, work as antioxidants, and improve immune response
Flavonoids (such as anthocyanins and quercetin)	Apples, citrus fruits, onions, soybeans and soy products (tofu, soy milk, edamame, etc.), coffee, and tea	May inhibit inflammation and tumor growth; may aid immunity and boost production of detoxifying enzymes in the body
Indoles and Glucosinolates (sulforaphane)	Cruciferous vegetables (broccoli, cabbage, collard greens, kale, cauliflower, and Brussels sprouts)	May induce detoxification of carcinogens, limit production of cancer-related hormones, block carcinogens, and prevent tumor growth
Inositol (phytic acid)	Bran from corn, oats, rice, rye, wheat, nuts, and soybeans and soy products (tofu, soy milk, edamame, etc.)	May retard cell growth and work as antioxidants
Isoflavones (daidzein and genistein)	Soybeans and soy products (tofu, soy milk, edamame, etc.)	May inhibit tumor growth, limit production of cancer-related hormones, and generally work as antioxidants
Isothiocyanates	Cruciferous vegetables (broccoli, cabbage, collard greens, kale, cauliflower, and Brussels sprouts)	May induce detoxification of carcinogens, block tumor growth, and work as antioxidants
Polyphenols (such as ellagic acid and resveratrol)	Green tea, grapes, wine, berries, citrus fruits, apples, whole grains, and peanuts	May prevent cancer formation, prevent inflammation, and work as antioxidants
Terpenes (such as perillyl alcohol, limonene, carnosol)	Cherries, citrus fruit peel, and rosemary	May protect cells from becoming cancerous, slow cancer cell growth, strengthen immune function, limit production of cancer-related hormones, fight viruses, and work as antioxidants

Source: American Institute for Cancer Research

Figure 9.17 Food rich in phytochemicals can improve health and decrease risks for certain diseases. *Why do you suppose the phrase "eat the rainbow" is used to describe a healthy eating pattern?*

Probiotics and Prebiotics

Probiotics are known as the "good" microorganisms found in foods that offer health benefits when eaten in sufficient amounts. These good microorganisms help to counterbalance the "bad" microorganisms in your intestinal tract. The evidence is not clear for all people, but for some, there is evidence that probiotics help boost the immune system. For others, bowel regularity may be improved. Evidence must be gathered to support other health claims, such as the possibility of lowering cholesterol. Yogurt, containing lactobacilli, is promoted as containing probiotics. Other foods with probiotics include miso (fermented soy), some types of sauerkraut and kimchi, and kefir (fermented milk smoothie). Bacteria in probiotic foods are killed when heated. Therefore, to reap any benefit from these foods, they cannot be cooked or canned.

Prebiotics are the nondigestible food ingredients that stimulate the growth of good microorganisms in the colon. The prebiotic serves as food for the good microorganisms. Prebiotics are found in foods such as whole grains, onions, bananas, garlic, asparagus, leeks, and artichokes (**Figure 9.18**).

Both probiotics and prebiotics are present naturally in some foods and beverages. They are also added to some foods and beverages. Probiotics are also available as dietary supplements. The health benefits result from the improved environment that results in the gastrointestinal tract (GI). If you think of the probiotic as a sunflower seed, the prebiotic is the water and plant food that is needed for the seed to flourish and become a flower. Foods high in probiotics and prebiotics are considered functional foods because they provide beneficial health effects beyond basic nutrition.

Research efforts continue on how functional foods can contribute to the health and wellness of consumers. As healthcare and food costs rise, people want to know how to take control of their health.

Vitamin Supplements

In the United States, people spend billions of dollars on vitamin supplements each year. Why? Is it necessary? Many people worry their diets are lacking in vitamins. Their schedules are busy and they may not have time to eat nutritiously.

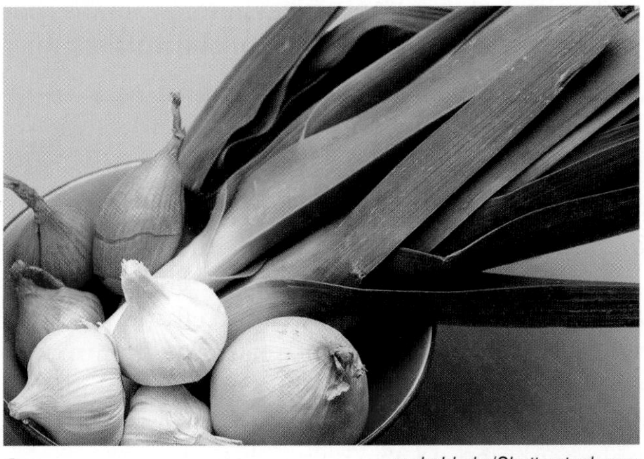

A *msheldrake/Shutterstock.com*

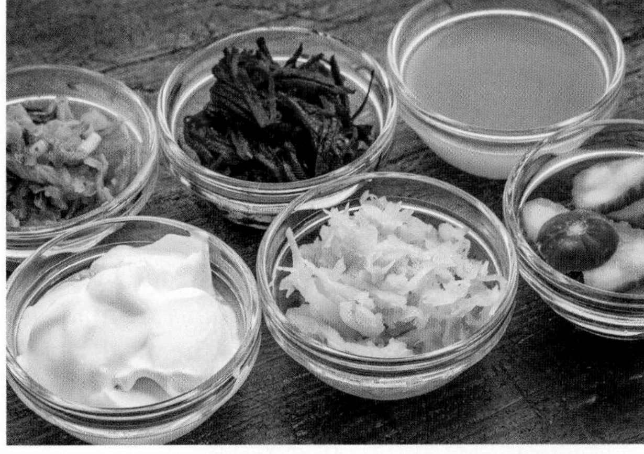

B *marekuliasz/Shutterstock.com*

Figure 9.18 The nondigestible fiber found in prebiotic foods (A) such as garlic, onions, and leeks serves as "food" for the good bacteria supplied by probiotic foods (B) such as sauerkraut, kimchi, pickles, and yogurt.

Others are convinced they have more energy when they take a vitamin supplement. However, these people may feel stronger or more energetic due to the placebo effect. The ***placebo effect*** is a change in a person's condition that is not a result of treatment given, but of the individual's belief that the treatment is working. The individual's expectation and belief cause the change in condition rather than the supplement.

Are Supplements Needed?

Those who sell vitamin supplements have profited from consumer concerns about health and nutrition. They promote numerous benefits of taking vitamin supplements to persuade people to spend more money. Contrary to some advertisements, vitamins are not "miracle cures" for everything from acne to AIDS. Vitamins cannot pep you up when you are feeling tired and run-down. They do not make you strong, attractive, or more popular. Supplements do not make up for poor eating habits, either. The only symptoms a vitamin supplement relieves are those caused by a lack of that vitamin. For example, a thiamin supplement relieves the symptoms of beriberi.

Some groups of people may need supplements to **augment** (increase) the vitamin content supplied by their diets. Doctors may advise pregnant and breast-feeding women to take supplements (**Figure 9.19**). Doctors may recommend supplements for infants, older adults, and patients who are ill or recovering from surgery. Doctors also occasionally prescribe large doses of vitamins for pharmaceutical purposes. For instance, large doses of vitamin A are sometimes prescribed to treat a particular eye disease. In addition, although vegans *can* consume vitamins via food sources, their beliefs prevent them from doing so. Few people outside these groups need vitamin supplements. A diet including the recommended servings from all the food groups supplies most people with the vitamins they need.

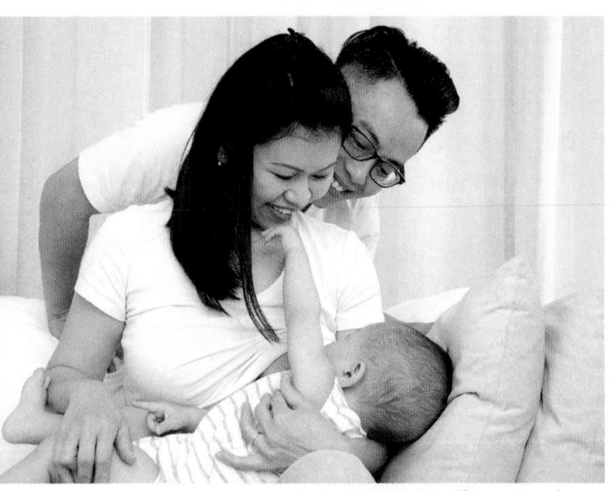

wong sze yuen/Shutterstock.com

Figure 9.19 Doctors often recommend vitamin supplements for breast-feeding women to help meet the extra needs caused by producing milk.

Taking more vitamin supplements than you need can cause health problems. The body can store toxic levels of fat-soluble vitamins. Excess water-soluble vitamins are normally excreted in the urine. However, large doses of some water-soluble vitamins produce negative effects for some people. For instance, too much vitamin C in the diet can irritate the gastrointestinal system. Additionally, an excess of one nutrient may affect how the body uses other nutrients.

Types of Supplements

People who decide to use supplements have a number of choices available. They may choose products in pill, liquid, or powder form. They may also choose between natural and synthetic vitamins. *Natural vitamins* are extracted from foods. *Synthetic vitamins* are made in a laboratory. Advertisers may claim natural vitamins are superior. Chemically speaking, there is no advantage of a natural vitamin over a synthetic vitamin. The body uses both types of vitamins the same way; however, synthetic vitamins are less expensive and are usually purer than natural vitamins.

People who choose to use supplements should also be aware that some supplements provide large doses of vitamins. Amounts may be many times higher than the recommended daily levels. Vitamins have specific functions and only very small amounts are needed for good health.

WELLNESS TIP

Hold That Supplement

Buying supplements is a costly way to get nutrients. In addition, vitamin supplements provide no fiber, energy, or taste. You cannot enjoy supplements as you do foods. Most nutritionists agree people benefit more from spending their money on a healthful food plan than on vitamin supplements.

Supplement Regulation

The Food and Drug Administration (FDA) regulates the sale of vitamin supplements. They require scientific research to back up health claims made on product labels or in advertising. Nevertheless, the FDA has little authority to regulate the amounts of vitamins supplements contain.

Preserving Vitamins in Foods

Eating vitamin-rich foods should ensure you are meeting your body's need for vitamins. Right? Wrong! Many vitamins are unstable. Careless food storage can destroy some vitamins. Cooking techniques can affect vitamin retention, too. In this section, you will learn how to select foods high in vitamins. You will also learn how to preserve the vitamins that are present in foods.

Selecting Foods High in Vitamins

Modern processing methods minimize nutrient losses. Therefore, canned, frozen, and dried foods are comparable to fresh in terms of vitamin content. Choose the form that is most convenient for you. However, be aware of products that contain large amounts of added fat, sugar, and sodium. Read Nutrition Facts panels to help you choose foods that are rich in nutrients.

Knowing signs of quality can help you avoid foods that may have suffered excessive vitamin losses. When buying fresh fruits and vegetables, choose items that have bright colors and firm textures (**Figure 9.20**). Avoid pieces with wilted leaves, mold growth, or bruised spots. When selecting canned products, do not buy cans that are dented or bulging. These signs may indicate a broken seal and possible contamination of the food.

Choose foods from the freezer case that are firmly frozen. Avoid frozen foods that have a layer of ice on the package. This indicates the food may not have been stored at a constant low temperature. Partial thawing can result in nutrient losses and a general decrease in quality. When buying dried foods, look for packages that are securely sealed.

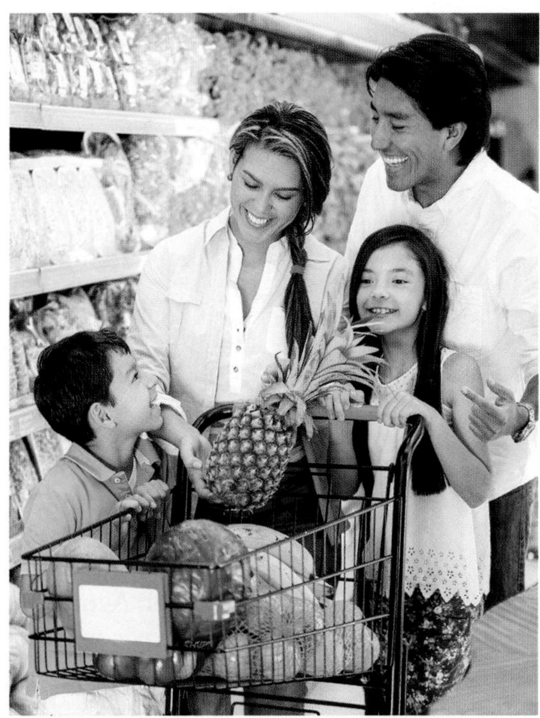

ESB Professional/Shutterstock.com

Figure 9.20 Buying fresh foods and eating them soon after they are purchased will help you get maximum vitamin value.

Storing Foods for Vitamin Retention

The way you handle food can affect its nutritional value. Exposing foods to air, light, and heat during transportation and storage causes vitamin losses. If fresh foods are not properly stored, they may have fewer vitamins than frozen or canned foods.

The following suggestions help to minimize nutrient losses during handling and storing of food:

- Keep freezer temperatures at zero degrees Fahrenheit or lower to retain vitamin content of frozen foods. Try to use frozen foods within several months. Avoid thawing and refreezing foods, which causes some vitamin losses.
- Store canned foods in a cool, dry storage area. The liquid in which foods are canned contains nutrients. Serve the canning liquid with the food or use it in cooking.
- Store milk in opaque containers to protect its riboflavin content. Riboflavin is destroyed by light.
- Heat and light can damage oils, particularly polyunsaturated ones. Keep them in cool storage or the refrigerator to avoid rancidity.
- Ripen fresh fruits and vegetables at room temperature away from direct sunlight.
- Store fresh vegetables promptly in a vegetable crisper in the refrigerator. The low temperature and high humidity of the crisper help preserve the vitamins in the vegetables.
- When storing cut foods, be sure to wrap them tightly. This prevents vitamins from being destroyed by oxidation. Storing foods promptly in the refrigerator reduces the action of enzymes that can break down vitamins.

Preparing Foods to Preserve Vitamins

Water, heat, acids, and alkalis used in cooking can all destroy vitamins. Knowing how vitamins respond to different cooking methods can help you preserve vitamins when preparing foods. The following guidelines may be helpful:

- To preserve water-soluble vitamins, do not soak fruits or vegetables in water. Instead, rinse fresh foods with water before cutting and serving. If foods are to be peeled, wash the food before peeling.
- Many vitamins are located just under the skin of fresh produce. Therefore, avoid paring and peeling fruits and vegetables, if possible.
- Limit exposing large amounts of surface area to light, air, and water by leaving food in large pieces.
- Cut up fruits and vegetables just before you are ready to cook or eat them (**Figure 9.21**). This reduces air and light exposure, which can damage vitamins.
- Choose steaming over boiling to help retain water-soluble vitamins. If you do boil vegetables, do not add them to cooking water until the water begins to boil. Use only a small amount of water and cook the vegetables just until tender. Avoid adding baking soda, which is an alkali, to vegetables. It can destroy some vitamins. Use cooking water in soups, gravies, or sauces.
- Use a pressure cooker or microwave oven to help preserve nutrients by reducing cooking times.

In general, keep cooking times short and use little water. Overcooking destroys heat-sensitive vitamins. Water-soluble vitamins leach into cooking water.

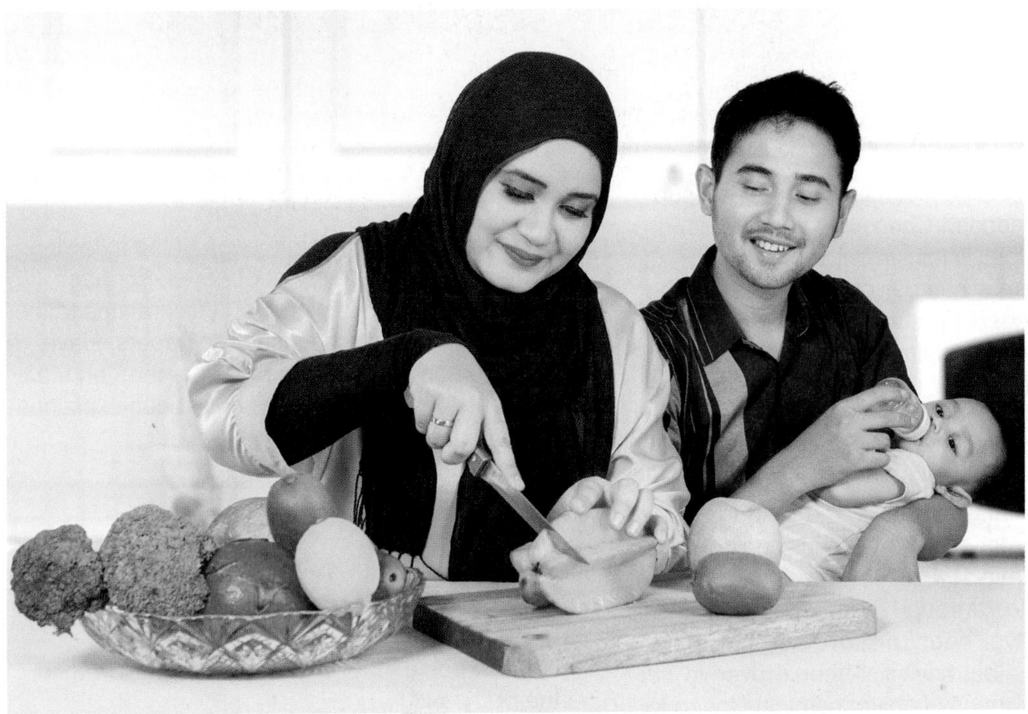

Creativa Images/Shutterstock.com

Figure 9.21
Cut fruits and vegetables as close to serving time as possible to limit exposure to air and light. *Why is it important to limit the time cut fruits and vegetables are exposed to air and light?*

RECIPE FILE

Baked Chicken with Potatoes

6 SERVINGS

Ingredients

- 4 chicken breasts, bone-in, skinless
- 4 chicken thighs, bone-in, skinless
- 1 lb. small Yukon gold potatoes, cut into quarters
- 1 large red onion, cut into eighths
- 1 head garlic, cloves separated and peeled
- 6 large sprigs thyme (or rosemary, sage, or marjoram)
- 1 lemon, quartered, seeds removed
- ¼ c. extra virgin olive oil
- 2 T. balsamic vinegar

Directions

1. Preheat oven to 450°F (232°C).
2. Place chicken, potatoes, onion, garlic, thyme, and lemon in a 12-inch × 16-inch roasting pan.
3. Whisk together oil and vinegar and drizzle over chicken and vegetables. Toss to combine.
4. Arrange chicken and vegetables in pan.
5. Roast until chicken reaches 165°F (74°C) and is golden brown, approximately 50 minutes.

PER SERVING: 307 CALORIES, 30 G PROTEIN, 20 G CARBOHYDRATE, 12 G FAT, 2 G FIBER, 94 MG SODIUM.

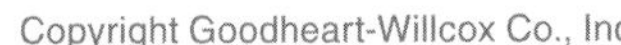

Chapter 9 Review and Expand

Reading Summary

Vitamins are essential nutrients. No one food supplies all the vitamins needed. Choosing a variety of foods is likely to supply all the vitamins most people need.

Vitamins perform a number of major roles in the body. They are needed to release energy from carbohydrates, fats, and proteins. They help maintain healthy body tissues. They are required for the normal operation of all body processes. They also help the body's immune system resist infection.

The fat-soluble vitamins are vitamins A, D, E, and K. They dissolve in fats and are found in foods containing fats. The water-soluble vitamins include the B vitamins and vitamin C. Excess water-soluble vitamins are generally lost through the urine.

Substances have been discovered that have vitamin-like qualities, but have not been proven to be vital to human life. Groups of phytochemicals found in foods are active beneficially at the cellular level and work to help prevent disease. Probiotics and prebiotics work together and yield health benefits when eaten in sufficient amounts.

Doctors may advise extra vitamin supplements for some people with special health or dietary needs. However, most people who use vitamin supplements should choose those that provide no more than the RDA or AI for each vitamin. Storing and preparing foods carefully helps preserve vitamins.

Chapter Vocabulary

1. **Content Terms** In teams, play *picture charades* to identify each of the following terms. Write the terms on separate slips of paper and put the slips into a basket. Choose a team member to be the *sketcher*. The sketcher pulls a term from the basket and creates quick drawings or graphics to represent the term until the team guesses the term. Rotate turns as sketcher until the team identifies all terms.

   antioxidant
   beriberi
   coagulation
   coenzyme
   collagen
   enriched food
   epithelial cells
   erythrocyte hemolysis
   fat-soluble vitamin
   fortified food
   free radical
   night blindness
   osteomalacia
   pellagra
   pernicious anemia
   phytochemicals
   placebo effect
   prebiotics
   probiotics
   provitamin
   rickets
   scurvy
   toxicity
   vitamin
   water-soluble vitamin

2. **Academic Terms** Write each of the following terms on a separate sheet of paper. For each term, quickly write a word you think relates to the term. In small groups, exchange papers. Have each person in the group explain a term on the list. Take turns until all terms have been explained.

   apt
   augment
   conclusive
   dilated
   surplus
   versatile

Review Learning

3. List five basic functions vitamins assist with in the body.
4. *True or false?* Most vitamins have several active forms, which have similar molecular structures.
5. What are two main causes of vitamin deficiency diseases?
6. List three differences between fat-soluble vitamins and water-soluble vitamins.
7. What form of vitamin A is provided by plant foods?
8. Why do some people need more vitamin D in their diet than others?
9. What is the main function of vitamin E in the body?
10. What is the main function of vitamin K in the body?
11. Name three deficiency symptoms shared by all the B-complex vitamins.
12. What is the name of the thiamin deficiency disease?
13. List three food sources of riboflavin.
14. *True or false?* Because niacin is water-soluble, it cannot build up to toxic levels in the body.
15. What is the RDA for pantothenic acid?
16. Why is adequate folate intake especially important to women of childbearing age?
17. What group of people has an increased need for vitamin C and why?
18. List two ways phytochemicals help prevent heart disease and some cancers.
19. Name three groups of people for whom doctors might recommend vitamin supplements.
20. Give three tips for selecting foods high in vitamins.
21. List five ways to prevent vitamin losses when storing and preparing foods.

Self-Assessment Quiz

Complete the self-assessment quiz online to help you practice and expand your knowledge and skills.

Critical Thinking

22. **Conclude** Continuing research has identified additional functions of Vitamin D. Draw conclusions about why you think many people are deficient in this vitamin. What might be some long-term effects of this deficiency?
23. **Assess** When you hear an advertisement about supplements, how can you tell if the information is credible? What sources can you use to verify data? Prepare a list of questions you would ask to evaluate the need for the advertised supplement.
24. **Analyze** Examine how well your daily food pattern meets vitamin needs. Complete a food journal listing all the foods you eat for a three-day period. Find diet analysis software online and use it to analyze your vitamin intake for each day. Which vitamin needs have you met and which are low? Identify foods you could add to your eating behaviors to increase intakes of needed vitamins.
25. **Evaluate** Compare the amounts of each vitamin listed on the labels to the DRIs for the various consumer groups being targeted. Include the same information for a generic multivitamin supplement. Note the price for each vitamin supplement. Organize your findings in a chart. Write a paragraph explaining your opinion whether the vitamin supplements with special claims are worth any difference in price.

Core Skills

26. **Writing** Use the Internet to research the relationship of vitamin K to successful surgery outcomes. Prepare a summary of current medical thinking on how to prepare for surgery to avoid excessive bleeding during and after surgery.
27. **Technology Literacy** Plan a blog about foods on the school lunch menu that are good sources of phytochemicals. First, consider who will be reading your blog and how to make the topic appealing to them. Next, identify three main points that you want to cover. Then, be sure to give your blog a clever title. After you finish writing, be sure to edit and revise your content before posting.
28. **Speaking** In small groups, debate the following topic: "Use the rainbow as a guide for choosing a healthy food plan." Support or refute the position that choosing colorful foods is enough for guiding the selection of a nutritious food plan.
29. **Science** Research how free radicals form in the body and how antioxidants may prevent free radical damage. Identify common sources of free radicals and antioxidants. Use presentation software to prepare and give an electronic presentation sharing your findings. Adjust the style and content of your presentation to your audience. Use digital media to add visual interest and improve understanding.
30. **Listening** Listen carefully as classmates deliver their presentations from the preceding activity. Take notes on important points and write any questions that occur to you. At the end of each presentation, ask questions to obtain additional information or clarification as needed.
31. **Reading and Writing** Learn about the genesis of functional foods. Write a paper summarizing the history of functional foods, future trends, and your opinion about the efficacy of these products.
32. **Math** When weighing small amounts using the metric system, weights are expressed in units called grams (g). Prefixes are used to identify units less than one gram. For example, the prefix micro (μ) means millionth. Therefore, one microgram is equal to one millionth of a gram. Other prefixes include
    - milli (m)—one thousandth
    - centi (c)—one hundredth
    - deci (d)—one tenth

    Subtract 900 micrograms from 7 grams.
33. **Career Readiness Practice** The ability to read and interpret information in context is an important workplace skill. Presume you work for a food manufacturer who typically fortifies its products with vitamins B and C. The company is considering adding vitamin D to some products, but wants you to evaluate and interpret some research on the additional need for vitamin D in the body. You will need to locate at least three reliable sources of information. Read and interpret the information on vitamin D. Then write a report summarizing your findings.

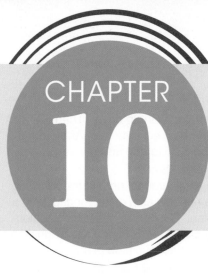

Minerals

Learning Outcomes

After studying this chapter, you will be able to

- **organize** minerals by classification;
- **explain** the major roles of minerals in promoting healthy growth and development;
- **identify** functions and sources of specific macrominerals and microminerals;
- **recall** symptoms of various mineral deficiencies and excesses; and
- **outline** guidelines for maximizing mineral absorption and availability in the body.

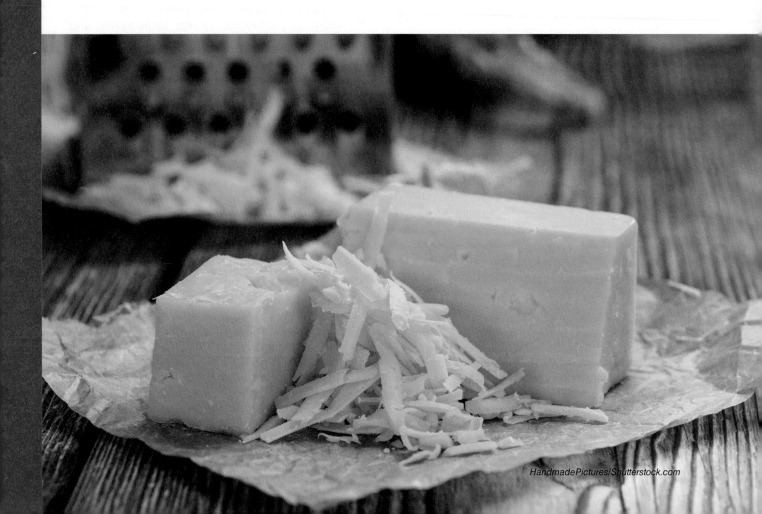

HandmadePictures/Shutterstock.com

Content Terms

acid
base
cofactor
cretinism
fluorosis
goiter
hemoglobin
iron-deficiency anemia
macromineral
micromineral
mineral
myoglobin
osmosis
osteoporosis
pH
thyroxine

Academic Terms

hinder
liberate
negligible
provoke
transmit

What's Your Nutrition and Wellness IQ?

Take this quiz to examine how much you already know about minerals. If you cannot answer a question; pay extra attention to that topic as you study this chapter.

- Identify each statement as *True*, *False*, or *It Depends*. *It Depends* means in some cases the statement is true; in some cases it could be false.
- Revise false statements to make them true.
- Explain the circumstances in which each *It Depends* statement is true and when it is false.

Nutrition and Wellness IQ

	Statement			
1.	Minerals are different from vitamins because they do not contain carbon.	True	False	It Depends
2.	If an essential mineral is missing from an eating pattern, health problems occur immediately.	True	False	It Depends
3.	Macrominerals are more important for good health than microminerals.	True	False	It Depends
4.	Once bones reach their peak mass, calcium foods are less important to consume.	True	False	It Depends
5.	Calcium is to osteoporosis as sodium is to hypertension.	True	False	It Depends
6.	A low-sodium eating plan is a sure way to avoid high blood pressure.	True	False	It Depends
7.	Whole foods (for example, an apple) are a better source of minerals than processed foods (for example, applesauce).	True	False	It Depends
8.	The same foods that provide iron in the diet also provide many other microminerals.	True	False	It Depends

While studying this chapter, look for the activity icon to

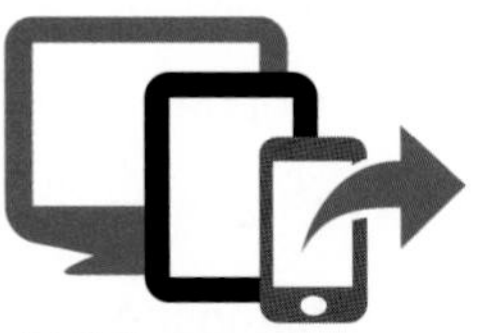

- **build** vocabulary with e-flash cards and interactive games;
- **assess** what you learn by completing self-assessment quizzes and completing review questions; and
- **expand** knowledge with interactive activities and activities that extend learning.

www.g-wlearning.com/foodsandnutrition/

Like vitamins, ***minerals*** are nutrients needed in small amounts to perform various functions in the body. Also like vitamins, minerals provide no calories. Vitamins are organic compounds. This means they are made of different elements bonded together, and one of the elements is carbon. In contrast, minerals are *inorganic elements*. This means a mineral is not a compound, and does not contain carbon.

Minerals in nutrition are the same inorganic elements listed on the periodic table of elements found in most chemistry classrooms. Nutritionists know a number of minerals, including calcium, phosphorus, zinc, and iron, are vital to good health. However, they are still studying the roles and functions of other minerals, such as tin, lead, and lithium. This chapter will discuss the minerals most researchers believe to be essential in the diet.

How Minerals Are Classified

Minerals are found in the soil and water where plants grow and animals feed. You absorb the minerals from the food you eat. At least 21 mineral elements are currently known to be essential to good health. Dietary Reference Intakes have been established for 15 of the minerals. These minerals can be classified into two major groups. The first group is ***macrominerals***, which are also called *major minerals*. These are minerals required in the diet in amounts of 100 or more milligrams per day. The second group is ***microminerals***, or *trace minerals*. These are minerals required in amounts of less than 100 milligrams per day. Microminerals are just as important for health as macrominerals.

Some microminerals can be found in the body in extremely small amounts and are referred to as *ultratrace minerals*. For example, the ultratrace mineral, boron, is needed in amounts of 1–13 milligrams per day. Others are needed in amounts known as *nanograms* (ng), which are units of one billionth of a gram. The biological function of ultratrace minerals in humans remains unclear. More research may show their increased importance for maintaining good health (**Figure 10.1**).

Classification of Minerals		
Macrominerals (Major Minerals)	**Microminerals (Trace Minerals)**	**Other Microminerals (Ultratrace Minerals)**
Calcium	Iron	Arsenic
Phosphorus	Zinc	Boron
Magnesium	Iodine	Nickel
Sulfur	Fluoride	Silicon
Sodium	Selenium	Vanadium
Potassium	Copper	
Chloride	Chromium	
	Manganese	
	Molybdenum	

Figure 10.1 Minerals are classified based on the daily amount that is recommended for good health.

All the minerals in your body combined make up only about four percent of your body mass. Although your mineral needs are small, meeting those needs is critical to good health. Minerals serve a variety of complex functions, which include

- helping enzymes complete chemical reactions
- becoming part of body components
- aiding normal nerve functioning and muscle contraction
- promoting growth
- regulating acid-base balance in the body
- maintaining body fluid balance

Studying key minerals will help you understand their specific functions, and their importance for good health throughout the life span.

The Macrominerals at Work

The macrominerals include calcium, phosphorus, magnesium, sulfur, sodium, potassium, and chloride. Each of these minerals serves specific functions in the body. Learning about food sources and daily needs will help you plan diets rich in minerals.

Calcium

The macromineral found in the largest amount in the body is calcium. Calcium represents about two percent of body weight. This means the body of a 150-pound person contains about three pounds of calcium.

You may have heard a parent say to a child, "Drink your milk." There is good reason for parents to be concerned about their children's dairy intake. Milk, cheese, and other dairy products are great sources of calcium for people of all ages. These parents know how important calcium is for normal growth.

Functions of Calcium

Nearly all the calcium in your body is stored in your bones and teeth. Calcium from the foods you eat is absorbed from your small intestine into your bloodstream. The blood then carries the calcium to your bones. Bones are always being rebuilt. Calcium is added to and removed from bones throughout life. The calcium in the bloodstream is maintained within a very narrow range. This balance is essential so that calcium is available for the many important jobs it performs in the body.

Calcium from your food intake is deposited in your bones to build and strengthen them. This process builds bone mass. *Bone mass* refers to the amount of minerals contained in a given volume of bone. Bone tissue at the ends of long bones looks something like a sponge covered by a shell layer. Healthy bone tissue is dense. The cells of the sponge are small, and the walls of the cells are thick. The shell layer is hard (**Figure 10.2**). When sufficient calcium is available for bone building, you are more likely to achieve your full growth potential. Peak bone mass occurs in the late 20s or early 30s when bone development ends. In a similar way, calcium is used to build strong teeth.

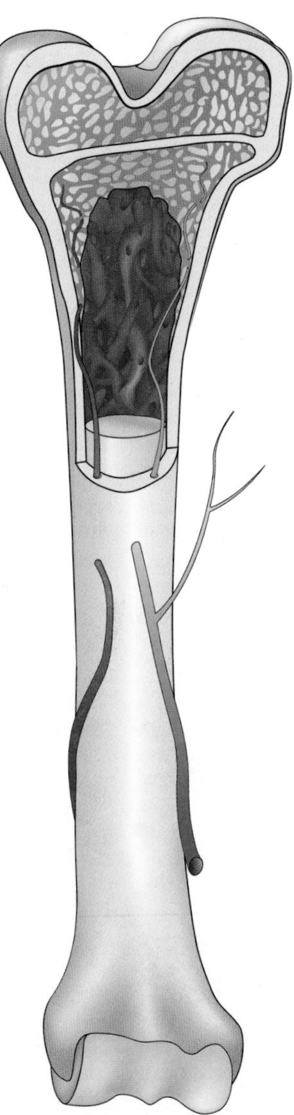

Yoko Design/Shutterstock.com

Figure 10.2 Bone tissue at the ends of long bones looks like sponge covered by a shell layer.

Many people associate calcium with bones and teeth. They often overlook the fact that a tiny amount of calcium is found in every cell of the body. This calcium plays many vital roles. It helps muscles contract and relax, and assists in blood-clotting processes. Calcium also helps **transmit** (relay) nerve impulses.

Amount of Calcium Needed

The Recommended Dietary Allowance (RDA) for calcium for males and females ages 14 through 18 is 1,300 milligrams per day. At age 19, the recommended amount decreases to 1,000 milligrams per day. The RDA increases again for women over age 50 and men over age 70.

Adequate calcium intake coupled with physical activity is particularly important during the preteen, teen, and early adult years. During this stage, your body requires more calcium to build bones to keep up with your body as it grows. Weight-bearing exercise helps build strong, dense bones.

Many teens and young adults fail to recognize the importance of eating good food sources of calcium. Including adequate amounts of calcium in the food you eat at this stage protects your bone health in the future. NIH (National Institutes of Health) reported only 10 percent of older teen girls met their daily need for calcium. Males in this age range fared better with 42 percent meeting their need for calcium.

Teenage males may get more calcium than teenage females simply because the males eat more food. Many teen women limit their food intake to lose weight. Some consume less than 300 milligrams of calcium per day. Individuals who are restricting calories should remember there are foods that are low in calories and rich in calcium.

Sources of Calcium

Foods found in MyPlate's dairy group are your primary sources of calcium. Consuming the recommended daily amounts will help you meet your calcium needs.

Relying on the dairy group may be difficult for people who are lactose intolerant. However, they still have a number of options for meeting their calcium needs. They can add the enzyme lactase to fluid milk to aid digestion. Some people experience digestive problems with milk, but may tolerate cheese, yogurt, and soy products as calcium sources. These products often contain much less or no lactose. They can also choose calcium-rich foods from other food groups.

A variety of nondairy foods supplies calcium. Leafy green vegetables, legumes, tofu, and sardines eaten with the bones all provide calcium (**Figure 10.3**). Some foods are processed with added calcium. For instance, orange juice is sometimes fortified with calcium, making it a good mineral source. Read food labels to identify calcium-fortified products.

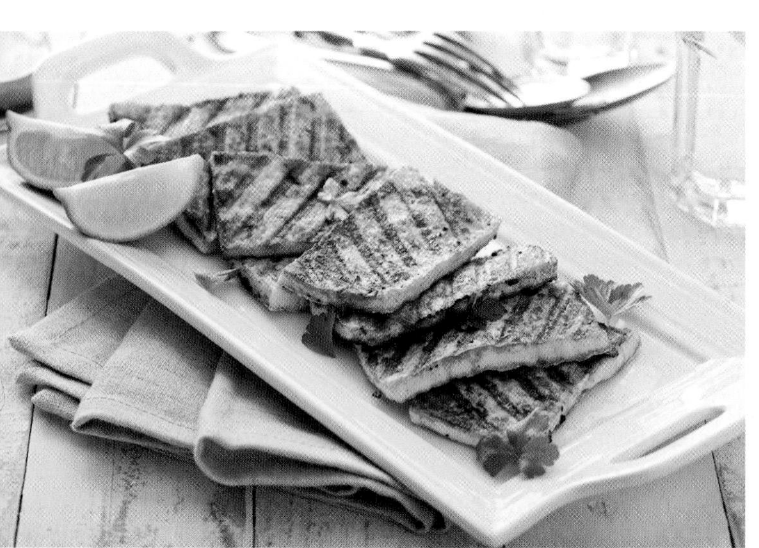

Elena Veselova/Shutterstock.com

Figure 10.3 When calcium salt is used in the production of tofu, it is an excellent source of calcium. *Why is tofu a good alternative for people who experience digestive problems when they consume milk?*

EXTEND YOUR KNOWLEDGE

Boning Up on Bones

The number of people with osteoporosis is increasing in the United States primarily due to an aging population. The main goal of treating people with this disease is preventing fractures. Along with a diet containing foods rich in calcium and vitamin D, some doctors prescribe medications. These medications are designed to reduce bone loss and increase bone density especially in the hip and spine. Many of these drugs belong to a group of drugs called *bisphosphonates*. People who take such drugs should ask their doctors about the side effects and the risk of a rare type of fracture in the thigh bone associated with some drugs. What other treatments are available for osteoporosis? Research such reliable websites as the National Institutes of Health and the Centers for Disease Control for more information.

People on low-calorie food plans sometimes avoid dairy products thinking they are too high in fat and calories. If you are restricting calories, consider choosing fat-free milk and yogurt, reduced-fat cheese, and other low-fat or nonfat dairy products. These foods are good sources of calcium and low in fat and calories.

Effects of Calcium Deficiencies and Excesses

Cells get the calcium they need from a supply found in the blood. Your life depends on the maintenance of normal blood calcium levels at all times. If your diet is calcium deficient, your blood pulls calcium from your bones. When bones lose calcium, they become less dense. The cells of the tissue become larger and the walls of the cell become thinner. The outer layer of the bone becomes brittle.

Calcium deficiencies are more likely to occur when the body's need for calcium is high. People have greater demands for calcium during certain stages of the life cycle. For example, infants and adolescents are in peak growth periods. Their calcium needs are high because their bones and teeth are developing. If their calcium needs are not met, their bones and teeth may not develop normally. Pregnant and breast-feeding women need calcium to meet their babies' needs in addition to their own. If these women do not consume enough calcium, the calcium stored in their bones is used.

Although low calcium intakes are common, calcium excesses from dietary sources are relatively rare. Excesses are generally the result of taking too many supplements. Possible problems from excess calcium intake include kidney stones, constipation, and gas.

Calcium and Bone Health

People who fail to eat a calcium-rich diet through their young adult years do not reach maximum bone mass. This increases their risk of problems due to bone loss later in life. Conversely, people who achieve a higher bone density in their youth are less likely to experience problems as they age. To illustrate this point, think about a bone that lacks mass as a toothpick. Think about a bone that has reached maximum mass as a 2-inch by 4-inch board. Suppose both "bones" lose the same amount of calcium. The one that started out as a toothpick is much more likely to break.

By age 40, many people begin to gradually lose bone density if they are inactive and consume too little calcium. Excessive use of tobacco and alcohol can contribute to decreased bone mass and should be avoided at any age.

A gradual loss of bone mass that continues for many years may lead to ***osteoporosis***. Osteoporosis is a condition that results when bones become porous and fragile due to a loss of calcium. The signs of this bone loss usually appear only after many years as the bones become fragile and lose their strength.

With older adults, breaks of wrist and hip bones are frequently the result of osteoporosis. A loss of mineral density and mass causes the bones to be less strong. Tooth loss may occur due to weakening of the jawbone. Bones in the spinal area can compress, causing height to decrease by several inches (**Figure 10.4**).

Genetics and body frame size also play a role in bone health. Some people have greater bone density than others. These individuals may have built more bone density when they were young or inherited a family trait for greater bone density.

Preserving Bone Health

Loss of bone mass is not always age-related. It is also linked to diet and exercise. People who eat calcium-rich diets and engage in weight-bearing exercise do not lose much bone mass as they age. On the other hand, even teens can lose bone mass if they follow extreme diet and exercise practices. Excess sweating that occurs with athletes can lead to calcium losses. Low calcium intakes compound these problems.

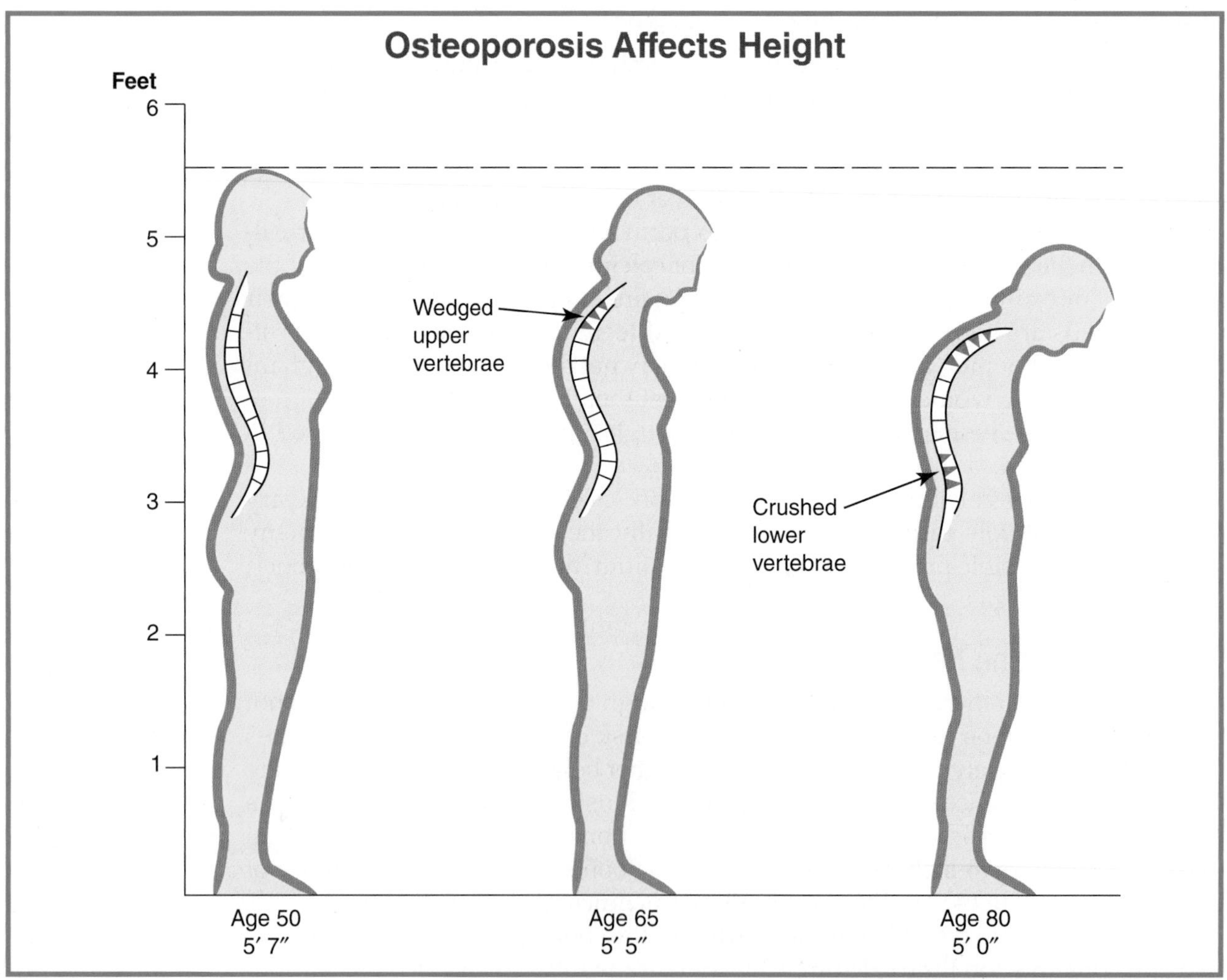

Goodheart-Willcox Publisher

Figure 10.4 Compression of bones in the spinal column due to osteoporosis results in a decrease in height.

Eating an energy-balanced diet that is rich in calcium and vitamin D can protect bones and teeth. Moderate exercise that places weight on the bones can also help keep bones dense and strong over a lifetime. Lifestyle choices of physical activity to reduce bone loss include walking, dancing, and jogging (**Figure 10.5**). The effects of bone loss will depend partly on the amount of calcium you store in your bones now.

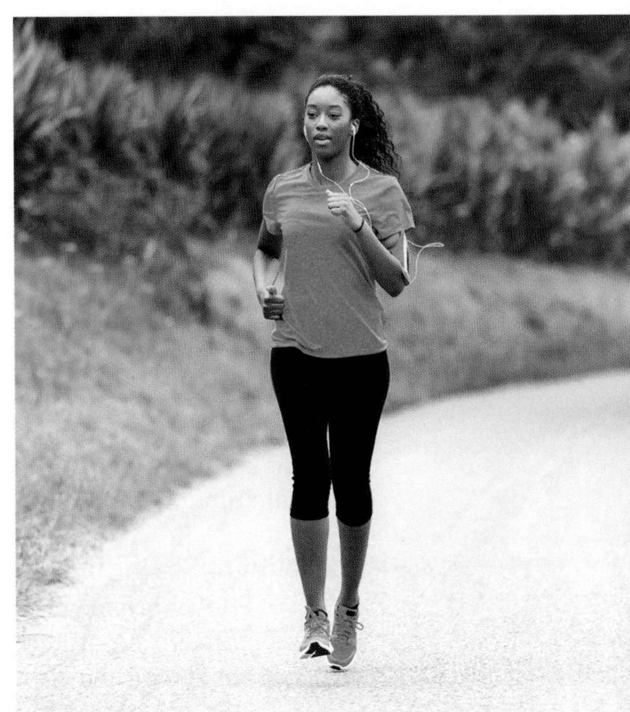

Samuel Borges Photography/Shutterstock.com

Figure 10.5 Weight-bearing exercise, such as running, helps increase bone density. *What are other examples of weight-bearing exercise?*

Calcium Supplements

One out of two women will face osteoporosis at some point in their lives. With the common problem of poor calcium intake and the effects of inactivity, you may wonder about the value of calcium supplements. Calcium supplements can benefit some people, especially those who cannot consume dairy products.

A number of types of calcium supplements are available. The body can absorb some types better than others. For instance, compounds of concentrated calcium, such as calcium carbonate, calcium phosphate, and calcium citrate are the best choices. Supplements made from powdered calcium-containing materials, such as bones and oyster shells, are not recommended. They may contain contaminants, such as lead or other impurities.

CASE STUDY

CASE STUDY

Fast-Food Choices

Jerry, a 16-year-old male, is at a fast-food restaurant with his friends. He has just read the chapter in his textbook about the need for calcium for strong bones and good health. Last week, he read about the importance of protein for muscle growth. He learned that milk is a source of both calcium and protein. Jerry thinks this is perfect because he loves milk shakes and ice cream sundaes!

However, Jerry is on the wrestling team and the coach has reminded him he must make his weight category. Strong muscles and bones are important in wrestling. Jerry realizes he must pay more attention to his food choices. He wants to meet his calcium needs, but he is concerned about too many calories from saturated fats. He has learned saturated fats can negatively affect weight and health. He looks at the menu to see his choices.

Case Review

1. What are several food choices commonly found on fast-food restaurant menus that will help Jerry meet his calcium and protein needs, and are also low in saturated fats?
2. Do you think Jerry should rely on fast-food restaurants to meet his daily calcium needs? Why?

People (usually older adults) who produce little stomach acid should take supplements with meals. This is so any acid produced during digestion can aid calcium absorption.

Calcium supplements often combined with vitamin D help reduce the risk of osteoporosis. Along with this advantage, taking calcium supplements can have some disadvantages. Calcium supplements can also **hinder** (prevent) the absorption of some other nutrients, such as iron and zinc. Most nutritionists agree getting calcium from food sources is preferred to using supplements. Avoid calcium intake greater than the recommended Tolerable Upper Intake Level (UL).

Phosphorus

Phosphorus is the mineral found in the second largest amount in the body. It makes up one to one and one-half percent of your body weight. Phosphorus and calcium together represent more than half of all the mineral weight in your body.

Functions of Phosphorus

Phosphorus works with calcium to help form strong bones and teeth. It helps maintain an acid-base balance in the blood. It is part of ATP (adenosine triphosphate), which is the source of immediate energy found in muscle tissue. Phosphorus is also in cell membranes and is part of some enzymes. Like calcium, it is part of every cell.

Meeting Phosphorus Needs

The RDA for phosphorus for males and females ages 14 through 18 is 1,250 milligrams daily. Phosphorus is easily found in the diet and is absorbed efficiently. Therefore, typical U.S. diets supply adequate amounts of phosphorus.

Phosphorus is found in protein-rich foods including milk, cheese, meats, legumes, and eggs. Peas, potatoes, raisins, and avocados are good sources, too. Baked products, chocolate, and carbonated soft drinks are also sources of phosphorus.

Effects of Phosphorus Deficiencies and Excesses

Phosphorus deficiencies are virtually unknown. However, too much phosphorus in the diet can hinder the absorption of other minerals. For example, excess phosphorus can contribute to bone loss and reduce calcium absorption and utilization.

The typical eating habits of a U.S. teen include roughly two to four times more phosphorus than calcium. A high protein diet combined with additives found in baked goods and other processed foods increases the chances of calcium-phosphorus imbalance. Carbonated soft drinks with phosphoric acid are a high source of phosphorus (**Figure 10.6**). Teens who replace milk with soft drinks may have insufficient intakes of calcium and vitamin D. Such a diet greatly increases the risk of less than optimal bone density. Researchers have noted that the imbalance can cause calcium to be drawn from the bone into the blood to neutralize the acidic effect of phosphorus. Too much phosphorus with insufficient calcium and vitamin D are contributing factors for osteoporosis, and gum and teeth problems.

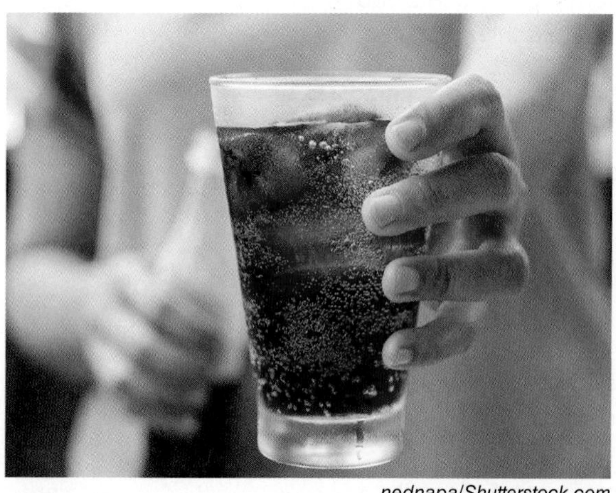

nednapa/Shutterstock.com

Figure 10.6 An excess of carbonated soft drinks may contribute to decreased bone density.

Magnesium

Like calcium and phosphorus, most of the magnesium in the body is in the bones. Additional magnesium is found in muscle tissue. However, the amount of magnesium is much smaller than the amounts of the other two minerals. The magnesium content in the body of an adult is less than two ounces.

Functions of Magnesium

Magnesium is involved in over 300 enzymatic reactions in the body. Magnesium makes the enzymes active and lets them work more efficiently. Magnesium also activates the ATP in your body so it can release energy. It helps the lungs, nerves, and heart function properly. Magnesium is also tied to your body's use of calcium and phosphorus and therefore important for bone health.

Meeting Magnesium Needs

The RDA for magnesium is 360 milligrams per day for women ages 14 through 18. For men in the same age group, the RDA is 410 milligrams per day. Many people in the United States consume less than the RDA for magnesium.

Good sources of magnesium include leafy green vegetables, potatoes, legumes, seafood, nuts, dairy foods, and whole-grain products (**Figure 10.7**). Hard water, which has a high concentration of minerals, is also a source of magnesium.

Effects of Magnesium Deficiencies and Excesses

Few Americans are deficient in magnesium. The body can store magnesium, so deficiency symptoms develop slowly in most people. Magnesium deficiencies are often the result of other health problems. For instance, starvation or extended periods of vomiting or diarrhea can cause low magnesium levels. Alcohol increases magnesium excretion. Therefore, alcoholics are at an increased risk of magnesium deficiency. Deficiency symptoms include weakness, heart irregularities, disorientation, and seizures.

Too much magnesium in the blood occurs mainly when the kidneys are not working properly. Excess magnesium from food sources is not considered a health concern. However, daily intakes of over 350 milligrams of magnesium from supplements may produce toxicity symptoms in teens and adults. Lower intakes from supplements may produce toxicity symptoms in children. Magnesium toxicity can cause weakness and nausea.

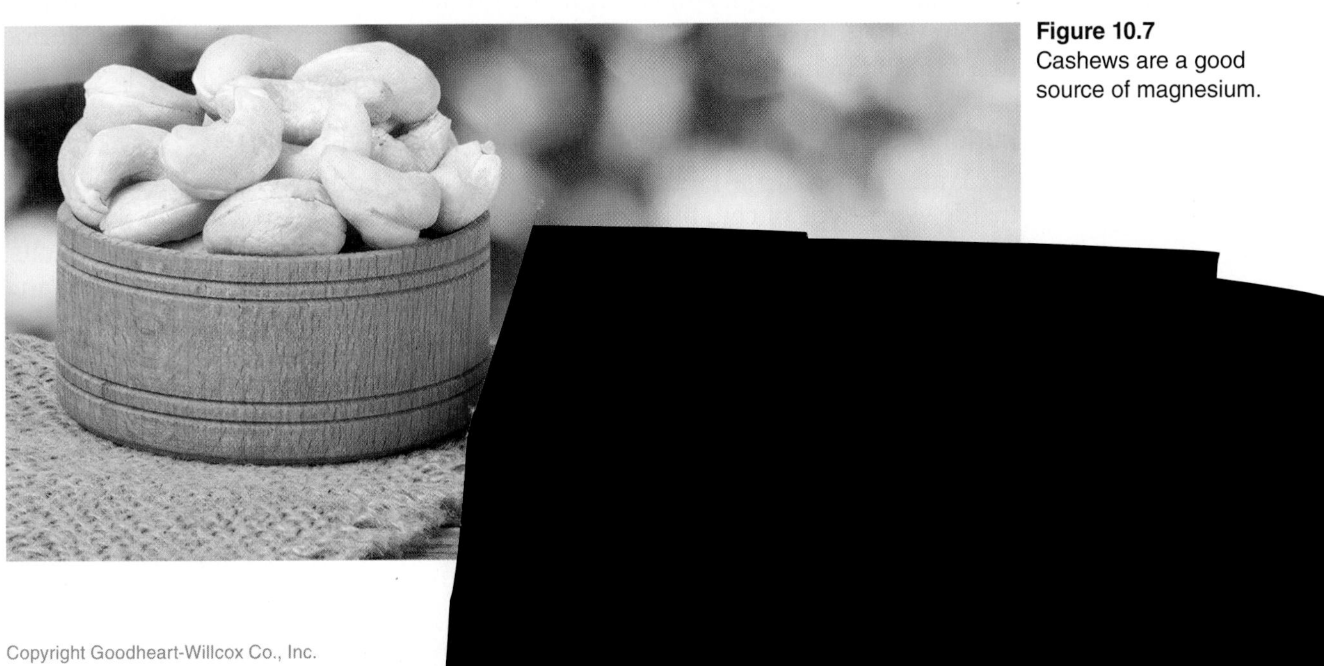

Figure 10.7 Cashews are a good source of magnesium.

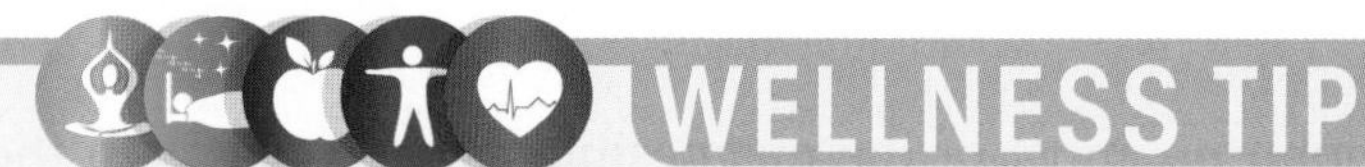

Support Bone Health—Limit Soft Drinks

Recent research shows that teens today consume more carbonated soft drinks than milk. Daily consumption of these beverages (high in phosphoric acid) can put teens at greater risk of bone fracture, especially teen females. Drink water to quench thirst. Protect your bone health by limiting soft drinks to special occasions and consuming milk and other calcium-rich foods to support bone health.

Sulfur

Sulfur is present in every cell in your body. Sulfur is in high concentrations in your hair, nails, and skin. If you have ever burned your hair, you may have recognized the sulfur smell.

Functions of Sulfur

Sulfur is part of the protein in your tissues. It is also part of the vitamins thiamin and biotin. It helps maintain a normal acid-base balance in the body. It also helps the liver change toxins into harmless substances.

Meeting Sulfur Needs

There is no RDA for sulfur. You can easily meet your sulfur needs through diet. You get sulfur from protein foods and sources of thiamin and biotin.

Effects of Sulfur Deficiencies and Excesses

Sulfur presents no known deficiency symptoms. There is no danger of toxicity associated with sulfur from food sources.

Sodium, Potassium, and Chloride

Sodium, potassium, and chloride are grouped together because they work as a team to perform similar functions. (Chloride is the form of the mineral chlorine that is found in the body.)

Functions of Sodium, Potassium, and Chloride

Water makes up a large percentage of your body weight. There is water inside every type of cell, from muscle to bone. There is also water in the spaces
is found in the fluids outside the cells.
ells. Chloride is found both inside and

he right amount and type of fluid, they
fluid imbalance occurs, it can cause a
eart failure. Sodium, potassium, and
lls and body compartments.
in your body is *semipermeable*. This
mbrane but particles, such as miner-

When the mineral concentrations on each side of the membrane are different, water is drawn across the membrane. Water moves from the side with fewer particles to the side with more particles. This helps equalize the concentrations of mineral particles on each side of the membrane. This movement of water across cell membranes is known as ***osmosis*** (**Figure 10.8**).

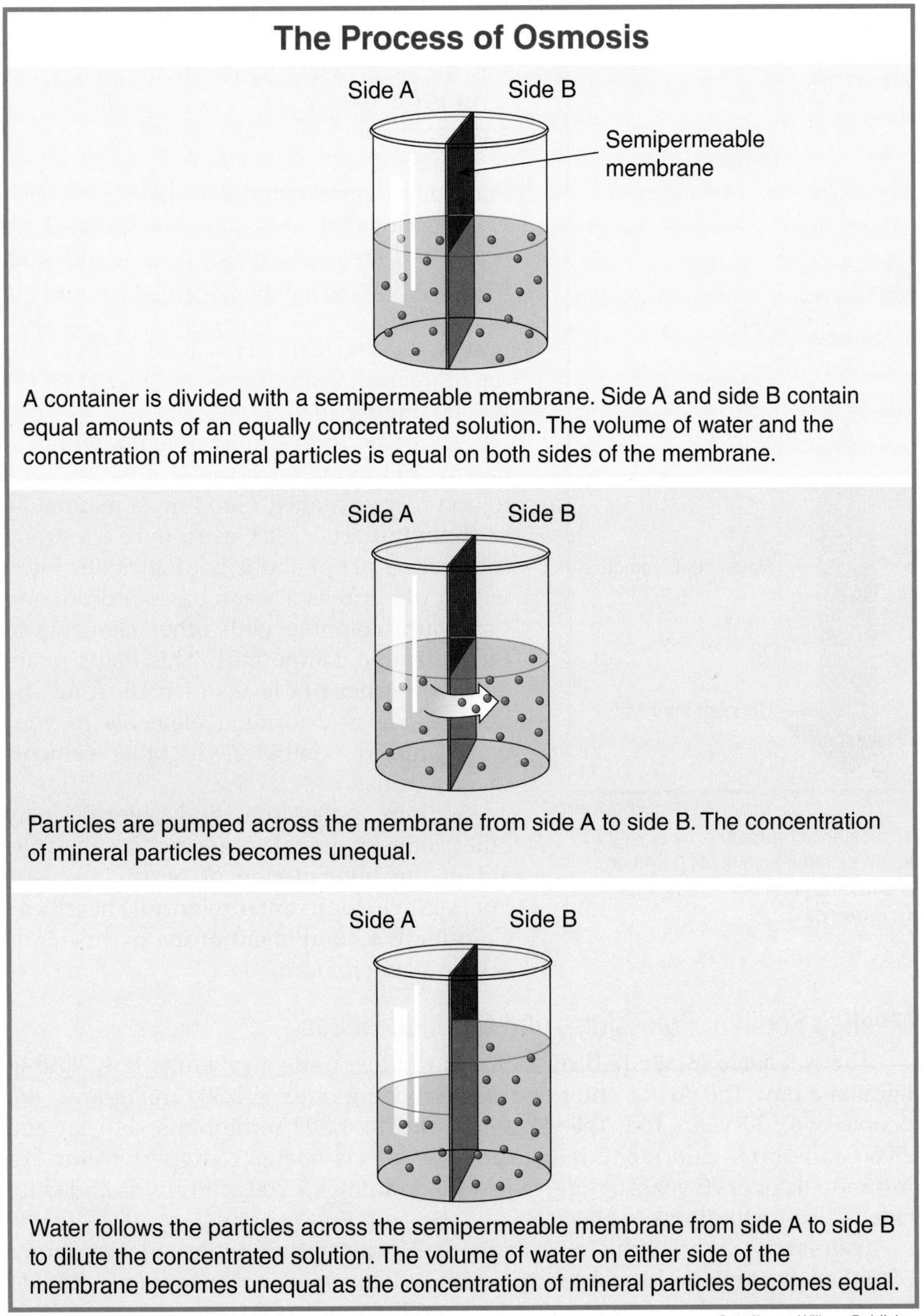

The Process of Osmosis

Side A Side B

Semipermeable membrane

A container is divided with a semipermeable membrane. Side A and side B contain equal amounts of an equally concentrated solution. The volume of water and the concentration of mineral particles is equal on both sides of the membrane.

Side A Side B

Particles are pumped across the membrane from side A to side B. The concentration of mineral particles becomes unequal.

Side A Side B

Water follows the particles across the semipermeable membrane from side A to side B to dilute the concentrated solution. The volume of water on either side of the membrane becomes unequal as the concentration of mineral particles becomes equal.

Goodheart-Willcox Publisher

Figure 10.8 Osmosis helps balance the concentration of fluid inside the body's cells with fluid that surrounds the cells. *What prevents minerals from being able to move freely in and out of the cells?*

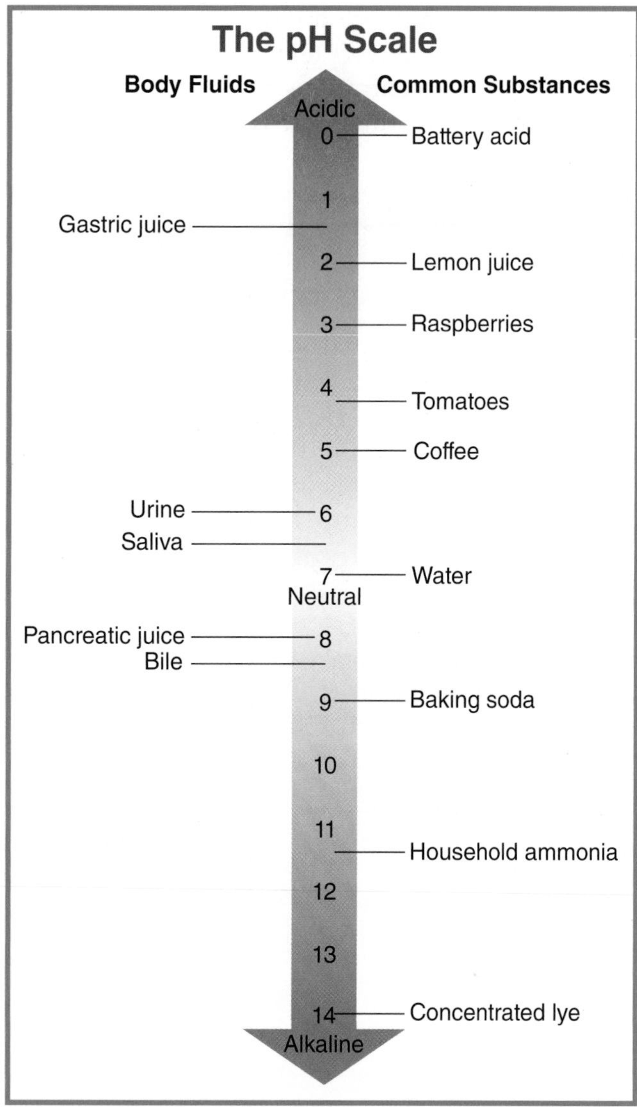

Goodheart-Willcox Publisher

Figure 10.9 The pH of a substance represents its acidity or alkalinity. On the pH scale, an extreme acid is pH 0 and an extreme alkali is pH 14. The neutral point is 7. *Are raspberries more or less acidic than coffee?*

Pumping mechanisms help draw potassium into body cells and sodium out of body cells. This controls the flow of water in and out of cells as the water moves to balance mineral concentrations.

Controlling osmosis is not the only function of sodium, potassium, and chloride. They also play an important role in maintaining the acid-base balance in the body. The term ***pH*** is used to express the measure of a substance's acidity or alkalinity. This measure is expressed on a scale from 0 to 14. Water and other neutral substances have a pH of 7. Compounds that have a pH lower than 7 are acidic and are called ***acids***. Compounds that have a pH greater than 7 are alkaline and are called *alkalis* or ***bases***. The more acidic a solution is, the lower its pH will be. Conversely, the more basic a solution is, the higher its pH will be (**Figure 10.9**).

All body fluids must remain within a narrow pH range for essential life processes to occur. For instance, blood must maintain a near-neutral pH of 7.4. Gastric juice is a strong acid with a pH of about 1.5. Pancreatic juice, with a pH of 8, is a weak base. Sodium and potassium combine with other elements to form alkaline compounds. This helps maintain the proper pH levels of body fluids by neutralizing acid-forming elements in your body. Chloride combines with other elements to form acids.

Sodium, potassium, and chloride play other important roles in the body. They aid in the transmission of nerve impulses. Potassium helps maintain a normal heartbeat. Chloride is a component of the hydrochloric acid in your stomach.

Meeting Sodium, Potassium, and Chloride Needs

The Adequate Intake (AI) of sodium for adolescents and adults is 1,500 milligrams a day. The AI for chloride for these age groups is 2,300 milligrams. For people over 50 years old, the AI is reduced to 1,300 milligrams sodium and 2,000 milligrams chloride to reduce adverse effects related to hypertension. For individuals over 70 years of age, the AI for sodium is 1,200 milligrams and chloride is 1,800 milligrams.

Sodium occurs naturally in many foods. However, the primary dietary source of both of these minerals is table salt, which is chemically known as *sodium chloride*. One teaspoon of salt equals roughly 5,000 milligrams: 2,000 milligrams of sodium and 3,000 milligrams of chloride.

Much salt in the typical U.S. diet is added to food during cooking and at the table. However, you may not realize the majority of salt in the diet comes from processed foods. Some experts estimate as much as 75 percent of sodium in the diet comes from processed foods. Salt is often added during processing to enhance flavors and preserve foods. Pickles, cured meats, canned soups, frozen dinners, and snack items are among the foods that are often high in sodium. Because salt contains chloride as well as sodium, foods containing added salt are also sources of chloride (**Figure 10.10**).

Many people in the United States consume well over 3,000 milligrams of sodium per day. For this reason, the *Dietary Guidelines* recommends reducing daily sodium intake to less than 2,300 milligrams. The recommendation is further reduced to 1,500 milligrams for individuals who have prehypertension or hypertension.

The Nutrition Facts panel on food labels can help you identify sources of sodium in your diet. A percent Daily Value of five or less is a low-sodium food. A percent Daily Value of 20 or greater is considered a high-sodium food.

The AI for potassium for adolescents and adults is 4,700 milligrams per day. Fresh fruits and vegetables are rich sources of potassium. Milk and many kinds of fish are also good sources.

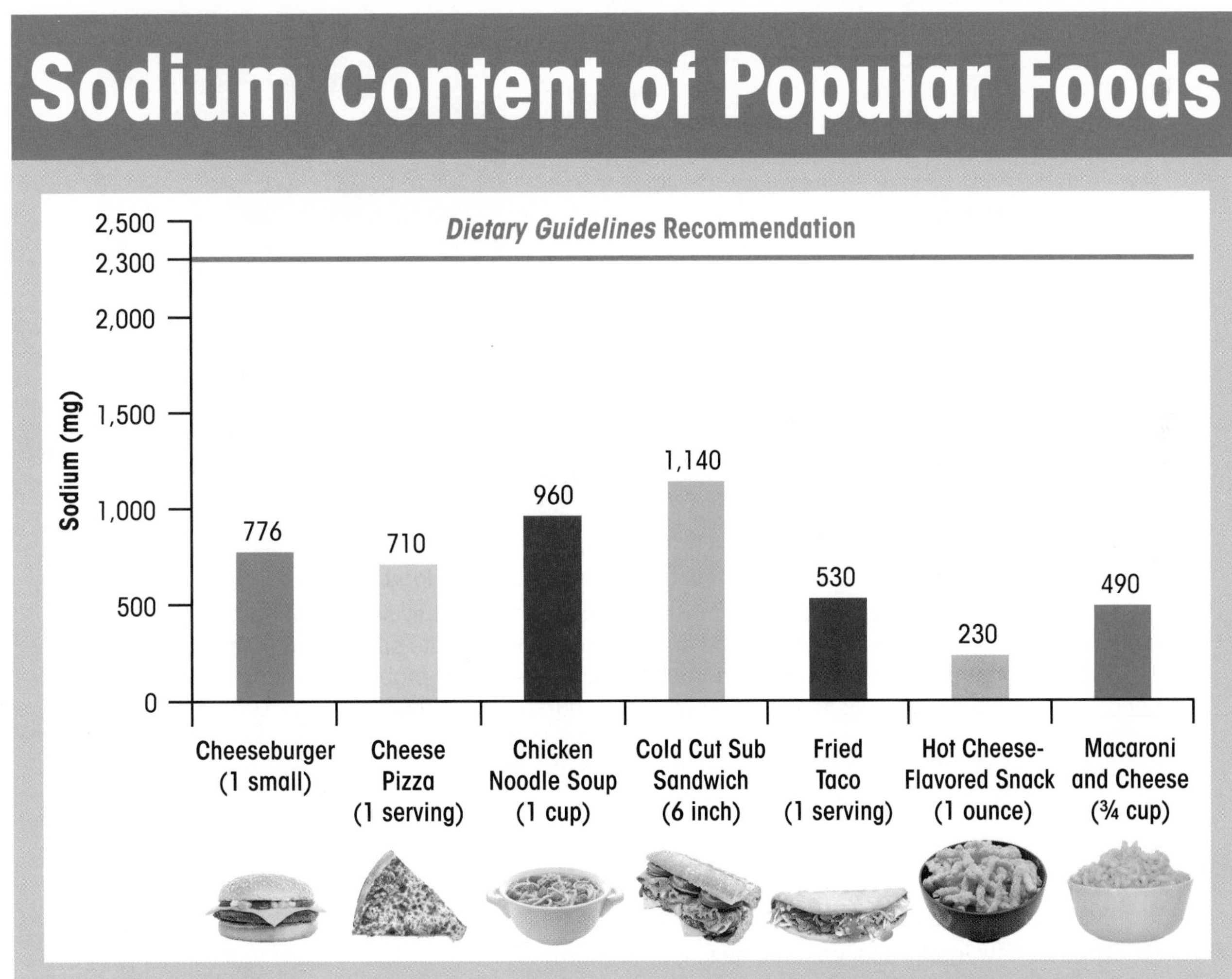

Left to right: EggHeadPhoto/Shutterstock.com; Hong Vo/Shutterstock.com; Danny Smythe/Shutterstock.com; Olga Nayashkova/Shutterstock.com; Duplass/Shutterstock.com; Mariontxa/Shutterstock.com; Michael C. Gray/Shutterstock.com

Figure 10.10 Many popular foods contain large amounts of sodium. *What percent of the* Dietary Guidelines *recommendation for sodium intake does one serving of cheese pizza supply?*

Effects of Sodium, Potassium, and Chloride Deficiencies and Excesses

Deficiencies are rarely the result of too little sodium in the diet. More often, fluid losses, such as vomiting or diarrhea, cause a drop in the body's sodium level. The kidneys respond to these losses by increasing retention of sodium and water. A typical diet soon makes up for these sodium losses. Increased fluid intake is needed to replace missing water. Sodium deficiency can cause muscle cramps, nausea, vomiting, and perhaps even death. If a person is on a very low-calorie diet and loses body fluids through sweat, symptoms will occur.

FOOD AND THE ENVIRONMENT

Food Waste: Is It a Problem?

One-third to one-half of all food produced, processed, and transported is never consumed. It is wasted. Another way of looking at the problem is one in four calories planned for consumption is lost to waste. In addition, food waste is expected to rise by 2020. The Food and Agricultural Organization (FAO) reports that food discarded by retailers and consumers would be enough to feed the entire world's hungry people.

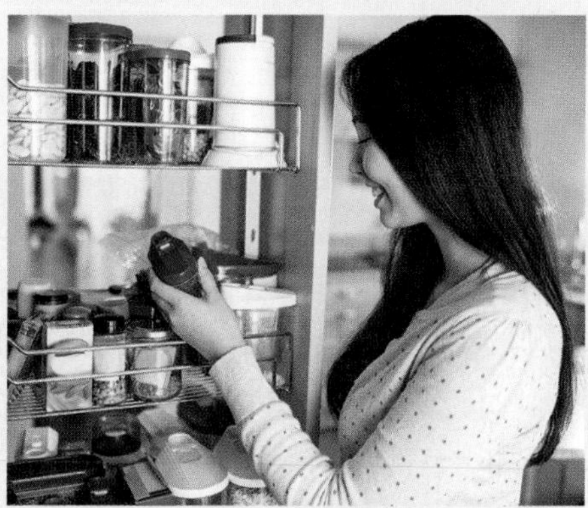
wavebreakmedia/Shutterstock.com

Another concern is the amount of organic waste added to landfills across the country. Organic food waste produces methane gas, a potent greenhouse gas, which contributes to global warming. Although it is not the largest source of greenhouse gas emissions, this gas adds to the problem.

What can be done to reduce food waste? Here are a few examples:

- Buy only the amount of food that you can eat and store it properly to avoid spoilage. Don't throw food away just because the sell-by date has expired.
- Repurpose leftovers or freeze them to eat later.
- Do not discard food just because it is overripe or aesthetically imperfect. Instead, freeze fruits and vegetables for later use in a smoothie, soup, stir-fry, or baked good.
- Save cracker crumbs and bread heels for use as breading or for casserole topping.
- Organize refrigerators and storage cupboards to rotate older food products forward.

Food producers and manufacturers must also be encouraged to seek ways to reduce waste. Individuals can donate food, organize food drives, and help distribute supplies to those in need.

Several organizations work to raise public awareness of the problems of food waste. World Food Day encourages people to donate foods rather than discarding edible items. Gleaning organizations work to recover and donate food before it is lost to waste. Feeding America is an organization that captures wholesome food via food drives and donations from food growers, grocery stores, and restaurants, and then delivers it to the hungry.

Think Critically

1. Evaluate food waste at your school and formulate a plan to reduce it.
2. Analyze how food waste contributes to global warming and draw a web chart to illustrate your findings.
3. Consider ways to incentivize producers, food manufacturers, and consumers to help stop food waste.

Sodium losses through perspiration during normal exercise are usually **negligible** (slight). If you lose more than three percent of body weight through perspiration, however, you may need to replace sodium. Adding salt to your food can restore your sodium levels. Some sports drinks and nutritional energy bars may contain extra sodium. There is no need to take salt tablets—you may be consuming more sodium than you lost in sweat. The additional sodium could cause stomach cramps.

The average person in the United States consumes several times the AI for sodium each day. In most healthy people, the kidneys filter excess sodium from the blood and excrete it in the urine. However, about 10 to 15 percent of the population is *sodium sensitive.* In these people, the kidneys have trouble getting rid of extra sodium.

Potassium needs must be kept in balance for a healthy heart. Too little potassium can cause the heart to malfunction. Other symptoms of potassium deficiency include muscle cramps, loss of appetite, constipation, and confusion. Like sodium, potassium can be lost with body fluids during bouts of vomiting and diarrhea. Fluid losses that happen with the use of some high blood pressure medications can also lead to potassium deficiencies.

Due to the quantity of chloride provided by salt in the typical diet, chloride deficiencies are rare. Deficiency symptoms are similar to those for sodium and are likely to appear under the same circumstances. Excess chloride in the diet does not normally produce toxicity symptoms.

Sodium and Hypertension

Too much sodium in the blood can **provoke** (bring about) hypertension in sodium-sensitive people. Someone who has hypertension has excess force on the walls of his or her arteries. Sodium draws water into blood vessels, causing the volume of blood to expand. Arteries are elastic. They stretch as blood volume expands. However, an excess of sodium causes blood volume to expand too much. This puts increased pressure on the arteries. If arteries are overstretched too often, they weaken, lose their elasticity, and may become damaged. If left untreated, hypertension can lead to heart attack or stroke.

Factors other than eating habits, including heredity, overweight, smoking, inactivity, and stress, affect the development of hypertension. Sodium-sensitive people can reduce their blood pressure by decreasing their salt intake (**Figure 10.11**).

Ways to Reduce Sodium in Your Diet
• Taste foods before adding salt during cooking or at the table.
• Use pepper, lemon juice, and herbs and spices in place of salt to flavor foods.
• Choose fresh fruits, vegetables, meats, fish, and poultry often. They generally contain less sodium than processed products.
• Check the Nutrition Facts panel on processed foods, frozen foods, and canned foods. Choose those products that provide the least amount of sodium per serving.
• Use cured and processed meats, such as hot dogs, sausage, and luncheon meats, sparingly.
• Use condiments, such as soy sauce, catsup, mustard, chili sauce, pickles, and olives, sparingly.
• Choose low- or reduced-sodium versions of foods when they are available.
• Limit intake of salty snack foods.

Figure 10.11
Following these tips can help you reduce the amount of sodium in your diet.

Also, the chance of becoming sodium sensitive increases with age. Therefore, experts recommend all people in the United States choose and prepare foods with less salt.

The DASH (Dietary Approaches to Stop Hypertension) eating plan is designed to help people reduce the risks of cardiovascular disease. DASH is high in vegetables, fruits, low-fat dairy products, whole grains, poultry, fish, beans, and nuts and is low in sweets, sugar-sweetened beverages, and red meats. It is low in saturated fats and rich in potassium, calcium, and magnesium, as well as dietary fiber and protein. It also is lower in sodium than the typical American diet, and includes menus with two levels of sodium: 2,300 or 1,500 mg per day. Healthy adults can follow DASH, along with daily exercise and stress reduction, as a way to delay hypertension during the aging process. Health professionals recommend people have their blood pressure checked yearly.

The Microminerals at Work

There are at least nine microminerals needed by the body. These include iron, zinc, iodine, fluoride, selenium, copper, chromium, manganese, and molybdenum. Several other trace minerals may also play a role in human nutrition. They include arsenic, boron, nickel, silicon, and vanadium, which currently do not have established known human needs. Trace minerals present a high risk for toxicity. A pile containing all the microminerals from your body would fit in the palm of your hand. However, these tiny amounts perform a variety of important functions.

Trace mineral research is one of the newest areas in the science of nutrition. Much of what nutritionists know about trace minerals has been identified in just the last 30 years. Many questions about trace minerals still remain. Could the average diet be low in some essential, yet unidentified mineral? Are trace minerals that occur naturally in foods removed when foods are refined and processed? Can trace mineral supplements serve as a safety net for people who fail to eat nutritious diets? Researchers will continue to seek the answers to these and other questions about how microminerals can affect wellness.

The two values used for daily micromineral recommendations are based on scientific knowledge that is available at this time. When research is inconclusive, daily recommendations are given as AIs. RDAs are given when research is more conclusive.

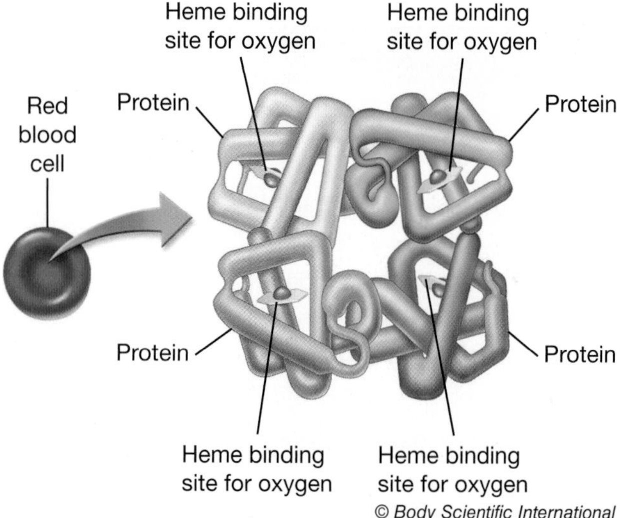

Figure 10.12 Iron plays an important role in transporting oxygen throughout the body.

Iron

The total amount of iron in your body is about one teaspoon. This may seem to be a trivial amount. However, iron plays a critical role in maintaining your health.

Functions of Iron

Most of the iron in your body is found in your blood as a part of hemoglobin. ***Hemoglobin*** is a molecule that includes a large protein called *globin* and an iron molecule called *heme*. Hemoglobin helps red blood cells carry oxygen from the lungs to cells throughout the body (**Figure 10.12**). It is what makes blood red. Hemoglobin also carries carbon dioxide from body tissues back to the lungs for excretion.

Another iron-containing protein is ***myoglobin***. This protein carries oxygen and carbon dioxide in muscle tissue.

Bone marrow stores some iron in the body, which is used to build red blood cells. The liver releases new red blood cells into the bloodstream. Red blood cells perform their oxygen delivery and carbon dioxide removal duties for three to four months before they die. Then the liver and spleen harvest the iron from the dead red blood cells. They send the iron back to the bone marrow for storage until it is recycled into new hemoglobin molecules.

In addition to carrying oxygen, iron helps the body release energy from macronutrients. It is also needed to help make new cells and several compounds in the body.

THE MOVEMENT CONNECTION

Jump for Bone Health

Why

Calcium accounts for almost 2% of body weight! All of the calcium contained in your body is stored in your bones, but there is a tiny amount of calcium in every cell in our bodies. If a diet is deficient in calcium, blood will pull the calcium from the bones which, over a lifetime, can lead to osteoporosis. With older adults, height can decrease due to wedged and crushed vertebrae in the spine.

In addition to a balanced diet including sufficient calcium, weight-bearing activities are necessary to promote bone health and avoid bone density loss.

Apply

Find a partner and sufficient space to perform this activity. Select an area where you won't bump into any objects or other students. When performing the jumps for this activity, follow these guidelines to avoid injury:

- Start with slightly bent knees and arms slightly behind you.
- Straighten legs as you push off the floor and use your arms to drive you in a small, upward movement.
- Land as softly and quietly as possible, with bent knees.
- Land evenly on feet from heel to toe.

If you are performing a hop, use just one leg and follow the same guidelines. Now, compete against your partner to see who can complete the "jumping pyramid" first.

Jumping Pyramid

Begin with

3 jumps both feet
3 hops right foot
3 hops left foot

Next,

2 jumps both feet
2 hops right foot
2 hops left foot

And finish with

1 jump both feet
1 hop right foot
1 hop left foot

Compete for the best of three rounds! How has this activity affected your energy level?

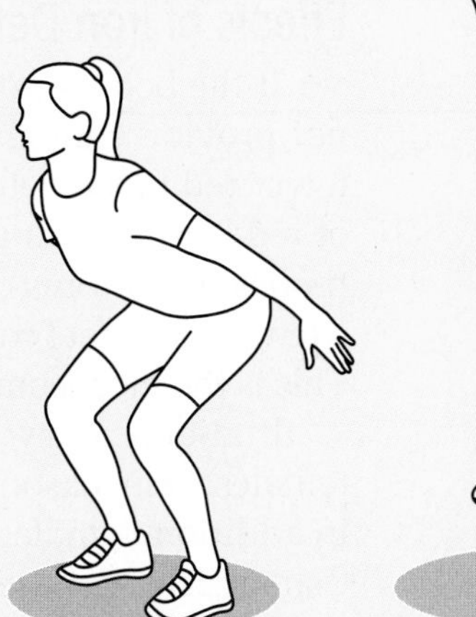

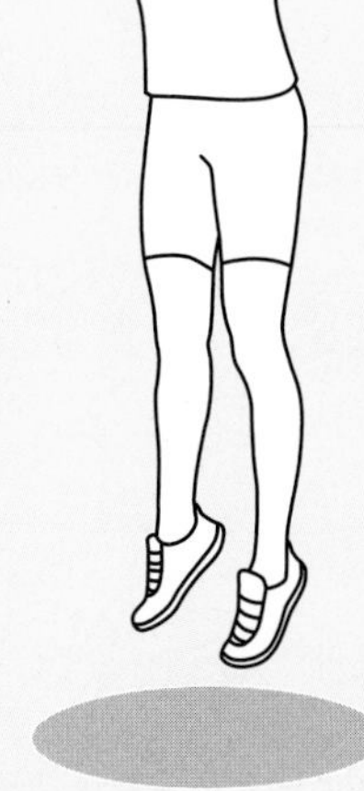

Meeting Iron Needs

The RDA for iron for males ages 14 through 18 is 11 milligrams per day. During these growth years, males have a significant increase in muscle mass. Extra iron is needed as myoglobin carries more oxygen and carbon dioxide in growing muscles. After age 19, the body is no longer growing, so the iron RDA for males drops to 8 milligrams daily. Maintaining muscle does not require as much iron as building new muscle.

Because iron is part of red blood cells, whenever blood is lost, iron is lost. Females lose blood every month through menstruation. Therefore, the RDA for iron for females ages 14 through 18 is 15 milligrams per day. Iron needs increase to 18 milligrams per day for females ages 19 to 50. Iron needs drop to 8 milligrams daily for women over 50, who are assumed postmenopausal.

Iron in foods is found in two forms—*heme* and *nonheme*. Heme iron is found in the hemoglobin and myoglobin of animal foods. Nonheme iron is found in plant and animal foods. The body can absorb heme iron more easily than nonheme iron. Vegetarians must pay attention to having adequate iron levels.

Red meat, fish and shellfish (clams, oysters), poultry, and organ meats (liver) are excellent sources of iron. Legumes, dark-green leafy vegetables, and whole grains are also good iron sources. Many bread and cereal products are enriched with iron. Acidic foods, such as tomatoes, also become good sources when they are cooked in iron pans. The acid helps **liberate** (set free, release) some of the iron from the cookware. This liberated iron remains in the food (**Figure 10.13**). Consuming good sources of vitamin C along with iron-rich foods will increase iron absorption. This is because vitamin C helps the body absorb iron.

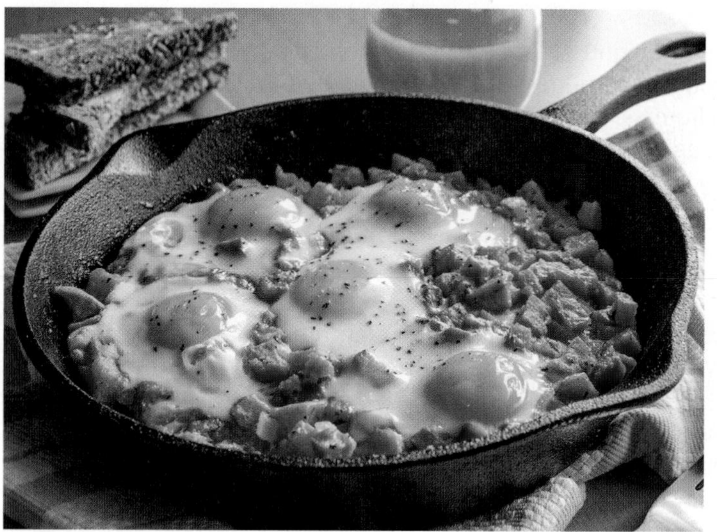

Teri Virbickis/Shutterstock.com

Figure 10.13 Cooking some foods in iron cookware can help increase their iron content.

Milk is a very poor source of iron. This is why infant formulas and cereals are fortified with iron. The addition of iron has helped reduce the number of iron deficiencies among young children.

Effects of Iron Deficiencies and Excesses

If the body's iron stores become depleted over time, and the food intake does not provide enough iron, an iron deficiency occurs. In this case, the body makes fewer red blood cells, and each cell contains less hemoglobin. The smaller number of red blood cells means the blood has a decreased ability to carry oxygen to body tissues. Symptoms of this condition include pale skin, fatigue, loss of appetite, and a tendency to feel cold. A person who has this condition has ***iron-deficiency anemia***. This is the most common type of anemia found worldwide.

Iron-deficiency anemia is common during the teen years, especially among females. One reason for this is iron needs increase during the teenage growth spurt. In addition, females are beginning their menstrual cycles and losing iron supplies that must be replaced. Females also tend to eat less than males and, therefore, have trouble getting enough iron in their diets.

The problem of low iron stores persists into adulthood for many women. In times of illness or pregnancy, the likelihood of an iron shortage increases. Doctors advise some women to take an iron supplement to help meet their daily needs.

Some people have an inherited disorder that causes them to absorb too much iron. This results in a condition called *iron overload*. The consequent buildup of iron is toxic and can damage the liver. Iron toxicity can also result from overdoses of iron supplements. This is a leading cause of accidental poisoning among children in the United States. Besides liver damage, iron toxicity can cause infections and bloody stools.

Zinc

Zinc is an amazing trace mineral that plays many important roles in the body. It is involved in most every physiological human function.

Functions of Zinc

Zinc serves a wide variety of functions. It aids in body growth and sexual development (**Figure 10.14**). It serves as a cofactor for many enzymes. A ***cofactor*** is a substance that acts with enzymes to increase enzyme activity. Zinc is also necessary for the successful healing of wounds and acid-base balance. It affects the body's storage and use of insulin. Zinc helps with the metabolism of protein and alcohol. Zinc also performs an important role in the body's resistance to infections.

Meeting Zinc Needs

Zinc is particularly important during periods of rapid growth and sexual development. The RDA for zinc is 9 milligrams per day for females ages 14 through 18.

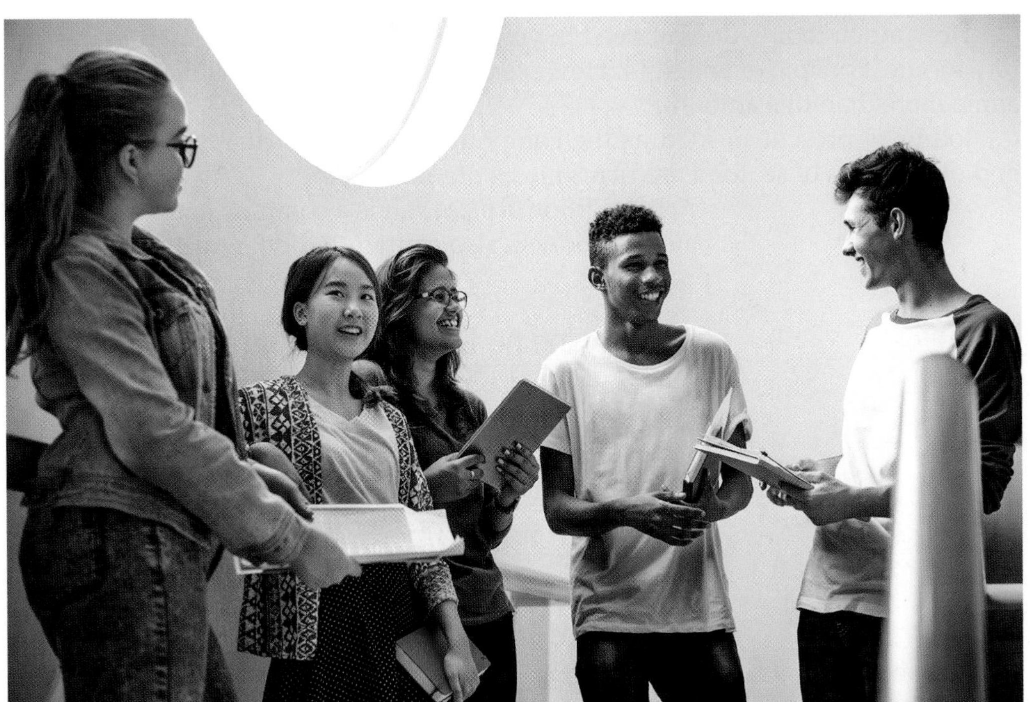

Rawpixel.com/Shutterstock.com

Figure 10.14
Zinc is especially important during the teen years and other periods of rapid growth.

The RDA is 8 milligrams per day for all females over age 19. The RDA for zinc for all males over age 14 is 11 milligrams per day.

A protein-rich diet, including seafood and red meats, is rich in zinc. Good plant sources include whole grains, legumes, and nuts.

Effects of Zinc Deficiencies and Excesses

A zinc deficiency will hinder a child's growth and sexual development. A number of other deficiency symptoms may appear. These include loss of appetite, reduced resistance to infections, and a decreased sense of taste and smell.

People are unlikely to get too much zinc from a nutritious diet. Excess zinc, resulting in toxicity, is most often due to the use of supplements. Zinc supplements are often used to reduce the symptoms of the common cold. There is no clear data to show they are effective. The danger is associated with excess, long-term use of zinc reducing the body's ability to absorb iron and copper. Large doses of zinc may impair the immune system and reduce good cholesterol (HDL) levels. Toxicity symptoms include diarrhea, nausea, vomiting, and impaired functioning of the immune system.

Iodine

The percentage of children with intellectual disabilities and growth delay is greater in countries where malnutrition is widespread. This is because women in these countries are often unable to obtain adequate sources of an essential mineral during pregnancy. This mineral is iodine.

Function of Iodine

Most of the iodine in your body is concentrated in one area: the thyroid gland. The thyroid produces a hormone called ***thyroxine***. This hormone helps control your body's metabolism. As part of thyroxine, iodine plays a role in metabolic functions.

Meeting Iodine Needs

How much iodine do you need in your diet? The RDA is 150 micrograms per day for most people over age 14. However, many people in the United States consume more than this amount.

Iodine is present in food as the compound iodide. Lobster, shrimp, oysters, and other types of seafood are rich sources of iodide.

In addition, *iodized* salt is a common source. Milk and bakery products also contain iodide, which is a result of processing.

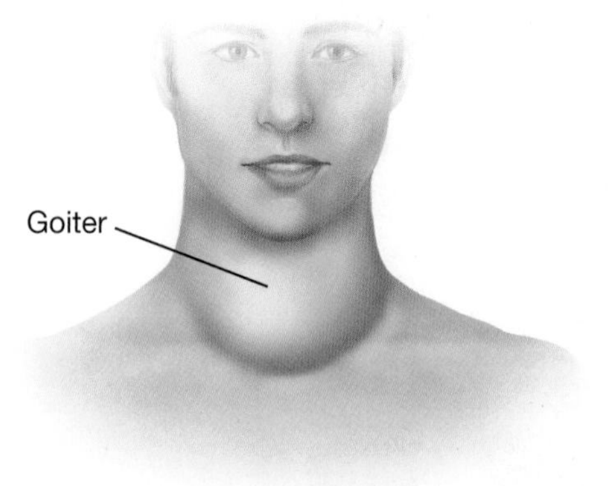

© Body Scientific International

Figure 10.15 Iodine deficiency can result in an enlargement of the thyroid gland called a *goiter*.

Effects of Iodine Deficiencies and Excesses

Iodine must be available for the thyroid gland to make thyroxine. When iodine levels are low, the thyroid gland works harder to produce the hormone. This causes an enlargement of the thyroid gland called a ***goiter*** (**Figure 10.15**). Other symptoms of iodine deficiency include weight gain and slowed mental and physical response.

Fortunately, iodine deficiency is less of a problem worldwide. Iodine is more commonly added to the salt people use. If a woman's diet is iodine-deficient during pregnancy, the development of the fetus may be impaired.

The child may have severe intellectual disabilities and impaired physical growth. This condition is called ***cretinism***.

A goiter is not only a symptom of iodine deficiency; it is also a symptom of iodine excess. Iodine is toxic in large amounts.

Fluoride

Fluoride is important for strong, healthy bones and teeth. Some scientists suggest it may help prevent the onset or decrease the severity of osteoporosis. Fluoride also helps prevent tooth decay. Children who drink fluoridated water have a much lower incidence of dental caries.

The AI for fluoride is three milligrams per day for all females over age 14. For males ages 14 through 18, the AI for fluoride is three milligrams. Adult males should consume four milligrams per day.

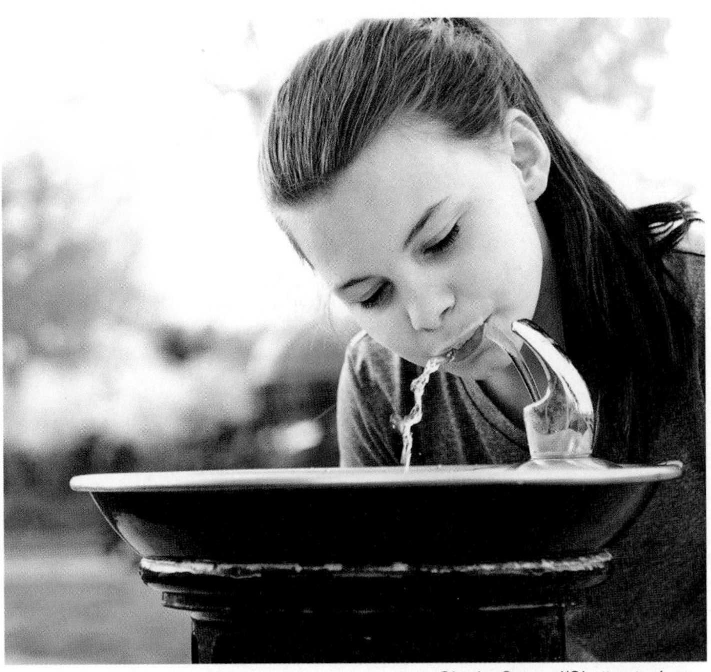

CharlesOstrand/Shutterstock.com

Figure 10.16 Fluoridated drinking water is a primary source of fluoride for many people in the United States.

Tea, seaweed, and seafood are the only significant food sources of fluoride. Fluoride occurs naturally in some water. Many communities add fluoride to their drinking water (**Figure 10.16**). In the United States, most people get fluoride from fluoridated water.

There is no evidence fluoridating water is harmful. A very high fluoride intake can cause teeth to develop a spotty discoloration called ***fluorosis***.

Selenium

Selenium works with vitamin E in an antioxidant capacity. It assists an enzyme that helps reduce damage to cell membranes due to exposure to oxygen. Antioxidants have been shown to play a role in the prevention of certain cancers. However, there is no clear evidence selenium will reduce the production of cancer cells.

The RDA for selenium is 55 micrograms daily for all males and females 14 years and older. Most teens in the United States have little trouble getting this amount.

Selenium is found in meats, eggs, fish, and shellfish. Grains and vegetables grown in selenium-rich soil are also good sources of the mineral.

A deficiency of selenium causes heart disease. Too much selenium is toxic, producing such symptoms as nausea, hair loss, and nerve damage.

Other Microminerals

Several other minerals have been identified as having important roles in the body. Each has varying and specific functions. Without them, health suffers. Many of the minerals are connected to energy metabolism and the body's ability to recover after expending great amounts of energy.

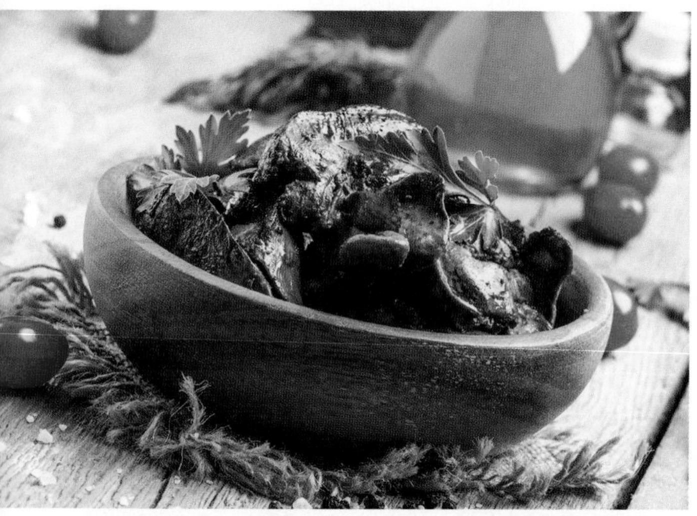

5PH/Shutterstock.com

Figure 10.17 Organ meats such as chicken liver are a rich source of copper.

Copper helps the body make hemoglobin and collagen. It also helps many enzymes work. The RDA for copper is 890 micrograms daily for all teens ages 14 through 18. Rich sources are organ meats, seafood, seeds, nuts, and beans (**Figure 10.17**). Deficiencies are uncommon but can result in anemia. Excesses can cause liver damage.

Chromium works with insulin in glucose metabolism. The AI for chromium is 35 micrograms daily for males ages 14 through 18. The AI is 24 micrograms daily for females in this age group. Chromium is found in meat, poultry, fish, and some cereals. Deficiencies lead to impaired glucose metabolism. Excesses can cause kidney failure.

Manganese helps many enzymes work. It plays a role in carbohydrate metabolism and in normal skeletal development. The AI for manganese is 2.2 milligrams for males ages 14 through 18 and 1.6 milligrams for females ages 14 through 18. Excesses of this mineral can be toxic.

Molybdenum is an essential part of several enzymes. The RDA for males and females ages 14 through 18 is 43 micrograms daily. Beans, whole grains, and nuts are good food sources. Excess molybdenum in the diet may affect the reproductive system.

FEATURED CAREER

Soil Scientist

Soil scientists study how soils help plants grow. They also study the responses of various soil types to fertilizers, tillage practices, and crop rotation. Many soil scientists conduct soil surveys, classifying and mapping soils. They provide information and recommendations to farmers and other landowners about the best use of land and plants to avoid or correct problems, such as erosion. They work to ensure environmental quality and effective land use.

Education

Most jobs in soil science require a bachelor's degree, but a master's or Ph.D. (doctoral) degree is usually required for university research positions. Soil scientists take courses including plant pathology, soil chemistry, entomology, plant physiology, and biochemistry. Some states require soil scientists to be licensed to practice.

Job Outlook

Job growth among soil scientists should be about as fast as average for all occupations. They also will be needed to balance increased agricultural output with protection and preservation of soil, water, and ecosystems.

Do not attempt to self-diagnose mineral deficiencies. If you have symptoms you suspect are due to a mineral deficiency, discuss them with a doctor. If he or she diagnoses a deficiency, a registered dietitian can help you evaluate your diet for good mineral sources.

Minerals and Healthful Food Choices

Information from this chapter can help you make healthful decisions about foods. You can put the facts you have read about minerals and their functions into practice at a personal level.

Mineral Values of Foods

The mineral content of plant foods depends on the soil, water, and fertilizers used to grow them (**Figure 10.18**). Thus, it is difficult to determine exactly how much of a mineral a given plant food will provide. Because animals eat plants, the mineral content of foods from animal sources is also hard to determine.

Most minerals in grains are located in the outer layers of the grain kernel. Most minerals in fruits and vegetables are located near the skin. Therefore, for maximum mineral value, choose whole grains and avoid peeling fruits and vegetables.

Generally, the most concentrated food sources of minerals are meat, fish, and poultry. Plant foods are rich in minerals; however, they provide a less concentrated source of minerals. People who eat no animal foods may be low in some minerals. They need to plan their diets to include mineral-rich foods of plant origin.

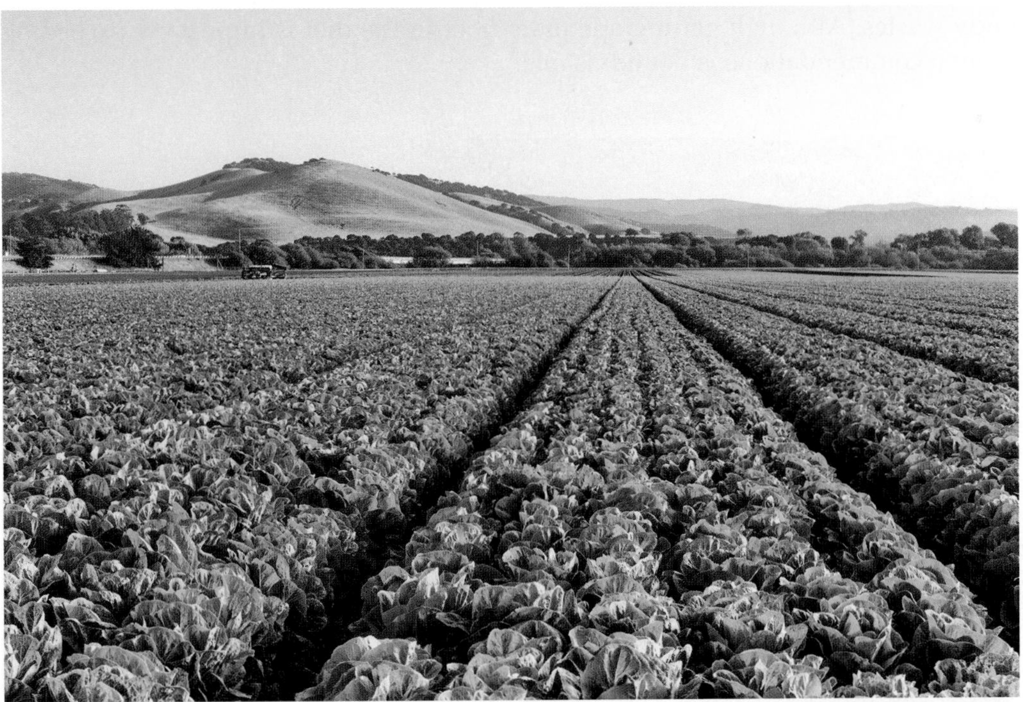

Ken Wolter/Shutterstock.com

Figure 10.18 The mineral content of soil will affect the mineral content of foods grown in it. *Do you think a farmer has a social responsibility to manage his or her soil wisely?*

Processing tends to decrease the mineral value of many foods. You are likely to find more minerals in whole foods than in processed foods. Fresh fruits and vegetables, whole grains, meat, poultry, and dairy products are rich sources of minerals. Fats, sugars, and refined flour are low in essential minerals.

Mineral Absorption and Availability

You take in minerals when you consume food and beverages. These minerals are absorbed into the bloodstream mostly through the small intestine. Your body does not absorb all the minerals you consume. In fact, most adults absorb less than half of the minerals they consume through food. Only the amounts of minerals your body absorbs are available to perform important functions. Unabsorbed minerals will be excreted with other body wastes.

Your body's ability to absorb many minerals increases with your need for those minerals. This is a lifesaving defense in times of starvation or illness. It also helps the body meet increased mineral demands, such as those that occur during growth spurts and pregnancy (**Figure 10.19**).

What can you do to maximize absorption of minerals needed for growth and regulation of body processes? You should learn what dietary factors decrease and increase the availability of minerals for absorption. Aside from being toxic, an excess of some minerals can interfere with the absorption of others. For instance, excess zinc can hinder the absorption of iron and copper. Absorption problems usually occur when people take supplements. Therefore, avoid taking mineral supplements unless a doctor or registered dietitian advises you to do so.

Fiber Affects Absorption

High-fiber diets can decrease absorption of some minerals, including iron, zinc, and magnesium. Fiber binds these minerals and the minerals are excreted with body wastes. Although getting adequate fiber in the diet is important, exceeding daily recommendations is not advisable.

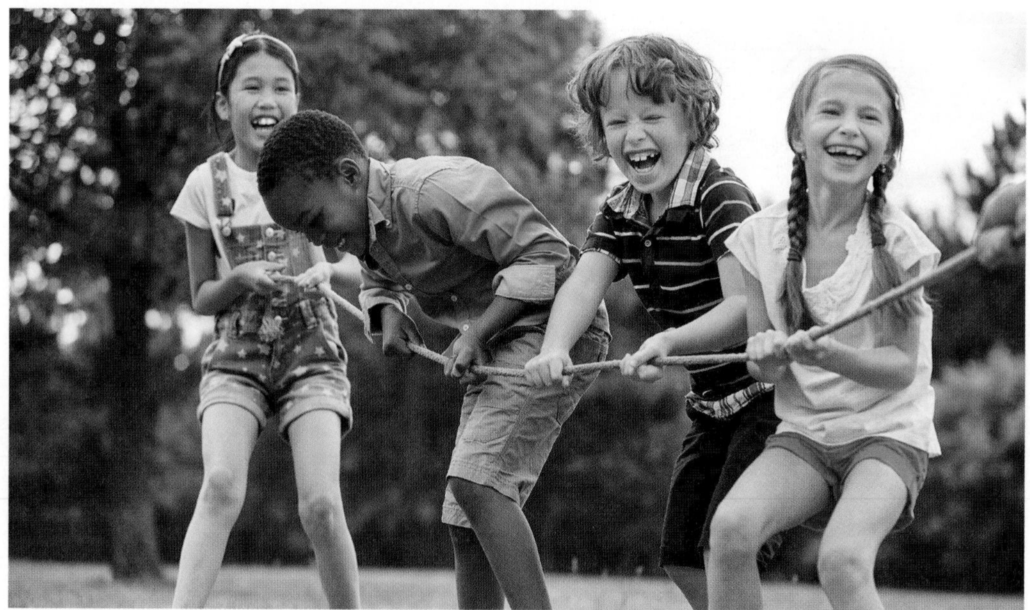

Robert Kneschke/Shutterstock.com

Figure 10.19 The body absorbs many nutrients very efficiently during the childhood years when growth is occurring rapidly.

Medications and Caffeine Affect Absorption

Some medications and caffeine can affect the availability of minerals in many complex ways. If you are taking prescription medication, ask your doctor about any effects they may have on mineral absorption.

Caffeine increases urinary output for some people depending on the amount, preparation method, and the individual's body mass and tolerance. Adolescents should avoid excess caffeine and energy drinks to eliminate unintended negative side effects.

Vitamins Affect Absorption

The presence of certain vitamins can promote the absorption of some minerals. For example, the presence of vitamin D improves calcium and phosphorus absorption. In addition, foods high in vitamin C increase iron absorption.

Conserving Minerals in Food During Cooking

Minerals are not as fragile as vitamins. Minerals are unaffected by heat or enzyme activity. However, minerals can be lost when foods are washed or cooked in liquid. Therefore, to preserve mineral content, avoid soaking foods when cleaning them. Also, cook foods using the smallest amount of water possible. Retain the minerals that have leached into cooking liquid by using it to make sauces, soups, and gravies.

RECIPE FILE

Asparagus and Blistered Cherry Tomato Pasta

6 SERVINGS

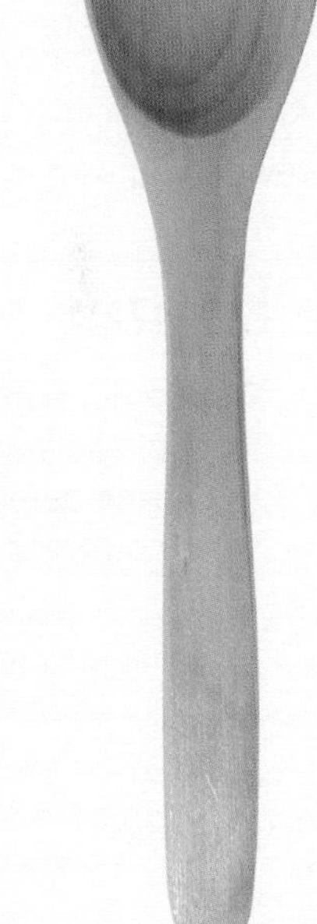

Ingredients

- 1 lb. whole-wheat pasta, penne or rotini
- 1 bunch fresh asparagus
- 1 T. olive oil
- 2 garlic cloves, minced
- 1 lb. cherry tomatoes, halved
- 1 c. reduced-fat Parmesan cheese, shredded

Directions

1. Fill a 5-quart pot with water and place over high heat.
2. Bring to a boil and add pasta. Cook pasta to al dente according to package directions, approximately 9 minutes.
3. Wash asparagus. Break off tough ends and discard. Cut the remaining asparagus stalks in half.
4. Sauté garlic in oil in a large skillet for about 30 seconds.
5. Add asparagus and sauté for about 6–7 minutes.
6. Add cherry tomatoes and sauté until they begin to blister, about 1 minute.
7. Drain pasta and add cooked pasta to the skillet.
8. Gently toss with parmesan cheese and serve.

PER SERVING: 313 CALORIES, 15 G PROTEIN, 49 G CARBOHYDRATE, 5 G FAT, 7 G FIBER, 248 MG SODIUM.

Chapter 10 Review and Expand

Reading Summary

Minerals are inorganic elements that can be divided into two classes. The macrominerals, or major minerals, include calcium, phosphorus, magnesium, sulfur, sodium, potassium, and chloride. The microminerals, or trace minerals, include iron, zinc, iodine, fluoride, selenium, copper, chromium, manganese, and molybdenum.

Although you need only small quantities of minerals, getting the right amounts is a key to good health. Without adequate intakes, deficiency symptoms can occur. At the same time, you need to avoid mineral excesses, which can be toxic.

Each mineral plays specific roles in the body. The vital functions of minerals include becoming part of body tissues. Many minerals help enzymes do their jobs. Some minerals help nerves work and muscles contract. Minerals also promote growth and control acid-base balance in the body. They help maintain fluid balance, too.

Minerals are widely found throughout the food supply. Selecting fresh and wholesome foods is preferred over the use of supplements. A health problem, such as osteoporosis, may require the use of a supplement. Choose a variety of plant and animal foods. Limit your use of highly processed foods. Eat the recommended daily amounts from each group in MyPlate. Following this basic nutrition advice should provide you with most of your mineral needs.

Chapter Vocabulary

1. **Content Terms** In teams, create categories for the following terms and classify as many of the terms as possible. Then, share your ideas with the remainder of the class.

acid	macromineral
base	micromineral
cofactor	mineral
cretinism	myoglobin
fluorosis	osmosis
goiter	osteoporosis
hemoglobin	pH
iron-deficiency anemia	thyroxine

2. **Academic Terms** With a partner, create a T-chart. Write each of the following vocabulary terms in the left column. Write a *synonym* (a word that has the same or similar meaning) for each term in the right column. Discuss your synonyms with the class.

hinder	provoke
liberate	transmit
negligible	

Review Learning

3. *True or false?* Because they are needed in larger amounts, macrominerals are more important for health than microminerals.
4. Where is nearly all the calcium in the body stored?
5. Which food group from MyPlate is the primary source of calcium?
6. Explain why women are at greater risk for developing osteoporosis than men.
7. What is the relationship of adequate phosphorus intake to good health?
8. What are five dietary sources of magnesium?
9. Where are high concentrations of sulfur found in the body?
10. What process helps equalize the fluid balance inside and outside of body cells?
11. What is the pH of a neutral substance, such as water?
12. What minerals are contributed by table salt?
13. What is the primary source of salt in the diet?
14. What organ is affected by potassium deficiencies and excesses?
15. What mineral is involved in carrying oxygen throughout the body?
16. Give two reasons why iron-deficiency anemia is common among teenage females.
17. What is the most likely cause of zinc toxicity?
18. Where is most of the iodine concentrated in the body?
19. What is the importance of fluoride in the body?
20. What is the main function of selenium?
21. Name two microminerals other than iron, zinc, iodine, fluoride, and selenium and give a function of each.
22. What are three factors that affect the mineral content of plant foods?
23. *True or false?* An excess of some minerals can interfere with the absorption of others.

Self-Assessment Quiz

Complete the self-assessment quiz online to help you practice and expand your knowledge and skills.

Critical Thinking

24. **Analyze** What evidence can you give to support eating whole, fresh foods rather than taking mineral supplements to obtain needed minerals?
25. **Evaluate** What human behaviors are detrimental to absorption of essential minerals?
26. **Apply** Write a one-day menu that meets the RDA for calcium for a friend who refuses to drink milk. Your friend is not lactose-intolerant and likes cheese and other dairy products.
27. **Recognize** Print a copy of the periodic table of elements. Circle the essential elements found in food and name a food source for each element that you circled.
28. **Apply** Using the information you learned in this chapter, make a list of actions you could take to improve the mineral content in your eating plan.
29. **Explain** Select one of the minerals discussed in this chapter. Research the health benefits associated with consumption of that mineral. Using the information from your research, write and produce a public service announcement (PSA) video promoting the benefits and sources of the mineral you selected.
30. **Analyze** What are the potential consequences to the health of consumers if farmland is not managed in a sustainable fashion?
31. **Conclude** The DASH (Dietary Approaches to Stop Hypertension) eating plan promotes foods that are good natural sources of potassium. Explain how increasing potassium in the diet might affect an individual's hypertension.

Core Skills

32. **Science** Use litmus paper to identify the pH of 10 food items and record your findings in a chart. Then investigate why eating acidic foods does not drastically affect the pH of your digestive tract. Share what you learn in a brief oral report.
33. **Math** The label on a can of tomatoes states the entire contents of the can contain 525 milligrams of sodium. The can contains 3½ servings of tomatoes. What percent of the AI for sodium does one serving of tomatoes contain?
34. **Speaking** Working in pairs, role-play a discussion between two people—one loves fruits and vegetables and the other does not. The fruit and vegetable lover must convince the other person of the importance of foods rich in minerals and vitamins to good health. Provide evidence to support your argument.
35. **Math** Keep a one-day food journal of all the food and beverages you consume. Include amounts of any salt added to your food at the table. Use food labels, Appendix C, or the USDA nutrient database online to determine the total milligrams of sodium consumed. The *Dietary Guidelines* recommendation is not to exceed 2,300 milligrams of sodium in one day. Calculate your intake as a percent of the recommended maximum intake of 2,300 milligrams.
36. **Reading and Writing** Read about the discovery of iodine. Who discovered it? Was that person searching for an essential mineral when he or she discovered iodine? Develop a time line showing who, when, where, and how iodine was identified as an essential mineral. Include the time line in a short paper sharing your findings. Cite your sources.
37. **Science** Use a reliable anatomy and physiology resource to investigate the urinary system's role in regulating fluid-electrolyte balance in humans. Write a brief summary describing the role of the various system organs.
38. **Speaking** Plant foods are a low source of essential minerals compared to animal sources. In a presentation, make a case supporting technological advances that will increase bioavailability of minerals in plants.
39. **Career Readiness Practice** Presume you are a dietitian. Your interpersonal skills—your ability to listen, speak, and empathize—are great assets when working with clients. Lilly is your latest client. She was recently diagnosed with osteoporosis. She is 75 years old. In addition to the medicine her doctor prescribed, Lilly was instructed to seek nutrition counseling about ways to increase the calcium in her diet. What calcium-rich foods would you recommend to Lilly? How much should she have daily?

Water

Learning Outcomes

After studying this chapter, you will be able to

- **identify** four main functions of water in the body;
- **differentiate** between the two levels of fluid balance in the body;
- **summarize** the effects of fluid imbalance on the body; and
- **compare** tap water with bottled and fortified waters.

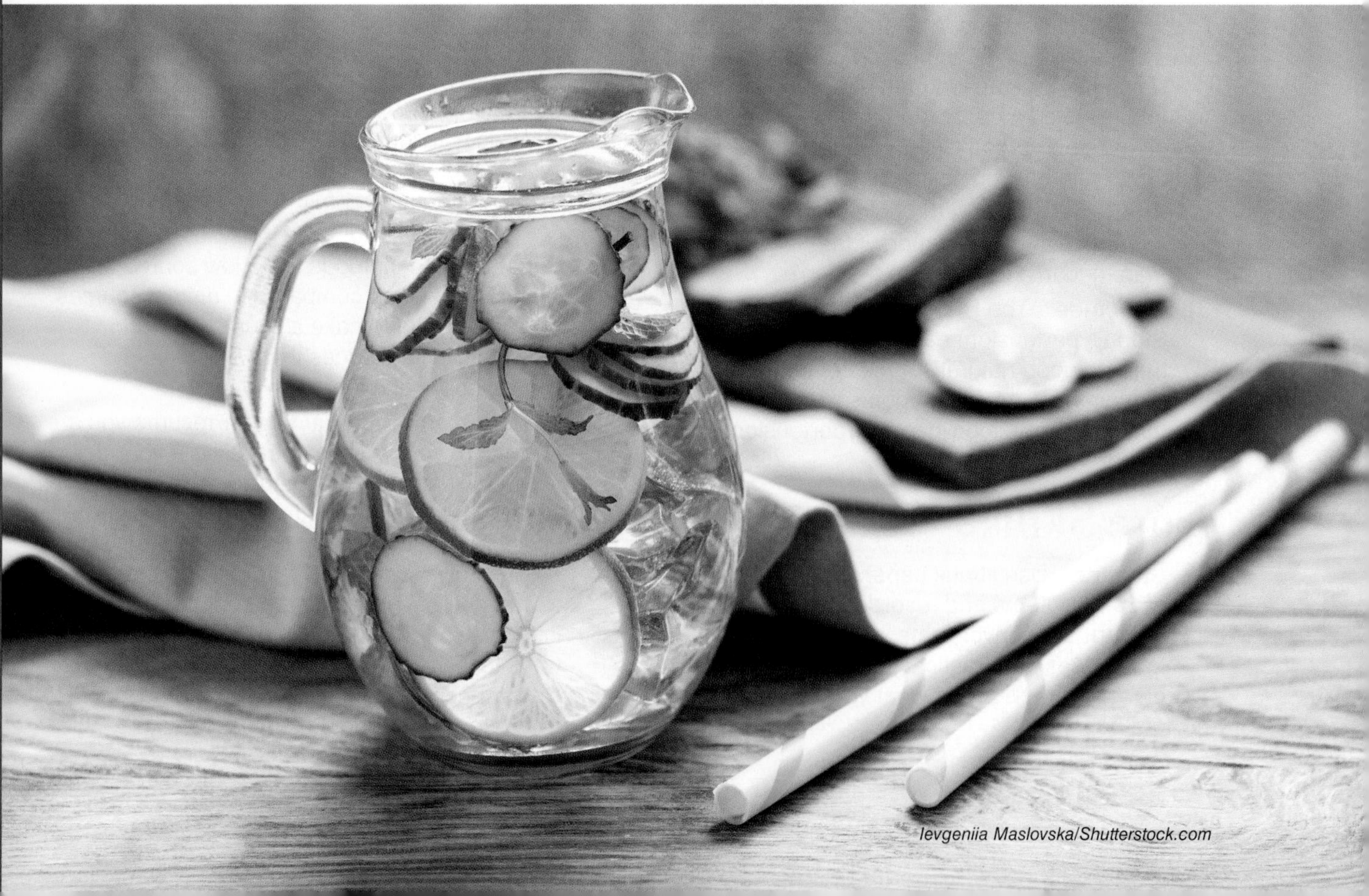

Ievgeniia Maslovska/Shutterstock.com

Content Terms 

dehydration
diuretic
enhanced water
extracellular water
intracellular water
lubricant
reactant
solvent
water intoxication

Academic Terms 

constrict
dissipate
rupture
stationary
viscous

What's Your Nutrition and Wellness IQ?

Take this quiz to examine how much you already know about water. If you cannot answer a question, pay extra attention to that topic as you study this chapter.

- Identify each statement as *True*, *False*, or *It Depends*. *It Depends* means in some cases the statement is true; in some cases it could be false.
- Revise false statements to make them true.
- Explain the circumstances in which each *It Depends* statement is true and when it is false.

Nutrition and Wellness IQ 

	Statement			
1.	The amount of water a person needs each day can vary.	True	False	It Depends
2.	Water is found in some—but not all—of the body's cells.	True	False	It Depends
3.	Hydration is important to help regulate body temperature.	True	False	It Depends
4.	Intracellular water flows out of cells to achieve cellular water balance.	True	False	It Depends
5.	During vigorous exercise, the body loses water to regulate body temperature.	True	False	It Depends
6.	The greater the loss of body fluids, the greater the number of electrolytes lost.	True	False	It Depends
7.	Sports drinks are the best fluid choice for all athletes.	True	False	It Depends
8.	The foods you eat help meet the body's need for fluids.	True	False	It Depends

While studying this chapter, look for the activity icon  **to**

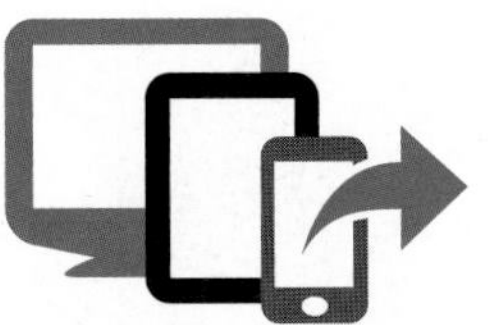

- **build** vocabulary with e-flash cards and interactive games;
- **assess** what you learn by completing self-assessment quizzes and completing review questions; and
- **expand** knowledge with interactive activities and activities that extend learning.

www.g-wlearning.com/foodsandnutrition/

Carbohydrates, fats, proteins, vitamins, minerals, and water are the six major nutrients you need for survival. Of these, water is the one that is most often overlooked. This is odd considering you could make a good argument for viewing water as the most critical nutrient.

Water is an essential nutrient that must be replaced every day. Depending on your state of health, you may be able to survive 8 to 10 weeks without food. Without water, however, you can survive only a few days. This chapter will highlight the vital role water plays in promoting health and wellness.

The Vital Functions of Water

Water is in every cell in the body. In fact, the presence of water determines the shape, size, and firmness of cells.

For most adults, body weight is about 50 to 75 percent water, or roughly 10 to 12 gallons (38 to 46 L). Fat tissue is about 20 to 35 percent water, whereas muscle tissue is about 75 percent water. Therefore, the total percentage of body weight from water depends on the ratio of fat to lean body tissue. This ratio varies from person to person. People who have a higher percentage of lean tissue have a higher percentage of water weight. Men typically have a higher percentage of lean tissue and, therefore, more water weight than women. Young people usually have a higher percentage of lean tissue and water weight than older people.

Body fluids include saliva, blood, lymph, digestive juices, urine, and perspiration. Water is the main component in each of these fluids. Your diet must include adequate amounts of water to allow your body to form enough fluids. Otherwise, body fluids will not be able to perform their functions normally. For example, in the absence of sufficient water intake, you will be unable to produce enough sweat to cool your body. A buildup of heat in the body can cause such symptoms as headache, nausea, dizziness, and loss of consciousness. If body temperature is not reduced, death can result (**Figure 11.1**).

Water performs a number of functions in the body. It helps chemical reactions take place. It carries nutrients to and waste products from cells throughout the body. Water is the substance that reduces friction between surfaces. It also controls body temperature.

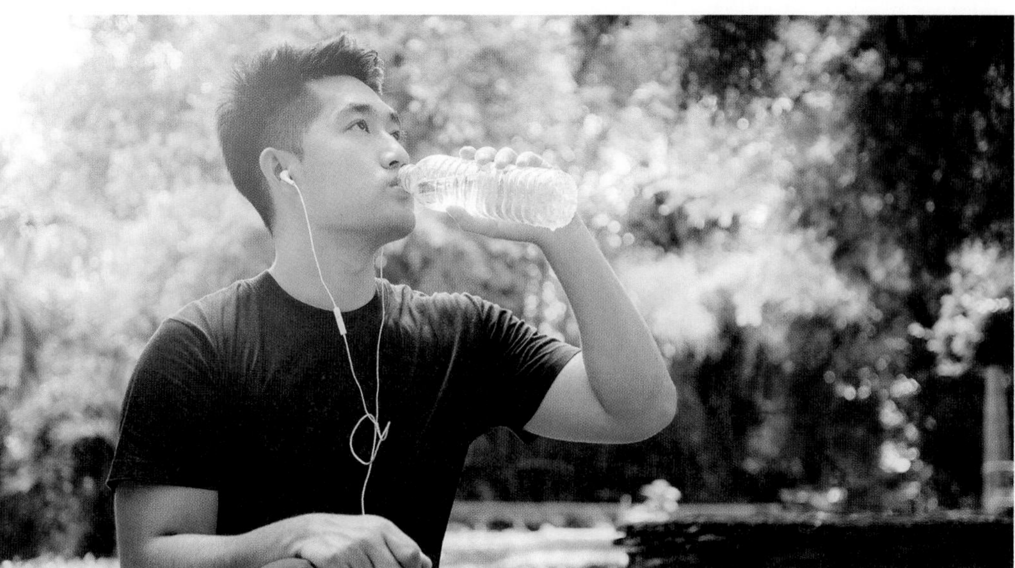

Figure 11.1
Much more than a thirst quencher—water is a vital nutrient.

TM_SALE/Shutterstock.com

Facilitates Chemical Reactions

Most chemical reactions in the body require the presence of water. This includes the reactions involved in breaking down carbohydrates, fats, and proteins for energy. It also includes reactions that result in the formation of new compounds, such as the creation of nonessential amino acids. Water seems to help some enzymes perform their functions. It also dilutes concentrated substances in the body.

Water is a reactant in many chemical reactions in the body. A ***reactant*** is a substance that enters into a chemical reaction, and is changed as a result. For example, digestion and energy production require water to break down starches into glucose. Remember that starch is a chain of glucose molecules bonded together. Water splits the bonds in the starch chain. The elements of the water molecules are hydrogen and oxygen. These elements become part of the separate glucose molecules (**Figure 11.2**).

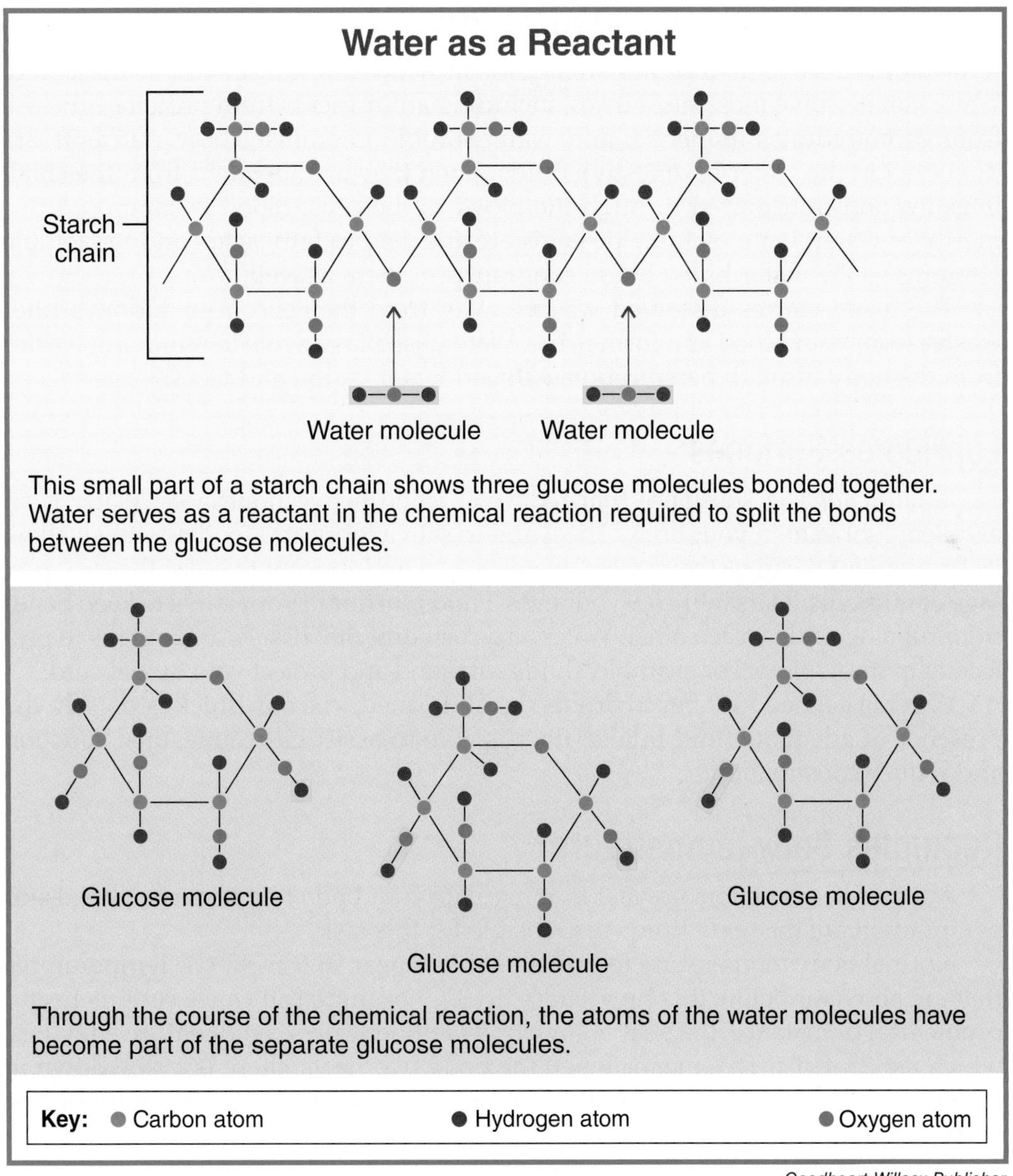

Water as a Reactant
Starch chain
Water molecule
Water molecule
This small part of a starch chain shows three glucose molecules bonded together. Water serves as a reactant in the chemical reaction required to split the bonds between the glucose molecules.
Glucose molecule
Glucose molecule
Glucose molecule
Through the course of the chemical reaction, the atoms of the water molecules have become part of the separate glucose molecules.
Key: Carbon atom
Hydrogen atom
Oxygen atom

Goodheart-Willcox Publisher

Figure 11.2 The water molecules (highlighted in yellow) react with the starch chain to break it into smaller units. *How does water's role as a reactant affect the digestive process?*

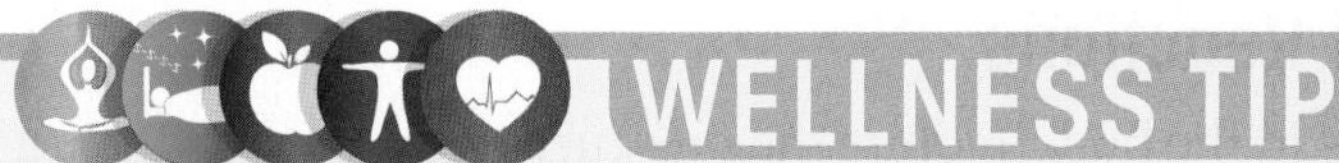

Emergency Preparedness

The Federal Emergency Management Agency (FEMA) program called "Do 1 Thing" encourages individuals, families, businesses, and communities to be prepared for emergencies and become disaster resilient. One easy "thing" you can do to prepare for an emergency is to stock and store three days' worth of drinking water in your home. This water should be a sufficient amount to cover household needs. Plan about one gallon of water per person per day to address household needs. Be sure to rotate your water supply about every six months to ensure water is fresh and drinkable.

Transports Nutrients and Waste Products

Water is a solvent. ***Solvents*** are liquids in which substances can be dissolved. Water can dissolve most substances, including amino acids from proteins, glucose from carbohydrates, minerals, and water-soluble vitamins. These nutrients are dissolved in the water of digestive fluids. Then they are absorbed from the small intestine and transported through the blood to the cells. Blood is composed primarily of water. Water-soluble proteins are attached to fatty acids and fat-soluble vitamins so the water-based blood can transport them as well.

The blood carries dissolved wastes away from the cells. Your kidneys filter wastes from your blood and form urine. Water also plays a role in removing wastes from the body through perspiration, exhaled water vapor, and feces.

Lubricates Surfaces

A ***lubricant*** is a substance that reduces friction between surfaces. Water is an excellent lubricant in your body. The water in saliva lubricates food as you swallow it. Throughout the digestive system, water acts like a lubricant to assist the easy passage of nutrients. Tears lubricate your eyes. Fluids surround your joints to keep bones from rubbing against each other. Water also cushions vital tissues and organs to protect them from injury. For example, fluids surround and protect your spinal cord.

Water is needed for fiber to produce well-formed, **viscous** (thick) stools. In the presence of adequate fluid intake, fiber is able to assist gastrointestinal function and reduce constipation.

Regulates Body Temperature

Another key function of water is to regulate your body temperature. Blood and perspiration are the body fluids responsible for this task.

Normal body temperature for most people is near 98.6°F (37°C). Temperatures that are above or below this by 5°F (2°C to 3°C) or more can cause serious health problems. For instance, the heat of high body temperatures can denature enzymes, which are proteins. This means when the body overheats, there is a slowdown in the chemical reactions promoted by enzymes in the body. Extremely high or low body temperatures can result in death.

Imagine you are riding a **stationary** (not movable) bicycle. Although you are using only your leg muscles, your entire body becomes hot. This is because blood distributes body heat. Your body uses this distribution system to regulate body temperature.

As blood flows near the surface of your skin, your body releases heat into the air. When you become warm, the blood vessels near your skin surface dilate. This happens when you are exercising or have a fever. The expanded blood vessels allow blood to flow more slowly and nearer the skin surface, causing heat to be lost.

At the same time, your sweat glands begin producing perspiration. The perspiration transmits heat from your body through pores in your skin surface. The evaporation of water in perspiration helps cool your body (**Figure 11.3**). The slowed evaporation of perspiration is what causes you to feel uncomfortable when the humidity level is high.

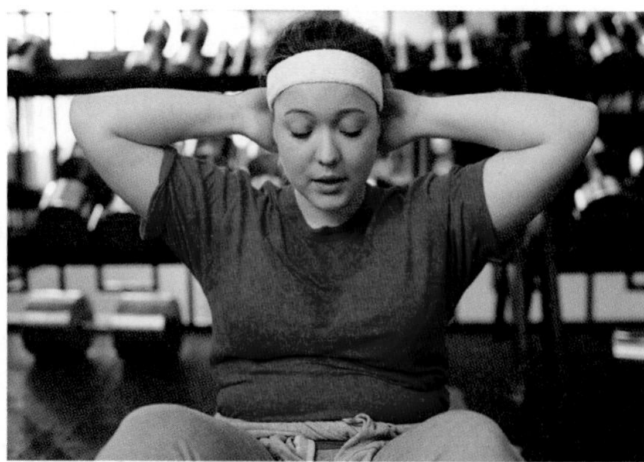

Pressmaster/Shutterstock.com

Figure 11.3 Perspiring during exercise helps reduce body temperature.

FOOD AND THE ENVIRONMENT

Practice Water Conservation as You Garden

Backyard gardens are a great source of fresh, tasty, nutrient-rich vegetables, but vegetables need water to grow. Unfortunately, gardeners cannot control when and how much it rains. Sometimes rainfall alone is not sufficient to maintain a healthy garden.

Many vegetables require about an inch of water per week. This water may come from the dew, rainfall, or from the water that you collect. To water a four-foot by eight-foot garden with one inch of water would require approximately 20 gallons of water.

Since water is such an important and valuable resource, it is important to use it responsibly. What can be done to reduce waste while watering plants? For example, when plants are established, it is better to water heavily once or twice a week rather than watering lightly every day.

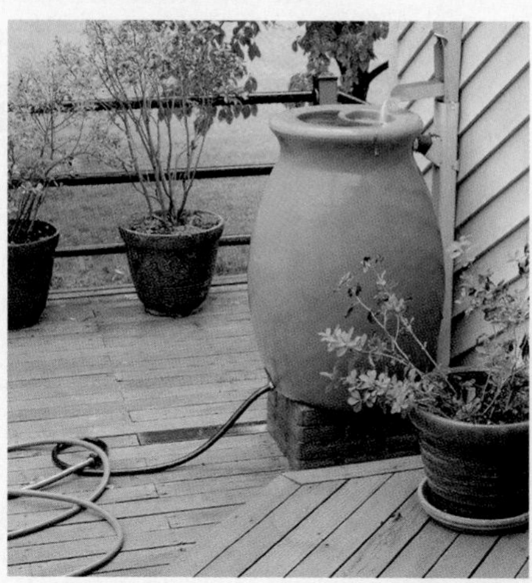

JuneJ/Shutterstock.com

Other ways you can help to conserve water while producing a thriving garden include the following:

- Add mulch to reduce evaporation
- Learn how to make and use compost to hold moisture and add nutrients
- Water plants during the morning or early evening when it is cooler
- Water when there is little or no wind
- Shape the area around the plant to slow down water runoff
- Use a drip or soaker hose
- Collect rainwater in containers, such as barrels, and use it to water your garden

Contact your local county extension agent from the Cooperative Extension office for more advice about growing vegetables and water use—the resource is free!

Think Critically

1. Why is it important to practice water conservation?
2. Can you think of other ways to conserve water and grow your garden?

When your body temperature drops, your body takes steps to conserve heat. It **constricts** (shrinks) the blood vessels near the surface of your skin. This restricts the amount of blood flowing near the surface of your skin, so less heat is lost.

Keeping Water in Balance

You can think of water balance at two levels. At the cellular level, there needs to be a balance between the water inside cells and the water outside cells. At another level, the body requires a balance between water intake and water loss.

Cellular Water Balance

Cells are like balloons that maintain their shapes. As with balloons, cells do not have an infinite ability to expand. If too much water flows into a cell, it could **rupture** (burst). Conversely, if a cell does not contain enough water, it could collapse. However, the body has mechanisms that keep the balance of water inside and outside the cells constant. These mechanisms prevent cells from bursting or collapsing.

There are two categories of water in the body. ***Intracellular water*** is the water inside the cells. ***Extracellular water*** is the water outside the cells. Water can move freely across cell membranes. The concentration of sodium, potassium, and chloride particles inside and outside the cells determines the movement of water. Health experts call these minerals *electrolytes*.

Water Intake

Thirst is the body's first signal that it needs water. Therefore, if you feel thirsty you should drink liquids. Thirst goes away automatically when you consume liquids. Deciding how much to drink is a lifestyle choice you can make that affects your state of wellness.

How Much Water?

If you are like most people, you need to increase your fluid intake. The Adequate Intake (AI) of fluid for females and males ages 14 to 18 is 2.3 liters and 3.3 liters. This represents about 2½ to 3½ quarts of fluids per day to replace lost body fluids. Your fluid needs are met through the liquids you drink and the foods you eat. To remain fully hydrated, about 9 to 13 cups per day should come from water and the other beverages you drink. Water is your best source for hydration. A small amount of water is produced in the body as a by-product of nutrient metabolism.

The color of your urine will help you determine if you are drinking enough water. Urine that is dark yellow indicates it is highly concentrated with wastes. This is stressful to your kidneys. When fluid intake is too low, the kidneys must work harder to eliminate wastes. Light-colored urine shows you are drinking enough to keep wastes flushed out of your body. Drinking plenty of water while you are young may lessen your chances of kidney problems in later years.

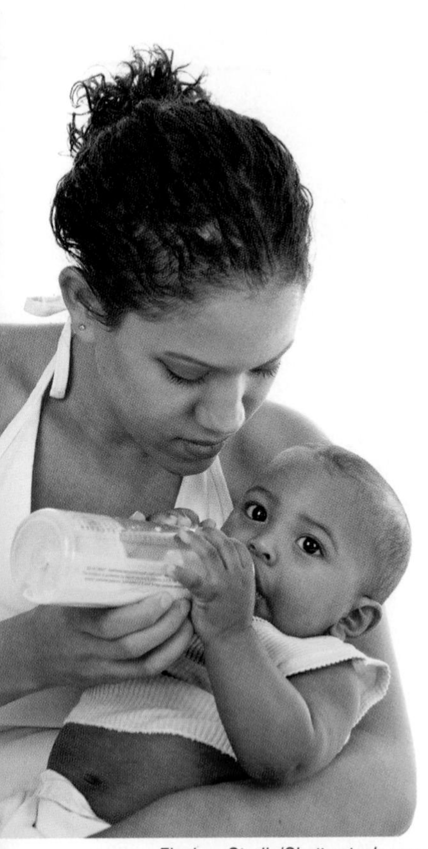

Flashon Studio/Shutterstock.com

Figure 11.4 Breast milk or infant formula normally supplies enough water to replace an infant's fluid losses.

Needs Across the Life Span

Some groups of people have above-average needs for water. An infant's immature kidneys are not as efficient as an adult's kidneys at filtering waste from the bloodstream. Therefore, infants excrete proportionately more water than adults to rid their bodies of waste. This increases their fluid needs (**Figure 11.4**).

Other groups who have above-average water needs include older adults, who lose some of their water-conserving abilities. Pregnant women need extra liquids because they have an increased volume of body fluids to support their developing babies. Lactating women need fluids to produce breast milk. People on high-protein diets require extra water to rid their bodies of the waste products of protein metabolism. A buildup of these waste products can cause kidney damage.

Older adults have the same need for fluids as young adults. The thirst mechanism of older adults can change and fluid intake can be affected. Some older adults choose to limit water intake if they have urinary incontinence problems. This requires medical treatment to avoid dehydration. Adequate fluid intake is necessary for continued good health through older adulthood.

Supplying the Body's Water Needs

Drinking liquids generally supplies the greatest amount of fluids. Of course, plain water is a pure source of this vital nutrient. However, milk, juices, broth, tea, and other liquids also have high water content.

You may be surprised to learn foods supply almost as much of your daily water needs as liquids. Most foods contain some water. Some foods are higher in water content than beverages. As an example, summer squash is 96 percent water, whereas orange juice is only 87 percent water. Even foods that look solid are a source of water. For instance, bread is 36 percent water. Butter and margarine contain water, but cooking oils and meat fats do not (**Figure 11.5**).

Metabolism meets roughly 12 percent of your water needs. The breakdown of carbohydrates, fats, and proteins in the body releases water. Your body can then use this water in other chemical reactions.

Your sources of water replacement may vary greatly from day to day. When you eat many water-loaded fruits and vegetables, you may not drink as much liquid. When you eat dry foods, you are likely to consume more liquids.

Water Loss

Water loss, referred to as water output, occurs naturally as you carry on regular activities throughout the day. On average, you lose about two to three quarts of fluid each day.

There are several paths by which water leaves the body. Most body fluids are lost through urine. Your kidneys regulate the amount of urine lost. Kidneys can retain some water, but they must also produce urine to rid the body of wastes.

Water Content of Common Foods

Food	Percent Water Content*
Lettuce	96
Salsa	92
Fat-free milk	91
Carrots, raw	90
Orange juice	87
Tomato soup	85
Potato	80
Egg	75
Milk shake	74
Tuna, water pack	74
Pasta, cooked	66
Apple	65
Chicken breast, roasted, skinless	65
Cantaloupe	57
Ground beef, lean	53
Pizza	48
Whole-wheat bread	38
Cheddar cheese	37
Butter	16
Chocolate chip cookie, homemade	6
Jelly beans	6
Cornflakes	3
Peanut butter	1
White sugar	<1
Corn oil	0

*percent of total weight

Figure 11.5 Approximately 20 percent of your fluid needs are provided by the foods you eat. *Can you think of other foods that have high water content?*

The volume of your urine varies with the amount of water you drink. If you produce less than 2½ cups (625 mL) of urine per day, the urine will be concentrated with waste products. This increases the risk of kidney stones. *Kidney stones* are hard particles of mineral deposits that form in the kidneys. They can cause tremendous pain when they pass from the kidneys to the bladder and out of the body. A healthy urine output is one to two quarts per day or more.

You lose body water through three routes other than urine: through your skin as you sweat, in your breath as you breathe, and small losses through bowel wastes.

A number of factors can affect water losses. Environmental conditions, level of physical activity, medications, and health status influence amount of water loss and replacement needs. Being aware of these factors can help you determine your fluid replacement needs.

Weather Conditions and Altitude

Hot and humid weather, as well as warm work or living environments can cause larger losses through sweating. Dry climates increase water losses through quick skin evaporation (**Figure 11.6**). Such climates include the atmosphere on airplanes and in buildings when heating systems are operating. The low oxygen pressure at high altitudes increases water losses for people not used to these altitudes. For example, people living in mile-high areas breathe harder to draw more oxygen into their bodies. They have a greater output of water vapor and must pay careful attention to the need for fluid replacement. When the weather is hot, you should make an effort to increase your fluid intake.

Physical Activity

Physical activity causes increased water loss. The body's energy production takes place in the fluid environment of the blood and muscles. The release of chemical energy generates much heat. Sweat **dissipates** (loses) the heat to avoid dangerous increases in body temperature. Most fluid is lost through sweat. The more energy you expend, the more you sweat, and the more water you need. Vigorous physical activity can cause the loss of a quart of water in an hour. Long-distance runners, such as marathon runners, can lose up to 13 pounds of water weight during a 26-mile race. To help maintain the body's fluid balance, athletes should plan to consume adequate liquids before, during, and after competition.

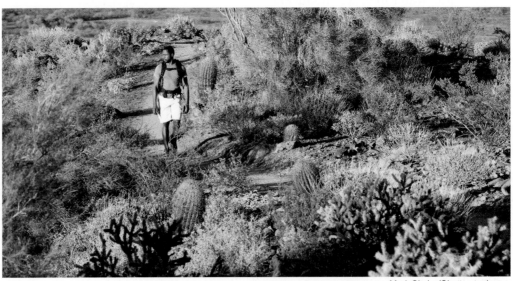

Mark Skainy/Shutterstock.com

Figure 11.6 Dry climates contribute to increased water loss because perspiration evaporates from the skin rapidly.

CASE STUDY

Losing the Hydration Game

Taryn is a 15-year-old girl who lives in Denver, Colorado—also known as the "Mile High City." Taryn loves to spend many hours playing basketball outside in the summer months. It is hot, sunny, and dry in the summer. There is a water fountain in a building near the basketball court, but she does not bother to take the time to drink. Her friends tell her to bring a water bottle with her. She usually forgets the water and thinks it is not that important anyway. Sometimes she remembers on her way to the game and buys a can of soda from a vending machine.

Taryn is often disappointed with her game. She finds that she runs out of energy by mid-game and often gets a headache. She wants to improve so that she can make the high school team next year.

Case Review

1. What do you think is contributing to Taryn's disappointing performance on the basketball court?
2. Why do you think Taryn believes that water is not important?

Use of Diuretics

Using diuretics promotes water losses. ***Diuretics*** are substances that increase urine production. Doctors often prescribe diuretics for patients with high blood pressure or body fluid imbalances. Alcohol and energy drinks act as diuretics, too. For this reason, you need to use care when choosing liquids to replace body fluids. Coffee or soft drinks that contain caffeine may not be the best options for fluid replacement. Liquids such as water, mineral water, or diluted fruit juices may be better choices for restoring fluid losses. Distilled water has natural minerals removed and is not recommended to replace plain water.

Illness

Vomiting, diarrhea, bleeding, and high fever are all conditions that can cause fluid losses. Tissue damage caused by burns also affects the body's fluid balance. The more severe these conditions are, the greater the water losses will be. Medical supervision and treatment may be necessary to correct these water losses.

During illness, you may not always feel thirsty; drinking plenty of liquid, however, is important to replace increased water losses. Consuming fluids also helps flush the products of drug metabolism from your body.

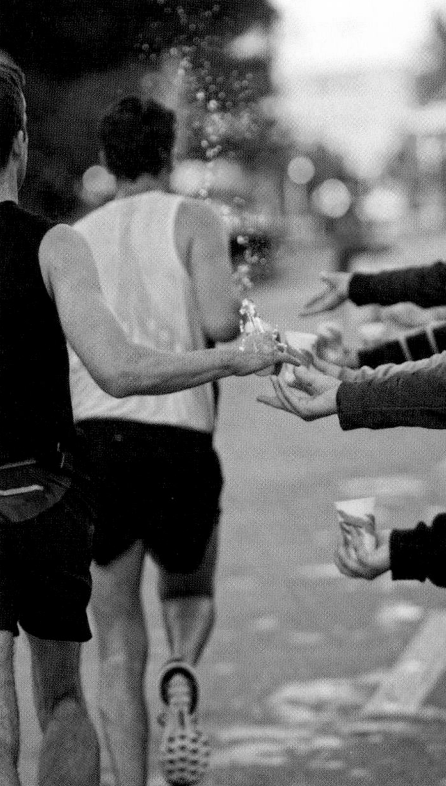

Daniel Korzeniewski/Shutterstock.com

Figure 11.7 Long-distance runners often train themselves to drink by schedule rather than by thirst.

Fluid Imbalance

The thirst mechanism is not always a reliable indicator of fluid needs. During hot weather or heavy exercise, the body may lose a fair amount of fluid before signaling thirst (**Figure 11.7**). When the body either loses or takes in too much water, fluid imbalances result.

THE MOVEMENT CONNECTION

A Fluid Spine

Why

Water requires daily replacement in our bodies due to the many ways we lose it, such as through sweating, urinating, and even breathing. Water is responsible for facilitating chemical reactions, transporting nutrients and waste, lubricating surfaces, and regulating body temperature. A whole chain of events in our bodies cannot take place when we are dehydrated. Just as a chain has many links, your spine has many small vertebrae. Your spine acts as a pillar, protecting and supporting your spinal cord.

The following stretch helps warm up your spine and keep it fluid.

Apply

- Stay seated in your chair with both feet on the floor and good posture.
- Place your hands on your knees or the tops of your thighs.
- As you inhale, arch your spine, rolling shoulders back and down.
- As you exhale, round your spine and drop your chin to your chest and bring your shoulders and head forward.

Repeat 10 times.

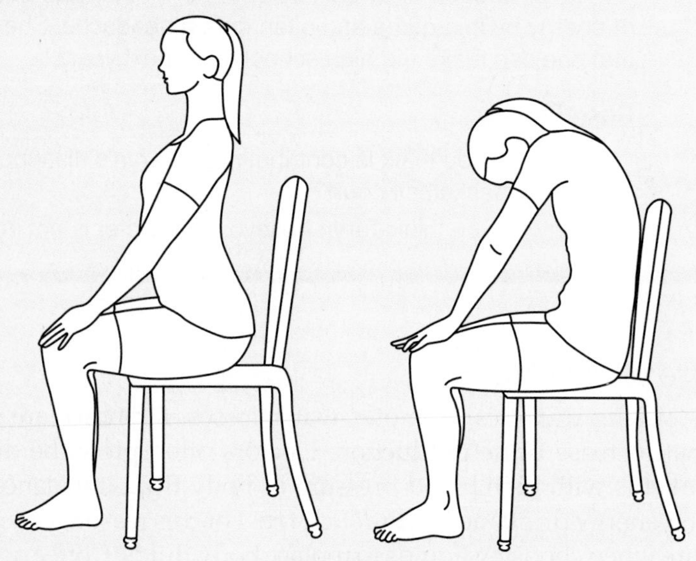

Effects of Water Loss

Because fluids make up a high percentage of your body weight, when you lose water, you also lose weight. Someone who wants to drop a few pounds may think this is good news. The weight you want to lose is fat, however, not water. Water weight is quickly regained when you replenish body fluids.

Even a small percentage of weight dropped due to water loss will make you feel uncomfortable. When you lose two percent of body weight in fluids, you will become aware of the sensation of thirst. Both the brain and the stomach play a role in making you aware there is a water imbalance. If you do not replace water losses, you may become dehydrated. ***Dehydration*** is a condition resulting from excessive loss of body fluids.

When dehydration occurs, the body takes steps to help conserve water. Hormones signal the kidneys to decrease urine output. Sweat production also declines. As the volume of fluid in the bloodstream drops, the concentration of sodium in the blood increases. The kidneys respond to the higher blood sodium level by retaining more water. These water-conserving efforts cannot prevent all fluid losses from the body. If fluids are not replaced, the damaging effects of dehydration will begin to take their toll.

Some older adults do not always recognize the thirst sensation. In cases such as these, it is important not to wait for the thirst signal to begin consuming liquids. Older adults may need to make a point of drinking even when they do not feel thirsty.

Replacing lost water is important for peak athletic performance. Athletic performance levels decline after a 3 percent loss in water weight. When water is lost from working muscles, blood volume decreases. The heart must pump harder to supply the same amount of energy. Mental concentration is affected as fluid losses increase. Some clear signs of dehydration are fatigue and lack of energy. Other symptoms may include dizziness, headache, muscle cramping, and reduced muscle endurance. A 10- to 11-percent drop in body weight due to water losses can result in serious organ malfunctions.

Can You Drink Too Much Water?

You may wonder if it is possible to drink too much water. The answer is yes. The result is a rare condition called ***water intoxication***. Water intoxication is caused by drinking too much water and consuming too few electrolytes.

Athletes who sweat heavily can experience water intoxication. After heavy excessive sweating, dehydration problems can occur. As a result, an imbalance of blood-sodium concentration occurs because body fluids are depleted. Sodium is lost with fluid perspiration losses. Sodium must be replaced to maintain an electrolyte balance. If the athlete drinks only plain water, the electrolytes are not replaced. If electrolyte levels stay low, early symptoms of water intoxication, such as headache and muscle weakness, may appear. Water intoxication can cause death when electrolyte imbalance is severe.

In some cases, there can be a psychological disorder of drinking excessive amounts of water on a daily basis. This can also cause a type of water intoxication. The electrolytes become imbalanced because gallons of water are consumed rapidly.

The greatest danger of water intoxication is when infants are given plain water after experiencing vomiting, diarrhea, or both. Diarrhea and vomiting pull electrolytes as well as water from the body. When fluid losses are excessive, electrolytes and fluids must be replaced. Electrolyte imbalance can happen to people of all ages. However, infants are at greater risk. They can lose body fluids more easily than people in other age groups.

FEATURED CAREER

Hydrologist

Hydrologists often specialize in either underground water or surface water. They examine the form and intensity of precipitation, its rate of infiltration into the soil, its movement through the earth, and its return to the ocean and atmosphere. Hydrologists use sophisticated techniques and instruments to monitor the change in regional and global water cycles. Some surface-water hydrologists use sensitive stream-measuring devices to assess flow rates and water quality.

Education

A bachelor's degree is adequate for a few entry-level positions. However, most hydrologists need a master's degree for most research positions in private industry and government agencies, and a PhD is typically required for advanced research and university positions.

Job Outlook

Employment growth for hydrologists is expected to be about as fast as the average for all occupations. Spurring this demand is the need for environmental protection and responsible water management.

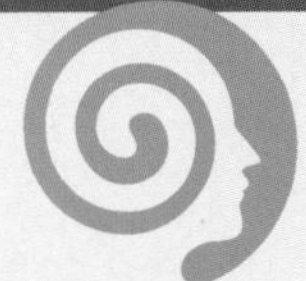

EXTEND YOUR KNOWLEDGE

The Cost of Hydration

Make a list of drinks commonly enjoyed by teens, such as bottled water, carbonated drinks, sports drinks, powdered drink mixed with water, fruit juices, and energy drinks. Gather information on the cost per gallon of the listed drinks. Use your family water bill to calculate the cost per gallon your family pays for tap water. Organize your findings in a table. Rank order the drinks by cost per gallon from most costly to least costly. Which drinks are most economical for hydration purposes?

Better Water?

In recent decades, sales of bottled and enhanced waters have increased dramatically. The cost of these waters can be several hundred times higher than the cost of tap water (**Figure 11.8**).

Bottled Water Versus Tap Water

Why do people buy bottled water? The reasons vary. Some think bottled water contains miracle minerals that promote health. Research does not confirm this. Others want the convenience of carrying bottled water when they are traveling or at work. For added convenience, they choose to buy disposable water bottles rather than a safe, reusable bottle.

Many people claim bottled water tastes better than local water supplies. Dissolved minerals give water its taste. Depending on where you live, the water from the tap might taste of iron deposits, sulfur, or other minerals. People who object to such mineral tastes might buy bottled water even though tap water is safe and clean.

Some bottled-water drinkers are concerned tap water contains contaminants. Purity of tap water depends on the area in which you live. Public drinking water is treated to meet federal health standards. Water from a private well is more likely to contain microorganisms. People who are concerned about the safety of their water can have it tested for the presence of contaminants.

Water sold in bottles is not always safer, cleaner, or purer than tap water. In fact, bottled water comes from the same sources as water from the faucet. Bottled water sold across state lines must meet the FDA federal standards for purity. Check the label for the "IBWA" trademark. This organization supports the FDA regulations for purity and sanitation. Not all states enforce bottled water sanitation rules.

For most people, fluoridated community water systems are the chief source of fluoride—an element that prevents tooth decay. Because most bottled waters have little or no fluoride, people who replace part or all of their drinking water with bottled water may be at greater risk for tooth decay.

Some people choose to use filtration systems to treat their tap water at home. These systems vary in cost and require upkeep or filter replacement from time to time. They also vary in terms of what they filter from the water. Some systems remove certain harmful contaminants. Some systems remove fluoride. Others may do little more than make water taste better.

Enhanced Water

Bottled sports, health, and energy drinks are a fast-growing industry. These beverages known as ***enhanced waters*** contain added ingredients such as artificial flavors, sugar, sweeteners, vitamins, minerals, amino acids, caffeine, and other "enhancers."

Cost of Tap Water Versus Bottled Water

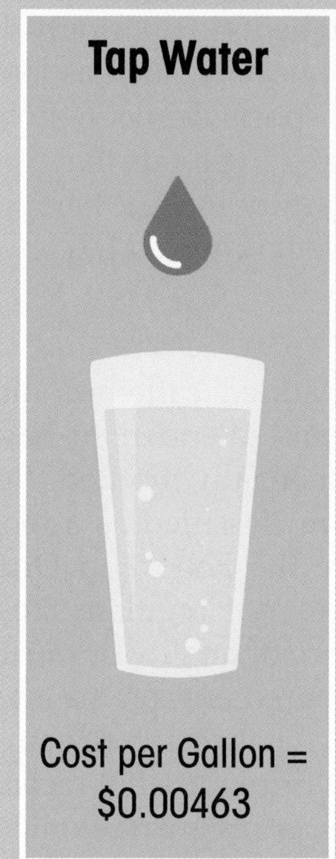
Tap Water
Cost per Gallon =
$0.00463

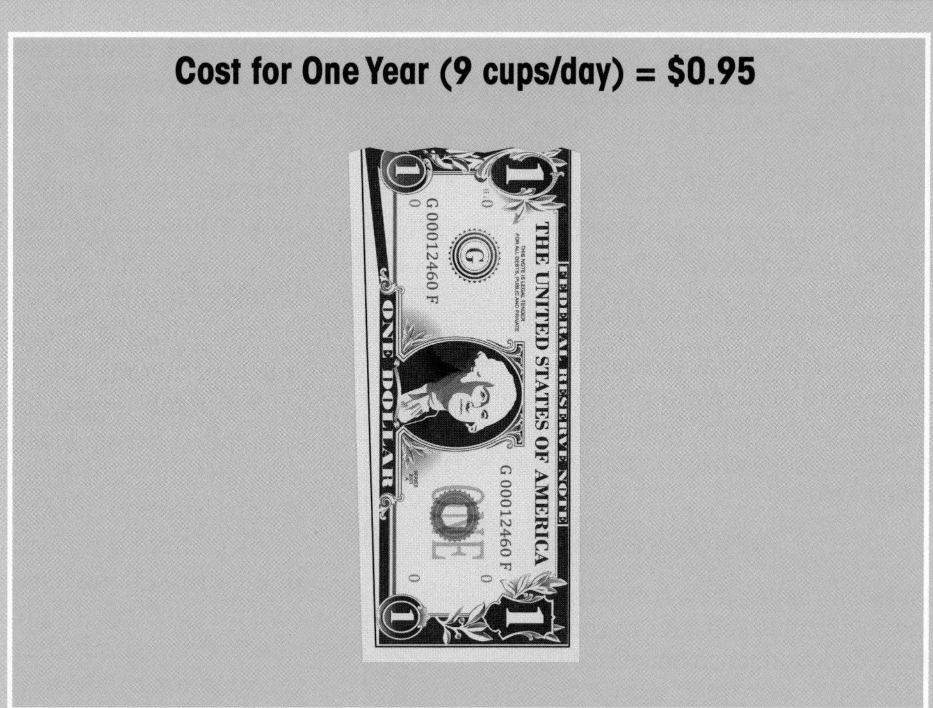

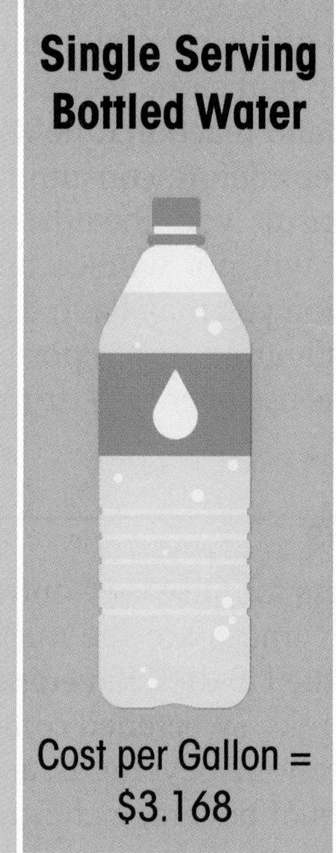
Single Serving
Bottled Water
Cost per Gallon =
$3.168

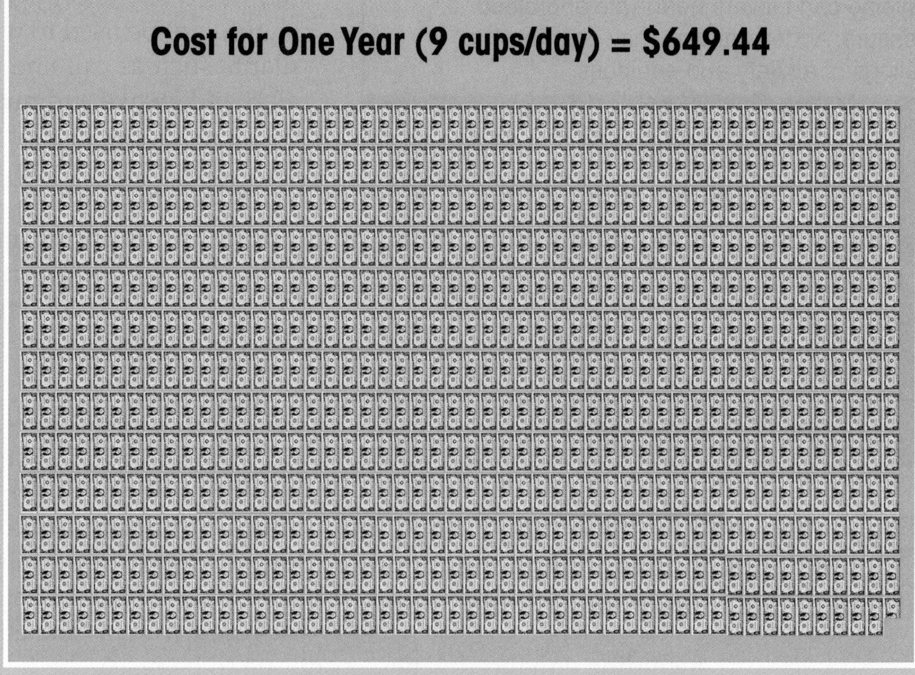

Water glass and bottle: OnD/Shutterstock.com; Dollar: mart/Shutterstock.com

Figure 11.8 The difference in cost between tap water and bottled water is significant. *How much do you spend on bottled water each year?*

Considering a Performance-Enhancing Drink? Check It Out...

✔ Type of Sugar

Added sugars may slow absorption of the water. Look for a combination of sucrose and glucose, which are easily digested and absorbed quickly.

✔ Amount of Sugar

Lower sugar concentration is easier to digest. Look for 6% or less (14 g or less sugar/8 oz. of water).

✔ Amount of Added Salt

Higher sodium content (100–200 mg sodium/8 oz. of water) for endurance athletes.

✔ Added Vitamins and Minerals

No research finds that energy levels or physical performance are improved by sports drinks with added vitamins and minerals. A daily vitamin may be more economical than vitamins supplied in bottled water.

✔ Added Protein

Drinks with added protein may cause an upset digestive system and have not been proven to add health or performance benefits.

✔ Added Caffeine

Caffeine can elevate heart rate and blood pressure. Added caffeine may contribute to feelings of anxiety and edginess.

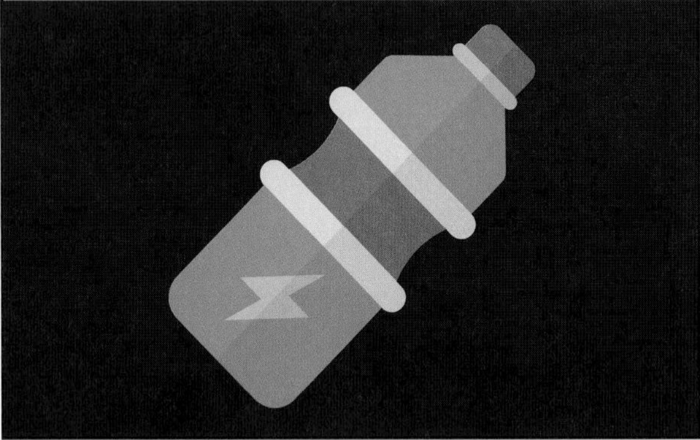

Bottle: jiunn/Shutterstock.com

Figure 11.9 Make sure you understand how the ingredients in an enhanced water may affect your body before you consume it.

Sports Drinks

A *sports drink* is a beverage with added electrolytes and sweeteners intended to improve and sustain energy. There are many types of sports drinks available on the market. Sports drinks may be high in added sugar and calories. The costs of these drinks vary and contents can be confusing. Sports drinks, used for fluid replacement, are recommended to be used sparingly. In cases where athletes sweat heavily, such as long sports events or hot days, sports drinks may be helpful. Most often, simply eating foods that contain salt, such as pretzels, salty energy bars, or tomato juice may be sufficient (**Figure 11.9**).

Energy Drinks

Energy drinks contain added caffeine, vitamins, or herbal supplements intended to have a stimulant effect. Commercially bottled fluids, called *energy drinks*, are classified as a food supplement, and therefore the Food and Drug Administration (FDA) does not regulate these drinks. There is no assurance of quality or purity of the drink. Long lists of ingredients on the label can mean there is greater chance for negative effects on the body. Energy drinks are not recommended for children, teens, or pregnant women.

The FDA cautions consumers that products marketed as "energy shots" or "energy drinks" should not be used to ward off sleep. While stimulants such as caffeine may make one feel more alert and awake, judgment and reaction time will be impaired by lack of sleep. Before consuming one of these products, consult your healthcare provider to ensure its use will not worsen any underlying medical condition you may have. The FDA is interested in investigating any reported adverse effects related to the use of energy drinks and supplements.

Sources of Added Sugars

According to the Centers for Disease Control and Prevention (CDC), beverages are the major source of added sugars in the US diet. Beverages include soft drinks, fruit drinks, sweetened coffee and tea, energy drinks, alcoholic beverages, and flavored waters. The effects of beverage choices, including enhanced waters, continue to be researched; however, excessive intake of added sugars is known to increase health risk outcomes.

When selecting a beverage to hydrate your body, read the label to determine if the ingredients will be harmful or helpful and then consider water.

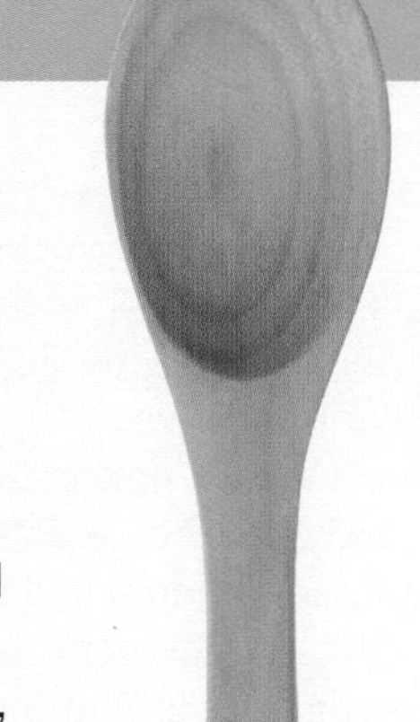

RECIPE FILE

Tortilla Turkey Meatball Soup

6 SERVINGS

Ingredients

- 2 large red bell peppers
- 6 garlic cloves, minced
- ¼ c. + 1 T. plain whole-grain bread crumbs
- 1 lb. ground turkey breast
- 2 egg whites
- 1 chipotle chile, canned in adobo sauce, minced
- 1 T. olive oil
- 2 c. chopped onion
- 2 c. red or white potato, 1-inch cubes
- 1 c. carrots, sliced ½-inch thick
- 5 c. low-sodium chicken broth
- 2 ears corn on the cob, husk and silk removed, each cob sliced into 3 equal pieces
- 4 each corn tortillas (6-inch diameter), cut into ½-inch wide strips
- cooking spray as needed
- ¾ c. low-fat, extra-sharp cheddar cheese, shredded
- ½ c. fresh cilantro, chopped

Directions

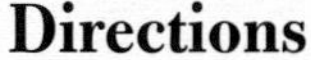

Peel Peppers

1. Place red bell peppers on the grate over a stovetop burner set on medium. When skin begins to char, turn with tongs. Continue until all the skin has been charred.
2. Place peppers in a paper bag and fold 2–3 times to close, or place in a sealed airtight container. Let stand for 15 minutes.
3. After 15 minutes, remove peppers from bag and chop. Set aside.

Meatballs

4. Place one garlic clove, bread crumbs, ground turkey, egg whites, and chipotle chile in a large bowl and mix to combine.
5. Shape mixture into about 40 tablespoon-size meatballs. Wet your hands if the mixture becomes too sticky to handle.
6. Heat olive oil in a 5-quart stockpot over medium-high heat.
7. Add meatballs to pot and sauté for 7 minutes, browning well on all sides. Remove from pan and set aside.

Soup

8. Add onion, potato, and carrots to the pot and sauté for 5 minutes.
9. Add remaining 5 garlic cloves and corn. Sauté for 1 minute.
10. Add peppers and broth and bring to a boil. Reduce heat and simmer for 20 minutes, or until vegetables are tender.
11. Add meatballs and cook 10 more minutes, or until meatballs are done.

Tortilla Strips

12. Cut tortillas into ¼-inch strips.
13. Place tortilla strips in a single layer on a baking sheet lined with foil and sprayed with cooking spray.
14. Broil for 3 minutes, or until golden brown.

Serve

15. Ladle 1½ cups soup into each bowl. Make sure each bowl has one piece of corn on the cob.
16. Top each serving with one tablespoon cheddar cheese, two teaspoons cilantro, and tortilla strips.

PER SERVING: 381 CALORIES, 34 G PROTEIN, 46 G CARBOHYDRATE, 8 G FAT, 6 G FIBER, 283 MG SODIUM.

Chapter 11 Review and Expand

Reading Summary

Water is a vital nutrient you must replace daily. It is in every cell in your body and is the main component in all body fluids. Water makes up over half of your body weight.

Water performs a number of functions in the body. It plays a role in chemical reactions. It transports nutrients to cells and carries wastes away from cells. Water acts as a lubricant and helps regulate your body temperature.

The fluids in your body need to remain in balance. There needs to be a balance between intracellular and extracellular water. There also needs to be a balance between your total water input and output. You receive water through the liquids you drink and the foods you eat. You also get water as a byproduct of metabolism. You lose body fluids through urine, sweat, vapor in your breath, and bowel wastes. Hot weather, warm environments, dry climates, high altitudes, and use of diuretics can all increase water losses. Illnesses and exercise increase water losses too.

When you do not replace water losses, you can become dehydrated. Greater levels of fluid loss can cause a decrease in physical performance and a lack of mental concentration. An excessive drop in body fluids can result in serious organ malfunctions.

Bottled and enhanced waters are more expensive options for hydration than tap water. People buy bottled water for a variety of reasons including convenience, taste, and purity. However, bottled waters are not always safer or more pure than tap water. Enhanced waters have specific nutrients or supplements added that are intended to improve health or performance. Research is not yet clear on the benefit or harm from these fortified fluids. Reading food labels will help identify amounts of added sugars and other ingredients in bottled water.

Chapter Vocabulary

1. **Content Terms** On a separate sheet of paper, list words that relate to each of the following terms. Then, work with a partner to explain how these words are related.

   dehydration
   diuretic
   enhanced water
   extracellular water
   intracellular water
   lubricant
   reactant
   solvent
   water intoxication

2. **Academic Terms** Individually or with a partner, create a T-chart on a sheet of paper and list each of the following terms in the left column. In the right column, list an *antonym* (a word of opposite meaning) for each term in the left column.

   constrict
   dissipate
   rupture
   stationary
   viscous

Review Learning

3. Name five body fluids composed mainly of water.
4. How does water's function as a solvent play a role in human nutrition?
5. How does water help the body release excess heat?
6. What three minerals control cellular fluid balance?
7. Name three groups of people who have increased fluid needs.
8. Name three foods that are more than 50 percent water.
9. List four factors that affect body water loss.
10. How does physical exercise increase water losses?
11. Describe the steps the body takes when it needs to conserve water.
12. *True or false?* Sports drinks are recommended to be used sparingly.

Self-Assessment Quiz

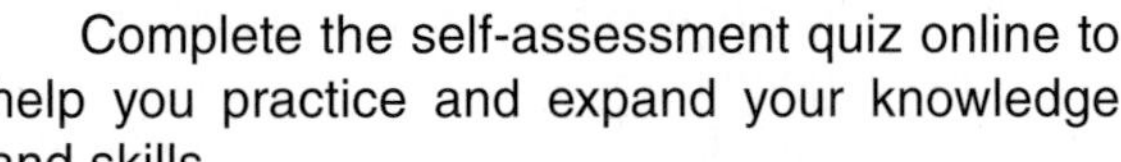

Complete the self-assessment quiz online to help you practice and expand your knowledge and skills.

Critical Thinking

13. **Evaluate** Suppose you have a friend who decides to go on a weight-loss diet and is delighted to have lost two pounds in a day. You know this weight loss is likely due to water loss. What evidence can you give your friend to show that restricting food and fluids can negatively influence health?

14. **Compare** With advertisers' push for bottled and fortified waters, people may be confused about what choices to make for good health. Compare tap water to bottled and fortified waters. Form an opinion about which drink is the best choice.
15. **Evaluate** For one day, avoid all beverages except water. Evaluate your satisfaction with water as your primary source of fluids. Include your personal evaluation in a written report on the advantages and disadvantages of choosing only water as a beverage.
16. **Create** Working in small groups, evaluate how the media influences people's choice of beverage for hydration. Prepare a public service announcement (PSA) to combat the media's influence and promote the merits of drinking tap water.
17. **Plan** Suppose you are planning a 10-day hiking trip in the Grand Canyon. Because you will be carrying all your supplies in a backpack, you will not be able to bring sufficient drinking water for the entire trip. Use reliable sources to make a plan for meeting your water needs during your trip. Determine how much water you will need and how you will source it. Make sure to consider the environment and the level of physical activity as you determine your needs. What sources of water are available to you in the Grand Canyon? Is it potable? What will you need to do to produce safe drinking water? Write a brief paper describing your plan.

Core Skills

18. **Listening** Interview a sports coach to learn what advice coaches give athletes regarding fluid intake before, during, and after a game or competition. Prepare for the interview by developing a list of questions to help you better understand the topic. These questions will also encourage the exchange of information. If you are unclear about any answers, be sure to seek further explanation. Prepare a brief critique of the interview. Consider what aspects of the interview went well and how you could improve your interview skills for the future.
19. **Technology Literacy** Research online to understand how the body regulates the need for water. Create an electronic presentation to share the process with classmates. Use diagrams to show which body systems are involved in the thirst response. Make strategic use of audio, visual, or other elements to add interest to your presentation and enhance understanding.
20. **Research** Learn what your state is doing about source water protection. Use the Internet to find your state's source water protection website. How does your state maintain the purity of tap water? Then check out the EPA website to learn more about what individuals can do to protect the quality of their drinking water. Share your findings with your class members.
21. **Math** Use Internet resources to learn the percent body weight that water comprises for a baby, a teen male or female, an obese male or female, a person over age 80, and a competitive athlete. Prepare a bar graph using spreadsheet software to display the results.
22. **Math** Design a blind taste test comparing a variety of waters such as tap, bottled, and mineral water. Create a rating system and have class members rate the taste of each water type. Calculate and report the results of your taste test.
23. **Speaking** The Great Lakes represent 18 percent of the fresh surface water on the planet. Research the Great Lakes Basin Compact to learn the purpose of the compact. Prepare a speech to share your findings with the class.
24. **Science and Technology Literacy** Plan and write three entries for a blog that promotes safe drinking water. The blog should highlight the importance of drinking water to health, threats to drinking water, and what we can do to protect it. First, consider the audience who will be reading your blog. What does your audience want and need to know about this topic? Then, determine the content and how you will organize it. Select three main points that you want to address each day. Next, create an appealing title to capture your reader's attention. Write each blog entry, providing supporting facts for each main point. Consider providing a tip or action item for each entry.
25. **Career Readiness Practice** As a teacher and wrestling coach, you are keenly aware of the importance of water to health and wellness. It has come to your attention that a number of athletes are limiting their water intake as they prepare for competition. Several wrestlers on the team became extremely dehydrated and sick during the last meet. You decide to e-mail a reminder to the athletes and their parents about the need for proper hydration. Draft a message about the importance of proper hydration before, during, and after a meet.

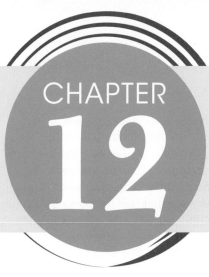

CHAPTER 12 Energy Balance

Learning Outcomes

After studying this chapter, you will be able to

- **explain** how the amount of energy in food is measured;
- **calculate** the three components of your energy expenditure;
- **identify** the outcomes of energy deficiency and excess;
- **differentiate** between body weight and body composition; and
- **use** various tools to assess healthy weight.

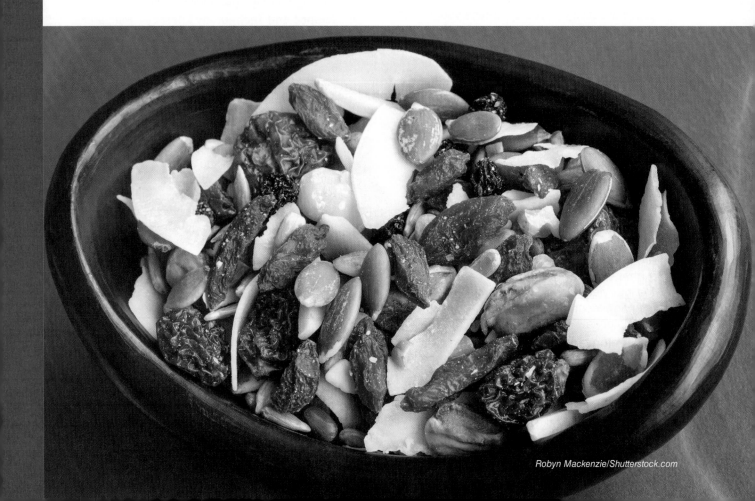

Robyn Mackenzie/Shutterstock.com

Content Terms

basal metabolic rate (BMR)
basal metabolism
bioelectrical impedance
body composition
body mass index (BMI)
calorie density
energy
healthy body weight
ketone bodies
ketosis
obese
overweight
resting metabolic rate (RMR)
sedentary activity
skinfold test
subcutaneous fat
thermic effect of food (TEF)
underweight

Academic Terms

apparatus
atrophy
buoyant
depress
fluctuation
longevity

What's Your Nutrition and Wellness IQ?

Take this quiz to examine how much you already know about balancing energy. If you cannot answer a question, pay extra attention to that topic as you study this chapter.

- Identify each statement as *True*, *False*, or *It Depends*. *It Depends* means in some cases the statement is true; in some cases it could be false.
- Revise false statements to make them true.
- Explain the circumstances in which each *It Depends* statement is true and when it is false.

Nutrition and Wellness IQ 

Statement			
1. Energy output is the same for sedentary and active teens.	True	False	It Depends
2. The inability to balance energy is related to obesity problems at any life stage.	True	False	It Depends
3. The amount of energy found in carbohydrates, fats, and proteins is the same.	True	False	It Depends
4. A person's basal metabolic rate is the same throughout life and cannot be changed.	True	False	It Depends
5. The body mass index (BMI) is a reliable tool for measuring body fat for all ages, shapes, and levels of fitness.	True	False	It Depends
6. The greater the amount of physical activity a person does, the larger the needs for energy intake.	True	False	It Depends
7. Age has no effect on basal metabolic rate.	True	False	It Depends
8. Belly fat appears naturally as people age.	True	False	It Depends

While studying this chapter, look for the activity icon 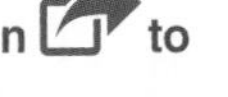 to

- **build** vocabulary with e-flash cards and interactive games;
- **assess** what you learn by completing self-assessment quizzes and completing review questions; and
- **expand** knowledge with interactive activities and activities that extend learning.

www.g-wlearning.com/foodsandnutrition/

Your body is using energy as you sit and read this page. ***Energy*** is the ability to do work. There are many different forms of energy. You cannot create or destroy energy; however, you can change or transfer energy from one form to another. When you eat, you take in chemical energy stored in food. Your body spends this energy when you move, to fuel body processes, and even to process the food itself. Through various activities, your body also generates heat, which is another form of energy.

Understanding energy balance is the key to weight management. Balancing energy requires consuming an amount of energy from food that is equal to the amount of energy you are using, or

Energy in = Energy out

The energy in foods is measured in units called *calories*. Therefore, the energy balance equation can also be expressed in calories (**Figure 12.1**). When energy in and energy out are in balance over time, body weight does not change.

Balancing energy does not need to be complicated. This chapter will help you understand the relationships between calorie intake, use of energy, and weight gain or loss.

Energy Intake

One side of the energy balance equation includes the foods and drinks you consume. Three nutrient groups provide food energy—carbohydrates, fats, and proteins. (Although alcohol provides calories, it is not considered a nutrient. Alcohol is a drug.) For most people in the United States, approximately 43 to 58 percent of daily calories comes from carbohydrates. About 30 to 45 percent comes from fats, and about 12 percent comes from proteins. The metabolism of these nutrients is the source of chemical energy in your body.

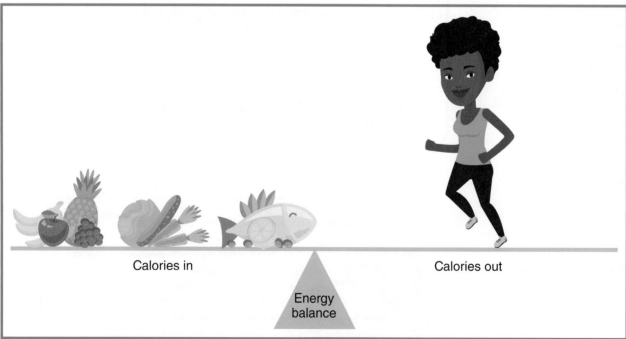

Food: wowomnom/Shutterstock.com; Person: Visual Generation/Shutterstock.com

Figure 12.1 The energy balance equation can also be expressed in calories. ***Is the person depicted in this illustration in energy balance?***

Measuring Energy in Food

Did you ever wonder how people know how many calories are in a spoonful of sugar? Researchers have determined the energy value of foods by burning them and measuring the amount of heat they produce. This technique for measuring energy is called *direct calorimetry* because it measures the heat produced directly by the food. To take this measurement, a piece of food is first precisely weighed. Then it is placed in a closed, insulated device called a *bomb calorimeter*. A container holding a kilogram of water surrounds the chamber holding the food. After the food is burned completely, the change in water temperature is precisely measured. Each degree of increase on a Celsius thermometer equals one calorie of energy given off by the food (**Figure 12.2**).

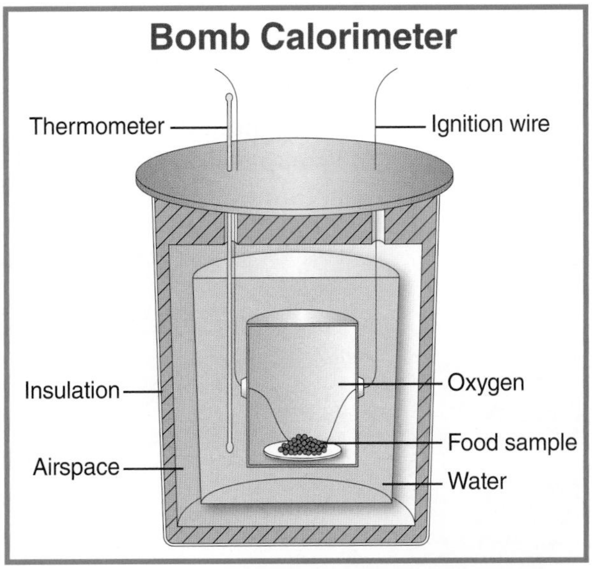

Bomb Calorimeter

Goodheart-Willcox Publisher

Figure 12.2 A food's calorie value is a measure of the heat it gives off when it is burned in a bomb calorimeter.

Using direct calorimetry, researchers have measured the calories in the wide range of foods listed in food composition tables. They have also determined the energy yield of one gram of a pure nutrient. As you have already learned, one gram of pure carbohydrate or protein yields 4 calories. One gram of pure fat yields 9 calories. This means fats produce more than twice the energy of the other two nutrients.

Consider Calorie Density

Being aware of the calorie density of foods can help you balance energy. ***Calorie density*** refers to the concentration of energy in a food. Fats are a concentrated source of energy. Therefore, foods that are high in fat are calorie dense. On the other hand, foods that are high in water lack calorie density because water yields no energy.

Comparing 100-gram portions of two different foods helps clarify the relationship between fat content and calorie density. For example, lettuce has high water content and no fat. 100 grams (3½ ounces) of lettuce supplies 13 calories. In contrast, mayonnaise has little water content and is high in fat. 100 grams (20 teaspoons) of mayonnaise supplies the body with 714 calories. Mayonnaise is clearly the more calorie-dense food.

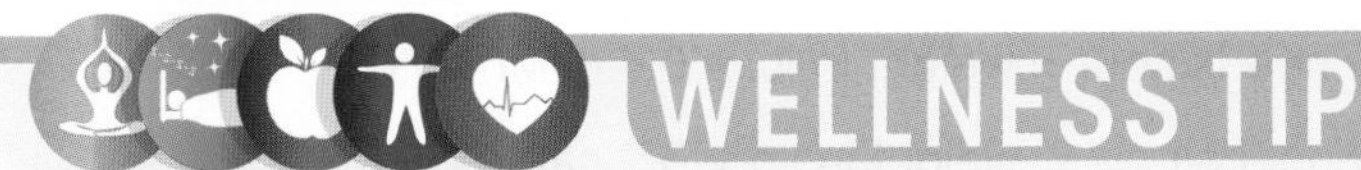

Keep a Food Journal

Keeping a food journal can help you evaluate your daily energy intake as well as your nutrient intake. Examine the number of calories per serving of foods listed in your diary. Those high in calories are energy dense. You can analyze other aspects of food intake by using the Supertracker at the ChooseMyPlate website.

Energy Output

The other side of the energy balance equation looks at the calories you burn throughout the day. Researchers have determined energy is used for basal metabolism, physical activity, and the thermic effect of food. Together, these three factors account for the calories you expend each day, called your *energy needs*, or output.

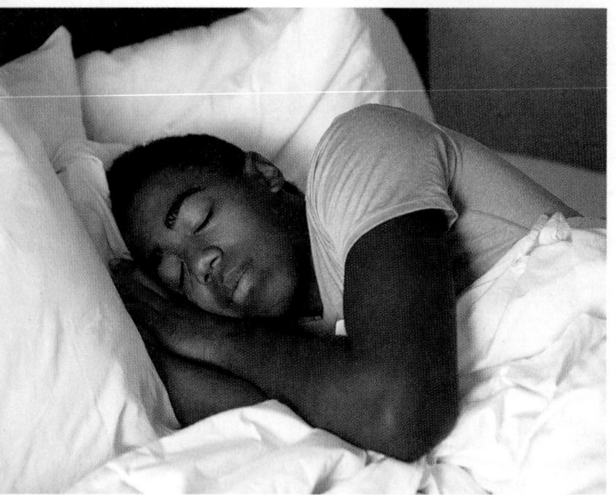

pixelheadphoto digitalskillet/Shutterstock.com

Figure 12.3 Even during sleep, the body needs energy to maintain the functions of its various systems. *What are some functions that require energy while the body is sleeping?*

Basal Metabolism

No matter how still the body is—even during sleep—internal activity continues (**Figure 12.3**). ***Basal metabolism*** involves all of the ongoing functions in the body that sustain life. This includes breathing, circulating blood, and maintaining nerve activity. Secreting hormones, maintaining body temperature, and making new cells are also part of basal metabolism. Energy fuels all of this internal activity. For instance, the brain and liver require about 40 percent of the total energy used to support basal metabolism.

Measuring Energy Use to Support Basal Metabolism

Basal metabolic rate (BMR) is the pace at which the body uses energy to support basal metabolism. In general, women have a lower basal metabolic rate than men (**Figure 12.4**). You may be surprised at the amount of calories necessary to support basal needs. Basal metabolism is the largest part of energy output for most people.

Resting metabolic rate (RMR) is another method used to measure the body's resting energy expenditure. It can be used nearly interchangeably with BMR. RMR measures are slightly higher. The difference stems from the method used to collect the data. RMR data is collected four hours after food has been eaten or significant physical activity. This is different from the BMR data collection method. BMR data collection occurs after a 12-hour fast in a controlled environment for a specific time while the individual is resting. Since RMR data is easier to collect, it is more frequently used as a research tool and in sports nutrition or health clubs to help determine caloric needs.

Figure 12.4 Basal metabolic energy needs are different for men and women.

Basal Metabolic Energy Needs
For Adult Women
Basal energy needs/hour = weight in lb. × 0.4 calories/lb.
(Basal energy needs/hour = weight in kg × 0.9 calories/kg)
Basal energy needs/day = basal energy needs/hour × 24 hours/day
For Adult Men
Basal energy needs/hour = weight in lb. × 0.5 calories/lb.
(Basal energy needs/hour = weight in kg × 1.0 calories/kg)
Basal energy needs/day = basal energy needs/hour × 24 hours/day

What Affects BMR?

Many factors affect a person's BMR. Body structure, body composition, and gender affect BMR and the amount of energy used for metabolism. A taller person will have a higher BMR than a shorter person. This is because the taller person has more body surface area through which heat is lost. ***Body composition*** refers to the percentage of different tissues in the body, such as fat, muscle, and bone. A person with a larger proportion of muscle tissue will have a higher BMR than someone with more fat tissue. This is because it takes more calories to maintain muscle tissue than fat. Males generally have a slightly higher BMR than females because males have more lean body mass and greater oxygen consumption for their body mass.

Temperature, both inside and outside the body, can affect BMR. Fever increases BMR. Adjusting to cold or hot temperatures in the environment increases BMR as well.

The thyroid gland secretes the hormone *thyroxine*, which regulates basal metabolism. An overactive thyroid produces too much thyroxine and increases BMR. Conversely, an underactive thyroid secretes less thyroxine and decreases BMR. This is why a thyroid disease can affect a person's body weight.

BMR tends to decline with age. There is an approximate five percent decrease in BMR every 10 years past age 30, mostly due to loss of muscle mass. People over age 50 must reduce their energy intake up to 200 calories per day to avoid weight gain. Older people who remain active and maintain lean body mass do not experience as much of a decline in BMR (**Figure 12.5**).

A very low-calorie diet decreases BMR about 10 to 20 percent. The body responds as it would during a famine. It makes adjustments to preserve life as long as possible. By lowering BMR, vital functions can be maintained even when fewer calories are available. Someone restricting calories to lose weight will have a harder time reaching his or her goal due to this factor. Stress in people's lives raises BMR. Stress releases hormones that affect BMR.

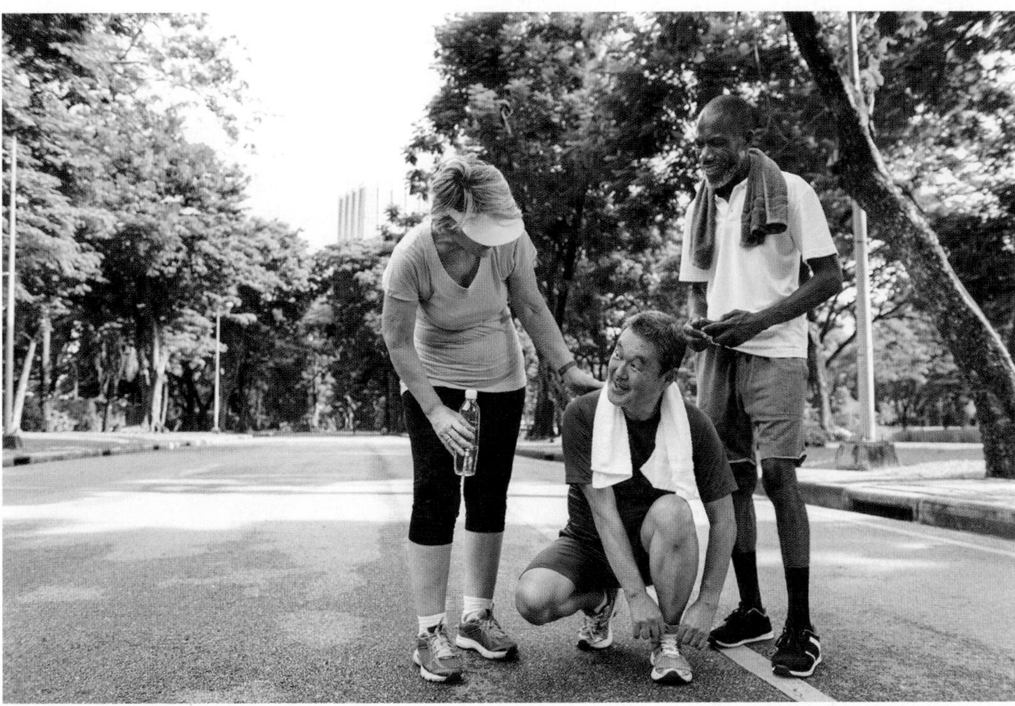

Rawpixel.com/Shutterstock.com

Figure 12.5
Staying physically active helps older people maintain a higher BMR.

BMR is higher during periods of growth. Therefore, infants, children, and teens have a higher BMR than adults. Women have a higher BMR during pregnancy. Meeting the basal energy needs for growth and maintenance of cells is critical for body development. This is why infants, children, teens, and pregnant women should not reduce their calorie intake unless advised by a doctor. These groups of people need the nutrients provided by a variety of foods. If children and teens are having trouble balancing energy, increasing physical activity is a more healthful choice than reducing calories.

Some of the factors described are temporary. Fever and pregnancy temporarily increase BMR. When these conditions end, BMR drops back to its normal level.

Changing BMR

Many of the factors that affect BMR cannot be changed. Therefore, the impact of these factors on BMR cannot be changed either. However, BMR can be changed by increasing muscle tissue. A regular exercise program helps develop muscle tissue and increase BMR. Generally, the greater the proportion of lean muscle tissue in your body, the higher your BMR will be and the more calories your body will use for metabolism.

THE MOVEMENT CONNECTION

Spinal Twist

Why

When the calories you consume are equal to the calories you expend, energy balance is achieved. Likewise, an imbalance in flexibility or strength from one side of the body to the other can lead to injury or discomfort.

As with calories, flexibility and strength should be balanced for optimal health. The spinal twist stretch helps restore balanced flexibility.

Apply

- Sit on floor with both legs in front of you and back straight.
- Bend your right knee and place right foot on the ground outside of your left thigh.
- Turn torso to the right and place right hand on the ground behind your lower back.
- Wrap your left arm around your right leg and breathe throughout the stretch.
- Hold for 10 seconds before releasing.
- Begin seated on ground with both legs in front of you and back straight.
- Bend your left knee and place left foot on the ground outside of your right thigh.
- Turn torso to the left and place left hand on the ground behind your lower back.
- Wrap your right arm around your left leg and breathe throughout the stretch.
- Hold for 10 seconds before releasing.

Repeat 3 times on both sides.

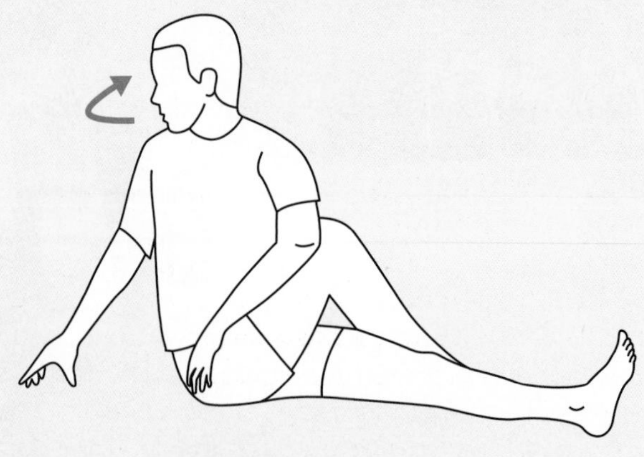

Physical Activity

The second category of energy needs is the energy used for physical activity. During physical activity, energy is needed to move muscles. Energy is also needed for the extra work of breathing harder and pumping more blood.

What Affects Energy Output During Physical Activity?

Energy output varies depending on body size. The larger the body size, the greater the amount of energy needed to make the muscles work to move the body. In other words, a 180-pound (82-kilogram) person burns more calories while walking than a 120-pound (55-kilogram) person walking at the same pace.

The actual amount of muscle movement also affects energy output. Therefore, more calories are burned if you swing your arms while walking than if you keep your arms still.

Sedentary activities are activities that require much sitting or little movement. Watching television, studying, working in an office, driving, and using a computer are all sedentary activities. People who spend most of their days being sedentary need to make a point of including more physical activity in their daily lives.

Physical activity can be increased by simply looking for more energy-intensive ways to complete daily tasks, like the following:

- taking the stairs instead of an elevator
- swinging your arms when walking
- standing rather than sitting when possible
- walking or riding a bicycle instead of riding in a car; or
- parking the car farther from your destination and walking the last block or two (**Figure 12.6**).

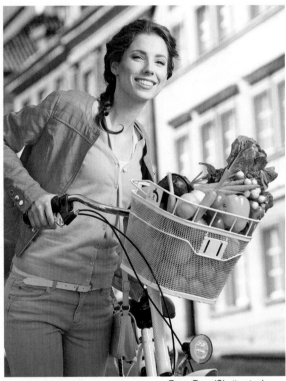

Zoom Team/Shutterstock.com

Figure 12.6 Biking to the supermarket can add physical activity to your daily routine.

Determining Calorie Needs for Physical Activity

Researchers commonly measure the number of calories burned from physical activity using *indirect calorimetry*. This measurement technique requires a person to wear an **apparatus** (equipment with a purpose) while performing a specific activity. The apparatus measures the person's oxygen intake and carbon dioxide output. (Oxygen consumption is required to burn calories. That is why you breathe harder when running or working hard.) The researchers then use mathematical formulas to convert the gas exchange into calories used.

Figure 12.7 on the next page lists ranges of calories used per hour for various common activities. These ranges include energy expended for basal metabolism as well as energy used for activities. By comparing activities, you will soon know which ones are high-energy users and which ones demand little energy. For instance, studying may seem like hard work. Unfortunately, studying burns no more calories per hour than watching television.

Figure 12.7
Body size and degree of muscle movement affect the specific number of calories a person burns through physical activity.

Energy Use for Various Activities

Activity	Calories Used per Hour
Sleep	60
Sedentary activities—reading, eating, watching television, sewing, playing cards, using a computer, studying, other sitting activities	80–100 (average 90)
Light activities—cooking, doing dishes, ironing, grooming, walking slowly, more strenuous sitting activities	110–160 (average 135)
Moderate activities—walking moderately fast, making beds, bowling, light gardening, standing activities requiring arm movement	170–240 (average 205)
Vigorous activities—walking fast, dancing, golfing (carrying clubs), yard work	250–350 (average 300)
Strenuous activities—running, bicycling, playing football, playing tennis, cheerleading, swimming, skiing, playing active games	350 or more

Use **Figure 12.7** to estimate how many calories you burn from physical activity. Begin by keeping an accurate record of all your activities for a typical 24-hour period. Note the amount of time spent on each activity. Use the following formula to compute your approximate energy use for each activity:

Calories used per hour × Hours of activity = Energy expended

Using this equation, you can calculate that you burn about 480 calories during 8 hours of sleep. You can also estimate that you use about 150 calories when you ride your bicycle for 30 minutes. Add the figures for all your activities in a 24-hour period to determine the total energy expended for the day.

Thermic Effect of Food

The third source of energy expenditure is the ***thermic effect of food (TEF)***. The thermic effect of food is the energy required to complete the processes of digestion, absorption, and metabolism. Think of it as the energy required to extract the energy from food.

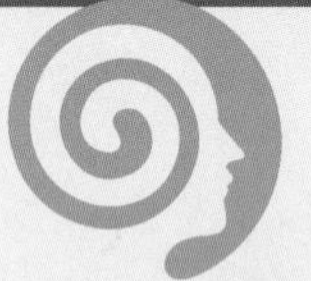

EXTEND YOUR KNOWLEDGE

"NEAT" Information

In addition to intentional physical activity, you expend calories through all the activities of daily living called *NEAT (non-exercise activity thermogenesis)*. NEAT refers to the energy expended during those times when you are not sleeping, eating, or participating in planned exercise. For example, NEAT activities might include walking to school, using the keyboard, sitting in a chair, blow-drying your hair, or fidgeting while taking a test. The cumulative impact of energy expenditure due to nonexercise activities is believed to be a significant factor in a person's ability to maintain a healthy weight.

Research to learn factors that might affect NEAT. What percent of an individual's energy expenditure might be from NEAT?

Types and amounts of foods eaten may affect the thermic effect of food slightly. Nonetheless, it generally equals 5 to 10 percent of your combined basal metabolism and physical activity energy needs. The calorie ranges from **Figure 12.7** that you used to calculate your energy needs for activity included basal metabolism. Therefore, simply multiply your calculated total energy expenditure for the day by 0.1 (10 percent). This will give you a reasonable estimate of energy used for the thermic effect of food. Someone using 2,200 calories for physical activity and basal metabolism would spend about 220 calories for the thermic effect of food.

For most people, approximately 60 to 65 percent of energy output is for basal metabolism. About 25 to 35 percent is for physical activity. For athletes, a lower percentage of energy output is for basal metabolism and a higher percentage is for physical activity. Five to 10 percent of energy output is for the thermic effect of food (**Figure 12.8**).

Calculating exact total energy needs is difficult for many people, but estimates can help determine whether energy intake is in balance with energy output. If weight is stable, energy balance has been achieved and the calories being eaten are balanced with the calories being used.

Energy Imbalance

Many factors can cause the energy equation to be out of balance. *Energy imbalance* occurs when a person consumes too few or too many calories for his or her energy needs. Over time, either of these conditions can lead to negative health consequences. Temporary weight **fluctuation** (change) is normal. Small weight changes that occur from one day to the next are mostly the result of water changes in the body.

A regularly occurring energy imbalance will cause a change in body weight. People who are trying to lose or gain weight intentionally create an energy imbalance in their bodies. People who pay little attention to their eating and activity habits may unintentionally create an energy imbalance.

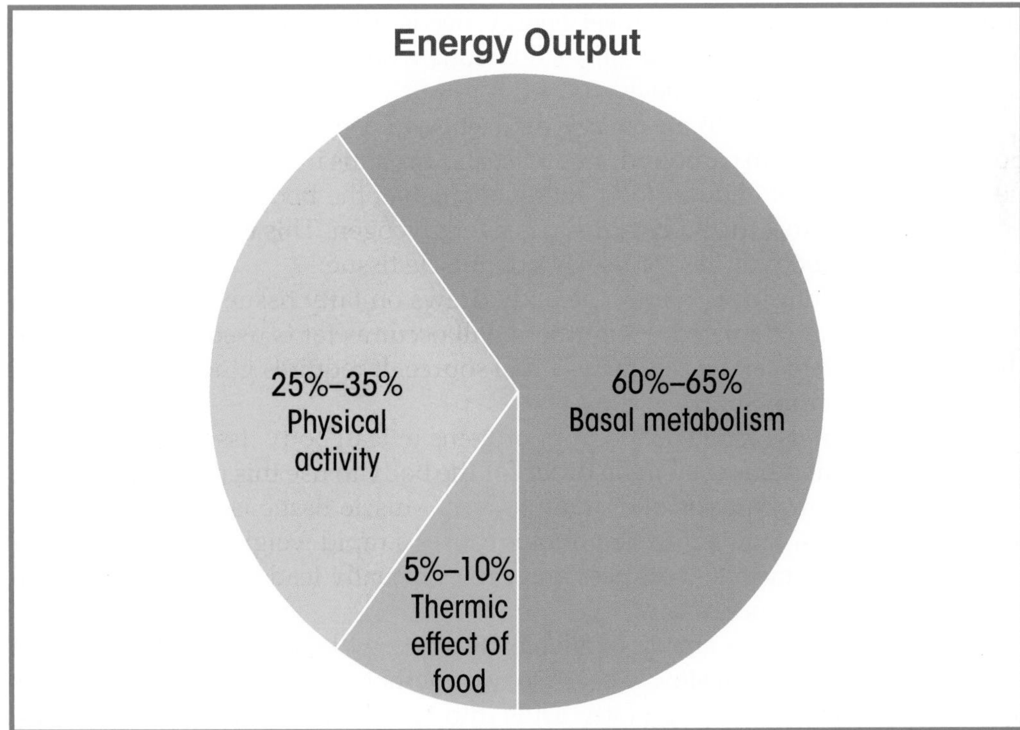

Figure 12.8
The majority of energy needs support basal metabolism, with a significant amount of energy also needed for physical activity.

FEATURED CAREER

Fitness Trainer

Fitness trainers lead, instruct, and motivate individuals or groups in exercise activities, including cardiovascular exercise, strength training, and stretching. They work in health clubs, rehabilitation centers, country clubs, hospitals, universities, resorts, and clients' homes. Fitness workers also are found in workplaces, where they organize and direct health and fitness programs for employees.

Education

Increasingly, most employers require fitness workers to have an associate's degree or a bachelor's degree in a field related to health or fitness, such as exercise science or physical education. Some employers allow workers to substitute a college degree for certification, but most employers who require a bachelor's degree also require certification. Some workers receive specialized training if they teach or lead a specific method of exercise or focus on a particular age or ability group.

Job Outlook

Jobs for fitness trainers are expected to increase about as fast as the average for all occupations. This is because more people are spending time and money on fitness. Likewise, businesses are recognizing the benefits of health and fitness programs for their employees.

Energy Deficiency

Energy deficiency occurs when energy intake is less than energy output. Several factors can result in an energy deficiency. In cases of poverty and famine, food sources may be too scarce to meet energy needs. Illness may **depress** (reduce) appetite or hinder energy metabolism. Someone who purposely eats a low-calorie diet creates an energy deficiency.

The body responds to an energy deficiency in a number of ways. First, the body uses energy from carbohydrates, fats, and proteins in food to meet its energy needs. If there is not enough food energy available, the body draws on stores of energy. The first store the body turns to is liver glycogen. This is the stored form of glucose from carbohydrates for use by nonmuscle tissue.

After about four to six hours, the body draws on fatty tissue for energy when glycogen stores are depleted. Weight loss will occur as fat is used. Unfortunately, the nervous system cannot use fat as a fuel source. It requires glucose, which cannot be obtained from fat.

The body can use amino acids from proteins in lean body tissues to make glucose to feed the nervous system. In order for the body to use this protein, however, it has to break down muscle and organ tissues. Muscle tissue is 75 percent water. Therefore, breaking down muscle proteins causes a rapid weight loss due to water loss. It also causes muscle weakness and can eventually lead to a number of dangerous health consequences.

When carbohydrates are not available, the body will take steps to limit muscle **atrophy** (wasting). It will slowly begin to use another method to feed the nervous system. The body will change fatty acids into compounds called ***ketone bodies***.

The nervous system can use ketone bodies to meet some of its energy needs. Ketone bodies reach the nervous system through the bloodstream. An abnormal buildup of ketone bodies in the bloodstream is a condition known as ***ketosis***. This condition can be harmful because it changes the acid-base balance of the blood.

Carbohydrates are always important in the diet because they are the preferred fuel for nerve and brain cells to function. Nutritionists do not recommend following very high-protein, very low-carbohydrate diets for extended periods. These diets cause muscle tissue to be broken down and large amounts of ketones to form. Instead, nutritionists suggest including enough carbohydrates in the diet to fuel the brain and central nervous system. Carbohydrate intake should also be sufficient to preserve muscle tissue. This will cause the body to use fat stores, rather than pull protein from muscle, for energy. Weight loss will result from the loss of fat, not muscle (**Figure 12.9**).

Energy Excess

Energy excess occurs when energy intake is greater than energy output. Excess calories from carbohydrates, fats, proteins, and alcohol can all be stored in adipose tissue. The body can use this stored energy when there is not enough food intake to meet immediate energy needs.

If energy excess occurs on a regular basis, weight gain will result. Scientists have calculated that an excess of 3,500 calories in the diet leads to one pound (0.45 kg) of stored body fat. The amount of weight gained and the speed with which weight is gained depends on the amount of energy excess.

Most overweight people have gained weight slowly over a period of years. Consuming an extra 25 calories each day adds approximately 2½ pounds (1.2 kg) each year. Just this small energy excess could cause a healthy-weight 20-year-old to be 25 pounds overweight by age 30.

Excess adipose tissue, as well as the location on the body where it is stored, is a health concern. The greater the amount of fat carried on the body, the greater the risk for related health problems.

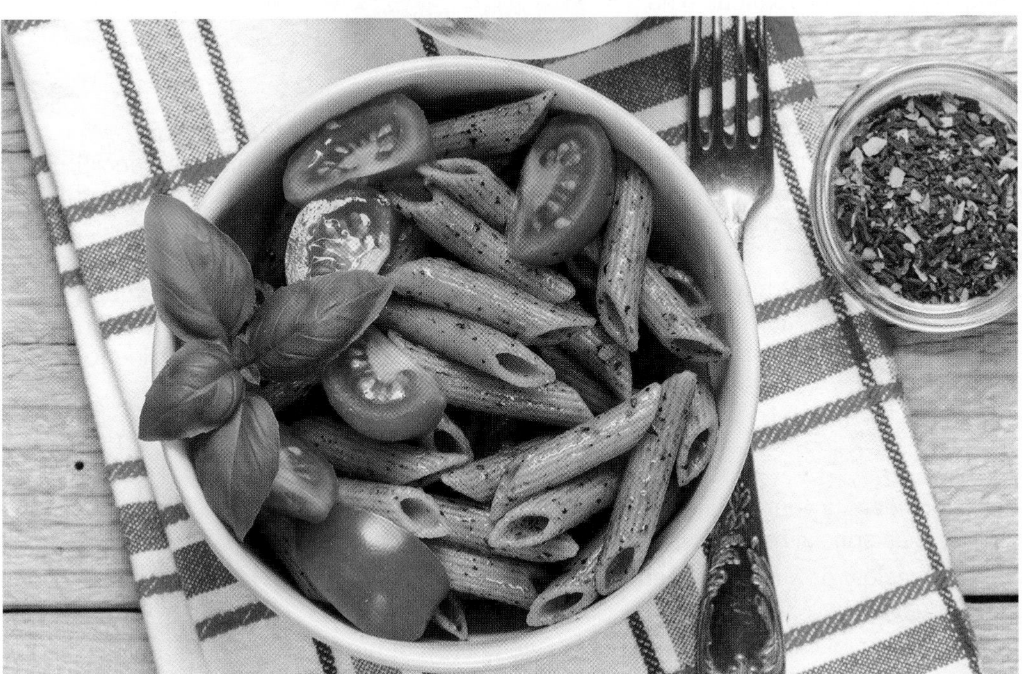

Viktory Panchenko/Shutterstock.com

Figure 12.9 Including whole-grain sources of carbohydrates in an energy deficient diet will result in weight loss without damage to body protein tissues.

Determining Healthy Weight

There are health risks associated with both too little and too much body fat. Maintaining a healthy body weight will help limit these health risks. Body weight is an individual's total mass measured in pounds or kilograms. ***Healthy body weight*** is a body weight specific to gender, height, and body frame size that is associated with health and **longevity** (long life). This may not be the weight that matches the media's image of a "perfect body." Instead, it is a weight at which body fat is in an appropriate proportion to lean tissue. *Body composition* is the term used to identify the proportion of lean body tissue to fat tissue in the body.

COMMUNITY CONNECTIONS

Pairing with an Individual with Special Needs

One way to give back to your community is to volunteer with a program that supports children with special needs. *Special needs* is a general term used to describe a wide array of diagnoses. Some children with special needs may have mild learning disabilities. Others may have severe cognitive impairment, food allergies, or a terminal illness. Physical developmental delays are common. Occasionally a child with special needs may experience a panic attack or show indications of more serious psychiatric problems.

As a volunteer, you might be helping a family with a special needs child or volunteering in a nonprofit organization serving children with special needs. To prepare, you should learn more about living with the particular disability and how it affects family and community life. You should receive an orientation before beginning your volunteer experience.

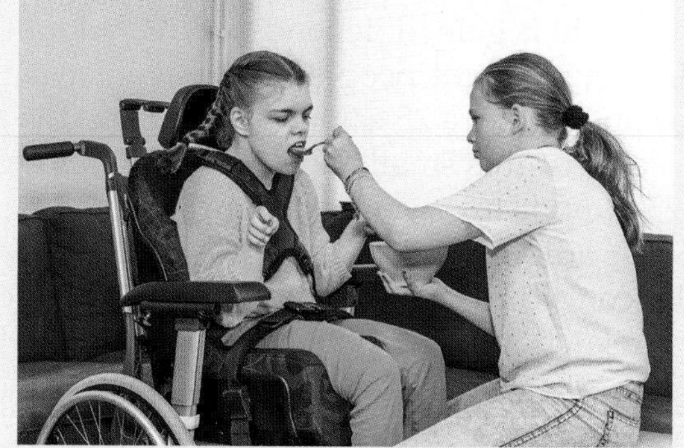

martin bowra/Shutterstock.com

Volunteering with children with special needs requires a willingness to be observant, flexible, consistent, positive, and patient. The child may be unable to communicate his or her needs, so you must be observant and anticipate them. Teaching new skills may require being flexible in your approach. Being consistent and positive inspires trust and motivates learning.

One example of a teen volunteer experience is a cooking program for children with special needs. The teen volunteers focus on kitchen safety, cleanliness, and handwashing. They teach kitchen skills such as mixing, measuring, and nutrition. Other programs, such as Special Olympics, focus on physical activity skills.

Some volunteer programs may have minimum age requirements and require a background check for safety reasons. To learn more about available opportunities for volunteering with children with special needs, visit with the staff of your school's special needs program or search online for programs that coordinate teen volunteers and children with special needs.

Think Critically

1. In group discussion, identify your feelings and perceived challenges about working with a young person who has special needs.
2. In what ways does society give fair treatment to children and youth with special needs? Where does unfairness exist?
3. What are the rewards of volunteering with a special needs child or program?

A healthy body weight requires a healthy body composition (**Figure 12.10**). Having a healthy body weight reduces the risk of a number of serious medical problems.

There are several ways to assess healthy body weight:

- estimate amount of body fat based on height and weight using a mathematical formula;
- use a body composition measurement technique; and
- identify body fat distribution patterns.

Each of these methods has advantages and disadvantages. However, they can all be useful approaches for evaluating weight status.

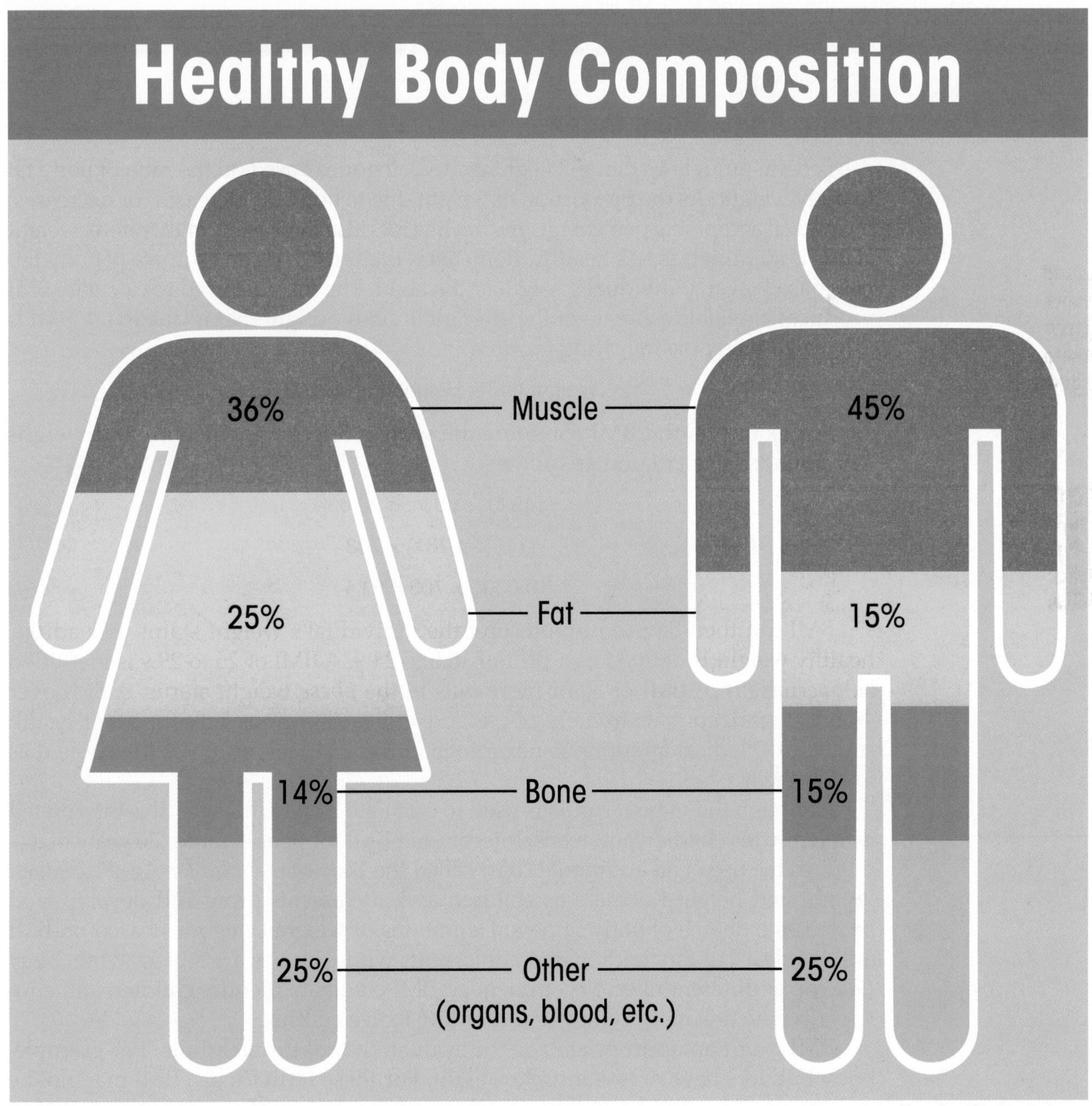

pockygallery/Shutterstock.com

Figure 12.10 Body composition can vary due to gender, age, level of physical activity, and genes. *Is healthy weight without healthy body composition possible?*

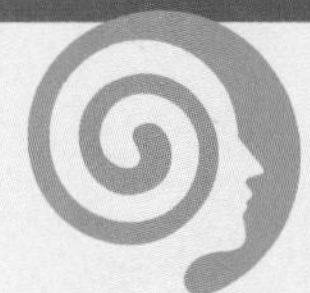

EXTEND YOUR KNOWLEDGE

Normal-Weight Obesity

Researchers have found that more than half of American adults with normal-weight BMIs (18.5–24.9) have high percent of body fat. Obesity is defined as having excess body fat. Normal-weight obesity carries the same serious health risks as obesity. A BMI measurement does not measure body fat. Thus, the need for applying other assessment tools, in addition to just weight and BMI, can help determine an individual's health status. Adding other measurements of percent body fat and body fat patterns can be beneficial. Percent of body fat mass, not weight, is often considered a better measure of your health and fitness.

Research the recommendations for individuals with normal-weight obesity to reduce the risks of metabolic disturbances linked to heart disease and diabetes.

Using Body Mass Index

Federal guidelines define weight status categories based on the ratio of body fat to body weight. As the proportion of weight due to body fat increases (or decreases) beyond an acceptable percentage, the health risks also increase, and therefore, weight status is identified as less healthy. ***Body mass index (BMI)*** is an estimate of body fatness based on an individual's height and weight. The formula used to calculate BMI produces a reliable estimate of the amount of body weight that is due to fat. BMI is calculated using the following formula:

$$\text{Weight (lb.)} \div \text{Height (in.)}^2 \times 703$$

For example, the BMI for someone who is 5 feet 9 inches tall and weighs 145 pounds is calculated as follows:

$$(145 \text{ lb.} \div 69 \text{ in.}^2) \times 703$$

$$(145 \div 4{,}761) \times 703$$

$$0.0305 \times 703 = 21.4$$

BMI can then be used to interpret the individual's weight status. For adults, healthy weight is defined as a BMI of 18.5 to 24.9. A BMI of 25 to 29.9 is identified as ***overweight***. A BMI of 30 or more falls in the ***obese*** weight status. A BMI over 40 is categorized as extremely obese and indicates serious risk for other health problems. Medical attention is recommended. A BMI below 18.5 is interpreted as ***underweight***.

Although the same formula is used to calculate BMI for all ages, it is interpreted differently for children and teens. Interpreting BMI for people under 20 years of age requires the use of an additional chart called the *Body Mass Index-for-Age Percentiles.* Weight and height fluctuate as children and adolescents grow and develop, and so does the degree of body fatness. Definitions of weight categories based on BMI are less clear-cut for children and adolescents whose bodies are still growing. They develop at different rates. Recommended BMI cutoffs to identify children and adolescents who are overweight vary according to age and sex.

BMI is not an appropriate weight evaluation tool for all adults. For example, body builders have excess muscle weight. For these individuals, BMI may not be an accurate gauge of body fatness. Older adults, pregnant women, and lactating mothers have unique BMIs because the amount of body fat changes with age and these physical conditions.

Measuring Body Composition

Analyzing body composition is another way to judge weight, or more importantly, health status. The components of the body can be divided into two categories—fat and fat-free. Fat tissue is located throughout the body. Some body fat is essential for normal body function. The *fat-free mass (FFM),* otherwise referred to as *lean tissue*, found in the body includes the water, protein, and minerals found in organs, muscle, and bone.

Interpreting Body Fat Percentage

A higher percentage of FFM indicates stronger bones and a larger proportion of skeletal muscle tissue. As the percent FFM increases, the percent body fat decreases. According to the American Council on Exercise (ACE), body fat greater than 25 percent is considered excessive for young adult males. A more desirable fitness range is 14 to 17 percent. For women, over 32 percent body fat is excessive. A range of 21 to 24 represents fitness. Acceptable ranges for good health are 18 to 24 percent for males and 25 to 31 percent for females.

Measuring Body Fat Percentage

How is percentage of body fat determined? One of the most accurate ways for measuring body fat is underwater weighing. Breath is exhaled and the person is submerged under water. The process is based on the principle that lean tissue is denser than fat tissue. A person with more lean tissue has a denser body. Water volume is measured to determine amount of body fat mass. A person with more body fat weighs less under water and is more **buoyant** (capable of floating). Few people, however, have access to an exercise physiology lab to have this test performed. Other acceptable, less expensive methods are available to provide data on fat and lean body composition.

A more common way to assess body composition is to do a ***skinfold test***. This test uses a special tool called a *caliper* to measure the thickness of a fold of skin (**Figure 12.11**). An estimate is made about how much of the thickness is due to ***subcutaneous fat***. This is the fat that lies underneath the skin, which accounts for about half the fat in the body. Skinfold measurements are often taken on the thigh, upper arm, abdomen, and/or back. The amount of subcutaneous fat in these areas reflects the total amount of fat throughout the body. As people become more physically fit, body fat measurements will reflect more lean body tissue and less fat tissue.

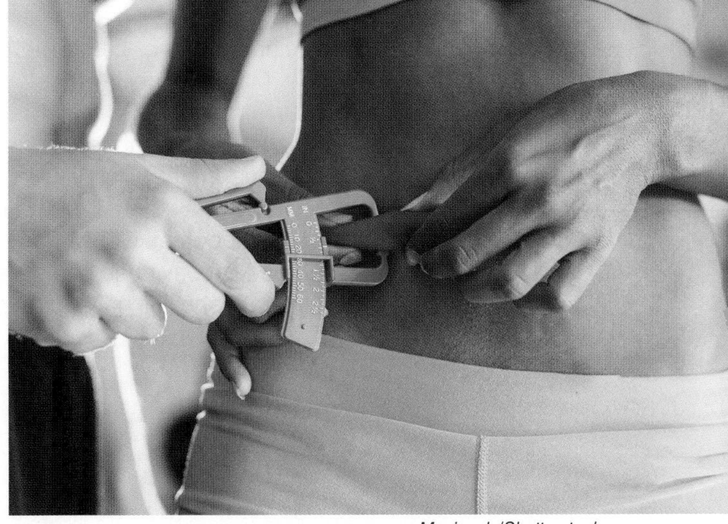

Myvisuals/Shutterstock.com

Figure 12.11 Skinfold measurement is an easy, inexpensive method for measuring body composition.

Another method for measuring body fat is ***bioelectrical impedance***. This process measures the body's resistance to a low-energy electrical current. Lean tissue conducts electrical energy, whereas fat does not. The more fat a person has, the more resistance there is to the flow of the electrical current. The measure of resistance is then converted to a percentage of body fat.

Newer methods continue to be developed to give fitness trainers an indication of percent fat mass and fat-free tissue mass.

For example, *infrared light beams* are being used to measure percent body fat. A fiber-optic probe is positioned at the mid-biceps (upper arm) and an electromagnetic radiation wave is sent out. This light beam is monitored as it enters subcutaneous fat and muscle. The reflection off the bone is read by the monitor. The amount reflected estimates body composition.

Measurements of body fat mass are estimates. The accuracy of the various methods used to measure percent body fat can differ significantly.

Location of Body Fat

Recent evidence suggests the location as well as the amount of body fat affects health. Fat stored in the abdomen, sometimes called *belly fat*, poses a greater health risk than fat stored in the buttocks, hips, and thighs. Fat stored in the abdomen also surrounds important internal organs. As a result, there is increased production of low-density lipoproteins by the liver, which is a risk factor for heart disease. High blood pressure and type 2 diabetes are other risk factors associated with excess belly fat.

Men and older women are more likely to accumulate fat in the abdominal area. They have what is sometimes referred to as "apple-shaped" bodies. Younger women more often store excess fat in the hips and thighs. They have what may be called "pear-shaped" bodies. You may have limited control over where your body stores excess fat. However, if you maintain a healthy weight, avoid sugary drinks, and exercise regularly, your fat stores should not pose a health problem.

CASE STUDY

Healthy Weight: A Simple Matter?

Jackie is 16 years old and barely 5 feet tall. After learning about the importance of maintaining healthy weight in her health class, she decided to learn more about her weight status. She used a BMI chart and discovered she is considered overweight for her age. Jackie knows being overweight increases her health risks. However, she is not experiencing any health problems now and feels alert and strong. She enjoys being active and is on her school's soccer team. She often lifts weights with her brother in the basement of their home.

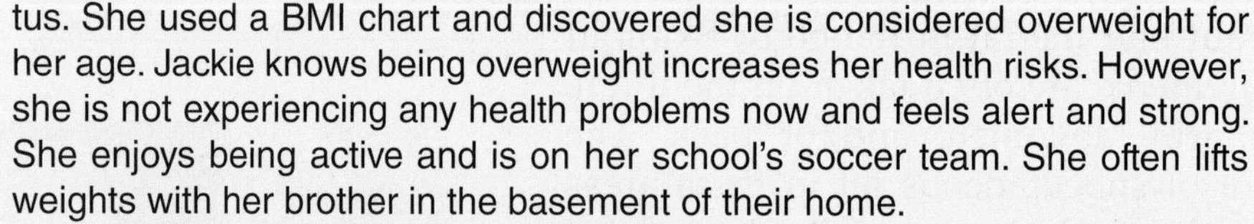

Malia is Jackie's best friend. Malia hates to exercise, eats junk food all day, and is tall and thin. Malia told Jackie that her BMI is in the middle of the healthy weight range. Jackie doesn't understand how Malia could be healthier considering her lifestyle.

Jackie's family likes being outdoors, but they also enjoy preparing good meals together. Cooking is a hobby that gives Jackie great satisfaction. Now, Jackie is convinced she must change her lifestyle to improve her health. She is afraid she will have to give up everything she enjoys.

Case Review

1. Decide if Jackie's assessment of her health and weight status is complete and accurate.
2. Do you agree that Malia is healthier than Jackie?
3. What advice would you give to Jackie to help her stay fit and healthy?

Measuring waist circumference is a method used to evaluate body fat distribution. Waist circumference is the distance around your natural waist (just above the navel) (**Figure 12.12**). The goal for waist circumference is less than 40 inches for men, and less than 35 inches for women. People with more weight around their waist are at greater risk of lifestyle-related diseases such as heart disease and diabetes.

When you evaluate your weight, avoid media-promoted stereotypes of how you should look. Try not to be concerned about every pound on your body and every calorie you eat every day. Plan a nutritious diet, be mindful of fats, added sugars, and sodium intake, and follow a program of regular exercise. These lifestyle choices will help you maintain your energy balance and support wellness.

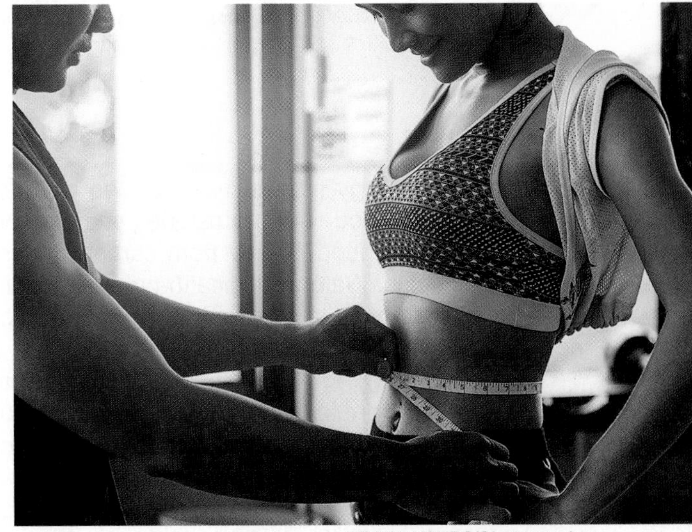

BRAIN2HANDS/Shutterstock.com

Figure 12.12 Waist circumference is an indication of how fat is distributed in the body.

RECIPE FILE

Turkey Pumpkin Chili

6 SERVINGS

Ingredients

- 2 T. olive oil
- 1¼ c. onion, chopped
- 2 jalapeño chiles, seeded and chopped fine
- 2 cloves garlic, minced
- 1 lb. ground turkey breast
- 1 can (14 oz.) crushed tomatoes
- 1 can (15 oz.) pureed pumpkin
- 1 c. chicken broth
- 1 T. chili powder
- 1 t. ground cumin
- ½ t. salt
- pepper, to taste
- 1 can (15 oz.) kidney beans, drained and rinsed
- 2 t. apple cider vinegar

Directions

1. Heat oil in a large pot over medium-high heat.
2. Add onion, chiles, and garlic. Sauté until tender, about 5 minutes.
3. Add turkey and cook until browned.
4. Add tomatoes, pumpkin, broth, chili powder, cumin, salt, and pepper. Bring to a boil.
5. Add beans and reduce heat to medium-low.
6. Cover and simmer, stirring occasionally for 30 minutes.
7. Add apple cider vinegar and stir well.
8. Ladle chili into bowls and serve.

PER SERVING: 313 CALORIES, 15 G PROTEIN, 49 G CARBOHYDRATE, 5 G FAT, 7 G FIBER, 248 MG SODIUM.

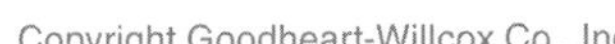

Chapter 12 Review and Expand

Reading Summary

Balancing energy means matching the calories you take in from food with the calories you expend each day. You get food energy from carbohydrates, fats, and proteins. Water is a health-promoting fluid for metabolism processes to occur. Knowing the calorie density of foods can help you balance energy.

You use energy for basal metabolism, physical activity, and the thermic effect of food. Basal metabolism is the energy needed to support basic body functions, such as breathing, blood circulation, and nerve activity. The rate at which the body uses energy for basal metabolism (BMR) is affected by many factors.

If you consume too few or too many calories for your energy needs, energy imbalance results. Energy deficiency occurs when there is not enough food energy available to meet the body's needs. Energy excess occurs when there is more food energy available than the body needs. Both energy deficiency and energy excess can lead to negative health consequences.

To avoid risks from too little or too much body fat, you need to maintain a healthy body weight. You can estimate healthy weight using body mass index (BMI), fat measuring techniques, and assessing body fat distribution. Excess fat in the abdomen seems to pose a greater health risk than fat in the buttocks, hips, and thighs. You can maintain a healthy weight by balancing energy through wise food choices and regular exercise.

Chapter Vocabulary

1. **Content Terms** Work with a partner to write the definitions of the following terms based on your current understanding before reading the chapter. Then join another pair of students to discuss your definitions and any discrepancies. Finally, discuss the definitions with the class and ask your instructor for necessary correction or clarification.

basal metabolic rate (BMR)	ketosis
basal metabolism	obese
bioelectrical impedance	overweight
body composition	resting metabolic rate (RMR)
body mass index (BMI)	sedentary activity
calorie density	skinfold test
energy	subcutaneous fat
healthy body weight	thermic effect of food (TEF)
ketone bodies	underweight

2. **Academic Terms** Write each of the following terms on a separate sheet of paper. For each term, quickly write a word you think relates to the term. In small groups, exchange papers. Have each person in the group explain a term on the list. Take turns until all terms have been explained.

apparatus	depress
atrophy	fluctuation
buoyant	longevity

Review Learning

3. *True or false?* High-fat foods yield the same amount of heat as high-protein foods when measured in the bomb calorimeter.
4. How much energy does a pure gram of each of the energy nutrients yield?
5. Name three additional internal body functions of basal metabolism besides breathing, blood circulation, and nerve activity.
6. What are known factors that affect a person's BMR? Name six.
7. Give three examples of ways to increase energy expenditure while completing daily tasks.
8. Explain how to estimate how many calories a person burns from physical activity.
9. Which of the three areas of energy expenditure accounts for the smallest percentage of calories burned?
10. Why do nutritionists avoid recommending very high-protein, very low-carbohydrate diets?
11. How many excess calories are stored in one pound (0.45 kilogram) of body fat?
12. What methods are used to assess healthy body weight?
13. What is the relationship of BMI to body fat and health risks?
14. Why does fat stored in the abdomen pose a greater health risk than fat stored in the buttocks, hips, and thighs?

Self-Assessment Quiz

Complete the self-assessment quiz online to help you practice and expand your knowledge and skills.

Critical Thinking

15. **Conclude** Some experts believe the thermic effect of food plays an insignificant role in total energy expenditure. Others believe the calories used for thermic effect can add up and contribute to leanness over a lifetime. Use Internet or print resources to research these views. Draw your own conclusions based on your findings and write a brief summary describing your opinion. Cite sources to support your opinion.
16. **Compare and Contrast** Compare and contrast the various methods for determining healthy body weight. Why is it beneficial to use more than one method in determining healthy weight?
17. **Apply** Use the formula given in the chapter to compute your basal energy needs for one 24-hour period. Keep an accurate record of your activities for 24 hours. Note the amount of time spent on each activity. Use the formula given in this chapter and Figure 12-7 to compute your approximate energy use for each activity. (Remember the ranges in the chart include energy expended for basal metabolism as well as for the activities.) Calculate your total energy expenditure for the day. Then calculate your energy needs for the thermic effect of food. Finally, compute the percentages of your total energy expenditure used for basal metabolism, physical activity, and thermic effect of food.
18. **Cause and Effect** Create a visual representation to explain how the body responds to an energy deficiency.
19. **Analyze** Find "My Daily Checklist" at ChooseMyPlate.gov. Enter your age, sex, weight, height, and physical activity level to obtain your "MyPlate Daily Checklist" and recommended calorie level. Use the "Food Tracker" on the SuperTracker website to record the foods you eat for one day. Compare your results to your Daily Checklist. Are you in energy balance?
20. **Compare and Contrast** Use a school-approved, global, social networking website to become an e-pal with someone from another country. Ask your e-pal what his or her country does to support the health of its citizens. Learn about the opportunities to participate in sports and other types of physical activities in his or her community.
21. **Create** Prepare a database of information and resources to help people improve their BMR over their life span.

Core Skills

22. **Math** Use the formula from the chapter to calculate the BMI for a 22-year-old woman who is 5 feet 5 inches and weighs 132 pounds. Check your answer with a BMI chart. What is this woman's weight status?
23. **Speaking** Debate whether television, computer, and video gaming have a negative or positive influence on the health of teens. Cite reputable sources to support your arguments.
24. **Research** Select a group of people to study who lived in the 19th century or earlier, such as medieval peasants, Victorian-era middle-class women, or child laborers during the Industrial Revolution. Research to learn about the physical demands of daily life and the typical diet these people experienced. Compare the intensity of their daily work and life with that of an American high school student today. Compare the average calorie intake of each group. Prepare to discuss how lifestyles affected the health of each group in small group discussions.
25. **Math** Compute how many hours of moderate fast walking (205 calories/hour) you would need to equal energy consumed from a large size hamburger, French fries, and a soda (1,290 calories).
26. **Technology Literacy** A mother asks you to help compute her six-year-old son's BMI. The boy is 4 feet tall and weighs 59 pounds. Use the Centers for Disease Control and Prevention (CDC) website to compute the child's BMI. Explain to the mother what the results mean. Explain health recommendations.
27. **Career Readiness Practice** Imagine you are a fitness trainer at a rehabilitation facility that specializes in rehab for workplace injuries. You work closely with several physical therapists at the facility. A number of clients have expressed interest in a class you lead on learning how to balance their energy requirements for a healthy lifestyle. What topics would you use in the class? How would you help people develop a fitness routine for balancing energy? How would you use your leadership skills to motivate, inspire, and persuade your clients to make fitness and energy management a goal for life?

CHAPTER 13 Healthy Weight Management

Learning Outcomes

After studying this chapter, you will be able to

- **summarize** health risks of obesity and underweight;
- **recognize** factors that influence a person's weight status;
- **estimate** your daily calorie needs and compare with your daily calorie intake;
- **state** why some rapid weight-loss plans are dangerous and ineffective;
- **explain** guidelines for safe ways to reduce body fat; and
- **list** tips for safe weight gain.

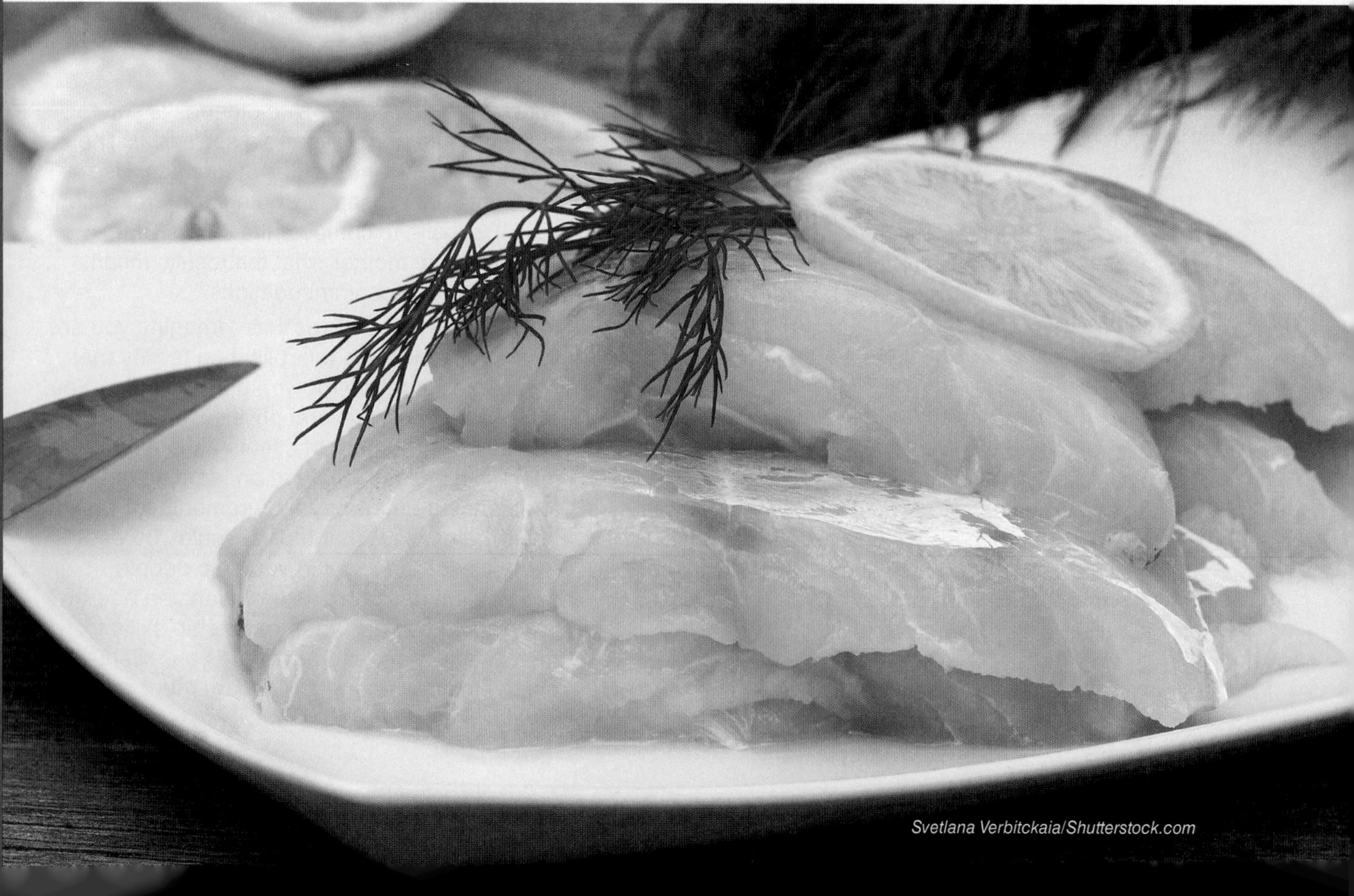

Svetlana Verbitckaia/Shutterstock.com

Content Terms

environmental cue
fad diet
fasting
habit
metabolic syndrome
weight cycling
weight management

Academic Terms

destine
fallacy
recidivism
sated
stigma

What's Your Nutrition and Wellness IQ?

Take this quiz to examine how much you already know about healthy weight management. If you cannot answer a question, pay extra attention to that topic as you study this chapter.

- Identify each statement as *True*, *False*, or *It Depends*. *It Depends* means in some cases the statement is true; in some cases it could be false.
- Revise false statements to make them true.
- Explain the circumstances in which each *It Depends* statement is true and when it is false.

Nutrition and Wellness IQ

Statement			
1. Healthy body weight is more important for teens than for older adults.	True	False	It Depends
2. To maintain healthy body weight, it is more important to count calories than it is to be physically active.	True	False	It Depends
3. Overweight and obesity have only one major health risk and that is the added risk for diabetes.	True	False	It Depends
4. Smelling popcorn in the movie theater is an environment cue for eating.	True	False	It Depends
5. Physical activity level, gender, and height affect how many calories are needed to maintain healthy weight.	True	False	It Depends
6. A good weight-loss goal would be to lose five pounds a week.	True	False	It Depends
7. A weight-loss plan should encourage physical activity as part of the plan.	True	False	It Depends
8. A balanced, nutrient-dense food plan is necessary for healthy weight loss or gain.	True	False	It Depends

While studying this chapter, look for the activity icon to

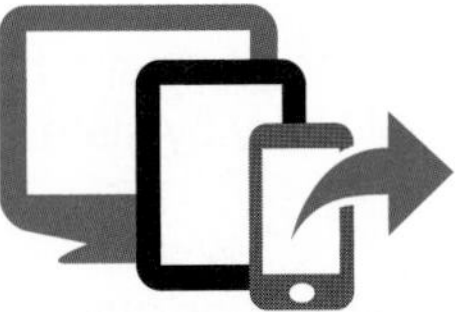

- **build** vocabulary with e-flash cards and interactive games;
- **assess** what you learn by completing self-assessment quizzes and completing review questions; and
- **expand** knowledge with interactive activities and activities that extend learning.

www.g-wlearning.com/foodsandnutrition/

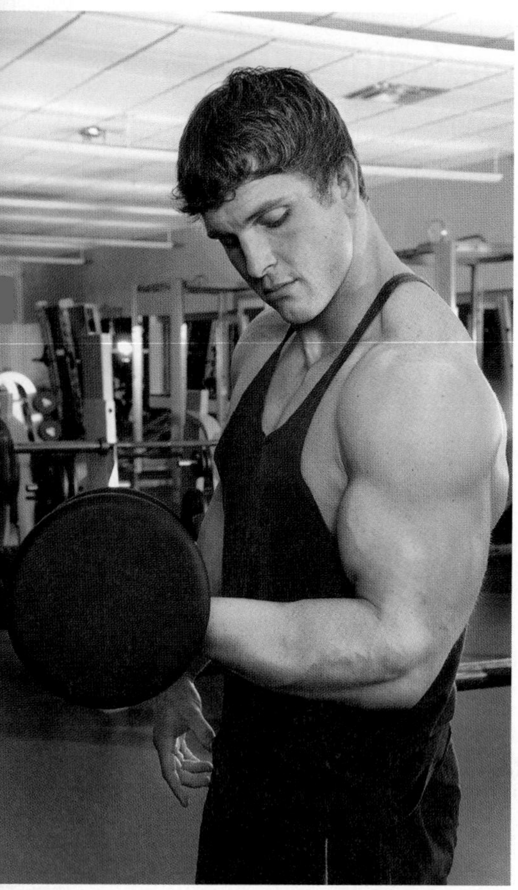

Gino Santa Maria/Shutterstock.com

Figure 13.1 Athletes who are overweight due to a high proportion of lean muscle tissue may be considered healthy weight.

Have you ever tried to lose or gain weight? If you have, you have much company. Millions of people every year take steps to try to adjust their weight. ***Weight management*** means attaining healthy weight and maintaining it throughout life.

In this chapter, you will examine health risks associated with too much and too little body fat. You will identify factors that affect your weight status. You will also learn to follow the guidelines of good nutrition and exercise as you learn to manage your weight.

Healthy Weight Is Important

Reaching a healthy body weight and body composition and maintaining them throughout life are important wellness goals. Having a healthy weight can improve your total sense of well-being and reduce your risk of many diseases.

Instead of discussing *weight* management, it may make more sense to discuss *body fat* management. Not everyone who is overweight has excess body fat. Overweight can also be due to muscle development. Athletes, for example, often have high weights for their heights. However, the weight is due to muscle, not fat. This type of excess weight is not a health problem. Problems associated with overweight and obesity arise when the weight is due to excess fat rather than excess muscle (**Figure 13.1**).

With so much attention focused on overweight, problems associated with underweight are often overlooked. In the United States, the number of people who are underweight is much smaller than the numbers who are overweight. However, both groups are at increased risk of health problems.

FEATURED CAREER

Sports Nutrition Consultant

Sports nutrition consultants work under contract with healthcare facilities or in their own private practice. They perform nutrition screenings for their clients and offer advice on diet-related concerns related to sports nutrition. Some work for wellness programs, sports teams, and coaches.

Education

Sports nutrition consultants need at least a bachelor's degree. Licensure, certification, or registration requirements vary by state.

Job Outlook

Applicants with specialized training, an advanced degree, or certifications beyond the particular state's minimum requirement should enjoy the best job opportunities. Employment is expected to increase.

Overweight and Obesity Increase Health Risks

In the United States, overweight and obesity have become more common in recent years. Most alarming is the increase in overweight and obesity in children. Childhood obesity in the 1960s was about 4.5 percent. In most recent years, the rate of obesity in children is near 18 percent. Many more are overweight.

An adult with a body mass index (BMI) of 25 to 29.9 is considered *overweight*. A BMI score of 30 or more is considered obese. Currently, over 60 percent of the people in the United States have BMIs greater than 25. Obesity is linked to many health risks (**Figure 13.2**). For this reason, reducing the occurrence of obesity in the United States is a national health goal. The more excess fat a person carries, the greater the health risks.

Obesity is a risk factor for metabolic syndrome. ***Metabolic syndrome*** is a term used to describe a cluster of conditions. According to the National Institutes of Health (NIH), a metabolic syndrome diagnosis is warranted when three or more of the following criteria are present:

1. A large waist circumference (40 inches or more for men and 35 or more for women) with excess fat stored in the abdominal area.
2. A blood triglyceride level that is 150 mg/dL or greater.
3. An HDL cholesterol level less than 40 mg/dL in men and less than 50 mg/dL in women. (HDL—the "good" cholesterol—helps remove cholesterol from your arteries.)
4. High blood pressure (130 mm Hg or greater systolic blood pressure and 85 mm Hg or greater diastolic blood pressure).
5. A fasting glucose (blood sugar) equal to or greater than 100 mg/dL or greater. This could be an early sign of diabetes.

Metabolic syndrome increases a person's risk of heart disease, stroke, and diabetes. Metabolic syndrome is both preventable and treatable. Positive health gains are possible if excess pounds are lost.

Health Risks of Obesity
• Heart disease
• Type 2 diabetes
• Cancers (endometrial, breast, kidney, and colon)
• Hypertension (high blood pressure)
• High total cholesterol or high levels of triglycerides
• Stroke
• Liver and gallbladder disease
• Respiratory problems
• Osteoarthritis (a degeneration of cartilage and its underlying bone within a joint)
• Gynecological problems (abnormal menses, infertility)
• Complications during surgery and pregnancy

Figure 13.2 The Centers for Disease Control and Prevention (CDC) reports that overweight and obesity are related to increased risks for certain health conditions.

Health Risks of Underweight

Having too little body fat can have serious effects on health. Underweight people may lack nutrient stores. When fat stores are needed, such as during pregnancy or after surgery, underweight people may have problems. Underweight people may also feel fatigued and have trouble staying warm.

Severely underweight people are urged to gain body fat as an energy reserve. Females with low body fat may stop menstruating. A number of other health risks result from underweight due to eating disorders.

Social and Emotional Health Risks

Unhealthy weight can be a source of social and emotional problems as well as physical ones—especially for children and teens. For years, mass media have overvalued a thin body as a standard of beauty. People are sometimes portrayed negatively simply because of their weight status. Because overweight and obesity are more prevalent in the United States, these conditions receive more attention. Nonetheless, individuals who are underweight also experience weight **stigma** (shame).

Some people can be very cruel to those who are overweight or obese. Childhood obesity can be particularly cruel as it relates to the development of their self-image. People who are obese may face isolation and discrimination in school. Adults may face difficulties at work and in other social settings. To add to the problem, excessive body fat may cause people to shy away from fitness activities.

Faulty media images and ill treatment from others add to stress among people who are obese. These factors can also cause people who are obese to form low opinions of themselves. People who are overweight often have the mistaken belief they are less worthy than people who have healthy body weights. Some weight-management programs work to dispute this misconception. They use counselors to help clients realize that personal value is not based on body weight.

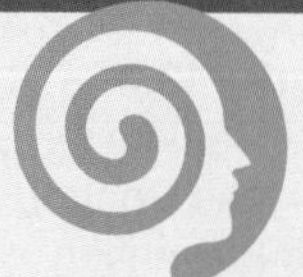

EXTEND YOUR KNOWLEDGE

Brown Fat Cells and White Fat Cells

Did you know that humans have different types of fat cells in their bodies? Humans have both white fat cells and brown fat cells. Brown cells are usually located around the upper back, side of neck, and shoulder area along the spine. Until recently, it was believed that infants had brown fat cells at birth, but that these cells mostly disappeared by adulthood. However, researchers have been able to detect brown fat cells in some adults, more often in active, healthy adults. Brown cells are metabolically active, or burn energy, compared with white fat cells, which store energy. The brown cells burn energy to produce heat. Cold temperatures seem to cause brown cells to be more active. White fat cells, on the other hand, are found under the skin and around internal organs. They help to insulate the body and cushion the organs, but they are not metabolically active. White fat cells store energy, but are relatively inert.

Adults have many more white fat cells than brown fat cells; however, people with greater amounts of brown fat cells tend to have lower body mass indexes (BMIs). These discoveries have inspired researchers to consider how this knowledge could be used in the prevention or treatment of overweight and obesity. Researchers are looking for ways to increase the amount of brown fat tissue as a means to boost energy production and possibly prompt weight loss.

Factors Affecting Your Weight Status

Your weight status is the product of many factors. A combination of these factors is responsible for the increase in overweight and obesity in this country.

What causes people to gain excess weight or maintain a healthy weight is very complex. There are factors inside your body (genetic, metabolic, and hormonal) and factors outside your body (environmental and psychological) that influence your weight status. Your physical activity level also has a major impact on your weight status.

Heredity

Genes set the stage for body shape (**Figure 13.3**). The size of bones and the location of fat stores in the body are inherited traits. Nonetheless, healthy body weight can be found in a variety of body shapes. Heredity also affects basal metabolic rate and how efficiently your body uses calories.

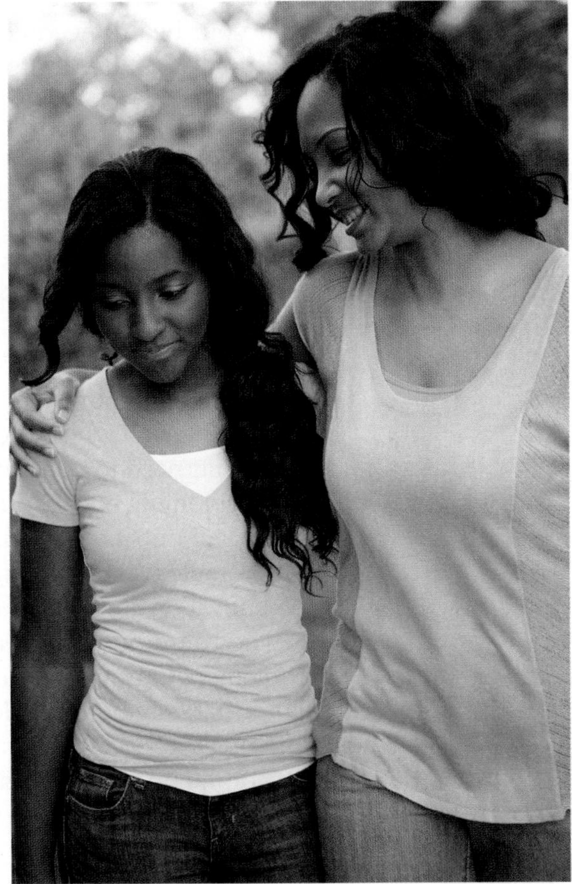

digitalskillet/Shutterstock.com

Figure 13.3 You are likely to have a body shape and size similar to your parents' because genes influence these factors.

Hormones and Weight Status

The human body has a complex system of hormones that interact in many different ways. Some research indicates certain genes may be linked to obesity. These genes are believed to be connected to hormones that influence appetite and energy expenditure.

Two hormones involved in appetite regulation and energy expenditure are *leptin* and *ghrelin*. Leptin is produced in the body fat cells. As the number of fat cells in the body increases, more leptin can be produced. The circulating leptin enters the brain and triggers a reduction in appetite. However, people who are obese can become resistant to the hormone leptin. Appetite becomes hard to manage. More food is eaten than needed when leptin functions at a reduced level.

Ghrelin is a hormone produced in the stomach. People who are overweight produce higher levels of ghrelin. This hormone stimulates the appetite. Ghrelin also encourages fat production and body growth. During periods of fasting, ghrelin is produced and hunger occurs. For people of healthy weight, ghrelin helps to stabilize body weight. People who are obese may develop a different sensitivity to ghrelin that promotes overeating.

These hormones may begin to explain why people differ in their tendency to gain weight. However, the genes linked to these hormones are not a recent development in humans and cannot be solely responsible for the rise in obesity. Other factors, such as calorie-dense foods and decreased activity, are likely contributing to the problem as well. Further research in the genetics and possible causes of obesity is still needed.

Can Heredity Be Overridden?

A family history of obesity does not necessarily **destine** (make unavoidable) a person to be obese. However, weight management may be more complex for people who inherit genes that promote obesity. Following a healthy lifestyle, increasing physical activity, and choosing nutritious foods will help overweight people work toward a healthy weight. Similarly, someone who has numerous thin relatives has no guarantee of a thin body. However, some people are genetically prone toward thinness. Their bodies store fat less readily than others. People who inherit this trait may find it hard to gain weight.

Heredity and genes play a role in making you special. They also help define what your health needs might be. Some inherited traits have minimal impact on your quality of life, and others may require a lifetime of medical attention.

Eating Habits

Weight trends within families are the result of more than just genetics. Eating habits affect weight status by influencing the "calories in" side of the energy balance equation. A ***habit*** is a routine behavior that is often difficult to break. For example, eating buttered popcorn at the movies can become a habit.

People begin to form eating habits early in life. Eating behaviors of children are based largely on the foods parents or caregivers offer them (**Figure 13.4**). They develop patterns in the kinds and amounts of foods they choose. They also form habits related to when and why they eat.

Parents need to be aware that children and teens who are obese have an increased risk of becoming obese adults. Parents can plan meals and snacks around appropriate portions of nutritious foods. This will help children establish healthful eating habits that promote weight management. Children who develop eating behaviors based on good nutrition are more likely to practice healthful eating habits throughout life.

The common pattern of eating meals away from home contributes to weight problems. "Eating out" usually means choosing from a menu of foods that are high in fat, sugar, and calories. Portions are often "supersized" to appeal to consumers. Fast-food restaurants promote big portions which have little relationship to recommended amounts for healthy eating. In addition, the age of television and computers often involves snacking on foods in a mindless manner.

Figure 13.4
Eating habits form early in life. ***How can parents and caregivers instill healthy eating habits in children?***

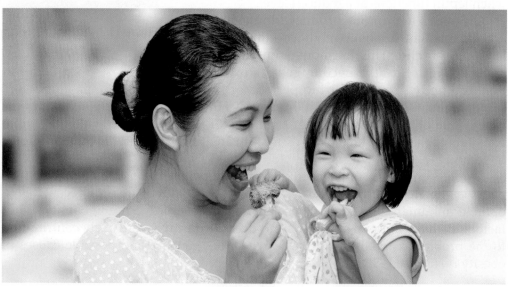

all_about_people/Shutterstock.com

As children grow up, some of their eating habits are likely to change. During the teen years, people begin to have more control over what foods they eat. Busy schedules, peers, and weight concerns often influence food choices. Many teens form the habit of frequently eating fast foods that are high in fat, sugar, salt, and calories. Others adopt patterns of skipping meals.

Eating habits continue to change through adulthood. Work and family obligations often impact food choices and eating behaviors. Adults who commute to work may eat on-the-go. Adults with children sometimes develop the habit of finishing leftovers from their children's plates. These habits may lead to calorie imbalance.

Environmental Cues

Some eating habits are responses to environmental cues. An ***environmental cue*** is an event or situation around you that triggers you to eat. The sight, taste, and smell of foods are common cues that stimulate eating. The time of day, such as lunchtime, is an environmental cue for many people. Social settings, such as parties, can be environmental cues (**Figure 13.5**).

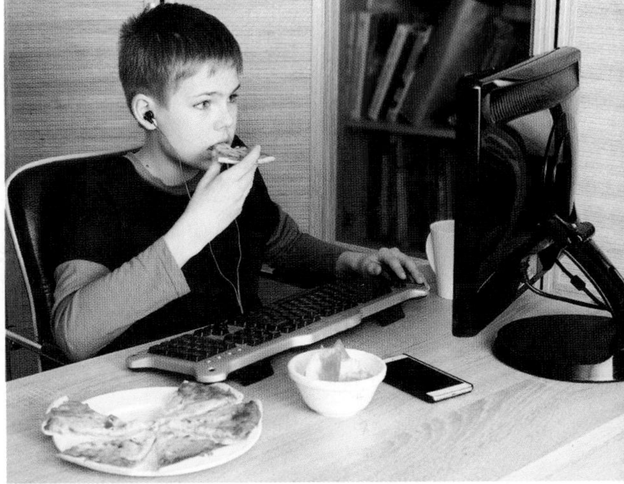

p_ponomareva/Shutterstock.com

Figure 13.5 For many people, most sedentary activities are environmental cues to eat.

Appetite and hunger usually work to make sure people eat enough to supply the fuel their bodies need. However, sometimes cues in the environment cause people to eat mindlessly even when they are not hungry or the food is not healthful. For example, a vendor calling "Hot dogs!" may prompt you to eat at a ball game. This type of eating behavior often causes people to consume more calories than they need.

Media and promotional campaigns can be environmental cues. These campaigns try to stimulate interest in buying the advertised food products. The campaigns appear on television, in movie theaters, in malls, and online, often promoting snack-type foods and beverages. These products are usually high in sugar, salt, and saturated fats. The visuals and aromas become environmental cues that encourage you to buy the foods sold in movie theater lobbies and mall food courts. These factors act to override your ability to interpret your body's cues regarding satiety or hunger.

WELLNESS TIP

Are Diet Sodas a Better Choice?

Some studies have suggested that consuming products with low-calorie sweeteners, such as diet soda, can help with weight loss. But other studies support the notion that diet beverages may lead to weight gain. The rationale behind the weight gain theory is that consuming intensely sweet foods (the body perceives diet soda as "intensely sweet") becomes a trigger for craving more sweet foods. The extra energy from the increased consumption of sweet foods is stored as fat. A different theory suggests that people who drink diet sodas reason that they have avoided enough calories to have a second helping of food.

The effectiveness of using artificially sweetened beverages for dieting purposes is not clear. Moderation in consuming added sugars and sweeteners is recommended. Water is the preferred fluid for weight management.

Overconsumption of these types of foods is a factor associated with the overweight and obesity crisis in America (**Figure 13.6**).

Being aware of when and why you eat is important. This will help you realize when you are responding to environmental cues rather than hunger. Developing this awareness of your eating habits can help you avoid overeating. When a cue triggers eating, replace your eating response with a response that makes you feel good about yourself. For example, coming home from school may be an environmental cue to have a snack. Families can help provide healthy cues for you. Seeing fruit on the table, rather than cookies or chips, may be just the cue you need to make a healthier food choice. To avoid the sedentary habit of playing video games after school, you could change your response to this cue and go outdoors for a social game of basketball.

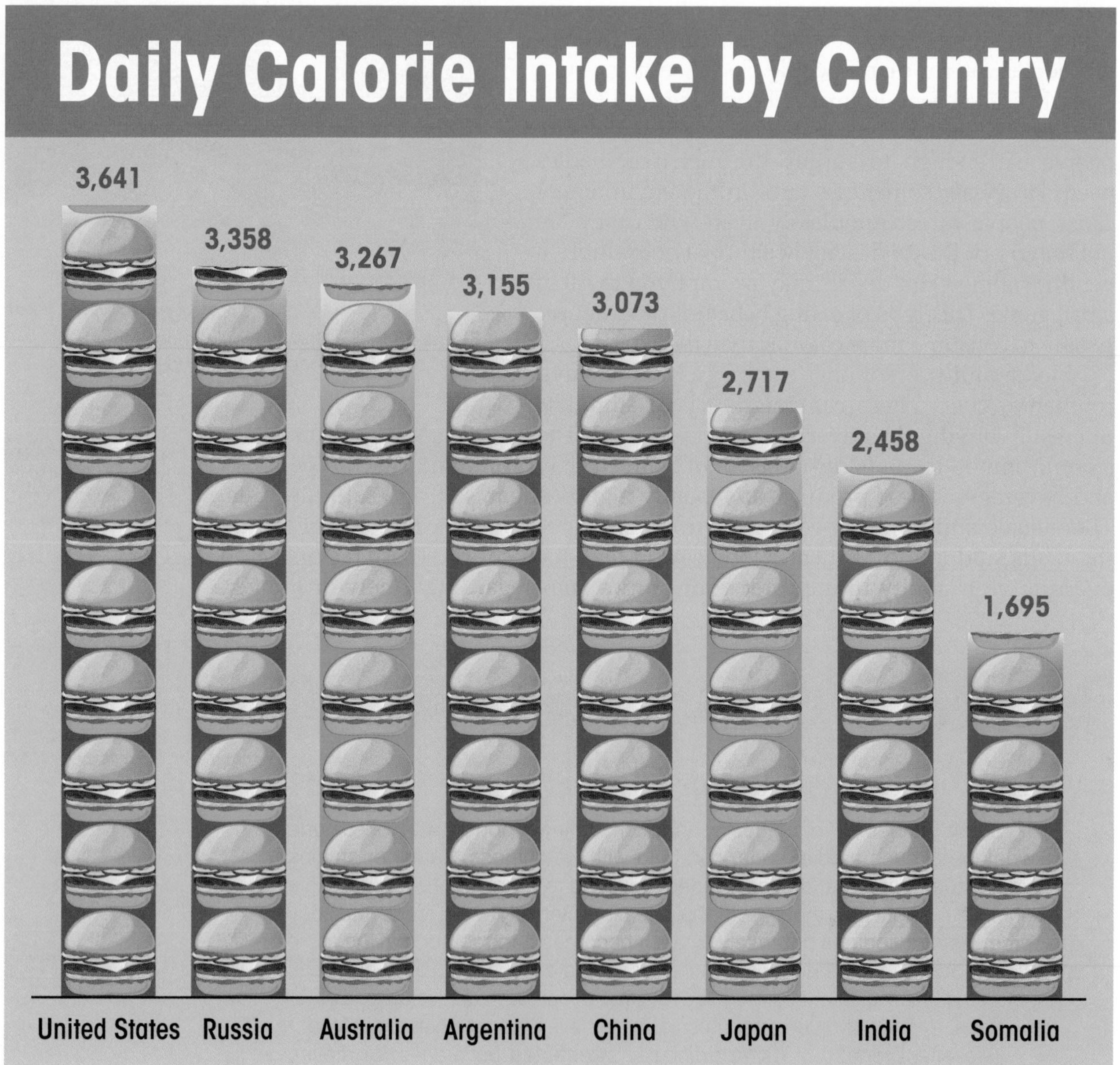

Alfazet Chronicles/Shutterstock.com

Figure 13.6 Average daily calorie consumption in the United States is greater than that of most other countries. *What factors do you think contribute to this excess calorie intake?*

Psychological Factors

Have you ever noticed your emotions influencing when and how much you eat? Eating habits are sometimes responses to psychological factors. Boredom, depression, tension, fear, and loneliness may all lead to irregular eating patterns. Some people respond to such feelings by overeating—others respond by failing to eat.

Good nutrition can help you maintain good health, which is an important tool in handling emotional challenges. Try to notice which emotions affect your eating behaviors. Look for appropriate ways to deal with these emotions while following a nutritious diet. For instance, if you find yourself reaching for food when you are bored, consider going for a walk instead. This will promote your total state of wellness.

Mindful Eating

Simply being more aware while you are eating may be a way to combat the environmental cues and psychological factors that contribute to overeating. This strategy is referred to as *mindful eating* and is being proposed as an approach to eating that could help with weight management.

This strategy suggests focusing all your attention on the food as you are eating to combat the "mindless" eating that often occurs. Mindful eating requires removing all distractions during mealtime or any other time food is being consumed. Additionally, it involves considering the work and resources that went into growing and preparing the food. Mindful eating encourages eating more slowly while giving thought to the color, texture, aroma, and flavor of the food. This strategy promotes being attentive to your body as you are eating and recognizing when your appetite has been **sated** (fully satisfied).

Activity Level

Physical activity levels affect weight status by influencing the "calories out" side of the energy balance equation. If you burn the same number of calories you consume, you will maintain your present weight. If you burn fewer calories than you consume, you will gain weight. If you burn more calories than you consume, you will lose weight.

One of the ways your body burns calories is through physical activity. As you become more active, you need more calories for energy.

For some people, an energy excess is the result of overeating. For many people, however, an energy excess is due to physical inactivity. Many people in today's society spend much time doing sedentary activities. They ride in a car instead of walking. They watch television, play video games, or use electronic devices and the Internet to connect with friends instead of taking part in physical activities (**Figure 13.7**).

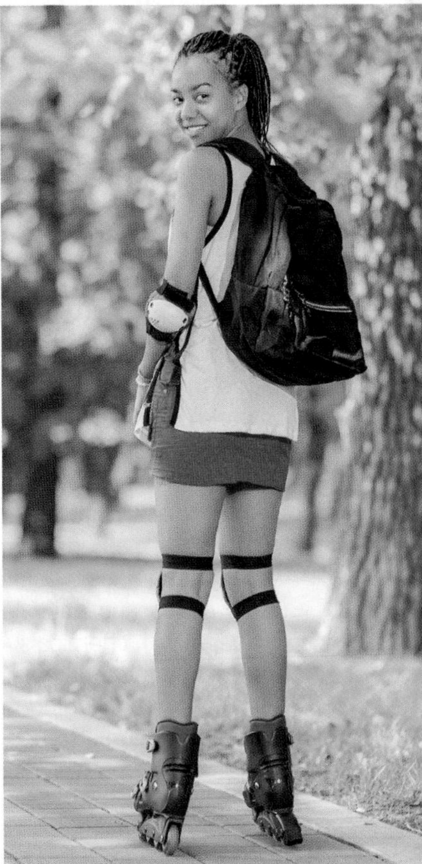

Dmitry Morgan/Shutterstock.com

Figure 13.7 Daily physical activity can be increased by choosing to skate or ride a bike to school instead of taking the bus or driving.

Losing Excess Body Fat

People who are overweight due to excess body fat would improve their health by reducing their fat stores. Creating an energy imbalance is required for weight loss. Numerous strategies for accomplishing this goal are promoted in books, magazines, and online. Some of these strategies are safe and effective, while others are dangerous. Knowing some basic information can help overweight people make sound weight-management decisions.

Consider Health Status

People should consider several factors when thinking about beginning a weight-loss program. One factor is health status. Women should not try to lose weight during pregnancy. Nutritious foods and a minimum weight gain are required to ensure the health of a developing fetus. People who are ill should avoid restricting calories to lose weight. The body needs an adequate supply of nutrients to restore health. Meeting these nutrient needs is difficult when calories are severely restricted.

Consider Age

Age is another issue to keep in mind when considering a plan to reduce body fat. Weight loss is not recommended for children and teens who are still growing. Losing weight could permanently stunt their growth. The recommendation for children and teens is to hold weight steady and grow in height without gaining weight. If a child is extremely obese, then healthcare supervision is needed.

FOOD AND THE ENVIRONMENT

Environmental Sustainability Through Mindful Eating

Mindful eating is a term often used by weight-management counselors to remind people to think carefully about their food choices and food portions before consuming food. Being mindful means being aware of your surroundings—physically, emotionally, mentally, and environmentally.

Mindfulness can also be applied to practicing environmentally sustainable eating. First, think about how much food you need in relation to how hungry you are. Acquiring more food than you need means you may be contributing to environmental food waste. Think about where the food you are eating comes from and the effects on Earth's resources. Responsible growing, harvesting, selling, preparing, and eating of foods plays a central role in the world's ability to preserve Earth's water, land, and air.

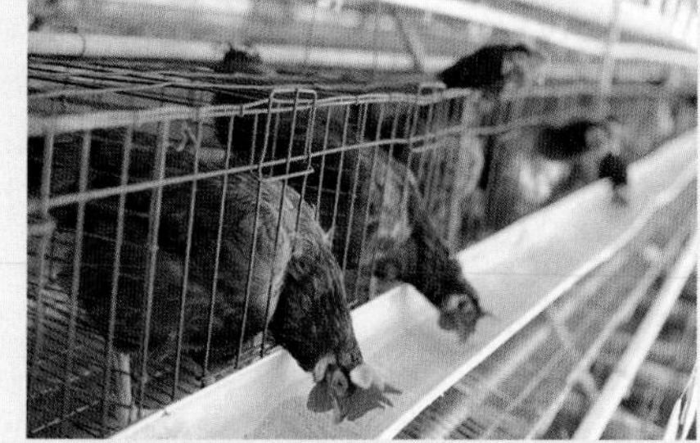

Aumsama/Shutterstock.com

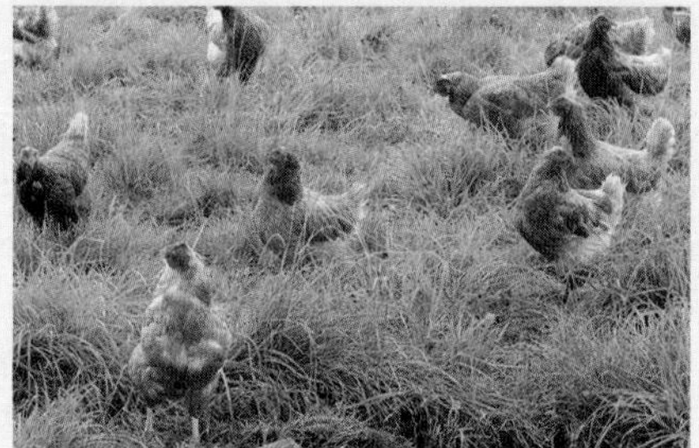

TFoxFoto/Shutterstock.com

For instance, mindful eating may cause you to question the type of fish you are consuming. Is that species being overfished? What methods are being used to catch the fish? Are these methods damaging the environment? Are livestock treated humanely before they are slaughtered for food? Are the plants and animals from which your dinner is sourced treated with chemicals that might harm human health?

As a mindful consumer, you might want to know where foods are grown, and how much transportation, packaging, and refrigeration was involved in putting your food on the table. Mindfulness enables people to connect with and fully appreciate the food they eat in a way that is healthy for themselves as well as the environment.

Think Critically

1. What challenges to practicing mindful eating can you identify? How can these challenges be overcome?
2. Remember a particular food choice you made in the past week. Propose an alternate, more mindful food choice you could have made.

Fad Diets and Other Weight-Loss Gimmicks

New weight-loss schemes turn up every day. These schemes show up on teen or sports magazines and websites. You will likely find descriptions of eating plans promising rapid weight loss. Such plans that are popular for a short time are often referred to as ***fad diets***.

Pills, body wraps, gels, and other weight-loss gimmicks are also widely available. These products are often advertised with words like *fast-working*, *incredible energy*, *inexpensive*, *painless*, and *guaranteed*. However, the advertising is often more effective than the products. Consumers spend millions of dollars on dubious weight-loss products every year.

You may read advice such as, "Eat all the protein you want, but avoid fattening carbohydrates." You might hear of a plan that suggests you "eat only rice for 10 days, and lose a pound a day." With all the slick advertising, separating dieting truth from **fallacy** (falsehood) can be difficult.

Research on several kinds of anti-obesity pills reported that people still remained obese with the use of the drugs. The truth is anyone can make a claim about how to lose or gain weight. Many people who promote dieting schemes lack medical or nutrition training. These people may be more interested in your money than your health.

Perhaps you assume that federal agencies will protect you from weight-loss frauds and the hucksters who promote them. However, the FDA and FTC take action only when false claims are made about particular products or foods.

The best way to deal with diet fads is to arm yourself with nutrition knowledge. Consult a registered dietitian nutritionist or qualified nutrition educator if you have questions about the claims of a particular dieting scheme (**Figure 13.10**).

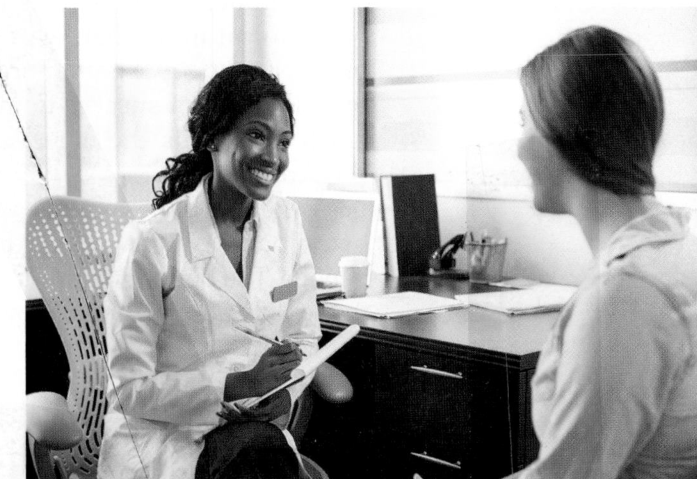

Monkey Business Images/Shutterstock.com

Figure 13.10 Consult a health professional if you are unsure about the efficacy of a weight-loss scheme.

Dangers of Rapid Weight-Loss Plans

Weight-loss diets that provide fewer than 1,200 calories per day are sometimes referred to as *crash diets*. Such diets lack essential nutrients. ChooseMyPlate.gov should be used to guide weight loss to ensure that recommended amounts from each food group are eaten.

Fasting is a form of crash dieting. ***Fasting*** means to refrain from consuming most or all sources of calories. Fasting over an extended period can create health problems. Within 24 hours of beginning a fast, the body's carbohydrate stores will be depleted. After this, the body will slowly begin breaking down lean tissues, including muscles and organs, to produce energy. The body will also convert fatty acids from body fat into ketone bodies that can fuel the nervous system. An abnormal buildup of ketone bodies in the bloodstream, which is known as *ketosis*, can be dangerous. Ketosis affects the acid-base balance of the blood.

Ineffectiveness of Rapid Weight-Loss Plans

Crash diets seldom produce long-lasting weight-loss results and have high rates of **recidivism** (relapse). Crash dieting may produce some dramatic initial weight loss; however, most of this weight loss is due to fluid loss. When the diet ends, fluid levels in the body readjust and water weight is quickly regained.

Losing weight too fast will reduce glycogen stores used for energy and protein stores found in muscle tissue.

Fad diets often have several drawbacks that make them ineffective for weight loss. Very low-calorie diets trigger the body to lower BMR, which makes it harder to lose weight. Fad diet plans usually tell people exactly how much and what they can eat. This gives people no control over their food choices. Fad diets require eating patterns that are radically different from most people's normal eating habits. This causes many people to give up on the diet because they miss the foods they are accustomed to eating. Fad diets teach people nothing about better eating behaviors. These diets are not designed to help people maintain their new weights. After completing the diet, most people return to their old eating habits and the lost weight quickly returns.

For some people, crash dieting leads to weight cycling. ***Weight cycling*** is a pattern of repeatedly losing and gaining weight over time. Weight cycling is sometimes referred to as the *yo-yo diet syndrome*. Following the diet, people begin to eat more than ever simply because they feel starved and deprived of food. Some people gain more weight than they lost by dieting. Discouragement over the lack of success in maintaining weight loss causes them to try another crash diet. This dieting cycle may be repeated many times throughout life (**Figure 13.11**).

Weight cycling may create feelings of stress and greater dissatisfaction with body looks. Weight loss for individuals who are overweight or obese is a health benefit. The better goal for losing weight is to commit to a lifelong pattern of permanent, healthy eating and activity behaviors.

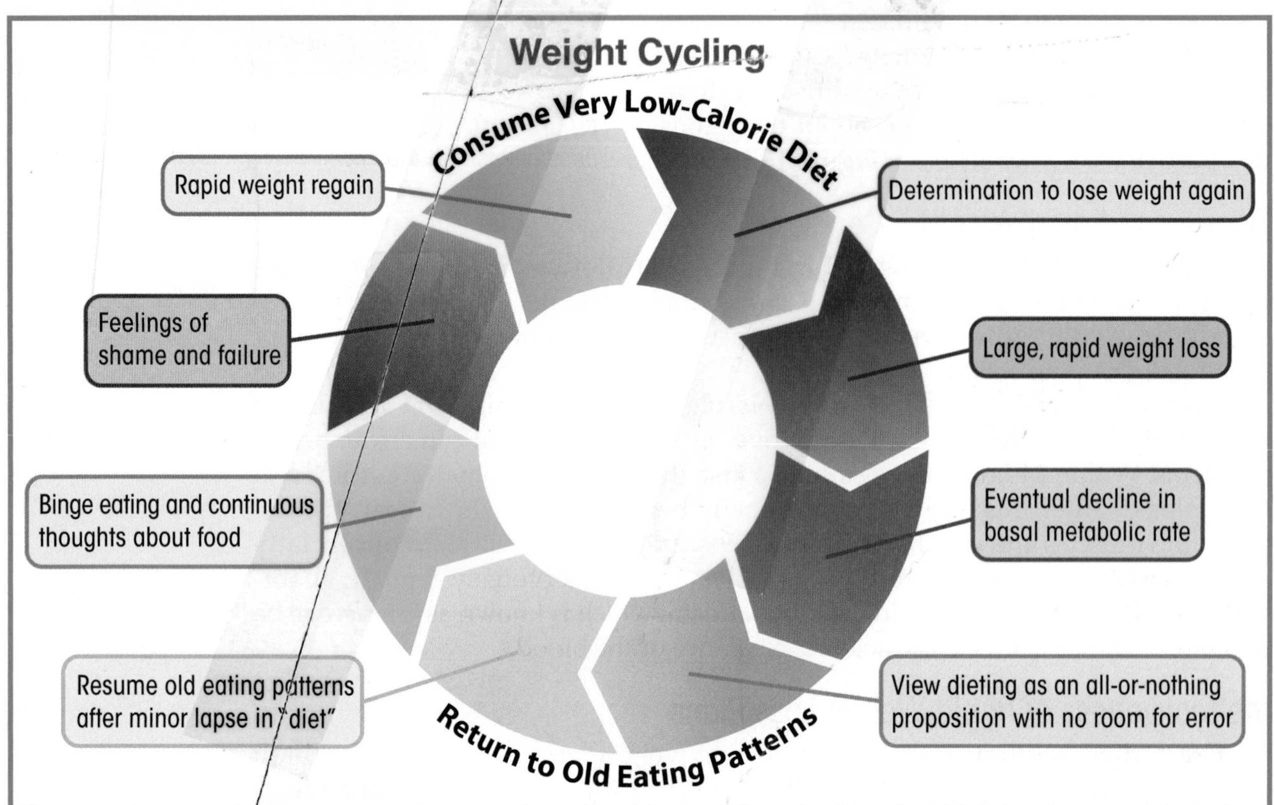

Figure 13.11 Failing to make permanent, sustainable changes in eating and physical activity habits most often results in a cycle of weight loss followed by regaining the weight.

Safe Fat-Loss Guidelines

Weight-management experts often advise people not to think of losing weight as "dieting." Likewise, they suggest not viewing food as an enemy to fight. Instead, they recommend thinking of losing weight as managing calorie and fat intake. Foods do not need to be eliminated, but rather chosen with fitness and health in mind. Experts also remind people that food is meant to be enjoyed. It just needs to be enjoyed in moderation.

People with health problems should talk to a doctor before beginning a weight-management program. A medical checkup is always recommended before children and teens begin a program. A checkup is also advised for people in other age groups who are trying to lose excess pounds.

Having correct information can help people be sure their weight-management efforts are safe and effective. The following guidelines for changing eating habits promote wellness through the loss of excess body fat.

Evaluate Programs Carefully

Evaluating a weight-management program's effectiveness and related risks can be rather confusing. If a weight-management program sounds too good to you, be sure to read the information carefully. Always be wary of schemes that encourage unsound eating patterns. Registered dietitian nutritionists can counsel people about sensible weight management.

Choose a weight-management program that is nutritionally sound. For greatest success, it should produce weight loss at a slow rate. It should also include a component of moderate exercise. A healthy weight-management program should

- provide all the needed nutrients for your age and gender;
- be agreeable with your food tastes;
- not result in extreme hunger or fatigue;
- allow participation in your typical social routine (**Figure 13.12**);
- be sustainable for the rest of your life; and
- stress regular physical activity.

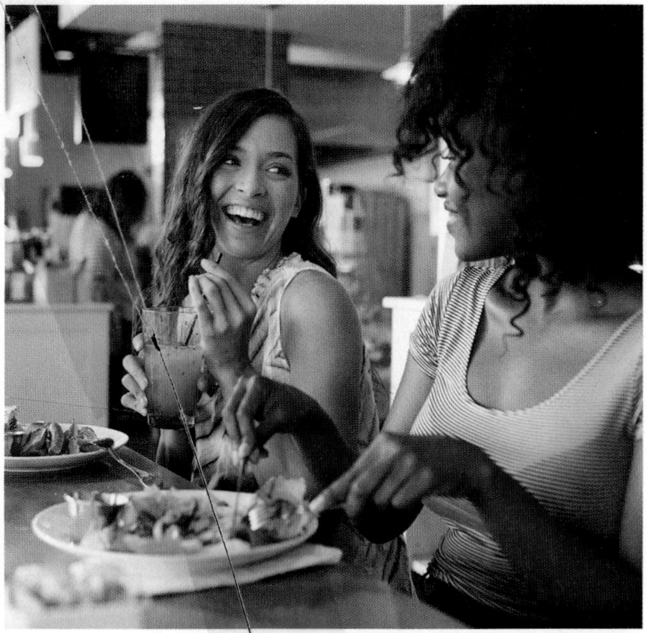

Monkey Business Images/Shutterstock.com

Figure 13.12 An effective weight-loss plan is one that can be followed in social settings as well as at home. *Why is this important?*

Avoid weight-management programs that stress the eating of single food items. For instance, a diet that suggests eating only bananas does not reflect normal eating behaviors. Such a diet may be dangerous because it is not nutritionally balanced. Remember, a nutritious diet includes foods from all the major food groups in the MyPlate system.

Beware of plans that restrict which foods you can eat. This includes diet plans that stress eating mostly one macronutrient, usually protein. These eating plans may lack important vitamins, minerals, and phytochemicals that are abundant in fruits and vegetables. Diets high in saturated fats increase blood cholesterol levels and add to the risk of heart disease.

Avoid diet plans that require the use of pills. Many diet pills are ineffective and the long-term effects are unknown. No known pill can eliminate body fat. Some pills can help suppress appetite or prevent fat absorption, but they cannot correct poor eating habits. Some diet pills may be addictive; others produce a variety of side effects.

Avoid weight-management programs that suggest fasting or modified fasting. Liquid diets and other programs that are very low in calories may cause fatigue, irritability, nausea, and digestive upsets. They can also affect heartbeat rhythm and the acid level of the blood.

Be wary of weight-loss plans that promise large weight losses in a short time. Dieters who constantly follow the "latest and greatest" diet scheme often find only short-term successes. People who lose weight slowly are more likely to maintain a healthy weight once they reach it. Losing weight slowly also reduces health risks.

Through a combined eating and exercise plan, a person should attempt to lose no more than one to two pounds a week. Teens who are growing taller should modify this advice by maintaining weight throughout their growth. Gradual weight loss gives the body time to adjust. Remember, it takes time to gain excess weight. It will also take time to lose it without jeopardizing health.

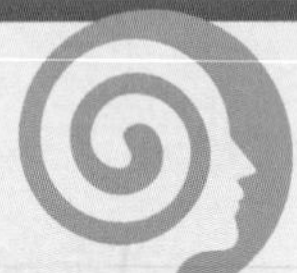

EXTEND YOUR KNOWLEDGE

Heavily-Processed Foods and Weight Gain

Many forms of food processing are beneficial. Processing techniques such as freezing, fermenting, canning, and drying have been used for hundreds of years to preserve food.

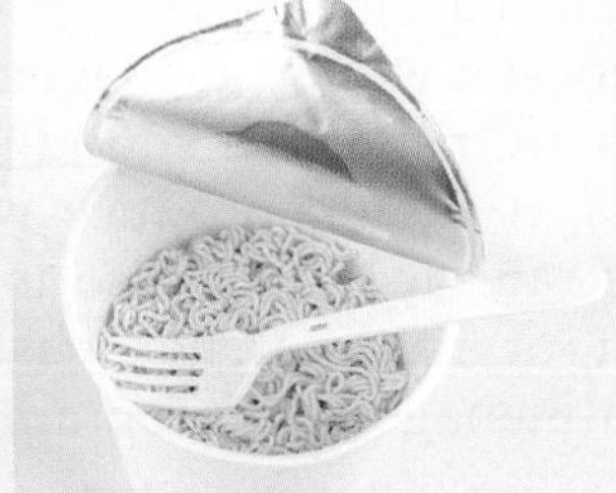

anaken2012/Shutterstock.com

When only a few basic ingredients are added, it is considered minimal processing. In more recent years, foods found on store shelves are processed with a complex formulation of ingredients and are called *heavily-processed foods*. Heavily-processed foods are food products that are generally cheap, ready-to-eat, and include added salt, sugars, and solid fats in addition to substances not used during typical food preparation. These ingredients are added to enhance flavors and textures, and to preserve the shelf life of the product. Examples of heavily-processed foods include soft drinks, packaged baked goods, reconstituted meat products, instant noodles and soups, and sugary cereals.

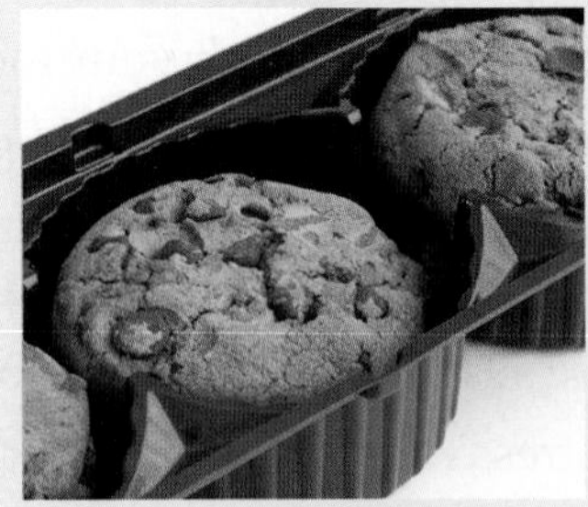

Moving Moment/Shutterstock.com

Many of the calories in heavily-processed foods come from added sugar. The number of calories per serving can be higher than for the same food in its fresh or minimally processed form. Additionally, these foods are often low in health-promoting nutrients such as fiber, vitamins, minerals, and phytochemicals.

Consuming these foods as a major part of an eating pattern is a factor that many nutrition researchers associate with the overweight and obesity epidemic in America. The overconsumption of these foods is rapidly increasing in the United States and around the world. Heavily-processed food products are vigorously advertised and considered very profitable. Exactly how these foods are contributing to the global epidemic of obesity continues to be evaluated.

What strategies would you suggest to encourage people to consume fewer heavily-processed foods and more whole, unprocessed or minimally processed foods? What role should government and the food industry play to help solve the obesity crisis?

Plan Food Choices

Your food choices determine the number of calories you consume. The following suggestions for selecting foods may help you manage calories:

- Reduce calories from saturated fats (**Figure 13.13**).
- Eat more vegetables and whole-grain foods. Make them the main dishes instead of the side dishes in your menus.
- Choose fresh fruits as an alternative to snack foods and desserts that are high in added sugars and saturated fats.
- When eating out, choose steamed, baked, or broiled foods rather than fried items. Ask for sauces and salad dressings on the side. Consider splitting an entrée with a friend, or take part of your food home for a later meal.
- Select recipes that are low in saturated fats. For instance, you might sauté vegetables in olive oil instead of butter or simply cook them in broth for added flavor.
- Use healthy food preparation methods. For example, microwave or steam vegetables and season with lemon juice instead of butter and salt.

Following these basic guidelines will help you maintain good health and a healthy weight while enjoying a delicious diet.

Substitutions to Reduce Calories from Saturated Fats

Replace...		With...
Sour cream	→	Nonfat yogurt
Cream or nondairy creamers	→	Evaporated fat-free milk
Whole or 2% fat milk	→	Fat-free or 1% fat milk
Mayonnaise	→	Avocado slices
Regular cheese	→	Reduced-fat cheese
Ice cream	→	Low-fat or nonfat dairy desserts
Butter cake, mousse, or fruit pie	→	Angel food cake, sponge cake, gelatin, or fresh fruits
Cream soups	→	Broth-based soups
Butter, lard, or stick margarine	→	Olive oil or reduced-fat margarine in tubs
Doughnuts, pastries	→	Whole-grain bagels, English muffins, or toasted bread
Chips or other fried snacks	→	Pretzels, air-popped popcorn, or saltines
Chocolate chip cookies	→	Graham crackers, vanilla wafers, or gingersnaps

Figure 13.13 A healthier eating pattern can be achieved by reducing calories from saturated fats. *Can you think of other substitutions for saturated fats in your eating pattern?*

Change Eating Habits

A food journal is a key weight-management tool. It can help you identify eating habits shaped by environmental cues and psychological factors. When completing your journal, list the time of day, the location, who you are with, and what you are doing. Record your state of mind at the time as well.

Analyze your completed food journal to better understand your eating patterns. Do you snack while watching television? Do you eat after school? Do you skip any meals? Do you tend to eat more when you are alone or with friends? Answering questions like these may help you learn where and why you might be consuming excess or unhealthy calories.

Once you recognize problem eating behaviors, you can explore ways to change them. For example, you may realize the snack counter at the movies tempts you to eat. As a solution, you may decide not to bring money for snacks when you go to the movies. Your new habits should not be temporary adjustments until you lose a few pounds. View your eating and activity habits as permanent changes that will help you maintain a healthy weight status throughout your life.

Knowing how emotions affect your eating behaviors can help you manage these behaviors. You may find you eat when you feel lonely or bored. If so, prepare a list of activities you can do instead of eating when these feelings overtake you. For instance, when you feel lonely, call a friend. If you are bored, try working on a hobby (**Figure 13.14**).

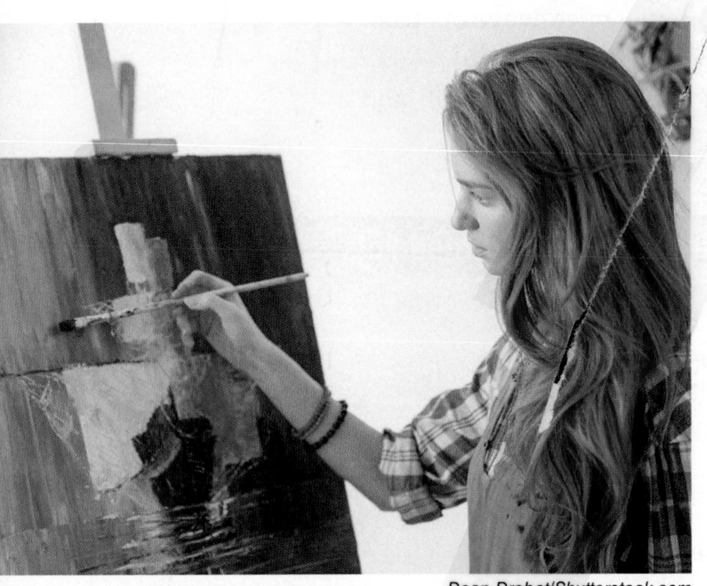

Dean Drobot/Shutterstock.com

Figure 13.14 Working on a hobby will take your mind off food when you are bored or lonely.

Modifying your behavior involves finding ways to change your responses when overeating is a concern. For instance, suppose a friend invites you to an after-school study session at his home. The friend sets out a bowl of potato chips and dip. How can you change this environmental cue so you do not overeat? You could move away from the bowl of chips. This may prevent you from responding to their sight and smell. You might also bring some fruit or cut vegetables to share with your friend while you study. Eating a healthy snack can help satisfy your desire to nibble.

Use a Behavior-Change Contract

One way to change an eating habit is to write a behavior-change contract. This is an agreement with yourself about the methods you will use to reach a personal goal. Written contracts seem to work better than mental or verbal contracts. In the contract, write what you plan to do. You might write, "I will always choose water to drink instead of getting a soft drink when I see a vending machine." Your food journal can quickly show you if you are achieving your goal. After you reach one goal, you can celebrate success and move on to another goal.

Do not be discouraged if you fail to live up to your contract. You may have set a goal that was unrealistic. Evaluate the methods you are using and your ability to reach your goals. Rewrite your contract if necessary. With practice, you will be able to use behavior-change contracts to improve your eating habits.

Use a Point System

Another technique some people find helpful for modifying eating habits is a point system. Give yourself a set number of points for healthful eating behaviors. For example, snacking on carrot sticks instead of corn chips might be worth a point. Skipping a rich dessert might be worth two points. After collecting a set number of points, treat yourself to a reward such as a movie or a new music download. Avoid giving yourself a reward that involves food.

Increase Levels of Daily Activity

Besides making careful food choices, you need to focus on your level of physical activity. Try to complete one hour a day of physical activity at a moderate and enjoyable pace. Many studies show people lose weight faster and maintain weight loss longer when physical activity is increased along with calorie restriction. Exercise speeds the body's metabolism as body composition changes to a higher proportion of muscle. Exercise also curbs short-term hunger for some people.

THE MOVEMENT CONNECTION

Quadriceps Stretch

Why

Just like eating habits, physical activity habits are often difficult to break. If you perform the Movement Connection activities in this text (whether at home or in class), you are on your way to changing your physical activity habits.

Homework and studying can add up to many hours sitting. Break up long periods of study with activity such as this quadriceps, or "quad" stretch. This can help you refocus and reenergize while providing physical benefits.

Apply

- Push your chair into your desk and stand centered behind it. Place your left hand on the back of the chair for balance.
- Standing with good posture, raise the heel of your right foot back toward your hamstring (back of your thigh).
- Grasp the top of your foot (where your shoelaces are) and hold it to the count of 30.
- Slowly lower your foot to the floor.
- Repeat with your left foot.
- Repeat three times for each leg.

Modification

- For an added challenge, as you stretch your right quad, lift your left arm straight up toward the ceiling.
- Keep your core engaged throughout the stretch to maintain your balance.

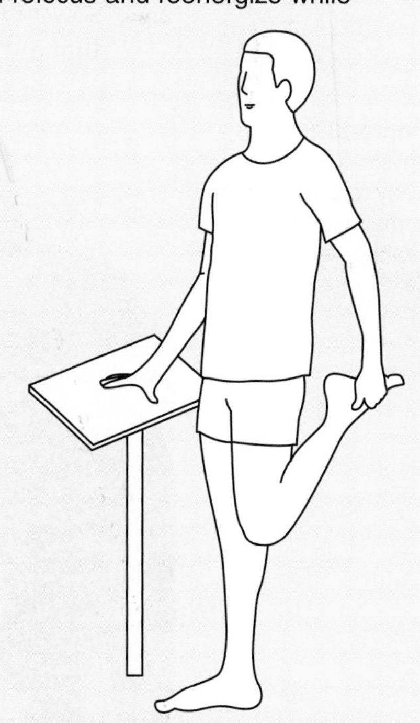

Simply changing food habits is not enough for weight loss. Physical activity is an especially important weight-loss strategy for children and teens. Young people need energy from food to support their growth. With moderate daily activity, they can lose weight without reducing their intake of nutritious foods (**Figure 13.15**).

Tips for Healthy Weight Loss

If you have trouble achieving or maintaining a healthy weight, try the following tips:

- Avoid eating a large amount of food at any one time of the day. Spread the day's calories over all your meals. Eat at least three regularly planned meals throughout each day.
- Measure your food and keep portion sizes moderate.
- Plan your meals and snacks to avoid snacking binges which may lead to weight gain.
- Make breakfast a habit. It gets you through the morning without experiencing extreme hunger. If you become exceedingly hungry, you are more likely to overeat.
- Keep a "lean" refrigerator and cupboard. Focus on stocking nutritious foods that are nutrient dense. Select foods that make you feel full when you eat them. Carrots, apples, plums, and whole-grain breads have food bulk to help you feel full. Keep foods that are high in calories and low in nutrients out of sight most of the time.
- Avoid eating after 7:00 p.m. Studies indicate that eating excess calories in the evening increases your chances of weight gain.
- Eat slowly. Lay your fork down between bites of food. You will feel full with less food. Set a timer and spend at least 20 minutes eating your meal.
- Avoid talking on the phone or watching TV during meals to avoid mindless eating and to focus on the food you are eating.
- Drink a glass of water before a meal. This may help you feel a little fuller, so you will eat less. Reduce amounts of soft drinks, sodas, or fruit punches that are calorie dense.

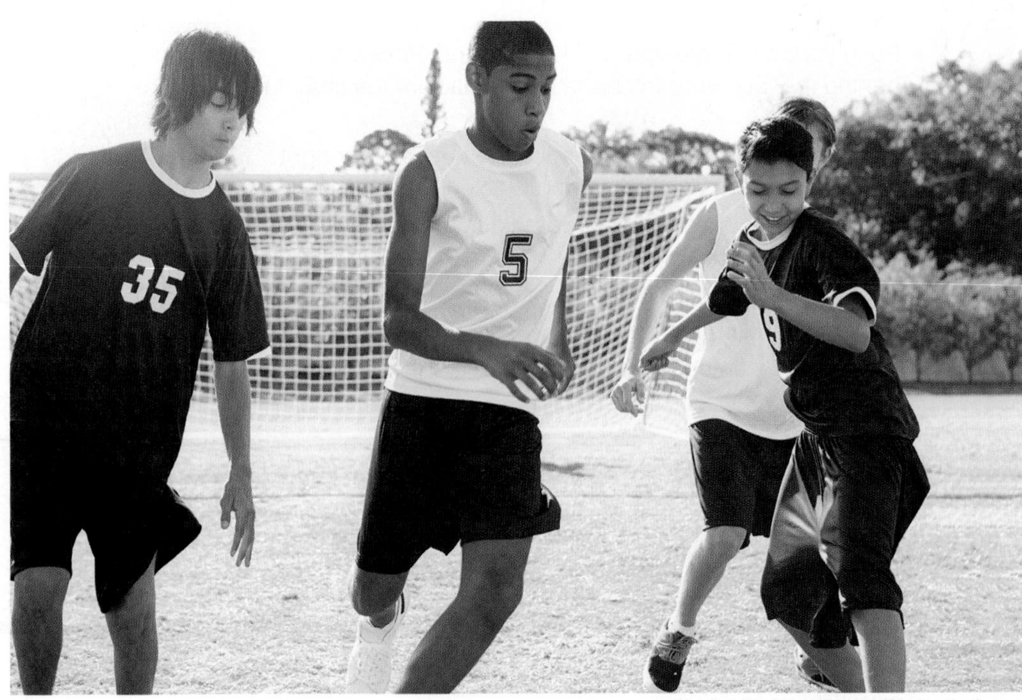

Figure 13.15 Physical activity plays a key role in reaching or maintaining a healthy weight.

Monkey Business Images/Shutterstock.com

- Avoid feeling the need to finish leftover foods. Store leftovers promptly and eat them at another meal.
- Use a smaller plate to manage portion sizes. Moderate portions look larger on a small plate.
- Avoid taking second helpings of foods. Serve yourself one plate. Avoid having all the food placed in serving dishes on the table.
- When eating out, try to decide what you will have before other people order and stick with your decision. This will keep you from being swayed by the power of suggestion if your companions order unhealthy foods.
- Avoid weighing yourself more than once or twice a week. If you are following a healthful weight-loss plan, you will be losing no more than two pounds per week. Therefore, frequent weight checks are unlikely to show much progress and may result in discouragement.
- Maintain regular sleep patterns and get about eight to ten hours each night. Research reports say that sleep loss can lead to overeating and snacking on energy-dense foods (**Figure 13.16**).
- Be physically active. In addition to burning calories, you cannot eat while you are being physically active.

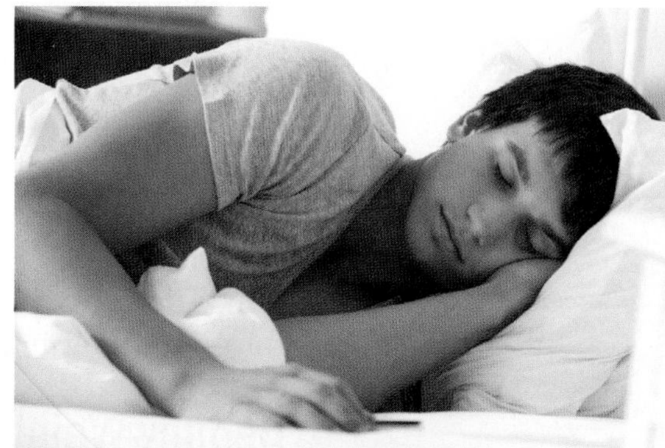

Monkey Business Images/Shutterstock.com

Figure 13.16 Teens who get sufficient sleep and maintain regular sleep patterns are more likely to be a healthy weight.

Maintain Weight Loss

Losing excess weight is quite an accomplishment for individuals who are overweight or obese. Health benefits are gained. Unfortunately, many individuals who lose weight have great difficulty maintaining their new weight status. Maintaining a new weight status requires different responses to food than before the weight loss. If the individual resumes former eating patterns and physical activity behaviors, the result is a rather quick return of unwanted pounds.

The following tips are some of the common characteristics among people who have successfully improved and maintained their weight status.

- Follow a healthy eating pattern. Several studies have shown that your body will need fewer calories to maintain weight than before weight loss was achieved. Your resting metabolism is lowered and hunger hormone levels have changed. Without some professional assistance, your body may be driving you toward your old weight status.
- Maintain a consistent eating pattern, even if your routine changes. When eating out or visiting friends, try to follow your same food eating plans.
- Eat breakfast every day. Eating breakfast is a common trait among people who have lost weight and kept it off.
- Engage in 60 to 90 minutes of moderate intensity physical activity most days of the week. Some people may need to talk to their healthcare provider before participating in this level of physical activity.
- Continue to maintain a food and physical activity journal. You will be able to track your progress and identify problems.
- Check your weight regularly. If you have gained a few pounds, get back on track quickly.
- Request support from family, friends, and others. Sometimes having a friend or partner who is also losing weight or maintaining lost weight can help you stay motivated.

Gaining Weight

For some people, managing their weight status might require adding pounds to body weight. Health issues are not as severe for moderately thin people as for people with obesity. However, being underweight may hamper a person's ability to feel strong and healthy. Underweight may also increase a person's susceptibility to infectious diseases such as colds and flu. A BMI of 18.5 and under may indicate malnutrition. The causes of underweight should be medically determined. Anyone who has unexpected weight loss should have a physical exam. A doctor can make sure there are no health problems causing the weight loss.

Gaining weight is as hard for someone who is underweight as losing weight is for someone who is overweight. Healthy weight gain should be due to a combination of fat stores and muscle tissue. Some people seem to inherit a tendency to be thin. They have difficulty storing body fat. However, they can add muscle mass through strength training exercises, such as weight lifting.

Healthy Weight Gain Plan

As with weight loss, weight gain requires a plan (**Figure 13.17**). Gaining weight means consuming more calories than the body expends. The goal is to gain lean body mass, not simply fat tissue. To build lean body mass (muscle), physical activity is necessary. Registered dietitians often recommend that people trying to gain weight consume 500 extra calories per day to gain an extra pound of body weight per week. Depending on your level of physical activity, 700 to 1,000 calories extra may be appropriate.

Figure 13.17 When trying to gain weight, additional calories should come from healthy food sources more often.

Tips for Healthy Weight Gain
• Choose calorie-dense foods containing healthy fats such as the mono- and polyunsaturated fats found in avocadoes, peanut butter, olives, and nuts.
• Snack on dried fruits which are nutrient- and energy-dense choices.
• Add small amounts of calorie-dense toppings, such as salad dressings, croutons, and dessert sauces.
• Try eating larger, more frequent meals.
• Consume snacks between meals, such as sandwiches, puddings, and thick vegetable soups.
• Add juices, milk, and low-fat milk shakes as fluid sources in addition to water.
• Carry snacks such as granola bars, trail mix, cheese and crackers, vegetables and dip, and dried fruit.
• Avoid drinking extra fluids before eating or during your meal.
• Add a weight-lifting or resistance training program to help increase lean body mass and body weight.
• Sleep between 8 and 10 hours per night.

Of course, the source of these calories should be nutritious foods. Added calories will create an energy excess over what is needed for the increased level of activity. Using a slow, steady approach to weight gain is the safest, most effective way to put on pounds. Gaining one-half to one pound per week is acceptable.

Avoid Unhealthy Strategies

A teen who has a distorted body image may be driven to build a very muscular body. When a teen perceives his or her body as too thin or lacking muscles, a harmful interest in shaping very large muscles may result. Sometimes this leads to use of drugs and other harmful strategies for weight gain and muscle building.

People who are trying to gain weight need to avoid fads and gimmicks. Many bodybuilding magazines and websites advertise products that promise to help people "bulk up" fast. These products may not provide a proper balance of nutrients. They will not help people establish long-term healthful eating habits. Some of these products may also have harmful side effects.

RECIPE FILE

Salmon Burgers

4 SERVINGS

Ingredients

- 1 lb. salmon fillet, no skin
- 1 clove garlic, crushed
- 6 sprigs fresh oregano
- 2 scallions, chopped finely
- 2 t. reduced-fat mayonnaise
- ¾ c. panko bread crumbs, divided
- 1 t. lemon zest

Directions

1. Examine salmon for small bones and remove.
2. Finely chop salmon and place in large bowl.
3. Flatten garlic on cutting board with side of a chef's knife until it resembles a paste. Add to salmon.
4. Remove leaves from oregano stems and chop finely. Add to salmon.
5. Add scallions, mayonnaise, ½ cup of the bread crumbs, and lemon zest to the salmon. Mix gently until combined.
6. Form into four patties (¾-inch thick).
7. Press salmon patties into remaining ¼ cup bread crumbs.
8. Heat 2 teaspoons olive oil in large skillet over medium-high heat.
9. When oil is hot, add bread crumb-coated salmon patties.
10. Cook 3–4 minutes, until browned on bottom, then turn and cook 3–4 minutes more, until browned and reaches 145°F (63°C). Patty will be springy in the center when pressed.
11. Remove patties from pan to a paper towel-lined plate.
12. Serve with Arugula Corn Salad (recipe found in Chapter 14).

PER SERVING: 251 CALORIES, 25 G PROTEIN, 15 G CARBOHYDRATE, 9 G FAT, 1 G FIBER, 229 MG SODIUM.

Chapter 13 Review and Expand

Reading Summary

Weight management means achieving a healthy weight and maintaining it throughout life. People who are either underweight or overweight are at increased risk of health problems.

Several factors affect your weight and your ability to put on and take off pounds. These factors include your heredity, eating habits, and level of physical activity. Environmental cues and psychological factors can influence your eating habits.

People who want to lose weight should first evaluate their health and consider their motivation. They need to estimate their current daily calorie needs and daily calorie intake. Comparing these two calorie figures can help them determine an appropriate daily calorie limit to maintain or lose weight.

People trying to lose weight should carefully evaluate the nutritional quality of any weight-loss plan they are considering. Healthful weight loss involves controlling calorie intake through planned food choices. Effective weight loss also demands a plan of daily physical activity.

Weight gain can be just as difficult as weight loss. People who are trying to gain weight need to include more calorie-dense foods in their diets.

Chapter Vocabulary

1. **Content Terms** With a partner, choose two words from the following list to compare. Create a Venn diagram to compare your words and identify differences. Write one term under the left circle and the other term under the right. Where the circles overlap, write two characteristics the terms have in common. For each term, write a difference of the term for each characteristic in its respective outer circle.

environmental cue	metabolic syndrome
fad diet	weight cycling
fasting	weight management
habit	

2. **Academic Terms** Individually or with a partner, create a T-chart on a sheet of paper and list each of the following terms in the left column. In the right column, list an *antonym* (a word of opposite meaning) for each term in the left column.

destine	sated
fallacy	stigma
recidivism	

Review Learning

3. *True or false?* A combination of social, emotional, and physical health risks are associated with overweight and obesity.
4. What are five added health risks associated with obesity?
5. What are two health problems associated with being underweight?
6. How does heredity affect a person's weight status?
7. Who has the greatest influence on eating habits formed early in life?
8. How can a person estimate his or her average daily calorie intake?
9. Why is a fasting diet plan dangerous?
10. What are two reasons fad diets may be ineffective?
11. What is a basic weight-management recommendation for a teenager who is overweight and still growing?
12. What information should be included in a food journal to help people identify factors that prompt them to eat?
13. What are general guidelines for safely losing body fat?
14. How many extra calories should a person who is trying to gain weight consume each day?
15. What are three tips for safe weight gain?

Self-Assessment Quiz

Complete the self-assessment quiz online to help you practice and expand your knowledge and skills.

Critical Thinking

16. **Conclude** What long-term consequences do you see as a result of rapid or ineffective weight-loss plans? Why do you think this is so?
17. **Analyze** Find your daily calorie needs based on your activity level. Keep a food and activity journal for three days. Use food composition tables or diet analysis software to figure your average daily calorie intake. Compare your daily calorie needs according to age, gender, and activity level (see Appendix C), with your totaled average daily caloric intake. How do the actual needs and computed

amounts compare? Consider healthy ways you can balance your energy equation.

18. **Evaluate** Find advertisements for weight-loss products in magazines or online. Create a bulletin board display of the ads. Next to each ad, post your brief evaluation of the product's safety and effectiveness. Cite any research that is available to suggest the product sold is safe or effective.
19. **Implement** Create a plan for adopting a more mindful approach to eating. Your plan should include at least three goals and the steps you are going to take to achieve those goals. Adhere to your plan for one week. Keep a journal to document your feelings during the experiment and any challenges you experienced. At the end of one week, write a summary describing the experience.
20. **Compare** Review the websites of authoritative health organizations such as Mayo Clinic, Cleveland Clinic, and WebMD. Compare the information each website provides about safe weight gain and loss, and how to build or maintain muscle mass. How does the information from each site compare? Share your findings with the class.

Core Skills

21. **Technology Literacy** Plan and write three entries about metabolic syndrome for the class blog. First, consider the audience who will be reading your blog. What does your audience want and need to know about this topic? Then, determine the content and how you will organize it. Select three main points that you want to address each day. Next, create an appealing title to capture your reader's attention. Write each blog entry, providing supporting facts for each main point. Consider providing a tip or action item for each entry.
22. **Speaking** The incidences of obesity, heart disease, and diabetes are increasing among young adults. Debate the following topic: All high school students should be required to take an exercise and nutrition class as a requirement for graduation. Address how this might affect students, the school, and the community.
23. **Math** Select two foods to compare such as raw baby whole carrots and potato chips. Using the serving size on each food's label, determine the weight of each food in grams using a food scale. Divide calories per serving (found on the label) by the weight in grams. Determine which food has the greater number of calories per gram. Identify other foods that have bulk (weight), but few calories per gram.
24. **Writing** Interview a psychologist to learn how behavior modification principles can be applied to weight-management goals. Perform additional research as needed. Write a news report to share what you learn. Write a headline for your report. Open your report with a short paragraph that provides the basic information of the report in a short, concise manner. Write the body of the report including more details, facts, and quotes. The report should be written in third person and convey information, not your opinion.
25. **Writing** Develop a position about the impact of fast foods on eating habits and health. Do the benefits of convenience and reliability outweigh the negative concerns of obesity and other health-related consequences? Write an argumentative paper supporting your position.
26. **Math** Jill weighs 130 pounds. She swims after school three days a week for one hour each of the three days. She learned that swimming at a speed of 20 yards per minute uses 0.058 calories per pound of body weight per minute. How many calories per week does she use swimming?
27. **Writing** Prepare a position statement either supporting or arguing against the need for a state tax on sodas and other sugary drinks as an obesity prevention effort.
28. **Career Readiness Practice** Presume the supermarket you work for is participating in a community health fair that will take place in six months. You are on the planning committee for the exhibit. Your exhibit at the health fair will focus on providing information on healthful foods for weight management. Demonstrations for preparing healthful foods are also being planned. With your committee (several classmates), set the goals for your exhibit. How will you take action on these goals in your exhibit booth? Consider using the U.S. Department of Health and Human Services website, *Healthfinder,* and the NIH *Weight-Control Information Network* website.

CHAPTER 14 Nutrition Across the Life Span

Learning Outcomes

After studying this chapter, you will be able to

- **explain** how nutritional needs are different for people of various ages and activity levels;
- **consider** how to avoid health and nutritional-related issues specific to each stage of the life cycle;
- **evaluate** food choices to best meet nutritional needs at each stage of the life cycle; and
- **critique** the role of activity in nutrition and fitness through the life cycle.

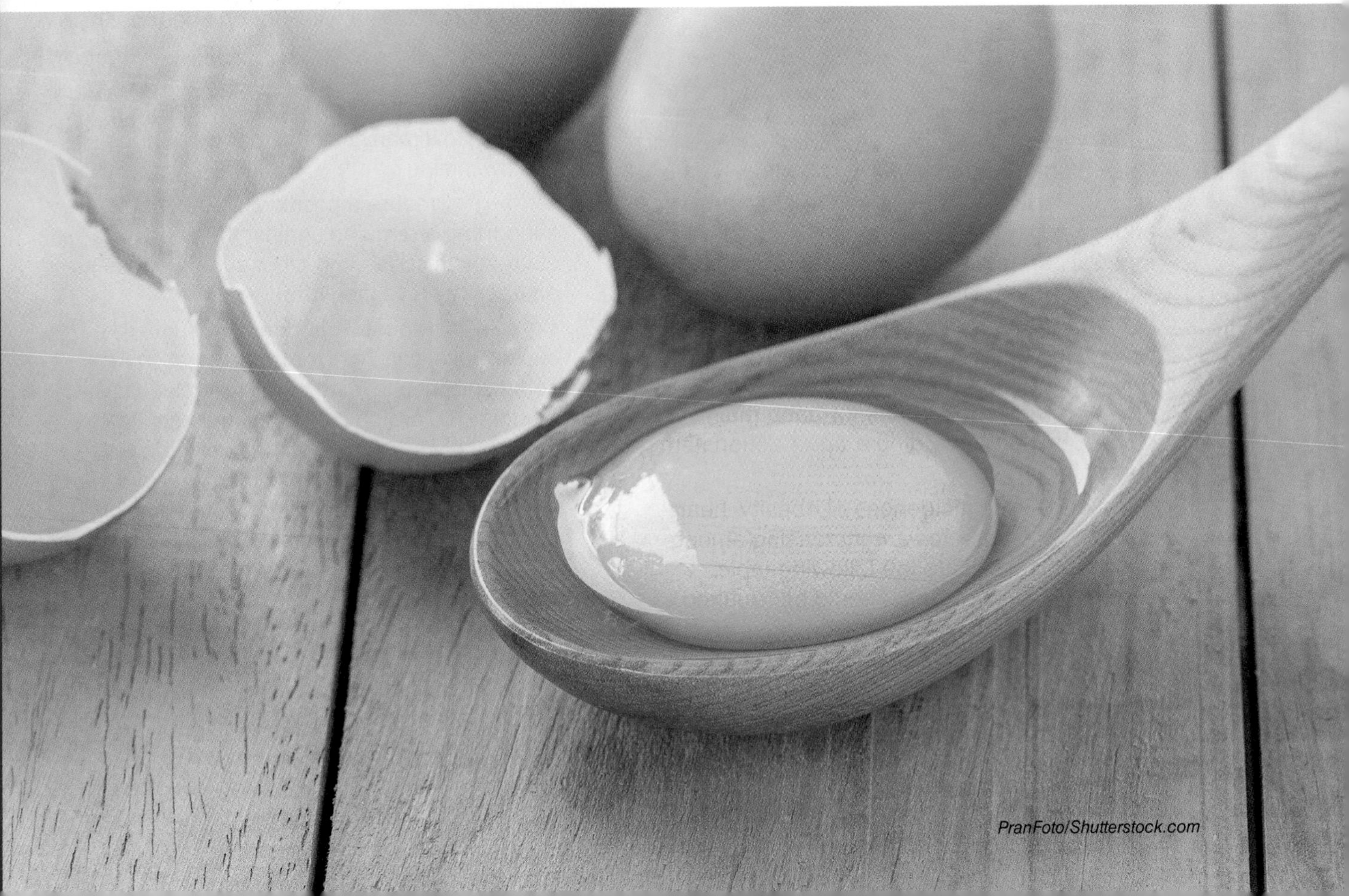

PranFoto/Shutterstock.com

Content Terms

adolescence
congenital disability
fetal alcohol syndrome (FAS)
fetus
growth spurt
infant
lactation
life cycle
low-birthweight baby
menopause
pica
placenta
premature baby
puberty
toddler
trimester

Academic Terms

exacerbate
manifest
necessitate
oversee
wane

What's Your Nutrition and Wellness IQ?

Take this quiz to examine how much you already know about nutrition across the life span. If you cannot answer a question, pay extra attention to that topic as you study this chapter.

- Identify each statement as *True*, *False*, or *It Depends*. *It Depends* means in some cases the statement is true; in some cases it could be false.
- Revise false statements to make them true.
- Explain the circumstances in which each *It Depends* statement is true and when it is false.

Nutrition and Wellness IQ 

	Statement			
1.	Nutritional needs vary depending on gender and age.	True	False	It Depends
2.	A woman's state of health before pregnancy has little or no effect on the health outcomes of her newborn baby.	True	False	It Depends
3.	During pregnancy, physical activity should be greatly reduced.	True	False	It Depends
4.	If a mother drinks alcohol, the uterine wall will protect a fetus from the influence of the alcohol.	True	False	It Depends
5.	Proportionately, young children require more of each nutrient per pound of body weight than adults.	True	False	It Depends
6.	Snack foods, such as whole grapes, raw carrots, and nuts should not be given to toddlers.	True	False	It Depends
7.	The eating patterns of an adolescent shape the health outcomes of the adolescent as an adult.	True	False	It Depends
8.	Physical activity has a greater health benefit for a young adult than it does for an older adult.	True	False	It Depends

While studying this chapter, look for the activity icon  **to**

- **build** vocabulary with e-flash cards and interactive games;
- **assess** what you learn by completing self-assessment quizzes and completing review questions; and
- **expand** knowledge with interactive activities and activities that extend learning.

www.g-wlearning.com/foodsandnutrition/

At the beginning of your life, you were smaller than the period at the end of this sentence. Then you grew. As an adult, you will be several million times bigger than you were at the start of your life.

The projected life span for an infant born today is between 76 and 81 years. During his or her life span, an individual's nutrition and fitness needs change. Although all humans need the same basic nutrients, certain stages of life may bring special nutritional concerns. This chapter will help you look more closely at nutritional needs as your body changes and you move through life.

Nutrient Needs Change

During an individual's life span, he or she progresses through a predictable pattern of changes called the *life cycle*. The ***life cycle*** is the series of growth and development stages through which people pass from before birth through death. The life-cycle stages include pregnancy and lactation, infancy, toddlerhood, childhood, adolescence, and adulthood. These stages are often further subdivided to reflect significant developmental changes. Each person's development is unique and the stages may vary from person to person (**Figure 14.1**).

Throughout their life span, people need adequate amounts of nutritious foods to build, repair, and maintain body tissues. The need for nutrients begins before birth. An unborn child's development depends on nutrients from the mother's bloodstream.

Each child's development is unique. Different parts of the body grow at different times and at different rates. Nonetheless, there are predictable growth patterns. For instance, bone and muscle growth are most rapid in infancy and adolescence. Nutritional requirements are especially high during these periods. Rapid bone growth increases the need for calcium. Rapid muscle growth increases the need for protein.

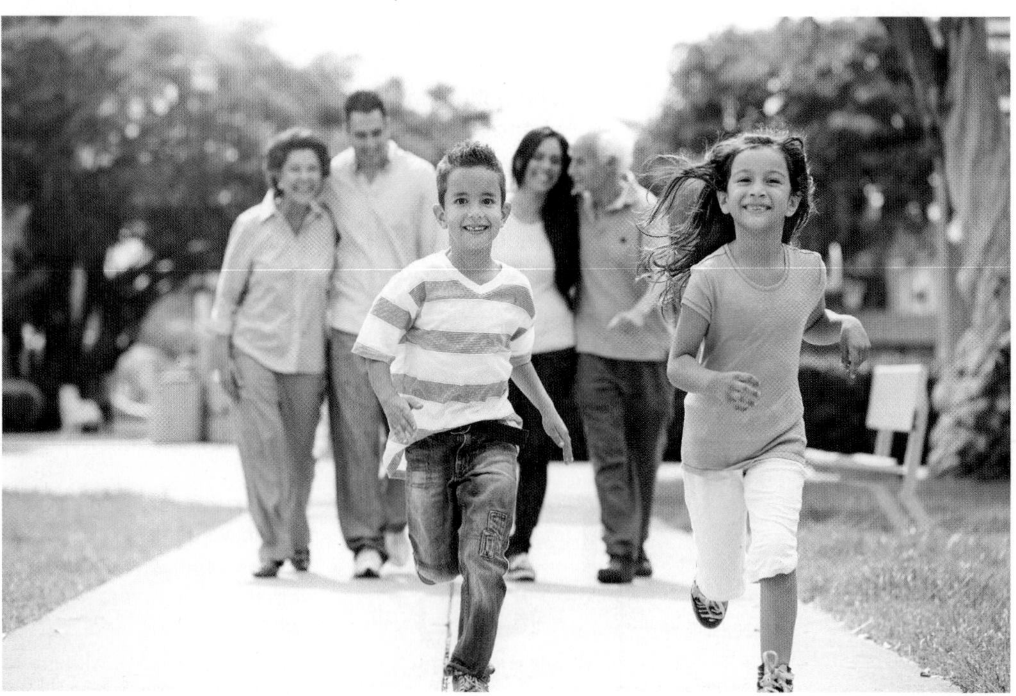

Monkey Business Images/Shutterstock.com

Figure 14.1
People need different amounts of nutrients in each stage of the life cycle.

Nutrient needs for adults decrease to a maintenance level. During the later years of life, the aging process affects nutritional status.

Some lifestyle choices such as participating in a sport or following a vegetarian diet can impact nutritional needs during the life cycle. These decisions contribute an additional level of nutritional need. However, these factors are choices and are not common to all individuals.

In addition to the life-cycle stages, a number of other factors influence the amounts of nutrients needed. These factors include body size and composition, age, gender, activity level, and state of health. These factors in combination with the demands of the life-cycle stage create a set of nutritional needs that are unique to each individual.

A relationship exists between an individual's nutrition and his or her life span. The quality of nutrition during each life-cycle stage can influence an individual's health across the life span. When good nutrition practices begin early in life, chances for optimal health in the future are improved.

The following sections focus on the nutrients the body needs during the various stages of life, beginning with pregnancy and ending with older adulthood.

Pregnancy and Lactation

The life cycle begins in a woman's body. During pregnancy, a woman's normal body functions change to take care of the developing baby. After conception, nourishment from the mother's body is necessary to support growth. Two weeks after conception, the developing human is called an *embryo*. From nine weeks after conception until birth, a developing human is called a ***fetus***. Following the birth of the baby, the mother's body begins producing breast milk. This is called ***lactation***. The demands of pregnancy and lactation placed on a woman's body affect her nutritional needs.

FEATURED CAREER

Lactation Consultant

A lactation consultant is a health-care professional with special training and experience in helping breast-feeding mothers and babies. These consultants may be on staff at a hospital or in a pediatrician's office or home health agency, or they may work in private practice.

Education

A Board Certified Lactation Consultant is required to take certain college-level classes plus a minimum number of hours working with breast-feeding mothers in a clinical setting. Many are registered or licensed in other health professions, such as nursing.

Job Outlook

There are far more mothers and babies that need help with breast-feeding than there are lactation consultants to work with them.

Health Needs Before Pregnancy

Women should be in good health before becoming pregnant. When planning a pregnancy, a woman should see a medical professional who can evaluate her health. The woman should visit a doctor again as soon as she thinks she is pregnant. The doctor needs to **oversee** (monitor) the woman's health throughout the pregnancy. This type of *prenatal* (before birth) care helps reduce the risk of health problems for the mother and fetus. Prenatal care also increases a woman's chances of delivering a healthy baby.

A woman's weight before pregnancy should be appropriate for her height. Obstetricians advise underweight and overweight women to attain a healthy weight before becoming pregnant. This helps ensure good health for the women and their babies.

Women who enter pregnancy 10 percent or more below healthy weight face a greater risk of having a ***low-birthweight baby***. This is a baby that weighs less than 5½ pounds (2,500 g) at birth. Low-birthweight babies have an increased risk of illness and death in early life. They are also more likely to have health problems that could affect them throughout life.

Women who are 20 percent or more above healthy weight are also more likely to experience problems during pregnancy. However, pregnancy is not an appropriate time for a woman to try to lose or maintain weight. A woman needs to gain a certain amount of weight for a healthy pregnancy and a healthy baby (**Figure 14.2**). A healthy eating plan can help an overweight woman achieve an appropriate weight gain during pregnancy.

Weight Gain During Pregnancy

Prepregnancy Weight	Total Weight Gain
Underweight	28–40 lb. (12.5–18 kg)
Normal weight	25–35 lb. (11.5–16 kg)
Overweight	15–25 lb. (7–11.5 kg)
Obese	11–20 lb. (5–9 kg)

Figure 14.2 Guidelines for weight gain during pregnancy for both teens and adults are based on prepregnancy weight.

Both underweight and overweight women are at greater risk of giving birth to a premature infant. A ***premature baby*** is a baby born before the 37th week of pregnancy. Premature birth is the leading cause of death among babies. Most premature babies have a low birthweight and are at risk for related health problems. Premature babies also have underdeveloped lungs. This increases their risk of respiratory problems throughout life (**Figure 14.3**).

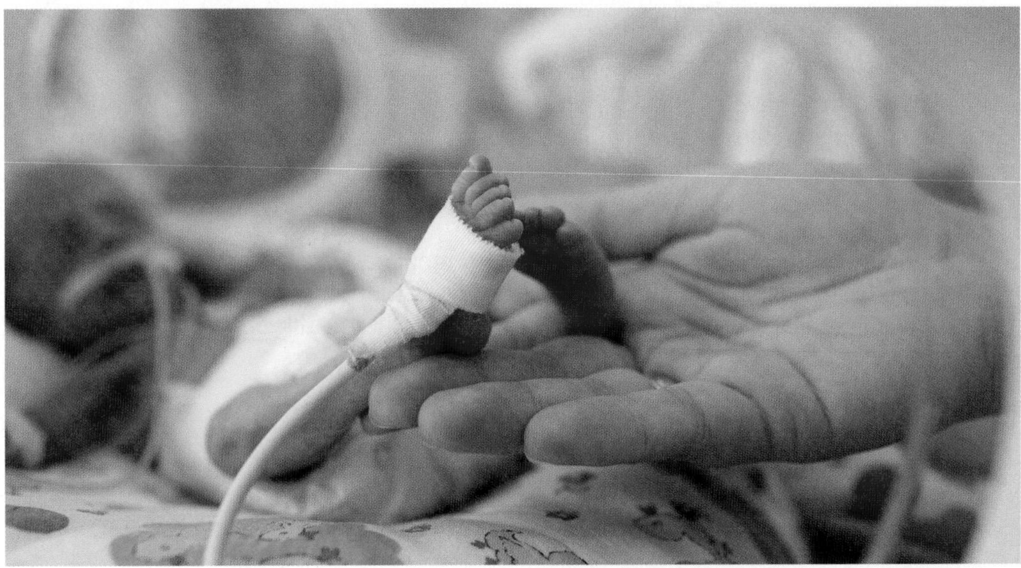

Kristina Bessolova/Shutterstock.com

Figure 14.3 Low-birthweight babies have a higher risk for health problems at birth and throughout their lives.

CASE STUDY

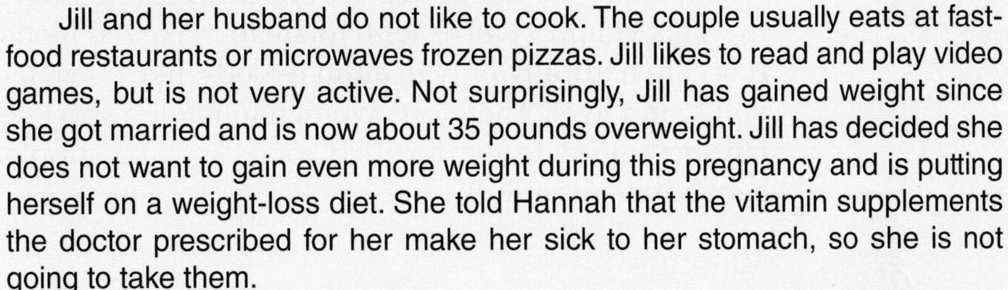

A Healthy Pregnancy

Hannah was excited to learn that her older sister, Jill, is pregnant. Hannah had health class last semester and learned a great deal about healthy pregnancies.

Jill and her husband do not like to cook. The couple usually eats at fast-food restaurants or microwaves frozen pizzas. Jill likes to read and play video games, but is not very active. Not surprisingly, Jill has gained weight since she got married and is now about 35 pounds overweight. Jill has decided she does not want to gain even more weight during this pregnancy and is putting herself on a weight-loss diet. She told Hannah that the vitamin supplements the doctor prescribed for her make her sick to her stomach, so she is not going to take them.

This baby will be Hannah's first niece or nephew and she plans to be a good aunt. However, Hannah is already worried for the health of her sister and the baby.

Case Review

1. Why do you think Hannah is worried about Jill and the baby?
2. What would you do if you were Hannah?

Nutrient Needs During Pregnancy

You may know a normal pregnancy lasts about nine months. When describing prenatal development, doctors refer to trimesters. A ***trimester*** is one-third of the pregnancy period and lasts about 13 to 14 weeks. A pregnant woman's nutritional needs vary a bit from one trimester to the next. This is because nutrients are critical in varying proportions for different aspects of a baby's development.

A woman needs extra amounts of many nutrients during pregnancy. One of the best ways to prepare for these increased needs is to form healthful eating habits before pregnancy. This approach benefits a woman in two key ways. First, a well-nourished female builds reserves of some nutrients. These reserves help her meet the increased nutrient demands of pregnancy and avoid deficiencies. Second, a woman who is consuming a nutrient-dense diet *before* pregnancy will understand how to select foods that benefit her nutrient intake *during* pregnancy.

Protein

Pregnant women need extra protein to help build fetal tissue. They also need extra protein to support changes in their bodies, such as increasing their blood supply and uterine tissue. Many women already consume more than enough protein. Therefore, most women do not need to adjust their diets to meet the protein needs of pregnancy.

Vitamins

A pregnant woman needs increased amounts of most vitamins. Folate is especially important at the beginning of the first trimester. This vitamin aids the normal development of the baby's brain and spinal cord during the first few weeks of pregnancy. This is before most women know they are pregnant. Therefore, health experts recommend all women of childbearing age consume 400 micrograms of folic acid

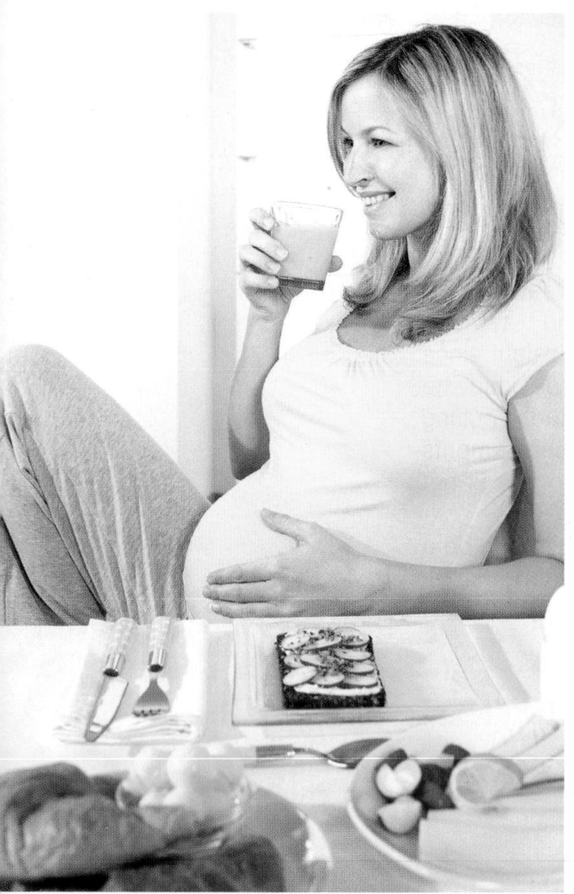

epicseurope/Shutterstock.com

Figure 14.4 Pregnant women may want to make fresh orange juice part of their daily diets. ***What nutrient does orange juice supply that women need in greater amounts during pregnancy?***

from fortified foods and supplements daily. During pregnancy, the recommendation is to consume 600 micrograms of synthetic folic acid from fortified foods (enriched grains, cereals, pastas, and rice) or supplements in addition to sources obtained from eating a varied diet (**Figure 14.4**). Meeting this recommendation will reduce the number of babies born with damage to the brain and spinal cord.

Pregnant women have an increased need for vitamin B_{12}. This vitamin works with folate to make red blood cells. It occurs naturally only in animal foods, like meat, fish, egg yolks, and liver. Therefore, women following strict vegetarian diets need to eat fortified foods or take supplements containing vitamin B_{12}.

Minerals

Women have some increased mineral needs during pregnancy. They need extra zinc to support the growth and development of the fetus. They need more magnesium to promote healthy fetal bones and tissues. Pregnant women require increased amounts of iron to provide reserves the infant will need after birth. They also need iron because their growing bodies are making more red blood cells. Pregnant women also need extra iodine. This mineral supports thyroid activity as basal metabolic rate increases in the second trimester.

The recommended daily intake for calcium does not increase during pregnancy. However, the calcium needed to form the baby's bones is pulled from the mother's bones. Therefore, it is critical that pregnant women consume the recommended 1,000 milligrams of calcium per day. This will help reduce the loss of minerals from their bones. Pregnant teens need 1,300 milligrams of calcium daily.

Hormonal changes affect the way a pregnant woman's body uses certain nutrients. For instance, when a woman is pregnant, her body absorbs and stores more calcium and iron. These changes help provide for some of an expectant woman's additional nutrient needs. However, many pregnant women have trouble meeting all their needs through diet alone. This is especially true for iron. Therefore, health professionals often prescribe vitamin and mineral supplements to help pregnant women meet their increased needs. Pregnant women should take supplements only with their doctor's recommendation.

A woman who fails to meet added nutrient needs during pregnancy can affect her health and the health of her baby. The woman may experience iron deficiency anemia. She is more susceptible to disease. She is even at an increased risk of death. Her baby is more likely to be born early or have a low birthweight. The newborn may not have the necessary nutrient reserves to draw on for growth. The baby may also be more susceptible to illnesses.

Calories

Along with extra nutrients, a pregnant woman needs extra calories to support fetal development. In the second trimester, an expectant woman needs to begin eating an extra 340 calories per day. In the third trimester, she needs to add another 110 calories to her daily diet.

Gaining enough but not too much weight during pregnancy is very important. The recommended weight gains result in the best chances of having a healthy baby. This weight reflects the weight of the developing fetus. It also allows for the growth of tissue and increase of body fluids in the mother (**Figure 14.5**). Most weight gain occurs during the second and third trimesters. With good eating habits and exercise, most women lose the majority of this weight within a few months after delivery.

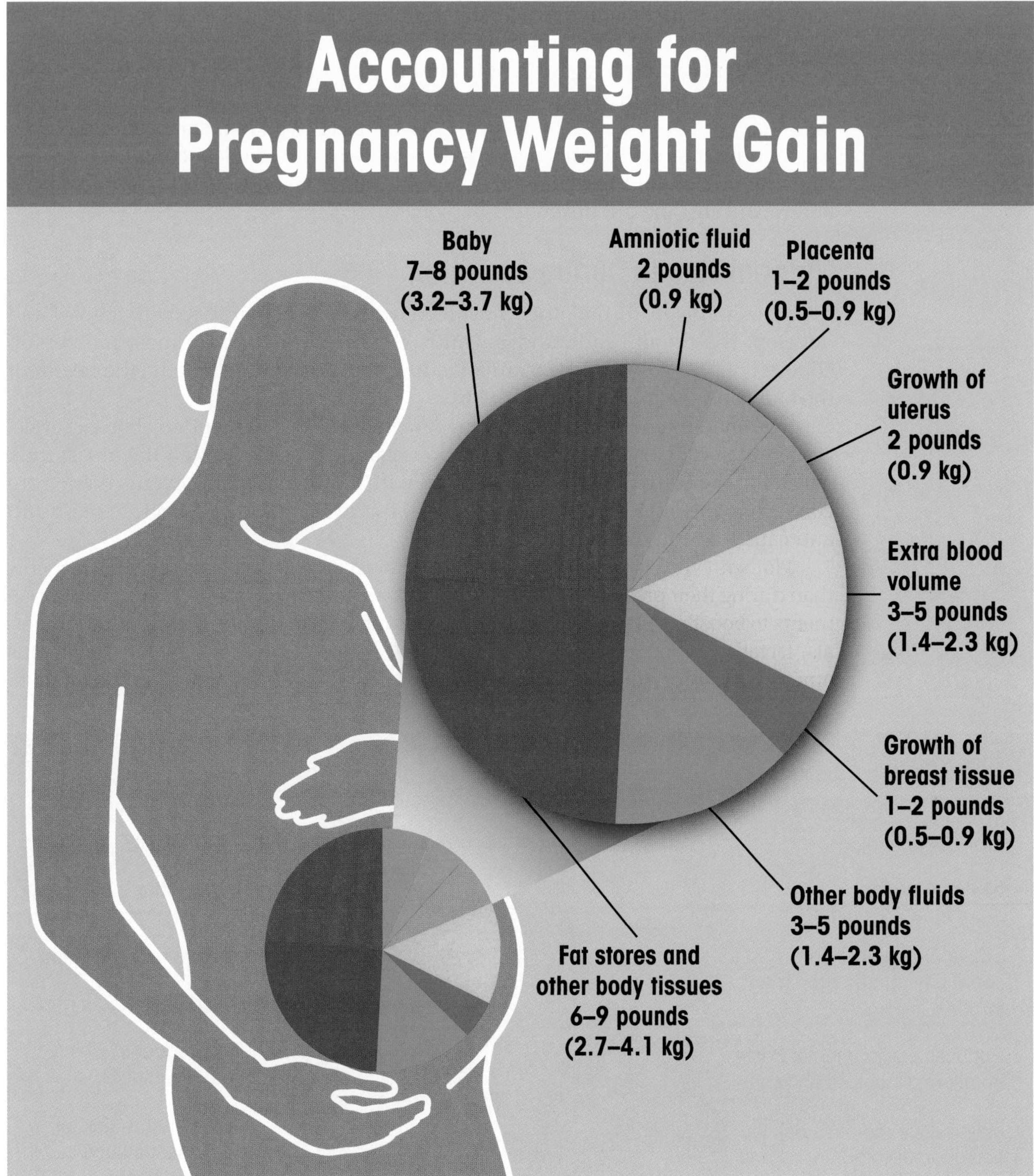

Avdeenko/Shutterstock.com

Figure 14.5 Factors other than just the weight of the fetus contribute to a woman's weight gain during pregnancy. *How much weight gain can be attributed to increased blood volume?*

Pregnancy and Physical Activity

A woman should follow a plan of regular exercise before, during, and after pregnancy. Physically fit women should stay physically active throughout their pregnancy. Staying active helps reduce stress, facilitates the process of labor, reduces the chances of gestational diabetes, and reduces the discomfort of pregnancy. Being physically active helps new mothers lose excess weight after pregnancy and begin to feel fit sooner after birth. Following a daily exercise program also smooths the transition to active parenthood. A woman should speak with her doctor to learn what types of physical activity are appropriate during pregnancy.

Caution is advised regarding the kind of physical activity chosen by pregnant women. Activities in which there is a chance of falling or being hit should be avoided. Low impact activities such as swimming, walking, stair climbing, rowing, and light strength training are safest. If there is a medical condition, professional advice should be followed. Care should be taken to drink plenty of fluid before, during, and after exercise.

Nutrient Needs During Lactation

After giving birth, a mother must feed her baby frequently to help it grow and develop. Nearly all health and nutrition experts strongly urge most mothers to choose breast-feeding over formula-feeding. Breast-feeding benefits the health of the baby and the mother (**Figure 14.6**).

In some situations, breast-feeding may not be recommended. For example, certain maternal diseases and medications can be passed through the breast milk and harm the baby. Some babies are born with a disorder that prevents them from converting the monosaccharide (galactose) found in milk. The galactose builds up and causes serious damage to the baby.

Mothers who choose to breast-feed need even greater amounts of some nutrients than during their pregnancy. Their doctors may prescribe vitamin and mineral supplements to boost nutrients found in a nutritious meal plan. Besides vitamins and minerals, lactating women need increased amounts of protein. They also need generous amounts of fluids and extra calories to produce the milk that nourishes their babies.

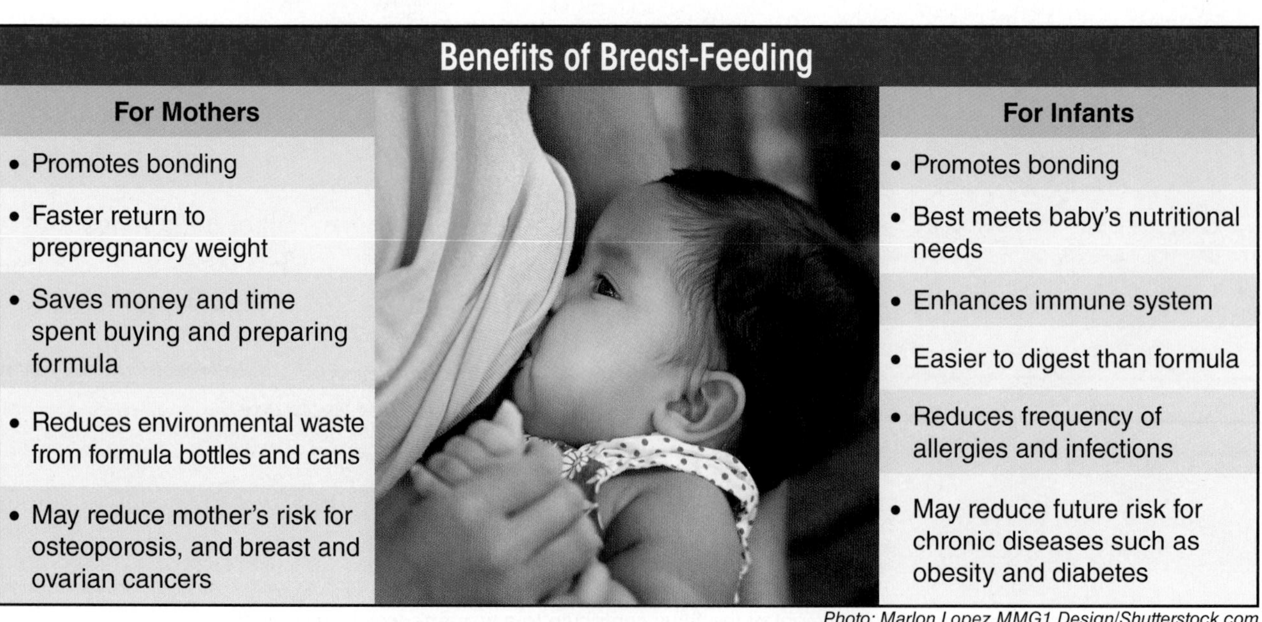

Benefits of Breast-Feeding
For Mothers
• Promotes bonding
• Faster return to prepregnancy weight
• Saves money and time spent buying and preparing formula
• Reduces environmental waste from formula bottles and cans
• May reduce mother's risk for osteoporosis, and breast and ovarian cancers
For Infants
• Promotes bonding
• Best meets baby's nutritional needs
• Enhances immune system
• Easier to digest than formula
• Reduces frequency of allergies and infections
• May reduce future risk for chronic diseases such as obesity and diabetes
Photo: Marlon Lopez MMG1 Design/Shutterstock.com

Figure 14.6 Breast-feeding benefits both the mother and baby.

Lactating women should drink at least two quarts of liquids per day and consume additional nutrient-dense calories as recommended by their doctor. The Dietary Reference Intakes (DRI) provide nutrient recommendations for women who are pregnant or lactating. For women who are obese or sedentary, the recommendations for added nutrient-dense calories may be too high. For underweight adolescent mothers who are still growing, more nutrient-dense calories may be needed.

Meals to Meet Nutritional Needs

Pregnant and lactating women are advised not to skip meals, especially breakfast. Eating regular meals and snacks provides them and their infants with a steady supply of needed nutrients.

Meals should offer a variety of nutritious foods. Whole-grain and enriched breads and cereals supply B vitamins and iron. Whole-grain products may also provide dietary fiber. Fruits and vegetables are good sources of vitamins, including the folate needed before and during early pregnancy. Fat-free and low-fat milk, soy milk, yogurt, and cheese provide protein and calcium. Limiting fat intake helps to reduce intake of problem amounts of cholesterol and too many calories. Lean meats, poultry, fish, and meat alternates supply protein, iron, B vitamins, and zinc. Eggs, soybeans, and beef are excellent sources of choline (**Figure 14.7**).

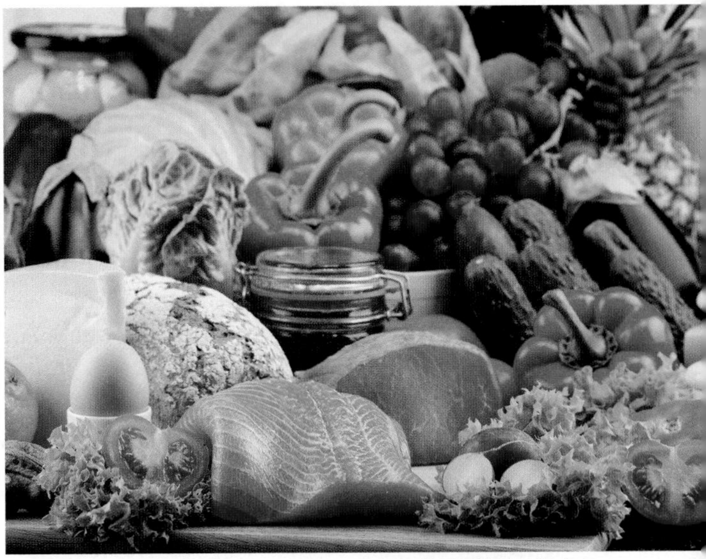

monticello/Shutterstock.com

Figure 14.7 Eating a variety of nutritious foods will help a woman meet the extra nutrient needs of pregnancy.

When planning meals, lactating women can include soups and fruit juices to help meet their fluid needs. Both during and after pregnancy, women can select fruits, vegetables, peanut butter, and low-fat yogurt and cheese as nutritious snacks. However, foods that provide little more than fats and sugars should be limited.

Pregnant or lactating women who follow vegetarian diets have an extra challenge when meeting nutrient needs. They should discuss their food patterns with a doctor or registered dietitian. Including good food sources of protein, such as nuts, seeds, whole grains, legumes, and tofu, is very important. Vegetarians must plan carefully to get enough iron, vitamin B_{12}, and folate for their important role in cell reproduction. Calcium, magnesium, iron, and zinc needs are high. Vegetarians may require supplements to meet their needs for iron. Vitamin B_{12} needs can be met by consuming supplements or fortified foods. Women who do not use dairy products may need calcium and vitamin D supplements as well. Protein supplements are not recommended and may be harmful.

Special Dietary Concerns

Certain conditions and foods can create special dietary concerns during pregnancy. Women should discuss these concerns with their physician or a registered dietitian nutritionist.

Craving Nonfood Substances

Women sometimes experience strange cravings during pregnancy that are not based on physiological needs. Most cravings are simply due to changed sense of taste and smell. They may also occur when women are low in some nutrients.

Women who practice pica during pregnancy may have specific dietary concerns. ***Pica*** is the craving for and ingestion of nonfood substances such as clay, soil, or chalk. These substances do not deliver any needed nutrients. In fact, they may interfere with the absorption of other nutrients the body needs or simply replace nutritious foods in the mother's diet. Eating these substances can have an adverse effect on the pregnancy.

Nausea

Nausea, often called *morning sickness*, may be a problem during the first months of pregnancy. Some women have morning sickness throughout their pregnancies. Many women feel nauseated at times other than morning. To relieve nausea, pregnant women are advised to eat whatever they believe will make them feel better. For some women, this may mean salty foods; for others it may mean bland foods. Eating frequent small meals may also help ease this condition.

Sometimes nausea and vomiting are extreme. Persistent vomiting can result in dehydration and poor weight gain. This condition is a health risk for both the mother and unborn baby. A woman experiencing this problem should inform her doctor.

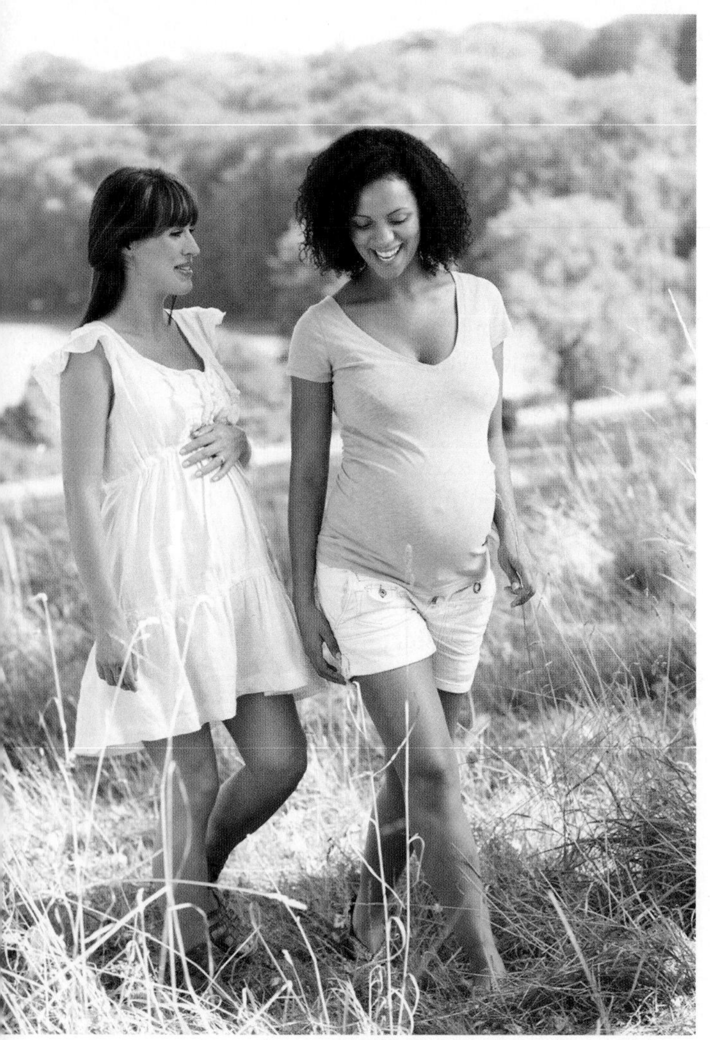

Monkey Business Images/Shutterstock.com

Figure 14.8 Physical activity during pregnancy is beneficial for a number of reasons.

Heartburn

Another common condition during pregnancy is heartburn. Heartburn is a burning feeling in the chest and throat that results when substances in the stomach move the wrong way and up into the esophagus. To decrease symptoms of heartburn, eliminate foods that **exacerbate** (make worse) the condition, postpone lying down for one hour after meals, and eat small, frequent meals.

Constipation

Constipation becomes a problem for many pregnant women, especially later in pregnancy. Hormones cause the intestinal muscles to relax, and the expanding uterus crowds the intestines. These factors decrease the rate at which the intestines are able to move waste through the body. The longer feces remain in the large intestine, the more water is absorbed from them. As feces lose water, they become hard, making bowel movements painful. Straining during bowel movements can increase the likelihood of developing hemorrhoids during pregnancy.

To avoid problems with constipation and hemorrhoids, pregnant women should be sure to drink plenty of fluids. Consuming an ample amount of fiber by choosing foods such as whole grains, fruits, and vegetables will help. Getting moderate daily physical activity also promotes regular elimination (**Figure 14.8**).

Diabetes and High Blood Pressure

Some women develop a form of diabetes or high blood pressure during pregnancy. These conditions can be serious and require careful monitoring by a doctor. They may also **necessitate** (require) some dietary changes. Fortunately, these conditions often go away after delivery.

Fish

Certain foods are a cause for concern for pregnant women. Certain types of fish contain high levels of a heavy metal called *mercury*. Mercury can damage the fetal brain and nervous system. To limit exposure to mercury, the FDA cautions women who are pregnant or may become pregnant, and women who are breast-feeding to

- avoid eating shark, swordfish, king mackerel, marlin, orange roughy, some tuna (big eye), or tilefish;
- consume no more than six ounces per week of albacore (white) tuna; and
- check with local authorities about the safety of fish caught in local waters.

Artificial Sweeteners

Most artificial sweeteners have been found to be safe during pregnancy. However, there is still some concern about the safety of saccharin. Most health professionals believe artificial sweeteners are safe when used in moderation. One exception is individuals who have a hereditary disease that prevents their body from breaking down the compound found in aspartame. They should not use aspartame. The best advice is to consult with a doctor and use artificial sweeteners in moderation or not at all. Instead, choose foods that are naturally sweet.

Pesticides

Pesticides may cause harm to unborn babies and children. Pregnant women should avoid contact with pesticides as much as possible. Wash and peel fruits and vegetables to remove pesticide residues (**Figure 14.9**). If pesticides must be applied in the home, all food and dishes should be removed from the area to be treated. Afterward, someone other than the pregnant woman should wash any food-contact surfaces.

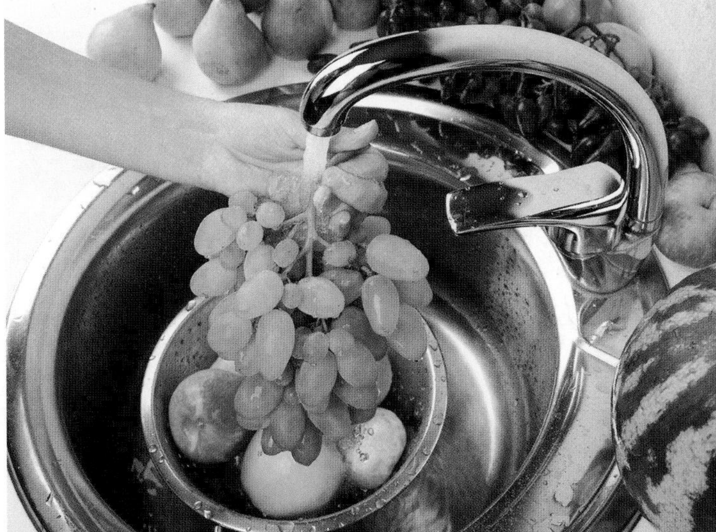

Africa Studio/Shutterstock.com

Figure 14.9 Fruits and vegetables should be washed to remove pesticide residues that could be harmful to unborn babies and children. *Does the fruit or vegetable need to be washed if you are going to peel it?*

Concerns Related to Teen Pregnancy

Pregnancy places extra stress on the body of a teenager. The adolescent body is still growing and, therefore, has large nutrient requirements. The nutrient needs of the fetus are then added to the teen's needs. Meeting these combined nutrient needs is very difficult for most teens.

Many adolescent females have poor diets. They fail to get enough calories, iron, folic acid, zinc, calcium, and vitamins A and D to help them grow to their optimum height and muscle development. Teens with poor nutritional status do not have the nutrient reserves needed to meet the demands of a developing fetus. If these teens lead an inactive lifestyle, they are also not at an ideal level of physical fitness.

These factors place teens at a much higher risk of complications during pregnancy than adult women. Teens are more likely to have miscarriages and stillbirths. They are also more likely to have premature and low-birthweight babies. Their babies are at higher risk for health problems and death.

When healthcare is received early in the pregnancy, health risks are reduced for both mother and baby. Being aware of the first signs of pregnancy can help teens determine when to seek prenatal care. These signs include a missed menstrual period, fatigue, nausea, swelling and soreness in the breasts, and frequent urination.

A pregnant teen must carefully follow the advice of her doctor. She needs to select an adequate number of servings of nutrient-dense foods each day. She must also take any nutrient supplements her doctor prescribes. This type of diet provides the nutrients needed by the teen and her developing baby. It helps her achieve recommended weight gain during her pregnancy. Taking these steps improves a teen's chances of avoiding complications and delivering a healthy baby.

Drug Use During Pregnancy and Lactation

During pregnancy, an organ called the ***placenta*** forms inside the uterus. In the placenta, blood vessels from the mother and the fetus are entwined (**Figure 14.10**). Materials carried in the blood can be transferred between the mother and the fetus through the placenta. Oxygen and nutrients from the mother's bloodstream are delivered to the fetus. Waste products and carbon dioxide from the fetus are transported to the mother for elimination.

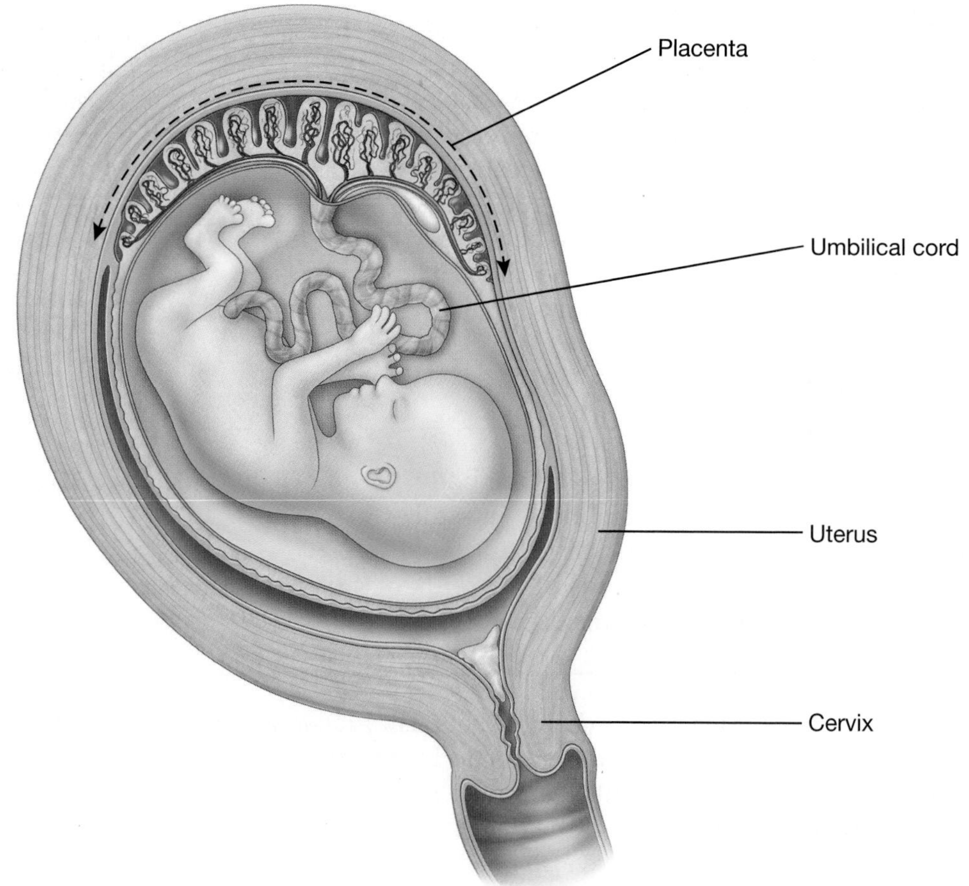

Figure 14.10
Substances in the blood are transferred between the mother and fetus via the placenta.

© Body Scientific International

Harmful Substances Are Transferred

Harmful substances such as alcohol and drugs from the mother's bloodstream can also be passed to the fetus through the placenta. The term "drug" describes a broad range of substances including caffeine, nicotine, over-the-counter and prescription medications, as well as illegal drugs.

When a woman uses a drug or alcohol, it enters her bloodstream. If she is pregnant, it can pass through the placenta to her unborn child. If she is lactating, the drug may be secreted in her breast milk. Therefore, any drug a woman uses affects not only her but also her baby.

Fetuses and infants have such little bodies that even a small amount of a drug can be harmful. They also have immature organs that cannot break down drugs efficiently. Therefore, the effects of drugs last longer in fetuses and infants.

Drugs present dangers to a fetus throughout pregnancy. However, they are of special concern during the first trimester of the pregnancy. This is the period when the vital organs and systems of the fetus are developing. Some drugs can also cause excessive bleeding during the last trimester of pregnancy. Some over-the-counter and prescription drugs are known to cause congenital disabilities. ***Congenital disabilities*** are conditions existing from birth that limit a person's ability to use his or her body or mind.

Doctors discourage pregnant women from using any types of drugs, even common nonprescription drugs, such as aspirin. Over-the-counter drug labels warn pregnant women to seek the advice of a health professional before using the product. A physician can recommend which over-the-counter drugs might be safe during pregnancy.

Substances to Limit or Avoid

Caffeine is a stimulant found in colas and many other soft drinks, coffee, tea, and chocolate (**Figure 14.11**). Caffeine is also in many over-the-counter and prescription drugs. Studies about the effects of caffeine on fetuses have led researchers to various conclusions. Further study is needed to settle the debate. However, many health professionals recommend that women limit foods and beverages containing caffeine during pregnancy. Health professionals also recommend limiting caffeine during lactation. This is because caffeine passes into breast milk and has been shown to cause irritability and restlessness in nursing babies.

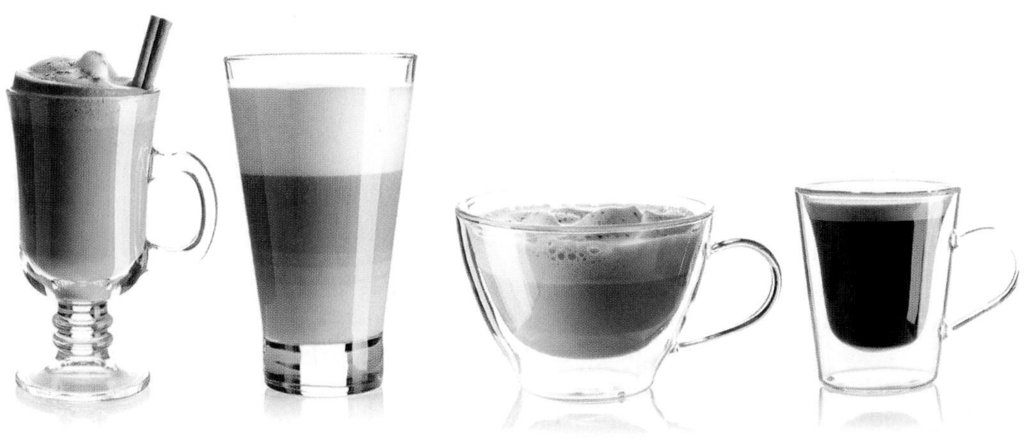

haveseen/Shutterstock.com

Figure 14.11
Many health professionals advise pregnant women to limit their use of coffee, tea, chocolate, soft drinks, and other products containing caffeine to no more than 200 mg per day. *How much caffeine do you typically consume each day?*

Smoking is not healthy for anyone. However, healthcare providers especially caution pregnant women against smoking. A pregnant woman who smokes is more likely to have a low-birthweight baby. Cigarette smoking decreases the oxygen delivered to the fetus and can endanger its health. In addition, smoking causes nicotine to circulate in the mother's bloodstream. The fetus can absorb this nicotine, which increases the risk of the fetus developing certain types of cancer in childhood.

Pregnant women should not drink alcohol, including beer and wine. Drinking even a small amount of alcohol during pregnancy can cause permanent damage to the fetus. A miscarriage or stillbirth may occur. Alcohol may damage the baby's developing organs such as the brain and heart. The head may not grow properly. The baby may die in early infancy or have intellectual disabilities. The baby may have sight and hearing problems, slow growth, and poor coordination.

Fetal alcohol syndrome (FAS) is a set of symptoms that can occur in newborns when a mother drinks alcohol while pregnant. Babies born with FAS suffer health effects throughout their lives. A baby born with FAS could have some or all the following symptoms:

- brain damage and below-average intelligence
- slowed physical growth
- facial disfigurement, including a flattened nose bridge, small eyes with drooping eyelids, and receding forehead
- short attention span
- irritability
- heart problems

Mothers should continue to refrain from drinking alcohol during lactation. If a lactating mother drinks alcohol, the alcohol can reach the baby through the breast milk. This may cause the baby to have developmental problems.

Infancy and Toddlerhood

Infants and toddlers have special nutritional needs and problems. An ***infant*** is a child in the first year of life. Children who are one to three years old are often called ***toddlers***. Nutritional care is very important during these periods.

Many parents receive nutritional advice from their children's doctors. Some doctors suggest parents consult a registered dietitian to better understand their children's unique nutritional needs.

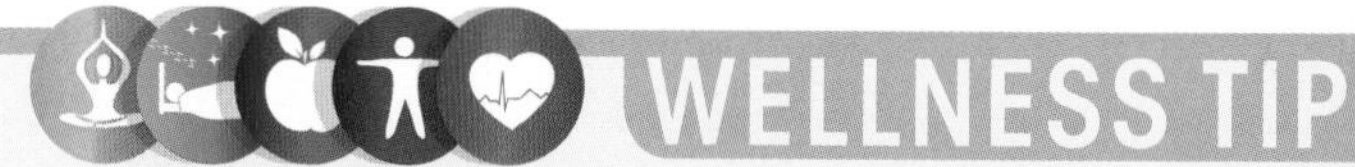

Preventing Infant Botulism

A spore called *Clostridium botulinum* causes infant botulism. These spores are all around you—in dirt, dust, and the air. Honey—pasteurized or unpasteurized—can be a source of these spores. To reduce the risk of infant botulism, do not feed honey or foods processed with honey (such as honey-coated cereals and honey graham crackers) to infants before one year of age.

Growth Patterns of Infants and Toddlers

Growth is more rapid during infancy than at any other time in the life cycle (**Figure 14.12**). The muscles, bones, and other tissues grow and develop at dramatic rates. The following growth pattern is typical for a healthy baby:

- Birth to 6 months–Baby grows about ½ to one inch per month and gains five to seven ounces per week. A baby should double his birth weight by age five months.
- Six to 12 months–Baby grows ⅜ inch per month and gains three to five ounces per week. A baby should triple his birth weight by one year of age.

The pattern of growth changes during the toddler years. The muscles of the legs and arms begin to develop more fully. Bone growth slows, but minerals are deposited in the bones at a rapid rate. This helps make the bones stronger to support the increasing weight of the toddler.

Nutrient Needs of Infants and Toddlers

Infants and toddlers need the same variety of nutrients as adults. However, growing, active children have *proportionately* greater nutritional needs than adults do. This means children require more of each nutrient per pound of body weight. For example, the Adequate Intake (AI) for calcium for a four-month-old infant is 200 milligrams per day. A 35-year-old adult needs 1,000 milligrams of calcium daily. Suppose the infant weighs 15 pounds and the adult weighs 150 pounds. This means the infant needs approximately 13 milligrams of calcium per pound of body weight. However, the adult requires only about 6.7 milligrams per pound of body weight. Proportionately, the infant needs more than twice as much calcium as the adult.

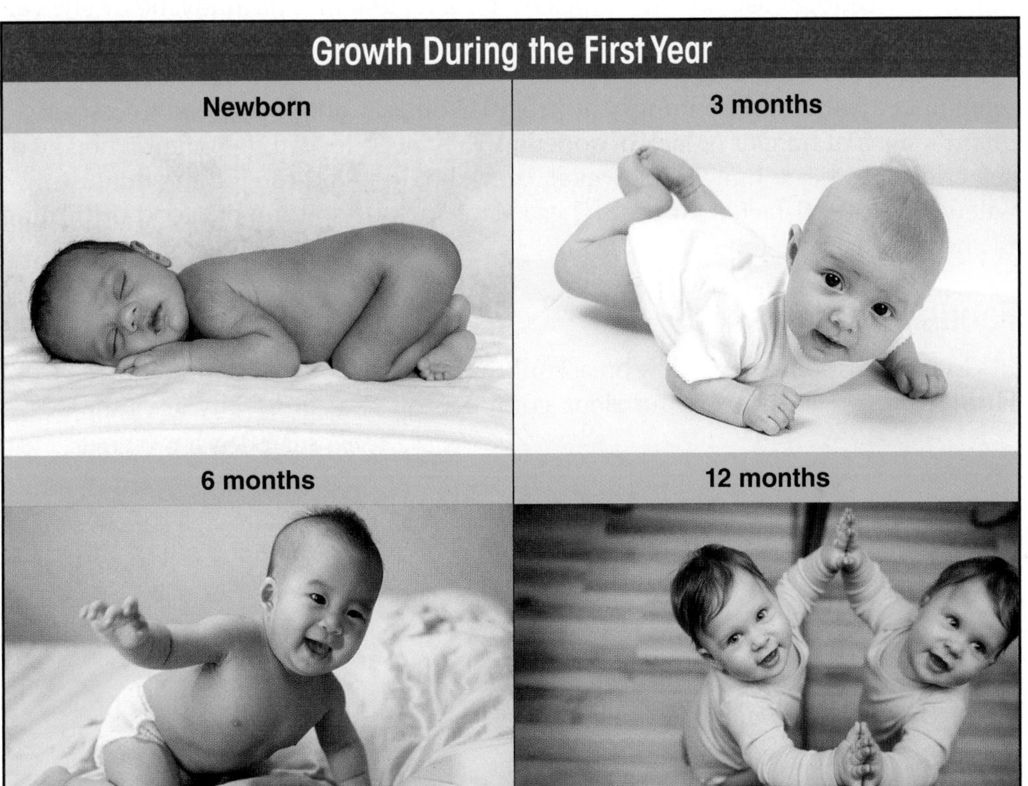

Top row: Anneka/Shutterstock.com; PHB.cz (Richard Semik)/Shutterstock.com; Bottom row: Nutpat Chaisinthop/Shutterstock.com; logoboom/Shutterstock.com

Figure 14.12 Babies grow and change rapidly during the first year of life. In addition to physical growth, they also develop the ability to use and control their muscles. A newborn can barely lift her head, but 12 months later is walking.

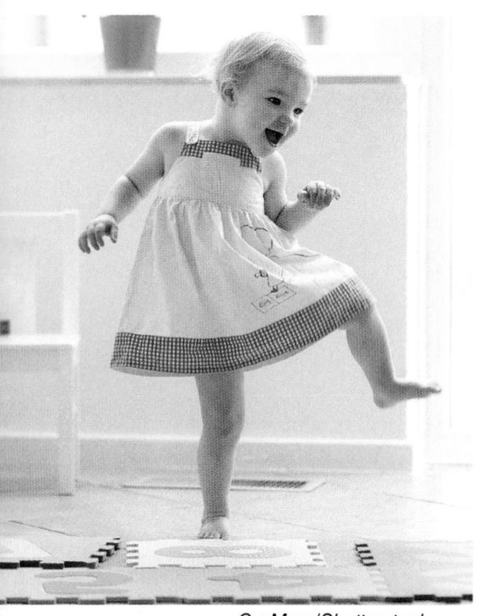

CroMary/Shutterstock.com

Figure 14.13 A toddler's diet must supply enough calories to support the toddler's high level of activity.

Infants born to healthy women who consumed adequate amounts of iron during pregnancy should have iron stored in their bodies. This stored iron should be enough to last until the infants are able to begin eating iron-fortified cereals. Infants also need high-quality protein to support the growth of muscles and other body tissues. An ample supply of calcium and phosphorous is essential for the development of teeth and bones. Breast milk or infant formula is designed to meet infants' needs for these and other nutrients. Breast milk or infant formula normally supply enough water to replace fluid losses. If rapid fluid losses occur due to diarrhea or vomiting, then extra electrolyte fluid for infants may be necessary. Consult with the baby's doctor for special care.

Infants grow fastest in the first six months or so of life. Growth slows during the second six months, and it continues to slow through the toddler years. Toddlers still need proportionately more nutrients than adults (**Figure 14.13**). However, their proportional needs are smaller than those of an infant.

Feeding Schedule for Infants

Proper feeding of an infant is critical to ensure normal growth. During the first few weeks, babies need to be fed every two to three hours. They are just learning how to eat, and their digestive tracts are immature. Therefore, newborns can handle only small amounts of breast milk or infant formula at each feeding.

After the first few weeks, babies usually want to be fed at regular times. Most babies require six feedings a day. Caregivers can plan a schedule to space feedings at four-hour intervals. Caregivers usually can reduce the number of daily feedings to five when the infant is around two months old. At around seven or eight months, four daily feedings usually are sufficient. By a child's first birthday, he or she can join family members for three daily meals with nutritious snacks in between meals.

Caregivers need to be flexible in following a feeding schedule. They need to remember a baby may be hungry at irregular times. Caregivers need to respect an infant's signs of hunger or lack of appetite. They need to feed the infant when he or she cries to indicate hunger. However, they should avoid forcing the infant to eat when signs of satisfaction appear. These signs include spitting out food or turning the head away from food.

Foods for Infants

Many nutrition experts view breast milk as the ideal food for infants (**Figure 14.14**). Human breast milk has a nutrient composition that is ideally formulated to

Figure 14.14 The stages that breast milk composition progresses through may vary slightly in length and timing for each mother.

Stages of Breast Milk

Stage	Time Frame	Characteristics
1st–Colostrum	First 3–5 days following birth	• creamy, yellow, thick milk • high in protein, vitamins, minerals, and antibodies
2nd–Transitional milk	Lasts about 2 weeks	• thinner, whiter milk • high in fat, lactose, and vitamins
3rd–Mature milk	Until baby is weaned	• 90% water for hydration • carbohydrate, protein, and fat needed for growth and energy

nourish humans. During the first few months following birth, breast milk changes to meet the changing needs of the infant. Composition of breast milk is quite different from cow's milk and infant formulas. Formulas include more of some nutrients than breast milk. However, more is not necessarily better. The smaller amount of protein in breast milk is easier for babies' immature systems to digest. Babies absorb the smaller amount of iron in breast milk more fully than they absorb the iron in formula. Breast milk also contains antibodies not found in formula. These antibodies help protect babies against diseases.

Infant Formula

The only alternative to breast milk recommended by the American Academy of Pediatrics (AAP) is iron-fortified infant formula. There are different types of these formulas including milk-based, soy-based, and some specialized formulas for specific health conditions. Most infants do well on milk-based formula, but some vegetarian parents may prefer to feed their baby a soy-based formula. The specialized formulas should only be used with a doctor's supervision. The nutrient composition of infant formulas must meet AAP standards. Iron fortification is important because an infant's iron stores at birth are enough to last only four to six months. A doctor can help parents find a suitable formula.

Formulas are usually sold in ready-to-feed, powdered, or liquid concentrate forms. Formulas must be prepared according to the directions. Food safety must be practiced when preparing or storing infant formulas (**Figure 14.15**). Practicing food safety is also essential when breast milk is being pumped and stored for later use. Formula or pumped breast milk that is improperly handled can result in a foodborne illness for the infant. This can be especially harmful because a baby's immune system is not fully developed.

Nutrients of Concern

Vitamin D is a nutrient of concern for infants. Doctors recommend that all infants get 600 IU of vitamin D every day. This includes infants who are breastfed as well as those on formula. The need for a vitamin D supplement should be discussed with a doctor.

Preparing Infant Formula

- Wash hands before preparing formula and feeding.
- Clean bottles in the dishwasher or follow manufacturer's instructions.
- Check that nipples are not clogged or torn. Discard any torn nipples.
- Mix formula according to directions on package and refrigerate until needed.
- Use refrigerated formula within 48 hours.
- Warm formula slowly in hot water. DO NOT boil or microwave formula. Test the temperature of the formula on your arm before feeding.
- Throw away any formula left in the bottle after feeding.

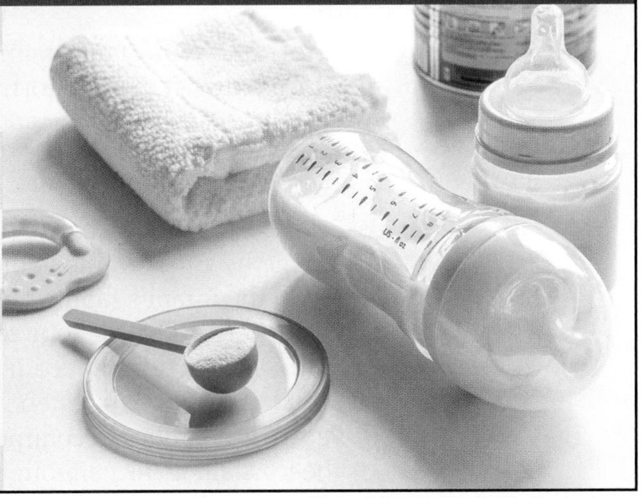

Photo: 279photo Studio/Shutterstock.com

Figure 14.15 Care must be taken during preparation and storage to ensure infant formula is safe and wholesome.

Babies should receive breast milk or iron-fortified formula for at least one year to ensure iron needs are met. Caregivers should not give infants cow's milk until they are one year old. Cow's milk does not provide sufficient iron and supplies too much calcium.

Solid Food

Caregivers should not add solid foods to infants' diets until they are around six months of age. Babies must be ready, physically and developmentally, to start solid foods. Before four months, infants have trouble swallowing solid foods. In addition, solid foods simply pass through because their immature GI tracts cannot absorb them. The Centers for Disease Control and Prevention (CDC) reported findings suggesting that feeding solid foods too early may be linked to increased risk of obesity, diabetes, and allergies.

Caregivers can watch for several signs to tell if infants are ready for solid foods. Infants should be able to sit with support. This provides a straight passage for solids to travel from the mouth to the stomach. Infants should no longer drool. This indicates they can control their mouths and tongues in a way that will permit swallowing of solids. Generally, infants should be double their birth weight, or weigh at least 13 pounds to begin solid foods. They should also show interest in eating solids by practicing chewing when they see others eating (**Figure 14.16**).

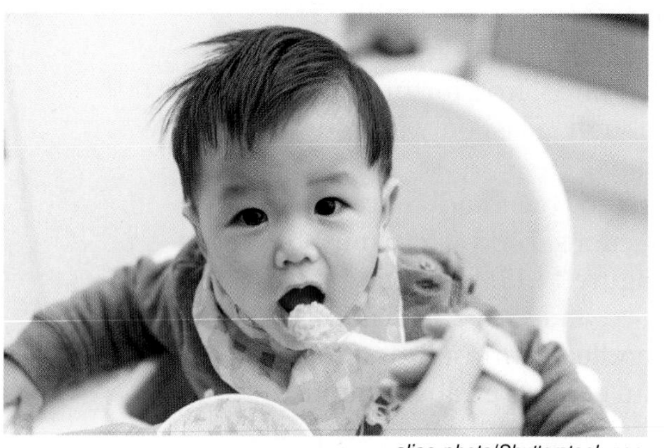

alice-photo/Shutterstock.com

Figure 14.16 A caregiver's attitude when feeding a baby can affect the baby's response to the food. *Does this baby appear to be receptive to the food being offered?*

Single-grain infant cereals are usually the first solid foods added to a baby's diet. Breast milk, formula, or water can be added to the single-grain cereal. These cereals provide iron in a form babies can easily absorb. After cereals, strained vegetables or fruits are introduced. Between six and nine months, meats can be offered. Meat provides a readily absorbed source of iron, zinc, and high-quality protein. By the end of the first year, a baby's diet should include a variety of foods; however, breast milk or iron-fortified formula should account for the major portion of an infant's diet during the first year.

Fluids

Before one year of age, babies should not be given juice. Until solid foods are introduced, breast milk or formula supply all the fluids a baby needs. When the baby begins on solid foods, water should be added to the diet.

Allergies and Intolerances

As the baby approaches one year old, continue to add food variety and textures. One by one, strained solid foods from each of the food groups should be offered. If the infant's family has a history of food sensitivities, introduce only one food at a time and wait four to five days before introducing another food. This way if an allergic reaction or intolerance occurs, the problem food can be readily identified. Allergic signs often include a rash, wheezing, diarrhea, or vomiting.

Pediatricians often recommend introducing infants to rice cereal first because it is the least allergenic, although oat cereal is also a good first cereal option. Wheat cereal is more likely to cause an allergic reaction, but may be offered by six months of age.

Eggs, dairy, fish, nuts, and orange juice can also cause allergic reactions; however, the American Academy of Pediatrics indicates there is no clear evidence that delaying the introduction of common allergenic foods prevents the development of allergies. In fact, guidelines became available in 2017 from the National Institutes of Health suggesting that offering a six-month-old these foods may reduce the risk of developing food allergies. Regardless, the infant's pediatrician should be consulted, particularly if there is a history of food allergies in the family.

A caregiver should be prepared to serve a new food a number of times despite the baby's repeated rejection. This allows the baby to learn to accept the food by growing accustomed to its new flavor and texture.

Commercially Prepared Versus Homemade Food

Baby foods can be purchased from the supermarket or made at home. Commercially prepared baby food is convenient and has a long shelf life. However, homemade baby food can be as nutritious as and less expensive than commercially prepared baby food (**Figure 14.17**). When preparing baby food at home, steps must be taken to ensure that the food is

- prepared and stored using safe food practices
- an appropriate texture for the child
- nutrient dense
- prepared without added sugar, salt, or spices

Preparing and Storing Homemade Baby Food
Preparation
1. Select good quality, fresh food. Avoid using leftover foods.
2. Wash, peel, seed, or trim foods as needed. Remove fat from meat.
3. Cook food until tender. Cook protein foods until well done.
4. Use a food mill or blender to process foods to appropriate texture. Foods can also be pushed through a fine-mesh strainer with a spoon.
5. Add cooking liquid, water, or fruit juice to thin puréed food if needed.
Storage
Foods that are not eaten immediately after cooking should be stored in refrigerator or freezer. Do not let the food sit at room temperature.
To Refrigerate
1. Place food in clean container with lid.
2. Label and date food.
3. Refrigerate immediately.
4. Discard food after 24 hours.
To Freeze
1. Place baby food into clean container. (Clean ice cube trays can be used to freeze food into baby-size portions.) Cover tightly with lid, plastic wrap, or foil.
2. Label and date food.
3. Place in freezer immediately.
4. Discard food after one month.

Figure 14.17 Always wash hands, equipment, and work area before you begin to prepare food.

Food Amount and Texture

Caregivers should avoid overfeeding infants to prevent the development of excess fat tissue. The amount of food infants willingly accept varies. The quantity consumed depends on age, sex, size, state of health, and characteristics of the food.

As infants develop teeth and the muscle coordination to chew, they can begin to eat mashed and chopped foods. They enjoy chewing crusts of hard bread, especially if they are teething. By the age of six or seven months, infants can pick up foods with their fingers. Holding foods with their hands, helps prepare infants to hold spoons.

Feeding Problems During Infancy

Though their nutrient needs are high, infants have small stomachs. Therefore, infants need frequent feedings.

Premature infants need special attention. They have greater needs for calories and all the nutrients. Premature infants do not have the iron reserves full-term babies have. They may also have trouble sucking and swallowing.

Problems can arise when caregivers have inappropriate expectations about when and how babies should eat. For instance, it is unrealistic to expect an infant to consume every drop of milk or spoonful of cereal. Infants will start eating less as their growth slows and their weight gain begins to **wane** (decrease). Caregivers must be patient and understanding about such normal infant behaviors.

Caregivers should not be upset when a child rejects a food. Rejecting a food is one of the few ways a baby has of showing independence. The child may accept the food if caregivers offer it again a few days later.

Pediatricians do not recommend forcing children to eat. Pleasant, happy eating conditions help children form positive feelings toward food and eating.

Babies are not born with food dislikes—they learn them. Caregivers must be aware of how they communicate their likes and dislikes to an infant. When a caregiver acts negatively toward a food, a child will notice this response. As a result, the child may learn to reject that particular food.

Foods for Toddlers

Foods for toddlers should be cut into bite-size pieces. Toddlers like foods they can pick up with their fingers. They also like colorful foods and soft textures that are easy to chew. Servings should be about one tablespoon of food for every year of age. The toddler's appetite should guide how much food he or she eats. Wait until the child asks for more food. The MyPlate food guidance system can be used to determine recommended amounts from each food group for older toddlers (**Figure 14.18**).

Dairy Group

Foods from the dairy group continue to be an important part of the toddler's diet. Some milk may be served as cream soups, pudding, yogurt, and cheese. Milk provides calcium as well as needed protein and phosphorus. It also supplies vitamins A and D, riboflavin, and some of the other B vitamins. Whole milk and milk products are recommended during the first two years of life. Fat is needed for calories and the normal development of organs such as the brain.

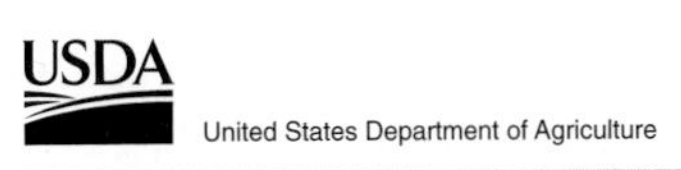

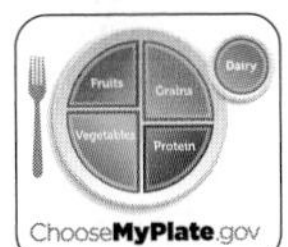

MyPlate Daily Checklist

Find your Healthy Eating Style

Everything you eat and drink matters. Find your healthy eating style that reflect your preferences, culture, traditions, and budget—and maintain it for a lifetime! The right mix can help you be healthier now and into the future. The key is choosing a variety of foods and beverages from each food group—*and making sure that each choice is limited in saturated fat, sodium, and added sugars.* Start with small changes—**"MyWins"**—to make healthier choices you can enjoy.

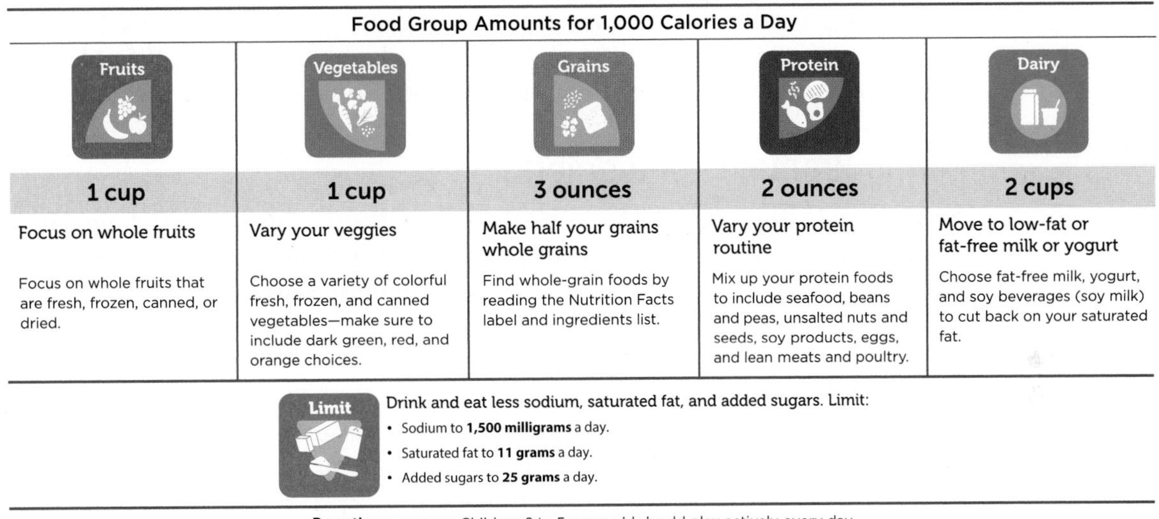

Food Group Amounts for 1,000 Calories a Day

Fruits	Vegetables	Grains	Protein	Dairy
1 cup	**1 cup**	**3 ounces**	**2 ounces**	**2 cups**
Focus on whole fruits	Vary your veggies	Make half your grains whole grains	Vary your protein routine	Move to low-fat or fat-free milk or yogurt
Focus on whole fruits that are fresh, frozen, canned, or dried.	Choose a variety of colorful fresh, frozen, and canned vegetables—make sure to include dark green, red, and orange choices.	Find whole-grain foods by reading the Nutrition Facts label and ingredients list.	Mix up your protein foods to include seafood, beans and peas, unsalted nuts and seeds, soy products, eggs, and lean meats and poultry.	Choose fat-free milk, yogurt, and soy beverages (soy milk) to cut back on your saturated fat.

Limit Drink and eat less sodium, saturated fat, and added sugars. Limit:

- Sodium to **1,500 milligrams** a day.
- Saturated fat to **11 grams** a day.
- Added sugars to **25 grams** a day.

Be active your way: Children 2 to 5 years old should play actively every day.

Use SuperTracker to create a personal plan based on your age, sex, height, weight, and physical activity level.

SuperTracker.usda.gov

USDA

Figure 14.18 This food plan is suitable for a two-year-old.

Protein Foods Group

Eggs, meats, peanut butter, beans, and peas are included in the protein foods group. Meat can be ground or cut into small pieces depending on the number of teeth the toddler has for chewing. Nuts are a choking hazard at this age and should be avoided.

Fruit and Vegetable Groups

The fruit and vegetable groups provide toddlers with vitamins, minerals, and fiber. At least one fruit serving per day should be a good source of vitamin C. Foods rich in vitamin C include citrus fruits, strawberries, cantaloupe, and tomatoes. Dark green and deep yellow fruits and vegetables are important for vitamin A. Potatoes and other starchy vegetables provide carbohydrates. Only 100-percent fruit juices should be offered and should be limited to no more than one-half cup per day. Too much juice might contribute to weight problems and leave little appetite for more nutrient-dense food choices. Sipping juice throughout the day or at bedtime can lead to tooth decay. For this reason, juice should be served in a cup and never a bottle.

Grains Group

Breads, cereals, rice, and pasta are included in the grains group. At least half of the grains in a toddler's diet should be whole grains. These foods supply carbohydrates, iron, and B vitamins to a toddler's diet.

Meals and Snacks

Toddlers can be served three meals a day with some between-meal snacks. Snacks are very important for toddlers. They have small stomachs and cannot eat enough at mealtime to carry them through to the next meal. Caregivers may choose the kind and amount of snack food to complement the foods a toddler eats at mealtime. Snack foods should contribute nutrients, not just calories from sugar and fat. Caregivers should avoid giving toddlers cookies, candy, and soft drinks as regular snacks. Instead, caregivers can offer fresh fruits, juices, milk, toast, and graham crackers. If snacks are eaten about two hours before a meal, they will not interfere with a child's appetite at mealtime.

Eating Problems of Toddlers

Several factors can lead to eating problems during the toddler stage. However, being aware of normal patterns of growth and development can help caregivers avoid many of these problems. Caregivers can help toddlers form food habits that promote good health and nutritional status.

Difficulty Chewing

Lack of teeth can be a source of eating problems for young toddlers. A one-year-old child may have only six to eight teeth. This can make chewing difficult and may lead to problems with choking. To make chewing easier, foods such as ripe fruit may be mashed into pulp or chopped into bite-size pieces. To prevent choking, caregivers should avoid feeding toddlers foods that contain seeds. Toddlers can also choke on nuts, corn, raisins, gristle in meat, marshmallows, pretzels, grapes, raisins, hard candy, and round slices of hot dogs and carrots.

Exploring While Eating

Some caregivers view toddlers' messy eating habits as a problem. Toddlers learn by using their senses to explore their environment, and food is part of that environment. Toddlers may involve their whole bodies in the eating process. They mash food with their hands to see how it feels. They place food in their mouths to taste it and feel the texture. They drop food on the floor to see what happens when they let go of it. By the end of a meal, toddlers may have applesauce in their hair and peanut butter on their elbows. Understanding how toddlers learn will help caregivers develop patience during this stage.

A toddler's developing sense of independence can sometimes lead to eating problems. When toddlers become physically able to use a spoon, they usually want to feed themselves. This can be time-consuming and messy. When toddlers learn to talk, they begin to ask for the foods they want. They may not always ask for the most healthful foods.

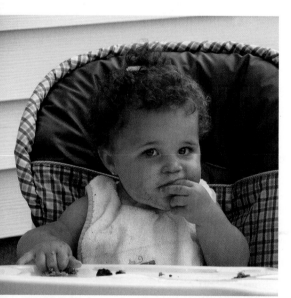

rSnapshotPhotos/Shutterstock.com

Figure 14.19 Young toddlers may make a mess when they feed themselves, but they are learning important skills.

Caregivers should encourage these steps toward independence. Allowing toddlers to feed themselves helps them develop hand-eye coordination (**Figure 14.19**). Offer finger foods, or foods not used with an eating utensil, to encourage eating independence. Allowing toddlers to choose between two nutritious foods helps them learn decision-making skills.

Short Attention Span

A toddler's short attention span can be another eating problem. Toddlers are often easily distracted from eating. They may find it difficult to sit through a meal with their families. They may want to get down on the floor to play. Children need to have regular mealtimes with few distractions. Turning off the television and keeping toys out of the eating area will help children focus on enjoying their food.

Picky Eating

Picky eating is a common problem among toddlers. A child may not want to eat a certain food for many reasons. The food might be too hot, cold, spicy, or bland. The toddler may want a special plate or cup and will not eat without it. The child may be tired or excited about something. He or she may not be hungry because of eating a snack too close to mealtime. The toddler may be coming down with an illness. Sometimes a toddler simply rejects food because of the attention he or she can gain from the rejection.

At times, a toddler may eat all the food on his or her plate and want more. At other times, the toddler may eat only part of the food. Children's appetites vary. Appetite tends to increase during a growth spurt and slow when growth slows.

Caregivers need to make mealtimes pleasant experiences for toddlers. Caregivers should offer familiar foods children like in small, attractive servings. They can help children develop interest in new foods by expressing positive attitudes toward new tastes. Caregivers should not force children to eat or fuss over whether they are eating. After a reasonable amount of time, caregivers can simply remove any uneaten food.

Parents often worry their toddler is not eating enough. Two indicators—normal growth and infrequent infections—can assure parents a child is getting adequate calories and nutrients.

Childhood

Nutritional needs change for children ages four to eight. Preschool and school-age children continue to eat the same basic foods they ate as toddlers. However, they need larger quantities to meet increasing energy needs.

Growth Patterns During Childhood

Growth rates vary among children. Every year brings unique changes. Illness, emotional stress, poor eating habits, and genetics can all affect growth patterns.

Growth is generally slower during childhood than it was in the first years of life. The chubby toddler becomes a taller, thinner preschool child. The child continues to grow and develop muscle control throughout the early school years (**Figure 14.20**).

Children are active during these years. Parents should encourage children to exercise through play activities. Exercise promotes wellness and helps children develop strong muscles and bones.

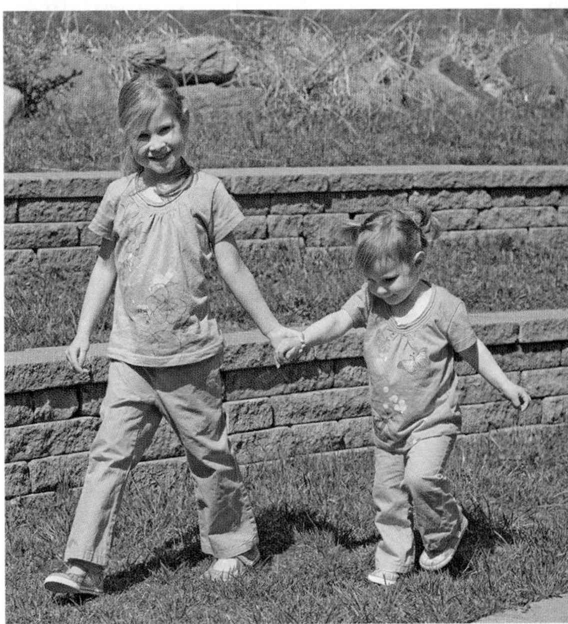

sonya etchison/Shutterstock.com

Figure 14.20 After toddlerhood, a child's body proportions become more like those of an adult.

Nutrient Needs During Childhood

Preschool and school-age children need more total calories than infants and toddlers due to their larger body size. You can use the tools on the ChooseMyPlate.gov to create nutritious food plans, meals, and snacks for children.

The daily requirements for high-quality protein and many vitamins and minerals increase for children ages four and over. An adequate supply of nutrients allows for growth and maintenance of new body tissue. Children should eat a variety of nutritious foods to meet their nutrient needs. Children's diets should contain enough calories from carbohydrates such as whole-grain cereals, breads, and pasta to spare protein for tissue building.

Most health professionals believe the best source of vitamins and minerals for healthy children is from foods in their diet. A doctor may recommend vitamin supplements for children who are at nutritional risk. For example, a doctor may determine that a child who is underweight, on a restricted diet, has a chronic illness, or has multiple food allergies may benefit from vitamin supplements.

Meals for Children

Good meal plans for children include eating meals throughout the day. One important meal is breakfast. It should contain carbohydrates and a small amount of fat. It should provide at least one-fourth of the daily requirements for calories and protein. Children who skip breakfast may have trouble concentrating and performing well in school. They may also have trouble meeting their daily nutrient needs. A nutrient-dense lunch improves performance in school and provides energy for after-school activities.

Children can supplement meals with snacks to help meet nutrient needs. Healthful snacking is easier if the kitchen is stocked with nutritious foods. Parents should keep such items as fruits, yogurt, raisins, carrot sticks, and fat-free milk on hand. They should limit snack foods that have a high salt, sugar, or fat content (**Figure 14.21**).

Too much snacking at the wrong times can decrease a child's appetite for regular meals. Caregivers can help children learn good snacking habits by offering appropriate amounts of snack foods. For example, caregivers can serve two graham crackers instead of offering children the entire box of crackers. They can give children a cup of plain popcorn rather than the bag.

Nutritional and Fitness Problems of Childhood

On the average, children today grow taller than children years ago. One reason for this is the availability of a healthful diet. However, children today are also more likely to be overweight or obese than their ancestors. Poor eating habits and lack of physical activity are the main causes of childhood weight problems.

Caregivers play an important role in preventing weight problems among children. By providing healthful foods, caregivers can help children learn healthy eating habits. Children should be offered water rather than sugar-sweetened drinks. Meals and snacks should be nutrient-rich foods. Caregivers can also limit the amount of time children spend in sedentary activities such as watching television or playing games on electronic devices. Children should spend 60 minutes or more per day being physically active—riding bikes, playing ball, or doing chores. Caregivers must promote healthy choices by explaining to children why it is important to eat right, be active, and get enough sleep each night.

Tooth decay is another nutrition-related problem that is common in childhood. The risk of dental caries, or cavities, is affected by the type of food and when it is eaten.

Meal and Snack Patterns

for a 1,600 calorie Daily Food Plan ...

These patterns are examples of how the Daily Food Plan can be divided into meals and snacks for a preschooler. There are many ways to divide the amounts recommended from each food group into daily meals and snacks.

Click on either pattern to see examples of food choices for meals and snacks.

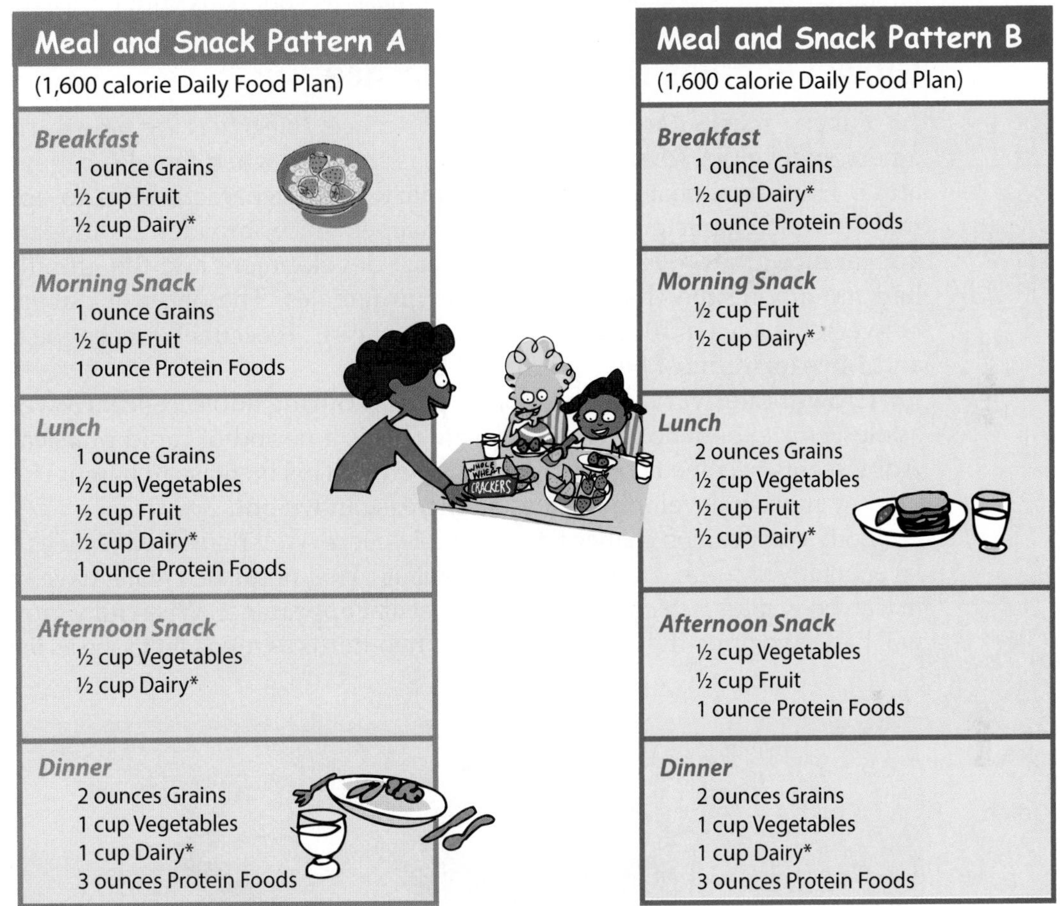

Meal and Snack Pattern A (1,600 calorie Daily Food Plan)	Meal and Snack Pattern B (1,600 calorie Daily Food Plan)
Breakfast 1 ounce Grains ½ cup Fruit ½ cup Dairy*	***Breakfast*** 1 ounce Grains ½ cup Dairy* 1 ounce Protein Foods
Morning Snack 1 ounce Grains ½ cup Fruit 1 ounce Protein Foods	***Morning Snack*** ½ cup Fruit ½ cup Dairy*
Lunch 1 ounce Grains ½ cup Vegetables ½ cup Fruit ½ cup Dairy* 1 ounce Protein Foods	***Lunch*** 2 ounces Grains ½ cup Vegetables ½ cup Fruit ½ cup Dairy*
Afternoon Snack ½ cup Vegetables ½ cup Dairy*	***Afternoon Snack*** ½ cup Vegetables ½ cup Fruit 1 ounce Protein Foods
Dinner 2 ounces Grains 1 cup Vegetables 1 cup Dairy* 3 ounces Protein Foods	***Dinner*** 2 ounces Grains 1 cup Vegetables 1 cup Dairy* 3 ounces Protein Foods

*Offer your child fat-free or low-fat milk, yogurt, and cheese.

***Daily Food Plan** (1,600 calories)*	***Total Amount for the Day***
Grains Group	5 ounces
Vegetable Group	2 cups
Fruit Group	1½ cups
Dairy* Group	2½ cups
Protein Foods Group	5 ounces

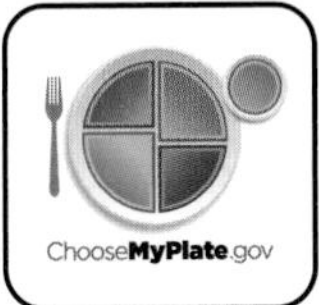

USDA

Figure 14.21 This sample meal and snack pattern is appropriate for a 6-year-old boy who is active 30 to 60 minutes per day.

Sticky, carbohydrate-rich foods eaten between meals are the chief promoters of this problem. However, sound nutrition and dental health practices help develop and maintain healthy teeth and oral tissues. Caregivers can help children prevent tooth decay by teaching them about good eating and dental care habits.

Adolescence

Adolescence is the period of life between childhood and adulthood. You and others who are in this stage of the life cycle are called *adolescents*. Adolescence is an important transition period. The body undergoes many changes during this time. Good food habits started in childhood need continued emphasis as your body continues to develop.

Growth Patterns During Adolescence

Puberty marks the beginning of adolescence. ***Puberty*** is the time during which a person develops sexual maturity. This is the time when females begin menstruating. Hormonal changes cause secondary sexual characteristics to appear. For males, these characteristics include a deeper voice, broader shoulders, and the appearance of facial and body hair. Breast development and the growth of body hair are among the changes that occur in females. The onset of puberty occurs between the ages of 10 and 12 years for most girls. It occurs between the ages of 12 and 14 years for most boys (**Figure 14.22**).

Growth rates vary from person to person during adolescence. However, most adolescents experience a ***growth spurt***. This is a period of rapid physical growth. Adolescents become taller as their bones grow. This increase in height is accompanied by muscle development and an increase in weight.

Body composition changes during adolescence. Well-nourished females develop a layer of fatty tissue that remains throughout life. Well-nourished males have an increase in lean body mass, which gives them a muscular appearance. When fully grown, males will have two times the muscle tissue and two-thirds as much fat tissue as females.

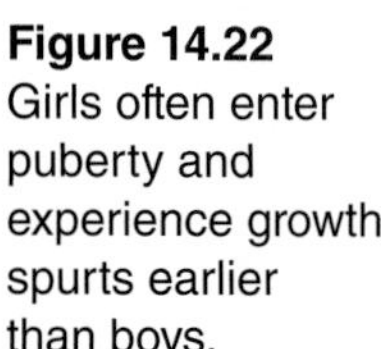

Figure 14.22 Girls often enter puberty and experience growth spurts earlier than boys.

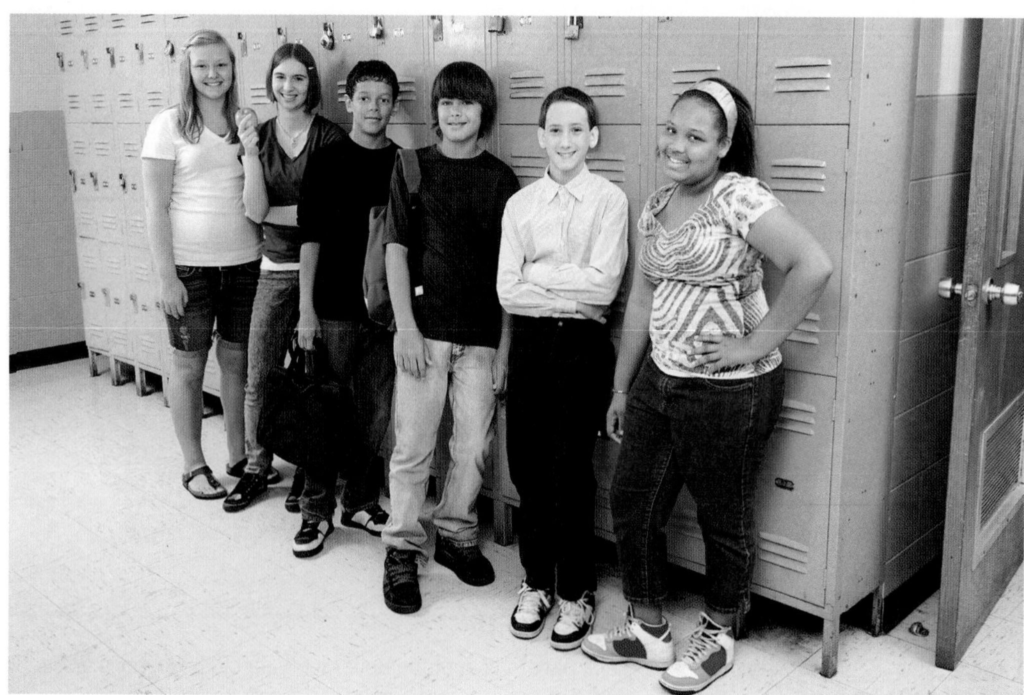

Lisa F. Young/Shutterstock.com

Nutrient Needs During Adolescence

Daily calorie needs in adolescence are higher than they are in late childhood. Specific needs vary with an adolescent's growth rate, gender, and activity level. The average caloric requirement for active 14- to 18-year-old females is roughly 2,300 calories a day. Males need more calories than females. This is partly because males have a higher percentage of lean body mass. The average daily requirement for active males 14 to 18 years old is about 3,100 calories. Teens of both sexes who are involved in intense physical activity have greater calorie needs. Likewise, teens who are less active have lower calorie needs.

Nutrient needs increase significantly for young people in the 9- to 13-year-old age group. Nutrient needs increase again for teens who are 14 to 18 years old. Teens in this group have needs equal to or greater than the needs of adults for most nutrients. Females need slightly smaller amounts of some nutrients than males.

Teens must consume adequate calories and nutrients to fulfill their growth potential.

Meals for Adolescents

The body functions better when it receives supplies of energy and nutrients at regular intervals throughout the day. A busy school, work, and social schedule may make you feel you do not always have time for regular meals. Some days you may skip breakfast. When you are in a hurry, you may be tempted to grab a candy bar instead of stopping for lunch.

You need to be aware of how irregular eating patterns can affect your overall wellness. Young people who skip meals tend to have more difficulty concentrating in school. They also become tired and irritable more easily and report suffering from more headaches and infections.

Breakfast Needs

Eating a good breakfast replenishes a teen's energy supplies after a night of sleep (**Figure 14.23**). Breakfast should provide about one-fourth of your daily nutrient and calorie needs. Any nutritious food helps get your body off to a good start in the morning. If you do not like cereal or eggs, try eating a peanut butter sandwich, yogurt, fresh fruit, fruit smoothies, or even pizza. There are important reasons for fitting breakfast into your daily schedule:

- Breakfast helps accelerate brain function. Your ability to focus and participate in memory and recall activities increases when energy level remains high during morning hours.
- Breakfast promotes healthy weight maintenance by reducing the likelihood of mid-morning snacking on unhealthy, energy-dense foods.
- Research shows that students who eat a healthy breakfast are more likely to choose healthier foods throughout the day. Regularly making healthy food choices affects long-term health and weight-management goals.

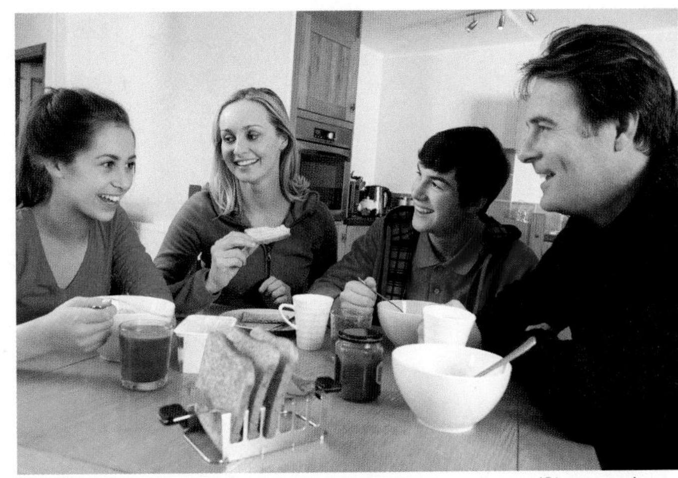

Monkey Business Images/Shutterstock.com

Figure 14.23 Students who eat breakfast perform better in school and have more energy.

Other Meals

Eating at least two other meals throughout the day should allow you to meet your remaining calorie needs. Carefully choosing the recommended daily amounts from MyPlate should supply you with your nutrient requirements. Between-meal snacks can help provide health-promoting nutrients.

Most teens eat some meals at fast-food restaurants. Foods such as pizza, hamburgers, and milk shakes provide nutrients; however, they also tend to be high in calories, sugar, saturated fats, and sodium. Therefore, eat these foods in moderation and balance them with other nutrient-dense food choices throughout the day (**Figure 14.24**). Many fast-food restaurants now offer nutrient-dense foods such as salads, whole-grain breads and pastas, low-fat dairy, and fruits.

Nutritional and Fitness Problems of Adolescence

Teens often have a reputation for having poor eating habits. Many young people do not deserve this reputation. Surveys suggest many adolescents get enough of most nutrients. However, some adolescent nutritional problems exist.

Anemia is an iron-deficiency disease that often occurs during the teen years. Adolescents need increased amounts of iron to support growth of body tissues. After age 14, females require more iron than males due to losses through menstruation. Some doctors prescribe iron supplements to help adolescent females make up for a lack of dietary iron. Red meat, legumes, dark green leafy vegetables, and whole-grain and enriched breads and cereals are good iron sources.

Weight problems are common among adolescents. Teens who are overweight need to adjust their food intake and increase their activity level. Teens who are underweight are at the other end of the weight management spectrum. These teens need to consume excess calories and exercise to build muscle. Many teens display eating disorders. Although an eating disorder is a mental illness, it often **manifests** (is made evident) as a weight problem.

Figure 14.24 Foods such as pizza, burgers, and tacos account for a large portion of the saturated fats and sodium in teens' diets. *How often do you eat these types of foods?*

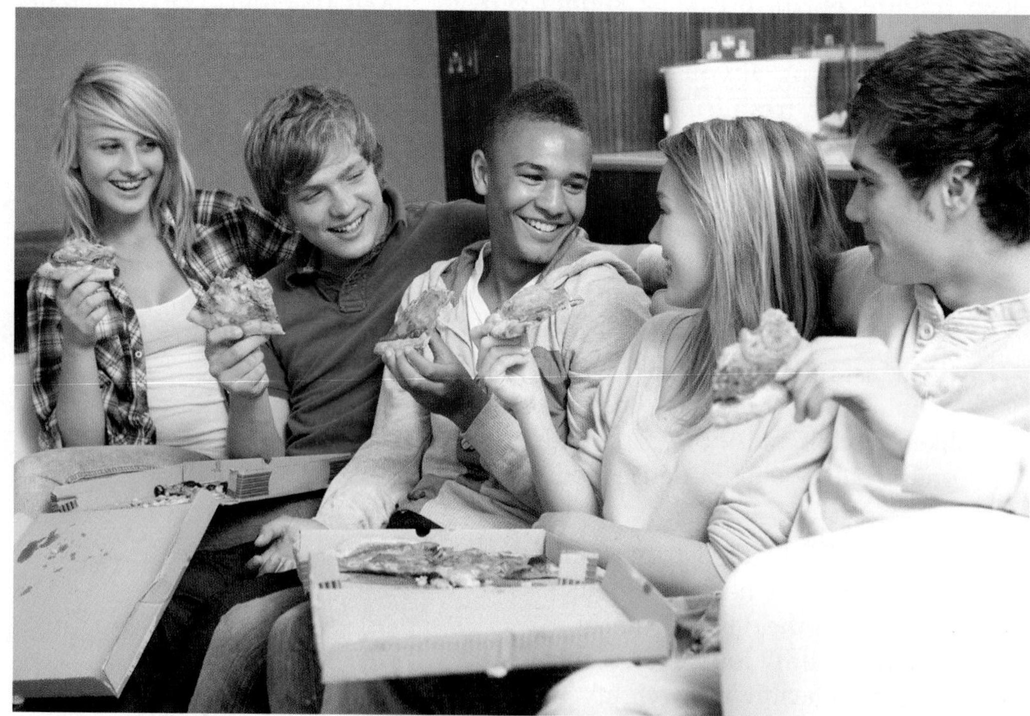

Monkey Business Images/Shutterstock.com

Smoking, consuming alcohol, and abusing drugs are habits that sometimes begin in adolescence. These lifestyle behaviors can affect nutritional status.

You need to be aware of the relationship between your diet during adolescence and your health as an adult. If your diet does not include enough calcium and vitamin D, your bones will not achieve maximum density. This lack of bone density will increase your risk of osteoporosis later in life. If you eat a diet high in sugar without proper dental hygiene, you are more likely to have dental caries. This increases your risk of gum disease and tooth loss in your later years. An eating pattern that includes too much saturated fat and calories raises your chances of developing chronic diseases, such as heart disease and some forms of cancer as an adult. Eating a healthful diet now can help prevent future health problems (**Figure 14.25**).

Adulthood

Young men and women move from adolescence into adulthood. This phase of the life cycle lasts until death. It covers the largest number of years.

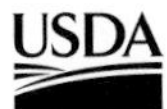

United States Department of Agriculture

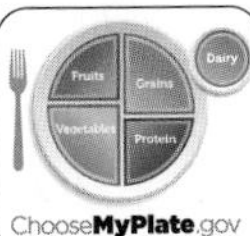

MyPlate Daily Checklist

Find your Healthy Eating Style

Everything you eat and drink matters. Find your healthy eating style that reflects your preferences, culture, traditions, and budget—and maintain it for a lifetime! The right mix can help you be healthier now and into the future. The key is choosing a variety of foods and beverages from each food group—*and making sure that each choice is limited in saturated fat, sodium, and added sugars.* Start with small changes—**"MyWins"**—to make healthier choices you can enjoy.

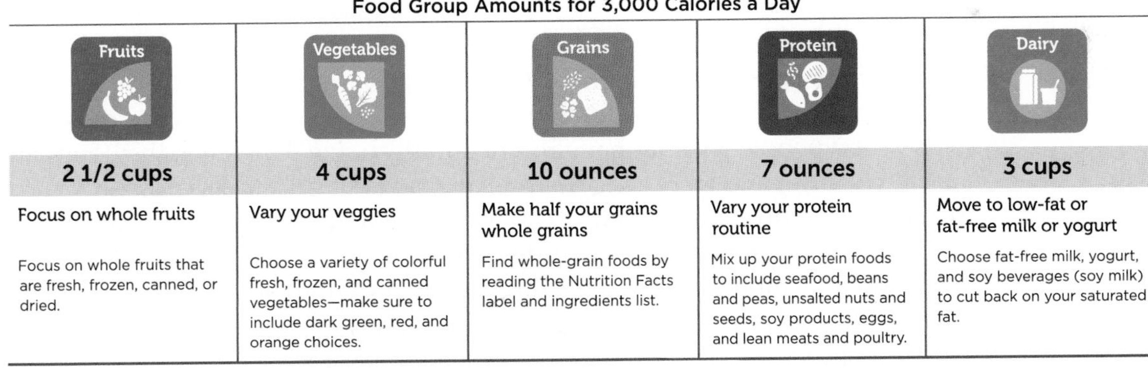

Food Group Amounts for 3,000 Calories a Day

Fruits	Vegetables	Grains	Protein	Dairy
2 1/2 cups	**4 cups**	**10 ounces**	**7 ounces**	**3 cups**
Focus on whole fruits	Vary your veggies	Make half your grains whole grains	Vary your protein routine	Move to low-fat or fat-free milk or yogurt
Focus on whole fruits that are fresh, frozen, canned, or dried.	Choose a variety of colorful fresh, frozen, and canned vegetables—make sure to include dark green, red, and orange choices.	Find whole-grain foods by reading the Nutrition Facts label and ingredients list.	Mix up your protein foods to include seafood, beans and peas, unsalted nuts and seeds, soy products, eggs, and lean meats and poultry.	Choose fat-free milk, yogurt, and soy beverages (soy milk) to cut back on your saturated fat.

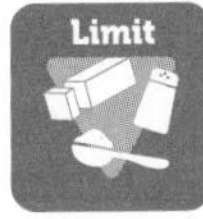

Drink and eat less sodium, saturated fat, and added sugars. Limit:

- Sodium to **2,300 milligrams** a day.
- Saturated fat to **33 grams** a day.
- Added sugars to **75 grams** a day.

Be active your way: Children 6 to 17 years old should move **60 minutes** every day. Adults should be physically active at least **2 1/2 hours** per week.

Use SuperTracker to create a personal plan based on your age, sex, height, weight, and physical activity level.

SuperTracker.usda.gov

USDA

Figure 14.25 This is a nutritious meal plan for an active 17-year-old male. *How does your daily diet compare with this meal plan?*

THE MOVEMENT CONNECTION

Body-Spanning Stretch

Why

Nutrition is important across the life span, not just for young infants or older adults. Similarly, it is important to stretch all your muscles rather than focus on just one area and ignore others.

This stretch will span your entire body to benefit all your muscles.

Apply

- Stand in front of your chair with good posture.
- As you inhale, raise arms straight up toward the ceiling. (Keep your shoulders relaxed down your back. Do not shrug your shoulders up to your ears.)
- As you exhale, lower your arms and sit back down.
- Come into a forward bend over the legs with your belly resting on the tops of your legs.
- Let your head hang heavy.
- Let your hands rest on the floor (if they reach).
- As you inhale, raise your arms back up over your head and come to a standing position.

Repeat 5 times.

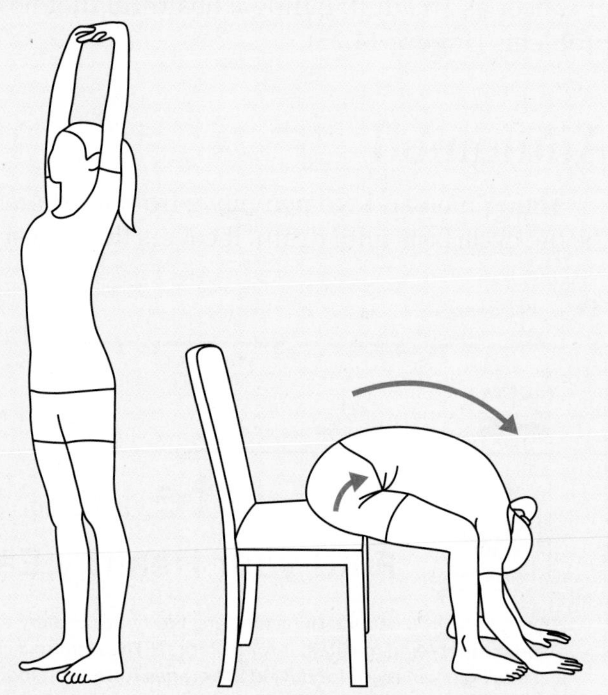

Nutritionists often divide adulthood into four stages. Early adulthood is the time from 19 through 30 years. By this stage, the rapid growth of adolescence has ceased and people's bodies have reached mature size. However, the bones are still storing calcium and increasing their density. Middle adulthood describes the years from ages 31 through 50. Some visible signs of aging begin to appear during this stage of life. Later adulthood includes people who are ages 51 through 70. Signs of aging become more apparent during these years. Older adulthood is over 70 years of age. People in this age group are more likely to develop special health and nutrition needs.

Signs of aging include graying hair, wrinkling skin, deteriorating vision, and slowing reflexes. These are natural changes that occur as the body gets older. However, many health problems that are more common among older people are not a natural result of aging. Research shows following a nutritious diet and exercising can help prevent such problems as heart disease and high blood pressure. This information has spurred many middle-aged adults to adopt good health habits. The earlier people make these habits part of their lifestyles, the more benefits they gain.

Nutrient Needs During Adulthood

Good nutrition is as important as ever during adulthood. The nutritional needs of adults are similar to those of adolescents. Adults need nutrients mainly to support vital body functions. Adult males need a bit more protein than adolescents. Because bones are no longer growing, adults need less calcium and phosphorus than adolescents need. However, the Recommended Dietary Allowance (RDA) for calcium increases for women over age 50 and men over 70 years old. The RDA for vitamin D increases for adults over age 70. In addition, doctors often recommend calcium supplements for older women to help maintain strong bones. The RDA for vitamin B_6 increases for older adults as well. Iron requirements drop for women following menopause.

Calorie needs gradually decrease in adulthood. For many adults, this is due to a decrease in the amount of energy their bodies need to operate. However, energy needs can remain at the levels seen in early adulthood if a person exercises and maintains lean body mass. Older adults require fewer calories to maintain their body weight. Some older people become less active, which causes physical abilities to change. This lowers the need for calories even more. Many adults gain weight as they age because they fail to stay active and match their calorie intake to their calorie output.

Adult Food Choices

Some adults find it hard to change the eating habits they established during childhood and continued in adolescence. In earlier life stages, people have high energy needs for growth. Some less nutritious food choices can fit more easily into diets at these stages. In adulthood, however, food choices need to be more nutrient-dense to meet nutrient requirements without exceeding calorie needs.

Many adults claim busy schedules and time pressures keep them from eating a nutritious diet. When they eat in a hurry, adults often choose foods that are high in saturated fat, sugar, and sodium.

The sample menu in **Figure 14.26** would provide a nutritious diet for a healthy adult female. This menu includes foods that are nutrient dense. Adults who require more calories to maintain a healthy weight can increase the number and size of portions. Adults who need fewer calories to maintain a healthy weight are encouraged to increase their activity levels.

Sample Menu for an Adult Female
Breakfast
1 whole-wheat English muffin 2 tsp. soft margarine 1 Tbsp. jam or preserves
1 medium grapefruit
1 hard-cooked egg
1 unsweetened beverage
Lunch
White bean-vegetable soup: 1¼ cup chunky vegetable soup ½ cup white beans
2-ounce breadstick
8 baby carrots
1 cup fat-free milk
Dinner
Rigatoni with meat sauce: 1 cup rigatoni pasta (2 ounces dry) ½ cup tomato sauce 2 ounces extra lean cooked ground beef (sautéed in 2 tsp. vegetable oil) 3 Tbsp. grated Parmesan cheese
Spinach salad: 1 cup baby spinach leaves ½ cup tangerine slices ½ ounce chopped walnuts 3 tsp. sunflower oil and vinegar dressing
1 cup fat-free milk
Snack
1 cup low-fat fruited yogurt

Figure 14.26 Adults need to choose nutrient-dense foods.

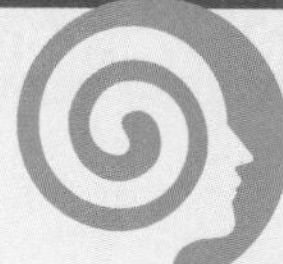

EXTEND YOUR KNOWLEDGE

Aging and Life Expectancy in the United States

The percent of the US population comprised of individuals age 65 or older is expected to be 20% by the year 2050. The 65 and older population is growing faster than the total US population. This represents over twice as many people in this age range as in the year 2000. Currently, people 90 and older now comprise 4.7 percent of the older population (age 65 and older), as compared with only 2.8 percent in 1980. By 2050, this share is likely to reach 10 percent. This aging trend in the population is due to an increase in average life span and an increase in fertility in the two decades following World War II, known as the "Baby Boom." Find the reports by the Administration on Aging (AoA) to study the projected future growth of the older population and the 65+ in the United States: 2010 on the US Census Bureau website to learn more about aging trends.

Nutritional and Fitness Problems During Adulthood

Maintaining a healthy body weight may be the biggest health-related problem affecting adults today. Overweight has been linked with type 2 diabetes, heart disease, and gall bladder disease. Avoiding overweight is wise because losing weight is hard for most adults. Adopting a healthy lifestyle including a nutritious diet and regular, moderate physical activity can help older people avoid becoming overweight. Adults are recommended to have 2 hours and 30 minutes (150 minutes) of moderate intensity aerobic activity (i.e., brisk walking) every week and muscle strenghening activities two or more days a week that work all major muscle groups (legs, hips, back, abdomen, chest, shoulders, and arms).

Constipation is a problem for some adults. Being physically active and choosing fiber-rich foods can help prevent this problem (**Figure 14.27**). Fruits, vegetables, legumes, and whole grains supply dietary fiber. Drinking at least six glasses of water a day can also help prevent constipation.

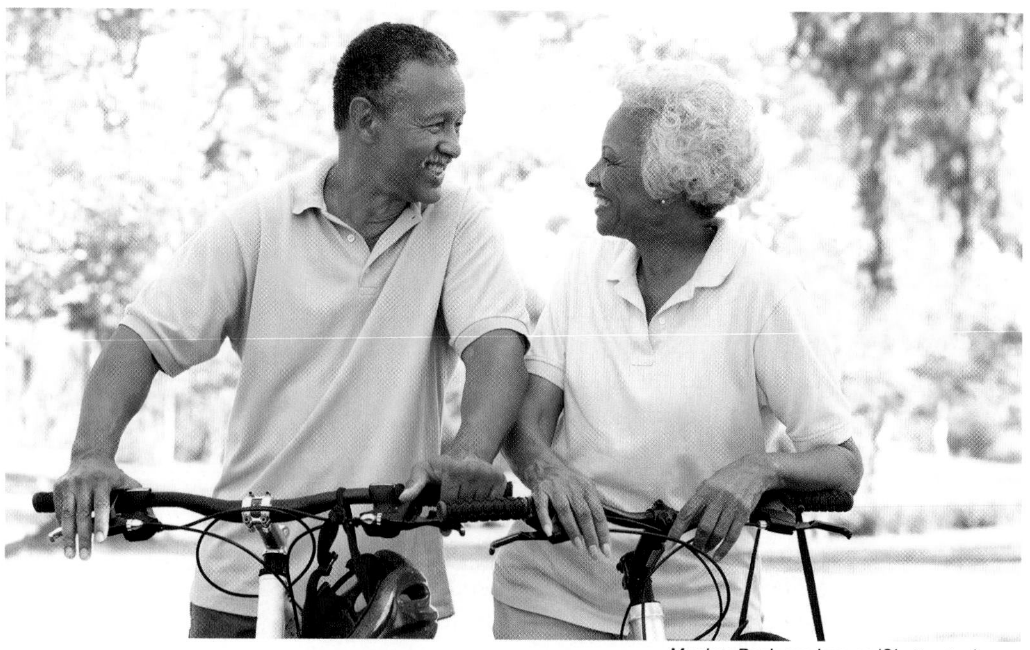

Figure 14.27 Remaining active can help adults over age 50 avoid problems associated with inactivity.

Monkey Business Images/Shutterstock.com

Many adult women fail to get enough calcium and vitamin D in their diets. This, along with hormonal changes of menopause and lack of weight-bearing activity, increases their risk of developing osteoporosis. At around age 50, women go through menopause. ***Menopause*** is the time of life when menstruation ends due to a decrease in production of the hormone estrogen. Among other functions, estrogen plays a role in maintaining bone tissue. Therefore, bone density loss occurs more rapidly in women after menopause due to the drop in estrogen levels.

COMMUNITY CONNECTIONS

Volunteer with Older Adults

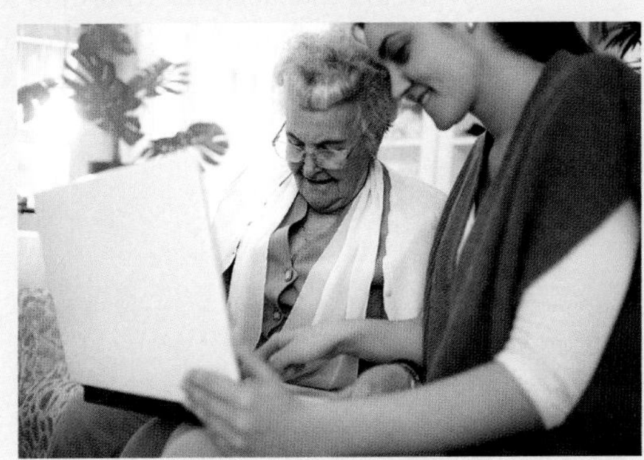
Cherries/Shutterstock.com

Many older adults have health problems that prevent them from leaving their homes and socializing. This isolation can contribute to a feeling of loneliness. Volunteers can help alleviate some of that loneliness and isolation by simply sharing their time. Opportunities to volunteer with older adults are numerous and rewarding.

Many teens have older adults in their life who would benefit from help. If you are interested in volunteering with older adults, you could begin with relatives or neighbors. Simply visiting on a regular basis to chat or play cards could make a big impact in their lives and yours. You could offer to perform household chores like raking leaves or shoveling snow.

Another option is volunteering in an assisted living facility or visiting a nursing home. Teen volunteers are often needed in organizations where the elderly live. You could bring a book to read aloud or perhaps share your musical talent by playing piano or guitar. Be sure to call the facility in advance to arrange your visit.

The connections you make with the elderly can add a rich experience to your life. You can learn a lot from listening to their life stories. It is interesting to hear what life was like when they were your age. For instance, join them at mealtime and discuss what foods were popular when they were young. Listening is an important part of this volunteer experience. Listen to their career success stories to gain insights on how to plan a successful career for yourself.

A teen who volunteers with the elderly may be assisting people with making crafts, participating in physical activity programs, teaching basic smartphone or computer skills, or simply preparing nutritious treats to share with a person. Take the opportunity to learn more about special diets served to the elderly who have health conditions. There is much for you to learn when working with the elderly.

Think Critically

1. What are the differences and similarities of working with the elderly as compared with working with other age group clients?
2. Research the steps required to find a volunteer position in a senior center in your community.
3. What do you think an older adult might want to know about teen life today?

Eating the recommended number of daily servings of milk, yogurt, and cheese can help women meet their calcium needs. However, as people age, their ability to absorb several important nutrients decreases. In addition, they may fail to get enough nutrients in their daily meals. Vitamin D, folate, and vitamin B_{12} are of special concern in the later years. Some physicians recommend supplements for people in this age group.

Special Problems of Older Adults

You may have friends or relatives who are in their later years. Some of these older people may be healthy and active. Others may have serious health problems and be confined to their homes.

Health Issues

Doctors recommend modified diets to help treat many diseases, including heart disease and diabetes. However, many other health problems can affect nutrient needs. For instance, recovering from surgery and some illnesses increases the need for protein. Recovery also increases the need for some vitamins and minerals, especially vitamin C and zinc.

Medications can affect a person's nutritional status, too. As an example, taking large daily doses of aspirin increases the rate of blood loss from the stomach. This can increase the need for iron. Use of tobacco and alcohol greatly increases older adults' health risks and can affect their nutritional status as well. Older adults may want to consult a registered dietitian nutritionist about how health problems and medications affect their nutrient requirements.

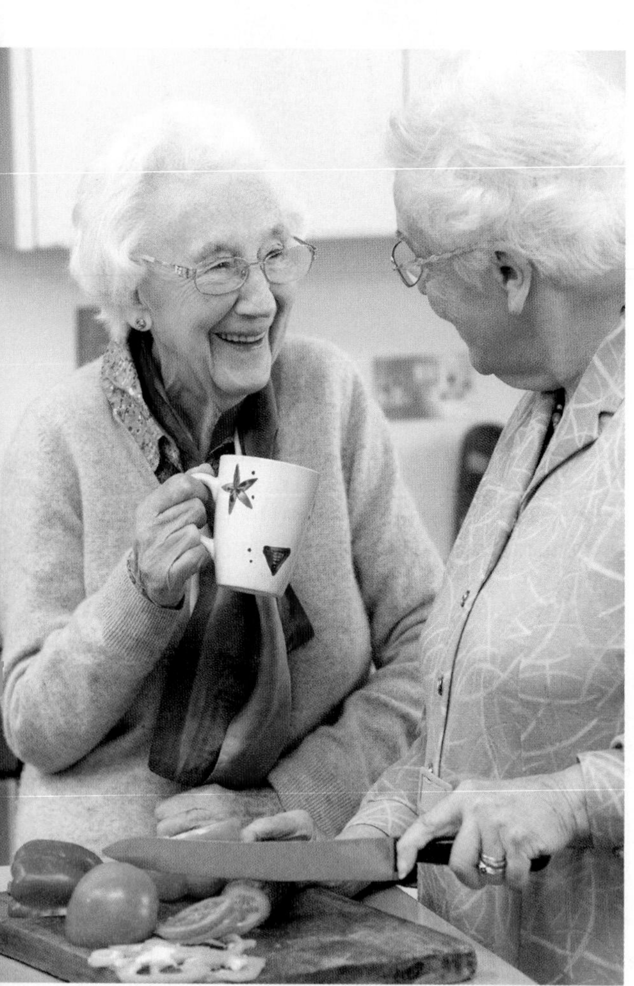

Monkey Business Images/Shutterstock.com

Figure 14.28 Companionship can motivate older adults to prepare and eat nutritious meals.

Digestive Issues

A number of factors can affect an older adult's desire and ability to eat. This, in turn, has an impact on the adult's nutritional status. A diminished sense of taste causes foods to seem bland to some older adults. Tooth loss may make chewing difficult. Digestive problems may result in stomach upset after eating.

Limited Income and Isolation

Limited income and lack of mobility can have an impact on food intake for some older people. Older adults with low incomes may choose to limit their food expenditures. Others may have trouble getting to a food market and carrying home bags of groceries. Buying, preparing, and serving a pleasing variety of foods for one or two persons may be a difficult task.

Isolation is another factor that affects the appetites of some older adults (**Figure 14.28**). A number of older adults live alone. They may be separated from family members and friends. Living alone may decrease their motivation to prepare and eat nutritious meals. Often fruits and vegetables are absent from meals. Some senior centers offer meals to help older people who are troubled by loneliness. Home meal-delivery services assist those who have difficulty getting out to shop for food.

Physical Activity in Older Adulthood

To stay healthy, older people should include physical activity in their everyday life. Regular physical activity helps older adults maintain good health. Activity reduces risks of health problems that come with aging. It helps muscles grow stronger to keep up with doing everyday activities. Health benefits increase with the more physical activity that occurs.

Even taking short walks throughout the day keeps muscles toned and improves blood circulation. A formal physical activity program may not be necessary, but joining a seniors' fitness program can be a motivator for fostering longevity and reducing the risk of Alzheimer's disease. Nutrition and fitness programs such as these help older adults maintain health through the years.

Nutrition and fitness programs for older adults often focus on strength training, aerobic activity, and flexibility and stretching exercises. The goal is to reduce the risks of falls and to continue with daily lifestyle activities.

RECIPE FILE

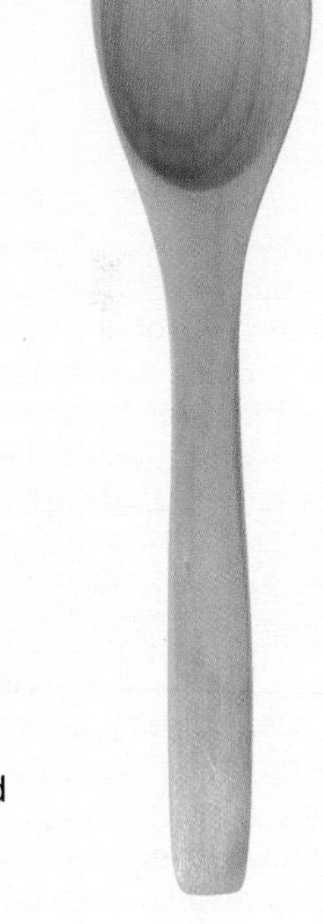

Arugula Corn Salad

4 SERVINGS

Ingredients

- 1 ear corn on the cob
- 2 T. olive oil
- 2 T. shallot, minced
- ½ lemon, juiced
- 1 bunch arugula
- 1 bag (10 oz.) baby spinach
- ¼ c. shaved Parmesan cheese

Directions

1. Cut corn kernels off the cob.
2. Heat 1 teaspoon of olive oil in a skillet over medium heat.
3. Sauté shallot and corn until shallot begins to soften, about 4 minutes.
4. In a small bowl, mix together corn and shallot, the remainder of the olive oil, and lemon juice.
5. Place arugula and spinach in a large bowl and pour shallot-corn mixture over and toss until combined.
6. Top with shaved Parmesan cheese.
7. Serve with Salmon Burgers (recipe in Chapter 13).

PER SERVING: 140 CALORIES, 6 G PROTEIN, 13 G CARBOHYDRATE, 8 G FAT, 4 G FIBER, 97 MG SODIUM.

Chapter 14 Review and Expand

Reading Summary

The life cycle is divided into stages. People in each of these stages require the same basic nutrients. However, the amounts needed vary due to special nutritional needs associated with each stage.

Good health and nutritional status before pregnancy helps ensure the health of mothers and their babies. Women require extra calories and nutrients during pregnancy to meet the needs of the developing fetus. Pregnant teens have especially high nutrient needs to support their development as well as their babies' development. Women who choose to breast-feed their babies also have increased nutrient needs. Eating a variety of nutritious foods is the best way to meet these needs. Smoking and using alcohol and other drugs during pregnancy may harm a developing fetus. These habits may also harm infants during breast-feeding.

Healthy babies grow rapidly during the first year of life. Toddlers, who are one to three years of age, grow more slowly. Infants and toddlers both need nutritious foods to support rapid growth. Breast milk or formula is the only food infants need for the first few months. Then a variety of strained foods is gradually added to the diet. Toddlers can eat small portions of most table foods. Being aware of normal infant and toddler development helps caregivers know what to expect when feeding young children.

Preschool and school-age children need more calories and nutrients each day than infants and toddlers. Healthful snacks can be an important source of nutrients for children at this age.

Bone and muscle growth are rapid during the adolescent growth spurt. Nutritional requirements are especially high during this period. Teens need to avoid poor eating habits, such as skipping meals or eating too many high-fat foods from fast-food restaurants. Such habits can cause nutritional deficiencies that may lead to health problems later in life.

By adulthood, the body has reached its mature size. Nutrient and energy recommendations for this age group are set at a maintenance level. However, many adults exceed these recommendations. This makes overweight the biggest nutrition-related problem affecting adults.

A number of physical, emotional, and social factors can place an older adult's nutritional status at risk. Consuming a good diet throughout the life cycle contributes to a state of wellness.

Chapter Vocabulary

1. **Content Terms** In small groups, create categories for the following terms and classify as many of the terms as possible. Then, share your ideas with the rest of the class.

   adolescence
   congenital disability
   fetal alcohol syndrome (FAS)
   fetus
   growth spurt
   infant
   lactation
   life cycle
   low-birthweight baby
   menopause
   pica
   placenta
   premature baby
   puberty
   toddler
   trimester

2. **Academic Terms** For each of the following terms, identify a word or group of words describing a quality of the term—an *attribute.* Pair up with a classmate and discuss your list of attributes. Then, discuss your list of attributes with the whole class to increase understanding.

   exacerbate
   manifest
   necessitate
   oversee
   wane

Review Learning

3. What are the six major stages of the human life cycle?
4. What factors other than life-cycle stage influence the amounts of nutrients needed by an individual?
5. In what two ways will forming healthful eating habits before pregnancy help a woman during pregnancy?
6. *True or false?* Mothers who choose to breast-feed need even greater amounts of some nutrients than they needed when they were pregnant.
7. What are two factors that place teens at a higher risk of complications during pregnancy than mature women?
8. What are three symptoms that might occur in a baby born with fetal alcohol syndrome?
9. Explain the statement "Children have proportionately greater nutritional needs than adults."

10. Why should caregivers introduce only one food at a time to an infant's meal plans?
11. Describe two factors that can lead to eating problems during the toddler years. Give a suggestion for dealing with each factor.
12. What are four examples of healthful snacks for school-age children?
13. What are two problems related to nutrition that are common in childhood?
14. Why do adolescent males need more calories than adolescent females?
15. Give two examples of how nutritional patterns during adolescence can affect health in adulthood.
16. Why do calorie needs decrease in older adulthood?
17. List four factors that can affect an older adult's desire and ability to eat.

Self-Assessment Quiz

Complete the self-assessment quiz online to help you practice and expand your knowledge and skills.

Critical Thinking

18. **Compare and Contrast** How are the nutrient needs of adolescents and adults similar? different?
19. **Predict Consequences** What health consequences might teens face later in life due to poor nutritional and fitness choices during adolescent years?
20. **Evaluate** Obtain school lunch menus from grammar, middle, and high schools. Evaluate whether each menu substantially meets the needs of the age group it serves. List any changes you would recommend.
21. **Create** Prepare two healthful snacks that would appeal to young children. Serve the snacks to a group of preschoolers and evaluate their reactions.
22. **Analyze** Create descriptions for two imaginary people. One should be a school-age child or younger and the other should be an adolescent or older. The descriptions should include the age, sex, level of physical activity, height, and weight. Visit ChooseMyPlate.gov and use your descriptions to create a MyPlate Daily Checklist for each of your imaginary people. Compare the daily amounts from each food group recommended for the young child to that for the adult. How do they differ?

Core Skills

23. **Math** Research and prepare cost estimates for breast-feeding versus bottle feeding for the first year of life. Present your findings in a graph or other visual format.
24. **Technology Literacy** Design a page for your school's website on the importance of physical activity in the life of teens and their parents or care providers. List examples of physical activities that are appropriate for each of the age groups.
25. **Science and Writing** Use a reliable biology resource to outline the stages of human gestation. Investigate to learn the impact of nutrition at each stage. Write a paper to share your findings. Provide citations for your sources.
26. **Listening** Conduct an oral history interview of a healthy older adult you know to learn about his or her diet and lifestyle. Ask what eating and activity patterns he or she believes have contributed to his or her well-being.
27. **Speaking** Debate the following topic: A healthy eating pattern combined with regular physical activity ensures longevity. Cite reliable sources to defend your assertion.
28. **Career Readiness Practice** As a nutrition educator at a family fitness center, you work with multigenerational families who find it difficult to meet nutrition needs economically and efficiently. One of your clients is a family with three children (ages 3, 7, and 12) whose parents hold full-time jobs. Living with them is a 75-year-old grandmother who has osteoporosis. Several nights per week involve a trip to the local fast-food drive through for the family meal. This is taking its toll on the family's budget and health. Write your responses to the following as you prepare to help this family:
    A. What appears to be the core problem for this family and what alternatives might solve it?
    B. How would you help the family develop an appropriate plan and take action on it?
    C. How would you help the family evaluate results?

Eating for Sports Performance

Learning Outcomes

After studying this chapter, you will be able to

- **compare** aerobic and anaerobic energy production systems;
- **recognize** the nutrient needs of athletes;
- **plan** meals and snacks for an athlete in training;
- **implement** recommendations for hydration before, during, and after an athletic event;
- **explain** how athletes can safely lose or gain weight for competition; and
- **recall** precautions related to performance aids marketed to athletes.

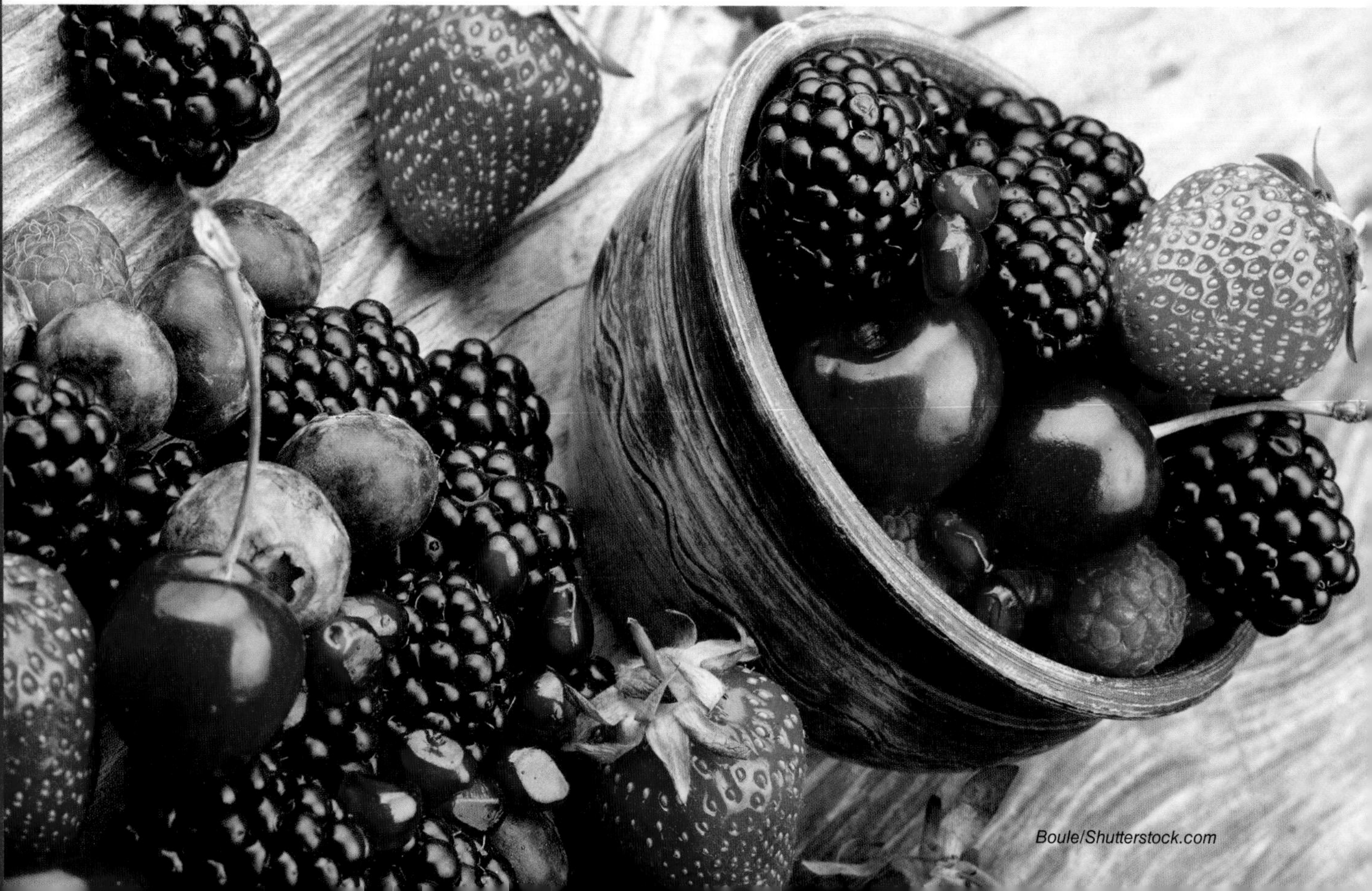

Boule/Shutterstock.com

Content Terms 

aerobic
anaerobic
carbohydrate loading
endurance athlete
lactic acid
recovery

Academic Terms 

convert
deplete
expend
lethargic
sustain

What's Your Nutrition and Wellness IQ?

Take this quiz to examine how much you already know about eating for sports performance. If you cannot answer a question, pay extra attention to that topic as you study this chapter.

- Identify each statement as *True*, *False*, or *It Depends*. *It Depends* means in some cases the statement is true; in some cases it could be false.
- Revise false statements to make them true.
- Explain the circumstances in which each *It Depends* statement is true and when it is false.

Nutrition and Wellness IQ 

1.	An athlete requires greater energy intake during training than during the off-season.	True	False	It Depends
2.	The body's aerobic energy production system requires the use of oxygen to break down glucose to produce energy.	True	False	It Depends
3.	Carbohydrate loading is recommended as preparation for all major athletic competitions.	True	False	It Depends
4.	Most athletes need to increase the amount of protein in their daily eating plans.	True	False	It Depends
5.	The best pre-event meal for an athlete is a steak and potato.	True	False	It Depends
6.	Water is always the best beverage for hydration purposes.	True	False	It Depends
7.	The best way to lose weight for a competition is to reduce fluid consumption for two days before the event.	True	False	It Depends
8.	The problem with performance aids is that they don't really work.	True	False	It Depends

While studying this chapter, look for the activity icon 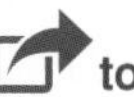 **to**

- **build** vocabulary with e-flash cards and interactive games;
- **assess** what you learn by completing self-assessment quizzes and completing review questions; and
- **expand** knowledge with interactive activities and activities that extend learning.

www.g-wlearning.com/foodsandnutrition/

Sports activities are an important part of everyday life. These activities provide health and wellness benefits for all who take part. They promote self-esteem and build physical skills. Through teamwork, sports also help people grow socially and emotionally.

Athletes often have an intense desire to excel. Team and partner sports are competitive. The focus is on beating an opponent. Individual sports present athletes with a challenge to surpass their previous best performance.

The drive for peak performance has led some athletes to seek a winning edge through their diet. Their search has fostered the spread of nutrition myths and misinformation. This chapter will help you sort the facts from the fallacies.

Fueling Muscle for Performance

Where do muscles get the energy needed to fuel activity? As you know, carbohydrates and fats are the main sources of energy for the body. Nutrients are supplied by the foods you eat and by your body's stores of fat and glucose. However, the body must first **convert** (change) these nutrients into an energy source that can be used by the muscle.

Energy Production in the Body

The energy that fuels muscle is produced either in the presence or absence of oxygen. One of the body's energy production systems is ***aerobic***, or requires the presence of oxygen. The body also has an energy production system that is ***anaerobic***, or takes place in the absence of oxygen. Each of these systems has benefits and drawbacks. The body uses them in combination to maximize the benefits.

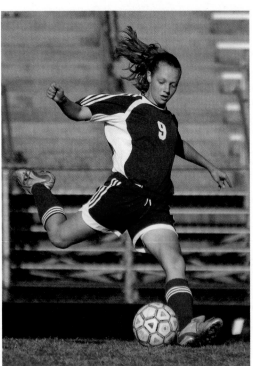

CLS Digital Arts/Shutterstock.com

Figure 15.1 Soccer players' muscles are fueled by both aerobic and anaerobic energy production systems.

The anaerobic energy production system is the first to supply energy when your body begins an activity. The first seconds of an activity are fueled by the very small but essential supply of energy that is stored in the muscle ready for immediate use. At the same time, the system begins converting the glycogen that is stored in the muscle to glucose. The glucose is then rapidly converted to an energy source the muscle can use (**Figure 15.1**).

The anaerobic system supplies energy quickly, but cannot sustain this rate of energy production for long. Therefore, the body turns to the aerobic energy production system for fuel. The aerobic system is slower to respond to the body's need for energy because it requires the presence of oxygen. The oxygen must be inhaled and transported through the blood to the muscle, which takes time. However, this system can supply energy to the body for hours. Unlike the anaerobic system, the aerobic system can access and utilize the energy stored in fat as well as that found in glucose.

In the absence of oxygen, an incomplete breakdown of glucose results in a buildup of a product called ***lactic acid*** in the muscles. The lactic acid changes the body's acid-base balance. As a result, you experience a burning sensation and fatigue in the muscles. For example, a cross-country athlete running at a fast pace becomes out of breath.

When this occurs, the athlete may need to slow down to allow breathing to catch up with the need for oxygen. As breathing improves, the needed oxygen is delivered to the bloodstream and the acid-base balance is restored.

Improving Energy Production

Both energy production systems can become more efficient with the use of appropriate training methods. For example, the anaerobic system can be improved with training that involves performing high-intensity exercises less than 10 seconds in duration separated by brief rest intervals. When hockey players train with repeated sprints across the ice and rapid direction changes, they are trying to improve their anaerobic energy systems.

Some sports require athletes, called ***endurance athletes***, to use their muscles for long periods. These endurance athletes may be involved in sports such as marathon bicycle and foot races or distance swimming. Endurance athletes must **sustain** (keep up) muscle efforts for several hours at a time. You might wonder how they can extend their muscle performance to avoid exhausting their glycogen stores and "hitting the wall." Improving the efficiency of the aerobic energy system is a goal for these athletes. Endurance athletes train to improve the ability of their heart and lungs to deliver oxygen to their muscles. Increased oxygen in the muscle improves the muscle's ability to use glucose. This allows the body to use more fat for fuel and conserve glycogen. Trained muscles also become more tolerant of lactic acid. Thus, soreness and fatigue will not occur as quickly.

Both the aerobic and anaerobic energy systems are always in use by the body. However, the nature of the activity and the fitness of the athlete influence which system is supplying more energy.

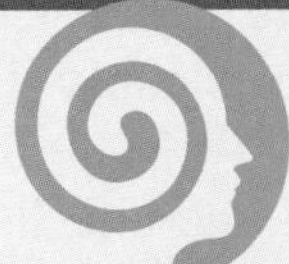

EXTEND YOUR KNOWLEDGE

Genes and Sports Performance

Your aptitude for sports may be the result of genetic factors. Genes affect your muscle strength, skeletal structure, tendon elasticity, and heart and lung size. Individuals perform at varying levels of endurance, speed, and power. Some athletes are naturally better at marathons, while others excel at 100-meter sprints.

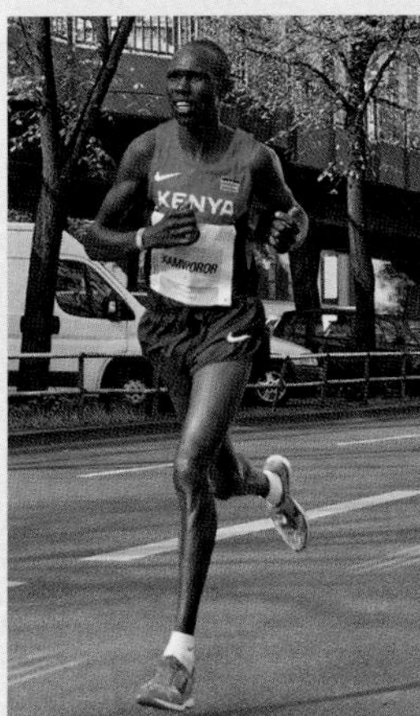

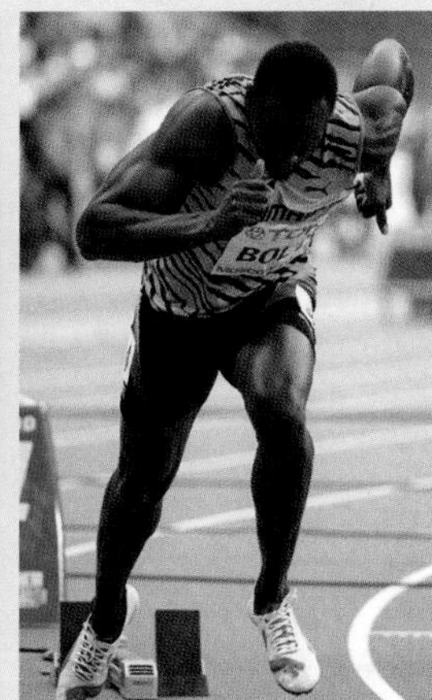

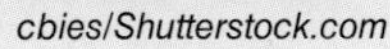

cbies/Shutterstock.com Kaliva/Shutterstock.com

For instance, an endurance athlete may have a cardiovascular system that is capable of delivering oxygen to working muscles more efficiently due to his or her genetic makeup. Genetic factors, such as height and body composition, affect the body's ability to maximize oxygen uptake and utilization. Athletes who are endowed with these genetic factors are more successful at endurance sports.

How does training factor into athletic success? Certain non-inherited factors also affect performance, such as social support, motivation, and specialized training. You can overcome the limitations you are born with, but it may take more effort. Which factor do you think most influences elite athletes' success, genes or training?

The Nutrient Needs of an Athlete

What should an athlete eat to ensure that his or her muscles are supplied with the energy needed to perform? What foods will improve his or her performance? Should athletes avoid certain foods before, during, or after athletic participation?

Carbohydrate

The *Dietary Guidelines* recommends 45 to 65 percent of total calories should come from carbohydrates. Competitive athletes should aim for 60 to 65 percent because carbohydrates are the major fuel source for energy, and help to meet the needs of the muscles and the central nervous system. However, an absolute amount of carbohydrates may be more useful to an athlete than a percentage. Body size and level of training intensity affect an athlete's carbohydrate needs, so these factors are used to calculate amounts of carbohydrate (**Figure 15.2**).

Carbohydrate loading, also known as *carb loading*, is a technique used to trick the muscles into storing more glycogen for extra energy. Carbohydrates are found in starches and sugars and are your body's main energy source. Both complex carbohydrates (legumes, grains, potatoes, peas, and corn) and simple carbohydrates (fruits and milk) are part of the diet. The carbohydrate loading strategy is used to improve the performance of endurance athletes, such as those who are marathon runners, swimmers, or cyclists. An endurance event usually lasts 90 minutes or more. The regimen is *not* intended for use by non-endurance athletes.

Carbohydrate loading involves eating a diet moderate in carbohydrates for a few days while in training. Then, during the three days before a sports event, an athlete consumes a high-carbohydrate diet (**Figure 15.3**). The increase in carbohydrates is coupled with a decrease in training intensity.

Some athletes have experienced side effects from carbohydrate loading. These problems have included water retention, digestion distress, muscle stiffness, and sluggishness. Athletes with chronic diseases such as diabetes are especially likely to have problems.

For most athletes, attempts to increase glycogen stores are not needed. If you are in a daily vigorous exercise program, eat a complex carbohydrate-rich diet and include a rest day in your schedule now and then. Such rest days will help build up the glycogen stores you need.

Figure 15.2
The recommended daily carbohydrate intake for an athlete is dependent on the activity intensity level and duration and the athlete's weight. *What range of carbohydrate intake would you recommend for a 154-pound (70 kg) athlete who runs 2 hours per day?*

Guidelines for Daily Carbohydrate Intake by Athletes

Exercise Intensity	Intensity Description	Daily Amount of Carbohydrate (per kilogram of body weight)
Light	Recreational activity (low-intensity or skill-based activities)	3–5 grams
Moderate	Moderate exercise program (~1 hour/day)	5–7 grams
High	Endurance exercise (1–3 hours/day moderate- to high-intensity exercise)	6–10 grams
Very high	Endurance exercise (>4–5 hours/day moderate- to high-intensity exercise)	8–12 grams

Source: Louise M. Burke, John A. Hawley, Stephen H. S. Wong & Asker E. Jeukendrup (2011): Carbohydrates for training and competition, *Journal of Sports Sciences*, 29:sup1, S17-S27

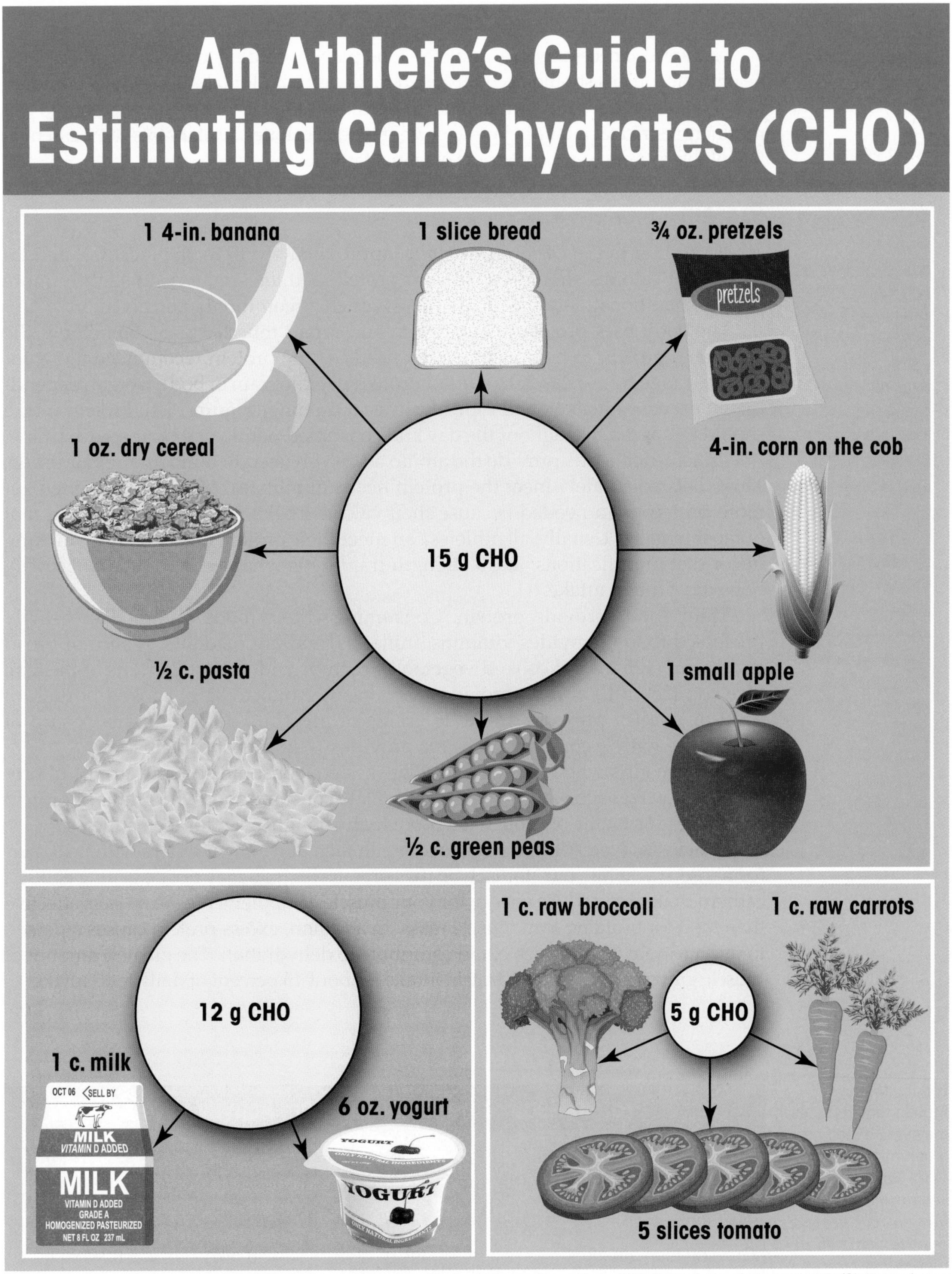

An Athlete's Guide to Estimating Carbohydrates (CHO)
1 4-in. banana
1 slice bread
¾ oz. pretzels
pretzels
1 oz. dry cereal
4-in. corn on the cob
15 g CHO
½ c. pasta
1 small apple
½ c. green peas
12 g CHO
1 c. milk
OCT 06 SELL BY
MILK
VITAMIN D ADDED
MILK
VITAMIN D ADDED
GRADE A
HOMOGENIZED PASTEURIZED
NET 8 FL OZ 237 mL
6 oz. yogurt
YOGURT
1 c. raw broccoli
1 c. raw carrots
5 g CHO
5 slices tomato

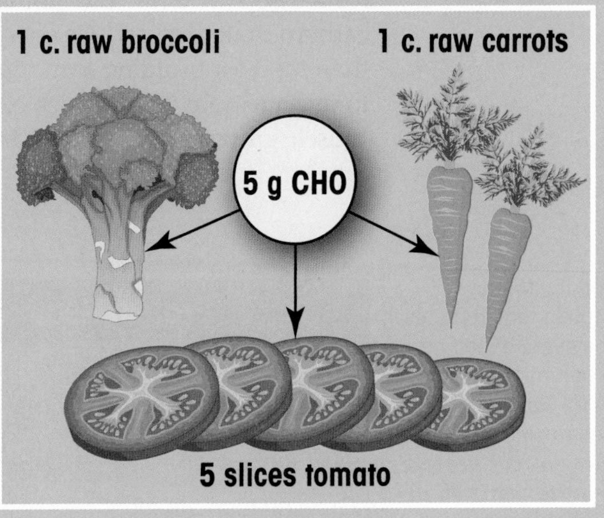

Top row: a_compot/Shutterstock.com; nicemonkey/Shutterstock.com; Shany Muchnik/Shutterstock.com; 2nd row: olegtoka/Shutterstock.com; La Gorda/Shutterstock.com; 3rd row: MightyRabittCrew/Shutterstock.com; TetianaMal/Shutterstock.com; Dioph/Shutterstock.com; bottom row: ybmd/Shutterstock.com; Gts/Shutterstock.com; broccoli: alekseyk/Shutterstock.com; carrot: Nikita Chisnikov/Shutterstock.com; tomatoes: Ansty/Shutterstock.com

Figure 15.3 With practice, estimating carbohydrate content of foods becomes easy.

Fat

Fats are also necessary in an athlete's food plan. According to the *Dietary Guidelines*, healthy fat sources should account for 20 to 25 percent of total calories and saturated fats should account for no more than 10 percent of total calories. Athletes should not routinely restrict fat intake below 20 percent of total calories. Dietary fats carry essential fat-soluble vitamins and contribute essential fatty acids.

Protein

According to the *Dietary Guidelines*, approximately 10 to 35 percent of an athlete's total calories should come from protein. Athletes may need slightly more protein than nonathletes need, but not as much as commonly perceived.

The body uses protein to strengthen and repair muscle tissue. Sometimes the body uses protein to help meet energy needs. Daily protein recommendations for athletes range from 1.2 to 2.0 grams of protein per kilogram of body weight, depending on exercise intensity and type of physical training (**Figure 15.4**). Protein intake should be spaced throughout the day and consumed within one hour after training.

Protein-rich foods provide the amino acids you need to build and repair tissue. Most diets adequately meet the protein needs of athletes. Male athletes often get more protein than needed because their calorie intake is simply larger than that of most females. Usually, all athletes can meet their protein needs without making major diet modifications. Extra strength training is what leads to muscle growth, not extra protein intake.

Many foods provide protein. Consuming whole foods, rather than heavily processed foods, provides vitamins, minerals, and antioxidants. A slice of bread and ½ cup (125 mL) of cooked vegetables each provide about 2 grams of protein. One cup (250 mL) of milk provides 8 grams. A 3-ounce (84 g) cooked portion of meat or poultry provides about 26 grams of protein. For vegetarians, ½ cup of brown rice with ½ cup of black beans provides 10 grams of proteins.

Teenage girls who follow the MyPlate system consume about 91 grams of protein per day. Teenage boys who follow MyPlate consume about 116 grams of protein daily. These amounts of protein are more than enough, even for teen athletes.

Protein supplements are not necessary. In fact, they may interfere with peak performance. If you fill your stomach on protein calories, you may not be getting enough carbohydrates to produce energy for your muscles. Supplements are *no more* effective than food for building lean muscle mass. In addition, excess protein causes a person to urinate more often, which could contribute to dehydration. The greatest amount of muscle growth occurs when protein intake is about 15 percent of daily food intake.

Figure 15.4
Protein requirements may vary based on a number of factors. *Why might a sedentary adult have lower protein requirements than a growing teen athlete?*

Protein Requirements for Different Activity Levels

If the Individual Is a(n)	Body Weight		Protein Needs		Total Protein
Sedentary adult	68 kg	x	0.8 g/kg	=	54 g
Growing teen athlete	68 kg	x	1.2–2.0 g/kg	=	82–136 g
Adult in strength/resistance training	68 kg	x	1.6–1.7 g/kg	=	109–116 g
Adult in endurance training	68 kg	x	1.2–1.4 g/kg	=	82–95 g

COMMUNITY CONNECTIONS

Recreational Activities/Sports Volunteer

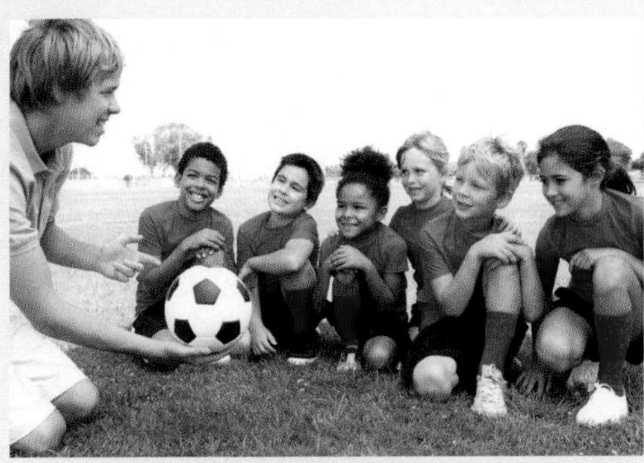

Monkey Business Images/Shutterstock.com

For students who love athletics, the experience of volunteering for sports events may be a way to learn more about a sports career field. Other volunteer teens may simply enjoy being active and participating in recreational activities.

Volunteers are often needed to assist with the coaching of youth basketball teams, assist staff with 5K runs by setting up or breaking down water stations, assist at golf tournaments, serve as scorekeepers or referees, and help at concession stands. You can learn about opportunities in your area by searching for sports volunteer matches online. Your community recreation center may also have volunteer opportunities.

Special Olympics volunteers or sports leagues for younger kids with disabilities need volunteers to help events run smoothly. Summer camp programs or after-school programs for kids also have opportunities for volunteering. Each opportunity gives you the chance to meet other people who share your interest in sports. Organizations usually post volunteer opportunities online along with volunteer application forms. Your qualifications will be reviewed and background screening performed before your name can be added to a database of volunteers.

As a volunteer, be prepared to be flexible. Job tasks may change as needs change. Be prepared to interact with many new people. Assertiveness may be needed while performing more uncomfortable tasks or redirecting people's actions. You may be required to follow a dress code.

The benefits are many. You are learning more about sports and recreational career options. You may meet people who can guide your career thinking. Through your volunteer contacts, you may obtain useful information to help you plan a career in a sports-related field. Most importantly, you have a chance to make a positive impact on others as a sports or recreational activity role model.

Think Critically

1. Where have you observed volunteers working at sports or recreational events? What emotions did the volunteers seem to express about their role?
2. What personality type do you think would most enjoy volunteering at a sports or recreational event?

Vitamins and Minerals

Athletes need to plan their diets around a variety of foods rich in vitamins and minerals. These nutrients are important for the conversion of carbohydrates, fats, and protein to energy. They promote growth and aid in nerve and muscle function.

Minerals, such as calcium, and vitamin D help maintain strong bones. Teens need 1,300 milligrams of calcium per day for calcium retention and bone mineral density. The health consequences of too little calcium can be poor formation of bone structure, stress fractures, and osteoporosis in later life. Athletes can boost calcium and vitamin D intake by choosing dairy products such as low-fat milk, yogurt, and cheese. Dairy products also supply protein and other vitamins and minerals.

WELLNESS TIP

Athletes and Vitamin D

What is your vitamin D status? Vitamin D is called the *sunshine vitamin* because it is produced in the skin when exposed to sunlight. There is growing interest in the role of vitamin D in muscle function and the possible effect on athletic performance. Vitamin D status has been associated with injury prevention and recovery, improved muscle function and size, lower risk for stress fractures, reduced inflammation, and decreased risk for illness.

Athletes who train primarily indoors, are conscientious about sunscreen, or have dark complexions are at greater risk for vitamin D deficiency. Athletes can improve their vitamin D status with careful, limited exposure to the sun—no more than half the time it takes for your skin to begin to burn. Athletes who are concerned about sun exposure can improve their vitamin D status by consuming good food sources of vitamin D such as fatty fish, beef liver, egg yolks, and vitamin D-fortified foods such as milk, orange juice, and cereals. A sports physician may recommend a vitamin D supplement if a deficiency is determined.

Many women do not get enough iron in their diet. Women with heavy menstrual cycles have increased loss of iron. When blood is lost, iron is lost and anemia can result. Symptoms of iron deficiency for athletes include fatigue and breathlessness. Anemia reduces athletic performance. If performance declines and cannot be explained in other ways, such as too much stress or lack of sleep, then iron-deficient anemia should be considered. Iron-rich foods, such as meat, fish, and poultry, help athletes meet their iron needs. Iron is also available in grains, peas, lentils, nuts, dark-green leafy vegetables, and nuts.

Vitamin and mineral supplements are an added expense and usually unnecessary. However, some athletes may benefit from a supplement. For example, a vegetarian athlete who avoids all dairy foods, fortified soy milk, and dark leafy vegetables would need a calcium supplement. Supplements that provide more than 100 percent of the RDAs or AIs are unnecessary. A multivitamin and mineral formula will meet most athletes' needs. Athletes with special dietary needs should consult a sports nutritionist.

Calories

Oftentimes, athletes **expend** (use up) many calories during training and competition. The number of calories athletes use is determined by their body weight and the types of activities they are performing. The amount of time spent training also affects the number of calories used. People who weigh more expend more calories during a given activity. More calories are used because more energy is required to move a greater body mass. Vigorous activities require more energy than less active sports. For instance, running requires more energy than jogging (**Figure 15.5**). The longer the workout lasts, the greater the calorie expenditure.

An athlete who burns more calories through training and competition than he or she takes in through food will lose weight. An athlete is more physically active than a nonathlete and, as a result, requires more daily calories to maintain a healthy body weight. Routine insufficient energy intake can affect not only the athlete's health, but also his or her performance. Chronic energy deficiency can affect metabolism, immune system function, and bone and heart health. It can have negative effects on an athlete's endurance, risk for injury, coordination, concentration, and muscle strength.

How Many Calories Do Athletes Burn?

Activity	Calories Burned per Minute by Body Weight				
	100 lb. (45 kg)	125 lb. (57 kg)	150 lb. (68 kg)	175 lb. (80 kg)	200 lb. (91 kg)
Aerobic dance	6.0	7.6	9.1	10.6	12.1
Baseball	3.1	4.0	4.7	5.5	6.3
Basketball, recreational	4.9	6.2	7.5	8.7	10.0
Bicycling, 10 mph	4.2	5.3	6.4	7.4	8.5
Canoeing, 4 mph	4.4	5.5	6.7	7.8	8.9
Dancing, active	4.5	5.6	6.8	7.9	9.1
Football, vigorous touch	5.5	6.9	8.3	9.7	11.1
Golf, carrying clubs	3.6	4.6	5.4	6.4	7.3
Hockey	6.6	8.3	10.0	11.7	13.4
Horseback riding	2.7	3.4	4.1	4.8	5.4
Ice skating	4.2	5.2	6.4	7.4	8.5
Jogging, 5.5 mph	6.7	8.4	10.0	11.7	13.4
Racquetball	6.5	8.1	9.8	11.4	13.0
Roller skating	4.2	5.3	6.4	7.4	8.5
Running, 8 mph	9.7	12.1	14.6	17.1	19.5
Skiing, cross-country, 4 mph	6.5	8.2	9.9	11.5	13.2
Skiing, downhill	6.5	8.2	9.9	11.5	13.2
Soccer	5.9	7.5	9.0	10.5	12.0
Swimming, crawl, 35 yd./min.	4.8	6.1	7.3	8.5	9.7
Table tennis	3.4	4.3	5.2	6.1	7.0
Tennis, recreational singles	5.0	6.2	7.5	8.8	10.0
Volleyball, recreational	2.9	3.6	4.4	5.1	5.9
Walking, 4 mph	4.2	5.3	6.4	7.4	8.5
Wrestling	8.5	10.6	12.8	14.9	17.1

Note: The energy costs in calories will vary. Values are approximate. Factors that influence calorie needs include wind resistance, ground levels, weight of clothes, and other conditions.

Figure 15.5
Locate the column closest to your weight for an activity you enjoy. Multiply the calories burned per minute by the number of minutes spent in the activity to figure total energy expenditure.

Women who train intensively while consuming insufficient calories for long periods may experience disorders with their menstrual cycles. Low weight and body fat can cause menstrual cycle abnormalities. Young athletes may experience a delay in the onset of menstruation beyond the normal ages of 11 to 15 years.

Women gymnasts who have very low amounts of body fat and weight have delayed *menarche*, a term used to describe when menstrual cycles begin (**Figure 15.6**). *Amenorrhea*, or loss of a menstrual cycle, has negative consequences. Production of important hormones involved in the development of strong bones is reduced. With amenorrhea, bone density can become extremely low. Tendon injuries and stress fractures become an increased risk. (See Chapter 16 for further discussion about chronic energy insufficiency and female athletes.)

Some athletes need more energy than they can comfortably consume through food. These athletes may find it helpful to consume energy in concentrated forms, such as dried fruits and nuts. Drinking high-energy liquids, such as yogurt shakes and fruit smoothies, may also be easier than eating solid foods. Supplements and special "power" foods are generally not needed and have not been shown to improve performance.

Planning Meals for the Athlete in Training

Sports nutritionists will tell you that healthy eating provides athletes with the foundation for peak performance. Meeting the athlete's energy needs through caloric intake and getting the necessary fluid replacements is critical for athletes.

Maintenance Eating Patterns

Eating meals and snacks on a regular basis throughout the day fuels your body for activity. Hydrating before, during, and after exercise is necessary to keep performance levels high. If you skip a meal and become too hungry, you may end up making poor food choices. Staying fueled throughout the day with nutritious foods and adequate fluids is necessary to support the demands of training and competition. Keep in mind that healthy eating is essential for optimal performance.

Eat breakfast to avoid an energy crash later in the morning. Skipping breakfast can reduce your energy levels for your workouts. Some people report feeling **lethargic** (lacking energy) for the rest of the day.

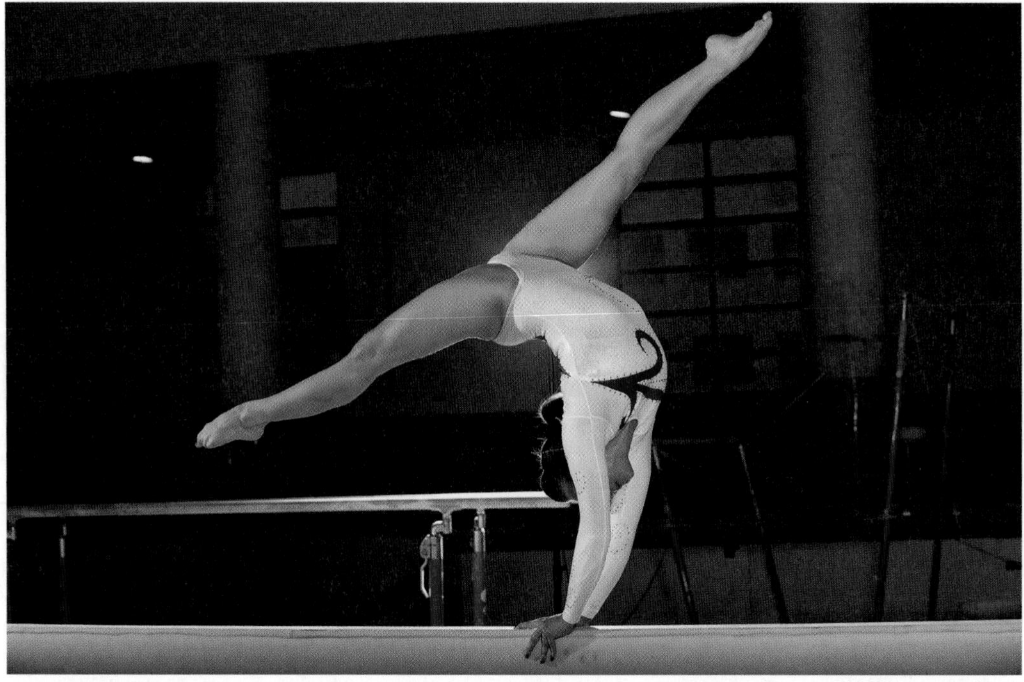

ITALO/Shutterstock.com

Figure 15.6 Although weight goals may be stressed in a sport such as gymnastics, female athletes should maintain 18 to 24 percent body fat.

CASE STUDY

Plan for Peak Performance

Nick is an aspiring athlete. He is 15 years old and wants to become a professional hockey player. He practices on the ice for hours several times a week. He was recently recruited by a league in his hometown. After his first practice with the team, Nick decides he needs to make some changes. During practice, Nick found that he became winded much sooner than his teammates and was often lagging behind on sprint plays. He also felt that he was being outmuscled. Nick decides he needs a plan to improve his performance on the ice.

The first part of Nick's plan involves building strength. His goal is to increase the size of his muscles. Nick decides the best way to build muscle mass is to increase the amount of protein in his diet. He has heard guys talking about protein powder so he buys some. He begins drinking protein shakes and eating three eggs per day. He also increases the serving size of protein foods at his normal meals. Nick finds that he is often too full to eat the bread, potatoes, or rice from his meal.

The other part of Nick's plan is to begin running. He sets his alarm an hour earlier than usual and runs two miles before school most mornings.

After following his plan for four weeks, Nick is a little disappointed with the results. He has not noticed much change in his muscle size. Although he doesn't seem to get winded as quickly, he still seems to be lagging behind on the fast plays. In addition, Nick is disappointed because, despite his plans to improve his performance, he feels less energetic most of the time.

Case Review

1. Are you surprised by the outcomes Nick is experiencing with his plan? Why?
2. What would you do differently if you were Nick?

Select nutritious snacks between meals. Snacks can make up 20 to 50 percent of your day's calories. These additional small meals add nutritional benefits and boost your energy. Be sure to plan snacks that add valuable nutrients and needed energy rather than nutrient-poor calories. Choose foods such as fruits, whole-grain bagels, popcorn, low-fat cheese, nuts, or vegetables (**Figure 15.7**).

Good nutrition is critical to top-level performance. Special sports nutrition products and supplements do not provide the same level of nutritional benefits that a healthy, well-planned meal pattern can supply.

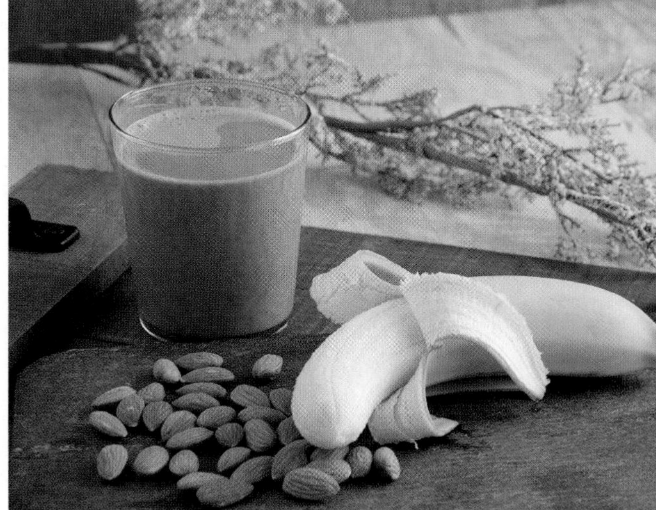

Dawn Damico/Shutterstock.com

Figure 15.7 Snacks contribute to an athlete's overall nutrition and should be nutrient rich. *What food groups are represented in this snack?*

Meal Management for Athletic Events

Meal and snack management for athletes is all about how food intake affects digestion and use of energy for top performance.

Meals Before an Athletic Event

The goals of the pre-event meal should be to provide appropriate amounts of energy and fluid. The meal should also help the athlete avoid feelings of fullness and digestive disturbances.

Very large meals before competition should be avoided. They require too much energy to digest. This does not mean you should go hungry. Hunger makes you feel tired and sluggish. For most sports events, the best diet plan includes a high-carbohydrate meal, with moderate amounts of protein, within 3 to 4 hours before competition. Avoid the high-protein, high-fat steak dinners that were once training table standards.

Carbohydrates have been found to have positive effects on performance. However, very sweet carbohydrates such as syrups and candy bars can cause water to pool in the gastrointestinal tract. Discomfort and diarrhea may result.

Athletes should avoid bulky and fatty foods on the day of competition. Too many high-fiber foods, such as whole-grain bagels and large portions of fresh fruits and vegetables, should be limited if you are prone to stomach aches. Also, avoid French fries, bacon, sausage, and other foods high in fat. Instead, choose foods such as spaghetti and meat sauce, peanut butter and jelly sandwich on white bread, pancakes, cooked rice, pasta or potatoes, fat-free milk, fruit juices, or other low-fat, low-fiber, and low- to moderate-protein foods (**Figure 15.8**).

Foods you have never eaten before are not recommended just before an athletic event. You cannot be sure how they will make you feel. Continue to drink water throughout the day.

Figure 15.8
A pre-event meal, eaten 3 to 4 hours before a competition, should be rich in carbohydrates that are easy to digest and moderate in calories.

Pre-Event Meals		
Foods	**Calories**	**Carbohydrates (grams)**
Pre-Event Breakfast		
Orange juice	112	27
Cornflakes with milk	152	30
Banana	104	27
Toast with jelly	103	22
Hard-cooked egg	78	1
Total	549	107 (78% of calories)
Pre-Event Lunch		
Pasta with meatless sauce	404	73
Roll	85	14
Applesauce	52	14
Fat-free milk	86	12
Total	627	113 (72% of calories)
Pre-Event Snack Ideas		
Bagel or crackers	Low-fat yogurt	Pretzels
Apples or bananas	Dried fruit	Low-fat granola
Popcorn	Pudding	

For some athletes, mental attitude can be just as important as the foods eaten. Suppose an athlete always eats pizza before a competition. For this athlete, it may be psychologically important to eat pizza to be ready to win. Follow the pattern that works best for you.

Snacks Before an Athletic Event

Snacks before exercise and pre-event meals should provide appropriate amounts of energy and fluid. Snacks are necessary to maintain energy. If your exercise takes place after school or work, you may not have the time for a meal before you are scheduled to perform. If there is a pre-event meal, avoid overeating to avoid feelings of fullness and digestive disturbances. Frequent smaller meals are better before performance events. Snacking on foods prior to exercise can help to boost your energy levels.

Most athletes can tolerate pre-event carbohydrate-rich snacks and drinks that are low in fiber and easily consumed. Examples of good pre-event snacks would include bananas, oranges, grapes, and low-pulp or pulp-free vegetable or fruit juices an hour before competition. The energy from the snack will be useful during the activity. Consuming foods high in fat, protein, or fiber may result in gastrointestinal discomfort during the event. If the activity is very intense, such as a time trial for a track event, you may be more comfortable competing with an empty stomach. Each athlete must learn what works best for his or her body in a given situation.

Eating During an Athletic Event

Eating small amounts of food during a long—lasting two hours or more—sports event can improve performance. For example, athletes like to eat small amounts of peanut butter crackers, fig bars, peanut butter and jelly sandwiches, or date snacks during triathlon events. Generally, the goal is to consume about 30 to 100 grams of carbohydrates per hour providing about 120 to 400 calories. Each athlete must learn what foods his or her body can tolerate without digestive disturbances. Any digestive discomfort will interfere with performance. Athletes can determine the energy source that works best for them by trying different foods during trial events. Foods in liquid form, such as food gels, high-nutrient shakes, and other energy drinks, may be easier to digest.

Fluid replacement is essential for avoiding dehydration and impaired performance (**Figure 15.9**). Some nutritionists recommend increasing salty foods in the diet for several days before an event. This depends on how much salt you tend to lose in sweat. Sports drinks are useful for long races such as marathons and triathlons. These drinks provide water, carbohydrates, and sodium.

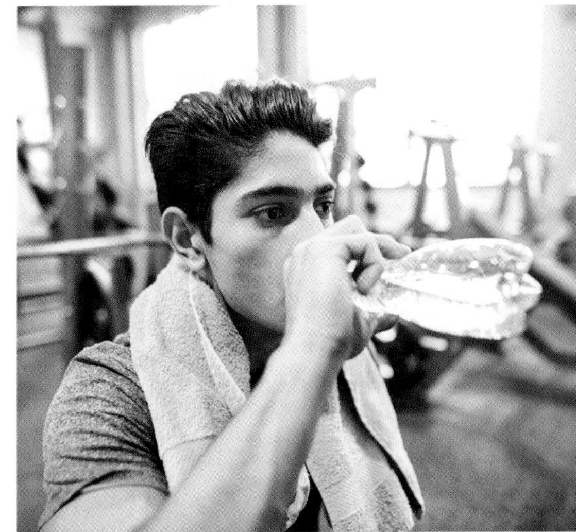

Halfpoint/Shutterstock.com

Figure 15.9 Athletes should maintain hydration for optimal performance.

Post-Athletic Event Nutrition

Recovery is the phase after exercise when glycogen stores are replenished to pre-exercise levels. Intense exercise takes a toll on your body and **depletes** (consumes) glycogen stores. Essential vitamins and minerals may be low or depleted. Training and competition cause physical and emotional stress to your body. Recovery and relaxation are important goals. Following an event, you will recover faster if you consume both carbohydrates and protein. Timing is important.

Eating within 15 to 60 minutes after an activity provides the best opportunity for replenishing muscle glycogen, body water, and electrolytes. Whole foods and water can supply essential nutrients. The most important nutrients to include in recovery nutrition are

- water for hydration;
- a carbohydrate with a high glycemic index that enters the bloodstream quickly, such as found in low-fat chocolate milk and other dairy products, fruits juices and smoothies, and cereals;
- a source of high-quality protein to help build and repair muscle tissue in recovery, including a turkey sandwich on whole-wheat toast, hard-cooked egg, tofu, nuts, or legumes; and
- sodium, found in tomato juice, nuts, pretzels, crackers.

Recovery drinks may be helpful if your body does not tolerate solid foods after an event. If you prefer recovery drinks, be sure to read the ingredients list. In some cases, nutrients are added such as saturated fats and added sugar that are not useful for recovery.

FEATURED CAREER

Athletic Trainer

Athletic trainers specialize in the prevention, diagnosis, assessment, treatment, and rehabilitation of muscle and bone injuries and illnesses. As one of the first health-care providers on the scene when injuries occur, they must be able to recognize, evaluate, and assess injuries and provide immediate care when needed.

Athletic trainers try to prevent injuries by teaching people how to reduce their risk for injuries. They also advise people on proper equipment use, exercises to improve balance and strength, and home exercises and therapy programs.

Applying protective or injury-preventive devices—such as tape, bandages, and braces—is another responsibility. Athletic trainers may work under the direction of a licensed physician or other healthcare provider. They may discuss specific injuries and treatment options with a physician or perform evaluations and treatments as directed by a physician.

Education

A bachelor's degree is required for most jobs as an athletic trainer. Master's degree programs are also common. Program education occurs both in the classroom and in clinical settings. Courses may include human anatomy, kinesiology, physiology, nutrition, and biomechanics. For college and university positions, athletic trainers may need a master's or higher degree to be eligible. Because some high school positions involve teaching along with athletic-trainer duties, a teaching certificate or license could be required.

Job Outlook

Employment is projected to grow much faster than average. Job prospects should be good in the health-care industry and in high schools, but expect competition for positions with professional and college sports teams. Employment is expected to grow for athletic trainers because of their role in preventing injuries and reducing health-care costs. Heightened awareness of long-term consequences of child athlete injuries (like concussions) and an increasingly active middle-aged and elderly population will also contribute to job growth.

After two hours, have a meal of mixed carbohydrates, fats, and protein. Hydration continues to be important. Light straw-colored urine is an indication that your fluid intake is adequate. Plan for adequate sleep to help your body fully recover.

Once the training season ends, you need to reduce calorie intake. If you continue with the same eating plan you followed during training, you will begin to gain weight. Balancing energy output with energy input may require adjustments to your eating pattern.

Eating Away from Home

Athletes often travel to participate in sporting events. Sometimes the activity may require that you travel hours or even days at a time. Meal schedules may be irregular. Athletes may be tempted to skip meals. Drinking enough water may be difficult if water is not carried by the athlete. Good food sources of carbohydrates may be harder to find. Fast-food restaurant menus feature many high-fat, high-protein foods. These foods are often low in carbohydrates, calcium, and vitamins A and C. When carbohydrates are inadequate, glycogen stores become depleted. Without enough water, dehydration may occur before an event begins. The effect on the athlete is reduced energy levels and performance.

The traveling athlete can improve performance by planning to include carbohydrates in the meals before an event. Choose restaurants that serve carbohydrate-rich foods such as pasta, burritos, baked potatoes, fruits, vegetables, and low-fat milk (**Figure 15.10**). These foods are common, inexpensive, and easily prepared by restaurants. The following tips will help you select nutrient-dense meals at restaurants:

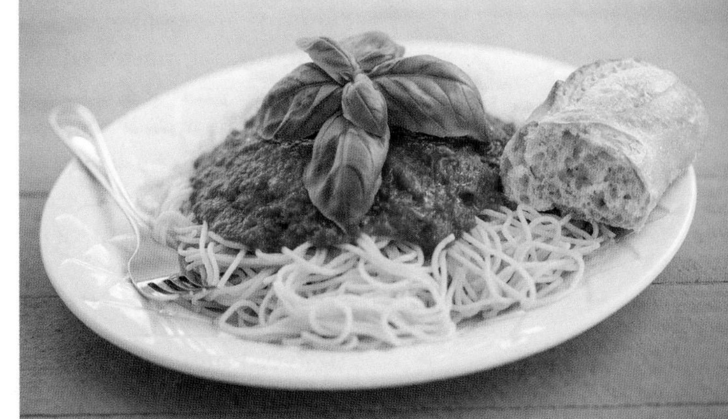

eurobanks/Shutterstock.com

Figure 15.10 Many restaurants offer carbohydrate-rich spaghetti on the menu. *What other carbohydrate-rich menu items do you see offered at restaurants?*

- Choose grilled sandwiches, hamburgers or cheeseburgers, or turkey subs on a whole-wheat bun. Avoid condiments that are high in saturated fats such as mayonnaise.
- Resist the temptation to order double burgers, large fries, and super-sized sodas.
- Limit high-fat salads and dressings, such as potato salad, marinated pasta, and vegetable salads, when eating at salad bars. Use restraint with high-fat toppings such as cheese and bacon.
- Request gravies, sauces, and salad dressings served on the side.
- Order pasta with tomato-based sauces and avoid cream or butter sauces.
- Choose salsa instead of sour cream or guacamole.
- Order stir-fried and steamed vegetables with rice or vegetarian pizzas with whole-wheat crusts.
- Avoid deep-fried foods such as fried fish, egg rolls, fried tortillas, and potato chips.
- Look for menu items that are steamed, boiled, broiled, roasted, or poached.

The Athlete's Need for Fluids

Drinking enough fluids may be the most critical aspect of sports nutrition. If fluid levels drop too low, dehydration results. Symptoms of dehydration include headache, dizziness, nausea, dry skin, shivering, and confusion. Dehydration also causes increases in body temperature and heart rate. Clearly, dehydration can impair performance.

Fluid Loss

During training or competition, athletes may not feel thirsty because exercise masks the sense of thirst. Sweating during moderate exercise causes you to lose about 1 quart (1 L) of water per hour. If the workout is vigorous, a loss of 2 to 3 quarts (2 to 3 L) of water per hour may result. Therefore, athletes need to drink regardless of whether they feel thirsty.

Athletes lose water during exercise even when the air temperature is comfortable. Water losses are greater when exercising in hot, humid weather. This makes heat cramps and heat exhaustion more likely. When exercising in these conditions, watching fluid replacement is even more critical.

Athletes can lose four to six pounds of water weight during a sports event. To determine how much water you lose, weigh yourself before and after an event (**Figure 15.11**). If you lose more than 3 percent of your body weight, your performance will deteriorate. For example, a 150-pound (67.5 kg) person should not lose more than 4½ pounds (2 kg) during an athletic activity.

Fluid Intake Guidelines

To avoid dehydration, athletes should drink water before, during, and after an event. Specific fluid hydration and replacement recommendations are dependent on an athlete's size, intensity of the physical activity, and temperature of the environment. All athletes need to be aware of fluid replacement guidelines.

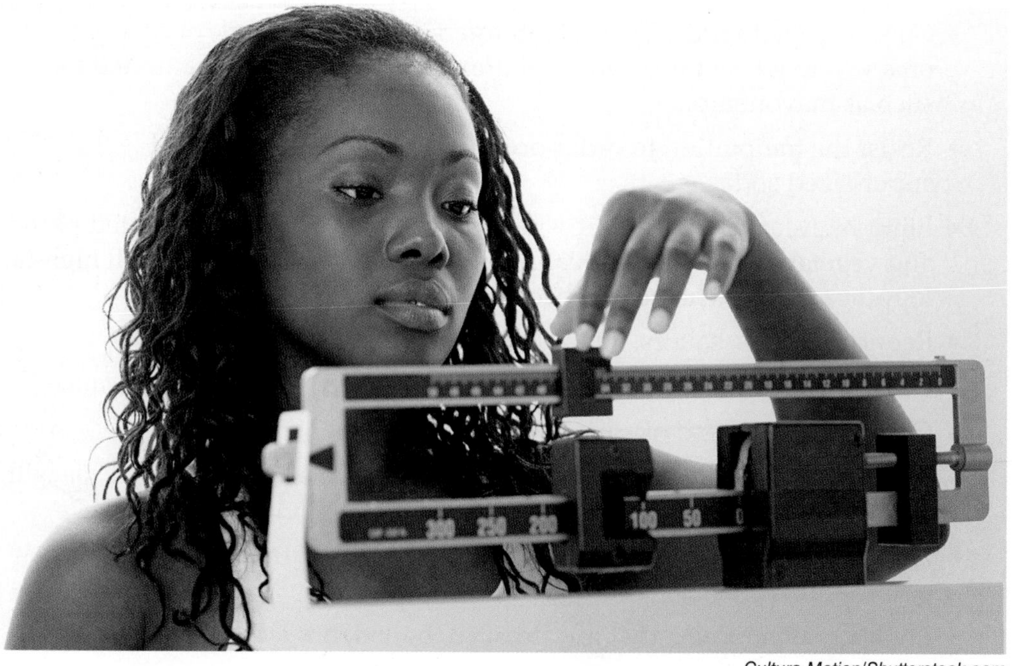

Figure 15.11
Athletes should weigh themselves before and after an activity to determine the amount of water loss.

Cultura Motion/Shutterstock.com

The National Athletic Trainers' Association (NATA) recommends the following guidelines for training and competition for athletes:

- 2–3 hours before event, consume 17–20 ounces (500–600 mL) fluid
- 10–20 minutes before event, consume 7–10 ounces (200–300 mL) fluid
- every 10–20 minutes during event, consume 7–10 ounces (200–300 mL) fluid
- within 2 hours following event, consume 20–24 ounces (600–700 mL) fluid for every one pound lost through sweat

Water is the preferred liquid for fluid replacement during a sporting event (**Figure 15.12**). Cool water (50°F–59°F) helps lower body temperature, and water empties from the stomach more quickly than any other fluid. The carbohydrates in some sweetened drinks can pull water from the body into the digestive tract causing cramps. The carbohydrates in most sports drinks are designed to be easily absorbed to prevent such cramping. Even so, if you choose a sports drink, you may want to dilute it with water or ice. Caffeine may increase body water loss. Alcohol is a depressant, has a diuretic effect, and is unhealthy for recovery. They should be avoided during physical activity.

Evaluating Beverage Choices for Athletes

Beverage	When Is It Effective?			Reason
	15–30 Minutes Pre-Event	During Event	After Event	
Alcohol	No	No	No	Undesirable, does not help performance, dehydrates cells and decreases muscle efficiency
Carbonated soft drinks	No	No	No	Carbonation may cause problems during an event and sugar may prevent fluids from quickly emptying the stomach
Coffee/tea	No	No	No	Caffeine pulls water from the body through increased urination; makes the heart work harder
Fat-free milk	No	No	Yes	Too difficult to digest for fluid use
Fruit juices	No	No	No	Sugar content is high; does not promote complete rehydration
Special sports drinks	Maybe	Maybe	Yes	Depends on content; may be high in sugar, which slows fluids in emptying from the stomach; salt content may be too high; consider diluting with water
Water (cool)	Yes	Yes	Yes	Best fluid for your system; regulates body temperature

Figure 15.12 Some beverage choices may have a negative effect on an athlete's performance. *According to this table, what is the best drink before, during, and after an athletic event?*

Fluid Loss and Sodium

Athletes also lose sodium when they sweat. Most athletes get enough sodium from the foods they eat. However, endurance athletes who compete in events lasting two or more hours may lose excessive amounts of water and sodium. These athletes may benefit from a sports drink that contains sodium, chloride, and potassium. Salting food a bit more liberally will also help them meet sodium needs.

Using salt tablets to replace sodium lost during physical activity is discouraged. They worsen dehydration and impair performance. They can also irritate the stomach and may cause severe vomiting. This is especially true when fluid intake is not adequate.

Weight Concerns of Athletes

Achieving optimum weight can positively affect your athletic performance. What is optimum weight? The answer depends on your percentage of body fat, or your body composition.

Knowing your percentage of body fat suggests whether you need to lose extra fat and/or build more muscle mass. Too much body fat increases energy needs. Energy needed for performance is used to move excess body weight instead. On the other hand, insufficient body fat hinders the body's ability to stay warm. Energy needed for competition ends up being used to maintain body temperature.

Lean body mass is especially valued by some athletes, such as gymnasts, distance runners, and body builders (**Figure 15.13**). For other athletes, such as discus throwers and baseball players, body composition may not matter as much. Most male athletes do well with 10 to 15 percent body fat. An acceptable level for most female athletes is 18 to 24 percent body fat. Most females stop menstruating when body fat drops below 17 percent.

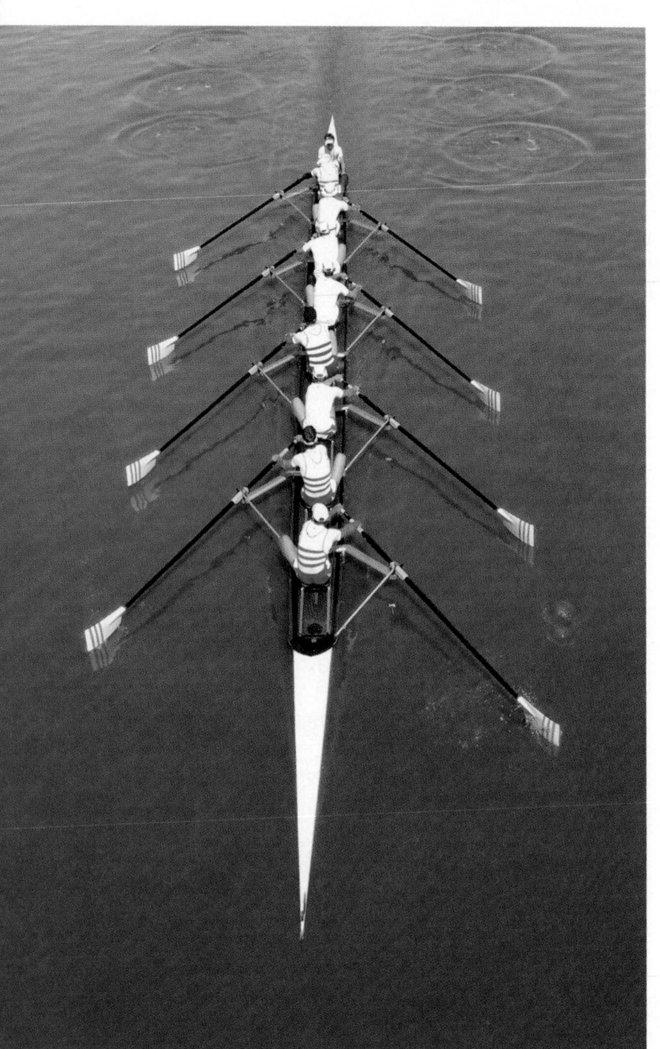

Danshutter/Shutterstock.com

Figure 15.13 Body composition is an important factor for rowers. *Can you think of other sports in which body composition is important?*

Losing Weight for Competition

Athletes in some sports, such as wrestling, boxing, and weight lifting, compete in specific weight classes. Some of these athletes use harmful methods to try to reduce their body weight quickly to compete in lower weight classes. They may try to skip meals or refuse to drink fluids one or two days before competition. Some use laxatives, diuretics, and emetics (substances that induce vomiting) to rid their bodies of food and fluids. Such practices can weaken an athlete's endurance.

Rapid weight loss can also harm an athlete's health. Severely restricting calorie intake while vigorously training can interfere with normal growth. The body will use energy to fuel activity rather than to support growth.

Weight management should begin long before the official training season begins. Athletes need to weigh themselves well before the start of their sports season. Then they will have ample time to reduce body fat and reach weight goals in a healthy manner before they begin competing.

Gradual weight loss is the best way to reduce pounds. Athletes need to set realistic goals for weight loss at a maximum of two pounds per week. Athletes who lose weight faster than this are probably losing more than fat. They are also losing body fluids and muscle mass.

To lose one pound of body fat, an athlete needs to consume 3,500 fewer calories than he or she expends. However, the athlete needs an adequate supply of nutrients to maintain strength and stamina while trying to lose weight. Most teen male athletes need at least 3,000 calories per day. Teen female athletes need a minimum of 2,200 calories daily. These amounts should be supplied by nutritious foods that provide the full range of vitamins and minerals. Eating more complex carbohydrates while reducing fats in the diet can help athletes limit calorie intake. Increasing energy expenditure by moderately extending workouts will help athletes gradually reach their weight goals.

Athletes who are trying to lose weight should work with a registered dietitian nutritionist. (Many coaches do not have adequate nutrition training to supervise an athlete's weight loss.) A dietitian can make sure athletes are meeting their daily calorie and nutrient needs for growth and training.

THE MOVEMENT CONNECTION

Neck Stretch

Why

Training for athletic performance requires you to use your head to make smart decisions. Your neck has the important job of supporting your head—so don't ignore your neck!

A head can weigh up to 10 pounds. Time spent looking down at a desk or smartphone adds pounds of force on your neck. This increases the work for your neck muscles and causes stress and tightness in your neck. It is important to take time to gently stretch and alleviate these problems.

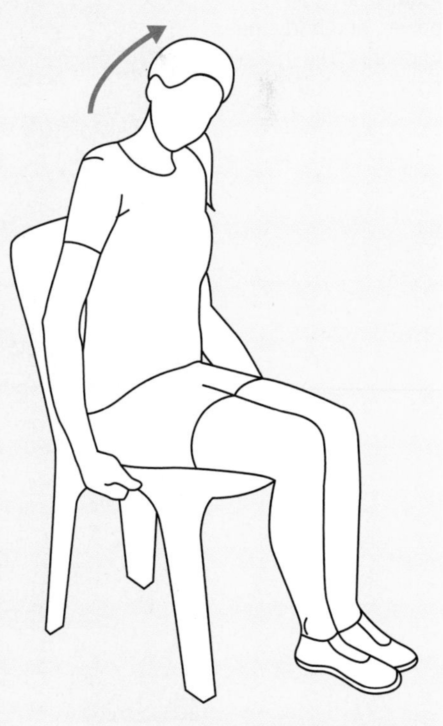

Apply

This stretch can be performed either sitting or standing.

- Assume good posture before beginning the move.
- Balance your head directly over your spine and keep your shoulders relaxed as you perform the stretch.
- Slowly lower your left ear to your left shoulder.
- Hold for 5 seconds, and bring your head back to a neutral, upright position.
- Repeat on the right side, lowering your right ear to your right shoulder.
- Repeat 3 times on each side.

Gaining Weight for Competition

Some athletes, such as football and hockey players, want to gain weight or "bulk up." Their goal is to gain size as well as strength. A large body mass will make them seem more formidable to their opponents (**Figure 15.14**).

For many athletes, gaining weight is difficult because they burn so many calories through long, hard workout sessions. Experts recommend athletes choose nutritious foods to add an extra 2,500 calories to their weekly intake. Some athletes may need to consume 5,000 calories or more per day to meet this recommendation.

High-fiber foods such as salads and whole-grain breads and cereals are discouraged in a weight-gain plan. These foods will cause an athlete to feel full too quickly. Athletes should include moderate amounts of monounsaturated and polyunsaturated oils because they are calorie dense; however, saturated fats should be limited.

Athletes who are trying to gain weight may wish to reduce the length and intensity of their regular workout sessions. They may also want to increase their rest and sleep time. These efforts will decrease the number of calories athletes burn for energy. However, an athlete's weight-gain program must include exercise, particularly weight training. An athlete's weight-gain goal is to add muscle, not fat. Simply increasing calorie intake does not build muscle. Weight gain without training will be fat gain, not muscle gain.

Athletes who consume coffee, tea, and colas should decrease their use of these products when trying to gain weight. The caffeine in these products tends to increase metabolic rates. Reducing caffeine consumption will help athletes burn fewer calories.

Figure 15.14
Football players require strength, power, and body mass to be effective in their sport.

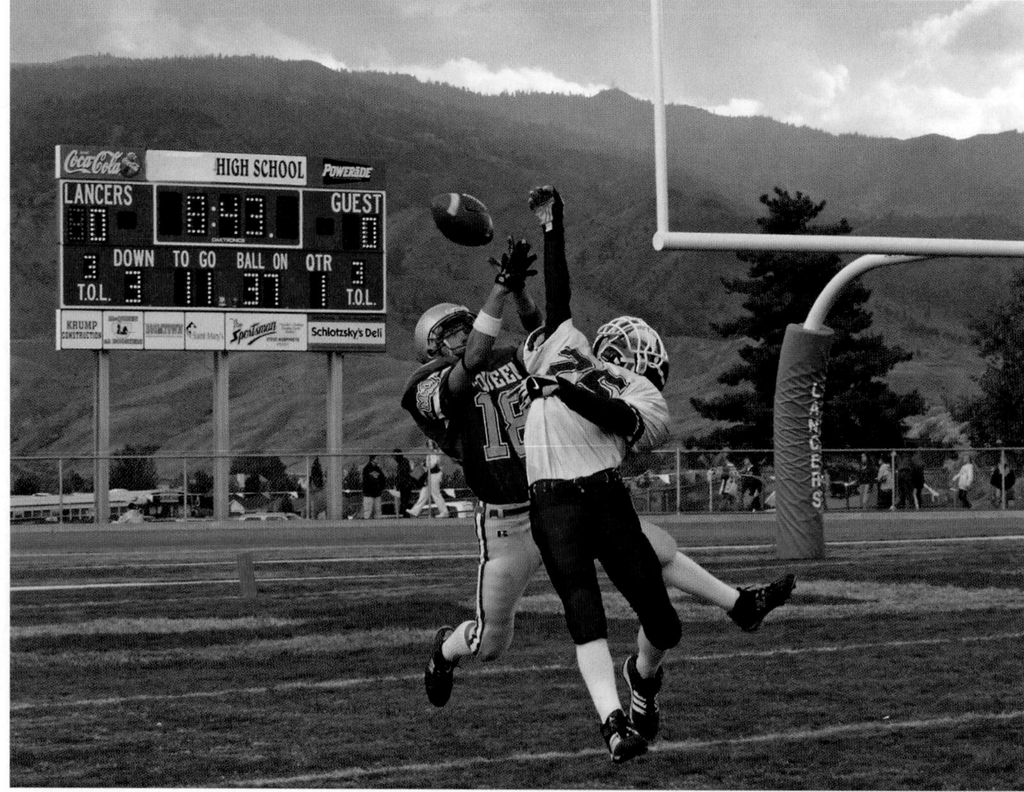

Bwilson/Shutterstock.com

Modifying eating and exercise patterns will help athletes gain about 1 to 2 pounds (0.5 to 1 kg) per week. Athletes trying to gain weight should work with a registered dietitian.

Harmful Performance Aids

Perhaps you have wished there were a special drink or pill that would make you stronger or faster. If only you could find some magic key to success, you would be sure to win—right?

Sports supplements (also called *ergogenic aids*) are products claiming to enhance athletic performance. Most of these products are a concoction of vitamins, minerals, amino acids, herbs, or other plant substances. You can generally buy them over the counter. As a dietary supplement, there is no US Food and Drug Administration (FDA) approval before these sports supplements come to market. Registered dietitians and sports nutritionists know these products are not the way to make an athlete stronger or faster. Likewise, no safe methods exist to add muscle weight quickly.

Schemes advertised by manufacturers promoting how to build muscle mass fast are often frauds. Some can negatively affect performance and health. Some contain a large amount of added sugar. They can even interfere with normal growth and development. The health effects of drugs and other substances can produce a range of symptoms. Mild symptoms include headache and nausea. Severe symptoms include liver disease, stroke, and death (**Figure 15.15** on the next page).

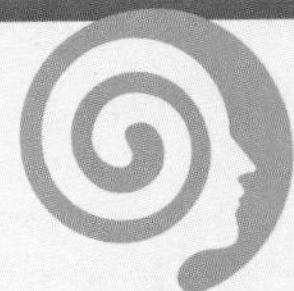

EXTEND YOUR KNOWLEDGE

Safety First

Many sports injuries occur during practice. Are measures in place in your school to ensure a student athlete's health and welfare?

A safe, well-run athletic program will have the following:

- a qualified individual on-site to care for injured athletes;
- a written plan of action if an athlete is injured;
- equipment that is in good working condition;
- effective helmets to limit risk for brain injury;
- adequate medical equipment for first response treatment including splints, spine boards, and an automatic external defibrillator (AED);
- personnel who are trained to provide cardiopulmonary resuscitation (CPR) and use medical equipment;
- current coaching credentials as required by the state and athletic conferences;
- clean, sanitary locker rooms and gyms to prevent the spread of bacterial, viral, and fungal skin infections;
- extreme weather policies that allow students to build up to training in hot weather;
- hydrating fluids available at all times; and
- policies that restrict athletes who are ill or injured from practicing or competing.

If you believe your school has a sports safety issue, discuss concerns with a trusted person such as a parent, guardian, school counselor, or administrator.

Harmful Effects of Performance Aids		
Performance Aid	**Reasons Used**	**Harmful Effects**
Anabolic steroids	A male sex hormone used to build strength and add muscle mass	Liver disorders, kidney disease, growth disorders, decreased level of HDLs (good cholesterol) and increased level of LDLs (bad cholesterol), high blood pressure, sexual problems, reproductive disorders (men—affects the production and functions of testosterone; women—growth of facial hair, baldness, menstrual irregularities, aggressiveness), unusual weight gain or loss, rashes or hives
Arginine (nitric oxide)	An amino acid supplement used to increase blood flow, improve exercise efficiency, and enhance performance	If taken in excess, may experience headache, nausea, and weakness; other side effects related to allergic reactions include diarrhea and stomach cramps. Doses greater than 30 grams are toxic.
Bicarbonate of soda or soft drinks (soda loading)	Used to avoid muscle fatigue	A form of doping, no confirmed benefits for game performance
Caffeine	A stimulant to the central nervous system used to increase endurance during strenuous exercise	May increase fluid losses; increases heart rate; can cause headaches, insomnia, and nervous irritability
Carnitine	An amino acid supplement used to improve endurance	Can cause muscle cramps, muscle weakness, and loss of iron-containing muscle protein
Human growth hormones	Used to build muscle and shorten recovery time	Thickening of bones, overgrowth of soft body tissues, possibility of grotesque body features
Pangamic acid (sometimes called vitamin B_{15})	Used to improve efficient use of oxygen in aerobic exercises	Ruled illegal by the Food and Drug Administration, unsafe for humans
Vitamin supplements	Used to feel better and provide a competitive edge	False promises, promotes "pill popping," costs more than food sources, individual becomes less concerned about eating a nutritious diet

Figure 15.15 These performance aids may appear to be quick fixes, but they may actually be harmful to your health.

New "performance enhancers" appear on the shelves of health-food stores every day. The sales pitches are creative, and the claims often sound miraculous. Remember, the goal of supplement advertisers is to make money by selling more supplements, and many claims may be misleading. As a careful consumer and serious competitor, you must evaluate claims carefully. Keep in mind that if a claim sounds too good to be true, it probably is. Most will not make you any stronger, and none will make you any faster or more skillful. Your time and money is better spent on a planned program of supervised training and nutritious eating as a safe and effective way to achieve peak performance.

RECIPE FILE

Spinach and Mozzarella Quiche

8 SERVINGS

Ingredients

- 1 unbaked 9-inch piecrust
- 1 medium onion, chopped
- 3 cloves garlic, minced
- 3 large eggs
- 3 large egg whites
- ¾ c. whole milk
- 1 c. frozen chopped spinach, thawed and drained well
- ¾ c. low-sodium, low-fat mozzarella cheese, grated
- ½ t. salt
- ½ t. black pepper

Directions

1. Preheat oven to 350ºF (177°C) for 9-inch pie or 375ºF (191°C) for tartlets.
2. Place the piecrust in a pie dish and set aside.
3. In a medium pan, sauté the onion and garlic until caramelized.
4. In a medium bowl, blend eggs and milk until evenly mixed.
5. Add the spinach, onion, and garlic to the egg and milk mixture.
6. Next add the cheese and mix well until evenly incorporated.
7. Add the salt and pepper and mix to combine.
8. Pour the mixture into the unbaked piecrust.
9. Sprinkle the top with a little more mozzarella if desired.
10. Place pie in oven and cook for 1 hour or until golden and puffed in the center.
11. If making tartlets, bake for 25–30 minutes.
12. Let the quiche sit for about 5 minutes before cutting.

PER SERVING: 220 CALORIES, 9 G PROTEIN, 17 G CARBOHYDRATE, 13 G FAT, 1 G FIBER, 360 MG SODIUM.

Chapter 15 Review and Expand

Reading Summary

Carbohydrates and fats are the main sources of energy for the body. The body uses both anaerobic and aerobic production systems to convert the nutrients into energy the muscles can use. In the absence of sufficient oxygen, the body's acid-base balance is changed. As a result, you experience a burning sensation and fatigue in the muscles.

Athletes have greater needs for energy and some nutrients than nonathletes. However, they can usually meet their calorie and nutrient needs through diet.

Athletes have high-energy needs to fuel their activity in training and competition. Most of this energy should come from carbohydrates in the diet. The diet should also provide moderate amounts of protein and fat. Athletes need vitamins and minerals to help metabolize the energy nutrients. Athletes need plenty of fluids before, during, and after sports events to avoid dehydration. Water is the preferred body fluid during vigorous exercise. Eating a high-carbohydrate diet a few days before an endurance event increases glycogen stores in the muscles. Athletes should avoid foods high in fat and fiber at pre-event meals.

Reducing excess body fat and increasing lean body mass improves performance in many sports. However, weight adjustments should be gradual. They should occur before the start of an athlete's training season. Body fat should stay within recommended limits.

Chapter Vocabulary

1. **Content Terms** On a separate sheet of paper, list words that relate to each of the following terms. Then, work with a partner to explain how these words are related.

aerobic	endurance athlete
anaerobic	lactic acid
carbohydrate loading	recovery

2. **Academic Terms** For each of the following terms, identify a word or group of words describing a quality of the term—an *attribute*. Pair up with a classmate and discuss your list of attributes. Then, discuss your list of attributes with the whole class to increase understanding.

convert	lethargic
deplete	sustain
expend	

Review Learning

3. Why does the body not use fat for energy during anaerobic activity?
4. *True or false?* Endurance athletes train to improve their anaerobic energy production systems.
5. What are three factors that affect the number of calories an athlete burns through activity?
6. Why are protein supplements not recommended for building muscle tissue and fueling activity?
7. Describe the type of athletic activity that is most likely to benefit from carbohydrate loading.
8. Explain two tips for planning a pre-event meal for an athlete.
9. List nutrients that are important to recovery after an athletic event.
10. How much liquid should an athlete consume after an event to replace fluid losses from the body?
11. What percentage of an athlete's body should be fat?
12. Why is exercise an important part of a weight-gain program for an athlete?
13. Why should athletes who are trying to lose or gain weight for competition consult with a registered dietitian nutritionist?

Self-Assessment Quiz

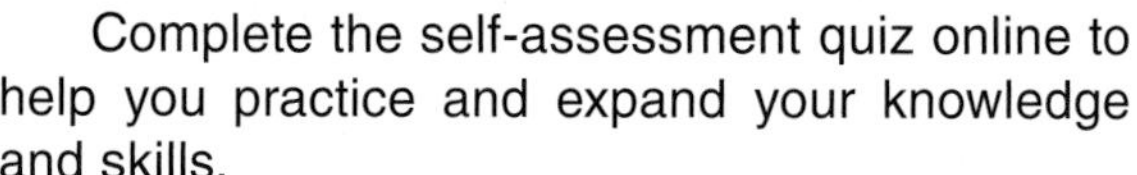

Complete the self-assessment quiz online to help you practice and expand your knowledge and skills.

Critical Thinking

14. **Apply** Presume you have decided to train for a triathlon that involves running, biking, and swimming. What decisions do you need to make regarding your meals for training and competition? Interview a triathlete living in your community. Learn the training methods and nutrition practices he or she uses to prepare for events. What are his or her trusted resources for training and nutrition information? Plan a day's meal and snacks appropriate for your training or competition needs.
15. **Conclude** After a week of practice with the new lacrosse team at your school, you have discovered that this new sport requires a lot of endurance and upper-body strength.

You want to build muscle strength quickly and a friend suggests a new "performance enhancing" supplement he found at the health food store. What evidence would you look for to determine whether this is a safe supplement? Why is healthful eating and an effective exercise plan the best way to get your desired results?

16. **Evaluate** Obtain menus from two restaurants you are likely to eat at when participating in an event away from home. Use the guidelines in this chapter to select foods that would benefit your athletic performance. Circle or highlight your menu choices.
17. **Create** Develop a recipe for a sports drink using ingredients you have at home. First, identify what needs you want your drink to fulfill. For example, do you want the drink to replace electrolytes, provide energy, and so on? Then, make a list of ingredients you can use to accomplish those goals. Begin experimenting with amounts and flavor combinations. Keep a record documenting each trial recipe and your assessment of each. Submit a recipe for your final product and consider making the recipe to share with your classmates.
18. **Plan** Prepare a lesson to inform on the relationship between a nutritious diet and athletic performance. Ask the coach of one of your school's athletic teams and a nutrition instructor to provide feedback. Create an electronic presentation to impart the lesson. Adjust the style and content of your presentation to your audience. Use digital media to add visual interest and improve understanding. Then share the presentation with a group of younger athletes.

Core Skills

19. **Technology Literacy** Plan a blog about a topic relevant to this chapter's content. For example, a topic on claims and effects of the newest performance enhancing supplements on the market or nutritional needs and concerns of cheer sports athletes. First, consider who will be reading your blog and how to make the topic appealing to them. Next, identify three main points that you want to cover. Then, be sure to give your blog a clever title. After you finish writing, be sure to edit and revise your content before posting.
20. **Listening and Writing** Interview an athlete in your school about what foods he or she eats before a sports event. Learn the reasons behind the food choices. Write a brief comparison of the athlete's practices with the recommendations for pre-event meals made in this chapter.
21. **Write** Research public health concerns regarding the need for further federal regulation of energy drinks or sports enhancing supplements. Prepare a summary of your findings. Write a letter to your lawmakers to get the FDA to regulate the contents of these products.
22. **Math** Use the chart shown in Figure 15.5 to calculate the approximate number of calories expended by a 175-pound athlete playing racquetball for 1½ hours.
23. **History and Writing** Learn about the dietary practices of ancient Olympians. Compare these practices with dietary practices of modern day Olympians. Write a summary comparing the two.
24. **Write** Contact one of the national associations for youth sports to find out their official position on weight requirements for various sports. Write an opinion paper agreeing or disagreeing with the association's position. Use a minimum of two references. Submit your paper to the school newspaper for consideration.
25. **Math** Use Appendix D to calculate total carbohydrates, total calories, and the percent of calories from carbohydrates supplied by the following pregame meal:

    3 4-inch pancakes

    2 tablespoons syrup

    1 large scrambled egg (milk and butter added)

    1 cup strawberries

    1 cup grape juice
26. **Career Readiness Practice** Imagine you are the health writer for your local newspaper and it has come to your attention that performance aids are being used excessively by local high school athletes. Your current assignment is to write a full-page public service announcement that captures student attention and warns athletes about the harmful effects of these performance aids. In your research, be sure to identify certain performance aids students are using and the harm these aids do to the human body.

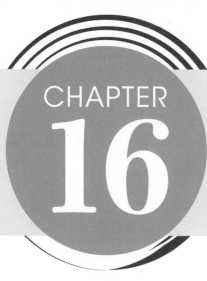

CHAPTER 16 Eating Disorders

Learning Outcomes

After studying this chapter, you will be able to

- **differentiate between** disordered eating and eating disorders;
- **recognize** characteristics and health risks associated with three common eating disorders;
- **analyze** possible causes of eating disorders;
- **assess** an athlete's risk for developing an eating disorder; and
- **summarize** methods of treatment for people with eating disorders.

Karissaa/Shutterstock.com

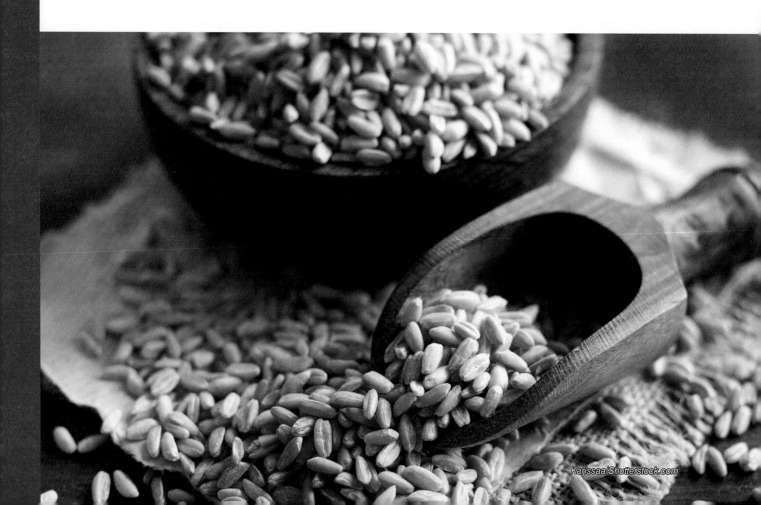

Content Terms

anorexia nervosa
antidepressant
binge-eating disorder
bingeing
bulimia nervosa
disordered eating
eating disorder
female athlete triad
outpatient treatment
purging

Academic Terms

compel
demeanor
disparity
dynamics
relapse

What's Your Nutrition and Wellness IQ?

Take this quiz to examine how much you already know about eating disorders. If you cannot answer a question, pay extra attention to that topic as you study this chapter.

- Identify each statement as *True*, *False*, or *It Depends*. *It Depends* means in some cases the statement is true; in some cases it could be false.
- Revise false statements to make them true.
- Explain the circumstances in which each *It Depends* statement is true and when it is false.

Nutrition and Wellness IQ 

	Statement			
1.	Disordered eating is typical teen eating behavior that is outgrown by adulthood.	True	False	It Depends
2.	All eating disorders increase the risk for serious health problems.	True	False	It Depends
3.	The cause for most eating disorders is clear and simple.	True	False	It Depends
4.	Disordered eating is more common in cultures that place value on physical appearance.	True	False	It Depends
5.	Treatment for anorexia nervosa can be successful.	True	False	It Depends
6.	A male with an eating disorder is likely to concentrate on exercise as a way to lose weight.	True	False	It Depends
7.	Teen athletes are at higher risk for an eating disorder than nonathletes.	True	False	It Depends
8.	If you notice unusual eating behavior patterns by your best friend, it is best to tell them you think they have a problem.	True	False	It Depends

While studying this chapter, look for the activity icon  **to**

- **build** vocabulary with e-flash cards and interactive games;
- **assess** what you learn by completing self-assessment quizzes and completing review questions; and
- **expand** knowledge with interactive activities and activities that extend learning.

www.g-wlearning.com/foodsandnutrition/

Have you ever overeaten at a buffet or skipped lunch to finish a school project? Neither of these behaviors may be the wisest choice from a nutritional standpoint; however, making an occasional unwise choice is not likely to risk your health. This is especially true if you balance such a choice with wiser choices throughout the day, but when do eating behaviors become unhealthy? This chapter will help to explain when eating patterns become a health concern.

Disordered Eating or Eating Disorder?

Our culture focuses much attention on food and body weight. Photos of meals and toned abdominal muscles occupy a great deal of space on social media platforms. People routinely lose weight simply to regain that weight and more.

The presence of any of the following behaviors may be an indication of disordered eating:

- habitual weight cycling, also known as *yo-yo dieting;*
- inflexible, unhealthy food and exercise practices;
- sense of guilt due to failure to maintain self-imposed food and exercise rules;
- uncontrolled or emotionally driven eating;
- persistent thoughts about food, body, and exercise that negatively affect your health and happiness; or
- use of extreme measures such as food restriction, exercise, or fasting to offset foods eaten.

This wide range of unhealthy eating behaviors can be an indication of ***disordered eating***. Disordered eating is a cause for concern because it increases the risk for serious health problems such as obesity, bone loss, digestive problems, and depression. Additionally, this pattern often turns into an eating disorder.

An ***eating disorder*** is a serious mental illness that is characterized by abnormal eating patterns focusing on body weight and food issues. A diagnosis of "eating disorder" requires that specific criteria be met. In contrast, disordered eating is a description rather than a diagnosis. Both disordered eating and eating disorders are treatable.

Characteristics of Eating Disorders

The emotional and physical problems associated with eating disorders can have life-threatening consequences. Eating disorders are diagnosed as mental disorders based on specific criteria. These disorders have the highest mortality rate of any mental disorder.

All ages, races, and socioeconomic groups are affected; however, eating disorders are most common among teenage and young adult women. Disordered eating is also more common in cultures that place value on physical appearance.

The three eating disorders commonly diagnosed are anorexia nervosa, bulimia nervosa, and binge-eating disorder (**Figure 16.1**). Certain behaviors are typical of each disorder, and all are harmful to health.

Anorexia Nervosa

Anorexia nervosa is an eating disorder characterized by self-imposed chronic and severe food restrictions, distorted body image, intense fear of weight gain, and refusal to maintain a healthy body weight. An individual with anorexia is likely to have a body weight 15 percent or more below recommended weight for age and height.

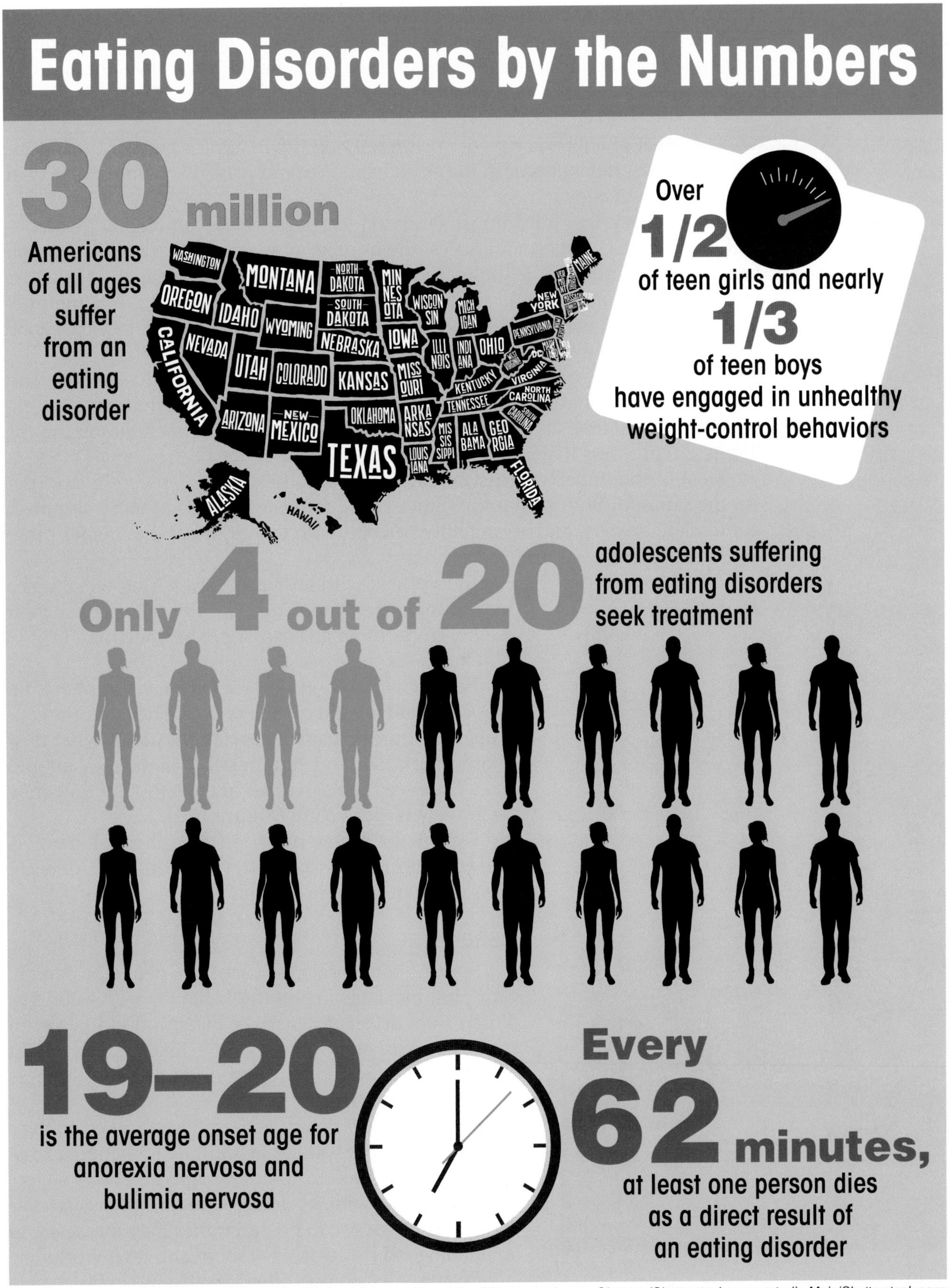

Eating Disorders by the Numbers

30 million Americans of all ages suffer from an eating disorder

Over **1/2** of teen girls and nearly **1/3** of teen boys have engaged in unhealthy weight-control behaviors

Only **4** out of **20** adolescents suffering from eating disorders seek treatment

19–20 is the average onset age for anorexia nervosa and bulimia nervosa

Every **62 minutes,** at least one person dies as a direct result of an eating disorder

Top to bottom: MJgraphics/Shutterstock.com; Forest Foxy/Shutterstock.com; Okuneva/Shutterstock.com; estudio Maia/Shutterstock.com; h0lyland/Shutterstock.com

Figure 16.1 It is likely that you know someone with an eating disorder.

The severe food restrictions practiced by individuals with anorexia nervosa can lead to illness, and social and emotional problems. The focus becomes weight loss, how to avoid food, and feelings of dissatisfaction with body weight.

Who Is Affected?

The onset of anorexia nervosa commonly occurs in adolescence or during the early twenties. It may occur in the adult years, but rarely begins before puberty or after 40 years of age.

Anorexia is the third most common chronic illness among adolescents. Although more common in females, the number of males with anorexia is growing. Ten percent of people diagnosed with anorexia nervosa are male. Males are more likely to concentrate on exercise as a way to lose body weight. Sometimes they choose to eat very low-calorie, low-fat diets that appear to be choices for good health, but actually are for weight loss.

Many males avoid seeking treatment for eating disorders due to fear and shame. The belief that anorexia is a female problem may prevent males from seeking help. By the time an eating problem is identified and treatment is sought, the illness can progress to dangerous levels.

Most of the underlying psychological factors that lead to an eating disorder are the same for both men and women. Low self-esteem, a need to be accepted, depression, anxiety, and an inability to cope with emotional and personal problems are common.

Individuals with anorexia view losing weight as a way to solve their problems. The ability to control their weight gives them a sense of power they may lack in other areas of their lives.

People with anorexia place excessive emphasis on the shape and weight of their bodies. They become consumed by unreasonable expectations about what they should look like and how much weight they should lose. They see themselves as fat even though they may be gravely underweight (**Figure 16.2**).

Except for amenorrhea, all the physical dangers and complications associated with eating disorders are the same regardless of gender.

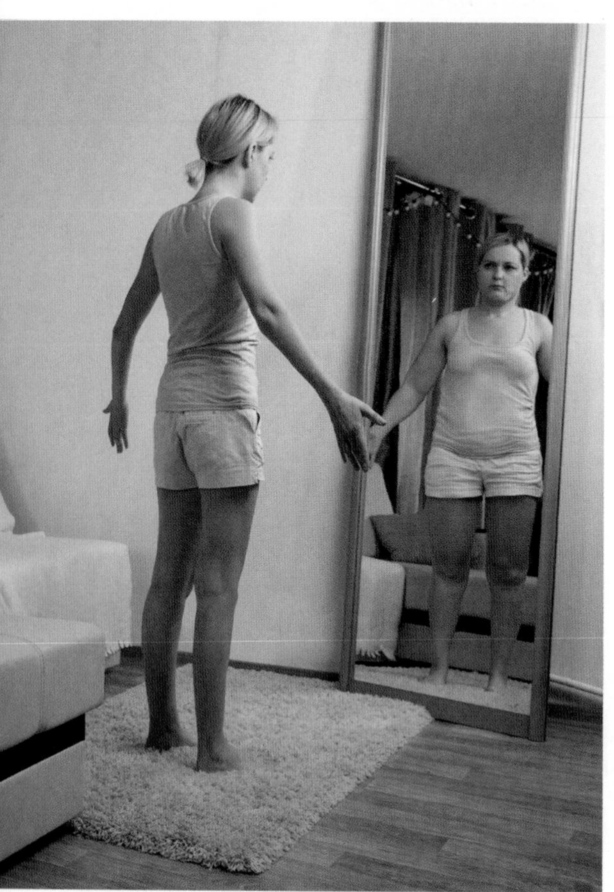

Tatyana Dzemileva/Shutterstock.com

Figure 16.2 Often, a person with anorexia nervosa sees a distorted body image when looking in a mirror.

Behaviors

Specific behaviors may vary from person to person. Skipping meals is a common behavior with anorexia. When they do sit down for a meal, individuals with anorexia are likely to eat very little. Instead, they might simply move the food around on their plates. Others will eat only in private.

Some people with anorexia choose to take laxatives or diet pills to lose weight. In addition to dieting, excessive exercise is used to control weight and body shape. They may jog, swim, or do aerobics for hours each day. However, the desire to be thin rather than the desire to maintain good health is what motivates their workouts.

People with anorexia often wear baggy clothes to hide their overly thin bodies. They may begin to withdraw from social events and exhibit a quiet, serious personality.

Symptoms

As anorexia nervosa develops, physical symptoms appear. A very low-caloric intake leads to a large drop in weight as a key symptom. Low body weight and body fat cause females to develop amenorrhea, or the cessation of menstrual periods.

The disorder causes stress, which may take the form of restlessness or irritability. Loss of insulation from the layer of body fat under the skin causes people with anorexia to feel cold. The body adapts to this loss of insulation by growing a covering of fine hair to trap heat. Rough, dry skin and hair loss are two other symptoms resulting from poor nutrient intake.

Anorexia nervosa takes a toll on health in many ways. Normal growth and development will slow down or halt. Muscle tissue wastes away along with body fat. Blood pressure and pulse rate drop and the body organs begin to shrivel. Bone density decreases and symptoms of osteoporosis may occur. Some people with anorexia die from starvation. Others fall into a deep depression and the risk of suicide increases.

Bulimia Nervosa

Some people suffer from an eating disorder known as ***bulimia nervosa***. This disorder involves two key actions. The first is ***bingeing***, which is uncontrollable eating of excessive amounts of food in a relatively short period. The second action can be one of several unhealthy practices used as attempts to prevent weight gain. These include purging, excessive exercise, prolonged fasting, and abuse of laxatives, diuretics, or enemas. For many people with this disorder, the second action is ***purging***. This means clearing the food from the digestive system. People with bulimia may purge by forcing themselves to vomit. Some abuse laxatives, diuretics, or enemas to rid their bodies of the food. Bulimia nervosa is two to three times more prevalent than anorexia nervosa.

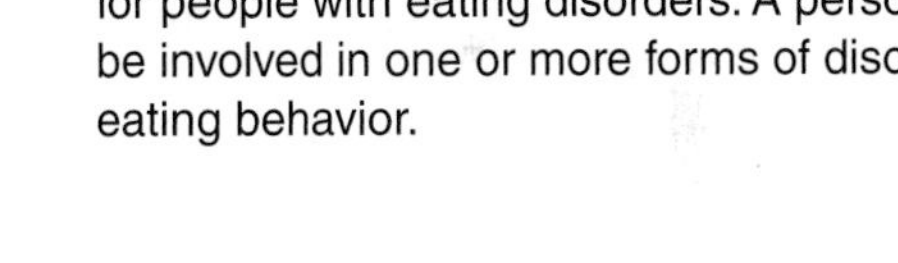

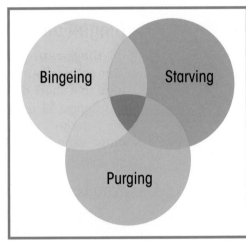

Goodheart-Willcox Publisher

Figure 16.3 Patterns of behavior may overlap for people with eating disorders. A person may be involved in one or more forms of disordered eating behavior.

Instead of purging, some individuals use excessive exercise or periods of fasting to prevent weight gain. Some people alternate between bulimic and anorexic behaviors (**Figure 16.3**).

People with this disorder repeat the cycle of bingeing and purging at least once a week for three months or more. Some repeat the cycle several times a day. Once the cycle begins, it is hard for many people to stop.

Who Is Affected?

Much like anorexia nervosa, the onset of bulimia nervosa commonly occurs in adolescence or during the early twenties. It peaks during young adulthood, and rarely begins before puberty or after 40 years of age. It is far more common in females than in males.

A person with bulimia often comes from a family and social group where weight and appearance are important. He or she usually possesses a low self-esteem.

Behaviors

As with anorexia, people with bulimia are always thinking about food. When bingeing, they consume thousands of calories in a few hours. Binge foods are often high in fats and carbohydrates. During a binge, someone might eat a whole cake, a dozen donuts, and an entire carton of ice cream. Choices about which foods and how much to eat are not related to hunger and satiety. Eating behaviors are out of control.

People with bulimia realize their eating patterns are not normal and are ashamed. They binge and purge in secret because they do not want others to be aware of their behavior. If a person with bulimia has an average body size, others may not notice the problem for a long time.

Symptoms

Individuals with bulimia nervosa are often normal weight or overweight. Females with this disorder may experience menstrual irregularities or amenorrhea.

Serious health problems are associated with bulimia nervosa. As the disorder becomes established, damage to the body becomes more severe and more difficult to reverse. Repeated vomiting can cause glands in the throat to swell. Acids from the stomach burn the esophagus. In addition, the acid can destroy tooth enamel. Vomiting can also cause a loss of water and minerals from the body. This can result in dangerous fluid and electrolyte imbalances. Problems with heart and liver damage can develop due to bulimia. Bulimia nervosa can be fatal.

Binge-Eating Disorder

Binge-eating disorder is the most common eating disorder in the United States. This eating disorder is characterized by repeatedly ingesting excessive amounts of food in a short time. The event may occur from as infrequently as once a week to as often as 14 times per week or more. Food is consumed in huge amounts until the person is uncomfortably full. The binge may last for one or two hours. With binge-eating disorder, there is usually no attempt to purge the food or burn off the excess calories through exercise.

Who Is Affected?

Binge-eating disorder is more prevalent among adults who are 18 years or older. Additionally, this disorder occurs with less **disparity** (difference) between males and females than either anorexia nervosa or bulimia nervosa (**Figure 16.4**). People with binge-eating disorder will likely—but not always—have problems with excess weight.

Figure 16.4
Unlike other eating disorders, binge-eating disorder is prevalent in females from a variety of races and ethnicities. It is also displayed by males more than other eating disorders. *What might account for a higher rate of males and nonwhite females engaging in this particular eating disorder?*

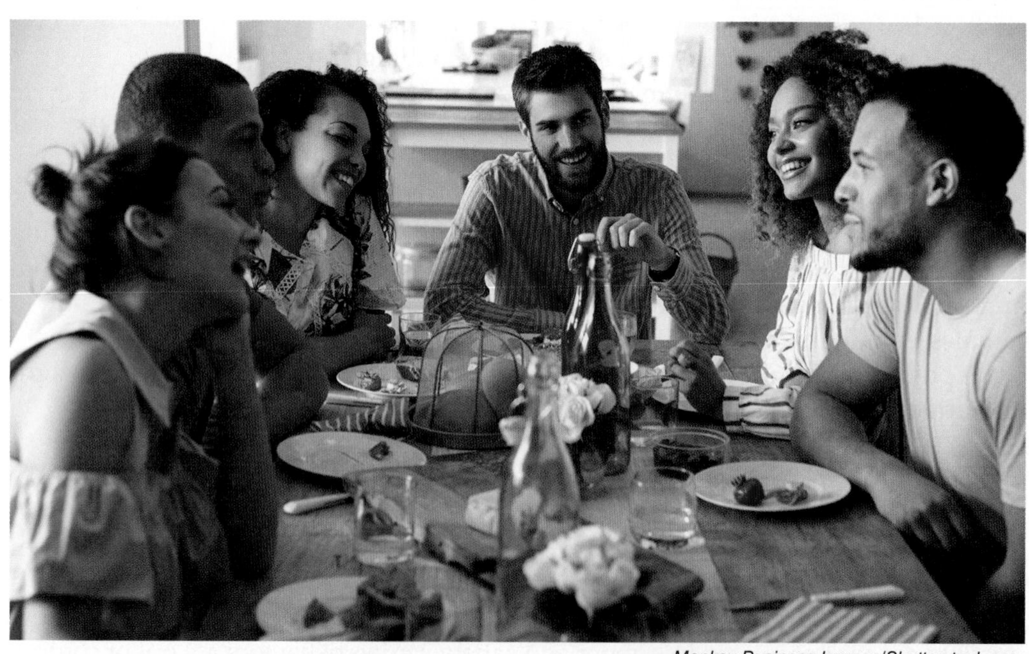

Monkey Business Images/Shutterstock.com

Behaviors

Triggers such as stress, hunger, or being alone may initiate a binge episode. The sense of helplessness to stop a binge can set off another binge. After the binge, the person often experiences feelings of depression, shame, or guilt. They may also have ongoing feelings of frustration and rejection. To be diagnosed with binge-eating disorder, binge frequency must be at least once a week for three months or more.

People with this disorder are likely to drop out of weight-loss programs due to emotional stress. A program might help them lose weight, but without psychotherapy and nutrition counseling, they are apt to repeat the cycle. Lost weight will be regained.

Symptoms

Individuals with binge-eating disorder often show no obvious physical symptoms other than overweight or obesity. Nevertheless, an indication of the disorder would include repeated attempts at dieting.

Other Eating Disorders

Many forms of eating disorders exist. Not all fit the criteria for a diagnosis of anorexia nervosa, bulimia nervosa, or binge-eating disorder. Regardless, these behaviors can be harmful to health and may develop into specific eating disorders.

For example, night eating syndrome is an eating disorder that is diagnosed. This syndrome is characterized by recurring episodes of excessive overeating after the evening meal or by waking from sleep to eat (**Figure 16.5**). In addition to nutritional concerns, the insomnia and sleep disturbances add risk for hormone disturbance problems.

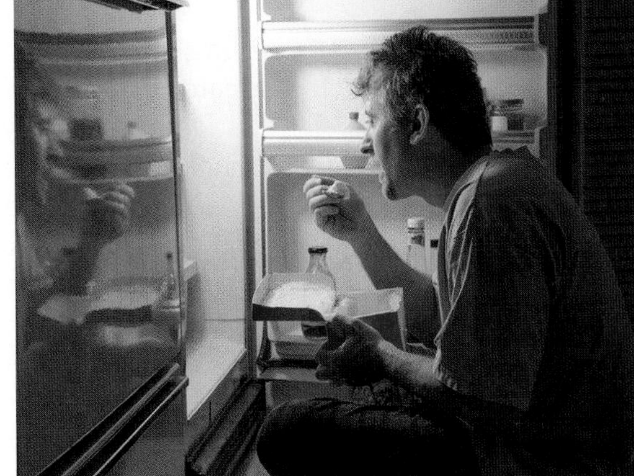

Mike Focus/Shutterstock.com

Figure 16.5 People with night eating syndrome are not sleepwalking; rather, they are fully aware they are eating.

Orthorexia is a form of disordered eating that does not have a diagnosis but can easily move into anorexia nervosa. People with orthorexia have an unhealthy obsession for "healthy" eating. If they hear unfavorable information about a particular food—whether from a reliable source or not—they eliminate it from their diet. Excessive time is needed to find the "right" foods to eat each day and can lead to social isolation. This leads to fewer and fewer foods that they "allow" themselves to eat. Eventually, food choices are so limited that their health begins to suffer.

Additional disordered eating behaviors include:

- obsession with physique and muscle size;
- fixation on a real or perceived flaw in appearance; or
- constant urge to eat or chew nonnutritive substances.

In general, any time an eating behavior causes personal emotional distress, shame, or discomfort, professional evaluation is needed. Leaving an eating disorder untreated can have serious health consequences.

Probable Causes of Eating Disorders

The probable causes of eating disorders are complex and often intertwined. A single factor may not lead to problem eating patterns. When several factors occur together, however, an eating disorder may be triggered. Risk factors vary for different eating disorders, but are usually emotional, environmental, or genetic and physiological in origin.

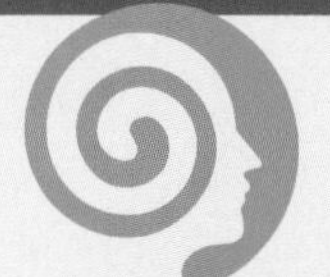

EXTEND YOUR KNOWLEDGE

When Is It No Longer Healthy Behavior?

Sometimes people are motivated by health, but the behaviors they adopt become unhealthy. *Orthorexia nervosa* is a term used to describe attempts to eat healthy that become so limiting that an individual's health is at risk. People who begin exercising to improve health or athletic performance may cross over into compulsive exercising. This disorder is known as *anorexia athletica*. Research online to find out more about these disorders. What are identifiable clues that behaviors cross the line and become potentially unhealthy?

Emotional

Children who exhibit obsessive behaviors have a greater likelihood of developing anorexia when they are older. People who have anxiety issues are also at greater risk for this eating disorder.

Depression, low self-esteem, weight-related issues, and social unease are emotional factors common to increased risk for bulimia nervosa.

Teens are especially vulnerable to feelings of rejection, worthlessness, and guilt. Their lives are in a state of physical, social, and emotional change as they approach adulthood. They seek reassurance from others. Some teens assume their appearance is the reason for any feelings of rejection they sense from others. They may feel worthless if they are overweight. They develop feelings of guilt because they cannot achieve society's standard of beauty.

Emotional change during the teen years may also create out-of-control eating patterns. Facing the challenges of physically growing up and separating from family and friends creates much stress for many teens. They may feel powerless over their lives. Such feelings lead some teens to become emotionally dependent on food. They use food as a source of comfort. They may also see food as one aspect of their lives over which they can have control. Such views of food can be harmful.

Some teens are reluctant to eat in public due to body image concerns. Simply enjoying a piece of pizza with a friend may result in feelings of low self-esteem. These teens may fear their friends will think they lack self-control for not turning down the pizza. Such fears may prompt these teens to eat alone. This can lead to a pattern of secretive eating, which is part of disordered-eating behavior.

Environmental

Anorexia nervosa is more likely to develop in people who grow up in a cultural environment in which thinness is valued. Careers, such as modeling, or athletics, such as gymnastics, place great emphasis on weight and physique. People involved in these activities are at greater risk for anorexia.

Social pressure to be thin prompts people to form unhealthful dieting patterns. Much of this pressure comes from the media. Recently, media has been making an effort to highlight the talents of overweight people; however, many overweight people are still portrayed as dull and dowdy. Thin celebrities shape society's concept of beauty. Many people feel they must be thin to be attractive and successful. They measure their self-worth by their body shape and weight. This **compels** (influences) them to diet. However, too many adolescents do not grasp the reality that most body types can never fit the model image.

Evidence suggests family **dynamics** (patterns) may be involved in the development of eating disorders. Family members of patients with eating disorders often show overt concern with appearance and high achievement. They may lack communication skills. They may also show a tendency to avoid conflicts within the family. Relationship problems can be a factor for people with eating disorders; however, the causes are different for every individual.

Severe trauma, such as sexual or physical abuse, is identified as a risk factor for bulimia nervosa.

FOOD AND THE ENVIRONMENT

Environmental Cues and Eating Disorders

People are influenced by environmental cues. These cues can trigger unhealthy eating behaviors in teens. For example, many female teens view the physical appearance of movie stars, social media celebrities, or fashion models as a standard to achieve. A typical runway model has a body mass index (BMI) of 16. The expectations of the fashion industry seem to encourage the near starvation required to achieve that BMI. According to the Centers for Disease Control and Prevention (CDC), a BMI below 18.5 is considered underweight and not a healthy weight. Public health professionals are arguing for regulations to make it illegal to employ runway models with a BMI less than 18.

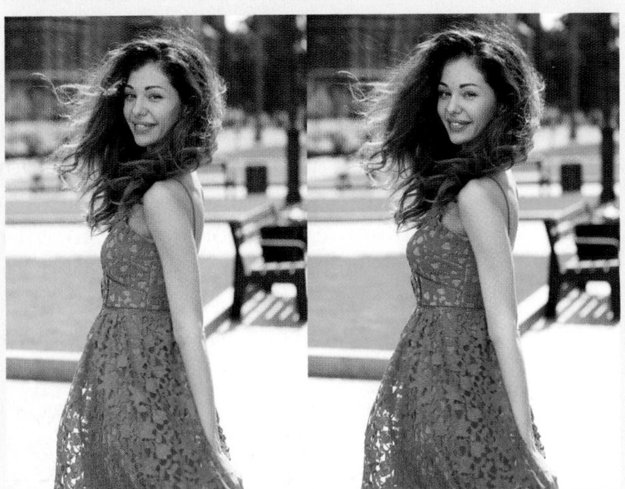

Andrey Arkusha/Shutterstock.com

There is also a movement to require that disclaimers accompany retouched photos. Photos of models and celebrities are often digitally altered to eliminate inches and imperfections. Unaware that the images are manufactured, young people participate in unhealthy eating behaviors in a vain attempt to achieve unrealistic body shapes.

Many male teens compare their bodies to the strong, muscular physiques promoted in the media. Media including television, films, video, billboards, magazines, movies, music, newspapers, fashion designers, social media, and the Internet bombards teens with unrealistic images every day. Most teens spend approximately six to seven hours viewing media daily. The impact on eating behaviors and body image can be damaging.

These environmental cues produce an unhealthy mindset for a teen about what body types are acceptable. Instead, media could help teens imagine a world where beauty is more than body shape and size. A broader definition of beauty and strength could help to inspire confidence and lead to greater human productivity, rewarding thoughts, and health-promoting behaviors.

Think Critically

1. When you see images of supermodels or muscular men, what effect does it have on you?
2. Have you ever been inspired to change your body based on images in the media?
3. Do you think the media has a moral obligation to promote realistic, unaltered images of people?

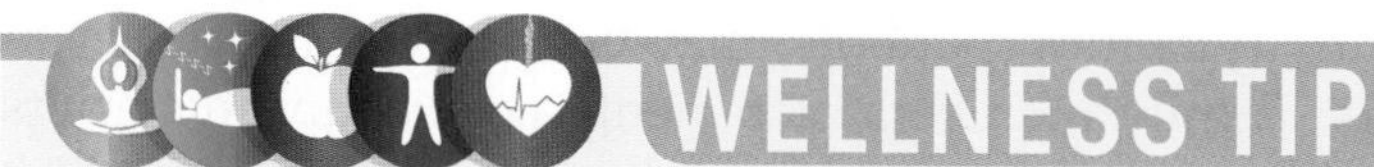

WELLNESS TIP

A Positive Body Image

People with a positive body image are confident and comfortable in their abilities to succeed and in their relationships with others. To increase your positive body image, focus on health and fitness rather than weight. Try keeping an affirmation list of things you like about yourself without focusing on your appearance. Add to your list on a regular basis and review it when you feel less positive.

Genetic and Physiological

Genetics are believed to play a role in the increased risk for eating disorders. Having a sibling or parent with an eating disorder adds to the risks of another family member having an eating disorder. Studies suggest certain chemicals produced in the brain may prompt people to overeat sweet, high-fat foods, and affect appetite preferences.

Early onset of puberty and childhood obesity increase the likelihood for developing bulimia nervosa.

Anorexia may start as a diet plan to lose a few pounds, which spirals out of control. People with this disorder tend to be highly achievement oriented. They feel a sense of control and pride when they reach their weight goals. They enjoy compliments from others about how nice they look. This inspires them to diet further to reach new, lower weight goals. As this dieting pattern continues, people with anorexia become more intent on losing weight. Feelings of pride turn into strong self-criticism. "I feel good about reaching my weight goal" becomes "I'm too fat. I have to lose more weight." Dieting becomes a life-threatening obsession; however, these individuals are usually unaware they have an eating disorder. Thus, denial becomes a serious obstacle to treatment.

Stressful events such as going away to college can also trigger disordered eating (**Figure 16.6**).

Risks for Athletes

Athletes are often prepared to do whatever is needed to excel. Their competitive **demeanor** (attitude) and above-average drive can make them not only highly successful in their sports, but also somewhat vulnerable.

Making Weight

Athletes are often at greater risk for eating disorders because many coaches focus on body weight during training. For instance, a wrestler knows he or she must compete within a weight class. A gymnast is told that his or her body size will affect balance. Constantly trying to achieve and maintain weight goals for their sports may lead athletes to develop eating disorders.

Males who compete in low-weight oriented sports such as jockeys, wrestlers, and runners are at an increased risk of developing an eating disorder. The pressure to succeed, to be the best, to be competitive, and to win at all costs also places

Factors Influencing Disordered Eating in Teens

Self-Image

Teens with negative views about their appearance are more likely to take drastic measures to change it.

Peers

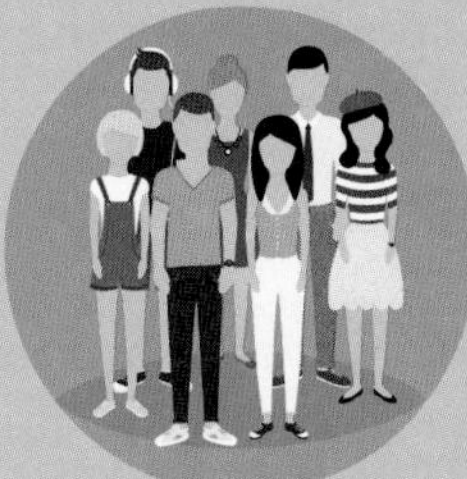

Teens may turn to disordered eating to alter their appearance to gain acceptance or to "fit in."

Bullying

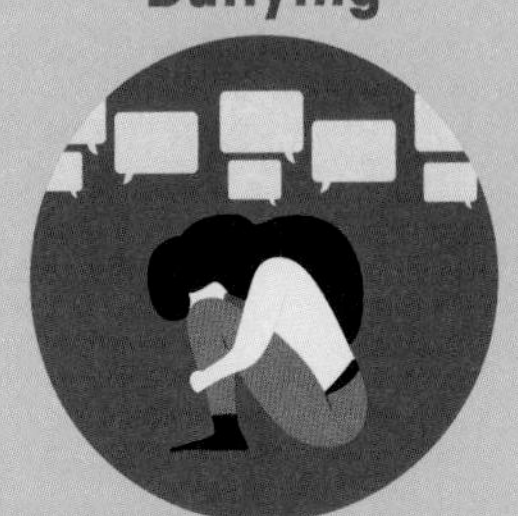

As much as 65% of people with eating disorders say bullying contributed to their development of an eating disorder.

Stress

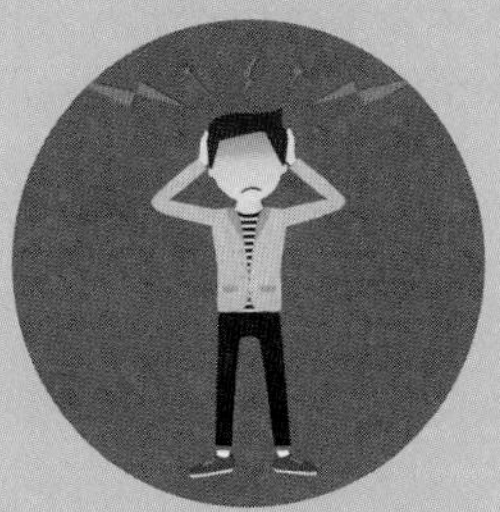

Excessive stress from school, work, extracurricular activities, or other responsibilities can lead to harmful food habits.

Social Media

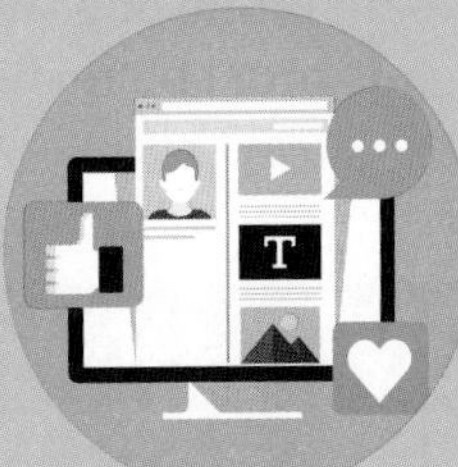

Research shows that social media influences body dissatisfaction due to the constant exposure to the "ideal body type" and the pressure to keep up appearances.

Societal Standards

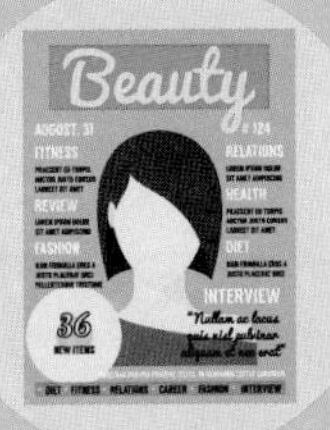

Not measuring up to the idealized body image commonly portrayed in magazines, TV, and movies may cause body dissatisfaction.

Psychological Factors

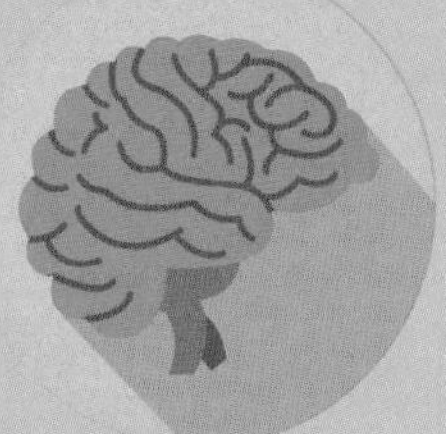

Feelings of rejection, vulnerability, worthlessness, guilt, or a need for control can trigger disordered eating.

Genetics

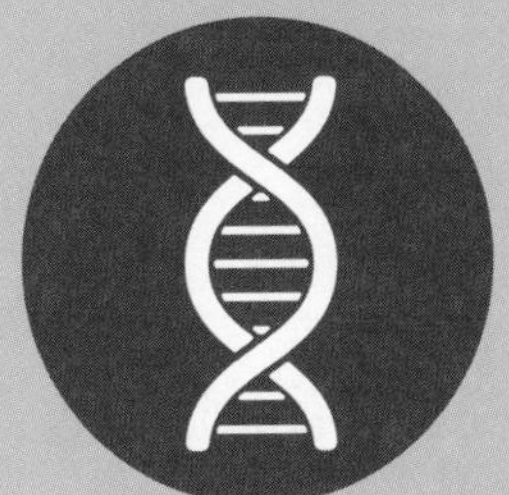

Studies indicate certain chemicals produced in the brain may prompt people to overeat and can affect appetite.

Unrealistic Goals

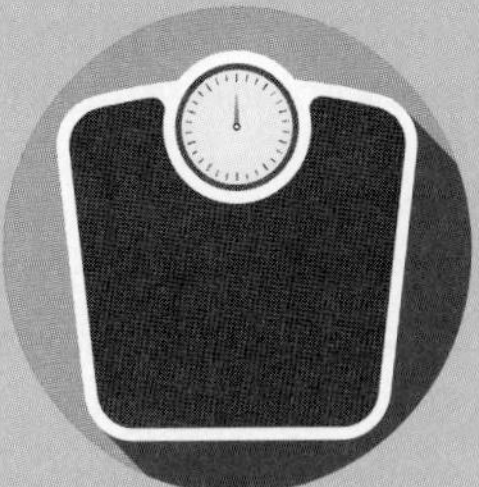

Some teens may wish to achieve a weight outside of the healthy range, and could turn to drastic habits in an attempt to reach their weight-loss goals quickly.

Top row: Pro Symbols/Shutterstock.com; Lesia_G/Shutterstock.com; mmstudiodesign/Shutterstock.com; 2nd row: Fancy Tapis/Shutterstock.com; howcolour/Shutterstock.com; Ira Yapanda/Shutterstock.com; bottom row: Rvector/Shutterstock.com; Vladvm/Shutterstock.com; lukpedclub/Shutterstock.com

Figure 16.6 Many factors can contribute to disordered eating in teens. *Why do you think the onset of most eating disorders occurs during the teen years?*

weight issues as a top concern. These issues combined with other pressures in their lives, such as family problems, friendship issues, or emotional or physical abuse, can contribute to the onset of disordered eating.

Athletes who train intensely may skip meals to train longer and harder. This can become the start of an eating disorder. Wrestlers in weight class events may choose to participate in a class below their normal weight. Disordered-eating patterns may be used to reach the desired weight class. During the off-season, athletes may gain back the weight. As the next season approaches, they may choose harmful ways to lose the weight once again. This weight cycling is dangerous for health and performance. The sports governing organizations do not approve of using harmful methods to "make weight."

Female Athlete Triad

Female athletes may be more prone to eating disorders than the general population. Performance stress and the desire to look perfect add to the desire to be slim. A girl may choose a particular sport to support or hide her eating disorder.

Coaches and trainers may advise an athlete to lose weight. Most students want to please their coaches. If you are given advice to lose or gain weight, ask for the necessary information on how to do so safely and effectively. The team may have access to a registered dietitian nutritionist who knows your sport and can assist with helping you set realistic and attainable goals.

Losing or gaining weight alone does not guarantee better performance. Weight and body composition goals must be realistic. Weight changes resulting from good

THE MOVEMENT CONNECTION

Heel Raise

Why

Treatment is crucial when dealing with eating disorders and must focus on the specific needs of the individual. With proper balance and help, eating disorders can be overcome.

Balance is also important while performing heel raises. The heel raise helps strengthen your calf muscles. Calf muscles are needed to move the body forward. They also play an important role in moving blood through the body.

Apply

- Assume a standing position behind your desk chair.
- Make sure your core muscles are engaged and you are standing with good posture.
- Slowly raise up on your toes and hold for two seconds.
- Lower your heels back to the ground.
- Repeat 10 times.

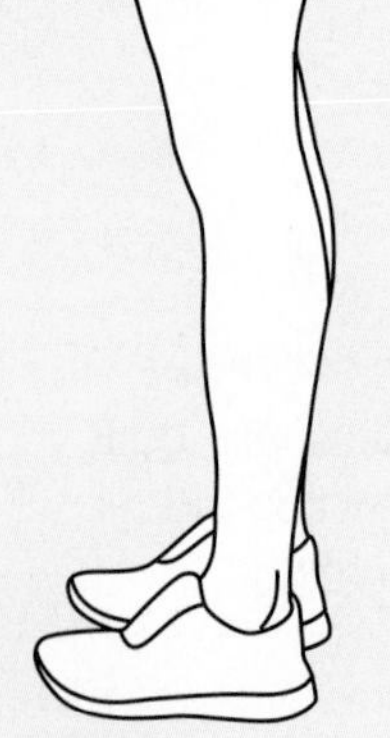

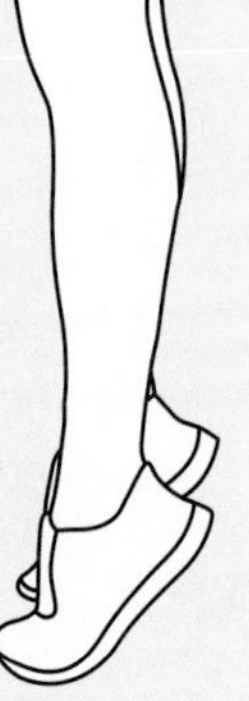

nutrition and appropriate training guidelines will offer long-term performance success (**Figure 16.7**).

Disordered eating among female athletes has become quite common. In fact, it is one of a trio of health problems many female athletes face. The second problem is amenorrhea. Amenorrhea has been linked with mineral losses from bone tissue. This leads to the development of the third health problem—osteoporosis. This set of medical problems has been given the name ***female athlete triad***.

One part of female athlete triad leads to another. The combination of the three disorders poses a greater threat to health than each of the individual disorders. A female athlete trains hard and eats little to maintain a weight goal. When body fat becomes too low, a woman stops menstruating. The resulting hormonal imbalance causes loss of bone mass. This puts her at greater risk of training and performance fractures. Lack of nutrients in the diet and minerals in the bones slows healing of fractures. This causes sports performance to deteriorate, which may foster feelings of low self-esteem and perpetuate the disordered-eating behaviors. If this cycle of problems continues, the young woman is at serious health risk.

Effective coaches put less pressure on women to be thin. They give more encouragement for balanced eating. This helps avoid problems that interfere with a female's normal physical development.

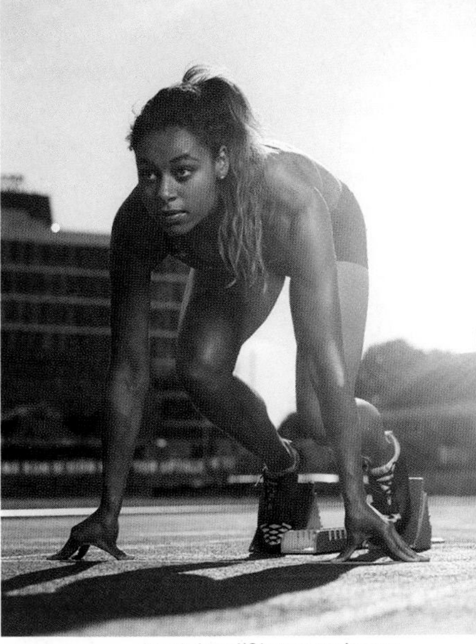

Jacob Lund/Shutterstock.com

Figure 16.7 A female athlete must maintain a nutritious diet to avoid health problems associated with female athlete triad.

CASE STUDY

The Model of Self-Esteem

Kathy is a 17-year-old high school senior and an excellent student. She wants to become an actress someday. Kathy takes great care in the way she presents herself. She spends much time on her clothes, hair, and makeup. Her body weight is healthy, but she sees herself as needing to look and be better. Kathy constantly thinks about food. Some days she doesn't eat at all in order to maintain her weight. Other days she cannot seem to stop eating. She eats when no one sees her. She quickly eats as much as she can. Sometimes she makes herself vomit. Kathy finds that she is unhappy with herself most days.

Kathy likes hanging out with her best friend, Abby. Kathy thinks Abby has it made. Abby doesn't obsess about her weight and figure like many girls their age. And Kathy has never heard Abby remark on someone else's appearance the way many girls do. Abby is easy to be around. Kathy has never heard Abby complain about her body—she seems very happy with the way she looks. Kathy feels better about herself when she is around Abby. Abby often admires Kathy's intelligence and her speaking ability. She assures Kathy that she will be great at whatever she decides to do.

Case Review

1. Why do you think Kathy feels better when she is with Abby?
2. Who do you think has healthier self-esteem? Why?

FEATURED CAREER

Clinical Psychologist

Clinical psychologists work with the assessment, diagnosis, treatment, and prevention of mental disorders. They are trained to use a variety of approaches aimed at helping individuals, and the strategies used are generally determined by their specialty. Clinical psychologists often interview patients and give diagnostic tests in their own private offices. They may design and implement behavior modification programs. Some clinical psychologists work in hospitals where they collaborate with physicians and other specialists to develop and implement treatment and intervention programs.

Education

Licensing and a doctoral degree usually are required for independent practice as a psychologist. Graduates with a master's degree and licensing can work under the supervision of a doctoral psychologist.

Job Outlook

Employment of clinical psychologists is expected to grow much faster than average for all occupations, to match the increased demand for psychological services in mental health centers, schools, hospitals, and social service agencies. Job prospects should be the best for people who have a doctoral degree from a leading university in an applied specialty, such as counseling or health. Master's degree holders will face keen competition.

Treatment for Eating Disorders

People need professional help to overcome eating disorders. Without medical care, people with eating disorders can suffer long-term health problems or even death. Treatment programs vary depending on the factors that led to the eating disorder. However, treatment must focus on the psychological roots of the disorder as well as its physical symptoms. The treatment is highly personalized and varies with each eating disorder.

The recovery rate for people with eating disorders is much higher if they get early treatment. Family and friends can help get someone with an eating disorder into a treatment program (**Figure 16.8**). However, they must recognize that an eating disorder is not just a passing phase.

Treatment for Anorexia Nervosa

Treatment for anorexia nervosa is neither quick nor simple. Therapy for this eating disorder can take many years.

Figure 16.8
These organizations can provide information about eating disorders.

Resources for People with Eating Disorders
• Academy for Eating Disorders (AED)
• National Association of Anorexia Nervosa and Associated Disorders (ANAD)
• National Eating Disorders Association (NEDA)
• Binge-Eating Disorder Association (BEDA)

Several approaches are used to treat anorexia. In some treatment programs, only the client is treated. In other programs, the family also becomes involved in the treatment. Sometimes programs require clients to stay in a hospital or treatment facility.

The first step in treatment is to attend to the physical health problems the disorder has caused. Care should be provided by a doctor trained in treating eating disorders. National help organizations can refer clients to treatment programs in their region.

Once a patient's physical condition has been stabilized, he or she can begin to accept psychological help. Clients explore attitudes about weight, food, and body image. They learn to think about and accept what a healthy body weight means. They receive nutrition counseling to help them gain weight and form healthful eating habits. They find out how to view their body shapes more realistically. They develop suitable exercise programs. As patients receive help to improve their self-images, their overall health also improves.

Clients are taught to build new controls into their lives. They practice verbal skills that help them relate better to their family members and friends. They learn stress-management techniques to use when responding to their emotions.

Family support helps ensure a patient will stick with a recovery program. Many professionals advise family therapy to improve relationships among all the family members.

Getting early treatment for anorexia improves the chances for healthy outcomes. Some people recover fully from anorexia nervosa. Most who recover do well in school and work. Nonetheless, some with this disorder continue to have problems. Studies show about 20 percent of adults who have a history of anorexia nervosa remain underweight. They may still struggle with bouts of low self-esteem and weight-image distortion.

Treatment for Bulimia Nervosa

As with anorexia, people with bulimia should be treated by healthcare professionals with specialized training. These professionals know how to fit treatment programs to the needs of the individual. Treatment for young patients often includes family members. Therapy for older patients may involve only the individual. In both cases, support from family members and friends is vital to the success of the treatment.

Unless a case is severe, people with bulimia usually receive ***outpatient treatment***. This is medical care that does not require a hospital stay. Sometimes physicians prescribe ***antidepressants*** as part of a treatment program. These are a group of drugs that alter the nervous system and relieve depression. They may be used to help the client control mood swings and avoid bingeing. Drugs can help control behavior; however, they cannot cure the mental problems at the root of an eating disorder. The use of antidepressants also involves risks and side effects. Doctors should discuss these issues openly with clients before prescribing medications (**Figure 16.9**).

iofoto/Shutterstock.com

Figure 16.9 Prescription medication cannot cure bulimia nervosa, but it is sometimes helpful in the treatment of this eating disorder.

Support groups can provide people recovering from bulimia with information and encouragement. Still, these groups cannot replace therapy.

Some studies show treatment helps about 25 percent of people with bulimia stop bingeing and purging. Recovery can take many years. With or without treatment, however, many people with this disorder have **relapses** (recurrences). Relapses most frequently take place during periods of stress or change. Counseling can help individuals prepare for and manage stressful events to avoid relapse.

Treatment for Binge-Eating Disorder

Like other eating disorders, binge-eating disorder requires treatment that focuses on emotional issues as well as eating problems. Counseling usually involves helping people with this disorder learn how to like themselves. It helps the clients analyze how their personal beliefs affect their actions. Counseling helps patients learn how to interact and connect better with family, friends, and other support systems. It gives clients the emotional tools to take control of their eating behaviors.

Treatment programs teach weight-management facts. They encourage people who binge eat to seek a healthier weight and form better eating habits. Therapy and the support of friends can help people with this disorder make sound lifestyle choices in many areas.

Questions to Ask a Therapist Before Treatment Begins

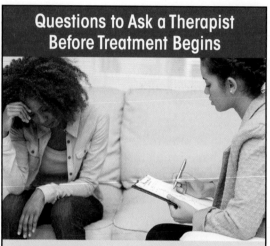

- How long have you been working with clients who have eating disorders?
- What are your professional credentials for treating people with eating disorders?
- What is your treatment philosophy?
- What types of treatment have you found most effective in treating eating disorders?
- What is your success rate in treating people who have eating disorders?
- What type of affiliations do you have with other support services, such as registered dietitian nutritionists, physicians, hospitals, clinics, educational programs, and community-based support groups?
- Do you provide family as well as individual counseling?
- How long does treatment generally last?
- Are you available for consultation if an emergency should occur?

Photo: ESB Professional/Shutterstock.com

Figure 16.10 When choosing an eating-disorder treatment program, have a list of questions to ask each potential therapist. Their answers will help you determine which is the best option for you.

Seeking Professional Services

Treatment for an eating disorder is likely to require the services of a team of healthcare professionals. If the disorder has affected physical health, a medical doctor will be part of this team. A psychologist can help a patient deal with the emotional issues at the root of the disorder. In most instances, a registered dietitian nutritionist will become part of the team. He or she can help the patient form healthful eating habits. An exercise specialist may help the patient plan a moderate exercise program. A treatment center may be recommended where the client is admitted for a period.

All these professionals should have special training in handling eating disorders. Some regions may not have many qualified professionals. However, most healthcare providers can refer patients to specialists or clinics that are equipped to address eating disorders.

For treatment to be effective, a client needs to feel comfortable with the members of the healthcare team. A concerned friend or family member can help someone with an eating disorder find out about a treatment program. He or she can call to ask about treatment methods, fees, and insurance coverage. If everything sounds agreeable, the friend or family member can schedule an appointment. He or she can go with the client to a screening interview. This face-to-face meeting will help the client decide if he or she feels at ease with the health professionals. Having a positive feeling about the treatment program will help the client recover from his or her disorder (**Figure 16.10**).

Helping a Friend with an Eating Disorder

What can you do if you suspect a friend has an eating disorder? The person may not admit he or she has a problem. Your friend may even get angry if you suggest he or she has a disorder.

Do not give up on your friend. Tell the person you are very concerned about him or her. If your friend is not receptive to your concern, you can seek help. Talk to a counselor or to your friend's parents. Tell them about the symptoms you have spotted that concern you.

You can also take steps to help prevent people from developing eating disorders. Be careful when encouraging someone to lose weight. Emphasize your acceptance of the person regardless of his or her weight. Show concern for the person's health and well-being. Encouragement, support, and acceptance may be just what your friend needs to help him or her reach healthy weight goals.

RECIPE FILE

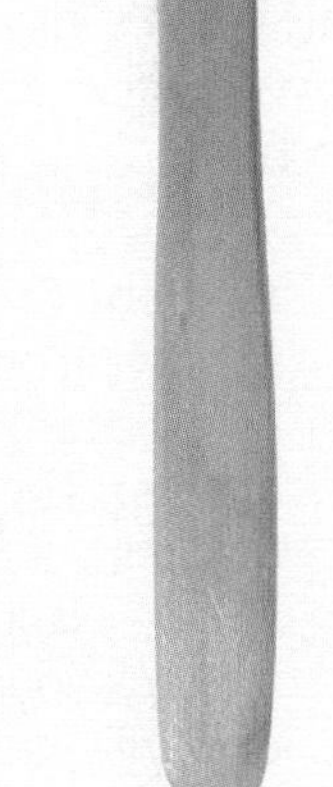

Asian Chicken Burgers

6 SERVINGS

Ingredients

- ¼ c. brown sugar, firmly packed
- ¼ c. low-sodium soy sauce
- 2 T. fresh lime juice
- ¼ t. dried crushed red pepper
- ¾ t. curry powder
- 2 lb. boneless, skinless chicken breasts
- 2 T. hoisin sauce
- 2 T. low-fat mayonnaise
- 1 jalapeño chile, seeded and minced
- 2 t. lime juice
- 1 clove garlic, minced
- 1–2 drops toasted sesame oil (optional)
- cooking spray as needed
- 6 whole-grain hamburger buns
- 1 large tomato, cut into 6 slices
- ½ c. cilantro, roughly chopped

Directions

1. Combine brown sugar, soy sauce, lime juice, crushed red pepper, and curry powder in a resealable plastic bag to make marinade. Reserve a small amount of marinade for basting chicken during grilling.
2. Cut chicken breasts into 6 equal pieces and add to bag with marinade.
3. Place chicken and marinade in refrigerator for at least 4 hours, or overnight. Turn bag several times to coat chicken.
4. Mix together hoisin sauce, mayonnaise, jalapeño (to your taste), and lime juice.
5. Place minced garlic on cutting board and crush with side of a chef's knife until paste consistency.
6. Add garlic and sesame oil (if desired) to mayonnaise mixture and place in refrigerator until ready to use.
7. Remove chicken and dispose of this marinade.
8. Spray grill grate with cooking spray. (If using a grill with an open flame, do not use cooking spray over flame.)
9. Place chicken on hot grill grate over medium heat. Close the lid.
10. Cook for 4 minutes and turn chicken over and close grill.
11. After a minute, baste chicken with the reserved marinade and cook for two more minutes.
12. Turn chicken and baste again with the reserved marinade.
13. Cook for two more minutes, or until chicken reaches 165°F (74°C) and is cooked through.
14. Place buns on grill, cut side down, until lightly browned.
15. Spread mayonnaise mixture on buns, place chicken on bun, and top with tomato and cilantro.

PER SERVING: 212 CALORIES, 22 G PROTEIN, 24 G CARBOHYDRATE, 2 G FAT, 2 G FIBER, 390 MG SODIUM.

Chapter 16 Review and Expand

Reading Summary

Disordered eating is a cause for concern because it increases the risk for serious health problems. An eating disorder is a serious mental illness characterized by abnormal eating patterns that focuses on body weight and food issues.

The causes of eating disorders are complex. Causes may be emotional, environmental, or genetic and physiological. Eating disorders are most common among teens and young adults. People who take part in sports or other activities where weight goals are rigid are most at risk.

Treatment for an eating disorder should be sought as soon as a problem is identified. Treatment must focus on the needs of the individual. It must address both psychological and physical characteristics of the disorder. This type of treatment generally requires the help of several professionals. Physicians, registered dietitian nutritionists, and psychologists may all be part of the clinical team.

Chapter Vocabulary

1. **Content Terms** Work with a partner to write the definitions of the following terms based on your current understanding before reading the chapter. Then join another pair of students to discuss your definitions and any discrepancies. Finally, discuss the definitions with the class and ask your instructor for necessary correction or clarification.

   anorexia nervosa
   antidepressant
   binge-eating disorder
   bingeing
   bulimia nervosa
   disordered eating
   eating disorder
   female athlete triad
   outpatient treatment
   purging

2. **Academic Terms** Write each of the following terms on a separate sheet of paper. For each term, quickly write a word you think relates to the term. In small groups, exchange papers. Have each person in the group explain a term on the list. Take turns until all terms have been explained.

   compel
   demeanor
   disparity
   dynamics
   relapse

Review Learning

3. List five behaviors that may indicate that disordered eating is occurring.
4. Compare eating disorders with disordered eating.
5. Which eating disorder is characterized by chronic caloric restriction, distorted body image, and intense fear of weight gain?
6. List six behaviors a person with anorexia nervosa might demonstrate.
7. What is the main difference between bulimia nervosa and binge-eating disorder?
8. *True or false?* Eating orders that do not fit the criteria of anorexia nervosa, bulimia nervosa, or binge-eating disorder are not harmful to health.
9. List the three categories into which causes for eating disorders fall and give an example of each.
10. Why are athletes at greater risk of developing eating disorders?
11. Describe the female athlete triad.
12. *True or false?* Treatment for eating disorders must focus on both psychological and physical aspects of the problem.
13. What factors contribute to successful recovery for people with eating disorders?
14. How can a person help prevent others from developing eating disorders?

Self-Assessment Quiz

Complete the self-assessment quiz online to help you practice and expand your knowledge and skills.

Critical Thinking

15. **Cause and Effect** What characteristics about eating disorders do you think might make people with diabetes prone to developing eating disorders? What effect might an eating disorder have on a person with diabetes?
16. **Consider** Suppose you have a friend who has either gained or lost a significant amount of weight in the past several months. What actions could you take to show caring support for your friend?

17. **Analyze** Write a journal entry answering the questions that follow. Use your journal to reflect on thoughts and feelings you were not aware you had. Once you are aware of issues, you can begin to work through them.
    A. How do I use food to reward or punish myself?
    B. What strong emotions might cause me to eat when I am not hungry?
    C. How do I feel about being hungry?
    D. How do I feel about myself when I eat too much at a meal or exercise excessively?
    E. How do I feel about myself when I turn down a snack or dessert?
    F. How do I feel about eating in front of other people?
    G. How do I feel about other people who eat too much food?
18. **Analyze** Write a journal entry answering the questions that follow. Use your journal to reflect on thoughts and feelings you were not aware you had. Once you are aware of issues, you can begin to work through them.
    A. Do I use exercise to reward or punish myself?
    B. What strong emotions might cause me to exercise for unusually long periods?
    C. How do I feel about myself when I exercise excessively to keep myself thin or muscular?

Core Skills

19. **Writing** Choose a year in history before 2000 CE. Research how under- and overweight people were portrayed in the media, advertising, and by celebrities that year. Learn what society considered "ideal body image" at that time. Write a paper examining body image then compared with the current body positive movement.
20. **Math** An estimated 2.6% of the US population has an eating disorder. Of those individuals with an eating disorder, 90% are women. If the population of the United States is 325,663,132 people, solve the following:
    A. Calculate the estimated number of people with an eating disorder.
    B. Calculate the estimated number of women with an eating disorder.
21. **Writing and Technology Literacy** Write and illustrate a short electronic book for children. Include age-appropriate font, graphics, and artwork. The theme of the short story is that beauty comes in different shapes, forms, and sizes. The book should emphasize how to appreciate your body. After your instructor's review, read your story to a group of young children. Reflect on any questions they have as a result of your story.
22. **Reading** Learn about the history of eating disorders. When were the first cases diagnosed? Why were the various terms used for the disorders? Who coined the term? Prepare a one-page summary of your findings.
23. **Speaking** Compose a script in which you discuss your concerns with a friend about his or her disordered eating. Role-play your conversation in class.
24. **Listening** Do an Internet search to find interviews or speeches made by people who have experienced eating disorders. Select one and listen to it in its entirety. Prepare a summary in which you analyze the following aspects of the interview: the intended audience, point of view, word choice, tone, points of emphasis, and organization.
25. **Science and Writing** Research how serotonin, a neurotransmitter in the brain, may be involved in eating disorders. Write a summary of your findings. Be sure to cite your sources.
26. **Career Readiness Practice** As a person who navigates life by firmly adhering to a strong code of ethics, you find yourself facing an ethical dilemma. A friend from school and work confides in you about her struggle with an eating disorder and makes you promise not to tell anyone about it. Over time, you have noticed your friend's work productivity declining. You are concerned about her health and quality of life. You are wondering if you should talk with your friend's parents or the school counselor about the symptoms of her condition. What should you do? What is the best way to practice integrity in this situation?

CHAPTER 17 Planning Healthy Meals

Learning Outcomes

After studying this chapter, you will be able to

- **identify** kitchen appliances, cookware, bakeware, and tools;
- **employ** flavor, color, texture, temperature, and shape and size to plan appealing meals;
- **recognize** resources for help planning healthy meals;
- **implement** strategies for managing time when preparing foods; and
- **apply** tactics for eating healthy meals away from home.

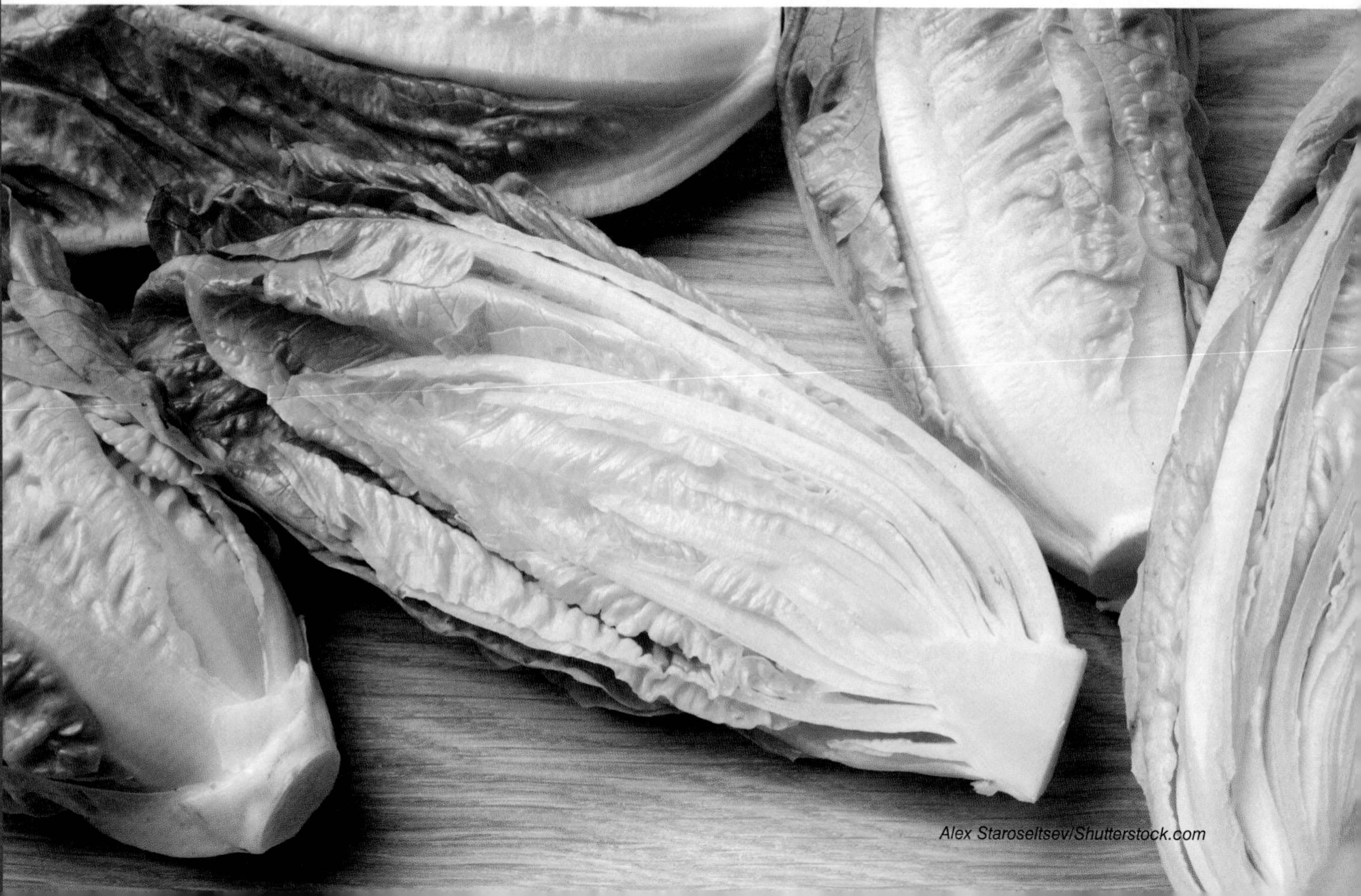

Alex Staroseltsev/Shutterstock.com

Content Terms

broiler
built-in oven
convection oven
cooktop
dishwasher
minimally processed food
perishable
pilot light
preheat
range
refrigerator-freezer

Academic Terms

homogenous
judicious
monochromatic
perforation
streamline
tepid

What's Your Nutrition and Wellness IQ?

Take this quiz to examine how much you already know about planning meals. If you cannot answer a question, pay extra attention to that topic as you study this chapter.

- Identify each statement as *True*, *False*, or *It Depends*. *It Depends* means in some cases the statement is true; in some cases it could be false.
- Revise false statements to make them true.
- Explain the circumstances in which each *It Depends* statement is true and when it is false.

Nutrition and Wellness IQ

1.	Kitchen equipment has little influence over meal planning.	True	False	It Depends
2.	A meal composed of similar color foods is most appealing to the eye.	True	False	It Depends
3.	Everyone requires the same nutrients, but the amounts people need may vary.	True	False	It Depends
4.	Individuals with special nutritional or health needs require a separate meal plan.	True	False	It Depends
5.	ChooseMyPlate.gov is a good resource for meal planning.	True	False	It Depends
6.	The best way to organize the kitchen is to store utensils in the lower cabinets and appliances in upper cabinets.	True	False	It Depends
7.	Some processed foods are healthy.	True	False	It Depends
8.	Eating at fast-food restaurants means eating unhealthy foods.	True	False	It Depends

While studying this chapter, look for the activity icon to

- **build** vocabulary with e-flash cards and interactive games;
- **assess** what you learn by completing self-assessment quizzes and completing review questions; and
- **expand** knowledge with interactive activities and activities that extend learning.

www.g-wlearning.com/foodsandnutrition/

At mealtime, do you find yourself opening the refrigerator and grabbing whatever is handy? Meals thrown together without planning often lack nutrition and appeal. With a little planning, meals can be healthy, appealing, and save you some money.

Planning Begins in the Kitchen

Before you begin planning meals, you must familiarize yourself with the kitchen and its contents. The types of equipment that your kitchen is stocked with influences the types of meals you can plan and prepare. To become a successful cook, you need to understand the appliances and tools that are most useful for preparing food.

Ingredient availability also influences the types of meals you can prepare. Certain ingredients are used on a regular basis. Planning a meal is much easier when the kitchen is always stocked with these ingredients.

Kitchen Appliances

Every kitchen has basic appliances. Each appliance has been carefully designed to perform a certain function with ease. In the kitchen, you will find major appliances and small appliances, each with a different function. Major appliances are large pieces of equipment powered by gas or electricity. They differ from small appliances because they are not portable. Every kitchen has several major appliances, such as a range, refrigerator-freezer, and dishwasher. There are numerous small appliances.

Range

A ***range*** is a large kitchen appliance that usually consists of an oven, cooktop, and broiler. Ranges may be powered by gas or electricity (**Figure 17.1**). A conventional oven is used to bake, roast, and broil food items. When baking or roasting, a heat source on the bottom of the oven cavity generates the heat.

Figure 17.1 Ranges may be powered by gas or electricity. *What reasons might influence your decision to purchase one type over the other?*

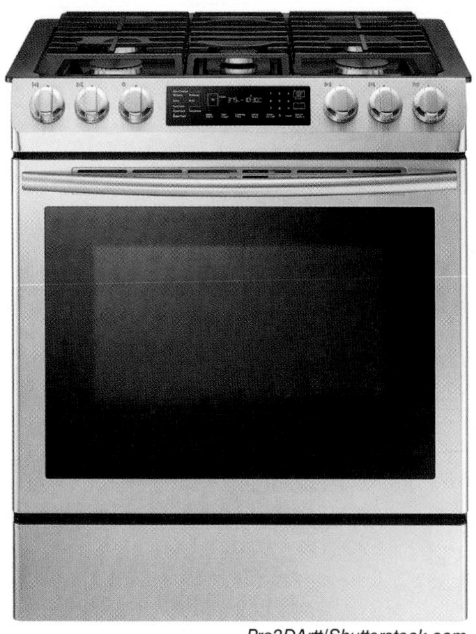

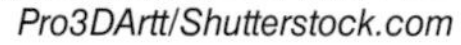

Pro3DArtt/Shutterstock.com

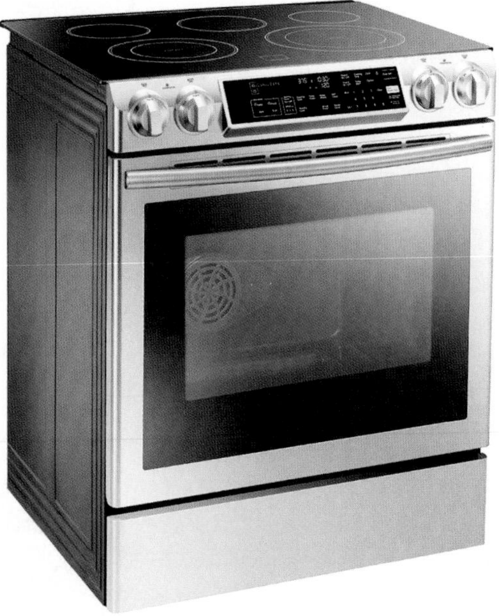

Pro3DArtt/Shutterstock.com

The heat flows to the top of the cavity because hot air rises. An oven must be ***preheated*** for at least 10 minutes to allow it to reach the selected temperature before baking or roasting. Once preheated, a thermostat maintains the desired cooking temperature.

When broiling, the heat source is located above the food. Inside a gas oven, a gas burner found on the bottom of the oven generates the heat for baking or roasting. When broiling, this same burner on the oven floor doubles as the heat source for the ***broiler*** found in a compartment below the main oven cavity. In recent years, the broiler has been moved into the oven cavity, where a dedicated gas burner is found on the ceiling of the oven. In an electric oven, metal heating elements generate the heat rather than gas burners.

In a ***convection oven***, a fan circulates hot air around the inside of the oven cavity, allowing foods to cook more evenly and quickly.

The ***cooktop*** consists of either gas burners or electric heating elements, controlled by knobs, or dials. On a gas cooktop, these knobs open a valve to release gas to the burner and regulate the size of the flame. A small gas flame called a ***pilot light*** burns continuously and lights the larger burner flame when needed. In modern gas ranges, an electronic spark ignition replaces the pilot light. The dials on an electric cooktop control the temperature of the heating element. Professional chefs prefer gas cooktops because they give instant heat when turned on and exceptional temperature control. An electric element must preheat for a short time before it reaches the desired temperature. Likewise, electric elements take longer to respond when the control dial is changed to a lower temperature.

Conventional freestanding ranges combine a cooktop with an oven all in one unit. However, some ovens are built into the cabinetry. Many times, ***built-in ovens*** have two ovens, or a double oven. Built-in ovens are paired with a separate cooktop that is built into the kitchen counter. These cooktops sit flush with the counter to give a sleek look.

Refrigerator-Freezer

The ***refrigerator-freezer*** is the cold storage center of your kitchen. The refrigerator portion holds beverages and perishable foods at safe temperatures above freezing but below 41°F. Full-size refrigerator-freezers range in size from 10 to 35 cubic feet. Most have two outer doors with the freezer located above, next to, or below the refrigerator. Some of the smaller models have one outer door and an inner compartment for the freezer. Compact, or mini, refrigerators range in size from one to four cubic feet and some have small freezers. They are much smaller than average refrigerators and take up very little space. They are easy to transport, making them perfect for dorm-type settings.

Dishwasher

Dishwashers have spray arms that distribute detergent and rinse water over, under, and around the dishes to loosen and remove soil. The dishwasher does this in several cycles, removing the dirty water from the machine after each phase of the cycle.

Contrary to popular belief, the dishwasher uses a relatively small amount of water, approximately 6 to 10 gallons, depending on the wash-level setting. The water temperature in a dishwasher should remain above 140°F to dissolve detergent, remove grease from dishes, and to sanitize. To ensure the water is hot enough, you should run water in the kitchen sink until it is hot before starting the dishwasher.

Dishwashers can be built into the cabinetry and hooked up to the plumbing. Portable and countertop dishwashers have hoses that attach to the kitchen faucet and drain into the sink. They have the same features as built-in dishwashers, only for smaller loads, and are convenient when space is limited.

Small Appliances

Small kitchen appliances are portable devices that can be moved easily. They generally sit on the countertop in the kitchen. Each one is designed to accomplish and simplify kitchen tasks (**Figure 17.2**).

A *handheld electric mixer* is a rotary mixing device with varying speeds, a motor, and removable beaters used to make batter, dough, frosting, and other ingredients. The mixer is held in your hand while in use.

A *stand mixer* is a heavy-duty electric mixer with a variety of attachments and a powerful motor. The mixer is attached to a base, so your hands remain free.

A *blender* is a tall glass, or plastic, container with a removable lid and motor-driven blades at the base, used to emulsify, liquefy, or puree, depending on the speed setting selected. These are commonly used for making smoothies, crushing ice, and pureeing soup.

A *food processor* is an all-purpose kitchen tool used to quickly and easily perform time-consuming jobs, like chopping, grating, mincing, blending, and slicing. Food processors come in various sizes and can come with a number of different blades for different tasks, including kneading dough.

An *immersion blender* is a hand-held utensil used for light- to medium-duty blending of small batches of food. This portable appliance can blend or puree soup while it is still in the pot.

An *electric skillet* is a countertop skillet that uses an electric element as its heat source, heats up quickly and evenly, and maintains the desired temperature without fluctuating. A lid helps retain heat and moisture.

A *slow cooker* is a countertop appliance consisting of a large stoneware bowl that fits inside a heating unit. Slow cookers have lids and come in different sizes. This appliance is used for cooking food at a low temperature for a long period. Food can be placed in the cooker before you leave in the morning and it is ready to eat when you return later in the day. Slow cookers are used to cook foods that benefit from long, slow cooking, like soups, stews, and tougher, less expensive cuts of meat.

A *pressure cooker* is a pot with a sealed lid that uses steam and pressure to cook food. The water inside the pressure cooker heats up and creates steam. When the steam cannot escape, pressure increases inside the pot. As the pressure rises, the temperature increases, which cooks food faster.

A *toaster* is a countertop appliance used to heat and brown a variety of breads and pastries. They commonly have two to four slots into which the bread is placed. When the bread slices are toasted to the selected level of browning, they will pop up in the slots. The browning level can be adjusted by a dial on the toaster.

A *toaster oven* is a small, countertop oven used to bake, brown, or reheat a wide variety of foods. When living in an apartment, the small size of this appliance makes it an excellent alternative to a full-size oven. It also produces less heat and uses less electricity than a full-size oven.

Coffeemakers are used to brew coffee with or without electricity. There is a variety of models. Brewing glassware, like the *French coffee press*, brew coffee by pouring boiling water over the grounds and allowing the grounds to float to the top. When the desired strength is achieved, the press, or plunger, pushes the grounds to the bottom of the container and prevents them from pouring out with the coffee. *Electric drip coffeemakers* come in a range of models with many

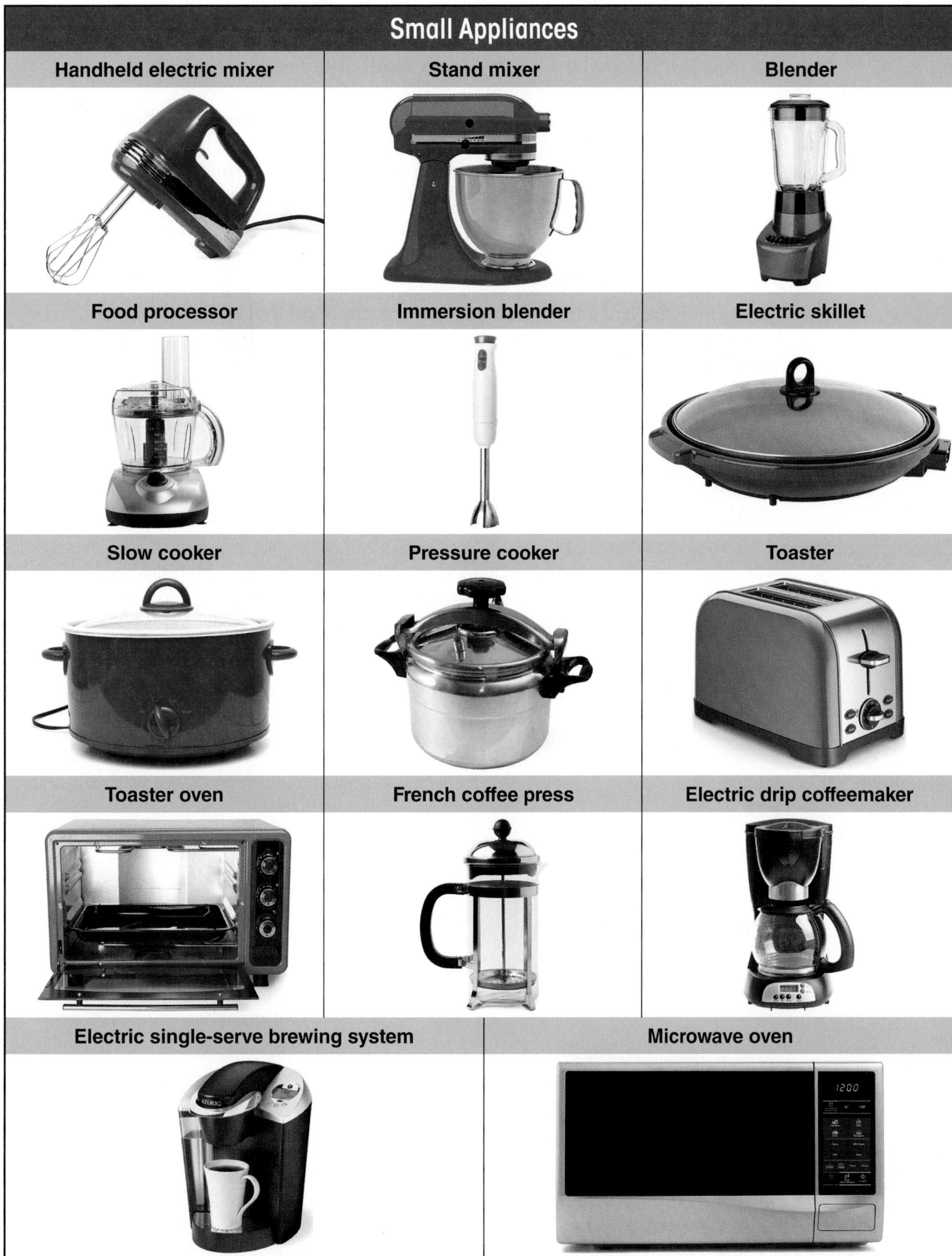
Small Appliances
Handheld electric mixer
Stand mixer
Blender
Food processor
Immersion blender
Electric skillet
Slow cooker
Pressure cooker
Toaster
Toaster oven
French coffee press
Electric drip coffeemaker
Electric single-serve brewing system
Microwave oven
KEURIG
12:00

Top row: Rae Alexander/Shutterstock.com; M. Unal Ozmen/Shutterstock.com; Danny Smythe/Shutterstock.com; 2nd row: Sean van Tonder/Shutterstock.com; iprachenko/Shutterstock.com; John Kasawa/Shutterstock.com; 3rd row: Quang Ho/Shutterstock.com; Konjushenko Vladimir/Shutterstock.com; Slavoljub Pantelic/Shutterstock.com; 4th row: Sergiy Kuzmin/Shutterstock.com; timquo/Shutterstock.com; Alexandru Nika/Shutterstock.com; bottom row: Keurig Green Mountain, Inc.; bergamont/Shutterstock.com

Figure 17.2 Small appliances save time and energy during food preparation.

different features, from a single on/off function to programmable timers, built-in bean grinders, and espresso, latte, or cappuccino options. *Electric single-serve brewing systems* are best for making an individual serving quickly and easily.

The *microwave oven* is a small appliance that defrosts, cooks, or reheats foods quickly. Countertop microwaves sit on the kitchen counter. Over-the-range microwaves mount over the cooktop, and have lights and exhaust fans to vent steam and odors. All microwave ovens present a fire danger if metal cookware is used. Use only microwave-safe cookware or bakeware with no exposed metal parts when cooking with a microwave.

Cookware and Bakeware

Cookware and bakeware are types of equipment that are used to cook and bake food items. These items are made from a variety of materials that have advantages and disadvantages (**Figure 17.3**).

Cookware

Cookware is used to prepare foods on the cooktop. Most cookware is either a *pot* or a *pan*. A pot is cookware that is taller than it is wide. A pan is cookware that is wider than it is tall. Each type of cookware has a different shape and size that makes it best suited for a particular cooking method (**Figure 17.4**).

A *saucepan* has a flat-bottomed pot with straight, vertical sides, and one long handle. It is used for heating and cooking food in liquid on the cooktop. Handles should be heat resistant to avoid burns. Saucepans come in a variety of capacities, but not greater than four quarts. For convenience, saucepans are often sold with matching lids.

Cookware and Bakeware Materials		
Material	**Advantages**	**Disadvantages**
Aluminum	• Lightweight • Conducts heat well	• Unless anodized (coated), will react with acidic foods
Cast iron	• Retains warmth • Distributes heat evenly • Resists sticking when seasoned • Can be used inside the oven or on the cooktop	• Heavy • Rusts quickly if not seasoned
Copper	• Conducts and distributes heat evenly	• Reacts with acidic and alkaline foods unless lined with other nonreactive material • Requires regular polishing and maintenance
Glass	• Can be used for both cooking and serving food • Can view covered food while cooking	• Conducts heat unevenly • Can chip or break
Nonstick finish	• Prevents foods from sticking • Can use less fat when cooking	• Requires the use of utensils that will not scratch the finish, such as wood or silicone • Finish is prone to scratching, rendering the finish useless
Stainless steel	• Resists corrosion, scratching, and denting • Does not react with acidic foods	• Conducts heat poorly, resulting in uneven cooking

Figure 17.3 Cookware and bakeware are available in a variety of materials.

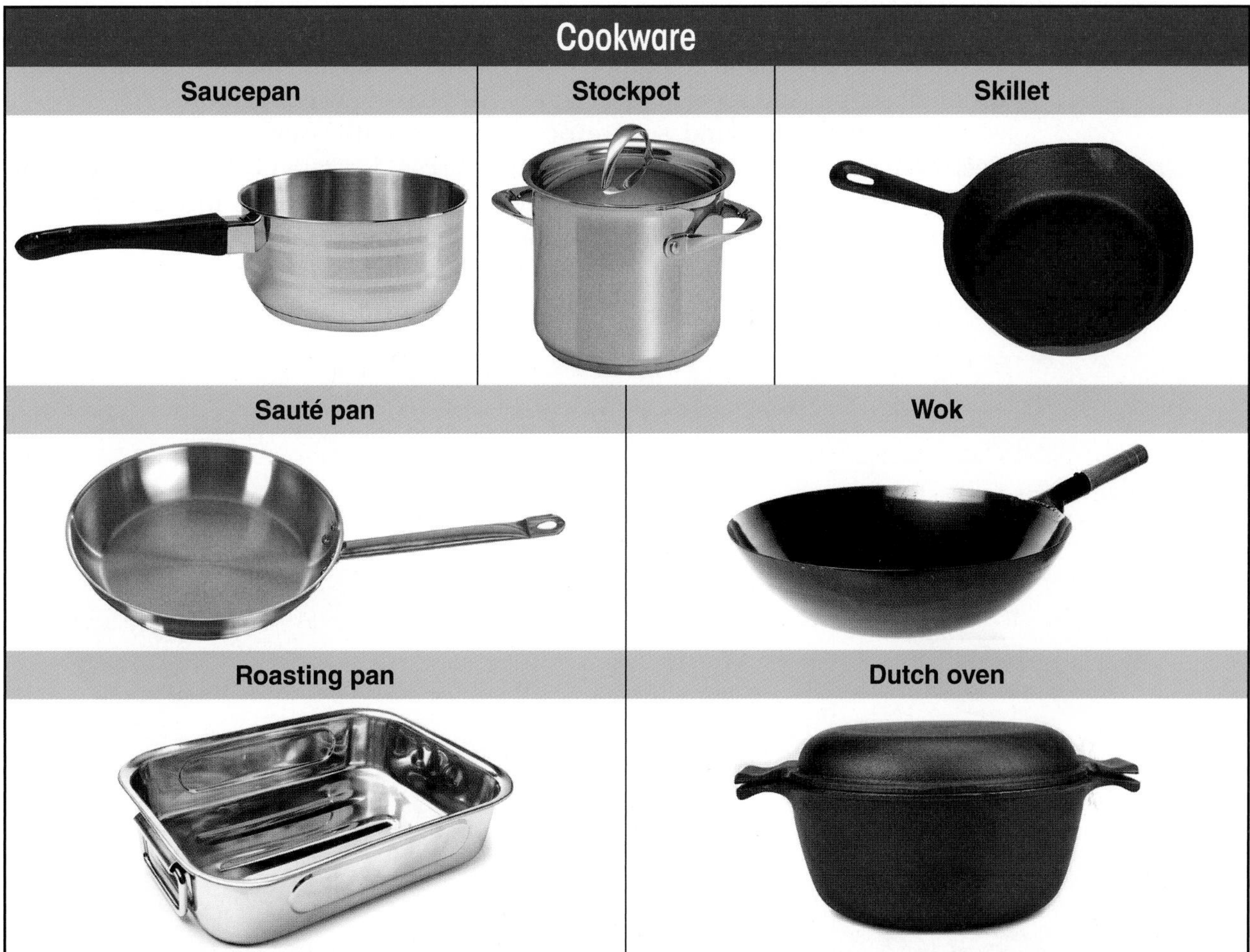

Top row: Luisa Leal Photography/Shutterstock.com; Zovteva/Shutterstock.com; Oleg Bezrukov/Shutterstock.com; middle row: urfin/Shutterstock.com; Early Spring/Shutterstock.com; bottom row: Olga Popova/Shutterstock.com; AVN Photo Lab/Shutterstock.com

Figure 17.4 Select the pot or pan that is best suited to the recipe and the cooking method being used. *What piece of cookware would you select to make a large batch of chili?*

A *stockpot* is a large, flat-bottomed pot with straight, vertical sides, and two small handles on opposite sides. These pots are used to cook large quantities of food in liquid on the cooktop. Stockpots come in a variety of sizes, usually four quarts or larger. They are typically sold with matching lids.

A *skillet* is a shallow, flat-bottomed cast-iron pan with one handle used to fry foods. Skillets may be sold with a matching lid.

A *sauté pan* is shallow, flat-bottomed pan used to cook foods using a small amount of oil over relatively high heat. Some sauté pans have sloped sides that makes it easy to flip and turn foods. Another type of sauté pan has straight sides. They are usually sold with matching lids.

A *wok* is a bowl-shaped pan with either one long handle or two small handles. It is used for a variety of Asian cooking techniques, such as stir-frying and steaming.

A *roasting pan* is a flat-bottomed pan with shallow vertical sides and two handles. It is used for roasting meats in the oven. Roasting pans often have a rack that suspends the meat above the juices that form during cooking. A roasting pan may or may not come with a lid.

Dutch oven is a thick-walled cooking pot with a tight-fitting lid. The Dutch oven is intended for use either on the cooktop or in the oven. Dutch ovens are usually made of cast iron, but other heatproof materials may be used.

Bakeware

Bakeware is used to cook foods in the oven. Bakeware includes pans of many different shapes and sizes to meet a variety of baking needs (**Figure 17.5**).

Cake pans can be round, square, or rectangular, and various sizes. A *tube pan* is a deep cake pan with a tube running through the center around which the cake forms.

A *muffin pan* is a baking pan with multiple indentations in which muffins and cupcakes are baked. Muffin pans are available in jumbo-, regular-, and mini-muffin sizes.

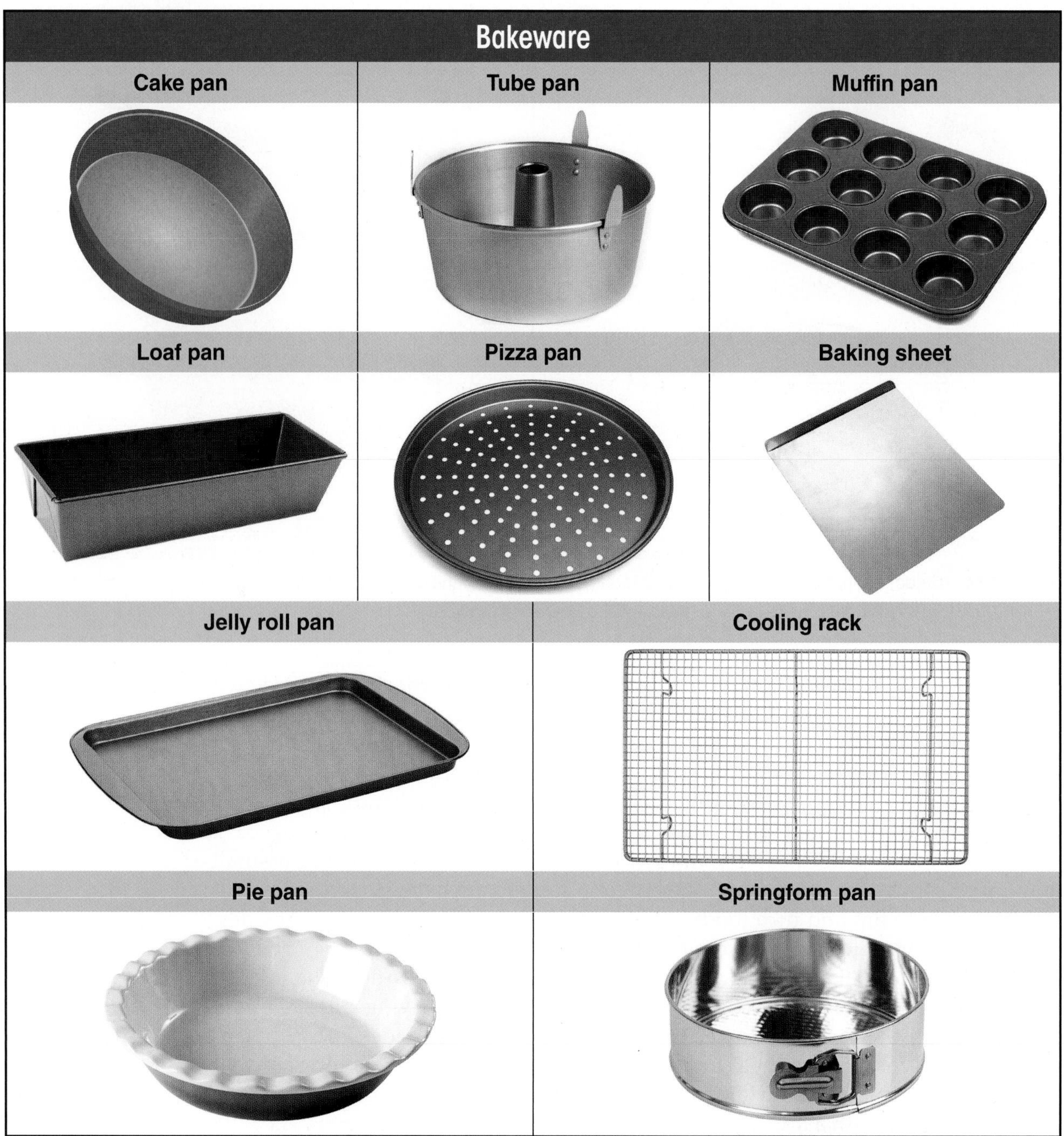

Top row: Constantine Pankin/Shutterstock.com; AnnapolisStudios/Shutterstock.com; ffolas/Shutterstock.com; 2nd row: kavring/Shutterstock.com; Joe Gough/Shutterstock.com; Goodheart-Willcox Publisher; 3rd row: cretolamna/Shutterstock.com; Kitch Bain/Shutterstock.com; bottom row: AS Food studio/Shutterstock.com; ffolas/Shutterstock.com

Figure 17.5 Bakeware comes in many shapes and sizes. *Which piece of bakeware would you use to bake banana bread?*

A *loaf pan* is a deep, rectangular baking pan used for baking wheat bread, quick bread, and meatloaf.

A *pizza pan* is a large, round baking sheet with **perforations** (holes) to make a crisp crust.

A *baking sheet* is a flat, rectangular sheet of metal used for baking biscuits, rolls, and pastries, as well as flat items like cookies. A *jelly roll pan* is a baking sheet with a short lip on all four sides.

A *cooling rack* is a raised wire rack that allows air to circulate around hot foods and let heat escape.

A *pie pan* is a round, shallow, sloped-sided dish with a flat or fluted edge to hold a piecrust. A *springform pan* has a removable bottom and a collar with a latch for easy removal. It is used to make cheesecakes, tortes, or other baked goods with a delicate bottom crust.

Kitchen Tools

Kitchen tools are small, handheld tools used during food preparation. Some are used for cooking food and others are used to prepare food for cooking. Each tool is designed to make a particular kitchen task easier. Kitchen tools include utensils and knives.

Utensils

Utensils are used to perform a variety of kitchen tasks, such as measuring, lifting, mixing, and cutting (**Figure 17.6** on the next page).

Liquid measuring cups are made from either glass or clear plastic, and are used when measuring quantities of liquids. They have a spout for pouring, a handle, and additional space at the top to prevent spilling.

FEATURED CAREER

Food Purchasing Agent

Food purchasing agents buy a vast array of food products for companies and institutions. They attempt to get the best deal for their companies—the highest quality at the lowest possible cost. These agents accomplish this by studying sales records and inventory levels of current stock and identifying foreign and domestic suppliers. Food purchasing agents also keep abreast of changes affecting both the supply of and demand for needed products.

Education

Requirements tend to vary with the size of the organization. Large stores and distributors prefer applicants who have a bachelor's degree with an emphasis in business. Many manufacturing firms put an even greater emphasis on formal training, preferring applicants with a bachelor's or master's degree in engineering, business, economics, or one of the applied sciences.

Job Outlook

Employment for purchasing agents is expected to increase slower than the average for all occupations. Job growth and opportunities will differ among different occupations in this category.

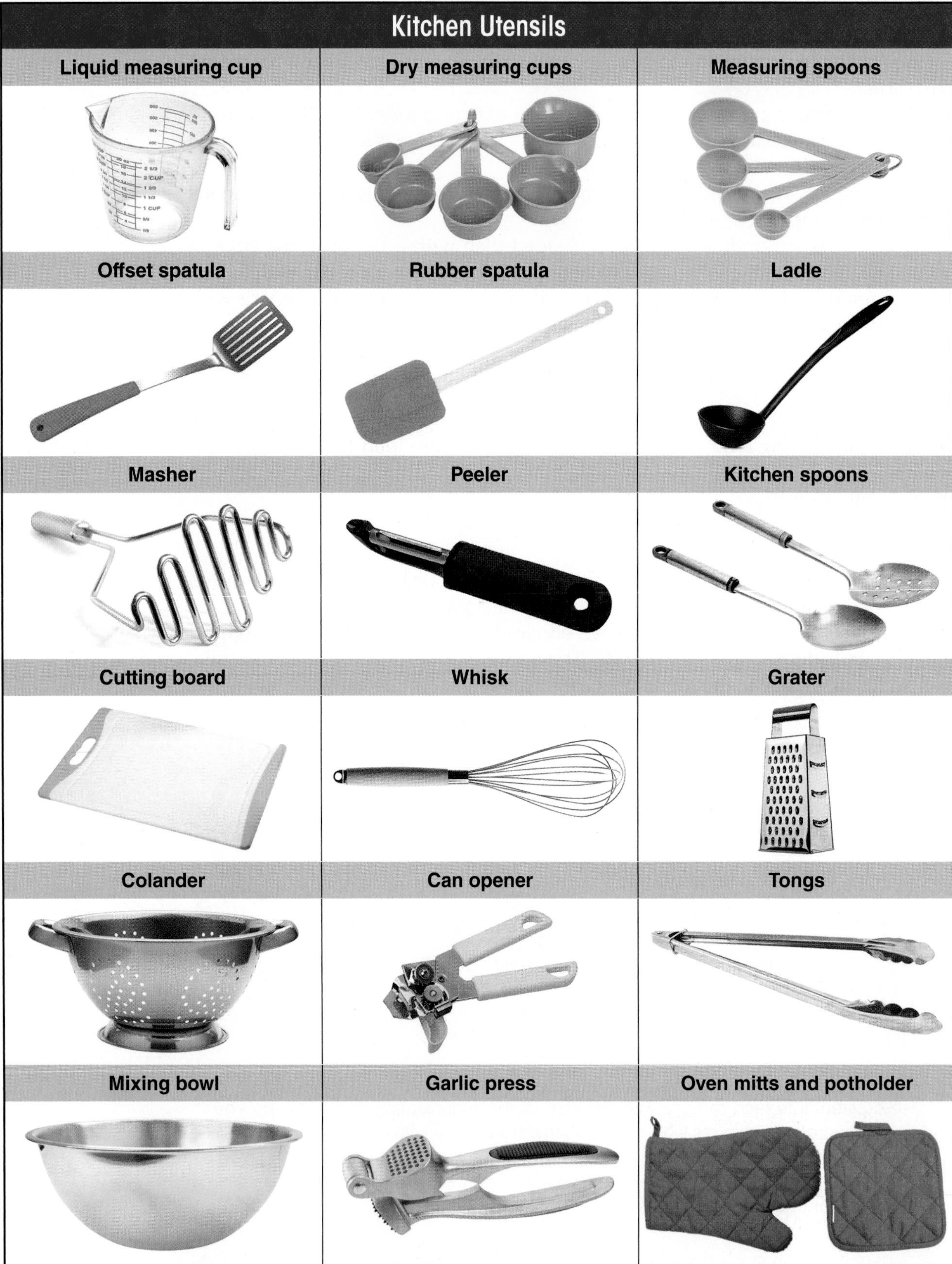

Top row: M. Unal Ozmen/Shutterstock.com; Laboko/Shutterstock.com; nuwatphoto/Shutterstock.com; 2nd row: Guru 3D/Shutterstock.com; Eaks1979/Shutterstock.com; Davydenko Yuliia/Shutterstock.com; 3rd row: Olga Popova/Shutterstock.com; Natan86/Shutterstock.com; nito/Shutterstock.com; 4th row: sevenke/Shutterstock.com; Sergey Skleznev/Shutterstock.com; Andrei Kuzmik/Shutterstock.com; 5th row: Danny Smythe/Shutterstock.com; ra3rn/Shutterstock.com; Gavran333/Shutterstock.com; bottom row: keerati/Shutterstock.com; mihalec/Shutterstock.com; Grygorii Lykhatskyi/Shutterstock.com

Figure 17.6 Kitchen utensils help you measure, lift, mix, and cut.

Dry measuring cups are used for measuring dry and solid ingredients such as flour and sugar. These cups are designed so ingredients can be leveled off for an accurate measurement.

Measuring spoons are used for measuring small amounts of liquid or dry ingredients. A set usually consists of four to six spoons, each with a different measurement: 1 tablespoon, 1 teaspoon, ½ teaspoon and 1¼ teaspoon; sometimes ½ tablespoon and ⅛ teaspoon are included.

An *offset spatula*, also called a *turner* or simply *spatula*, has a blade with an offset handle and is used for lifting and turning foods. The offset handle allows your hands to remain a safe distance from the heat.

A *silicone or rubber spatula* has a flexible blade used for scraping the contents from a container. Heat-resistant spatulas are used for cooking in nonstick pans.

Ladles have a long handle with a cup on the end for reaching to the bottom of pots or serving containers, and transferring liquids. They come in many sizes, ranging in capacity from 1 to 16 ounces.

A *masher* has a long handle attached to a head with a grid or zigzag pattern. It is used for mashing soft foods such as potatoes and avocados.

A *peeler* has a sharp, slit blade mounted on a handle and is used to remove the skins from fruits and vegetables.

Kitchen spoons have long handles with either solid or perforated bowls on the end. They are made from stainless steel or wood, and are used for mixing, draining, and serving.

A *cutting board* is a flat surface on which to cut food, usually made from plastic or wood and in a variety of sizes.

A *whisk* incorporates air into a mixture, blends ingredients, or folds one ingredient into another.

A *grater* is a metal surface with different-sized slots used to shred food. Different types of graters include box graters and flat graters.

A *colander* is a bowl-shaped utensil with holes or slots used to drain food such as pasta.

A manual *can opener* is a plier-type utensil with two small rotating circular blades that remove the lid from a can by turning a key.

Tongs are metal, plastic, or wooden pinching tools used to hold or turn food.

Mixing bowls are various size kitchen bowls in which ingredients are combined.

Garlic press is a utensil used to crush garlic cloves through fine holes.

Oven mitts and *potholders* are constructed of silicone or fabric and protect your hands when handling hot objects or kitchen equipment. An oven mitt is an insulated mitt worn like a glove and a potholder can be a piece of textile or silicone to wrap around the handle of a hot pan.

Knives

Knives are essential kitchen utensils. Knives are designed for specific cutting tasks. Using the best knife for the task makes the task easier and safer (**Figure 17.7**).

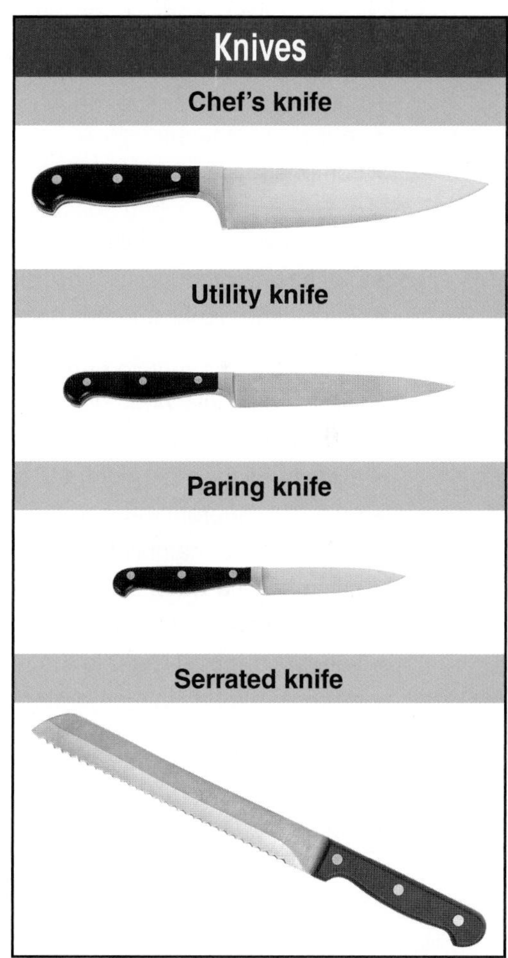

From top to bottom: Dron skm/Shutterstock.com; Dron skm/Shutterstock.com; Dron skm/Shutterstock.com; James Clarke/Shutterstock.com

Figure 17.7 Using the right knife for the task makes the work much easier.

A *chef's knife* is an all-purpose, versatile kitchen knife, measuring from 6 to 12 inches long. It is used for most types of chopping, dicing, slicing, and mincing, as well as for heavy-duty work with thicker cuts of vegetables and meats.

A *utility knife* is a small, lightweight knife that is slightly larger than a paring knife. It measure from 4 to 7 inches long, and is used for miscellaneous light cutting.

A *paring knife* is a small knife with a straight, sharp blade usually between 3 and 5 inches long. It is used for peeling and coring foods, and mincing or cutting small items.

A *serrated knife* has a 5- to 10-inch blade with a sawtooth edge. It is used for slicing through foods that are firm on the outside and soft on the inside, like breads and soft fruits or vegetables.

FOOD AND THE ENVIRONMENT

Conservation in the Kitchen

Most people don't think about the amount of resources that are used for food preparation. It is important to establish practices to conserve resources for future generations. The entire household should participate in conservation of resources on a daily basis. The Environmental Protection Agency (EPA) suggests individuals reduce, reuse, and recycle waste to conserve resources.

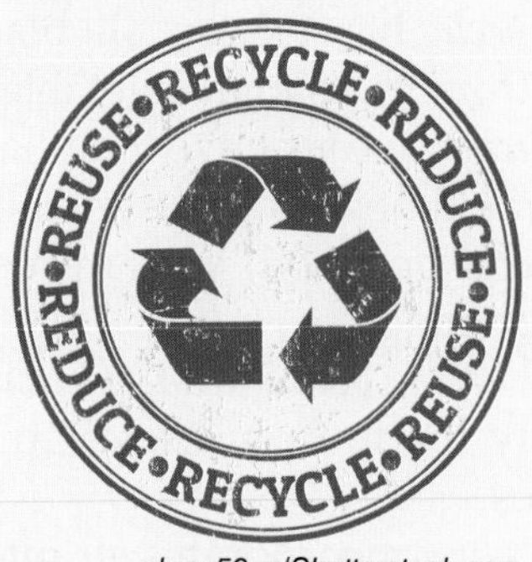

ducu59us/Shutterstock.com

Households can reduce the amount of trash thrown away by

- reusing containers,
- composting food scraps,
- recycling waste when possible and buying products made with recycled materials,
- purchasing products with as little packaging as possible, and
- using cloth napkins rather than disposable paper napkins.

Households can reduce energy and water use by

- turning off lights when not in use,
- running dishwasher only when full,
- allowing dishes to air-dry and skipping dishwasher's dry cycle,
- using the appropriate-size burner for the pot or pan,
- cleaning and maintaining refrigerators and freezers,
- using as little water as possible when cooking,
- scraping dishes (not rinsing) before placing in dishwasher,
- keeping drinking water in the refrigerator rather than running faucet water until it is cool, and
- defrosting foods in refrigerator overnight rather than in running water.

Think Critically

1. Discuss the challenges and benefits of composting food waste at home after visiting the Environmental Protection Agency's (EPA) website.
2. What actions are required to get your school on board with the three R's: reduce, reuse, and recycle?
3. You found leftover meal items in the refrigerator. The items are half of a turkey loaf, a bag of frozen peas, salad greens, a loaf of bread, and a bag of carrots. Consider a way to repurpose these items to create a new meal.

Staple Ingredients

Staple ingredients are used on a regular basis and should always be kept on hand. Some of these ingredients are ***perishable***, or prone to spoil and decay. Nonperishable ingredients are not apt to spoil and have a longer shelf life.

Some staple ingredients are universal; however, as a cook builds a recipe collection, he or she may identify additional ingredients to keep on hand. A well-stocked kitchen makes planning and preparing successful meals easier (**Figure 17.8**).

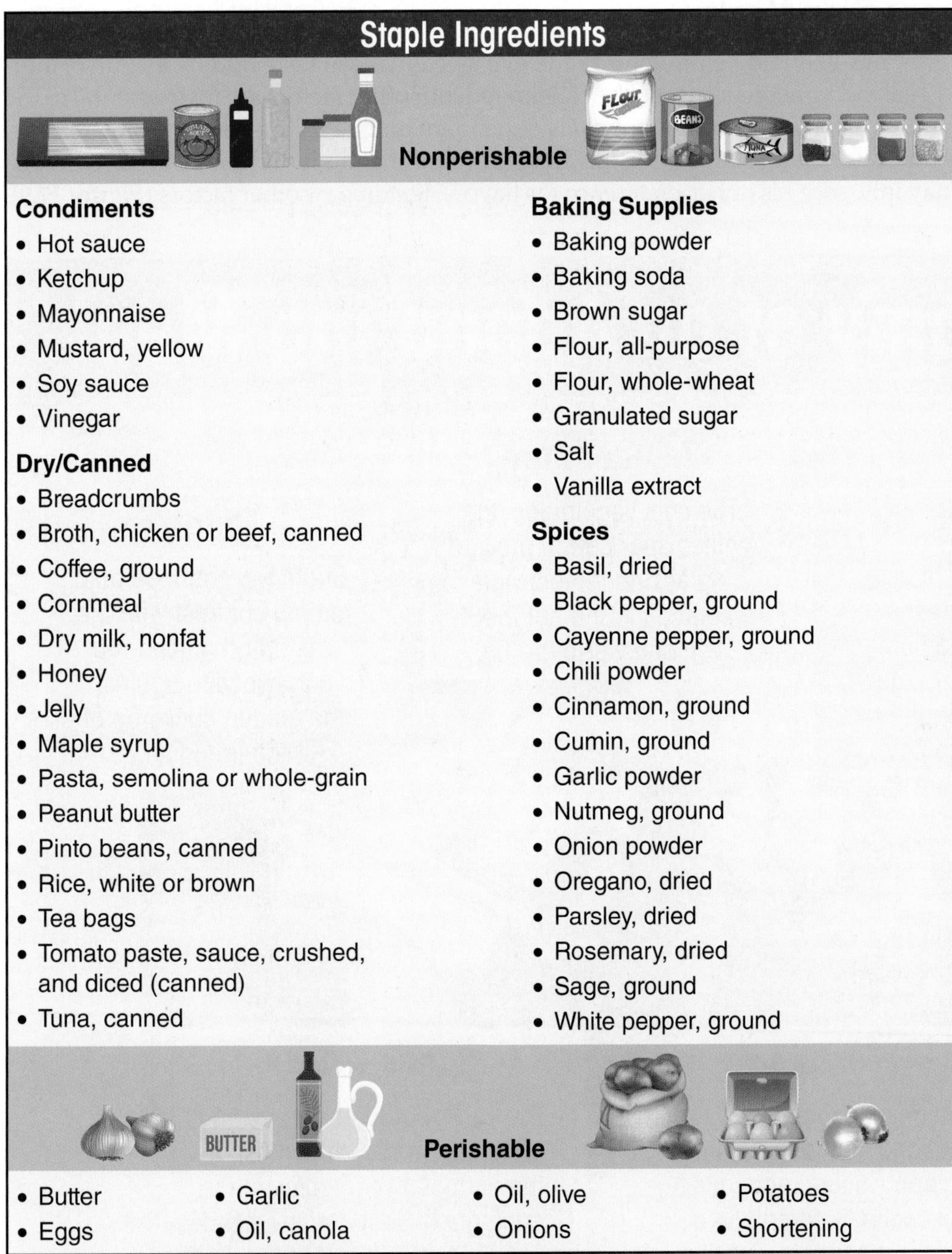

Staple Ingredients
Nonperishable
Condiments
• Hot sauce
• Ketchup
• Mayonnaise
• Mustard, yellow
• Soy sauce
• Vinegar
Dry/Canned
• Breadcrumbs
• Broth, chicken or beef, canned
• Coffee, ground
• Cornmeal
• Dry milk, nonfat
• Honey
• Jelly
• Maple syrup
• Pasta, semolina or whole-grain
• Peanut butter
• Pinto beans, canned
• Rice, white or brown
• Tea bags
• Tomato paste, sauce, crushed, and diced (canned)
• Tuna, canned
Baking Supplies
• Baking powder
• Baking soda
• Brown sugar
• Flour, all-purpose
• Flour, whole-wheat
• Granulated sugar
• Salt
• Vanilla extract
Spices
• Basil, dried
• Black pepper, ground
• Cayenne pepper, ground
• Chili powder
• Cinnamon, ground
• Cumin, ground
• Garlic powder
• Nutmeg, ground
• Onion powder
• Oregano, dried
• Parsley, dried
• Rosemary, dried
• Sage, ground
• White pepper, ground
BUTTER
Perishable
• Butter
• Eggs
• Garlic
• Oil, canola
• Oil, olive
• Onions
• Potatoes
• Shortening

Top row, l to r: wanpatsorn/Shutterstock.com; Tribalium/Shutterstock.com; Mountain Brothers/Shutterstock.com; BlueRingMedia/Shutterstock.com; BlueRingMedia/Shutterstock.com; BlueRingMedia/Shutterstock.com; OWLage/Shutterstock.com; AminaAster/Shutterstock.com; lukpedclub/Shutterstock.com; 2nd row, l to r: NotionPic/Shutterstock.com; Natykach Nataliia/Shutterstock.com; BlueRingMedia/Shutterstock.com; Natykach Nataliia/Shutterstock.com

Figure 17.8 Staple ingredients, such as spices and condiments, vary from person to person based on the types of foods he or she typically prepares.

Creating Meal Plans

Appealing, healthy meals do not just happen, they require planning. A meal may supply all the needed nutrients, but if it remains uneaten because it is unappealing, the nutrients serve no purpose. Learning to plan a meal that people want to eat and that meets their nutritional needs is not difficult and can be quite rewarding. Involving other family members in the meal planning process, including children, may create greater interest and enjoyment of the meals served.

Appealing Meals

A meal should be pleasing to the eye as well as the taste buds. Of course, individual food preferences must be considered, but other factors are instrumental in the success of a meal. A meal's appeal is dependent on five factors: flavor, color, texture, temperature, and shape and size. Keep in mind that an individual's life-cycle stage may influence his or her preference for flavors, textures, or other factors (**Figure 17.9**).

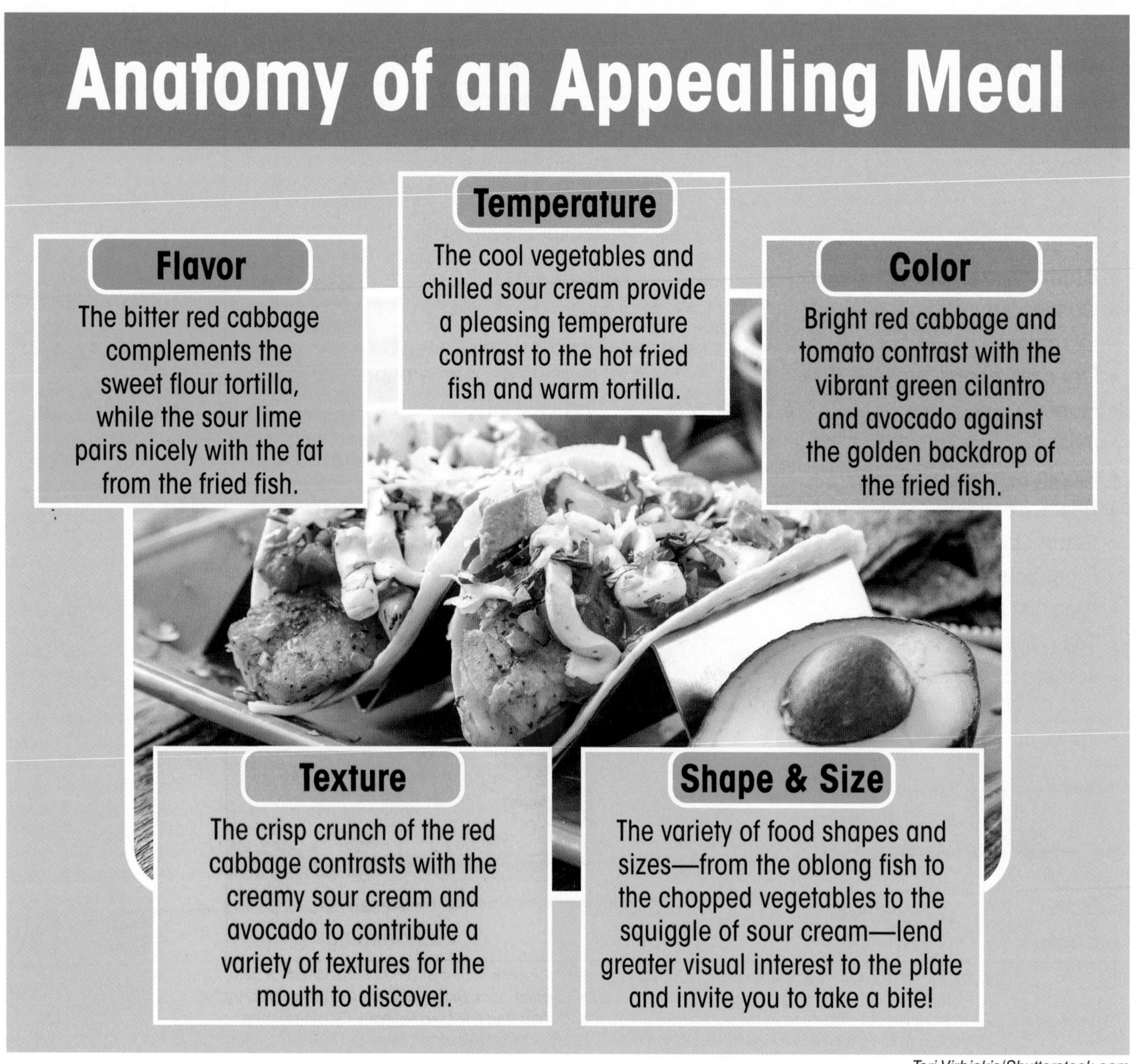

Anatomy of an Appealing Meal
Temperature
The cool vegetables and chilled sour cream provide a pleasing temperature contrast to the hot fried fish and warm tortilla.
Flavor
The bitter red cabbage complements the sweet flour tortilla, while the sour lime pairs nicely with the fat from the fried fish.
Color
Bright red cabbage and tomato contrast with the vibrant green cilantro and avocado against the golden backdrop of the fried fish.
Texture
The crisp crunch of the red cabbage contrasts with the creamy sour cream and avocado to contribute a variety of textures for the mouth to discover.
Shape & Size
The variety of food shapes and sizes—from the oblong fish to the chopped vegetables to the squiggle of sour cream—lend greater visual interest to the plate and invite you to take a bite!

Teri Virbickis/Shutterstock.com

Figure 17.9 A meal is guaranteed to be appealing if certain factors are addressed.

Flavor

Flavor gives food a distinctive taste. Use a variety of flavors in your meal planning. This means more than serving different dishes throughout the week. You need to include a variety of flavors in every meal. Think about a meal with tomato juice as an appetizer, tomatoes on the salad, and tomato sauce on the pasta. So much tomato flavor would make the meal seem rather boring. Substituting marinated peppers for the appetizer and toasted almonds on the salad would introduce variety.

Certain basic tastes complement each other and add interest to a meal. Consider some of these basic taste combinations when planning a meal:

- salty and sweet
- sweet and sour
- fat and sour
- bitter and sweet
- sour and salty

Make a point of balancing strongly flavored foods with those that are more subtle. For instance, you could complement a spicy burrito with some mild pinto beans. You might balance a dish of tart apple slices with a drizzle of sweet caramel topping.

When experimenting with flavor, consider the age of those who will be eating the dish. Children are often more sensitive to tastes than adults and may prefer milder flavors. Older adults or people with certain health conditions may have lost some of their sense of taste or smell. For these people, more highly seasoned foods may act to stimulate their appetites.

Color

Color appeals to the eye and stimulates appetite at all stages of the life cycle. Picture a meal of poached fish, scalloped potatoes, and steamed cabbage. These foods are **monochromatic** (similar color) and pale. Now envision how the plate would look if you top the fish with a mango and jalapeño salsa. Sprinkle the scalloped potatoes with bright red paprika. Replace the cabbage with deep green broccoli. By making a few changes, a bland-looking meal has become quite colorful.

Texture

Food texture refers to the properties of food that are sensed by the mouth. Texture variety makes meals more enjoyable to eat. How appealing is a meal of creamed turkey, mashed sweet potatoes, and applesauce? These foods have **homogenous** (similar) textures. They are all smooth, soft, and creamy. A meal that includes crunchy and chewy textures as well as soft would be more appetizing. You could introduce some different textures by changing the menu to roast turkey with mashed sweet potatoes. Then replace the applesauce with a salad of crisp apple wedges on a bed of fresh spinach.

Still, texture should not present a challenge to the person eating the food. Children and older adults may have difficulty with certain textures. Young children may be in the process of losing baby teeth and gaining permanent teeth. Loose or missing teeth can present challenges when eating. Older individuals are more likely to have dental issues that make chewing difficult as well. They may not be able to eat regular textures. Soft, cut up, ground, or minced foods may be necessary. Enhancing the flavor and appearance of texture-modified foods will help improve their appeal.

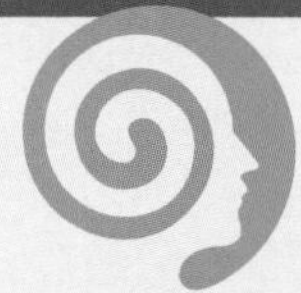

EXTEND YOUR KNOWLEDGE

The Fifth Basic Taste

Until recent years, the following four basic tastes were recognized: salty, sweet, bitter, and sour. In the year 2000, a fifth basic taste, umami, was officially established.

Nonetheless, the lack of official recognition did not prevent umami from being appreciated in many food preparations. People have enjoyed the taste in stocks, broths, aged cheeses, protein-rich foods, tomato products, dried mushrooms, and more. The flavors that umami elicits are described as savory, full-bodied, and meaty.

The umami taste is the result of interactions between your taste buds, aroma receptors, and specific compounds found in foods. Although these compounds occur naturally in many foods, some foods require processing of one form or another before the umami taste can be experienced. For instance, dehydration, fermentation, and aging help to liberate the umami taste.

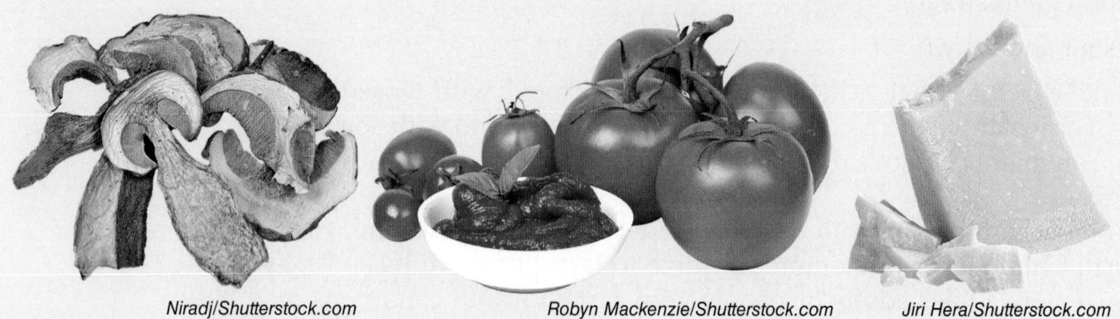

Niradj/Shutterstock.com *Robyn Mackenzie/Shutterstock.com* *Jiri Hera/Shutterstock.com*

Temperature

Most people enjoy a balance of hot and cold foods in their meals. Consider a breakfast of scrambled eggs, toast, warm fruit compote, and hot chocolate. These foods are all hot. Changing the fruit compote to a chilled fruit salad and the hot chocolate to cold chocolate milk adds temperature variety and interest to the meal.

Whatever foods are on your menu, be sure to serve them at the proper temperature. Few people enjoy **tepid** (lukewarm) soup or milk that is room temperature. They prefer their soup to be piping hot and their milk to be icy cold. Besides being more appealing, foods are safer when served at the correct temperatures. Keep hot foods hot, above 140°F (60°C), and cold foods cold, below 40°F (5°C). This will help prevent growth of bacteria and other pathogens that can cause foodborne illness.

Shape and Size

The shape and size of foods on your plate affect the visual appeal. Think about a plate filled with strips of pepper steak, French fries, and carrot sticks. These foods are all long, thin pieces. The plate would be more appealing if you served a baked potato and sliced carrots with the pepper steak. Creating food in fun shapes is particularly appealing to children.

The size of foods should also vary. For instance, a tuna and rice casserole is made up of little pieces. Green peas and coleslaw would not be good accompaniments for this casserole. They are also little pieces and would provide no contrast with the casserole. Snow peas and a salad of sliced tomatoes might complement the casserole better.

Healthy Meals

Meal planning is an opportunity to ensure that nutritional and health needs are met. No single food can provide all the needed nutrients; therefore, serving a variety of nutrient-dense foods is optimal.

Planning meals for individuals with special nutritional or health needs may require additional consideration. Many resources are available to help with planning meals that meet nutritional needs.

Address Special Needs

Everyone requires the same nutrients; however, the amounts of nutrients each person needs may vary. For instance, children need smaller amounts of nutrients, but they have greater proportional needs than adults. The age, sex, body size, and activity level of an individual affects his or her nutrient needs. Separate meals are not necessary to meet individual needs. All household members can usually enjoy the same meal, but in different portion sizes.

Older adults who are living on their own may experience problems with nutrition and meal planning. This group is more likely to be at nutritional risk due to health issues. Social isolation, poor mobility, or lack of income can contribute to problems with meal planning. A few simple tips can be used to improve meal planning for older adults (**Figure 17.10**).

Factors other than age can affect an individual's nutritional needs. Sometimes one or more members of a household follow a special diet due to a health condition. Someone with high blood pressure may follow a low-sodium diet. Individuals with food allergies need to avoid certain foods. A vegetarian chooses not to include eggs or meat products in his or her diet.

Adapting meals to the special needs of individuals helps them continue to enjoy good nutrition. These requirements must be considered when planning meals.

Meal Planning Tips for Older Adults
• Grocery shop with a friend and divide quantities that are too big for one person. For example, share a bunch of broccoli, bag of potatoes, or a melon.
• Cook extra and freeze to have healthy, easy meals on days when cooking is difficult.
• Keep frozen or canned vegetables, beans, and fruits on hand for quick, healthy additions to meals.
• Rinse canned vegetables under cold running water to lower their salt content. If fruit is canned in heavy syrup, drain the juice unless added calories are needed.
• Perk up bland-tasting foods with herbs, spices, and lemon juice rather than relying solely on salt or sugar.
• Set the table with a cheerful, clean cloth and flowers to make mealtime enjoyable.
• Eat regularly with someone whose company you enjoy.
• Learn about community programs in the area that serve or deliver meals to older adults.

Figure 17.10 Older adults have meal planning needs that can be addressed with a few adjustments or modifications. *Can you think of other tips to help older adults with meal planning?*

Use Resources for Planning Healthy Meals

A number of resources are available to help meet the nutritional needs of individuals. ChooseMyPlate.gov provides information on meal planning for many life-cycle stages including pregnant women, children, and older adults (**Figure 17.11**).

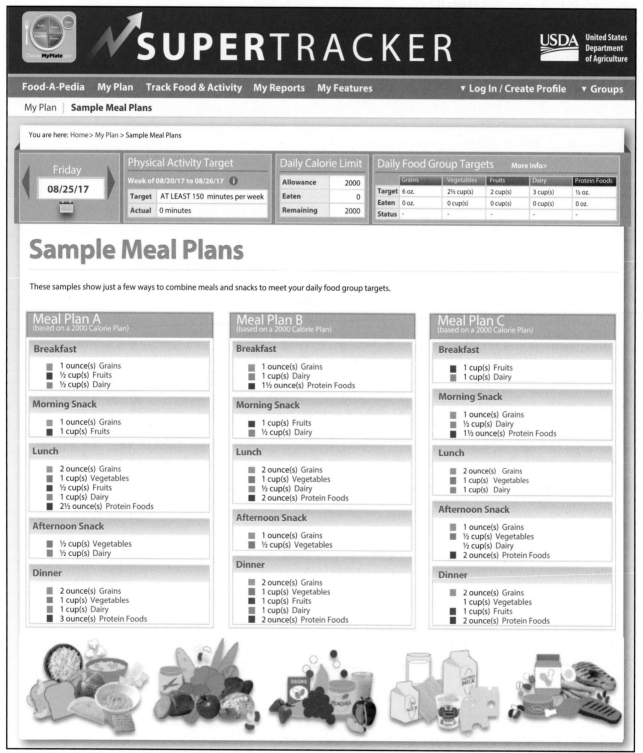

USDA

Figure 17.11 The SuperTracker website produces a variety of sample meal plans to meet your daily food group targets.

The *2015–2020 Dietary Guidelines for Americans* provides a Mediterranean-style eating pattern, a vegetarian eating pattern, and a healthy US-style eating pattern in the appendix. The DASH (Dietary Approaches to Stop Hypertension) eating plan is found on the National Institutes of Health (NIH) website along with other nutrition resources. The American Heart Association and the American Diabetes Association websites offer many meal-planning resources for individuals with heart disease and diabetes. In addition, a registered dietitian nutritionist is a good resource to learn about meeting the special needs of individuals when planning meals.

Technology resources make meal planning easier. Management and meal planning apps are available for download on smartphones and computers. Computer programs facilitate menu planning, recipe collection, shopping lists creation, and maintenance of food inventories.

Weekly Menu

It is inefficient to plan meals each day. Instead, create a menu for the week that will serve as your guide for shopping and food preparation. When deciding which meals to serve each day, begin by making a list of food you already have in your kitchen.

Next, create a menu worksheet with spaces for breakfast, lunch, dinner, and snacks for each day of the week (**Figure 17.12**). Consider making notes of any activities throughout the week that might affect meals. For example, if you have basketball practice after school on Tuesday and a club meeting that night, you will have less time to prepare and eat a meal. Therefore, plan to eat leftovers that night or to prepare a quick, simple recipe.

Sample Weekly Menu Worksheet

	Sunday	Monday	Tuesday	Wednesday	Thursday	Friday	Saturday
		4:15 p.m. dentist appt.		6:30 p.m. choir practice			
Breakfast	Scrambled eggs, toast, fresh berries, milk	Oatmeal, banana, milk, walnuts					
Lunch	Tuna salad sandwich, apple, carrot sticks	Turkey/ spinach wrap, grapes, carrots sticks, yogurt					Beef barley soup, banana, milk
Dinner	Roast chicken, sweet potato fries, broccoli, milk	Chicken stir-fry, brown rice, pineapple, milk	Chili with beans, avocado, corn bread, milk	Leftovers	Salmon burgers, arugula corn salad, grapes, milk	Tortilla turkey meatball soup, fruit salad, milk	Vegetable quesadilla
Snacks	Grapes, cheese cubes	Almonds, string cheese	Hummus, cucumber slices	Almonds, string cheese	Hummus, whole-grain pita chips	Peanut butter, apple slices	Popcorn, orange segments

Figure 17.12 Using a menu worksheet will save time and money.

As time goes on, you will collect more and more recipes that you like. Use your recipe collection along with the list of foods that you already have to write your menu. Consider planning leftovers into the menu. Rather than throwing away leftovers, plan ahead for their use in the menu. If roast chicken is on the menu for Sunday, plan chicken casserole for later in the week. Make the casserole with leftover chicken and any leftover vegetables from the week.

Consult resources for planning healthy meals discussed earlier to ensure that your menu meets the nutritional and health needs of those you are feeding.

Managing Time for Meal Preparation

Meal planning saves time and effort. Efficient use of time is important to people with busy schedules. Some people skip meals if they cannot prepare foods quickly and easily. For them, fast and simple meal preparations are essential to good nutrition.

A number of strategies can help you make the best use of your time in the kitchen. Organizing your work area, using a work schedule, and performing advance preparation help ensure meals are ready on time. Time-saving devices can **streamline** (simplify) cooking tasks. You can also use recipes and food products designed to speed your food preparation tasks.

THE MOVEMENT CONNECTION

Walking Meeting

Why

Healthy meals require planning, but healthy meals don't have to be boring. Use your creativity to make meals both healthy and enjoyable.

In addition to physical health benefits, studies have shown that the act of walking boosts creative thinking. Working with a partner, locate the SuperTracker Food Tracker feature online. (If you haven't already done so, create a meal plan for each partner using the My Plan feature on the SuperTracker website.) Enter each partner's favorite meal from the past week into the Food Tracker. Determine how the meals compare to the Daily Food Group Targets.

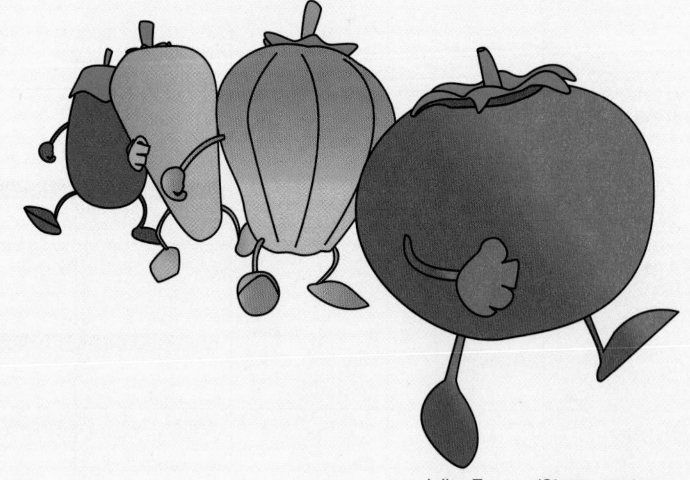

Julien Tromeur/Shutterstock.com

Apply

Take five minutes to hold a walking meeting in your classroom. During the meeting, discuss your findings. Use your creativity to propose ways the meals could be changed to make them healthier.

Organize Work Area

An organized work area prevents time wasted looking for a particular utensil, ingredients, or appliance. It also saves unnecessary steps.

Store kitchen utensils close to where you are likely to use them. For instance, you might store a pancake turner close to the range and a vegetable peeler close to the sink (**Figure 17.13**). Keeping cupboards and drawers neat makes it easier to find the items that are stored in them. Store appliances in handy locations. If appliances are difficult to get out and put away, you are less likely to use them.

Ingredients need to be on hand when you are ready to use them. Avoid running out of items by placing a dry-erase board or pad of paper in the kitchen for noting staple ingredients or supplies that need to be resupplied. This prevents last minute, unplanned trips to the store to pick up missing ingredients.

Create a Work Schedule

A successful meal is not only appealing and healthy, but also timely. Making sure all parts of a meal are ready at the allotted time requires a schedule. The schedule may be quite simple if the meal is simple, but meals that have more dishes and preparation steps require a more formal schedule.

Work schedules begin with the end in mind. In other words, the time you want to sit down to eat is when your work schedule starts and you work back from that time. For example, suppose you want the meal on the table at 6 p.m. If the chili you are serving takes 1½ hours to prepare, you should start preparing the chili at least 1½ hours prior to 6 p.m., or at 4:30 p.m. You need to perform this calculation for every dish you are serving. If you are the only person preparing the meal, you need to account for this in your schedule and start some dishes earlier.

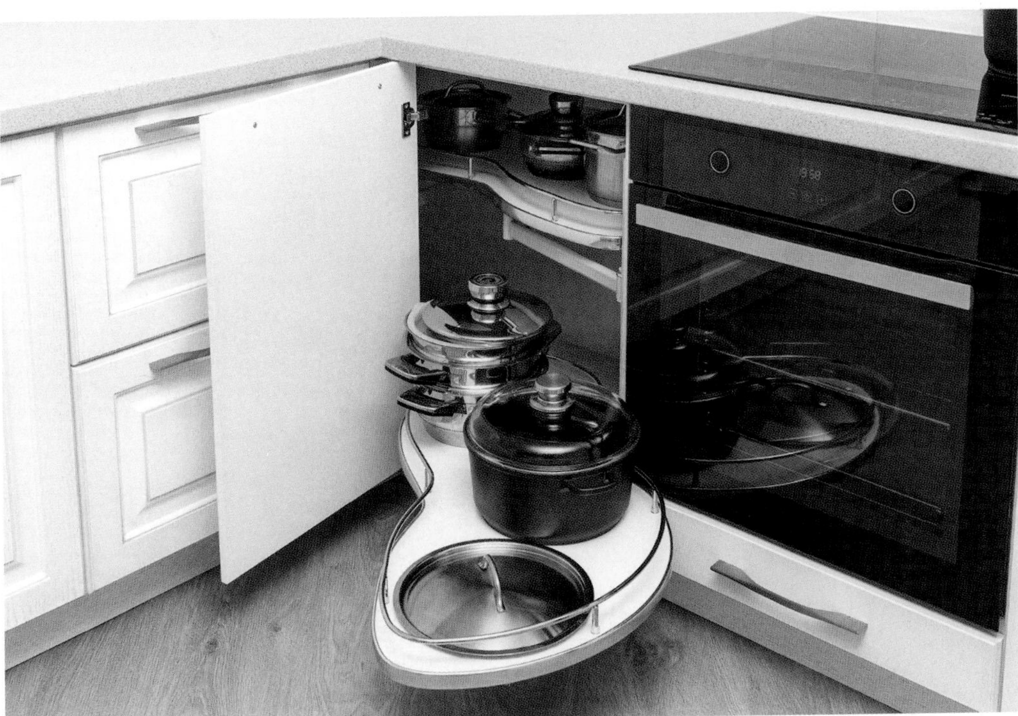

Raisa Suprun/Shutterstock.com

Figure 17.13
Store pots and pans near the range to save steps and time during food preparation. *What appliance could you store plates, cups, and eating utensils near to save time?*

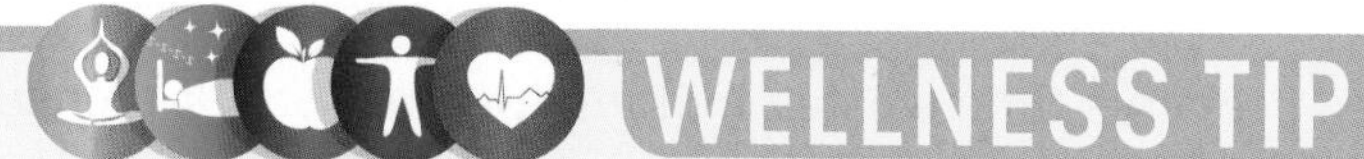

Healthful Quick Cooking

When planning meals for a busy week, choose healthful quick-cooking methods such as steaming, microwaving, and stir-frying to retain more nutrients. Use high-temperature cooking methods, such as deep frying, less often because they result in greater nutrient loss.

Prepare Items in Advance

As you write your weekly menu, consider items for recipes that can be prepared a day or two in advance. For instance, chopping green peppers and onions for the chili on Sunday when you have more leisure time will save time on Tuesday's meal preparation (**Figure 17.14**). Measure the dry ingredients for the corn bread on Sunday and keep them in an airtight container until you are ready to make the corn bread on Tuesday.

Carrot sticks for the week's lunches can be prepared on Sunday. Chop a week's worth of walnuts for the breakfast oatmeal and keep them in the freezer.

Use Time-Saving Devices

Many small appliances can save preparation and cooking time. Food processors can save time when chopping, grating, or mixing large portions of fruits, vegetables, or other ingredients. Pressure cookers reduce cooking time. Slow cookers and bread machines allow you to prepare foods in the morning and have them ready to eat at dinnertime.

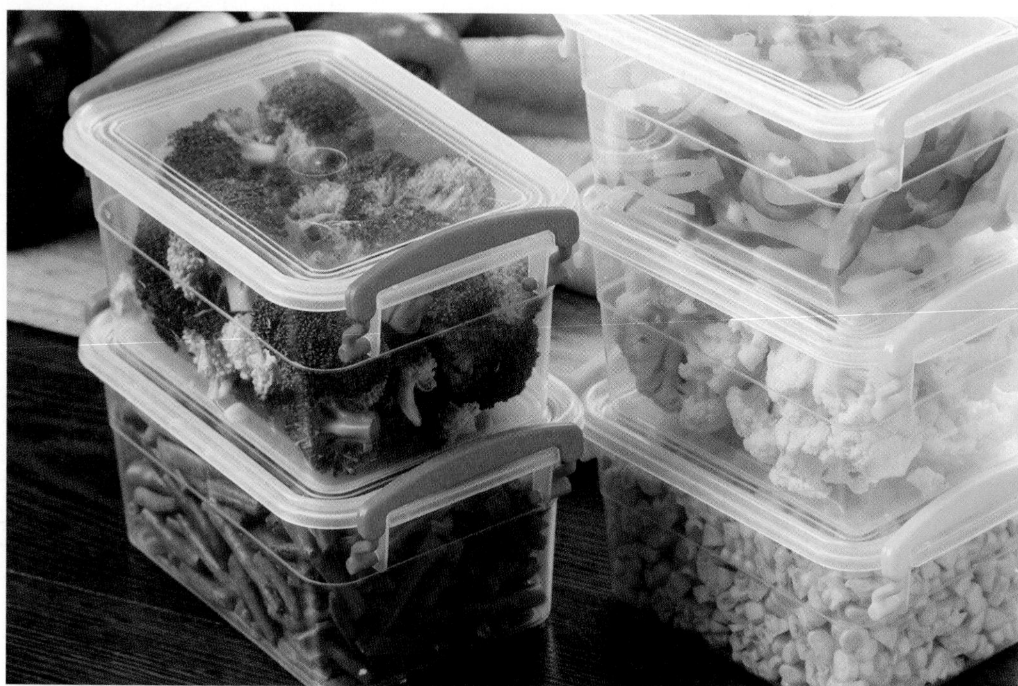

Figure 17.14 Many types of vegetables can be cut in advance to save time during meal preparation.

BravissimoS/Shutterstock.com

Microwave ovens are useful for reducing time when cooking and reheating leftovers. Using a microwave oven can also save serving and cleanup time. This is because many foods can be cooked, served, and stored in the same microwave-safe container.

Select Quick and Easy Menu Items

With planning, you can prepare many meals in 30 minutes or less. These meals can be as tasty and healthful as those that take more time and trouble to prepare.

Quick and easy meals begin with quick and easy recipes. Most simple recipes require only a few ingredients. Ingredients are generally foods that most people have on hand. These recipes have a small number of preparation steps and require only a few utensils. They usually rely on fast cooking techniques, such as microwaving and stir-frying.

Keep a file of simple, healthy recipes that you enjoy. Organize them into categories, such as main dishes, salads, and desserts. You might also want to keep a file of quick menu ideas for various types of meals. This will make it easy for you to prepare complete meals when you are in a hurry.

When you have time to cook, double recipes and store half in the refrigerator or freezer. In the time it takes to cook or reheat the stored portion, you can prepare accompanying menu items. In a matter of minutes, you will be able to serve a complete meal. Meat loaf, soups, and casseroles work especially well for this type of meal planning.

Consider Minimally Processed Foods

Heavily processed foods should be limited or avoided; however, minimally processed foods can save time and yield a healthy meal. A ***minimally processed food*** preserves most of its innate physical and nutritional properties. In fact, these foods are often as nutritious as their unprocessed versions. Examples of minimally processed foods include sliced fruits, chopped vegetables, bagged salad greens, or shelled nuts. Slightly more processed foods include items such as frozen fruits and vegetables or canned beans, tuna, fruits, and vegetables. Processed foods, such as salad dressings, jarred pasta sauce, and flavored yogurts, have ingredients such as oils, sweeteners, preservatives, or thickening agents added. Heavily processed foods include many ready-to-eat foods, such as breakfast cereal, crackers, and lunch meat, as well as frozen, canned, or boxed meals.

Not all processed food is bad. Consider whole-wheat flour that is the result of processing wheat berries (**Figure 17.15**). Even homemade whole-grain bread has been processed. The **judicious** (sensible) use of minimally processed or processed foods can save time and produce healthy meals.

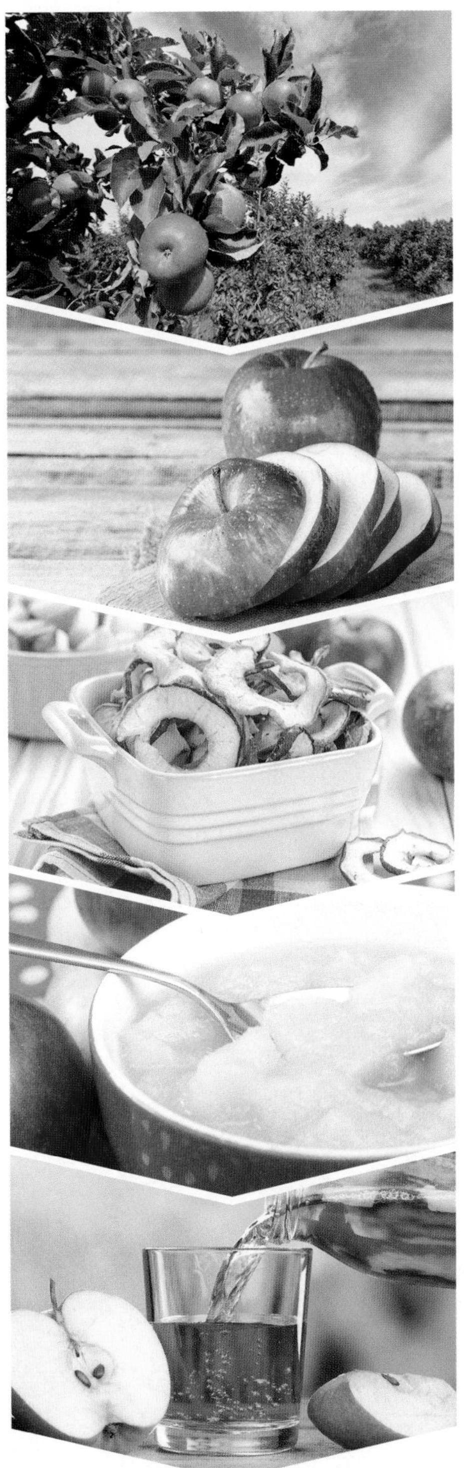

Top to bottom: Jorge Salcedo/Shutterstock.com; DomDew_Studio/Shutterstock.com; Sea Wave/Shutterstock.com; Shirinov/Shutterstock.com; Markus Mainka/Shutterstock.com

Figure 17.15 Apples can be processed to make many different foods. The foods shown illustrate a continuum of processing ranging from least processed—apples on the tree—to most processed—apple juice. *Can you think of another processed apple product?*

Processed foods often cost more than their unprocessed forms. You must decide whether the saved time, taste, and nutritional contributions of the processed products are worth the cost. Be sure to read nutrition labels when choosing processed products. Many are higher in sodium, fat, and sugar than foods you would prepare yourself using the unprocessed forms.

Home-delivery meal kits are a popular service that is a great time saver. These services deliver a box containing recipes and pre-portioned ingredients right to your door. As with other processed foods, time and money are factors when deciding whether to use this product.

Eating Healthy Meals Away from Home

Meals eaten away from home play an important role in meeting nutrient needs. These meals can also be costly and can quickly exceed planned food spending. Planning for these meals is just as important as planning for meals eaten at home.

Packing a Lunch

Many people carry meals from home to eat at school or the workplace. These meals are most often lunches.

Carrying a lunch from home has many advantages over purchasing food from a restaurant or vending machine. When you pack a lunch, you can include your favorite foods. In addition, you can use healthy, cost-effective ingredients.

Packing a lunch can also have a downside. There may be limitations to the types of food you can pack. For example, you will not want to pack leftovers that must be reheated if you will not have access to a microwave. Additionally, packing a lunch requires time and planning.

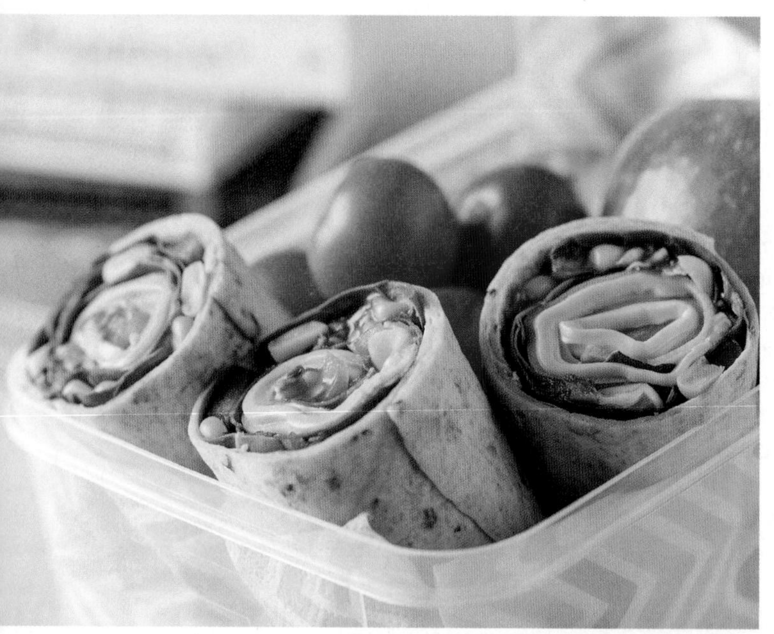

3523studio/Shutterstock.com

Figure 17.16 Whole-grain tortillas can be used to make sandwich wraps for a healthy lunch option. *What ingredients would you put in your wrap?*

Sandwiches are frequently the main course in a packed lunch. Look for new recipes if you like variety. You can add interest to sandwiches by using different kinds of breads and rolls and preparing various fillings (**Figure 17.16**).

When packing lunches, try to include a variety of foods from the five food groups. Limit snack foods, cookies, and cakes that are high in fats, sugar, and sodium. Choose some foods that are high in dietary fiber, such as whole-grain breads, and fresh fruits and vegetables.

Packing a lunch need not take much time. Many people pack lunches the night before and keep them in the refrigerator. When clearing the dinner table, store leftovers in serving-sized containers. Place them directly into lunch bags and refrigerate. Try setting up an assembly line to make sandwiches for the entire week. You can quickly complete each meal by adding a piece of fresh fruit. Packing a thermos of milk or a frozen box of juice will provide a cool drink with lunch.

Keep food safety in mind when packing lunches. Use food containers that will maintain foods at the proper temperatures until mealtime.

Choosing from a Menu

In the United States, many food dollars are spent on foods prepared away from home. This includes foods purchased from concession stands, vending machines, take-out counters, and all types of restaurants.

You have less control over the appeal, nutrient content, and cost of foods when eating out. However, you can control the foods you choose to order.

Many restaurants offer a variety of choices for their health-conscious customers. Most restaurants offer nutrition information for their menu items. Sometimes healthful options are marked by a special symbol on the menu. In addition, menu terms can help you identify foods that may be high in fat and sodium (**Figure 17.17**).

You may find healthful eating a bit more challenging when eating at fast-food restaurants. This is because many fast foods are high in sodium, fat, and calories. One large burger, French fries, and a milk shake can supply half a day's calorie needs for many teens. This meal is low in fiber and vitamins A and C. It contains approximately 1,400 milligrams of sodium, and over 50 percent of the calories come from fat.

You do not have to avoid fast-food meals. However, registered dietitian nutritionists suggest selecting foods wisely and adjusting other meals throughout the day to balance calorie and nutrient intake.

Menu Clues	
Terms Suggesting Higher Fat Content	
Au gratin or in cheese sauce	Hollandaise
Breaded	In its own gravy, with gravy, pan gravy
Buttered or buttery	Pastry
Creamed, creamy, or in cream sauce	Rich
Fried, French-fried, deep-fried, batter-fried, panfried	Scalloped
Terms Suggesting Higher Sodium Content	
Barbecued	Mustard sauce
Creole sauce	Parmesan
In a tomato base	Pickled
In broth	Smoked
In cocktail sauce	Soy sauce
Marinated	Teriyaki

Figure 17.17 Avoid menu items described using these terms. These foods will be higher in fat and sodium.

The following tips can help you meet your goals for good nutrition when eating out:

- Resist the temptation to order double burgers, large fries, and supersized drinks. Select regular-size menu items (**Figure 17.18**).
- Order half-size, appetizer, or children's portions or consider sharing an entrée with a friend.
- Limit high-fat creamy and oily salads, such as potato salad, tuna salad, and marinated pasta and vegetable salads.
- Request that gravies, sauces, and salad dressings be served on the side. Limit or avoid toppings such as cheese and bacon.
- Select salad dressings made with healthy fats, such as oil and vinegar, and use lemon juice on fish rather than tartar sauce.
- Avoid adding salt at the table.
- Trim fat from meat, skin from chicken, and breading from fish. Blot the oil on pizza with a napkin.
- Choose fruit or nonfat frozen yogurt for dessert.
- Order water, milk, or sparkling water instead of soda.
- Get exercise after eating. Walk home from the restaurant or plan other light activities to help burn a few calories.

Through planning, you can enjoy eating out. As people have become more nutrition conscious, restaurants have increased their offerings of healthful menu items. Many restaurants post the nutrition information for their menu items on their website and on their menus.

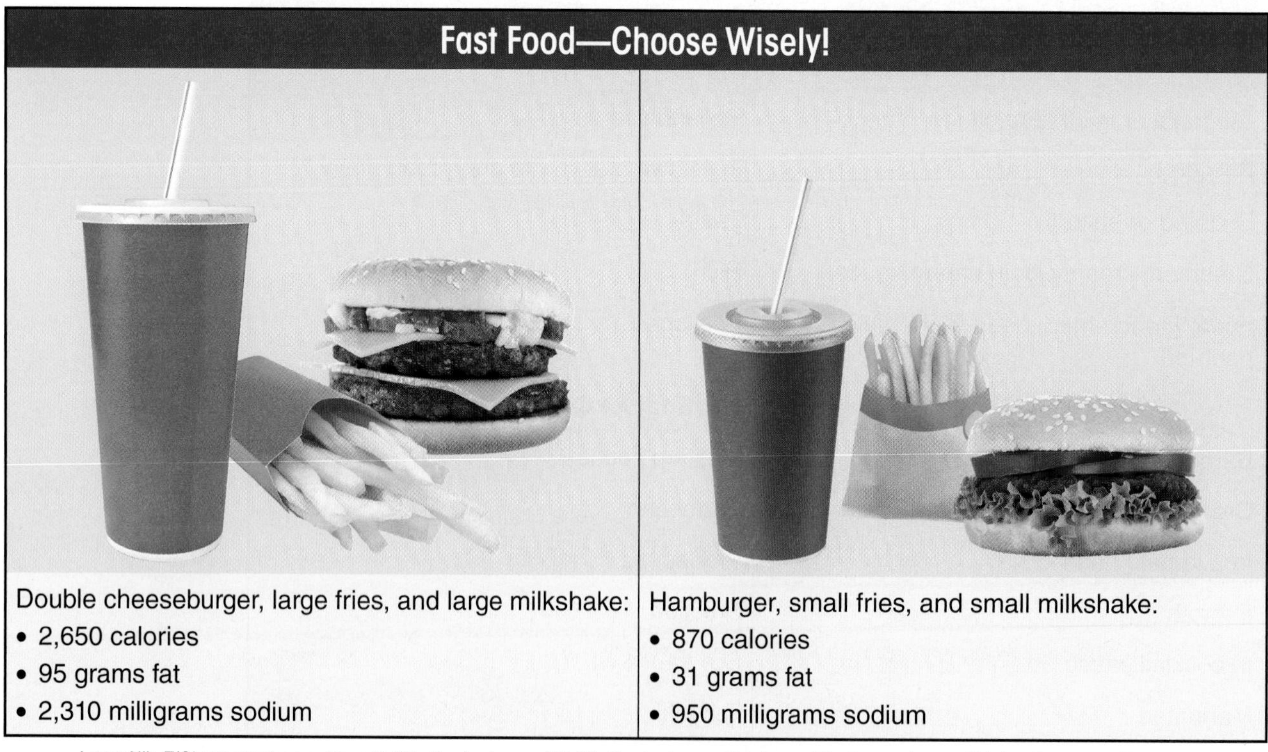

Fast Food—Choose Wisely!
Double cheeseburger, large fries, and large milkshake:
• 2,650 calories
• 95 grams fat
• 2,310 milligrams sodium
Hamburger, small fries, and small milkshake:
• 870 calories
• 31 grams fat
• 950 milligrams sodium

L to r: Nils Z/Shutterstock.com; Hong Vo/Shutterstock.com; Nitr/Shutterstock.com; Fotofermer/Shutterstock.com; Kristina Postnikova/Shutterstock.com; Lukas Gojda/Shutterstock.com

Figure 17.18 The meal on the left provides more calories than most people need for the entire day. The meal on the right contains one-third the calories, fat, and sodium.

CASE STUDY

Latrell's Lunch Makeover

Jada was on the phone with her brother Latrell one day. Latrell had recently moved into his own apartment closer to his new job in the city. He is trying to save money on food by packing his own lunch for work. He complains to Jada that he often runs out of time in the morning and is unable to make a lunch. He also states that he is bored with his lunches, and feels sluggish and tired most days.

Jada asks what he usually packs for lunch. Latrell says, "I pack the same lunch every day—a bag of potato chips, can of soda, and bologna and mayonnaise on white bread." Jada starts laughing and says, "No wonder you don't feel well! Your lunch needs a makeover."

Case Review

1. How could Latrell resolve the time crunch in the morning when making his lunch?
2. What do you think Jada means when she says Latrell's lunch needs a makeover?
3. What resources might be useful for Latrell as he plans his lunch?

RECIPE FILE

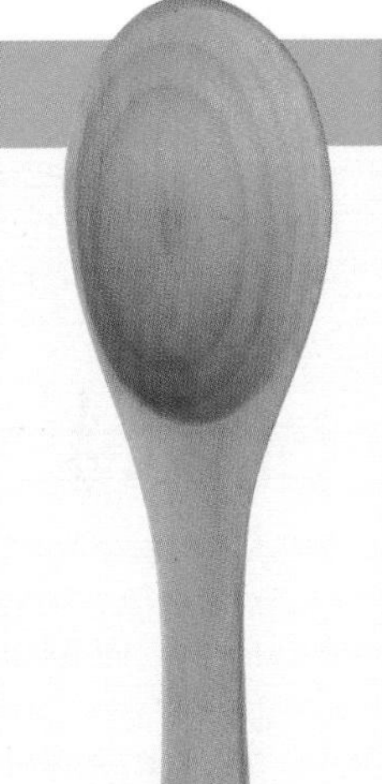

Meatballs

4 SERVINGS

Ingredients

- 1¾ T. egg (about ½ an egg), lightly beaten
- ¼ c. plain bread crumbs
- ¼ c. green onions, minced
- 1 clove garlic, minced
- 1 T. fresh parsley leaves, chopped
- 1½ T. Parmesan cheese, grated
- ¼ t. pepper
- 1 pinch each: garlic powder, onion powder, smoked paprika, pepper, dried oregano, and dried thyme
- 8 oz. ground turkey

Directions

1. Place all the ingredients, except turkey, in a large mixing bowl. Mix together just until combined.
2. Add turkey and mix until ingredients are blended into the turkey uniformly.
3. Form meatballs by rolling meat mixture into 1 tablespoon-size balls.
4. Place meatballs on a nonstick, foil-lined baking pan. (*Hint*: If your hands are slightly damp, the meatballs will roll more easily without sticking.)
5. Bake at 350°F (177°C) until meatballs reach 165°F (74°C), about 20 minutes. Turn meatballs once during cooking.
6. Serve with marinara sauce and whole-grain pasta, or sliced in a sandwich.

PER SERVING: 154 CALORIES, 15 G PROTEIN, 6 G CARBOHYDRATE, 6 G FAT, 0.5 G FIBER, 128 MG SODIUM.

Chapter 17 Review and Expand

Reading Summary

The types of equipment that your kitchen is stocked with influence the types of meals you can plan and prepare. Major kitchen appliances are usually powered by gas or electricity. Small appliances are portable and designed to accomplish and simplify kitchen tasks.

Cookware is used for preparing foods on the cooktop and bakeware is used to cook foods in the oven. Cookware and bakeware can be made from a variety of materials.

Successful meal planning results in appealing, healthy meals. Flavor, color, texture, temperature, and shape and size affect a meal's appeal. The special nutritional and health needs of each household member must be considered when planning meals. Many resources exist for planning healthy meals.

A number of strategies can be used to save time in the kitchen. Maintaining an organized work area and using time-saving appliances streamlines meals. Choosing quick and easy recipes and taking advantage of minimally processed foods saves time as well.

Include a variety of foods from the five food groups when packing meals to eat at school or the workplace. Keep food safety in mind when packing lunches. Read the nutrition information provided and select foods wisely when eating at restaurants.

Chapter Vocabulary

1. **Content Terms** In teams, play *picture charades* to identify each of the following terms. Write the terms on separate slips of paper and put the slips into a basket. Choose a team member to be the *sketcher*. The sketcher pulls a term from the basket and creates quick drawings or graphics to represent the term until the team guesses the term. Rotate turns as sketcher until the team identifies all terms.

broiler	perishable
built-in oven	pilot light
convection oven	preheat
cooktop	range
dishwasher	refrigerator-freezer
minimally processed food	

2. **Academic Terms** Individually or with a partner, create a T-chart on a sheet of paper and list each of the following terms in the left column. In the right column, list an *antonym* (a word of opposite meaning) for each term in the left column.

homogenous	perforation
judicious	streamline
monochromatic	tepid

Review Learning

3. List four small appliances used for mixing, blending, or processing food.
4. Compare cookware made from aluminum with cookware made from stainless steel.
5. List two kitchen tools that could be used to remove the skin from an apple.
6. *True or false?* Staple ingredients are rarely used ingredients that are purchased only when called for in a recipe.
7. Evaluate the following meal for appeal: baked cod garnished with toasted almonds; white rice; steamed cauliflower; fresh, chilled pear wedges; and milk. Identify the factor that was not considered when this meal was planned.
8. What resource provides a vegetarian eating pattern and a Mediterranean-style eating pattern?
9. Describe the process for planning a weekly menu.
10. List five strategies for making the best use of your time in the kitchen.
11. *True or false?* Some minimally processed foods can be as nutritious as their unprocessed versions.
12. What are two tips for saving time when packing lunches?
13. What are five tips for meeting the goal of good nutrition when eating out?

Self-Assessment Quiz

Complete the self-assessment quiz online to help you practice and expand your knowledge and skills.

Critical Thinking

14. **Analyze** Consider the meaning of the statement "Healthy eating begins in the kitchen." How do you interpret this statement? Do you agree with the statement? Write a paragraph summarizing your opinion.

15. **Conclude** What food choices do you make when you go out to eat with friends? Do you choose healthful options or go along with the crowd? Draw conclusions about ways that you can improve your food choices when you eat away from home.
16. **Evaluate** Find an image of a plated meal either from a magazine or a photo you took of a meal at a restaurant or at home. Attach the image to your evaluation of the meal's appeal. Describe how the meal addresses the factors of flavor, color, texture, temperature, and variety of shapes and sizes. What changes would you recommend and why?
17. **Apply** Write a one-day menu for your household. Use resources discussed in the chapter to help you. Be sure to note any special nutritional or health needs and how you addressed them in the menu.
18. **Determine** Select one meal from the menu you wrote in the previous activity. Make a list of the appliances, utensils, cookware, bakeware, and kitchen staples you would need to prepare the meal.
19. **Evaluate** Obtain a menu from your favorite restaurant or print a copy of the menu if you find it online. Select and highlight a healthy meal that you could order the next time you eat at that restaurant. Explain why your choices are health promoting.
20. **Analyze** Conduct an analysis of the school's cafeteria meals for one week. Prepare a rubric to evaluate the menus using the various factors that contribute to the appeal and health of a meal. Use the Food Tracker tool on ChooseMyPlate.gov to evaluate nutritional content of the menus.
21. **Assess** Make a list of 10 foods in your kitchen. Organize them in order of least processed to most heavily processed. Propose ways unprocessed food or minimally processed foods you could use in place of the heavily processed foods.
22. **Implement** Use the Food Tracker tool on the SuperTracker website to create a daily food menu for yourself. Enter your menu choices for the day and examine the data presented on the tracker. How well does the meal target recommended portions in each of the food groups? Do the calories meet your individual needs? What portion of the menu is considered empty calories? Reevaluate your menu plan and adjust to better target the goals of the food groups and calorie needs. Now, assume your menu will be used to feed a preschooler. Construct a profile for the preschooler and create an eating plan. Identify how you will need to adjust the menu to meet the needs of the preschooler.

Core Skills

23. **Reading** Read about meal planning in the 1930s. Prepare an electronic presentation comparing it to meal planning and preparation today.
24. **Science and Writing** Plan and conduct a small taste test to evaluate the effect of flavor, color, texture, shape, size, or temperature on food choices. Divide a batch of mashed potatoes in half. Color one-half blue and leave the other half unaltered. Ask people to taste both potatoes and tell you which they prefer and why. Next, have the same people wear blindfolds and sample the potatoes again. Note their responses. Perform the taste test comparing cheese at room temperature to the same cheese served cold. Summarize your findings and write a conclusion about factors that affect food appeal.
25. **Writing** Research the international Slow Food movement. Based on your findings, write a persuasive paper either in favor of or against the movement. Interview a member of a Slow Food chapter to lend support to your position.
26. **Math** Look online or in a store to find saucepans made from four different materials discussed in this chapter. Make sure the saucepans have the same capacity. Record the price for each pan. Make a bar graph to show how the prices compare.
27. **Career Readiness Practice** The ability to read and interpret information is an important workplace skill. Presume you work for a national supermarket chain that typically sells only food products. The company is considering adding a cookware line to its products, but wants you to evaluate and interpret some research on which cookware material is the best product for the best price. You will need to locate three reliable sources of the latest information on cookware. Read and interpret the information and then write a report summarizing your findings.

CHAPTER 18 Shopping for Food

Learning Outcomes

After studying this chapter, you will be able to

- **compare** options for where to shop for food;
- **implement** strategies for controlling food costs;
- **explain** factors that can affect consumer food choices; and
- **identify** your consumer rights and responsibilities.

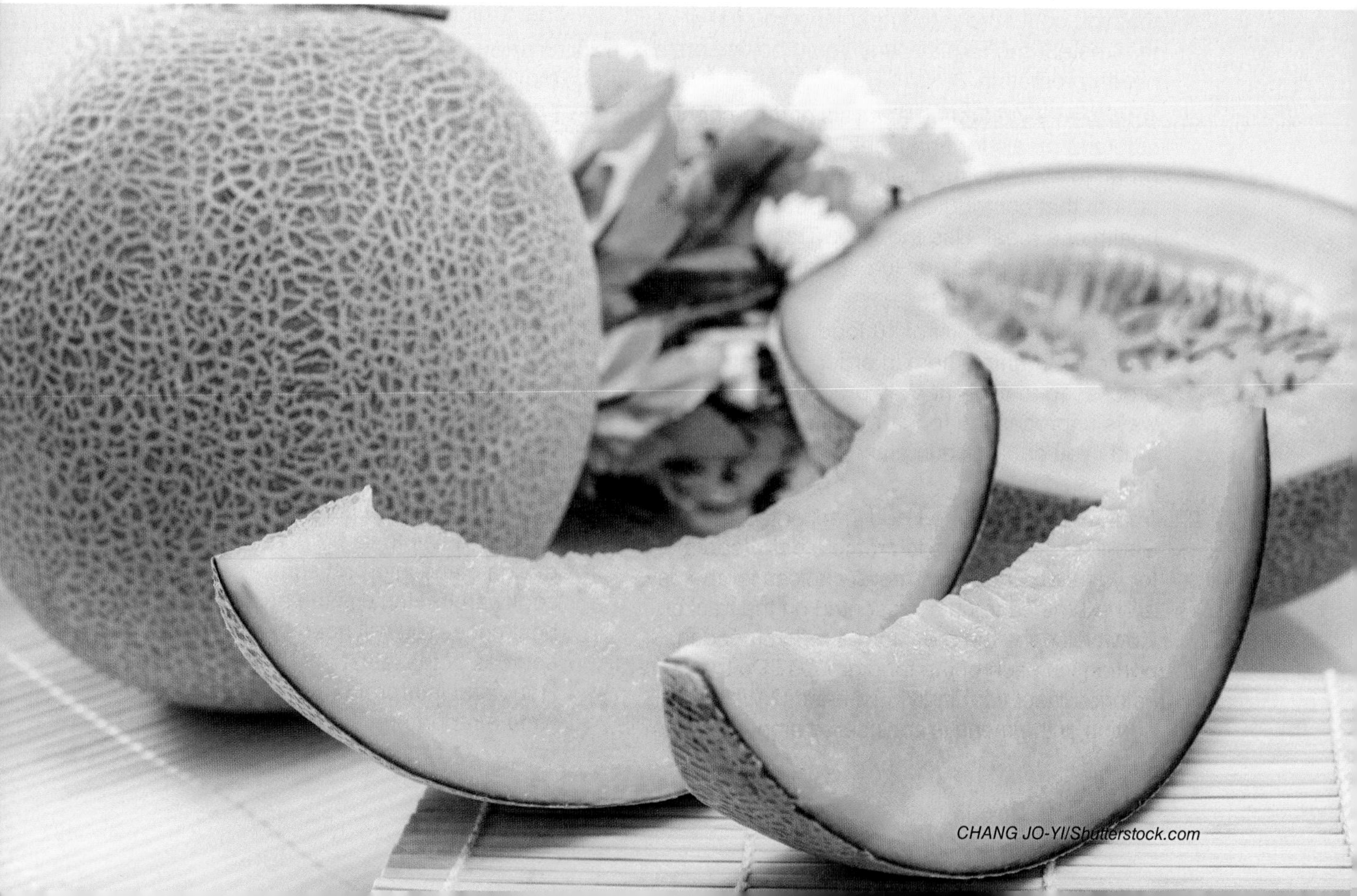

CHANG JO-YI/Shutterstock.com

Content Terms

budget
comparison shopping
congregate meal
consumer
food additive
food irradiation
food processing
generally recognized as safe (GRAS) list
generic product
impulse buying
national brand
organic foods
store brand
unit price

Academic Terms

entice
frugal
fundamental
suffice
verified

What's Your Nutrition and Wellness IQ?

Take this quiz to examine how much you already know about shopping for food. If you cannot answer a question, pay extra attention to that topic as you study this chapter.

- Identify each statement as *True*, *False*, or *It Depends*. *It Depends* means in some cases the statement is true; in some cases it could be false.
- Revise false statements to make them true.
- Explain the circumstances in which each *It Depends* statement is true and when it is false.

Nutrition and Wellness IQ 

	Statement			
1.	Supermarkets offer the lowest food prices.	True	False	It Depends
2.	The last step in the consumer complaint process is to contact a consumer protection office.	True	False	It Depends
3.	Unit pricing is an effective tool for comparing two different brands of canned pizza sauce.	True	False	It Depends
4.	Heavily processed foods have more additives than whole foods.	True	False	It Depends
5.	Irradiated foods are unsafe to eat.	True	False	It Depends
6.	Organically grown foods are more nutritious than nonorganic foods.	True	False	It Depends
7.	Generic canned peaches have lower nutrient content and quality than national brand canned peaches.	True	False	It Depends
8.	Using a spending plan helps control food costs.	True	False	It Depends

While studying this chapter, look for the activity icon to

- **build** vocabulary with e-flash cards and interactive games;
- **assess** what you learn by completing self-assessment quizzes and completing review questions; and
- **expand** knowledge with interactive activities and activities that extend learning.

www.g-wlearning.com/foodsandnutrition/

How do you decide which foods to buy and where to buy them? Are your decisions swayed by advertising? Do you base your food choices on the way products taste, their nutritional value, or their packaging? Perhaps you buy certain products out of habit. These and many other factors influence your market decisions.

This chapter will provide you with skills to control food costs and guidelines for handling problems in the marketplace.

Where to Shop for Food

How do you decide where to buy the foods you need? If you are like most people, one of the factors that affects your choice of stores is price. Nonetheless, price should not be your only consideration. If you drive from store to store to get the lowest price, you may end up losing money rather than saving it. This shopping strategy takes time and adds to your transportation costs.

It is more practical to shop at only one or two stores. Choose stores that give you the best overall price and quality. Look for stores with convenient locations. The stores should also be clean, offer customer services, and provide a variety of products.

Many different types of stores sell food products. These include supermarkets, warehouse stores and buying clubs, convenience stores, outlet stores, specialty stores, health food stores, food cooperatives, roadside stands and farmers' markets, and virtual stores that offer online shopping. Conveniences, type of service, food quality and selection, and cost are primary reasons for choosing one store over another. Each alternative offers particular advantages and disadvantages.

Supermarkets

Supermarkets offer a wide range of products. In addition to food, they carry household items, health and beauty products, clothes, and pet supplies. Many stores have bakery, deli, and meat departments. Some have pharmacies, bank branches, and cafeterias. Supermarkets offer consumers wide variety in product selection and parking convenience (**Figure 18.1**).

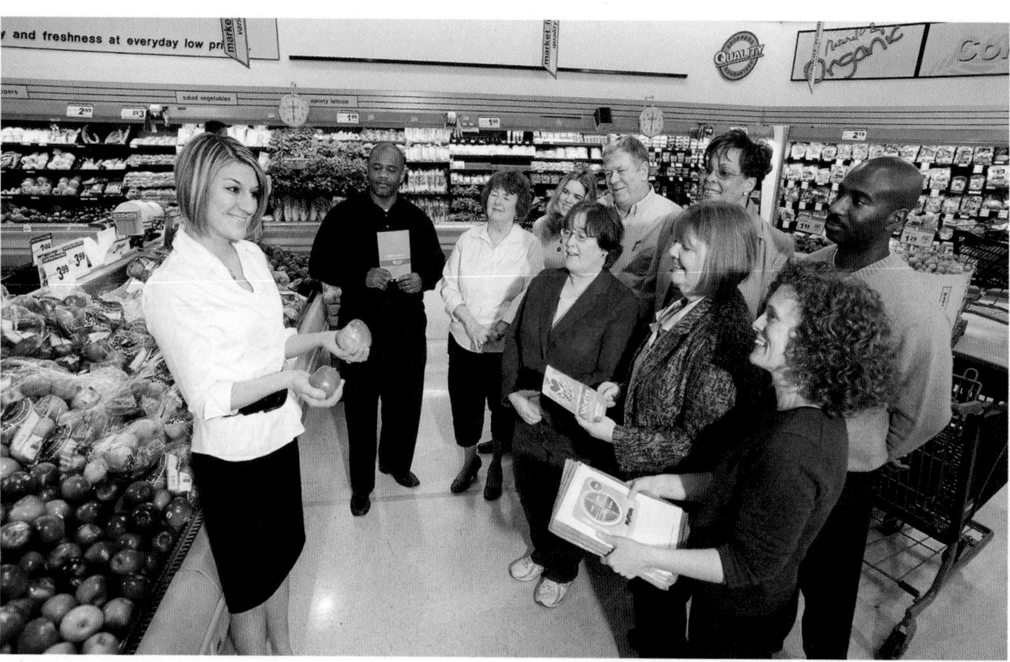

Figure 18.1 Many supermarkets employ dietitians to serve as nutrition resources for their customers. Supermarket dietitians teach cooking classes, educate about reading labels, or provide nutrition coaching.

Stephen Ausmus/USDA

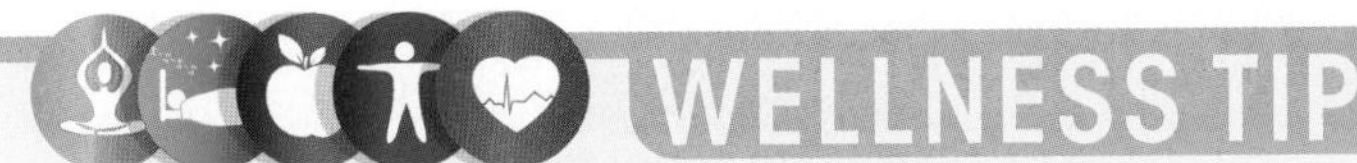

Wash Reusable Grocery Bags

Although reusable grocery bags are good for the environment, they can be bad for your health without proper care. Without regular washing, these reusable bags can be a breeding ground for foodborne bacteria. To keep your reusable grocery bags safe, clean them after every use. Wash fabric bags in your washing machine. Clean bags made of plastic-like materials in a sink filled with soapy water and one-fourth cup of distilled vinegar.

On the other hand, some shoppers have trouble finding the products they need in such large stores. Some supermarkets are open 24 hours a day and more are offering home delivery or pickup service.

Warehouse Stores and Buying Clubs

Warehouse stores and buying clubs offer a variety of products other than foods. Selections and variety may be limited. Many items are sold in large containers and multiunit packages. This can be a convenience for shoppers who like to stock up on food items or who plan to feed a larger number of people. Prices at warehouse stores can be lower than supermarket prices. Some warehouse clubs charge membership fees and may not accept coupons. These factors make warehouse prices less of a bargain.

Convenience Stores

These stores usually have longer business hours than other food stores. Many stay open around the clock. They are typically located on the way to or from workplaces. They stock a limited variety of food items and household essentials. They often sell a variety of sports drinks, snacks, and ready-to-eat foods, such as sandwiches and pizza. These stores are in locations that make it easy to pick up a few needed items quickly. Prices at convenience stores are often higher than supermarket prices.

Outlet Stores

Outlet stores usually sell products made by one food manufacturer and are sometimes located in outlet malls. Although these items are wholesome, some of them may not meet the manufacturer's standards for quality. For instance, bagels may be slightly misshapen or the frosting on a cake may be smudged. Products at outlet stores are usually sold at substantial discounts over retail prices. However, the consumer has no opportunity to compare and select competing brands.

Specialty Stores

Specialty stores include international markets, dairies, bakeries, cheese, meat, or fish markets. These stores specialize in selling one type of product. You may not be able to find the specialty food products in other supermarkets. Many gourmet food stores sell their products online. Their products are usually high quality and very fresh. Most specialty stores charge premium prices.

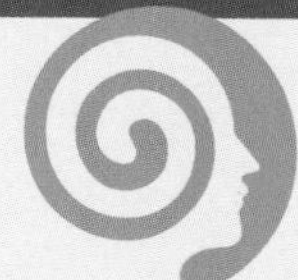

EXTEND YOUR KNOWLEDGE

Shopping for Fair Trade?

Are there ethical considerations when shopping for food and other items you purchase? What responsibility do you have for promoting equitable global trade of goods?

Fair Trade is a global business model that helps farmers and craftspeople in developing countries find customers for their products and experience financial success. Additional goals of the Fair Trade model include protecting the environment, safeguarding the rights of children, and ensuring fair wages and safe working environments.

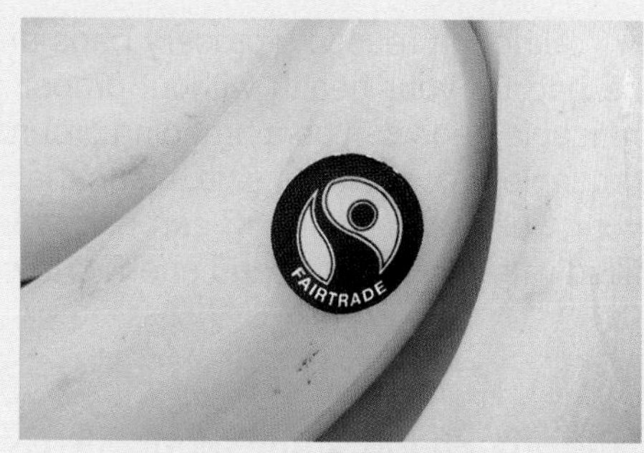

Thinglass/Shutterstock.com

Common Fair Trade foods include coffee, cocoa, beans, sugar, and spices. There are a number of different organizations that certify, label, and market Fair Trade foods and other products. How do you feel about the need to support Fair Trade practices? Try to find foods with Fair Trade labels next time you are at the supermarket.

Health Food Stores

Health food stores often emphasize natural foods, whole foods, organic foods, herbal and vitamin supplements, and may specialize in sports supplements and energy drinks. You may find health food choices not found in other stores, but prices may be higher than in supermarkets. Additionally, scientific research does not support claims regarding the benefit of using many of the health-promoting foods or food supplements sold at these stores.

Food Cooperatives

Most food cooperatives, or co-ops, are not open to the public. They are owned and run democratically by a group of consumers. Many co-ops choose to buy locally grown produce and building community is a shared value of most co-ops.

Only members of the group may take advantage of the discounted grocery prices. Food prices are low because the group buys foods in bulk and adds no charge for profit. Nonmembers may be allowed to shop, but do not receive the discounted pricing. Co-ops also save labor costs by requiring members to volunteer at the co-op for a few hours each month. Members may also need to pay an annual fee.

Roadside Stands and Farmers' Markets

Roadside stands and farmers' markets offer consumers the chance to buy fruits and vegetables fresh from the field. Roadside stands are operated by individual produce growers during the growing season. Farmers' markets sell produce from a number of farmers, often in a city location. Roadside stands and farmers' markets usually have limited hours. However, their produce is fresher, usually grown locally, and priced comparably or lower than supermarket produce.

Shopping Online

Shopping online eliminates the need for consumers to travel to a store. Food stores that provide online shopping allow customers to order food using their smartphones or home computers. Online shoppers can find a wide range of food and nonfood items to order and either pick up or have delivered.

After a consumer completes an order, he or she submits it to the online service provider. The customer's order is filled and delivered to the address provided. Electronic payment for services is usually completed before the delivery occurs.

Adding tips for delivery services adds to the cost of shopping online. Spending for online food shopping is expected to nearly triple by the year 2021.

How, when, and where you can shop is constantly changing and evolving (**Figure 18.2**).

Food Shopping Trends

- **Increased digital interaction with shoppers.** Digital signs and displays on store shelves will deliver messages, promotions, and product information. The use of mobile apps for virtual coupons will continue to grow. Augmented reality (AR) provides the shopper with images, video, and graphics while shopping in store or online.

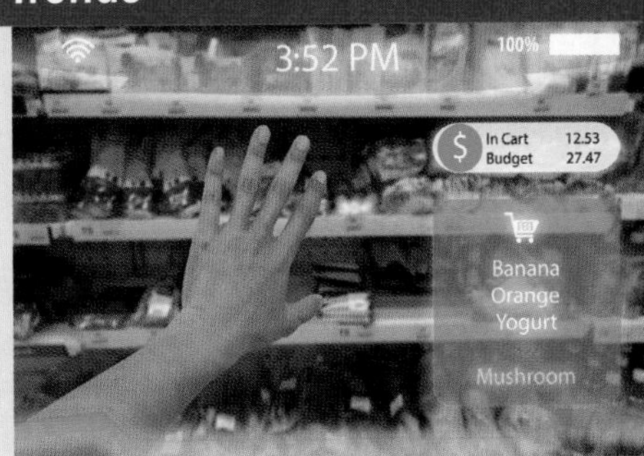

- **Competing with meal kits.** Supermarkets will stock meal kits to compete with online meal kit delivery services.
- **Enhanced access to product information.** Product labels will display barcodes or QR codes that link to more detailed product information including where the product was grown, food certifications, allergens, and more.

- **Faster ways to check out.** Shoppers may be using a mobile app to scan their purchases as they shop and then pay electronically.
- **Increased produce variety.** Stores will offer more varieties of organic fruits and vegetables, as well as more diverse food selections from around the world.
- **Greater focus on local products.** This approach appeals to customers who want fresh, tasty, nutritious products; like to support the local economy; and are concerned about environmental impact.

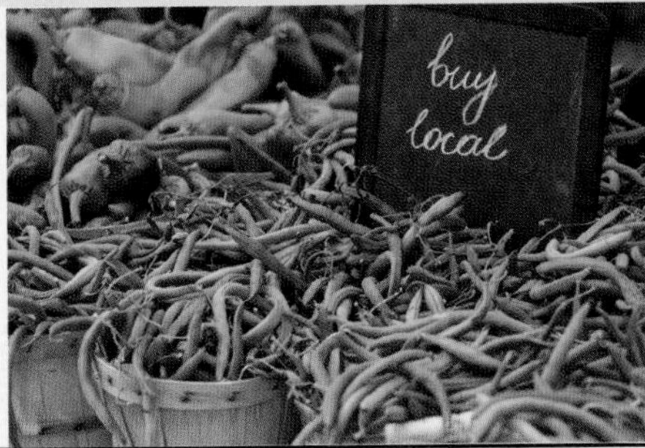

Top to bottom: ekkasit919/Shutterstock.com; Monkey Business Images/Shutterstock.com; Arina P Habich/Shutterstock.com

Figure 18.2 The food shopping experience is changing rapidly. *Have you used or observed any of these or other trends in your supermarket?*

Controlling Food Costs

Meal planning not only enables you to serve healthy meals, but also allows you to manage food costs. Food can be very expensive. Tools such as spending plans, shopping lists, price comparison, low-cost meal strategies, and food assistance resources can help you control food costs without sacrificing appeal or nutrition.

Follow a Spending Plan

To plan meals that stay within your financial limits, you first need to decide what those limits are. Preparing a ***budget***, or a spending plan, will help you establish those limits. A budget helps you plan how to use your sources of income to meet your various expenses. Many expenses occur on a monthly basis. Therefore, many people find it convenient to set up a monthly budget (**Figure 18.3**).

The **fundamental** (important) principle of budgeting is to spend only as much money as you receive. The amount of money you budget for food must allow you to pay other expenses. These include *fixed expenses*, such as housing, transportation, health insurance, and taxes, which are the same each month. You also have *flexible expenses*, such as clothing purchases, entertainment, and utility bills, which vary from month to month. The food category of a budget is considered a flexible expense.

To ensure that you stay within the established food budget, save all your food-shopping receipts for one week. In addition, keep a record of money spent eating away from home including restaurants, vending machines, and take-home meals. Total all the receipts to determine how much you have spent on food. If the amount exceeds one-fourth the monthly food budget (one week is roughly one-fourth of the month), you must make some adjustments.

Consider all the resources available to you as you plan for your food needs and look for ways to be more **frugal** (thrifty, economical). Eating out and having frequent dinner guests increases your food spending. You may need to cut back on these types of food purchases if you are unable to stay within your budget.

Monthly Household Budget (for one person)		
Income	$3,150	
Taxes	–567	
After tax income		$2,583
Expenses		
Housing and utilities	$1,200	
Food (at home and away from home)	260	
Transportation	480	
Health care	272	
Savings	60	
Other (telephone, clothing, entertainment, etc.)	311	
Total expenses		$2,583
Income minus expenses		0

Figure 18.3 Most people spend approximately 10 percent of their after-tax income on food.

Use a Shopping List

One of the best ways to control food spending is to prepare a shopping list. A shopping list can help you avoid ***impulse buying***, or making unplanned purchases. Impulse buying can cause you to spend money you had not planned to spend on items you do not need. A shopping list can also help you save the time required to return to the store for forgotten items (**Figure 18.4**).

To prepare your list, begin by reviewing the menus and recipes you plan to use. Write all the ingredients you do not have on hand on your shopping list. Keep the shopping list handy and add needed food items as supplies run low.

Organize your shopping list according to the way foods are grouped in the store. This will save you time and keep you from missing items you need. Your list might include such headings as *produce*; *canned foods*; *rice*, *beans*, and *pasta*; *baking needs*; *cereals*; and *breads*. Place the headings *meats*, *dairy products*, and *frozen foods* at the bottom of the list. You should pick up perishable foods in these categories last to reduce the chance of spoilage.

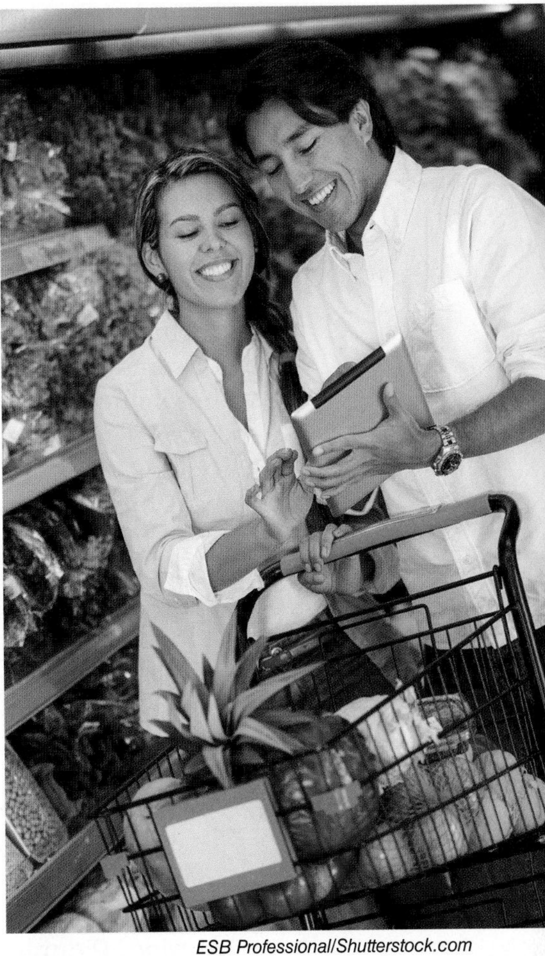

ESB Professional/Shutterstock.com

Figure 18.4 A shopping list helps you remember everything you need to purchase and helps you avoid unnecessary purchases. *What other strategies could you use to avoid impulse buying?*

Compare Food Prices

You are standing in the supermarket in the canned goods aisle. Canned tomatoes are on your shopping list, but there are five brands of tomatoes on the shelf! In addition, most of the tomato products are offered in two or three different can sizes. You want to choose the best price, but it is overwhelming.

Use comparison shopping to make the best choice and avoid overspending. ***Comparison shopping*** is assessing prices and quality of similar products. It enables you to choose the product that best meets your needs and fits your price range.

Use Unit Prices

Unit pricing makes it easy to comparison shop. A ***unit price*** is a product's cost per standard unit of weight or volume. For instance, the unit price for breakfast cereal is the cost in cents per ounce. The unit price for milk might be expressed in cents per quart. Unit prices for products such as eggs and paper napkins are based on count, for example cents per dozen.

Unit prices are usually posted adjacent to the products on the shelf. You can use unit pricing to compare different forms, sizes, or brands of products to find the best buy.

Compare unit prices of uncut and precut items, such as chunk versus shredded cheese or whole fruit versus fruit salad. Precut items tend to cost more. They may also spoil more quickly. Foods that are packaged in individual servings also have higher unit prices. Extra packaging adds to the cost of the product and places a strain on the environment.

Compare Brands

The product brand often affects the price and quality of a product. Therefore, when you are deciding which brand to buy, you need to compare both the price and the quality.

National brand products are distributed and advertised throughout the country by major food companies. These products are generally considered to be high quality. To cover the costs of nationwide advertising, the prices of these products are usually high.

Store brand products bear the name of the food store in which they are bought, and are sold only in those stores. These products are often of similar quality to national brand products. However, because they are not widely advertised, their prices are usually lower than national brands.

Generic products are unbranded and have no trade name. You can identify them by their plain, simple packaging. You may find generic products to be of somewhat lower quality. For instance, the size of generic green beans may not be uniform. However, the nutritional value of generic products is comparable to other products. They are usually less expensive than national or store brands.

Consider how you intend to use a food when choosing among national brands, store brands, and generic products (**Figure 18.5**). For example, suppose you are going to cut up canned peaches for a salad. Irregular shapes and sizes will not be noticeable in this type of dish. Therefore, you do not need to pay a high price for the top-quality national brand when a generic product will **suffice** (be adequate). Consider buying store brand or generic peaches instead. The nutritional quality will remain the same, and you will save money.

Adopt Cost-Cutting Strategies

Using some basic strategies during meal planning and shopping can help reduce money spent on food.

At Meal Planning

Build meals around low-cost foods in each food group. For instance, brown rice and fresh pasta are both in the grains group. You could use either as the basis of a tasty, nutritious casserole; however, fresh pasta costs about three times more than the brown rice. When planning meals, use less costly foods from all the food groups. From the fruit and vegetable groups, choose fresh produce that is in season. Frozen and canned fruits and vegetables are also good values. Avoid the fruit and vegetable products that include extra ingredients, such as sauces, because they are more costly.

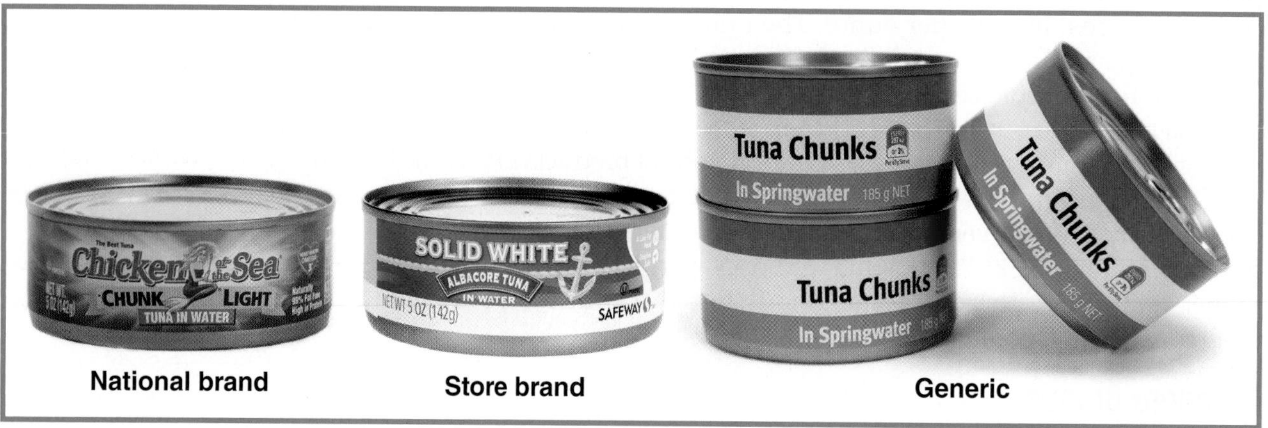

Left to right: Sheila Fitzgerald/Shutterstock.com; Jeffrey B. Banke/Shutterstock.com; Kitch Bain/Shutterstock.com

Figure 18.5 Your supermarket may offer a national brand and a store brand tuna, as well as a generic tuna. *If you were making tuna salad, which tuna product would you choose?*

FEATURED CAREER

Food Lawyer

Food lawyers focus on the most critical issues facing our food system today: sustainable food production and distribution, animal and human rights, immigration, GMO labeling, food safety, environmental concerns, trade, and more. They may do legal work for a variety of clients, such as chefs, local and federal government, farmers, or nonprofit corporations.

Education

Entry-level positions require a bachelor's degree and a juris doctor (JD). The JD is a professional graduate degree that prepares you to take the bar exam. Particularly helpful classes for this career are urban planning, public health, public policy, and nutrition.

Job Outlook

The demand for legal experts specializing in this field is currently high. Consumers, corporations, and government agencies are all taking a closer look at our current food system from GMO labeling to increased global demand for foods. Food lawyers study, use, and create the rules for this system, so career opportunities are increasing.

In the dairy group, you can save money by using nonfat dry milk in your menu plans. Dry legumes and peanut butter are the best buys in the protein foods group. You can use them to create high-fiber, low-fat meatless main dishes.

Plan menus that take advantage of advertised store specials. If broccoli is on sale, you might plan to serve it for several meals. You could use it in a salad one day and in a side dish another day.

Control the cost of your menu by planning the appropriate amounts of foods. Base the amount of food on individuals' nutrient needs—do not prepare more food than is needed. If you have an active teen male in the household, the menu plan will include more food than if you are feeding a school-age child (**Figure 18.6**).

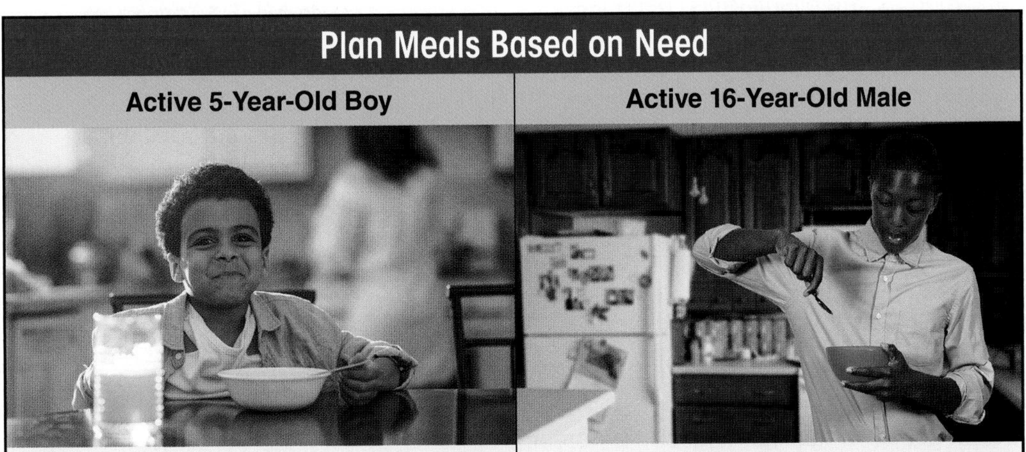
Plan Meals Based on Need
Active 5-Year-Old Boy
Active 16-Year-Old Male
Estimated daily calorie needs: 1,600 calories
Approximate weekly cost of food = $39.00
Estimated daily calorie needs: 3,200 calories
Approximate weekly cost of food = $70.00

Left to right: Joshua Resnick/Shutterstock.com; Rob Byron/Shutterstock.com

Figure 18.6 It costs nearly twice as much to feed a 16-year-old male as it does to feed a 5-year-old boy. Failing to adjust meal planning based on need can have a significant effect on a food budget.

During Shopping

Careful shopping can also help you save money when buying food. Try to avoid shopping when you are tired, hungry, or rushed. You are more likely to make unplanned purchases under these conditions.

Buy only what is on your shopping list and avoid impulse purchases. Store displays may **entice** (tempt) you to buy items not on your shopping list. For example, a display of toppings with the frozen desserts may encourage you to make an unplanned purchase.

Take advantage of coupon websites and apps to buy items you need or use regularly. Before you use a coupon, however, compare quality and prices of similar products. Even with coupons, some foods cost more than other brands. If you have the storage space, stock up on sale items that will stay fresh in your home. Canned and frozen foods may be more cost effective when purchased in larger quantities, if properly stored. Pay attention to expiration dates.

Prevent money lost due to spoiled food by returning home with food purchases immediately after shopping. Store foods properly to maintain their wholesome quality and extend their shelf life.

Consider planting a vegetable garden to save money spent on vegetables. Freshness is guaranteed when vegetables are just picked from the garden!

FOOD AND THE ENVIRONMENT

Sustainable Alternative Vertical Farming

Innovative farming methods are being used to meet the increasing global demand for nutritional foods as farmland is shrinking. Farmland is being lost to housing developments to meet the needs of a growing population. By 2045, the global population is predicted to increase by 2 billion to nearly 9 billion people.

One example of an innovative method is vertical farming. Vertical farming cultivates plant and animal food sources in vertical structures, such as tall buildings or skyscrapers. Sometimes old factories or warehouses are repurposed for vertical farming operations. Fast-growing crops, such as leafy greens, herbs, tomatoes, mint, and strawberries, are often farmed because they grow quickly and sell quickly.

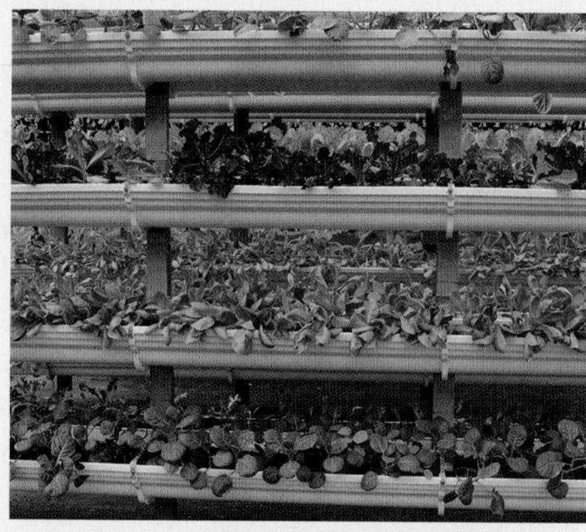

Aisyaqilumaranas/Shutterstock.com

The beds in which the plants are grown are stacked vertically in space that is environmentally controlled. Everything the plants need to grow—humidity, temperature, light, and nutrients—is provided and controlled. The growing mediums may be *hydroponic* (liquid nutrient solutions), *aquaponic* (water used to raise fish), or *aeroponic* (liquid nutrient solutions applied to roots by misting). Other nonsoil growing mediums may be used including coconut husks or peat moss. Use of these mediums helps overcome the limited land area needed for traditional farming methods.

Vertical farming also avoids the use of potentially harmful chemicals and pesticides. As usable farmland diminishes and over-farming of available land for production of crops continues, vertical farming may be a sustainable option for feeding a growing population.

Think Critically

1. Describe advantages of vertical farming for the farmer.
2. What types of crops would not be practical to grow using vertical farming? Why?
3. Discuss the potential impact of vertical farming on helping to solve world hunger issues.

Food Assistance Resources

Many people experience the need for assistance at some point in their life, whether it is due to old age, illness, or other reasons. The government offers a number of food programs to help people bridge these difficult times.

The following programs are available through the United States Department of Agriculture (USDA). Some of these programs are funded jointly by the states. These programs provide resources for eligible individuals at various life-cycle stages.

Supplemental Nutrition Assistance Program (SNAP)

The Supplemental Nutrition Assistance Program was formerly called the *Federal Food Stamp Program*. The focus is on nutrition and making healthy food accessible to low-income households. You apply for benefits by completing a state application form. Benefits are provided on an electronic card that is used like an ATM card. The card is accepted at most grocery stores, as well as some food cooperatives and farmers' markets (**Figure 18.7**). Through educational training programs, SNAP helps clients learn to make healthy eating and active lifestyle choices.

This assistance program supplements food needs for a family, but it is not enough to purchase a complete nutritionally adequate diet. Families must add money to their SNAP allotment to meet all their nutritional needs.

Child and Adult Care Food Program (CACFP)

The USDA's Child and Adult Care Food Program provides meals and snacks to children in family or group day care homes, as well as children residing in homeless shelters. It also provides meals and snacks to adults in adult day care centers.

National School Programs

The National School Lunch program provides nutritious lunches at reduced or no cost to eligible children. The lunches must meet the *Dietary Guidelines'* recommendations for the age group being served. Additional programs offered through schools include the Afterschool Snack, Seamless Summer, Summer Food Service, Fresh Fruit and Vegetable, School Breakfast, Farm to School, and Special Milk programs.

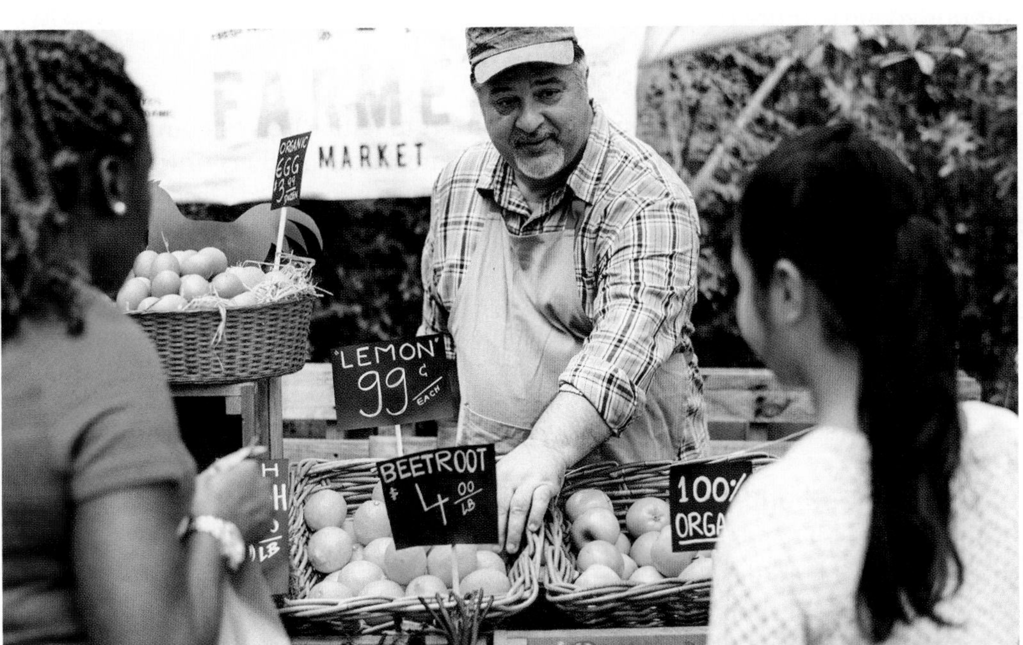

Rawpixel.com/Shutterstock.com

Figure 18.7
SNAP recipients can double their dollars when using the vouchers to purchase fresh produce at participating farmers' markets and supermarkets.

Special Supplemental Nutrition Program for Women, Infants, and Children (WIC)

The Special Supplemental Nutrition Program for Women, Infants, and Children (WIC) is intended to help children get a healthy start in life. It focuses on children up to age five and pregnant and lactating (breast-feeding) women. The program is designed to help low-income mothers and children who are at nutritional risk. WIC services provide vouchers for the purchase of specific nutritious foods. These foods supply nutrients to meet the nutritional needs of the WIC clients. The program also provides nutrition education, as well as referrals to other health and social services.

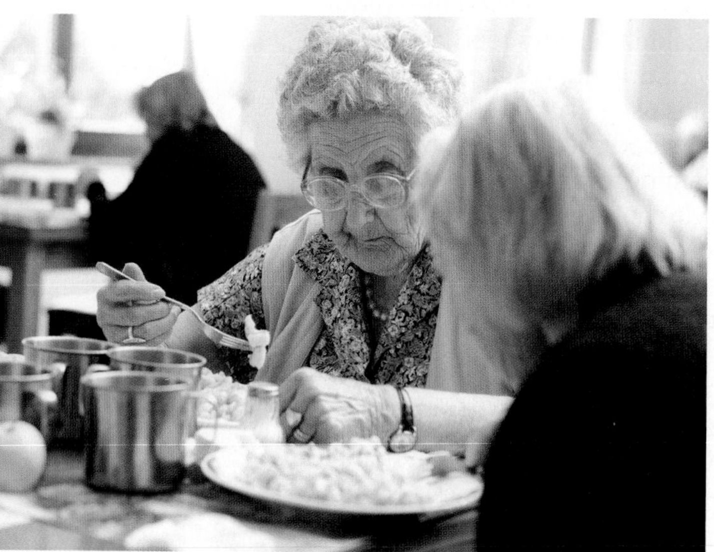

Kristo-Gothard Hunor/Shutterstock.com

Figure 18.8 In addition to nutrition, congregate meals provide an opportunity for social interaction.

Elderly Nutrition Program

The Elderly Nutrition Program provides funding to support nutrition services to older adults throughout the United States. The nutrition services include congregate and home-delivered meals. The meals must provide at least one-third of estimated required nutrients.

Congregate meals are designed to meet both the social and nutritional needs of people age 50 and older. A ***congregate meal*** is a group meal. Group meals are provided at local places of worship, community centers, or other facilities one or more days a week (**Figure 18.8**).

The Meals on Wheels program provides meals for individuals who cannot leave their homes and are unable to prepare their own meals. Volunteers deliver these meals to the individuals' homes.

The Senior Farmers' Market Nutrition Program (SFMNP) provides low-income seniors with coupons that can be exchanged for eligible foods (fruits, vegetables, honey, and fresh-cut herbs) at farmers' markets, roadside stands, and community-supported agriculture programs.

Commodity Supplemental Food Program

The Commodity Supplemental Food Program (CSFP) gives commodity food to low-income pregnant and breastfeeding women, new mothers, infants, children up to age six, and elderly people 60 years and older. A *commodity food* is a common, mass-produced item. This program often distributes foods such as instant dry milk, flour, sugar, and cornmeal. Perishable foods, such as butter, cheese, fruits, and vegetables, may also be issued.

Unlike some of the other food programs, CSFP distributes the food directly to individuals. Many of the individuals who qualify for SNAP and WIC will qualify for this program as well. Resources through this program may shrink as farm policies change and food costs continue to rise.

Expanded Food and Nutrition Education Program (EFNEP)

The Expanded Food and Nutrition Education Program (EFNEP) does not distribute food supplies. Instead, this program provides individuals with limited resources with the knowledge, skills, attitudes, and changed behavior needed to make healthy food choices. Participants attend a series of classes on food preparation, storage, and safety and sanitation. They will learn how to manage their food budgets effectively. The EFNEP also offers youth programs with topics including nutrition, health, and food preparation.

Factors That Affect Food Choices

A number of factors other than price affect the choices you make when you are shopping for nutritious and wholesome food. For instance, advertising may influence you to try a new product. Perhaps the level or type of processing used to produce a food product is important to you. On the other hand, maybe food additives are your concern. Maybe you feel strongly about buying organic foods or locally grown foods.

Food Advertising

Food advertising may influence your buying behavior more than you realize. Manufacturers spend billions of dollars each year promoting products. Their intent is to sway how you spend your food dollars. They want to convince you one product is different from or better than a competing product.

Advertisers use a number of methods to encourage consumers to buy products. *Informational advertising* tends to focus on facts, such as ingredients, price, and nutrients. This type of information can help you decide how products might fit into your meal planning. Special nutrients found in the product may be highlighted. Food labels may include QR (quick response) codes that can be read with an app on your smartphone. QR codes link you to more information about the food product. For example, if you are buying fish, the QR code information may tell you where and when the fish was caught. Other information might include nutritional information, ingredients, allergens, social compliance programs, usage instructions, advisories and safe handling instructions, and company or brand information.

CASE STUDY

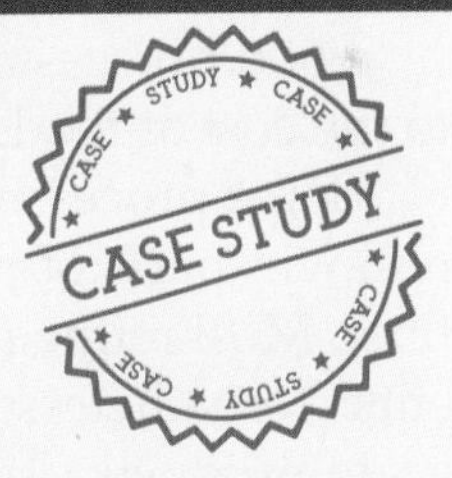

Healthy Party Snacks?

Abby returns home from school to find her favorite magazine *Teens Rock!* has arrived. She decides to flip through the magazine for ideas before writing her shopping list for the party she is planning.

Near the front of the magazine, she notices a colorful ad for a new food snack labeled "Organic Freezer Pops." The ad states the pops are "produced with Mother Nature's own hands!" The ad features a slim teen enjoying the snack while chatting with friends who are looking enviously at the pop. "Perfect," Abby thought, "I can order the package of 24 2-ounce pops for $25 online!"

Abby thought to herself, "My friends will be impressed when I tell them it is a healthy snack." She busily starts to sketch out a list of other snack needs for her after-school party next week.

Case Review

1. What kind of advertising is the food manufacturer using in this advertisement?
2. Do you agree with Abby that pops are a healthy snack? Why?

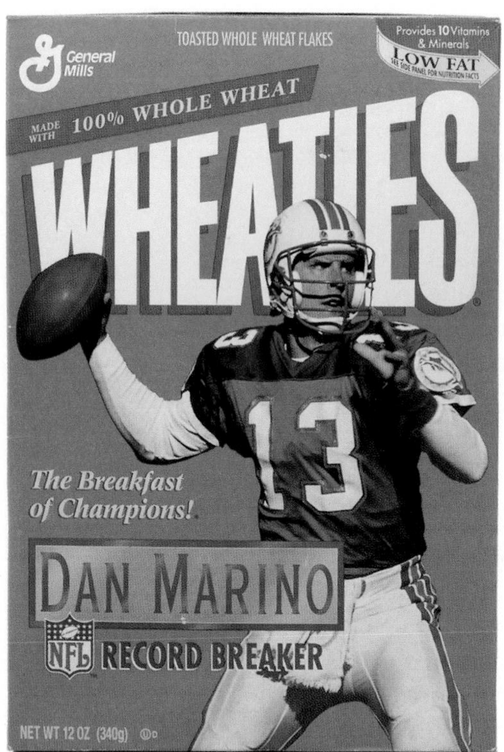

Perry Correll/Shutterstock.com

Figure 18.9 Sometimes both informational and persuasive advertising is used. *What kind of advertising can you identify on this cereal box?*

Persuasive advertising appeals to your human needs and desires for love, beauty, physical power, social approval, and happiness. Often, food is advertised for its impact on your life rather than for its nutritional value. For instance, an advertisement may imply you will be more popular if your friends observe you drinking the newest sports drink (**Figure 18.9**).

Be aware of how advertising is affecting your shopping decisions. Some ads are helpful, but others may cause you to overspend or buy items you do not need or want.

Food Processing

The degree to which foods are processed may influence some of your purchasing decisions. ***Food processing*** refers to any procedure performed on food to prepare it for consumers. Food processing is a continuum ranging from whole food (no processing) to heavily processed food.

Advantages

Some food processing offers consumers advantages. For instance, canning green beans preserves them for long-term storage. Pasteurizing milk kills harmful bacteria and makes the milk safer to drink. Washing, cutting, and boning chicken save consumers preparation time. Fortifying margarine makes it more nutritious. Some chemical and physical changes occur during processing (**Figure 18.10**). As you may realize from these examples, preparing meals without some processed foods is nearly impossible.

Disadvantages

Food processing also has some disadvantages for consumers. Processing adds to the cost of foods. The more processed a food is, the higher its price tends to be.

Some processing methods result in nutrient loss. For instance, refining grains removes parts of the grain kernel that are rich in vitamins, minerals, protein, and fiber. Most refined grain products are enriched to add back some of the lost nutrients. Nonetheless, enriched products do not match the nutrient levels of whole-grain products.

Some studies have shown that eating patterns consisting largely of heavily processed foods contribute to the potential for overweight and obesity. Heavily processed foods include snack-type foods, such as chips, cookies, fruit tarts, and frozen pizza. Soft drinks, instant noodle products, or chicken nuggets are also considered heavily processed. Heavily processed foods often include unrecognizable ingredients.

Weighing the Factors

Your shopping task is not easy. There are many factors to consider, such as convenience, cost, potential environmental impact from processing or packaging, and nutritional value. As you make your food choice, consider what has been added to the food during the processing. Perhaps large amounts of salt, sugar, and fats? Then think about what has been removed from the food during processing. Perhaps fiber, vitamins, minerals, and phytochemicals?

Effects of Food Processing	
Processing Technique	**Chemical and Physical Effects on Foods**
Canning	Canning involves heating foods in sealed containers to destroy organisms that can cause disease or produce toxins. Heat causes changes in texture, color, and nutritive value of food products. Canned foods maintain quality for 1 to 2 years.
Aseptic canning	This processing method may use temperatures as high as 302°F (150°C) to sterilize food in as little as one second. This short time minimizes changes to the food product. Sterilized food is then placed in sterilized packages within a sterile environment.
Dehydration	Dehydration preserves food by lowering its water content. This stops microbe growth and inactivates enzymes. As food loses water, its weight and size are reduced. Its texture may become leathery or brittle. Flavors often become more concentrated. Treatments used to prevent enzymatic browning may destroy some vitamins in the food.
Fermentation	Microbes are added to cause specific enzymatic changes in some food products. As enzymes break down components in the food product, by-products such as carbon dioxide, acidic and lactic acids, and ethanol may be released. These by-products can change the texture, flavor, and keeping quality of foods such as bread, cheeses, and pickles.
Freezing	Freezing increases shelf life of food by slowing the growth of microbes and the chemical reaction rate of enzymes. Most frozen foods maintain their quality for three to nine months. Rapid freezing right after harvesting is best for preserving food texture and nutrients. Treatment of fruits and vegetables before freezing helps prevent darkening.
Irradiation	Irradiation exposes approved foods to radiant energy that kills bacteria and parasites in the food. This improves food safety and increases shelf life. Irradiation does not change food's nutritional value or flavor.
Pasteurization	Pasteurization involves heating a food product to 161°F (72°C) for 15 seconds to reduce enzyme activity and destroy pathogens and some spoilage bacteria. This improves food safety and increases shelf life. Pasteurization can affect food flavors and destroy heat-sensitive nutrients, which may be replaced through fortification.
Ultrapasteurization	Ultrapasteurization heats a food product to a higher temperature (280°F, 138°C) for a shorter time (2 seconds) than pasteurization. This process also affects food flavors and destroys heat-sensitive nutrients, which may be replaced through fortification. Foods treated with this process can be stored at room temperature until opened.

Figure 18.10 Food processing may affect both the physical and chemical characteristics of food products.

Food Irradiation

In 1963, the FDA determined food irradiation to be a safe process. ***Food irradiation*** is the treatment of approved foods with ionizing energy. Ionizing energy creates positive and negative charges. Irradiation of foods is a useful method for

- food preservation
- food sterilization
- control of sprouting, ripening, and insect damage
- control of foodborne illness

THE MOVEMENT CONNECTION

Core Strengthening

Why

Many factors affect your food purchasing decisions. Food choices are the result of an internal decision about what to eat and why. Consistently choosing to eat healthy foods requires inner strength.

It's difficult to feel strong inside if you are not also physically strong. Developing your core strength is the foundation on which physical strength is built.

The following exercise targets not just your leg muscles, but also works your core muscles.

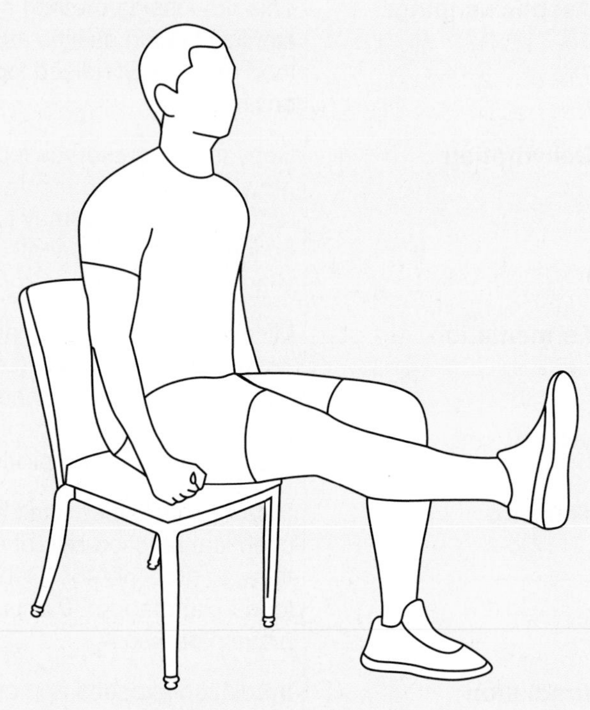

Apply

- Sit in your chair with good posture.
- Engage your core muscles as you straighten and lift your right leg until it is parallel to the floor.
- Hold this position for two seconds.
- Return your leg to the floor, and repeat the move with the left leg.
- Repeat 10 times on each side.

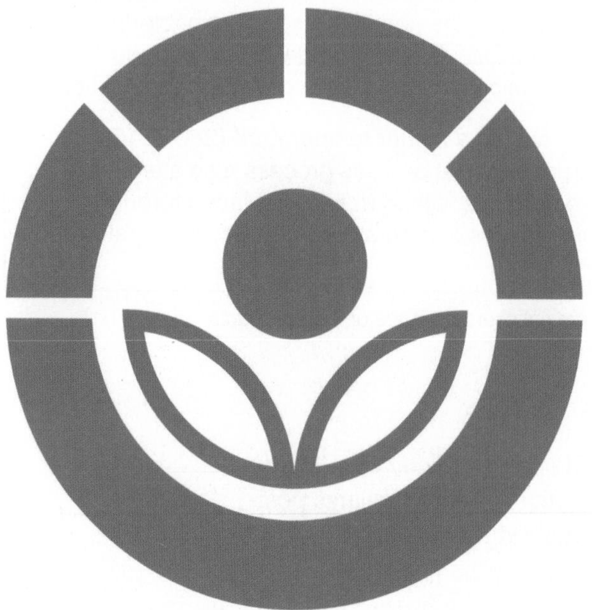

Lack-O'Keen/Shutterstock.com

Figure 18.11 The international symbol named *radura* is used to identify irradiated foods.

Irradiation improves food safety and extends shelf life by killing or inactivating organisms that cause food spoilage and decomposition. It kills harmful bacteria and parasites (not viruses) that can cause foodborne illness. Irradiation does not change the food itself in any way. It does not make the food radioactive. It is impossible to detect if food has been exposed to irradiation.

The first food approved for irradiation by the FDA was for US space program astronauts. If you have eaten any spices, you probably already sampled irradiated food. Spices are the most commonly irradiated food in the world. The other foods approved by the FDA for irradiation include fruits, vegetables, lettuce, spinach, wheat flour, potatoes, fresh shell eggs, pork, poultry, and red meat. The FDA requires a special symbol on the labels of irradiated food (**Figure 18.11**).

During irradiation, foods go through some slight chemical and nutritional changes. Electromagnetic waves strike molecules in the food product. The force breaks molecular bonds, and new compounds are produced, such as carbon dioxide, formic acid, and glucose. These substances are commonly found in all types of foods. No substances produced have been found to be harmful. Keeping food temperatures and oxygen levels in check during irradiation limits damage to nutrients. It causes little change in flavor, texture, or color of most foods.

Irradiation is a safe, effective, and thoroughly tested method for preserving food. Nonetheless, food irradiation does not protect against future contamination, and consumers are still expected to wash and refrigerate irradiated foods for safe use. Restaurants are not required to provide labeling for irradiated foods on the menu.

Food Additives

Food additives are substances added to food products to cause desired changes in the products. Substances added to foods during processing may affect some of your consumer choices.

The Food and Drug Administration (FDA) regulates the use of food additives. The FDA places food additives that have proven to be safe on the ***generally recognized as safe (GRAS) list***. The GRAS list includes sugar, salt, and hundreds of other substances. GRAS list substances are also called *ingredients* in processed foods. The FDA has reviewed substances on the GRAS list and removed those whose safety is suspect. Manufacturers can freely use any of the substances on the GRAS list.

Manufacturers must seek FDA approval to use any food additives other than those on the GRAS list. The FDA will not approve the use of any substance found to cause cancer in humans or animals. Aspartame, nitrites, and synthetic food colorings are among the hundreds of additives used in foods.

Most packaged foods contain additives to perform one or more of the following functions:

- preserve food
- enhance colors, flavors, or textures
- maintain or improve nutritional quality
- aid processing

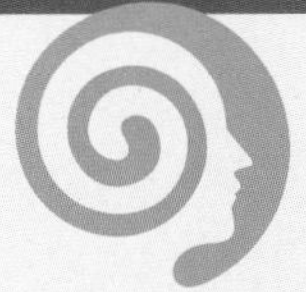

EXTEND YOUR KNOWLEDGE

The Delaney Clause

The Delaney Clause was included in the Food Additives Amendment of 1958 and the Color Additives Amendment of 1960. This clause stated that no food or color additives could be approved for use in foods if they were shown to cause cancer in humans or animals.

The intent of the clause was good, but it created some problems. Experts questioned whether results of experiments in which lab animals were fed extremely high levels of a substance over a lifetime were relevant to humans eating much smaller amounts. In addition, advances in technology made the zero-cancer-risk standard established by this clause impractical.

In 1996, US foods safety laws were reformed. As a result, a new safety standard was established limiting quantities of these substances in foods to levels that ensured reasonable certainty of no harm to consumers.

Food manufacturers must limit additive use to the smallest amount needed to produce a desired effect. Even so, some people have adverse reactions to certain food additives. Others want to limit their intake of food additives. Reading ingredient labels on food products will help people avoid specific additives if desired (**Figure 18.12**). As a wise consumer, you must weigh the costs and benefits of buying foods that contain additives.

Locally Grown

A growing number of people are interested in participating in sustainable living practices. Eating locally grown foods is an example of a sustainable living practice. People choose to shop for locally grown foods for many social and environmental reasons.

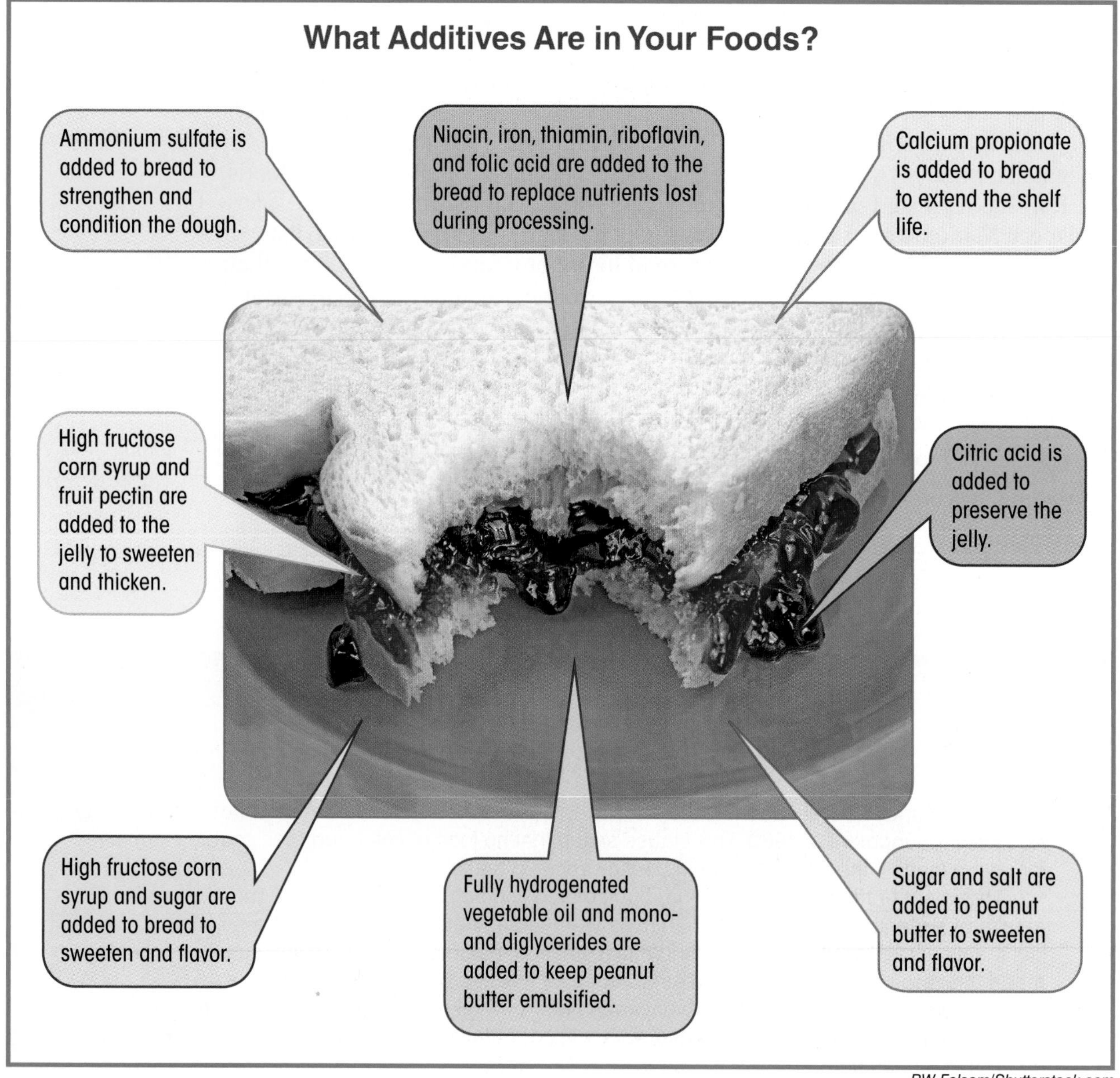

What Additives Are in Your Foods?
Ammonium sulfate is added to bread to strengthen and condition the dough.
Niacin, iron, thiamin, riboflavin, and folic acid are added to the bread to replace nutrients lost during processing.
Calcium propionate is added to bread to extend the shelf life.
High fructose corn syrup and fruit pectin are added to the jelly to sweeten and thicken.
Citric acid is added to preserve the jelly.
High fructose corn syrup and sugar are added to bread to sweeten and flavor.
Fully hydrogenated vegetable oil and mono- and diglycerides are added to keep peanut butter emulsified.
Sugar and salt are added to peanut butter to sweeten and flavor.

BW Folsom/Shutterstock.com

Figure 18.12 Even a simple peanut butter and jelly sandwich can contain many food additives. *What might be the outcome if all food additives were banned?*

When you hear "locally grown food" perhaps you imagine food that has been grown or raised on small, nearby family farms or greenhouses. However, the USDA has no strict definition for what makes a food locally grown.

In the absence of regulation, businesses have established standards that vary widely. Some retailers and restauranteurs define locally grown food as food grown within a 50-mile radius of the business. Others extend the range to as much as a 150-mile radius. Some businesses use the term *locally grown* solely for marketing purposes. Therefore, if you value eating locally grown foods, you should ask what definition the business is using.

How far food travels from the farm to your plate is called *food miles*. Some people believe food miles are the way to judge the food's impact on the climate. However, some studies have shown that transporting food accounts for only 11 percent of greenhouse gases related to food consumption. The majority of these gases result from the practices used to grow and harvest the foods. For example, it may be more efficient to transport lettuce from a warmer growing climate than to heat a greenhouse to grow lettuce locally.

Nevertheless, the benefits of eating locally grown foods are many (**Figure 18.13** on the next page). When the growers are local and accessible, you can ask questions about farming practices used to raise and harvest the crops or recommendations for how best to store and prepare the food.

Learning more about where your food is grown and who grew it contributes to mindful eating.

Organically Grown

Just as you may be concerned about the chemical additives in processed foods, you may also be concerned about the chemicals used to grow foods. If so, you may want to shop for organic foods. ***Organic foods*** are produced without the use of synthetic fertilizers, pesticides, antibiotics, herbicides, or growth hormones. Materials and farming methods are used that are designed to be in ecological balance. Organic farmers often use manure or compost to enrich the soil. They may hoe to control weeds and use natural pesticides to control insects.

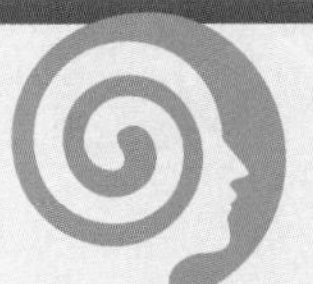

EXTEND YOUR KNOWLEDGE

Organic Labeling

When shopping for organic foods, look for the USDA organic seal. Food production is overseen by a USDA National Organic Program-authorized certifying agent. To qualify means following all USDA organic regulations. The label provides a seal on fresh or processed products that contain organic ingredients. Be familiar with the different levels of organic labeling:

- If the product is labeled "100 Percent Organic," the product must contain only organic ingredients, not including water and salt. Genetic engineering, ionized radiation, and use of sewage sludge is excluded.
- Products labeled "Organic" must contain at least 95 percent organic products, not including water and salt.
- Foods labeled "Made with Organic Ingredients or Foods" must contain 70 percent or more organic ingredients, not including water and salt. These labels cannot display the USDA Organic Seal.
- Products containing less than 70 percent organic ingredients can list organic ingredients in the ingredients statement, but cannot display the USDA Organic Seal.

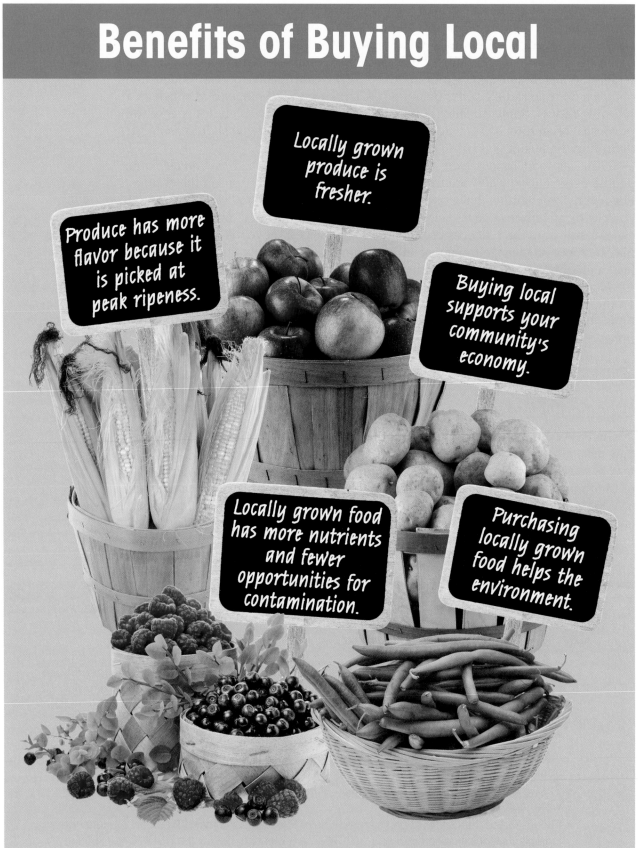

Produce has more flavor because it is picked at peak ripeness.
Buying local supports your community's economy.
Locally grown food has more nutrients and fewer opportunities for contamination.

Sign: nito/Shutterstock.com; Clockwise from top: Photoexpert/Shutterstock.com; Jamie Roach/Shutterstock.com; Hong Vo/Shutterstock.com; Madlen/Shutterstock.com; Alexander Iotzov/Shutterstock.com

Figure 18.13 In addition to farmers' markets, locally grown foods are being offered at restaurants and supermarkets.

The United States Department of Agriculture (USDA) established standards and a certification program for organic products sold in this country. The USDA organic seal on a product means the ingredients and production methods have been **verified** (confirmed) by a certifying agency as meeting or exceeding USDA standards for organic production (**Figure 18.14**). This seal assures consumers they are buying a product that is uniform and consistent with federal standards.

The organics food industry is growing. Sales of organic foods are expected to continue to increase. The average cost of organic foods is usually higher than similar nonorganic foods. Many organic farms are small although larger food manufacturers are also interested in a share of the organic food sales. Small organic farms cannot produce and ship foods as economically as large farming operations. Covering their production costs raises food prices.

Some health-conscious consumers prefer organic produce, eggs, milk, meats, and other products. They may think these foods are more nutritious. However, research has not yet found this to be the case. Many consumers who choose organics are also concerned about the pesticide residues on nonorganic fruits and vegetables. However, many residues can be removed from nonorganics by washing them in cool running water. Washing is an important step when preparing any fresh produce to remove soil, other debris, and insects.

Resolving Problem Purchases

As a consumer, you have power. A ***consumer*** is someone who buys and uses products and services. People who produce and sell products and services want to keep you happy. They want you to continue spending your money on the items they offer. For this reason, most businesses will try to resolve any problems you may have with a purchase. However, if a business is unable or unwilling to resolve an issue, you have a course of action. First, you must be familiar with your rights and responsibilities as a consumer.

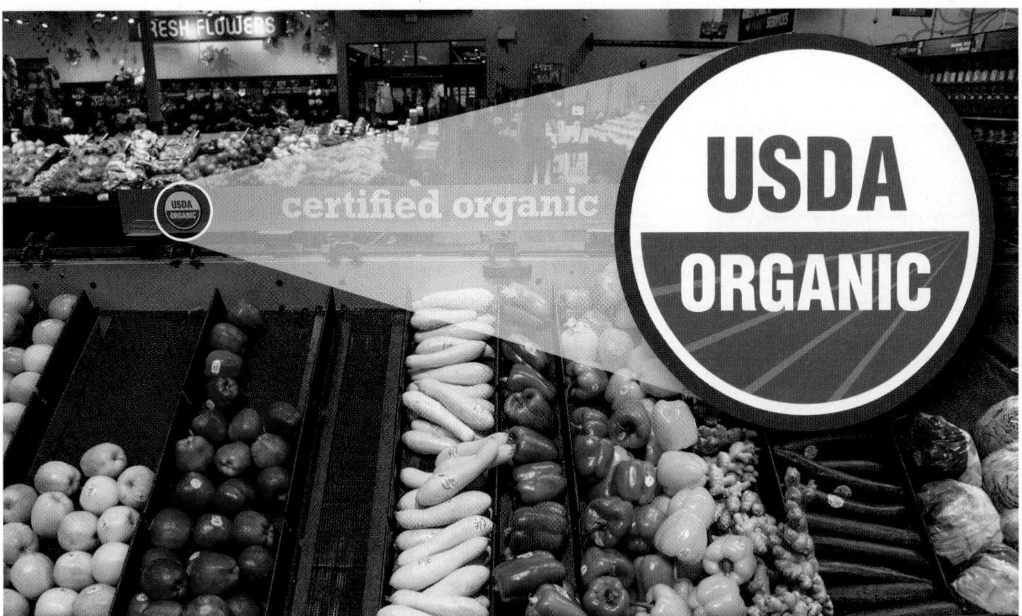

Photo: Trong Nguyen/Shutterstock.com; logo: USDA

Figure 18.14 Look for this seal when buying organic foods to be sure they have been produced in accordance with USDA standards.

Consumer Rights and Responsibilities

Consumers have specific rights, some of which are protected by federal laws. Consumers also have responsibilities. You must use your consumer power in appropriate ways when you have problems in the marketplace. Consumers have rights and responsibilities when buying food, services, and other products (**Figure 18.15**)

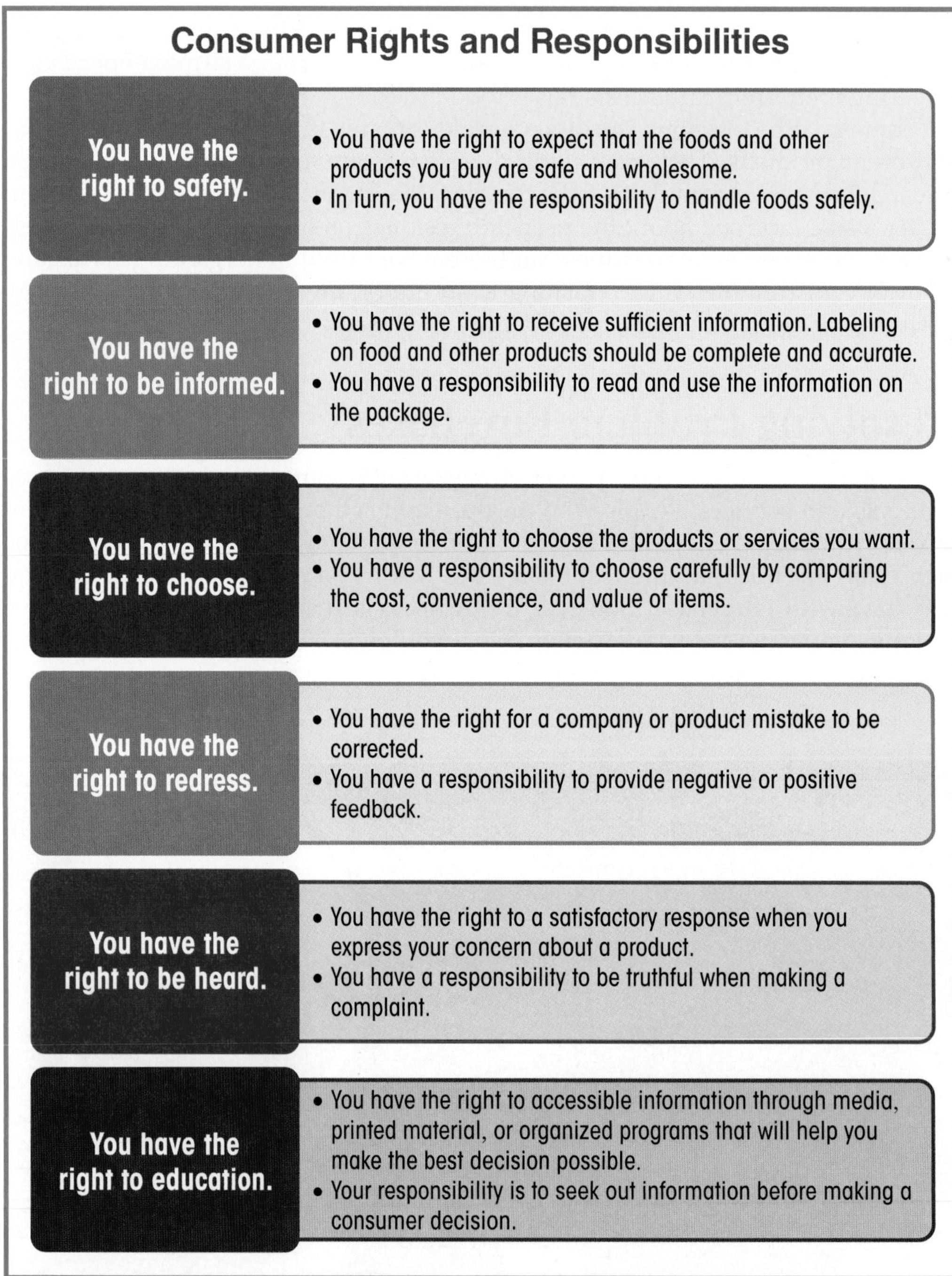

Consumer Rights and Responsibilities	
You have the right to safety.	• You have the right to expect that the foods and other products you buy are safe and wholesome. • In turn, you have the responsibility to handle foods safely.
You have the right to be informed.	• You have the right to receive sufficient information. Labeling on food and other products should be complete and accurate. • You have a responsibility to read and use the information on the package.
You have the right to choose.	• You have the right to choose the products or services you want. • You have a responsibility to choose carefully by comparing the cost, convenience, and value of items.
You have the right to redress.	• You have the right for a company or product mistake to be corrected. • You have a responsibility to provide negative or positive feedback.
You have the right to be heard.	• You have the right to a satisfactory response when you express your concern about a product. • You have a responsibility to be truthful when making a complaint.
You have the right to education.	• You have the right to accessible information through media, printed material, or organized programs that will help you make the best decision possible. • Your responsibility is to seek out information before making a consumer decision.

Figure 18.15 Consumer rights and responsibilities help to prevent a business from taking unfair advantage of a customer. *Is it possible for a customer to take unfair advantage of a business?*

Consumer Complaint Process

For one reason or another, you may find the need to make a consumer complaint. Perhaps you bought a package of cheese that was moldy when you opened it. For this and other reasons, a complaint may be in order.

To receive a satisfactory response to your complaint, you need to complain to the right party. If the product you bought came from a local store, your first step is to return the item. Bring your receipt to document when and where you bought the item. State your complaint to the manager. The manager may simply return your money or offer you a replacement product.

Sometimes it may be more appropriate to contact the manufacturer of a product. Look for a toll-free number, website, or e-mail address on the product package. You can use these resources to contact a consumer service representative. Clearly explain your problem. Have the product package handy to answer manufacturer queries regarding package code numbers and other identification information.

If a store or manufacturer cannot resolve your problem, you may want to contact an appropriate government office. State, county, and local consumer protection offices can settle complaints and conduct investigations. The FDA can help you with problems with food products. The US Consumer Product Safety Commission (CPSC) can help solve problems related to other types of products.

When you call, ask to speak to a consumer affairs officer. Again, clearly explain your problem. The officer may be able to take action on your behalf to find an acceptable solution.

RECIPE FILE

Roasted Broccolini

6 SERVINGS

Ingredients

- 1 bunch (about 1½ lb.) broccolini
- 2 t. olive oil
- 1½ T. Parmesan cheese, grated
- pepper to taste

Directions

1. Preheat oven to 435°F (224°C).
2. Line a baking sheet with foil and spray with cooking spray.
3. Spread broccolini on baking sheet and drizzle with olive oil.
4. Sprinkle with Parmesan cheese and pepper.
5. Roast for 20 minutes, or until broccolini is slightly crispy.

PER SERVING: 43 CALORIES, 3 G PROTEIN, 5 G CARBOHYDRATE, 3 G FAT, 2 G FIBER, 24 MG SODIUM.

Chapter 18 Review and Expand

Reading Summary

There are many types of food stores; each has advantages and disadvantages. The latest supermarket trends are geared toward making food shopping more convenient.

Food costs can be controlled by using tools such as a spending plan, a shopping list, price comparison, low-cost meal strategies, and food assistance resources. Cost-cutting strategies are applied both during meal planning and while shopping.

A number of factors affect your choices when shopping for food. You may be swayed by both informational and persuasive advertising. The level of processing, the amount of additives, or if food has been irradiated may affect your choice of foods. Perhaps purchasing locally grown or organic foods influences where you shop and what foods you buy.

As a consumer, you have a number of rights, which are protected by law. You must be aware these rights carry the weight of certain responsibilities. Going through proper channels to make a complaint can help you address problems in the marketplace.

Chapter Vocabulary

1. **Content Terms** In teams, create categories for the following terms and classify as many of the terms as possible. Then, share your ideas with the remainder of the class.

budget	generic product
comparison shopping	impulse buying
congregate meal	national brand
consumer	organic foods
food additive	store brand
food irradiation	unit price
food processing	
generally recognized as safe (GRAS) list	

2. **Academic Terms** Write each of the following terms on a separate sheet of paper. For each term, quickly write a word you think relates to the term. In small groups, exchange papers. Have each person in the group explain a term on the list. Take turns until all terms have been explained.

entice	suffice
frugal	verified
fundamental	

Review Learning

3. List five places people shop for food and give one advantage and one disadvantage of each.
4. Describe three supermarket trends that are intended to make shopping more convenient for consumers.
5. Compare informational advertising and persuasive advertising.
6. *True or false?* Irradiated foods kill harmful bacteria and parasites (not viruses) that can cause foodborne illness.
7. What reasons do people give for buying locally grown produce?
8. Why do organic foods tend to cost more than nonorganic foods?
9. _____ _____ products are distributed and advertised throughout the country by major food companies.
10. Give five food cost-cutting strategies.
11. How could impulse buying affect a food budget?
12. What is a definition of a food product labeled *organic*?
13. *True or false?* The first step in filing a consumer complaint is to speak with the appropriate government agency.

Self-Assessment Quiz

Complete the self-assessment quiz online to help you practice and expand your knowledge and skills.

Critical Thinking

14. **Compare and Contrast** Compare an organically grown food product with its traditionally grown counterpart for flavor, cost, and nutrient content. Display your findings in a visual format such as a bar chart or infographic.
15. **Conclude** What impact do you think food advertising has on consumer purchases? Provide examples of misleading food advertising. Draw conclusions on how food advertising influences consumers to purchase less-healthful food choices.

16. **Analyze** Select a national food store or manufacturer and research to learn the number of methods the company uses to distribute coupons to consumers. (For example, store flyers, coupon app, etc.) Why do you suppose the company chooses to spend money and effort with coupon offers rather than simply reduce prices? Prepare a brief summary of your findings and conclusion.

Core Skills

17. **Technology Literacy** Find QR (quick response) codes on a number of similar food products—for example, ground beef, ground turkey, ground chicken, and vegetable-based patties. What information was provided for each product? Which product provided the most useful information for consumer decision making? Prepare an electronic presentation to report your findings to the class.
18. **Math** Create a list of 10 food items that you purchase often. Visit three different food stores and record the prices for the 10 food items at each location. Prepare an analysis that includes the purchase price, pack size, and unit price for each item on the list and organized by store. Determine which stores in your community have lower food prices. (*Note:* A variety of food items may need to be selected for comparison to get an accurate outcome.) Share the results of your price comparison in a spreadsheet.
19. **Speaking** In small groups, debate the following topic: "Food irradiation should be used on more foods to improve the safety of the food supply." Each team should conduct research to support its arguments.
20. **Math** Select one food that is sold in different forms that vary in the level of processing, ranging from whole food to heavily processed. For example, a potato is sold whole, canned, dehydrated, French fries, or potato chips and so on. Visit the supermarket and record the price per serving for each product. Rank the products by their price per serving. Create a visual representation of your findings such as a bar chart. Include a brief paragraph explaining the cost variations with the bar chart.
21. **Writing** Select one of the food assistance programs discussed in the text or another one of your choosing. Research to learn how a person qualifies for the program, how long the typical recipient is on the program, what type of food or other resources the recipient receives, and any other information about the program. Write an informative paper about the program.
22. **Math** Lena wants to compare the unit price of frozen peas to canned peas. A 10-ounce box of frozen peas has 2½ servings and costs 79 cents. A 15-ounce can of peas has 3½ servings and costs 99 cents. Calculate the price per ounce for both the frozen and canned peas. Which has the lower unit cost?
23. **Listen** Interview a grocery store manager to learn about trends in food products. Prepare for the interview by developing a list of questions to help you better understand the topic. For example, you might ask the following: How does the manager decide where to place the new product and how much shelf space to allocate to the item? How does the manager predict consumer interest in the food item? These questions will also encourage the exchange of information. If you are unclear about any answers, be sure to seek further explanation. Prepare a brief critique of the interview. Consider what aspects of the interview went well and how you could improve your interview skills for the future.
24. **Research** Assume you just landed your first full-time job and are living on your own. Based on your current career goals, research to learn the income you could expect to receive from your first job. Consider where you will be living and research to learn about typical housing, utility, transportation, and other costs in that area. Learn how much you will be paying in taxes and deduct this from the amount of money that will be available for expenses. Find out what you might expect to pay for health insurance. Then prepare a budget including your expenses for food, savings, and entertainment.
25. **Career Readiness Practice** Imagine that you are a nutrition educator for a national supermarket chain. Your job responsibilities include giving supermarket tours focused on healthful eating, demonstrating recipes to customers, and writing articles for the supermarket's information center. This month you will write an article about how to choose the best quality, low-cost fresh foods. Focus especially on in-season produce, low-fat cuts of meat and poultry, quality fish, and low-fat dairy foods. Be sure to include a healthful recipe or two that use six or fewer ingredients.

CHAPTER 19 Preparing Food

Learning Outcomes

After studying this chapter, you will be able to

- **demonstrate** correct use of a recipe;
- **describe** the different food preparation techniques and their uses;
- **compare** the different cooking methods;
- **understand** the characteristics of common foods from each food group;
- **select** appropriate cooking method for different foods; and
- **create** a healthier recipe by modifying ingredients and cooking methods.

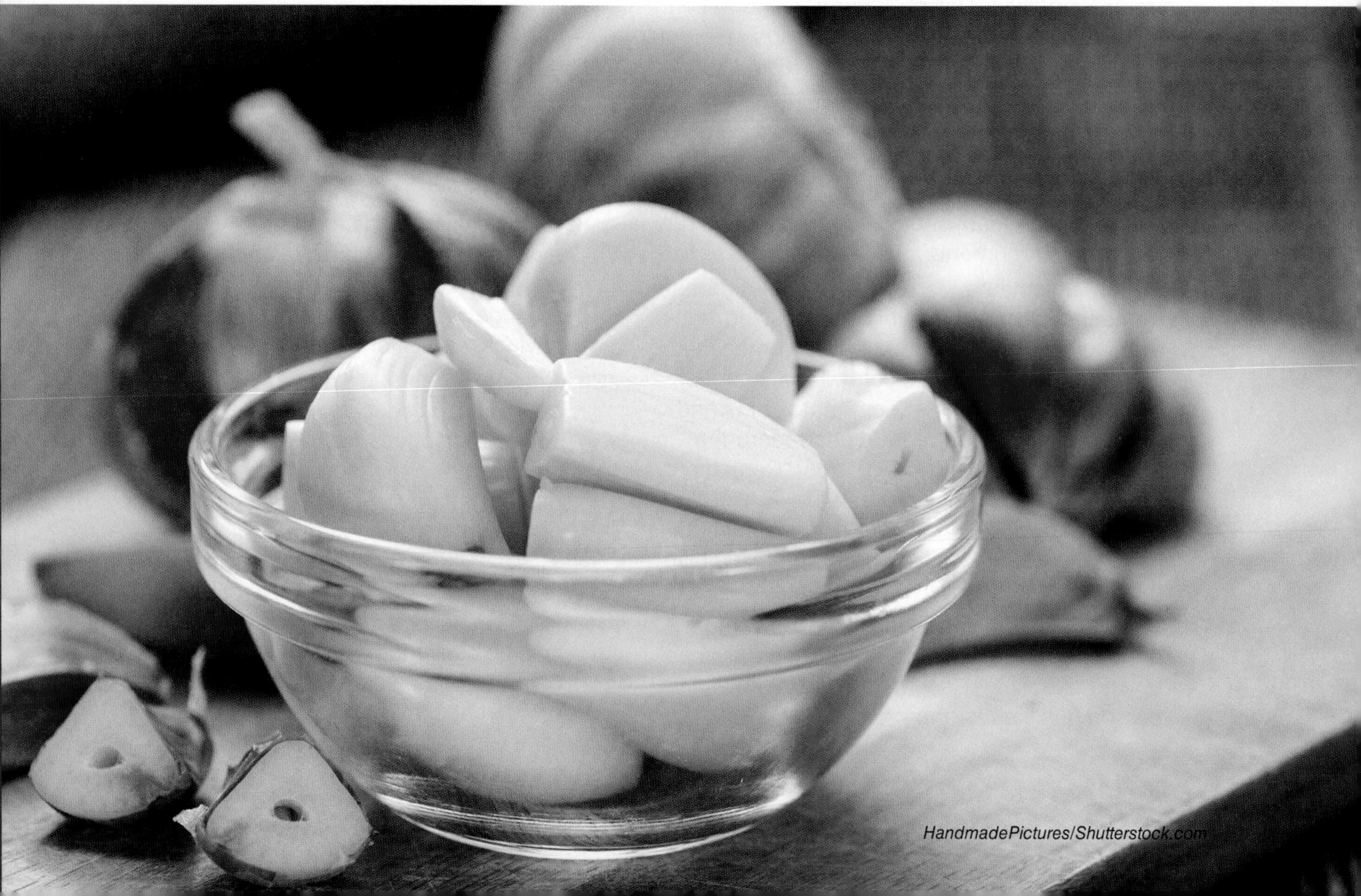

HandmadePictures/Shutterstock.com

Content Terms

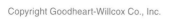

al dente
caramelization
combination cooking method
conduction
convection
conversion factor
curdle
dry-heat cooking method
elastin
gluten
homogenization
Maillard reaction
mise en place
moist-heat cooking method
pasteurization
radiation
recipe
scorch
sear
tempering

Academic Terms

medium
opaque
palatability
proximate
reconstitute
residual
translucent

What's Your Nutrition and Wellness IQ?

Take this quiz to examine how much you already know about food preparation. If you cannot answer a question, pay extra attention to that topic as you study this chapter.

- Identify each ent as *True*, *False*, or *It Depends*. *It Depends* means in some cases the statement is true; in some cases it could be false.
- Revise false statements to make them true.
- Explain the circumstances in which each *It Depends* statement is true and when it is false.

Nutrition and Wellness IQ

1.	It is unnecessary to read a recipe in advance of preparing it.	True	False	It Depends
2.	The teaspoon that you eat cereal with and the teaspoon in a measuring spoon set are interchangeable.	True	False	It Depends
3.	Dry ingredients and liquid ingredients are measured differently.	True	False	It Depends
4.	Simmering and boiling cooking methods are the same.	True	False	It Depends
5.	Metal conducts heat more effectively than liquid.	True	False	It Depends
6.	Refined grains typically require longer cooking times than whole grains.	True	False	It Depends
7.	Milk products are defined by their butterfat content.	True	False	It Depends
8.	It is best to use the freshest eggs possible when cooking.	True	False	It Depends
9.	Poaching and braising are healthier cooking methods than panfrying.	True	False	It Depends

While studying this chapter, look for the activity icon  **to**

- **build** vocabulary with e-flash cards and interactive games;
- **assess** what you learn by completing self-assessment quizzes and completing review questions; and
- **expand** knowledge with interactive activities and activities that extend learning.

www.g-wlearning.com/foodsandnutrition/

Every day—three times a day (or more)—you place food in your body. Common sense would tell you that something you do this often has a significant impact on your health. This logic supports the belief that good health begins in the kitchen, and this means that you hold the key to your future health.

By learning a few basic skills, you can positively influence your eating pattern and your future health. This chapter provides you with the basic knowledge you need to begin cooking.

Using a Recipe

Organization is essential for successful food preparation. The French term for this is ***mise en place (meez ahn PLAHS)***, meaning "everything in its place." In other words, all the necessary ingredients and utensils are available, equipment is in good working order, and the cook (you) understands the required preparation techniques. Mise en place begins with reading the recipe.

A ***recipe*** is a set of instructions for preparing a particular food item, including a list of ingredients and a preparation method. Most importantly, the measurements, temperatures, and cooking times listed in a recipe must be accurate.

Learning how to read a recipe is an important first step toward successful meal preparation. Although recipes can be written using one of several formats, all must include a few standard components.

Recipe Components

All recipes must include the following components: title, yield, list of ingredients, and directions (**Figure 19.1**). Some recipes also include a nutrition analysis. Most importantly, the measurements, temperatures, and cooking times must be accurate and all of the ingredients must be included.

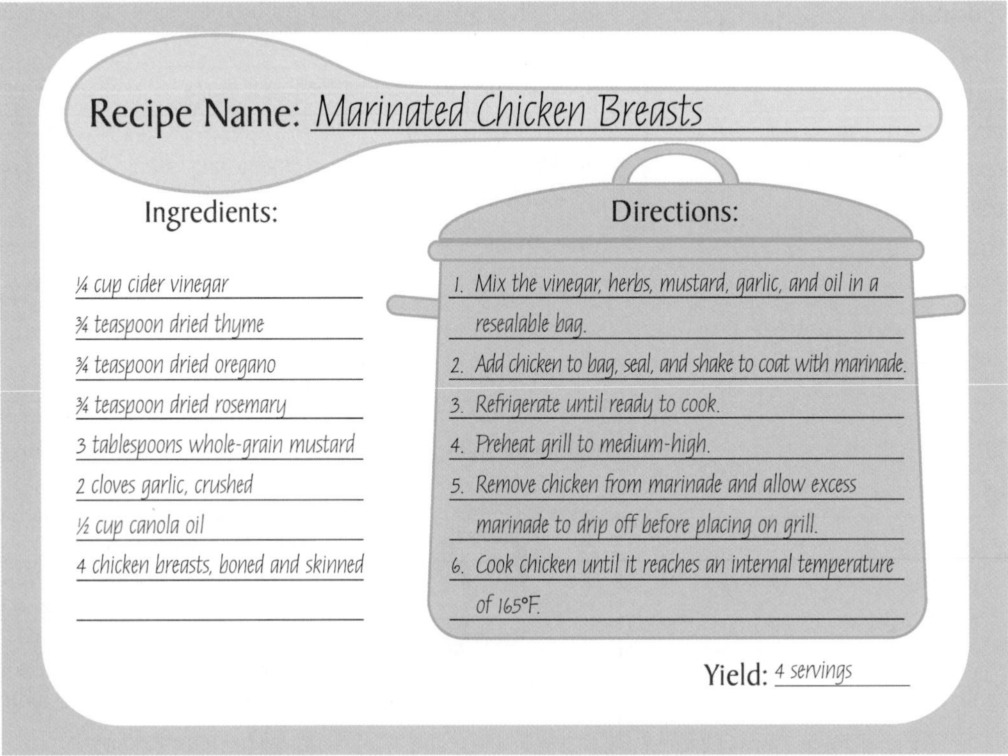

Recipe Name: Marinated Chicken Breasts
Ingredients:
¼ cup cider vinegar
¾ teaspoon dried thyme
¾ teaspoon dried oregano
¾ teaspoon dried rosemary
3 tablespoons whole-grain mustard
2 cloves garlic, crushed
½ cup canola oil
4 chicken breasts, boned and skinned
Directions:
1. Mix the vinegar, herbs, mustard, garlic, and oil in a resealable bag.
2. Add chicken to bag, seal, and shake to coat with marinade.
3. Refrigerate until ready to cook.
4. Preheat grill to medium-high.
5. Remove chicken from marinade and allow excess marinade to drip off before placing on grill.
6. Cook chicken until it reaches an internal temperature of 165°F.
Yield: 4 servings

Figure 19.1
Recipes may have different formats, but all should include a title, list of ingredients, directions, and yield.

Recipe graphics: ZenFruitGraphics/Shutterstock.com

The title is the name of the recipe. The yield is the amount of food the completed recipe produces. The yield may be listed as a number of servings, a quantity (e.g., two dozen cookies), or a volume (e.g., one quart). All recipes must include a complete list of ingredients and their required amounts. The ingredients are listed in order of their use.

Recipes also have a list of step-by-step directions that includes the cooking temperature, cooking time, and cooking methods. Some recipes identify the equipment needed to prepare the recipe and the size of cookware needed. More often, you must determine this based on the preparation methods used in the recipe and the amount the recipe yields. A nutritional analysis lists the amount of calories, protein, fat, sodium, fiber, or other nutrients in one serving of the recipe.

Measurement Units and Abbreviations

Understanding measurement units and their abbreviations is one of the most important skills necessary to read and prepare a recipe. Measurement mistakes can ruin a dish. Many recipes are written using measurement abbreviations. Understanding the meaning of each abbreviation is a basic skill necessary for a successful finished product (**Figure 19.2**).

Ingredient quantities may be expressed as a volume or a weight. Volume and weight are different units of measure and not easily interchangeable. For example, four ounces by weight of shredded cheese may yield one cup by volume. This may seem incorrect because one cup is equal to eight ounces. However, volume describes an amount of space the ingredient assumes and the weight describes how heavy it is.

Common Recipe Abbreviations	
approximate = approx.	ounce = oz.
cup = C. or c.	package = pkg.
dozen = doz.	pint = pt.
fluid ounce = fl. oz.	pound = lb. or #
gallon = gal.	quart = qt.
gram = g	tablespoon = Tbsp. or T.
kilogram = kg	teaspoon = tsp. or t.
liter = L	volume = vol.
milliliter = mL	weight = wt.

Figure 19.2 Recipes employ common abbreviations for consistency and clarity.

FEATURED CAREER

Personal Chef

Personal chefs work for individuals. They plan and prepare meals in private homes according to the client's tastes or dietary needs. They order groceries and supplies, clean the kitchen, and wash dishes and utensils. They also may serve meals. Personal chefs usually prepare a week's worth of meals in the client's home for the client to heat and serve according to directions. These chefs typically work full-time for one client, such as corporate executives, university presidents, or diplomats, who regularly entertain as a part of their official duties.

Education

Most personal chefs have some postsecondary training. Formal training may take place at a community college, technical school, culinary arts school, or a college with a degree in hospitality. A growing number of chefs participate in training programs sponsored by independent cooking schools, professional culinary institutes, or in the armed forces.

Job Outlook

Job openings for personal chefs are expected to be good. However, competition should be keen.

Consider a gallon jug filled with pennies and a gallon jug filled with feathers. Which would you rather drop on your toe? Although both are the same volume, a gallon jug of pennies can weigh 35 pounds, whereas a gallon jug filled with loosely packed feathers can weigh as little as 1½ ounces. Measuring ingredients by weight is far more accurate and that is why professional chefs measure by weight when cooking. However, home cooks often use both weight and volume.

In the United States, customary units of measure are used, whereas most other countries use metric units of measure. Customary units of volume include gallon, quart, pint, cup, fluid ounce, tablespoon, and teaspoon. Customary units of weight include pound and ounce. Metric units of measure use the liter as a base for volume and the gram as a base for weight (**Figure 19.3**).

Changing Recipe Yield

Sometimes you need more or less finished product than the recipe yields. When this happens, you need to change the ingredient amounts in your recipe to achieve the desired yield. To know how much to increase or decrease the amounts, you must determine the conversion factor. The ***conversion factor*** is the number used to adjust each original ingredient amount to achieve the desired yield. For example, if you need twice the yield, you will multiply every ingredient quantity by two. In this case, two is the conversion factor. However, the conversion factor may be more difficult to determine. For example, suppose you

Figure 19.3 Learning basic measurement equivalents will make reading recipes easier. *How many tablespoons are in ⅜ cup?*

Measurement Equivalents	
Volume (Metric measurements reflect typical metric measuring tool volumes.)	
1 Tbsp. = 3 tsp. = ½ fl. oz. = 15 mL	¾ c. = 12 Tbsp. = 6 fl. oz. = 175 mL
⅛ c. = 2 Tbsp. = 1 fl. oz. = 30 mL	1 c. = 16 Tbsp. = 8 fl. oz. = 250 mL
¼ c. = 4 Tbsp. = 2 fl. oz. = 50 mL	½ pt. = 1 c. = 8 fl. oz. = 250 mL
⅓ c. = 5 Tbsp. + 1 tsp. = 2.65 fl. oz. = 75 mL	1 pt. = 2 c. = 16 fl. oz. = 500 mL
½ c. = 8 Tbsp. = 4 fl. oz. = 125 mL	1 qt. = 2 pt. = 32 fl. oz. = 1 L
⅔ c. = 10 Tbsp. + 2 tsp. = 5 fl. oz. = 150 mL	1 gal. = 4 qt. = 128 fl. oz. = 4 L
Weight	**Fraction to Decimal**
1 oz. = 1/16 lb. = 28 g	⅛ = 0.125
4 oz. = ¼ lb. = 113 g	¼ = 0.250
8 oz. = ½ lb. = 227 g	⅓ = 0.333
12 oz. = ¾ lb. = 340 g	½ = 0.500
16 oz. = 1 lb. = 454 g	⅔ = 0.667
	¾ = 0.750

want enough crust to serve pastries to 20 guests you have invited for dinner. If your recipe yields four servings, multiplying each ingredient by two only increases the yield from four to eight servings. To find the conversion factor, use the following formula:

Desired yield ÷ Original yield = Conversion factor

Insert the original and desired yields into the formula.

20 servings ÷ 4 servings = 5 conversion factor

Then, apply the conversion factor to the ingredient using the following formula:

Original quantity × Conversion factor = New quantity

This formula must be applied to every ingredient in the recipe to change the recipe yield (**Figure 19.4**).

Once you have the new quantities, they must be converted to amounts that are more easily measured. It is more efficient to measure ingredients using the largest appropriate unit of measure. For example, the new butter quantity in Figure 19.4 is expressed using many smaller units of measure (tablespoons) that could be converted to a larger unit of measure (cup). This is performed using measure equivalents.

First, express the new butter quantity in tablespoons as follows:

New quantity = (1⅔ cups × 16 tablespoons/cup) + 10 tablespoons

New quantity = 26 tablespoons + 10 tablespoons = 36 tablespoons

Now, convert the tablespoons back to the larger cup unit of measure.

New quantity = 36 tablespoons ÷ 16 tablespoons/cup = 2¼ cups

Therefore, the new butter quantity should be expressed as 2¼ cups.

Substitutions

Sometimes it is necessary to substitute one ingredient for another in a recipe. Perhaps you forgot to purchase an ingredient, you want to lower the fat or sugar content, or someone in your family has an allergy. To exchange one ingredient for another successfully, you must know the basic properties of the ingredient and its function in the recipe. Substituting nonessential ingredients, like using cranberries instead of raisins, is not likely to ruin your finished product.

Changing Yield: Pastry Crust Recipe

Ingredient	Original Quantity	×	Conversion Factor	=	New Quantity
Flour	1½ cups	×	5	=	7½ cups
Butter	⅓ cup + 2 tablespoons	×	5	=	1⅔ cups + 10 tablespoons
Egg yolk	1	×	5	=	5
Sugar	2 tablespoons	×	5	=	10 tablespoons
Water	¼ cup	×	5	=	1¼ cups

Photo: Sharon Day/Shutterstock.com

Figure 19.4 Adjusting a recipe yield requires only basic math skills.

However, particularly in baked goods, the substitution of basic ingredients such as baking powder, sugar, flour, or eggs can affect the outcome of the recipe. See a list of common substitutions in the appendix.

Food Preparation Techniques and Terms

Food preparation has its own set of vocabulary. The techniques called for and the terms used in recipes have been created to produce a specific outcome. You must learn these terms and techniques to be a successful cook.

Measurement Techniques 

Ingredients may be liquid, dry, or fat. Different types of ingredients require different measuring techniques.

When measuring liquids, use a liquid measuring cup. For amounts less than one-fourth cup, use measuring spoons. Place the measuring cup on a flat, level surface and locate the desired measurement mark on the cup. Bend down until you are at eye level with the mark to make an accurate reading. Pour the liquid into the cup and fill until it reaches the desired mark. When using measuring spoons, carefully fill to the top.

When measuring dry ingredients, use dry measuring cups. For amounts under one-fourth cup, use measuring spoons. Spoon the ingredient into the cup. Overfill the cup and then level off the excess with a straight edge (**Figure 19.5**). When measuring flour, always spoon lightly into the cup or spoon. Do not pack the flour. On the other hand, brown sugar must be packed into the cup or spoon. Overfill the cup, pack it with the back of a spoon or a spatula, and level off the excess with a straight edge.

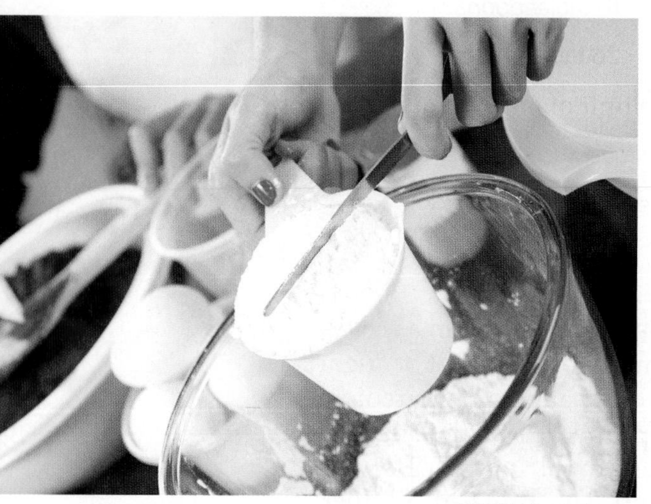

pedalist/Shutterstock.com

Figure 19.5 To measure dry ingredients, overfill the measuring cup and then level off with a straight edge.

Measure fat ingredients such as margarine, shortening, or peanut butter with the same measuring cups and spoons as you use for dry ingredients. Overfill the cup or spoon with the ingredient and press down to remove air pockets. Then, level off the excess with a straight edge. Other moist solids such as pureed pumpkin and tomato paste are measured in the same manner.

The *water displacement method* can also be used to measure solid fats, or other ingredients like baby carrots or olives. Fill a two-cup (or larger) liquid measuring cup to the one-cup mark. To measure ½ cup of either fat or other solid ingredients, add the ingredient to the water slowly until the water reaches the 1½-cup mark. Then carefully drain the water from the ingredient.

Knife Safety and Skills

Food preparation requires the frequent use of knives. To avoid injuries and save time, you must learn how to use the knife safely and correctly.

The first rule of knife safety is to maintain a sharp edge on your knife. Sharp knives slice through ingredients more easily, giving you more control over the knife. Sharp knives also reduce preparation time. Store knives in a drawer, on a magnetic strip, or in a knife block to help maintain their edge.

Set Up the Work Area

Before you begin using your knife, you must set up your work area. Always perform knife work on a clean, stable cutting board. Using a cutting board for knife work not only preserves your knife-edge, but also protects your countertop from cuts and stains. Position the cutting board on a counter that is a comfortable height for you. Then, place a wet dishtowel underneath the cutting board to ensure it will not slide or shift on the countertop while you are cutting. Be sure to clean and sanitize the cutting board after each use.

Grip the Knife

Next, you must learn how to hold the knife correctly. You hold a knife with your dominant hand (the hand you write with) using either the blade grip or the handle grip. To employ the blade grip, place your index finger and thumb on either side of the blade close to the handle. Then wrap the three remaining fingers comfortably around the handle.

All four fingers and your thumb are grasping the handle when using the handle grip. Although many beginning cooks use the handle grip, experienced cooks prefer the blade grip because it offers greater control and balance. Practice using these grips so you become comfortable and the knife becomes an extension of your hand (**Figure 19.6**).

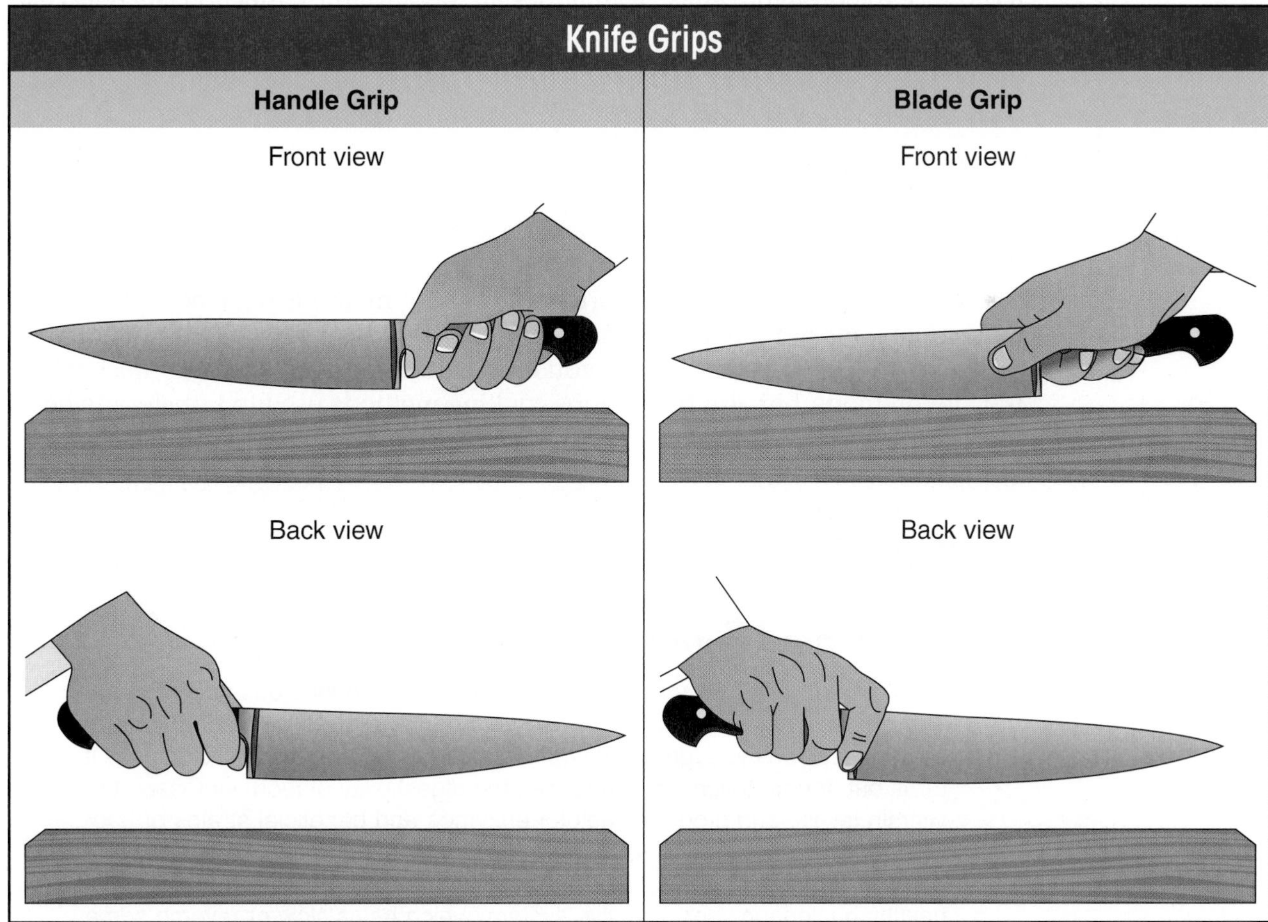

Goodheart-Willcox Publisher

Figure 19.6 Experienced cooks often prefer to use the blade grip when holding a knife. *Why do experienced cooks prefer the blade grip?*

Learn the Cutting Motion

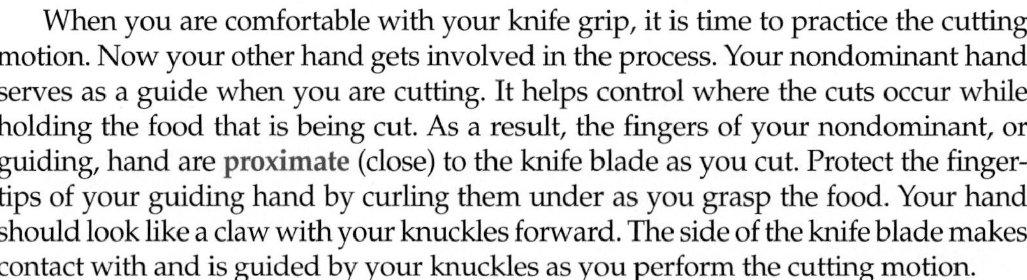

When you are comfortable with your knife grip, it is time to practice the cutting motion. Now your other hand gets involved in the process. Your nondominant hand serves as a guide when you are cutting. It helps control where the cuts occur while holding the food that is being cut. As a result, the fingers of your nondominant, or guiding, hand are **proximate** (close) to the knife blade as you cut. Protect the fingertips of your guiding hand by curling them under as you grasp the food. Your hand should look like a claw with your knuckles forward. The side of the knife blade makes contact with and is guided by your knuckles as you perform the cutting motion.

The cutting motion is a combination of rocking motion—front to back— as well as up and down. This movement should be a smooth, continuous motion. Practice this motion on the cutting board before you attempt it on a food item.

When cutting round or irregularly shaped foods, first trim the food to create a flat surface on one side. Position the food item so the flat surface rests on the cutting board. This will prevent the food from rolling while you are cutting it.

Preparation Techniques

Over time, people have discovered many ways to alter foods with the purpose of creating pleasing dishes. To promote communication and consistency, preparation techniques and terms were established. In this way, any cook could read a recipe and reproduce the desired results. Techniques are organized by function, such as coating, cutting, or combining. To be successful in the kitchen, it is necessary to become familiar with common food preparation terms and techniques (**Figure 19.7**).

Cooking Food

Cooking often involves the application of heat to food. Heat is transferred from the heat source to the food in a number of ways and each produces a recognizable effect on the food. Over time, a variety of cooking methods have been developed that employ one or more heat transfer methods.

To be successful in the kitchen, you must understand not only the effect of heat transfer on foods, but also the various cooking methods used to transfer the heat.

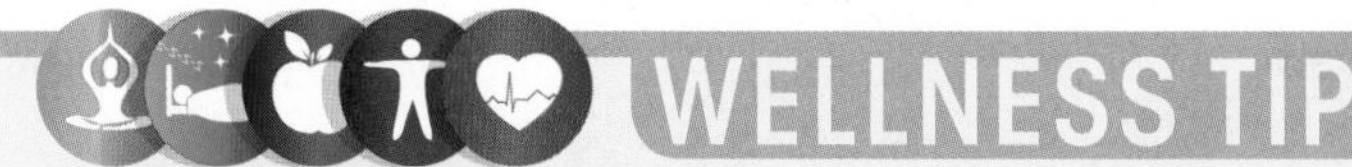

Fermented Foods

The process of fermenting foods has been around for thousands of years. The process was developed to preserve foods. During fermentation, natural bacteria feed on the sugars and starches in the food, creating lactic acid. As it turns out, fermentation also enhances the digestibility of food, increases the vitamin levels, and produces helpful enzymes and beneficial strains of bacteria, or probiotics. Eating fermented foods, like sauerkraut and kimchi, and drinking fermented drinks, like kefir and kombucha, promote the growth of healthy bacteria in your digestive system, which helps slow or reverse some diseases, improves bowel health, and helps you absorb more of the nutrients you eat.

Preparation Terms and Techniques	
Coating Techniques	
baste	Moisten food with pan juices, melted fat, or other liquid during cooking to keep the food moist and add flavor.
bread	Coat food with flour, then beaten egg, and finally bread crumbs or cracker crumbs.
brush	Apply sauce, melted fat, or other liquid to the surface of a food with a pastry brush.
dot	Place small pieces of butter or other ingredient over the surface of food.
dredge	Coat a food with flour, crumbs, or other dry ingredient.
dust	Lightly coat a food with dry ingredients.
flour	Sprinkle or coat with flour.
glaze	Apply a liquid on food to form a glossy coating.
Combining Techniques	
beat	Mix ingredients together with a rapid, circular motion using a spoon, whisk, rotary, or electric beater.
blend	Stir ingredients until they are thoroughly combined.
cream	Brisk mixing of softened fat with sugar to incorporate air.
cut in	Combine solid fat with flour using a pastry blender until the fat is in pea-size pieces and is coated with flour.
fold	Incorporate a delicate mixture into a thicker, heavier mixture with a gentle, lifting motion that moves ingredients from the bottom to the top.
knead	Work dough with a repeated pressing, folding, and turning action until it is smooth, elastic, and gluten develops.
mix	Combine two or more ingredients until evenly dispersed.
stir	Mix gently in a circular motion using a spoon, whisk, or other utensil.
toss	Flip or shake ingredients to combine.
whip	Beat quickly and vigorously with a whisk or whip to incorporate air.
Cutting Techniques	
chop	Cut into small pieces without concern for consistent size or shape.
dice Animation	Cut into small, equal-size cubes; dice cut may be small (1/4 inch), medium (3/8 inch), or large (5/8 inch).
flake	Break or separate off small layers of food; term often used with fish.
grate	Cut food into small pieces by rubbing against a rough surface.
julienne Animation	Cut food into thin, matchstick-size strips measuring 1/8 × 1/8 × 1/2 inches.
mash	Crush food with a spoon, masher, or ricer to produce a smooth pulp.
mince	Cut or chop into very fine pieces.
puree	Process food with a food mill, grinder, or blender to form a thick, smooth liquid.
shred	Cut or grate food to produce long, thin pieces.
snip	Cut into small bits with kitchen shears; often used with fresh herbs.

Continued

Figure 19.7 A glossary of food preparation terms and techniques.

Preparation Terms and Techniques *(Continued)*
Miscellaneous Techniques
deglaze Dissolve browned food bits stuck to the bottom of pan with liquid.
drain Separate solid food from liquid by pouring it through a colander.
marinate Soak a food item, such as meat, in a seasoned liquid to flavor or tenderize.
preheat Heat an appliance to desired temperature before use.
reduce Boil a liquid to decrease the volume by evaporation and intensify the flavor.
season Flavor a food by adding herbs, spices, or other ingredients; prepare a cooking utensil surface, such as a cast-iron skillet, to prevent or limit food from sticking.
shell Remove the tough, inedible outer coating of a food, such as nuts, eggs, or shellfish.
skim Remove a substance from the surface of a liquid.
steep Soak food in a hot liquid to extract flavor or to soften.
strain Separate solid particles from liquid by pouring through a strainer or a sieve.
thicken Increase the density of a liquid by adding a thickening agent, such as flour, cornstarch, or egg yolk.
vent Leave an opening for steam to escape while food is cooking.

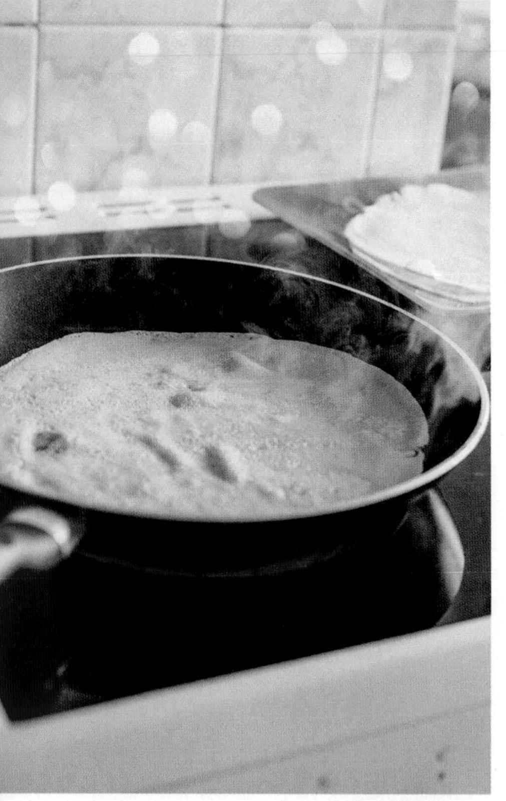

exousia/Shutterstock.com

Figure 19.8 Heat is transferred to food through conduction, convection, or radiation. *How is the heat being transferred to the pancake in this photo?*

Heat Transfer

When heat is transferred to food, it not only warms the food, but also changes the food at a molecular level. Heat also destroys microorganisms and makes food safer to eat. Heat releases the flavors and aromas that make food more pleasing. It also changes the texture and color of foods. For instance, a tough cut of meat may brown and become more tender. A red tomato may become brighter red. Sauces and gravies become thicker. Many foods are more easily digested when cooked, making the nutrients more accessible to the body.

On the other hand, if heat is applied for too long, at an excessive temperature, or with the wrong technique, the texture and nutrient content of food can suffer. For example, heat can destroy vitamin C and the B vitamins. A tender cut of meat can become tough and dry when overcooked. Brightly colored vegetables lose their color and become unappealing. The brown exterior that adds the pleasing flavor and color to a roast or French fries becomes bitter tasting.

Heat Transfer Methods

Heat transfer from the source to the food occurs in one of the following ways: conduction, convection, or radiation. In cooking, the heat source may be a cooktop burner, broiler, grill, or oven.

Conduction transfers heat by direct contact. For example, a cooktop burner conducts heat energy to the metal pan resting on it. The pan then transfers the heat to its contents (food) (**Figure 19.8**). The various **mediums** (substances) through which heat is conducted vary in effectiveness. Some metals conduct heat more effectively than others. Liquids and gases are less effective heat conductors than metal. Regardless of how heat is transferred to a food, the heat moves from the food's surface inward via conduction.

Convection is the movement of molecules from a hotter area to a cooler area in a liquid or gas. This movement transfers the heat as the molecules move. As heat energy is applied from the source, the molecules in the liquid or gas vibrate more quickly, which causes them to move farther apart. This makes the heated liquid or air less dense, causing it to rise. As these hot molecules rise, the molecules of the cooler, denser liquid or air sink to replace them. A circular flow occurs and transfers the heat throughout the product (**Figure 19.9**).

Radiation transfers heat through waves of energy that penetrate food and bump into the molecules of water and fat. These molecules then begin to vibrate, which creates friction. The friction produces heat.

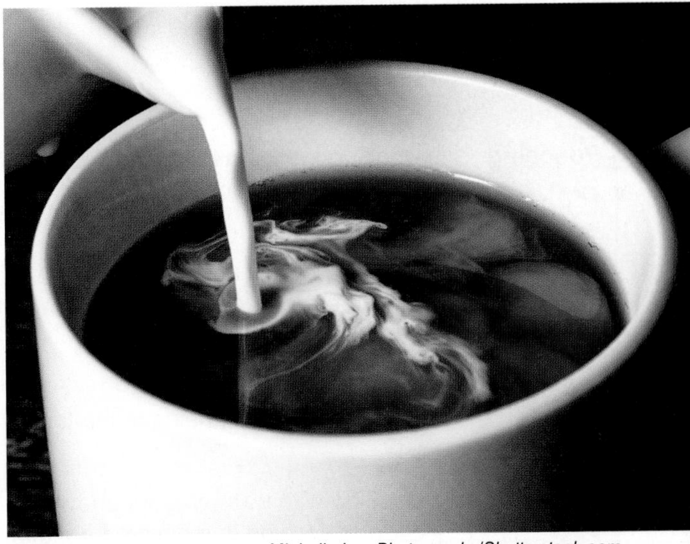

Michelle Lee Photography/Shutterstock.com

Figure 19.9 You can observe convection as currents of cream rise and fall in a cup of hot coffee. *What other heat transfer methods can you observe with a cup of hot coffee?*

Cooking Methods

Different cooking methods produce different effects because each varies in the form of heat transfer used and the medium through which the heat is transferred. Understanding how the various cooking methods affect foods will help you become a better cook and be more flexible with your recipes. A successful cook knows the best cooking method for each type of food.

Each cooking method—moist heat, dry heat, or combination—uses conduction, convection, radiation, or a combination of these to transfer heat to food. The medium through which the heat transfer occurs can be metal, air, fat, water, or steam.

A ***moist-heat cooking method*** uses liquid or steam to transfer heat to food at temperatures ranging from 160°F to 212°F (**Figure 19.10** on the next page). Cooking in flavored liquids like stock, broth, wine, or milk can add flavor to the food. In addition, a sauce can be made from the liquid that remains after cooking. Some moist-heat methods are suitable for inexpensive meat cuts because the moisture acts to tenderize tough fibers. On the other hand, some moist-heat methods are used to cook delicate foods like fish.

A ***dry-heat cooking method*** uses hot air or fat to transfer heat to foods. Dry-heat cooking methods use high temperatures, 300°F or higher (see Figure 19.10). A dry-heat cooking method is any cooking method in which heat is transferred to food in the absence of moisture.

Foods prepared using dry-heat methods are characterized by browning, which contributes a rich flavor. The ***Maillard (my-YAR) reaction*** is a chemical reaction between the amino acids and sugars in a protein food that occurs when dry heat is applied. This reaction is responsible for the browning, as well as the rich, complex flavors and aromas. For example, cooks ***sear***, or brown foods by cooking quickly over high heat, to produce the Maillard reaction and the accompanying flavors.

Cooking Methods	
Moist-Heat Cooking Methods	
Poaching Animation	Cooking food in a liquid between 160°F and 180°F. At this temperature, the liquid moves slightly but produces no bubbles. Flavored liquids are often used for poaching.
Simmering Animation	Cooking food in a liquid between 185°F and 205°F. At this temperature, the liquid shows movement with bubbles rising slowly. Flavored liquids are often used for simmering.
Boiling Animation	Cooking food in a liquid at 212°F. At this temperature, the liquid has a vigorous, rolling action with large bubbles rising to the top.
Steaming Animation	Cooking with water vapors above 212°F by suspending food over boiling water. Steaming is often performed in a covered pot to surround food with the vapor.
Dry-Heat Cooking Methods	
Roasting Animation	Cooking meat, poultry, or vegetables uncovered and surrounded by hot air in an oven at temperatures ranging between 300°F and 425°F.
Baking Animation	Cooking breads, pastries, fish, or casseroles surrounded by hot air in an oven at temperatures ranging between 300°F and 425°F.
Broiling Animation	Cooking with a heat source located above the food at temperatures between 425°F and 550°F.
Grilling Animation	Cooking food on a grate with a heat source located below at temperatures between 425°F and 550°F.
Sautéing Animation	Quickly cooking food in just enough fat to cover the bottom of a preheated pan, over high heat ranging between 320°F and 450°F. *Stir-frying* is similar to sautéing except food is cut in smaller pieces for quicker cooking.
Panfrying Animation	Cooking in a moderate amount of fat (usually enough to cover the food halfway) at temperatures between 325°F and 375°F.
Deep Frying Animation	Cooking by immersing food in hot fat ranging in temperature from 325°F to 375°F.
Combination Cooking Methods	
Braising Animation	Cooking large pieces of food (often less tender cuts of meat or poultry) by first browning in a small amount of fat, and then adding liquid and simmering in a covered container.
Stewing Animation	Cooking small pieces of food by first browning in a small amount of fat, and then adding liquid and simmering in a covered container.

Figure 19.10 Cooking methods.

Caramelization is a different browning process that occurs when heat is applied to sugars. Caramelization produces rich flavors and aromas similar to the Maillard reaction; however, amino acids are not present (**Figure 19.11**).

The ***combination cooking method*** uses both dry- and moist-heat cooking methods (see Figure 19.10). Combination methods are known for producing tender dishes that are rich in flavor.

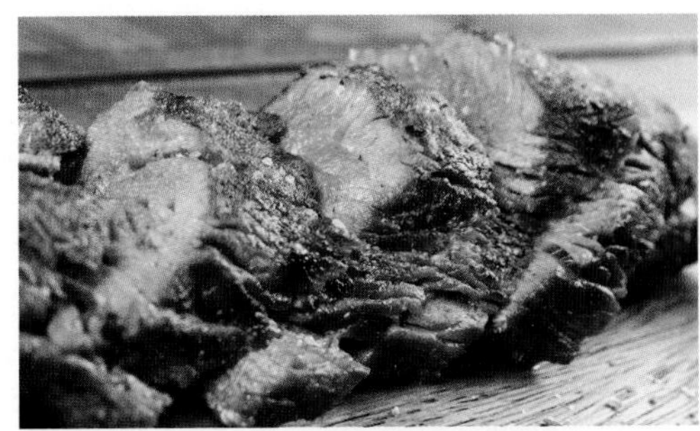

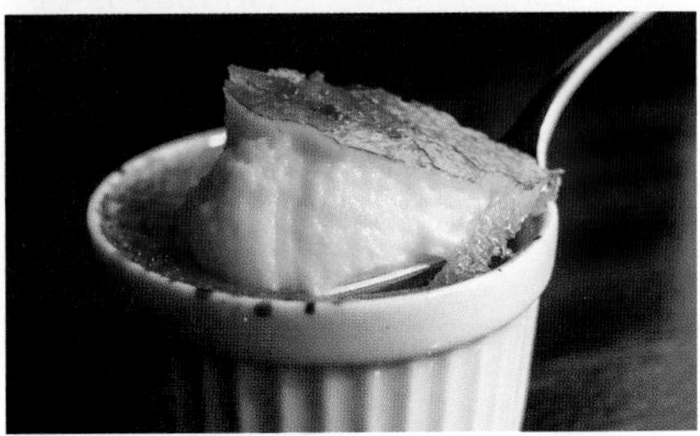

vsl/Shutterstock.com; pic0000/Shutterstock.com

Figure 19.11 The browned surface of the meat is the result of the Maillard reaction. The crunchy, browned surface of the crème brûlée is the result of caramelization of sugars sprinkled over the top of the custard.

Understanding Grains

All grains belong to the grass family and are commonly called *cereals*. Any food made from wheat, rice, oats, corn, rye, barley, or any other cereal is a grain product. Some foods, such as buckwheat, amaranth, and quinoa are mistakenly considered grains. Although these foods are similar to grains in many ways, they are the seeds of plants that are not grasses. Nonetheless, these foods are processed and cooked much like grains, and therefore, included in this discussion.

People prepare and eat grains in a variety of forms that have been processed to varying degrees (**Figure 19.12**).

Forms of Grains

Form	Amount of Processing	Cooking Time	Examples
Whole or Groat	Least processed; only the hull is removed	Longest cooking time	Wheat berries, brown rice, farro; used in salads, soups and baked goods, or side dishes
Pearled	Bran layers are removed	Cooks faster than a whole grain and is more tender	Pearled barley, pearled farro; used in soups, stews, and as side dishes
Grits or Steel-Cut	Cut into smaller pieces	Cooks much more quickly than whole grains	Steel-cut oats, corn grits; used as cereal or in baked goods
Rolled or Flaked	Steamed and rolled into flattened, or flaked kernels	Cooks much more quickly than whole grains	Rolled oats, rolled barley; used as cereal or in baked goods
Meal	Ground into a coarse, sandy texture	Cooks quickly	Cornmeal; used in breads, tortillas, and cereals
Bran	Removed from kernel and ground into a meal	Usually not cooked alone; cook time varies based on final product	Used as a supplement or added to foods
Germ	Removed from kernel and ground into a meal	Usually not cooked alone; cook time varies based on final product	Nutritional supplement added to foods
Flour	Ground and sifted into a powdered form ranging in texture from coarse to fine	Usually not cooked alone; cook time varies based on final product	Wheat flour, rye flour; main ingredient in pasta and baked goods

Figure 19.12 Grains that are less processed often require longer cooking time.

Common Types of Grains

Grains commonly prepared and consumed in the United States include corn, wheat, oats, and rice.

Corn

People consume corn in many different forms and foods. The sweet corn that is often eaten as corn on the cob is usually considered a vegetable. The corn that is harvested when the seeds are dry is considered a grain.

Hominy is produced by soaking dried corn in lye. This processing removes the germ and hull; therefore, hominy is not considered a whole grain. The hominy can be coarsely ground and prepared as grits or polenta. Some people find whole-grain grits less appealing due to the presence of dark specks that are pieces of the whole-grain kernel.

Dried corn kernels are ground to produce cornmeal. Cornmeal is used in many recipes, including corn tortillas, tamales, and corn bread. If the label states the cornmeal is from "whole corn" or "whole-grain corn," the cornmeal is whole grain.

Cornstarch is the endosperm of a corn kernel that is ground into a fine powder. It is used to thicken sauces and fillings, and lends a glossy sheen to the food.

Wheat

The most common grain products in the United States are made from wheat. The red-wheat variety has the slightly bitter flavor associated with whole-wheat baked goods. Whole white wheat, or albino wheat, has a mild flavor more appealing to those who are accustomed to refined baked goods. Wheat is refined to produce the white flour traditionally used in breads, cakes, and pastries.

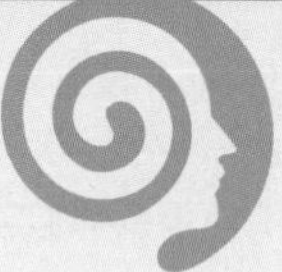

EXTEND YOUR KNOWLEDGE

Grind Your Own Flour

Have you ever thought about what is in the flour that you purchase at the grocery store? Or, what is *not* in it? When you grind whole-wheat kernels, the bran and the germ remain in the flour. The germ contains a small amount of oil, so the flour can go rancid quickly. Commercial flours have the bran and germ removed—along with the vitamins and fiber—to extend the shelf life.

If you grind your own flour at home, you can be sure that nothing has been added or removed, and it tastes better! You can use a mill to grind flour, but it is not essential. You probably have what you need in your kitchen right now. A food processor, blender, or coffee grinder works just as well. In addition, you can grind a wide variety of grains, beans, and seeds into flour at home, such as corn, mung beans, quinoa, or oats. You can also use an ancient grain, like spelt or kamut.

Be sure to start with a good-quality organic grain and only grind as much as you plan to use right away. Sift your flour afterward to remove any pieces of kernel that were not ground. Can you think of any other grains, beans, or seeds that you can grind into flour?

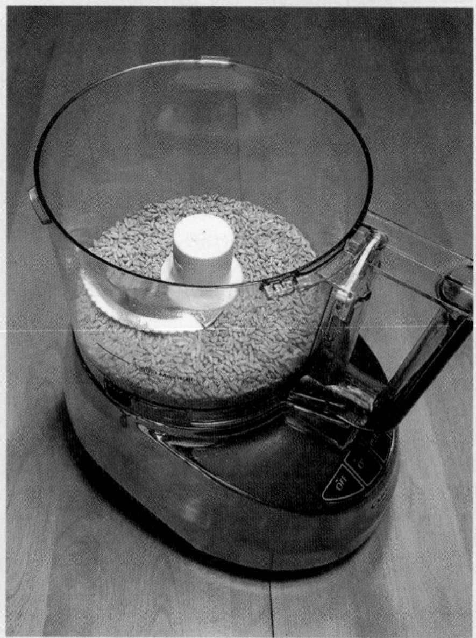

Goodheart-Willcox Publisher

Wheat berries, bulgur, and whole-wheat flour are all whole-grain forms of wheat (**Figure 19.13**). Wheat berries are simply raw wheat kernels that have had the hull removed. Wheat berries are precooked, dried, and chopped into pieces to make bulgur. Bulgur is a quick cooking whole-grain product that is popular in Middle Eastern dishes. The entire wheat kernel is ground to make whole-wheat flour.

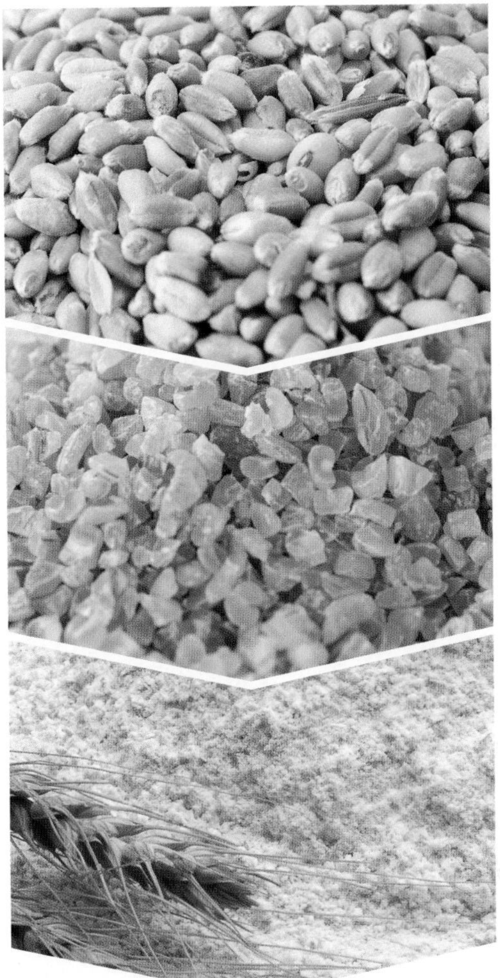

Lunik MX/Shutterstock.com; HandmadePictures/Shutterstock.com; M. Unal Ozmen/Shutterstock.com

Figure 19.13 Although all these products are whole grain, the wheat berries are less processed than the bulgur, and the bulgur is less processed than the whole-wheat flour.

Oats

Oats are used widely for human consumption as a cereal grain, but the vast majority of commercially grown oats are used for livestock feed. During processing, oats are hulled, but the bran and germ are left intact. The resulting product is a concentrated source of fiber and nutrients. Cooked oatmeal is a common breakfast food. Oats can be added to baked goods or ground into flour. People often add oat bran to food as a fiber supplement.

Rice

Both brown rice and white rice are available in different grain lengths: short grain, medium grain, and long grain. Short-grain rice is almost round and has the highest starch content; the grains stick together when cooked. Medium-grain rice is slightly longer than short-grain rice, and the cooked grains do not stick together as much as short-grain rice. The most common rice—long grain—is about three to four times as long as it is round. These grains do not stick together after cooking. Each rice has dishes it is better suited to than others. Wild rice, a close cousin of common rice, is also a good option as it is high in protein and dietary fiber.

Other Grains

Amaranth is a good source of plant protein, iron, calcium, and fiber. The tiny, brown kernels have a sweet, nutty flavor when cooked. Toasted amaranth can be sprinkled on food for added nutrients and crunch.

Barley is a staple ingredient in soups and stews. It is sold in both pearled and hulled forms; however, hulled is the whole-grain form. Buckwheat kernels, also called *buckwheat groats*, are high in magnesium and protein. The kernels can be cooked or ground into flour for use in noodles, pancakes, or breads. Toasted buckwheat kernels, called *kasha*, have a nutty flavor.

Millet, like barley, is sold pearled or in the whole-grain hulled form. These tiny yellow beads are high in manganese, magnesium, and phosphorous.

Quinoa has a mellow flavor and is high in magnesium, iron, and other minerals. Quinoa has the highest protein content of any grain. In addition, it is a complete protein, containing all nine essential amino acids. Quinoa must be rinsed well before cooking because it is covered with bitter tasting soap-like compounds called *saponins*. However, quinoa should never be soaked, because the saponins can leach into the seeds, leaving the finished product with an undesirable taste.

Pasta

Although pasta is a grain product and not a grain, it warrants discussion due to some unique aspects and its popularity with cooks. Typically, pasta is made from durum wheat that is processed into *semolina flour*. Semolina flour is used because it retains its shape and firm quality when cooked.

Pasta comes in different shapes and sizes. Different pasta shapes require different cooking times and are recommended for different recipes (**Figure 19.14**).

Cooking with Grains

Brown rice, whole-grain cereal, bread, and pasta can be simple, healthy, and economical additions to your eating plan at every meal. Grains can be served with vegetables or topped with sauces and served as main courses. Grains can also be served as side dishes to accompany meat or other proteins. They can also be added to soups and stews. Whole-grain cereals can serve as breakfast and baked goods can be prepared with whole-grain flours.

Basic Grain Preparation Techniques

Three techniques commonly used for cooking both whole and refined grains are boiling, simmering, and steaming. Depending on the grain type, you may also use additional cooking techniques, such as stir-frying and baking.

Figure 19.14 Pastas are made in a variety of shapes to serve different functions in dishes. For instance, pasta with ridges holds sauce, while tiny ball- or cylinder-shaped pastas work well in soups.

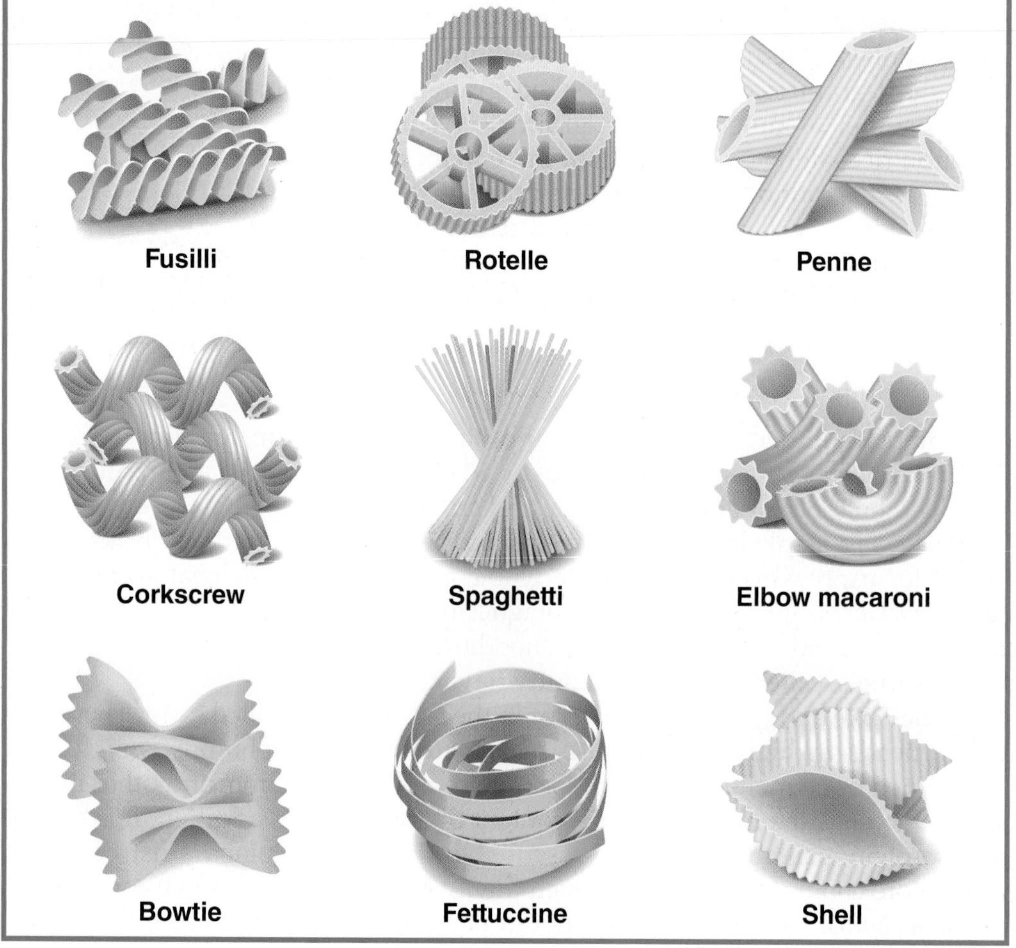

La Gorda/Shutterstock.com

Before cooking brown rice, and cracked or whole grains, always rinse them first. This removes excess starch and debris from the kernels. After rinsing, place the grain in a pan of water or broth and bring to a boil. Most commonly, the measurement ratio of liquid to grains is two to one, or two cups of liquid for every one cup of grain. Once the liquid begins to boil, reduce the heat to a simmer, cover the pan, and cook for the time directed. Whole grains such as brown rice typically take much longer to cook than refined grains. Unless stirring is suggested, do not open the lid because this disrupts the steaming process.

Oats come in several different forms: instant, quick-cooking, rolled or old-fashioned, steel-cut, and groats. Oats do not require rinsing before cooking, but they are cooked using a two to one ratio of liquid to grains. Instant oats are simply mixed with hot water to produce a smooth, creamy texture. Quick-cooking oats are similar to instant, but take one to two minutes to cook. Old-fashioned oats require roughly five minutes to cook. Steel-cut oats must be cooked for 20 to 30 minutes. Groats can take up to an hour to cook because they are the least processed.

Flour and Baked Goods

Wheat and other cereals contain the two proteins, *gliadin* and *glutenin*. During mixing, these two proteins combine to form the protein ***gluten***. When a gluten-containing flour is mixed with a liquid, the gliadin and glutenin become hydrated and flexible, much like strands of spaghetti when they are boiled. These two proteins begin to move about and link together to form gluten. Mixing or kneading causes more links to form and create a stronger, rubbery gluten. This structure has the capacity to stretch and rise with the action of leavening agents. It is responsible for the texture of bread and baked goods. Tender or flaky baked goods, like quick breads or piecrusts, require less developed gluten and overmixing can make the finished product tough. On the other hand, yeast dough requires extensive kneading to create a strong structure. For this reason, be sure to follow recipe instructions carefully.

Leavening agents are substances that release gases and cause the dough to expand, or rise. There are three types of leavening agents: biological, like yeast; chemical, like baking soda or baking powder; and steam from the evaporation of liquid, or air caused by the mechanical action of whipping or beating. When the gas is released, it creates little bubbles in the dough that expand without bursting, remaining trapped. While the dough cooks, it sets and the structure that the gluten created holds its expanded shape (**Figure 19.15**).

Different types of flours contain differing amounts of the proteins that create gluten. The bran in whole-wheat flour inhibits gluten formation; therefore, gluten is often added to a bread recipe when using whole-wheat flour. Bread flour has a high protein level and is favored for making bread where a strong structure is required. On the other hand, cake and pastry flours create less gluten, giving the finished products a tender texture.

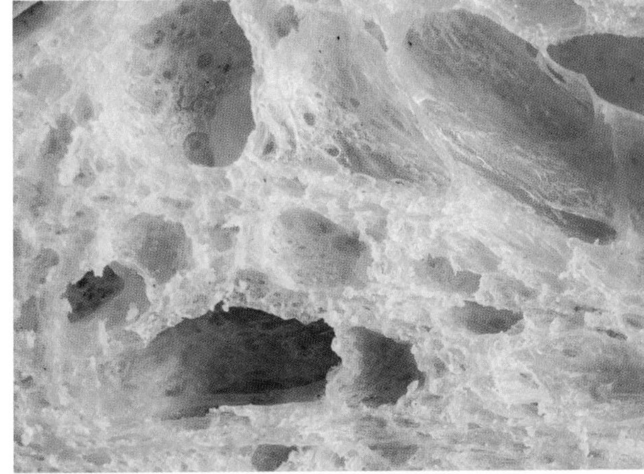

Lithiumphoto/Shutterstock.com

Figure 19.15 The texture of this bread clearly shows where gas bubbles formed and were trapped by the gluten structure as the dough cooked.

Pasta Preparation

Pasta should be cooked until tender, but firm, or ***al dente***. Al dente is an Italian term that means "to the tooth." Larger, fuller shaped pasta requires a longer cooking time to reach al dente than thinner, smaller varieties. Each shape differs in its ability to hold sauce and its cooked texture. These differences guide which pasta to use in a particular dish. Pasta shapes with holes or ridges, like wagon wheels or rotini, work well with chunkier sauces. Light, thin sauces work better with delicate pastas, such as angel hair or vermicelli. Thicker pasta shapes, like fettuccine, are used with heavier sauces.

The boiling technique is used to cook pasta. Generally, one pound of pasta requires one gallon of water with about one-half teaspoon of salt added. Bring water and salt to a boil in a large pot. Unlike other grains, the water must be boiling before you add the pasta. Add the pasta to the boiling water and stir gently to prevent sticking. Continue boiling, stirring a few times, until the pasta reaches al dente or as directed on the package. When finished cooking, drain pasta carefully. Position a colander in the sink and pour the boiling water and pasta from the pot into the colander (**Figure 19.16**). Serve immediately.

If cooked pasta must be held for a short time, toss with a small amount of oil to prevent sticking and place back in the pot and cover to keep warm. For salads, prepare pasta the day before and toss with a small amount of oil to prevent sticking and drying out. Store the cooked pasta covered in the refrigerator until ready to use.

Understanding Dairy Products

The dairy group consists of milk and milk products. Dairy is an excellent source of calcium and protein, and is included in many recipes. All forms of dairy products are made from milk; however, the animal from which the milk is sourced can vary. Milk is collected not only from cows, but also from goats, sheep, yaks, water buffalo, and other animals.

Milk is processed to varying extents to produce a range of products including butter, cream, concentrated milk, cultured products, frozen products, and cheese.

Milk and Cream

Federal law provides legal definitions for dairy products. These definitions identify required levels of fat content. Federal law also requires that all milk and milk products be pasteurized. ***Pasteurization*** is the process of heating every particle of the milk or milk product to a precise temperature for a specified time.

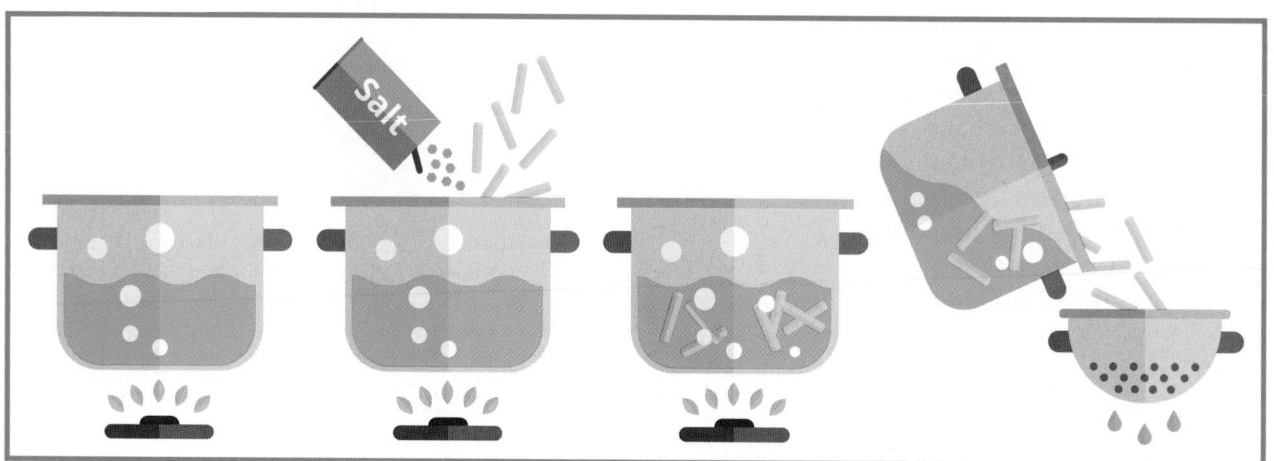

Graf Vishenka/Shutterstock.com

Figure 19.16 Be sure to use sufficient water so pasta can move freely and cook evenly.

This destroys enzymes and harmful bacteria present in raw, or unpasteurized, milk. Some believe that raw milk has greater health benefits than pasteurized milk; however, the possible presence of harmful bacteria in unpasteurized milk can cause serious illness.

Fresh, whole milk from the cow contains approximately 87 percent liquid and 13 percent milk solids. Milk fat, or butterfat, makes up a portion of the milk solids. Milk products are primarily defined by the amount of butterfat they contain. Milk is processed to adjust levels of butterfat in the final product (**Figure 19.17**).

In fresh milk, butterfat separates and rises to the top as cream. To prevent this, milk is processed to suspend the butterfat in the milk permanently. This process is called ***homogenization***. This prevents the butterfat, or cream, from rising to the top.

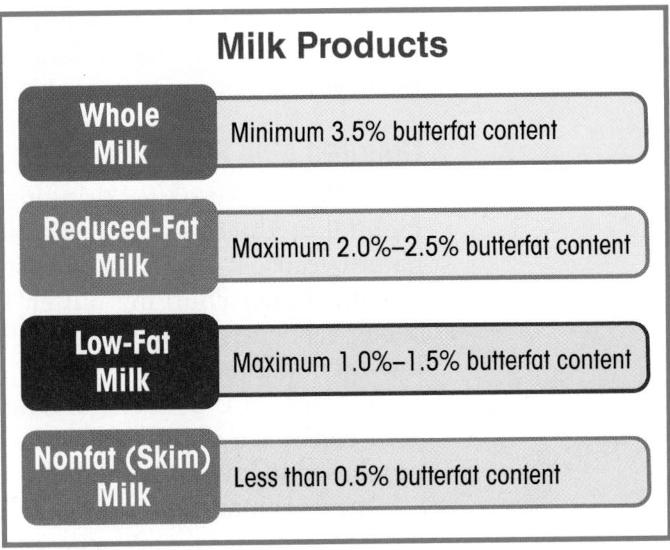

Figure 19.17 Milk products are defined by their butterfat content.

The butterfat that is removed during homogenization is not wasted. This butterfat is used to create high butterfat products, which are also defined by the amount of butterfat they contain (**Figure 19.18**).

Concentrated Milk Products

Water is removed from milk to produce concentrated milk products with increased levels of protein, sugars, and butterfat. These products are then canned or dried.

Removal of most of the fat and water from whole milk produces a product called *nonfat dry milk*. Water can be added to **reconstitute** (restore) the powder to fluid whole milk once again. *Evaporated milk* is whole, reduced fat, or nonfat milk from which 60 percent of the water is removed. This produces a thick, rich, cream-like product that is used in recipes or reconstituted to fluid milk by adding water.

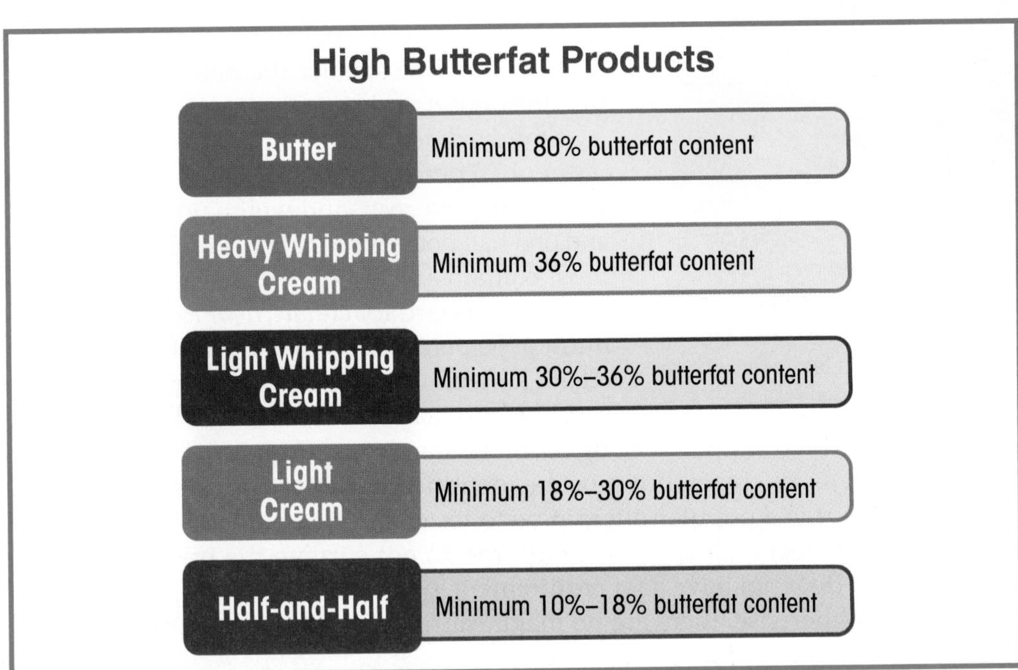

Figure 19.18 High butterfat products are required to contain minimum legal amounts of fat.

Sweetened condensed milk is whole or nonfat milk from which 60 percent of the water is removed and to which a large amount of sugar is added. The final product is a thick, very sweet product used in baking.

Cultured Milk Products

Buttermilk—used for drinking, cooking, and baking—is often thought to be a high-fat product because the word *butter* is in its name. However, it received this name because it originally consisted of the watery, sour tasting, low-fat liquid that remained after churning butter. In modern day, it is made by adding strains of bacteria, or cultures, to nonfat milk and allowing it to ferment. The result is a tangy low-fat milk product.

When strains of bacterial cultures are added to cream, it produces *sour cream*. Sour cream is a slightly thick, tart milk product used in recipes. It can be also be purchased in low-fat and nonfat varieties.

Yogurt is made by adding strains of helpful bacteria to warm milk and allowing it to ferment, creating a tangy, custard-like milk product. Yogurt contains more calcium and nutrients than regular fluid milk. It can be purchased in a variety of options including: whole, low-fat, nonfat, plain, and flavored. *Greek yogurt* is regular yogurt that has been strained. As a result, Greek yogurt is a denser and more nutrient-rich product than regular yogurt. It contains more protein, and less sodium and carbohydrates than regular yogurt. *Kefir*, a cultured milk beverage, is made by adding kefir grains to milk and allowing it to ferment. The resulting product tastes similar to yogurt. Kefir grains are not true grains, but the name for the live cultures of beneficial yeasts and bacteria used to make kefir.

Frozen Dairy Products

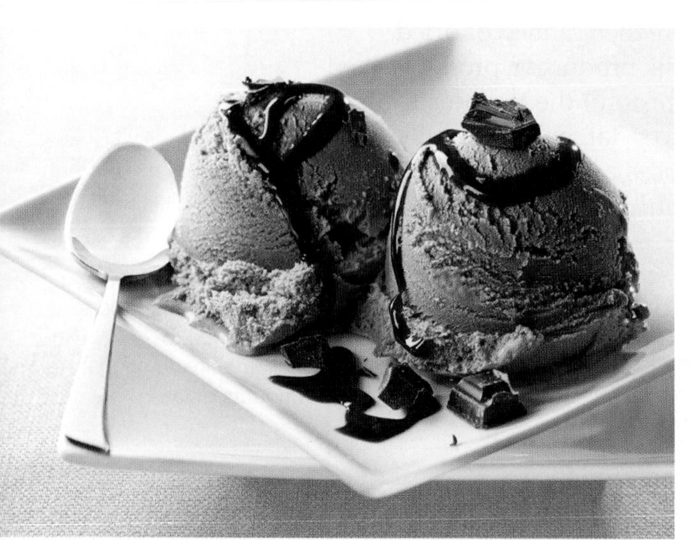

DUSAN ZIDAR/Shutterstock.com

Figure 19.19 More overrun produces an ice cream that is lighter and creamier than ice cream with less overrun.

Ice cream is a mixture of cream, milk, sugar, and stabilizers that is simultaneously frozen and whipped to create a light and fluffy texture. The amount of air whipped into the mixture is called *overrun* and is identified as a percentage (**Figure 19.19**). For example, if one gallon of ice cream mixture has 100 percent overrun, its volume increases by 100 percent to yield two gallons of ice cream. The smaller the percentage of overrun, the denser and heavier the finished product.

Standard ice cream must contain a minimum of 10 percent butterfat, have no more than 100 percent overrun, and weigh no less than four and one-half pounds per gallon. *Reduced-fat ice cream* must contain at least 25 percent less total butterfat than standard ice cream, *light ice cream* a minimum of 50 percent less total butterfat, low-fat ice cream a maximum of three grams of total fat per serving, and *nonfat ice cream* must have less than a half gram of total fat per serving. If these standards are not met, it cannot be legally labeled as ice cream, but must be identified as *frozen dairy dessert*.

Frozen yogurt is a popular alternative to ice cream that is made with cultured milk instead of cream, although the cultures do not survive the freezing process. Frozen yogurt does not have a fat requirement, but it is typically less than half that of ice cream. Otherwise, there are no major nutritional differences between the ice cream and frozen yogurt.

Sherbet, often confused with sorbet, is made from fruit, milk or cream, and sometimes egg whites. *Sorbet* contains no dairy, only fruit and sugar. Sherbet contains a very small amount of dairy compared to ice cream and only one to two percent butterfat.

Dairy Substitutes

For people with lactose intolerance or dairy allergies, or those who do not wish to consume dairy, there are many dairy substitutes available. Nut or grain milks, like soy, almond, cashew, or rice milk, make excellent substitutes for milk in recipes and drinking. For whitening coffee, there is nondairy creamer and substitute nondairy whipped topping for whipped cream. Margarines made with vegetable oils in stick form can make good substitutes for butter. Avoid vegetable oil spreads that contain less than 80 percent fat, however, as they do not substitute well for butter and can negatively affect the finished product.

Cheese

Cheese is a form of concentrated milk. It takes approximately 10 pounds of milk to produce one pound of cheese. All cheeses are made from the milk of animals such as cows, goats, and sheep. In the United States, cheese is usually made from cow's milk.

When an enzyme, like *rennet*, is added to milk, it causes the milk to coagulate and form a custard-like mass called a *curd*. The curd separates out and leaves behind a thin-bluish liquid called *whey*. The whey is drained from the milk solids, leaving only the curds. The curds are usually placed in a mold, sometimes pressed. Over time, the curds knit together to become cheese.

Cheese is categorized as either *unripened* (fresh) or *ripened* (aged). Unripened, or fresh, cheese is highly perishable and must be refrigerated and used within a few days. It is soft and has a mild flavor (**Figure 19.20**).

Fresh Cheeses		
Type	**Characteristics**	**Uses**
Chèvre	Made from goat's milk, slightly tangy, spreadable consistency	Spread on crackers and sandwiches, stuffed in meats and poultry
Cottage Cheese	Curds with milk or cream added; slightly tangy, mild flavor	Eaten plain, blended and substituted for ricotta in cooking
Cream Cheese	Smooth, creamy texture; mild, slightly tangy flavor; spreadable consistency	Used in baking, frostings, and cooking; spread over toast and bagels
Feta	Brined; salty, tangy flavor; crumbly texture; typically made with sheep's or goat's milk, but can be made with cow's milk	Used in Mediterranean cuisine, on salads, in wraps
Ricotta	Slightly grainy texture; sweet, milky flavor; spreadable consistency	Used in traditional Italian cuisine
Queso Fresco	Mild, slightly salty flavor; dry, crumbly texture	Used in traditional Latin cuisine

Figure 19.20
Fresh cheese has a short shelf life.

Aged cheese has ripening agents added, such as bacteria, mold, yeast, or enzymes. It is allowed to cure, or age, under controlled conditions (**Figure 19.21**). Aging conditions depend on the type of cheese desired and can last from weeks to years. Aged cheeses are categorized into four groups:

- **Soft**—very soft cheese with a white, edible rind.
- **Semisoft**—cheese with smooth, creamy interior and little or no rind; flavors range from mild to very pungent.
- **Firm**—a broad category of cheeses with textures ranging from elastic to hard; flavors range from very mild to sharp and pungent.
- **Blue-veined**—cheese to which a mold is added, creating a characteristic blue-green veining; distinctive flavor that ranges from mild to pungent with a strong odor.

Aged Cheeses		
Type	**Characteristics**	**Uses**
Soft		
Brie	Light yellow; buttery rich flavor; white, edible crust	Baked, spreads, snack
Camembert	Light yellow; buttery rich flavor; white, edible crust	Baked, spreads, snack
Neufchâtel	White; creamy texture; slightly tangy flavor; low-fat substitute for cream cheese	Spreads, baking, sandwiches
Semisoft		
Colby	Often orange in color; mild and creamy flavor; soft texture	Sandwiches, eaten plain, melted, used in cooking
Monterey Jack	Creamy white; smooth texture; mild flavor	Sandwiches, eaten plain, melted, used in cooking
Mozzarella	White; sweet, mild flavor; very elastic; melts well	Used in cooking, eaten plain, melted on pizza
Firm		
Cheddar	Creamy white to orange color; mildly pungent to extra sharp flavor; slightly crumbly texture	Sandwiches, eaten plain, melted, used in cooking
Parmesan	Light yellow color; crumbly, dense texture; sharp, salty flavor	Grated toppings for pasta and pizza, used in cooking
Swiss	Shiny pale yellow; savory-sweet, nut-like flavor; holes; firm texture	Sandwiches, eaten plain, melted, used in cooking
Blue-Veined		
Blue Cheese	Creamy white with blue veins; creamy, crumbly texture; sharp, salty flavor	Salads, salad dressings, used in cooking
Gorgonzola	Yellow with blue-green veins; crumbly, soft texture; mildly sharp flavor	Salads, salad dressings, used in cooking
Roquefort	Creamy white with blue-green veins; moist, crumbly texture; salty, sharp, tangy flavor	Salads, salad dressings, used in cooking

Figure 19.21 Cheese loses moisture and becomes more firm as it ages.

Cooking with Dairy Products

Several problems can occur when cooking with milk or cream. As milk is heated and water begins to evaporate at the surface, the milk solids and fat begin to form a skin. The skin traps steam and prevents it from escaping. Pressure builds underneath the skin and eventually the milk will boil over. Stirring the milk while it cooks or covering the pan will prevent the skin from forming.

Additionally, the heat transferred from the burner to the pan can cause the milk that is in contact with the bottom of the pan to overheat. This can result in curdling or scorching. Heat causes proteins in the milk to ***curdle***, or coagulate. The curdled protein sticks to the bottom of the pan and ***scorches***, or burns. Scorched milk turns brown and has a bitter flavor. To avoid scorching and curdling, wet the bottom of the pan with water before you add the milk to help discourage proteins from sticking to the pan. Also, use moderate heat for cooking milk or use a double boiler.

Curdling can also be caused by the addition of acidic foods. To prevent this, temper the milk or cream with the acidic ingredient. ***Tempering*** is the gradual addition of an ingredient to the milk, while stirring constantly. The acidic ingredient should be added incrementally in small amounts. Tempering is also used when adding milk or cream to a hot food like a gravy or sauce.

Cheese is a concentrated form of milk with high protein and fat content; therefore, care must be taken when cooking with cheese. Cheese should be cooked just long enough to melt it. When cooked for too long or at a temperature that is too high, cheese can become tough and rubbery or the fat can separate out into balls of grease. Grating cheese or cutting it into small pieces helps it melt more evenly and blend more quickly (**Figure 19.22**). When adding cheese to other foods, they should be precooked or only have a short cooking time left. When melting cheeses into sauces, it should be done over a low temperature.

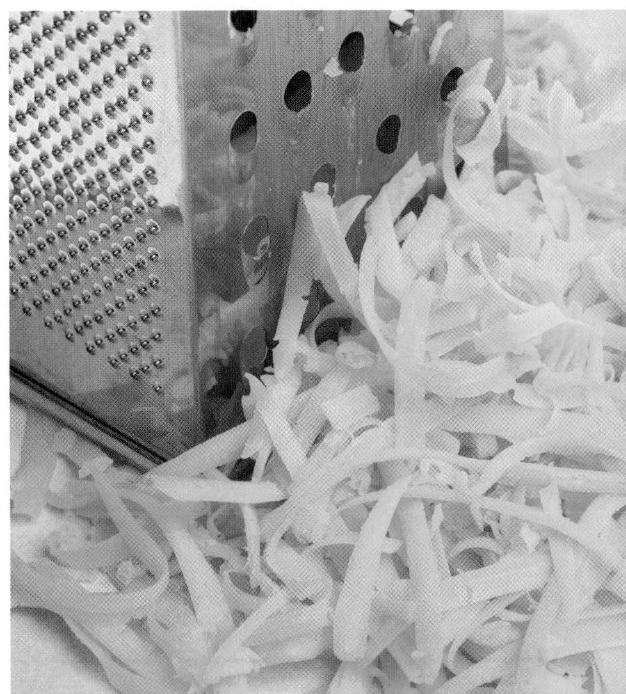

Joe Gough/Shutterstock.com

Figure 19.22 Grated cheese melts more evenly and blends more quickly.

Understanding Protein Foods

The protein foods group includes eggs, poultry, meat, fish and shellfish, as well as legumes, beans, and peas. Meals are often planned around the protein. Some proteins are quite economical and others quite expensive.

To be successful in the kitchen and maintain a food budget, you must know how to choose and prepare the foods in this group properly.

Eggs

Eggs are an excellent source of good quality protein, B vitamins, vitamins A and D, iron, and other minerals. Both the white and the yolk contain nutrients; however, most of the vitamins and minerals, and 60 percent of the protein is found in the yolk. Large eggs only contain about 70 calories each. Eggs are nutrient dense, cost effective, easy to prepare, and fit into a healthy diet.

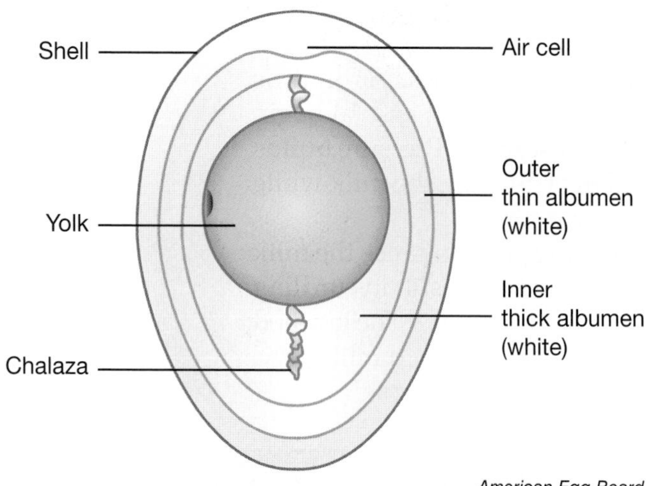

Figure 19.23 The chalazae are formed from the egg white and act to hold the yolk in place.

Egg Structure

The hard shell that surrounds an egg is porous; therefore, air and moisture can pass through its pores. It has a thin outer coating—the cuticle—that keeps out dust and bacteria. Eggshells may be brown, white, blue, or green, depending on the breed of the chicken. Other structures of the egg are not so easy to identify (**Figure 19.23**).

The egg's structure gives you some hints about its age. For example, the air cell forms as the egg cools after it is laid, and its size increases over time. As the egg ages, the albumen becomes thinner and the yolk flattens. In addition, a prominent chalaza is a sign of a fresh egg.

Egg Grades

There are three consumer grades for eggs—AA, A, and B. The USDA sets the grading standards based on the interior quality of the egg and the appearance of the shell. Grade AA eggs have thick, firm whites; high, round yolks; and clean, unbroken shells. This standard is modified just slightly for grade A eggs to state the whites are "reasonably" firm. Grade B eggs have thinner whites, flatter yolks, and may have stained shells.

Grades AA and A have thicker whites after cooking, and are the best choice when frying or poaching eggs. Grade B eggs are best used for baking, and in omelets or for scrambled eggs; however, these eggs are primarily used for liquid, frozen, or dried egg products.

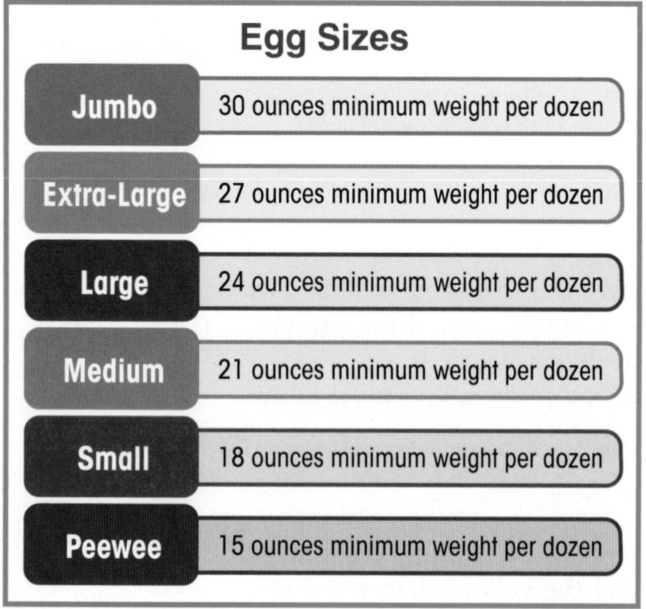

Egg Sizes

Jumbo	30 ounces minimum weight per dozen
Extra-Large	27 ounces minimum weight per dozen
Large	24 ounces minimum weight per dozen
Medium	21 ounces minimum weight per dozen
Small	18 ounces minimum weight per dozen
Peewee	15 ounces minimum weight per dozen

Figure 19.24 Egg sizes are defined by their minimum weight per dozen. *When would the size of the egg affect the dish you are preparing?*

Egg Size

Eggs are sold in different sizes—jumbo, extra-large, large, medium, small, and peewee. Egg size is based on their minimum weight per dozen and has nothing to do with quality (**Figure 19.24**).

When preparing eggs for the main dish, egg size may not be important; however, egg size matters when preparing baked goods. Standardized recipes require size large eggs, unless otherwise stated. Using a different size without making any adjustments can affect the outcome of your baked goods. See the Egg Size Conversion chart in Appendix B.

Egg Safety

Due to the concern about *Salmonella*, care must be taken when purchasing and storing eggs. At the store, check to make sure eggs are properly refrigerated and shells are intact. Take eggs home and refrigerate immediately after purchasing. Do not wash the eggs. Washing may remove the protective coating that protects the egg from contamination. Store eggs in their original carton in the coldest part of the refrigerator, not in the door. If a recipe calls for room temperature eggs, either remove eggs from the refrigerator 30 minutes prior to use or place them in a bowl of warm water. Condensation forms on a cold egg left out at room temperature, which can allow bacteria to move into the egg.

Do not freeze shell eggs. The shell may crack during freezing and the egg must then be discarded. Instead, whisk whole eggs just long enough to blend, place in a container, label, and freeze.

Egg Substitutes

As an alternative to regular eggs, various types of egg substitutes are available. You can find them in frozen, refrigerated, or dried form. Many commercial egg substitutes do not contain egg yolk. They are primarily pasteurized egg whites with added flavorings, vitamins, and thickeners. These types are an excellent substitute for those wishing to cut down on their intake of fat and cholesterol. These products are not appropriate for people with egg allergies or vegans. Egg substitutes can be used in the same way as regular eggs.

Egg Properties

Eggs have certain properties that make them useful in many different recipes. These properties are mainly due to their protein content. For example, eggs act as a *binder* in recipes by coagulating. When eggs are heated, their proteins coagulate and change from liquid to a semi-solid or solid (**Figure 19.25**). When eggs solidify, they bind ingredients to one another, such as in cookie dough, custards, or meatloaf. Egg yolks act as an excellent emulsifier. *Emulsifiers* prevent two liquids, like lemon juice and oil in mayonnaise, from separating.

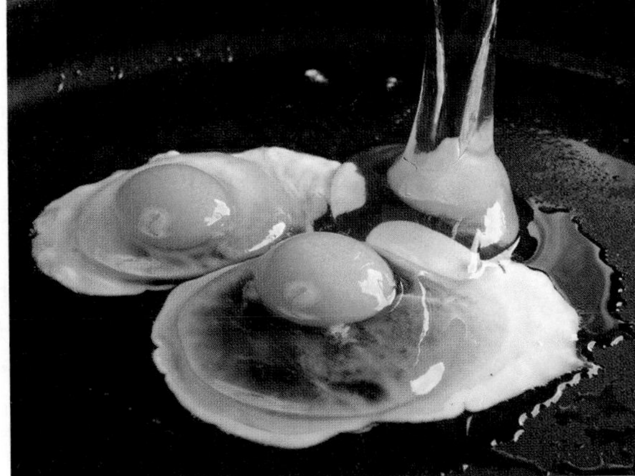

Fotokostic/Shutterstock.com

Figure 19.25 When eggs are heated, their proteins coagulate and change from liquid to semiliquid or solid. *How can you tell if the skillet in this photo is hot?*

Cooking Eggs

Eggs are a versatile food. They can be used as ingredients in a variety of main dishes and desserts, but they are also prepared as the main dish. Sometimes the entire egg is used and other times only parts of the egg are used.

Though care must be taken when preparing eggs, they can be simple to cook after learning a few techniques. Never eat raw or undercooked eggs because they may contain *Salmonella*. After handling raw eggs, always wash your hands and sanitize all cooking surfaces that have come in contact with them to avoid cross-contamination. Eggs and egg dishes should be cooked to 160°F, or until the white is firm and the yolk is thickened.

Separating the Egg

Before you can use an egg as an ingredient, you must remove it from its shell. Though it may seem daunting at first, with practice it becomes a simple task. Hold the egg in your dominant hand and tap the egg on the edge of a bowl or with a knife. Cracking the egg on the countertop, however, reduces the chance of getting shell in the bowl of eggs. Tap the egg with just enough force to crack it. Ideally, you would like to crack the shell at the egg's equator, or the center of the egg. Once the egg is cracked, carefully pull the egg open with your thumbs as if it is attached with a hinge on one side and let the egg drop into your bowl.

Sometimes you may need only the egg white or the egg yolk. In this case, you must separate the yolk from the white. If you have an egg separator, this process is just like cracking open an egg. Just follow the steps for cracking the egg and drop it into the egg separator that you are holding over a bowl. The yolk will remain in the egg separator while the white will flow down into the bowl. If you do not have a separator, you can use the two halves of the cracked eggshell. Hold the two shell halves over a bowl and pour the yolk back and forth between the two halves of the shell while allowing the white to flow down into the bowl. When finished, only the yolk remains in the shell. Cover the unused yolk or white and place it in the refrigerator to use at another time.

Beating Egg Whites

When egg whites are beaten or whipped, air is incorporated, proteins are broken down, and a *foam* forms. Continued beating causes the air bubbles to decrease in size and increase in number, which thickens and stabilizes the foam. This foam adds volume and lightness to foods like angel food cake and meringue.

If performed properly, beaten egg whites should be stable and hold their volume during the addition of other ingredients. Place the egg whites from fresh, room-temperature eggs in a clean metal or glass bowl. Make sure no yolk has fallen into the white because the yolk contains fat and fat prevents the eggs from reaching their full volume. Recipes often call for the addition of an acid like lemon juice, vinegar, or cream of tartar. The acid stabilizes the whites and increases volume.

To begin, beat egg whites at a low speed, gradually increasing to high speed. At first, the egg whites become foamy, primarily liquid with some bubbles. With continued beating, they develop *soft peaks*. Soft peak stage can be identified by lifting the beaters out of the eggs. If the mixture forms a peak that slumps over to the side, it is at soft peak stage. Further beating creates *firm peaks*. When the beaters are lifted out of the eggs at firm peak stage, the peaks stand up and do not fall over (**Figure 19.26**). If beating continues beyond this stage, the whites become over whipped, lose volume, liquefy, and are unsalvageable. Often recipes require egg whites that are beaten to the "soft peak" or "firm peak" stage.

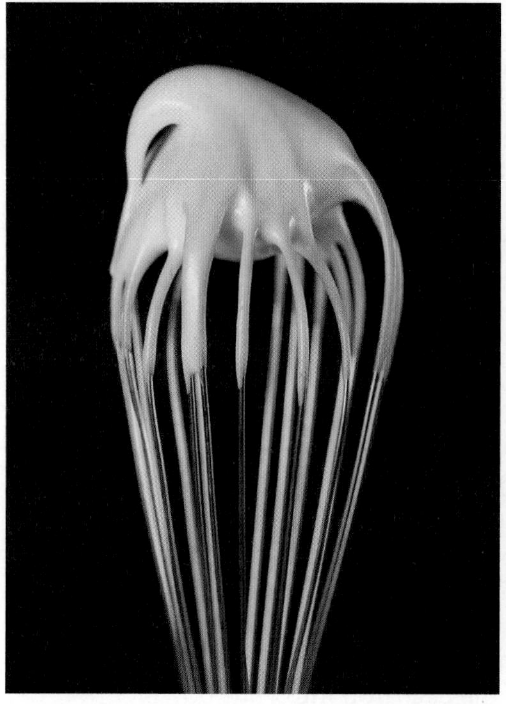

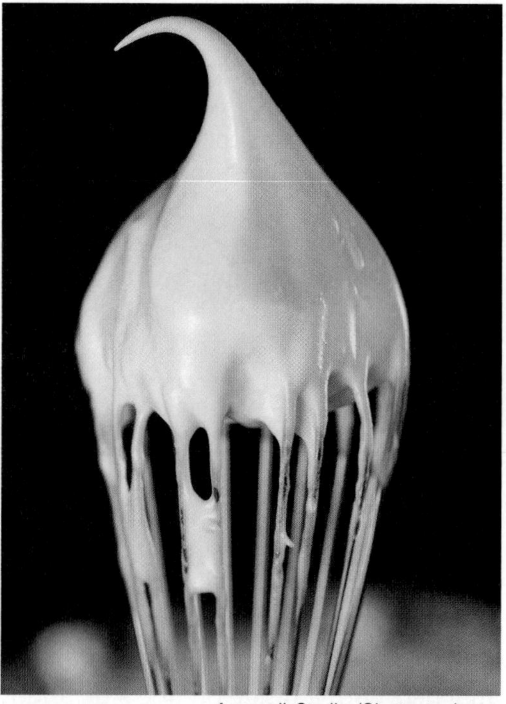

AnnapolisStudios/Shutterstock.com

Figure 19.26
Some recipes require egg whites whipped to soft peak stage, while other recipes require egg whites whipped to firm peak stage.

Cooking in the Shell

One of the simplest ways to prepare eggs is to cook them in their shell. To *hard cook* eggs, place them in a single layer in a saucepan. Adding another layer may cause the eggs to bump against one another and crack the shells. Add water to the pan until it is at least an inch above the eggs. Cover the pan and bring to a boil. As soon as the water begins to boil, remove the pan from the heat source to prevent further boiling. Let the eggs stand in the covered pan for approximately 12 to 15 minutes if they are large eggs; 9 minutes for medium eggs, 15 minutes for extra-large eggs. This cooks the eggs gently, producing a tender egg. Drain and serve hard-cooked eggs immediately, or cool them in cold water and refrigerate. Due to the cooking process, the protective layer has been removed from the outside of the shell, so hard-cooked eggs can only be refrigerated safely for up to one week.

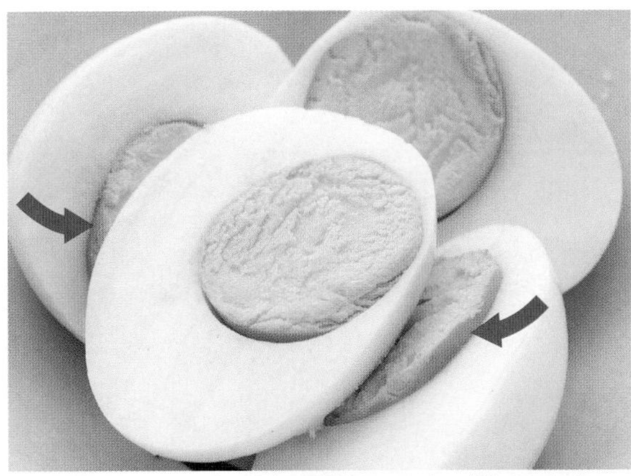

Suphaksorn Thongwongboot/Shutterstock.com

Figure 19.27 The greenish-gray ring that sometimes appears around the yolk is harmless, but unappealing. *How can you prevent this ring from forming?*

Sometimes, an unsightly, but harmless, greenish-gray ring may appear around the yolk (**Figure 19.27**). This is caused by a chemical reaction between the sulfur in the egg white and the iron in the yolk. Avoid this by adhering to cooking guidelines and cooling eggs quickly after cooking.

For hard-cooked eggs that are easy to peel, begin with eggs that are one week to 10 days old because very fresh eggs are difficult to peel. Be sure to cool eggs immediately after cooking. Additionally, eggs are easiest to peel right after cooling.

Cooking Without the Shell

A shelled egg that is cooked gently in liquid is called a *poached egg*. To poach an egg, fill a pan with two to three inches of water and bring to a boil. Reduce heat to a gentle simmer. Unless the eggs are very fresh, add one teaspoon of vinegar to the water to prevent the egg white from spreading out in the pan. Crack an egg into a small bowl, and then lower the bowl close to the surface of the liquid. Gently tip the bowl to slide the egg out into the simmering water. Simmer until the white is completely set and firm and the yolk is thick, approximately three to five minutes. Remove the egg from the pan with a slotted spoon and place on a paper towel to drain. Serve on toast or an English muffin.

Shelled eggs can also be fried. *Fried eggs* are cooked in a small amount of oil, butter, or margarine in a hot skillet. If using a nonstick pan, use nonstick spray. The skillet is hot enough to cook when a drop of water sizzles in the pan. Crack the egg into a small bowl and slide the egg onto the skillet. Cook until the white is set and the yolk is thick, approximately five to six minutes. To cook the top, carefully turn the egg or cover for the last two to three minutes of cooking. Fried eggs can be served in a sandwich or with vegetables.

Scrambled eggs are an easy way to prepare shelled eggs. Heat a small amount of fat in a skillet over low heat. Crack the desired number of eggs into a bowl. Use a fork or whisk to beat eggs with a small amount of water or milk. This incorporates air and the liquid into the eggs, which adds volume and fluffiness to the finished product. Once the pan is hot, add the eggs and allow them to stand for about a minute. When the eggs begin to thicken, stir gently to form large curds and to allow uncooked egg to make contact with the bottom of the skillet. Continue this process until the egg mixture is thickened and no liquid remains. The curds should be large and fluffy. Scrambled eggs can be served alongside toast and fruit, or inside a breakfast burrito with cheese, beans, and vegetables.

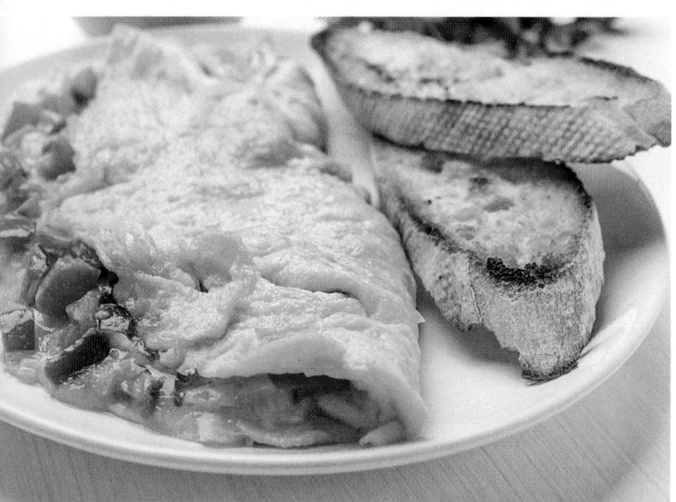

Olga Nayashkova/Shutterstock.com

Figure 19.28 Fill your omelet with vegetables to increase your daily vegetable intake.

An omelet can be a complete meal. Preparation of an *omelet* is similar to scrambled eggs, but the egg mixture is not stirred. Mix two to three eggs with about a tablespoon of water or milk. Heat a small amount of fat in a skillet over medium heat. When the pan is hot, pour the egg mixture into the pan, swirling and tipping the pan so the egg mixture completely covers the bottom. Allow eggs to set up for about 30 seconds. Gently pull thickened egg mixture back from the edge of the pan toward the center and tip the pan to allow the uncooked egg to flow into the space you have created. Continue this process until the top is thickened and no liquid remains. Place your desired fillings on one-half of the omelet and fold the other half over to cover them. Carefully slide the omelet out onto a plate and serve immediately (**Figure 19.28**).

Custard

Custard is a mixture of milk and eggs that can be baked or stirred on the cooktop. It is thickened by the coagulation of egg proteins. Custard can be sweet, as in pastry cream, or savory, as in quiche. Stirred custards tend to be sweet and thicker than baked custards, which can be sweet or savory.

Care must be taken when making custard due to the delicate nature of egg proteins. Custard should be cooked just long enough to set. Cooking custard for too long produces a curdled and runny product rather than a thick and creamy one. The temperature used to cook custard should not be too high.

To prepare stirred custard, bring milk and other ingredients, except the eggs, to a simmer over a low heat. Avoid curdling by tempering the eggs, or allowing them to adjust to the temperature of the mixture gradually. To do this, add a small amount of the hot liquid to the eggs before adding them to the hot mixture. Reduce heat to low and continue to cook, stirring frequently, until thickened, approximately 15 to 20 minutes.

To prepare a simple baked custard, mix all ingredients together as directed by your recipe and pour into custard cups. Fill a large baking dish halfway with water to create a *water bath*. When custards are prepared in the oven, they must be baked in a water bath. A water bath insulates the custard from the direct heat of the oven because the temperature of water cannot rise above 212°F. This allows the custard to cook evenly and not crack. Carefully, place custard cups in the water and baking dish. Bake as directed.

Poultry

Poultry are domesticated birds raised for food, including chickens, turkeys, ducks, geese, and Cornish game hens. Chicken and turkey are the most popular poultry consumed in the United States. US consumption of chicken has even surpassed beef.

Chicken and turkey have both light and dark meat. *Dark meat* is found in the part of the bird that gets the most exercise. Muscles that get frequent or strenuous exercise need more oxygen than those that do not. Oxygen is stored in *myoglobin*, a red-pigmented protein. Myoglobin is present in higher concentrations in dark meat since those muscles require more oxygen. The muscles that get the most exercise—the legs and thighs—are higher in myoglobin and considered dark meat. Domesticated chicken and turkey do not fly, so the muscles used for flight—the breast and wing muscles—do not contain high levels of myoglobin. This explains why breast and wing meat is lighter in color. These parts of the bird are considered *white meat*.

Both white and dark meat are an excellent source of protein, B vitamins, iron, and other minerals. They are also low in saturated fat. Since dark meat muscles require more energy and fat is the most efficient way to store energy, dark meat has higher fat content than white meat. However, dark meat also contains more nutrients than white meat, including B vitamins, iron, zinc, and other minerals.

Ducks and geese are all dark meat. They are high in fat and flavorful. They are best roasted because of their high fat content.

Types of Poultry

Chickens can be purchased in various forms and are divided into classes based on age and weight. Different cooking methods are preferred based on the age of the bird (**Figure 19.29**).

Other terms used to describe chickens include *free-range* and *kosher*. These terms indicate the conditions under which the birds are raised and slaughtered. Free-range chickens are not kept in cages. Some think that they have a better flavor because exercise develops their muscles. Kosher chickens are slaughtered according to Jewish dietary law. Free-range and kosher chickens are no less nutritious than other chickens or no less prone to *Salmonella* contamination.

Turkeys are larger than chickens and have a stronger flavor. The most common turkeys are hens and toms. *Self-basting turkeys* are injected with flavorings and fat to keep them moist while roasting.

Poultry

Type	Weight Range	Description	Cooking Methods
Chicken			
Cornish hen	< 2 lb.	Special breed of chicken, very tender and delicate	Sautéing, broiling, or frying
Broiler/fryer	3–4 lb.	Tender, young bird	Sautéing, broiling, or frying
Roaster	3½–7 lb.	Tender, more flavorful meat than broiler/fryer	Roasting
Stewing	4–7 lb.	Flavorful, but less tender	Braising, simmering
Capon	5–9 lb.	Tender, flavorful, high fat content	Roasting
Turkey			
Hen	8–16 lb.	Young female bird, tender flesh	Roasting
Tom	10–24 lb.	Male bird, reasonably tender flesh	Roasting

Figure 19.29 Poultry can vary significantly in weight and age.

Poultry Fabrications

Much of the chicken purchased today is already cut into parts: whole or half breasts, thighs, legs, wings, bone-in or boneless, with skin or skinless (**Figure 19.30**). These pieces can be baked, broiled, grilled, sautéed, or fried.

Turkey parts are also available. You can purchase breast, leg, thigh, wings, and necks. This is a convenience for small families. An entire turkey may be too much for an individual or small family to consume.

Chicken and turkey are often sold with the giblets. *Giblets* are the edible internal organs, including the liver, heart, and gizzard. Giblets can be sold separately, but are normally found in a bag located in the cavity of the whole bird. Always check the bird's cavity before cooking to be sure you do not roast the bird along with the bag of giblets.

Ground chicken and turkey can be excellent low-fat substitutes for ground beef, when substituted correctly. If you read the Nutrition Facts labels on ground chicken and turkey products, you will see the nutrient content vary widely. For example, regular ground turkey can have up to 17 grams of fat and 240 calories per serving, whereas ground turkey breast only has 1.5 grams of fat and 120 calories per serving. Ground turkey and chicken breast products are leanest, while ground thigh and leg products can have a much higher fat percentage. A package labeled "ground turkey" or "ground chicken" can be a mixture of white and dark meats, therefore higher in fat and calories.

Ground dark meat turkey and chicken products are best used when you desire a juicy and flavorful final product, like burgers and meatballs. Whereas, lean ground turkey and chicken are less juicy and work better in sauces.

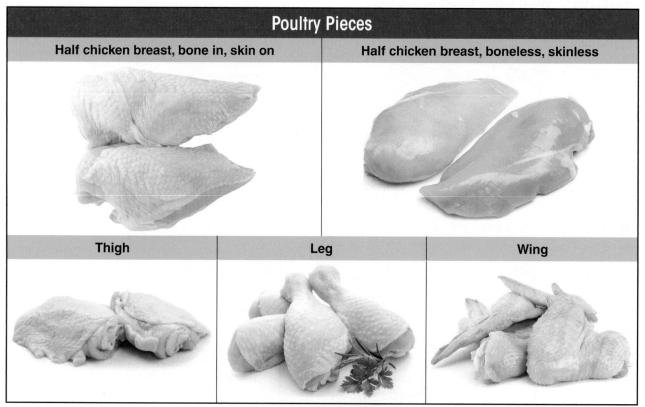

Top row, l to r: taro911 Photographer/Shutterstock.com; Joe Gough/Shutterstock.com; bottom row, l to r: Aedka Studio/Shutterstock.com; Alexander Raths/Shutterstock.com; De2marco/Shutterstock.com

Figure 19.30 Poultry pieces are usually more expensive than whole poultry. *Why do you think pieces are more expensive?*

Purchasing and Storing Poultry

The United States Department of Agriculture (USDA) grades and inspects poultry. Inspection is mandatory and grading is voluntary. Grade A is the highest grade. It indicates the poultry is juicy, tender, meaty, and virtually free from defects. Usually, only grade A poultry is sold in grocery stores.

When selecting poultry, look for poultry that is plump and meaty with creamy white to yellow skin. Avoid poultry with torn skin or leaking packages. Make sure there is no off odor and check the sell-by date. Do not buy a product that is close to the sell-by date unless you plan on using it or freezing it right away. To freeze poultry, wrap it tightly, seal, and write the date on the package. Whole frozen chicken or turkey can be frozen up to one year and chicken or turkey pieces can be frozen up to nine months if wrapped properly. Always defrost raw poultry in the refrigerator to avoid growth of *Salmonella* or other bacteria.

Due to possible *Salmonella* contamination, poultry must be handled with care. To avoid cross-contamination, always store raw poultry and meat on the bottom of the refrigerator, away from ready-to-eat items. Wash hands carefully after handling and sanitize all preparation surfaces that raw poultry contacts. Always make sure to cook poultry to an internal temperature of 165°F. When checking the temperature, be sure not to touch the bone with the thermometer. This will yield an inaccurate temperature reading.

Cooking Poultry

Select the cooking method that works best for the type and cut of poultry you are cooking. When using moist-heat cooking methods, like braising or stewing, the most economical choice is a whole broiler-fryer. When using poultry parts, bone-in, skin-on pieces are the most economical (**Figure 19.31**).

Most fat content in poultry is in the skin. To reduce fat when using moist-heat cooking methods to cook poultry parts, remove the skin and trim off visible fat *before* cooking. If using dry-heat cooking methods, remove the skin *after* cooking to help retain moisture while cooking. No matter which cooking method is used, bone-in poultry pieces take longer to cook than boneless pieces because the bone absorbs heat.

When using a whole chicken in soups or stews, take care to remove all the bones before serving. After cooking a whole chicken in liquid, the connective tissue has dissolved and the meat and skin fall off the bone. Small bones may also dislodge and remain in the soup or stew if you are not careful to remove them. To ensure no bones are present in the finished product, strain all the solids out of the liquid by pouring it through a strainer or scooping them out with a slotted spoon. Sift through the solids carefully to remove any small bones that remain.

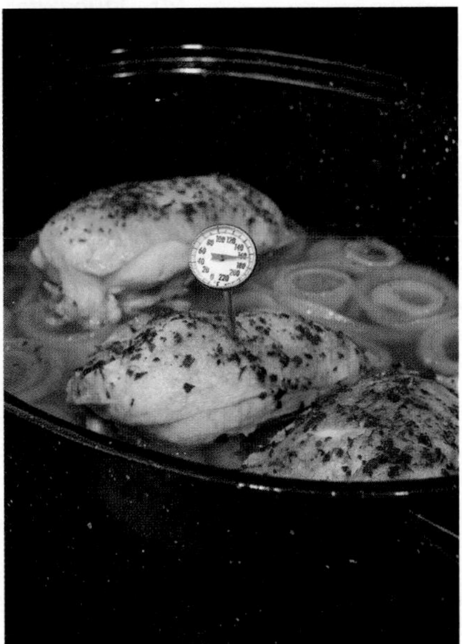

Carlos Yudica/Shutterstock.com

Figure 19.31 Moist-heat cooking methods are preferred for older types of poultry.

Many types of poultry—both parts and whole—roast well. Roast poultry uncovered and baste several times during cooking. Check for doneness by inserting a thermometer into the thickest part of the thigh of a whole bird, or the thickest piece when roasting parts. Avoid touching the bone with the thermometer when checking the temperature. The bone absorbs heat more readily than the flesh and produces an inaccurate reading.

When sautéing or stir-frying poultry, cook until it is no longer pink inside and the juices run clear. As soon as the meat becomes firm, cut a larger piece in half to check the color inside. White meat can dry out more quickly than dark meat, so pay particular attention when cooking with breast meat. Remove from pan or oven immediately when done.

Meats

Meat, commonly called *red meat,* is the edible muscle portion of domesticated animals raised for food, including cows, pigs, and sheep. Other edible portions of these animals are called *variety meats*. These include the liver, heart, tongue, brains, and tripe. Similar to poultry dark meat, red meat obtains its color from the high concentration of myoglobin. Red meat is also a major source of protein, B vitamins, iron, zinc, and other minerals.

Cuts of Meat

The carcass of the animal is divided into large sections called *primal cuts*. Primal cuts include chuck, brisket, rib, plate, loin, sirloin, flank, and round. These large cuts are divided into smaller cuts—such as roasts, chops, and steaks—that you see in the supermarket. When you buy a meat product at the store, the name will include the location on the animal from which the cut originates, for example, *sirloin steak, chuck roast*, or *brisket flat* (**Figure 19.32**).

Ground pork usually is made from pork shoulder and contains about 15 percent fat. Sausage-grade ground pork is about 25 to 30 percent fat. Ground lamb and veal contain lean meat and trimmings, and can originate from any primal cut area.

Ground beef is the most popular cut of beef in the United States. It is produced from muscle meat from any primal cut area, unless the label specifies a specific area. For example, if the label reads *ground sirloin,* the meat must only come from the sirloin primal cut. If the label simply reads *ground beef,* meat from several different primal cut areas may be ground together. Any type of ground beef must have no more than 30 percent fat and the fat must come only from the meat trimmings used to prepare the ground beef. In addition, it cannot contain added water, phosphates, binders, or extenders. *Hamburger* meat is similar to ground beef; however, hamburger meat can have added beef fat from a source other than the meat used to prepare the hamburger, as long as it does not exceed 30 percent.

Food Safety and Ground Meat

Burgers or other ground meats should be cooked until they are no longer pink inside and reach a temperature of 160°F. Rare meat, or meat that is still pink inside, has not yet reached a temperature high enough to destroy pathogens. Rare steak can be consumed because any pathogens remain on the outer surface of the meat and are destroyed during the cooking process. In contrast, the outer surface of the meat is mixed throughout the final product during the grinding process used to produce ground meats. Any pathogens on the surface are distributed throughout the ground meat, so the entire burger—inside and out—must reach a temperature high enough to destroy pathogens.

Types of Meat

Different types of meat come from different animals. *Beef* comes from adult cattle over one year old. It is a bright, deep red color with creamy white fat. *Veal* comes from calves. Veal calves are separated from their mothers at three days old and slaughtered at 16 to 18 weeks old. The meat is a light gray-pink color with little fat. *Pork* comes from pigs under one year old. Pork is tender with a gray-pink color and little fat. *Lamb* comes from sheep less than a year old. The meat is bright pink and has a unique, almost game-like flavor with white, brittle fat.

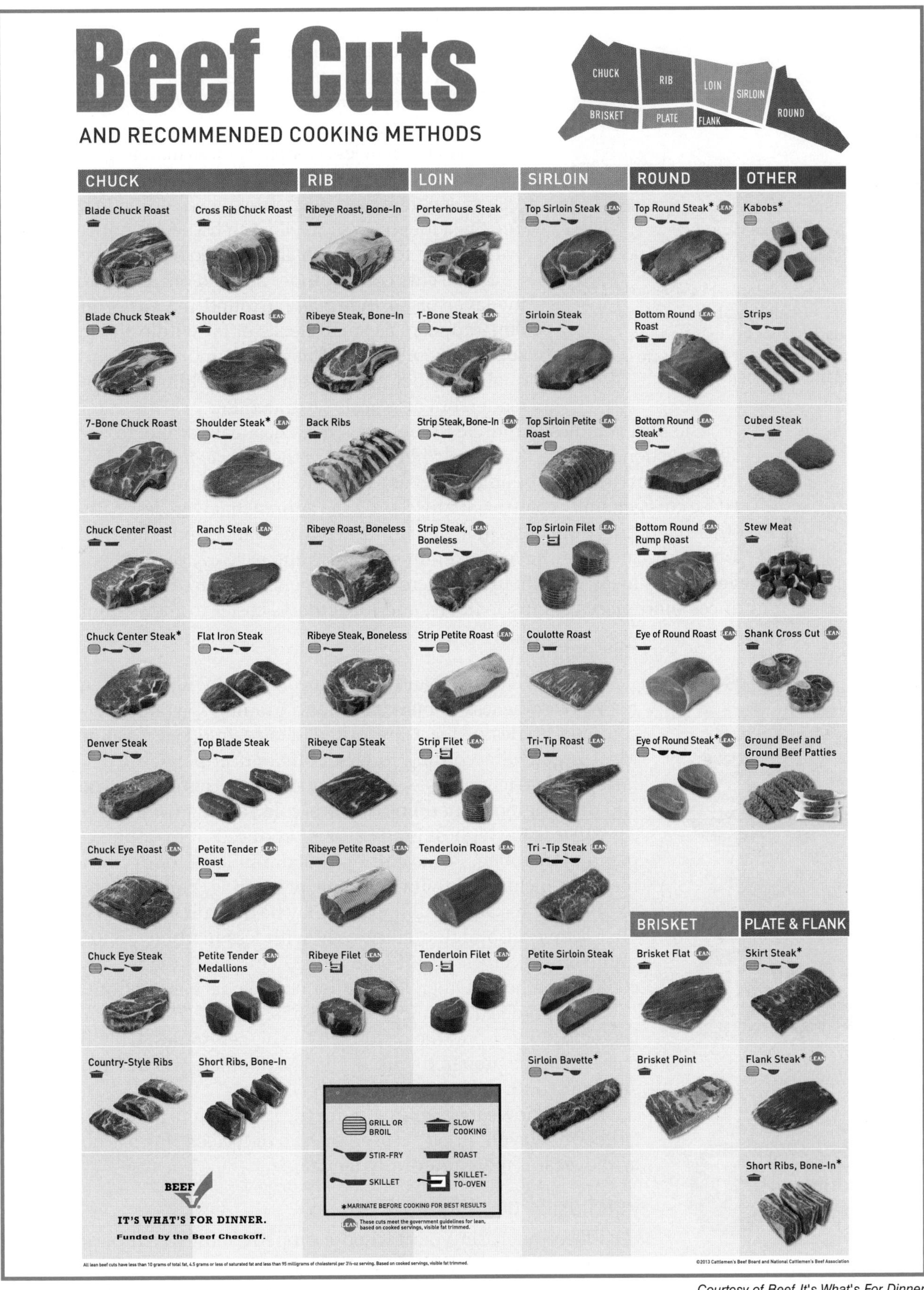

Courtesy of Beef. It's What's For Dinner

Figure 19.32 Knowing the part of the animal from which a cut originates will help you select the best cooking method to use.

Meat Composition

Meat is the edible muscle portion of the animal. Muscles are comprised of bundles of cells called *fibers*. Other components in muscle are *connective tissue*, such as *collagen* and *elastin*, and intramuscular fat, referred to as *marbling*. Connective tissue can make the meat less tender, whereas marbling makes meat more tender. *Collagen*, a transparent tissue between muscle cells, softens and becomes gelatin when cooked in moist heat. ***Elastin***, a tough, elastic, yellowish tissue, cannot be softened by heat; therefore, it is usually trimmed off before cooking.

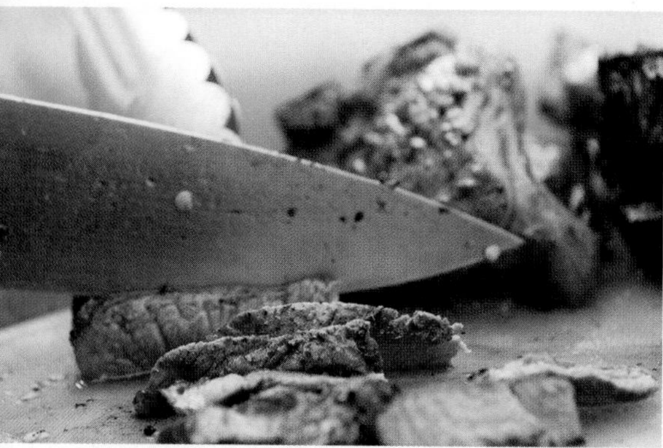

karanik yimpat/Shutterstock.com

Figure 19.33 Before you begin cutting a piece of meat, look for the muscle fibers running through the meat and cut across, or perpendicular to, the fibers.

Some cuts contain more fat than others. In addition to the layer of fat that may surround the cut of meat, marbling appears as small flecks of fat within the muscle tissue. Lean cuts of meat have little marbling, whereas high quality, tender cuts have more. Marbling makes the meat tender, but also adds saturated fat.

The fiber bundles of muscle tissue run across the meat parallel to one another. The direction in which the muscle fibers align is the *grain of the meat*. In expensive cuts of meat, the fiber bundles are very thin and do not form a significant grain. These cuts generally come from muscles on the animal that were less active. On the other hand, cuts from areas that were more active tend to be more flavorful, but are tougher because they have thicker muscle fibers and a clearly defined grain. When slicing this meat, you should cut across, or perpendicular to, the grain. This produces short pieces of muscle fibers, and meat that is easier to chew (**Figure 19.33**).

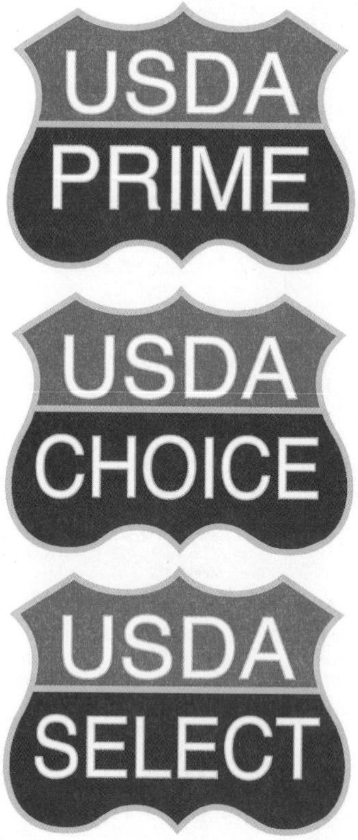

Inspection

The USDA inspects and grades meat. Just as with poultry, inspection for wholesomeness is mandatory and grading is voluntary. The most common grades of meat are prime, choice, and select (**Figure 19.34**). Meat is graded according to factors that affect **palatability** (agreeable taste), such as tenderness, juiciness, and flavor. This includes the amount and distribution of marbling, texture, color, and age of the animal.

Prime is the highest grade and is produced from young cattle with plentiful marbling. Prime cuts of meat are suitable for dry-heat cooking methods, including broiling, grilling, or roasting. This grade is normally reserved for restaurant dining and may be difficult to find in stores.

Choice is also high quality, only with less marbling, and normally found in grocery stores. Some choice cuts are suitable for dry-heat cooking methods. Other, less tender choice cuts benefit from braising.

Select grade cuts of meat have less marbling, and therefore may be less tender, juicy, and flavorful than the higher grades. Only the tender cuts should be prepared with dry heat. All others should be marinated and braised for the best results.

Lamb and veal are graded with the same prime and choice grades as beef; however, "good" is used instead of "select." Pork is not graded, as the meat is more uniformly tender.

USDA PRIME

USDA CHOICE

USDA SELECT

USDA

Figure 19.34 Meat is graded for quality based on tenderness, juiciness, and flavor.

Purchasing and Storing Meat

When purchasing meat, choose properly refrigerated packages that are not leaking. Remember to check the sell-by date so you know how soon you must prepare it. Choose cuts that are smooth with no ragged edges. The desired color of the meat depends on the cut and the animal.

Beef and lamb should be dark red with creamy white-colored fat. Pork and veal should be a pinkish-gray color. The texture should be smooth with tight, uniform grain fibers. The cut you are buying affects the desired amount of fat. For example, a rib eye should have abundant marbling, while a brisket cut should have a tighter, more visible grain with no marbling.

After shopping, take raw meat home and refrigerate it immediately. Place the meat on the bottom of the refrigerator away from ready-to-eat foods to avoid cross-contamination. If you are freezing the meat, wrap it tightly and mark the date on the package. Uncooked roasts, steaks, and chops can remain in the freezer for up to one year, while uncooked ground meat must be used within four months. Always defrost meat in the refrigerator and not at room temperature. Defrosting in the refrigerator takes longer, but avoiding the bacterial growth that can result from defrosting at room temperature is worth it.

Cooking Meat

Meat can be prepared using moist-heat cooking methods as well as dry-heat cooking methods. The cut and grade determine which cooking method should be used. On the other hand, if you have a specific recipe you are preparing, then the cooking method employed by the recipe should guide the selection of cut. More costly, tender cuts like tenderloin, flat iron, New York strip, porterhouse, or rib eye can be grilled, broiled, stir-fried, or roasted. However, less tender cuts like flank steak, top sirloin, and chuck are better braised, stewed, or prepared in a slow cooker. These cuts also tend to be more economical.

Regardless of which method you use, trim all visible fat from meat before cooking to reduce the fat content (**Figure 19.35**). An easy way to trim fat from meat is to place the meat in the freezer for 20 minutes before trimming. Fat is easier to cut when it is partially frozen. Partially frozen raw meat is also easier to cube or slice.

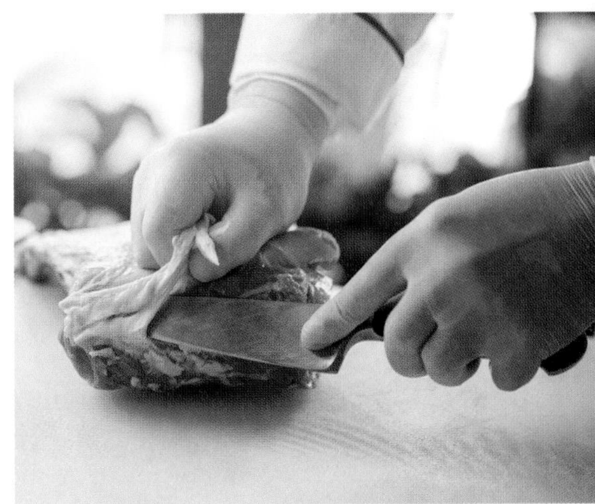

DenisProduction.com/Shutterstock.com

Figure 19.35 Trim visible fat from meat before cooking to reduce fat content.

Searing and Sautéing

When using moist-heat or combination methods, searing the meat first adds a rich and complex flavor. To sear, begin by drying the meat with a paper towel. Then, heat a skillet over medium-high heat until a water drop dances around the pan. Next, add a small amount of fat to the pan and swirl to coat the bottom of the pan with the fat. Add the meat to the skillet, taking care not to overload the pan. Placing too much meat in the pan will cause the pan to cool. The meat will steam in its juices rather than produce a beautifully browned surface.

When you place the meat in the hot pan, it will stick to the bottom. Shake the pan every minute or so to see if the meat releases. When it releases, it is finished searing on that side. Turn the meat over and repeat.

Sautéing is ideal for smaller, tender cuts of meat. This technique adds flavor and preserves the texture and moisture of the meat. The method used for sautéing is the same as that for searing.

Grilling, Broiling, and Roasting

Grilling and broiling are typically used on smaller cuts of meat. Roasting is better suited to larger cuts of meat.

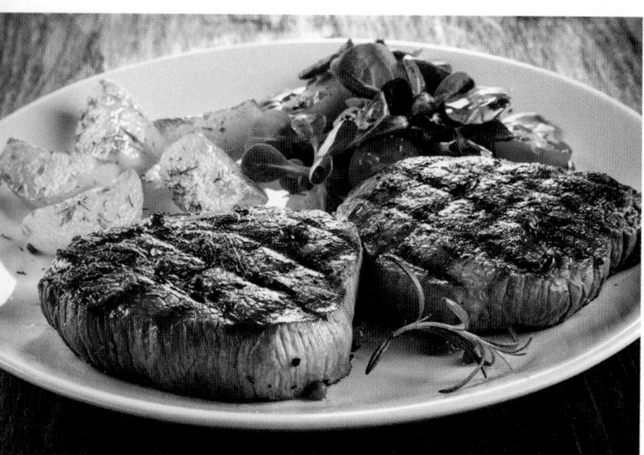

Jacek Chabraszewski/Shutterstock.com

Figure 19.36 These appealing grill marks are the trademark of a well-grilled meat and are created by rotating the meat 90 degrees to form a second set of marks.

When grilling or broiling, preheat the oven or grill. Clean the grill grate and brush a little oil on it. If broiling, oil the broiler pan grate. Place the meat over the heat source if you are grilling or under the source if you are broiling. Cook meat to the desired degree of doneness—rare, medium-rare, medium, medium-well, and well done. Halfway through the cooking process, turn the meat over (**Figure 19.36**). When done cooking, remove from the heat source, loosely cover the meat with foil, and allow the meat to rest for 10 to 20 minutes. Resting allows the juices to reabsorb into the meat. This step is essential for a flavorful, tender, juicy finished product. As it is resting, the meat continues to cook from **residual** (remaining) heat for a few minutes. This additional cooking should be factored into your decision about when to pull the meat from the heat source.

Meat is roasted uncovered in an oven at low, moderate, or high temperatures. Lower temperatures work better for larger roasts, and higher temperatures produce a nicely browned crust without overcooking smaller roasts. As with grilling and broiling, remove the meat from the heat source once the desired temperature is achieved. Loosely cover the roast in foil and allow it to rest for 10 to 20 minutes before serving.

Check for doneness in the same way you check poultry. Insert the thermometer in a thick part of the meat, taking care to avoid the bone.

Braising and Stewing

Braising and stewing methods are ideally suited to less tender, less expensive cuts of meat. A successfully braised meat begins with a good sear as discussed earlier. Once the meat is seared, it is moved to a Dutch oven or slow cooker and enough liquid is added to cover about 30 to 60 percent of the meat. The amount of liquid you add depends on how much sauce you want the dish to yield. The liquid—usually a flavored liquid such as a stock—is used to make sauce after the meat is cooked.

Braising is a long, slow cooking method often requiring a few hours depending on the size of the meat. The liquid should never be allowed to boil because this makes meat tough. To test for doneness, insert a large fork or skewer into the meat. If the meat easily slides off the fork or skewer, it is considered done. This is called *fork-tender*.

Stewing is essentially the same method as braising except it is performed on bite-size pieces of meat.

Fish and Shellfish

The USDA recommends consuming fish and shellfish twice a week. They are an excellent source of protein and one of the few sources of natural vitamin D. Fish and shellfish have B vitamins, iron, and other minerals, and are low in saturated fat. Fatty fish, like salmon, contain omega-3 fatty acids. Saltwater fish is a good source of natural iodine.

Unlike meat, fish has very little connective tissue. This means fish is naturally tender and cooks very quickly. Care must be taken not to overcook and dry out fish.

Types of Fish and Shellfish

Fish are divided into two categories, *lean fish* and *fatty fish*. Lean fish contain less than five percent fat by weight. Lean fish have white flesh with a mild flavor. Examples of lean fish include bass, catfish, cod, flounder, mullet, perch, sole, and tilapia. In contrast, fatty fish contain more than five percent fat by weight and are high in omega-3 fatty acids. Their flesh is usually a deeper color with a stronger flavor than lean fish. Some examples are anchovies, eel, herring, salmon, sardines, and whitefish. Although lean fish contain fewer calories, fatty fish contain more beneficial omega-3 fatty acids.

Shellfish have a mild sweet flavor. They are also divided into two categories, *crustaceans* and *mollusks*. Crustaceans have segmented limbs and are covered with shell. Some examples are crab, shrimp, and lobster. Mollusks have soft bodies covered with a very hard shell. Some examples are clams, oysters, scallops, and mussels.

Purchasing and Storing Fish and Shellfish

Fish can be purchased in several forms including: whole, drawn, dressed, fillets, or steaks (**Figure 19.37**). When choosing fish and shellfish, they should be as fresh as possible. Fish and shellfish should be properly refrigerated or displayed on a thick bed of ice, and have a slight fish or seaweed-like smell.

Select whole, drawn, or dressed fish with undamaged skin, flesh that springs back when touched, and bright, shiny color. For whole or drawn fish, the eyes should be clear and not cloudy or sunken, and the gills should be bright red. Select fillets or steaks with wet, glossy flesh. Darker meat flesh should be bright and white flesh should look **translucent** (see-through). Reject fish with a strong odor, pooled liquid in the package, mushy flesh, or cracks that run between the muscles and the *collagen sheaths* (the white lines running through the fish).

Some shellfish must be purchased live because they spoil rapidly after death. Lobsters and crabs should be active with leg movement. The shells of live clams, oysters, and mussels should not be cracked or broken and should be tightly closed. If the shells are slightly open, tap them. If they do not close when tapped, reject them. Scallops and shrimp are not alive when sold and should be properly refrigerated or stored on ice. Scallops are often sold without their shells and shrimp can be purchased with or without their shells. The flesh should be firm and moist, but not in liquid. The shells of shrimp should be translucent.

Bring freshly purchased fish and shellfish home and refrigerate immediately on the bottom shelf of the refrigerator. Store live shellfish in open containers with no water, covered with a clean, damp cloth in the refrigerator.

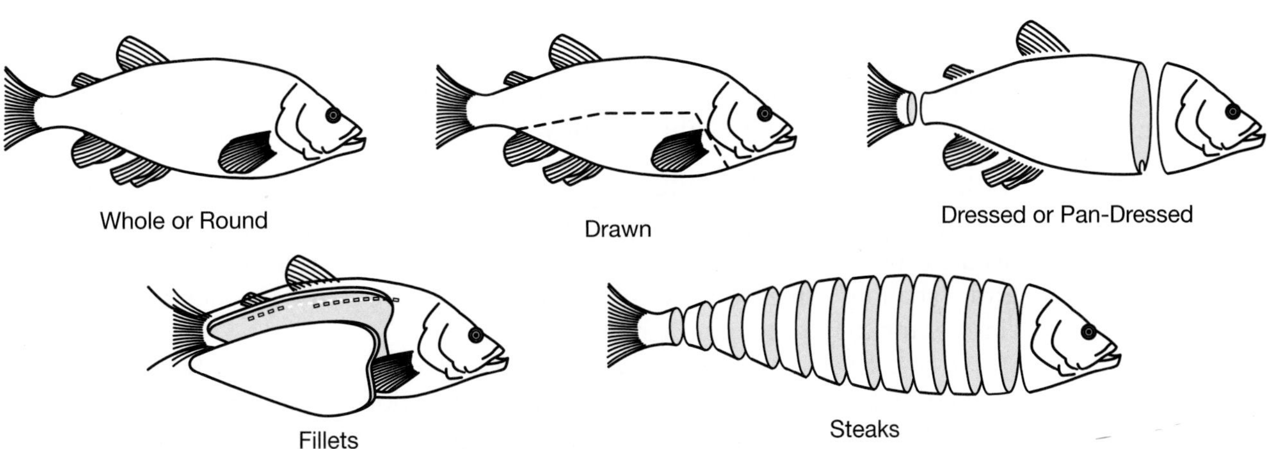

Figure 19.37 As with meat, fish can be purchased in a variety of forms.

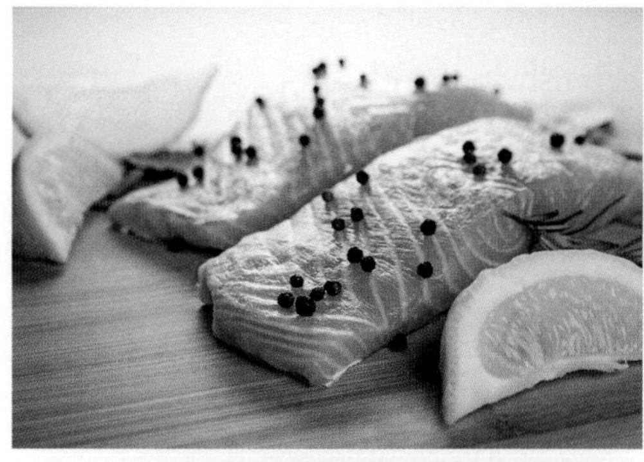

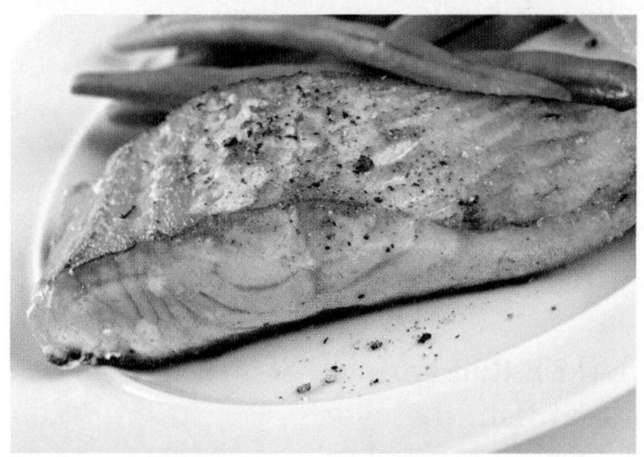

DwaFotografy/Shutterstock.com; Flashon Studio/Shutterstock.com

Figure 19.38 During cooking, muscle fibers in the fish coagulate and change from translucent to opaque.

Cooking Fish and Shellfish

Many people do not eat fish or shellfish because they do not know how to select or prepare it. In reality, fish and shellfish can be prepared in many simple ways. Fish can be prepared successfully using either dry- or moist-heat methods. However, moist-heat methods should be used to prepare lean fish due to their low fat content.

Fish cooks quickly because it has very short muscle fibers, unlike meat and poultry. When fish cooks, the muscle fibers coagulate and become **opaque** (not see-through) (**Figure 19.38**). In addition, the collagen dissolves quickly, causing the fish to separate into flakes. The largest concern when preparing fish is overcooking. The general rule when cooking fish is to cook 10 minutes per inch of thickness; however, this varies depending on the temperature and method. Properly cooked fish should be opaque, tender, and flaky, but not tough.

Dry-Heat Cooking Methods

Fish can be broiled or grilled easily. Thicker, firmer fish is easier to broil or grill; however, a thinner fillet or steak can also be broiled or grilled. To broil, place the fish on an oiled piece of aluminum foil and position it two inches below the heat source for every half-inch thickness of fish. For example, if the fish is one inch thick, place it four inches below the heat source. Halfway through the cooking time, turn the fish over.

To grill, make sure your grill grate is clean, and brush both the fish and the grate with a little oil. For thicker fillets or steaks, place them directly onto the grill grate. Delicate fillets or small shellfish can be grilled in a pouch made of aluminum foil or in a grill basket placed on the grate. Turn the fish midway through cooking. Sturdy fish and shellfish can be grilled on a skewer. Soak wooden skewers in water for 30 minutes before use to prevent them from burning. Thread the shellfish or pieces of fish on the skewers and lay the skewers directly on the grill grate.

Fillets and steaks can be fried in oil or butter. The fish can be breaded or plainly seasoned. Begin with a skillet heated over medium heat. When the pan is hot, add enough oil to cover the bottom of the skillet. Place fish in the skillet in a single layer. Turn fish halfway through the cooking time.

Whole fish, and large steaks and fillets bake well. Bake steaks and fillets uncovered, with skin side down in an oiled pan. Fish do not need to be turned with this cooking method. Whole, drawn, and dressed fish can be stuffed, placed in an oiled pan in the oven, and basted frequently.

Moist-Heat Cooking Methods

Either poaching or steaming works well for delicate and lean fish. The liquid used for poaching or steaming can be water, broth, or milk. Pour enough liquid into a shallow skillet to fully cover the fish and bring to a simmer. Add fish and simmer for 10 minutes per inch of thickness.

To steam fish, you will need a rack suspended over boiling water. Put one inch of water or broth into a pot or steamer. Bring to a boil. Place fish on a rack that has been coated with oil or nonstick spray. Place the rack with the fish over the boiling liquid, making sure the liquid does not touch the rack. Cover and steam for four to eight minutes, depending on the thickness of your fish.

Live shellfish are often boiled or steamed. Mollusks and shrimp can also be poached, baked, or sautéed. When done, crustacean shells turn bright red and the flesh is opaque. When mollusks are done cooking, their flesh also becomes opaque and their shells open.

Understanding Fruits and Vegetables

Fruits and vegetables are nutrient dense, full of fiber, and very low in sodium and fat. They can be eaten raw or cooked. A healthy eating pattern includes a variety of fruits and vegetables every day. The MyPlate food guidance system recommends that half of every meal be comprised of fruits and vegetables.

Types of Fruits and Vegetables

Fruits develop from the flower of a plant and ripen to a sweet, tender, appealing food. Fruits are sometimes called "nature's candy." All the other parts of the plant—leaves, roots, stems, seeds—are consumed as vegetables. Fruits are divided into six groups—pomes, drupes, berries, melons, citrus, and tropical. Vegetables are categorized based on what part of the plant they are (**Figure 19.39**).

Fruits and Vegetables			
Fruits			
Group	Description	Group	Description
Pomes	Fleshy fruit; edible skin; central core with several seeds Examples: apple, pear	**Melons**	Large, round fruit; hard, thick rind, or outer skin; sweet and juicy; many seeds Examples: watermelon, cantaloupe, honeydew
Drupes	Fleshy fruit; thin skin, central stone (often called a pit) containing the seed Examples: apricot, peach, plum	**Citrus**	Juicy flesh divided into segments; thick rind; grown in warm regions Examples: orange, grapefruit, lemon, lime
Berries	Small juicy fruit; thin outer skin; brightly colored Examples: blueberry, raspberry, blackberry	**Tropical**	Grown in tropical climates; differing characteristics Examples: banana, pineapple, guava, papaya

Continued

Top to bottom: Artem Kutsenko/Shutterstock.com; Kovaleva_Ka/Shutterstock.com; Volosina/Shutterstock.com; COLOA Studio/Shutterstock.com; Amero/Shutterstock.com; MRS. Siwaporn/Shutterstock.com

Figure 19.39 Fruits and vegetables are all plant-based foods, but vary greatly in appearance, flavor, and nutritional value.

Fruits and Vegetables *(Continued)*			
Vegetables			
Part of Plant	**Description**	**Part of Plant**	**Description**
Root	Serves as plant's food supply storage; mostly starchy vegetables; most must be cooked, some can be eaten raw Examples: radish, carrot, sweet potato	**Leaf**	Edible leaves; some grow individually and some form heads; most are eaten raw, others need light cooking Examples: spinach, lettuce
Tuber	Edible modified underground stem; mostly starchy vegetables; most must be eaten cooked Examples: potato, jicama	**Flower**	Reproductive part of plant; firm vegetables; some can be eaten raw Examples: artichoke, broccoli, cauliflower
Bulb	Short, edible, underground stem surrounded by fleshy leaves; can be eaten raw or cooked Examples: onion, garlic, shallot	**Fruit**	Botanically identified as fruits; often harvested for culinary use as vegetables; most can be eaten raw, others need light cooking Examples: tomato, eggplant, squash
Stem	Edible stems that grow above ground; tender vegetables; some require light cooking, some can be eaten raw Examples: asparagus, celery	**Seed**	Grows into a new plant; some seed vegetables are also classified as a protein Examples: beans, corn, peas

Top to bottom: Nattika/Shutterstock.com; Quang Ho/Shutterstock.com; Kittikun/Shutterstock.com; Binh Thanh Bui/Shutterstock.com; Binh Thanh Bui/Shutterstock.com; Binh Thanh Bui/Shutterstock.com; bergamont/Shutterstock.com; matkub2499/Shutterstock.com

Choosing and Storing Fruits and Vegetables

Each fruit and vegetable has a growing season when it is at its peak and more plentiful. As a result, fruits and vegetables are reasonably priced at this time. When fresh, seasonal produce is not available, frozen fruits and vegetables are a great option. Frozen fruits and vegetables are usually frozen within hours of being picked. Sometimes frozen produce can be just as nutritious as fresh. Canned fruits and vegetables are another option; however, some canned goods contain large amounts of added sugars and sodium. To avoid added sugar, select canned fruits that are packed in water or 100 percent juice, rather than syrup.

For canned vegetables, read the label to learn the sodium content. Purchase low sodium options, and when possible, rinse canned vegetables to remove some of the sodium.

When choosing fresh fruits and vegetables, choose only those that have bright color and firmness. Avoid those that have bruises, spots, wilted leaves, blemishes, or are misshapen. Purchase only the amount that can be eaten within five days. With the exception of potatoes and onions, fresh produce is highly perishable.

Many cities host farmers' markets. Farmers bring the produce directly from their fields to the consumer. Most often, the produce is allowed to ripen on the vine before harvesting, and is brought to market the next day. Supermarket produce is picked before maturity because it must be shipped across the state, the country, or around the world. It may take a week or more to arrive at the store. During this time, the produce may ripen but it also loses nutrients.

Since fruits and vegetables are highly perishable, they must be refrigerated. Potatoes and onions are an exception to this rule. Potatoes should be stored in a cool (not cold), dry, dark place. Onions should be stored in a cool, dry area. Place other vegetables in plastic bags or the refrigerator crisper. Do not wash the vegetables until you are ready to prepare them. Bananas and citrus fruits can be kept at room temperature. Ripe fruits, cut fruits, and berries should be refrigerated. Cut fruits should be stored in an airtight container. All other produce can be stored in an uncovered container or a perforated plastic bag. Unripe fruits must be kept at room temperature to ripen. Once they are ripe, they can be stored in the refrigerator.

Cooking with Fruits and Vegetables

Though most fruits and vegetables can be eaten raw, you can also cook them using any method. Before cooking, you must wash them to remove dirt, contaminants, wax coatings, and pesticide residue. Some fruits and vegetables are associated with foodborne illness. Even if you will be peeling the fruit or vegetable, it must be washed first or you risk transferring the contaminants from the outside to the inside (**Figure 19.40**). Wash fruits and vegetables by holding them under cold running water and gently rubbing. Submerge more delicate fruits and vegetables under cold water and allow them to drain. Studies have shown washing produce with just water can remove 98 percent of bacteria.

Cooking fruits and vegetables breaks down the cellulose in the cell walls and makes them more tender. This increases their digestibility and the body is better able to absorb the nutrients.

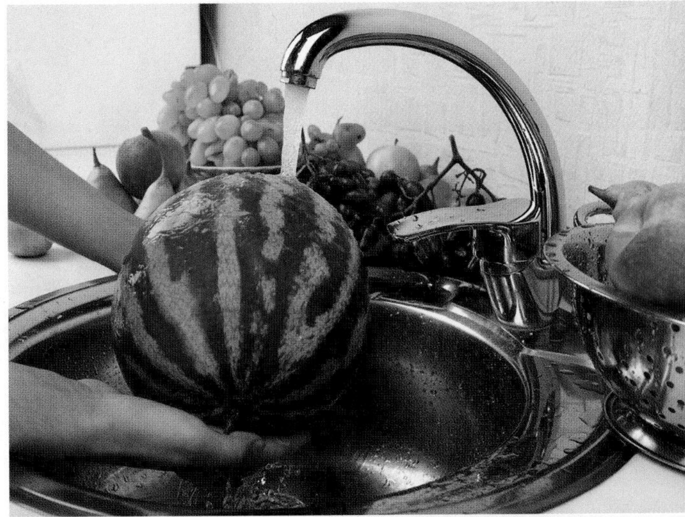

Africa Studio/Shutterstock.com

Figure 19.40 Even fruit whose rind or skin you will not be eating must be washed before cutting to avoid contaminating it with substances on the outer surface of the fruit as you cut. *Can you think of other fruits that should be washed before preparing?*

Dry-Heat Cooking Methods

Dry-heat cooking methods produce a desirable texture, as well as interesting flavor due to browning and caramelization. Many fruits and vegetables can be roasted, baked, grilled, broiled, sautéed, or fried. Some foods are better suited to certain cooking methods than others.

Baked vegetables and fruits are also referred to as *roasted*. Prepare the fruit or vegetable as needed. For example, you may want to peel inedible skin before cooking. You may want to cut or slice vegetables for more uniform cooking or simply for appearance. Toss cut vegetables in a small amount of oil and seasonings. Then simply place the prepared fruit or vegetable on a baking sheet lined with foil. Spread in one layer on the baking sheet. Roasting time will vary depending on the oven temperature, the size and type of vegetable or fruit, and if you prefer a tender, moist or a dry, crispy product. Soft vegetables cook more quickly than the firmer ones. Therefore, cut firmer vegetables into smaller pieces when roasting soft and firm vegetables together, so the vegetables finish at the same time. You can test the vegetable for doneness with a fork or the tip of a knife.

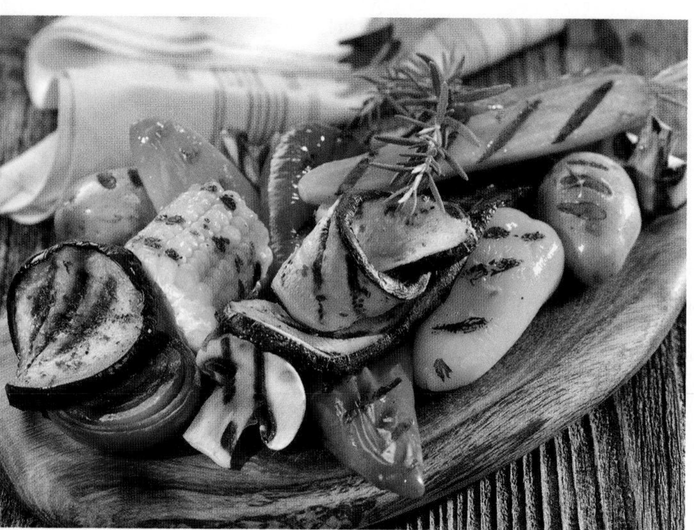

Karl Allgaeuer/Shutterstock.com

Figure 19.41 Grilling can make vegetables more appealing for people who do not typically like vegetables.

Fruits and vegetables are easy to grill (**Figure 19.41**). Cut the food to be grilled in uniform-size pieces for even cooking. Pieces must be large enough that they will not fall through the grate or smaller pieces can be placed on a skewer. Preheat a clean grill grate and rub some oil on it to prevent sticking. Turn the pieces or skewers halfway through cooking to produce attractive grill marks on both sides. Grill the fruit or vegetable until soft, watching carefully that they do not overcook.

Sauté fruits and vegetables over moderate heat. Add oil or butter to a preheated pan and swirl to cover the bottom of the pan. Add vegetables or fruit, season, and cook to desired doneness.

Some fruits and vegetables can be dipped in batter or dredged in flour and fried. Some vegetables may need to be partially cooked before frying.

Moist-Heat Cooking Methods

Boiling and steaming can be performed on most vegetables. Prepare vegetables by trimming, peeling, or cutting as needed. Bring a pot of water to a boil and add vegetables. Return water to boil. Cook green vegetables and strong-flavored vegetables uncovered. All other vegetables can be covered during cooking.

The movement of water during boiling can cause delicate vegetables to break up or become mushy. For these types of vegetables, steaming may be preferable. To steam, place vegetables in a basket or on a rack suspended over boiling water and cook covered. Be sure to arrange vegetables in a single layer for even cooking. Cook to desired doneness.

Legumes

Legumes, such as beans and peas, are the protein-rich seeds of plants and are counted in both the vegetable and protein foods groups. Green peas and green beans are not considered legumes because their nutrient profile is much different. Although legumes are considered vegetables, they are unique in both their nutrient profile and cooking method from most vegetables, so they are being discussed separately.

When legumes are harvested as dry products, they are called *pulses*. Examples of pulses include black-eyed peas, pinto beans, black beans, lentils, chickpeas, and split peas (**Figure 19.42**). Pulses are rich in fiber and protein, and fat free.

Soybeans and peanuts are also legumes, but they contain fat and are processed in different ways than pulses.

Cooking Legumes

Legumes—beans, peas, and lentils—are sold in both dried and canned forms. Canned legumes are ready to use. Rinse them first to remove the added sodium. To prepare dried legumes, begin by sorting through them to remove any rocks, broken or shriveled legumes, or other foreign matter. After sorting, rinse legumes under running water. Next, the dried legumes need to be rehydrated; however, split peas and some lentils do not require this step.

To rehydrate, cover the dried legumes with three cups of water for every one cup of dried legumes. Complete rehydration in one of the following ways:

- soak legumes overnight
- boil in water for two minutes and allow to stand for one hour (called the *quick-soak method*)

Discard the water after soaking. Add fresh cold water to cover legumes by one to two inches. Place pot on cooktop and bring to a boil. Reduce the heat, cover, and simmer until the legume is tender. The amount of cooking time varies from one hour to three hours depending on the legume. Do not add salt or acidic ingredients until the legumes are nearly done cooking. These ingredients may prevent the legumes from becoming tender.

Recipe Makeover

How do you know if a recipe is healthy? A very basic way is simply to look at the list of ingredients and the cooking method. Knowing which ingredients and cooking methods are healthy helps you select healthy recipes. You can also use this knowledge to perform a recipe makeover and make your recipe healthier.

Healthy meals result when healthy ingredients are prepared using healthy cooking methods. Once you are able to recognize healthy ingredients and cooking methods, you can adjust recipes to create healthier versions.

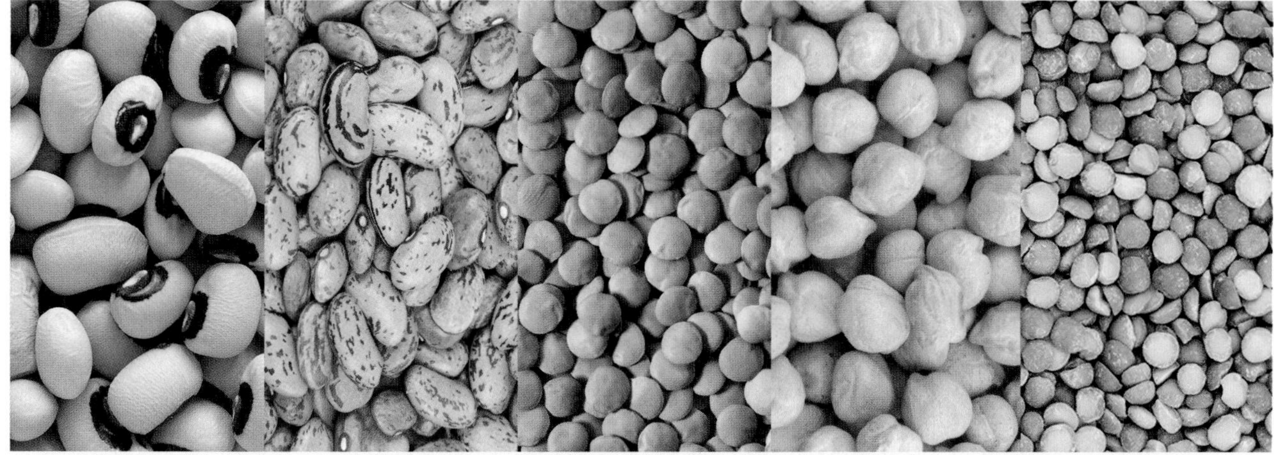

L to r: D. Pimborough/Shutterstock.com; Ilizia/Shutterstock.com; Alaettin YILDIRIM/Shutterstock.com; Flipser/Shutterstock.com; Enlightened Media/Shutterstock.com

Figure 19.42 These black-eyed peas, pinto beans, lentils, chickpeas, and split peas are a small sampling of the many types of legumes.

Healthy Ingredients

To prepare a healthy meal, you must start with healthy ingredients. Luckily, healthy ingredients can be found in all the food groups and oils.

The *Dietary Guidelines* recommends making at least half of the grains you eat be whole grains. Incorporating whole-grain ingredients into recipes and meals will result in a healthier meal. Substitute whole-grain flour for a portion of the refined flour in baked goods. Use whole-grain pastas for salads and casseroles. Mix brown rice in with white rice. Over time, gradually increase the proportion of brown rice to white as individuals adjust to the change in texture and flavor.

Use low-fat dairy products in place of full-fat products. For example, try substituting fat-free milk when a recipe calls for whole milk. Some cheeses are naturally lower in fat than others. Parmesan cheese contains about 25 percent less fat than cheddar cheese. Feta cheese contains approximately two-thirds the amount of fat found in cheddar cheese.

Use healthier protein ingredients for meals. Try leaner cuts of meat. Cuts of red meat that include "round" or "loin" in the name are considered lean. Look for ground meats or poultry with less than five percent fat content. Trim visible fat off meat before cooking. Nuts, seeds, and dried beans and peas are good alternate sources of protein. Top salads with garbanzo beans or add walnuts to oatmeal. Combining these foods with whole grains will provide your body with all the essential amino acids. For example, peanut butter on whole-wheat bread, red beans and rice, or pinto beans in a corn tortilla will provide the needed amino acids.

Whole, unpeeled fruits and vegetables generally retain more of their nutrients. Therefore, if you have the time to wash and trim produce yourself, avoid buying precut produce. Use a variety of fruits and vegetables in meals to benefit from the different nutrients each supplies. Make vegetables a bigger portion of the meal or recipe. Add a vegetable ingredient to a recipe that lacks vegetables. Adding broccoli to a chicken rice casserole recipe improves color appeal and adds nutrients.

Select healthier fats. Use more oils which contain unsaturated fats and avoid solid fats such as butter, lard, and shortening. If the recipe says to panfry the chicken in butter, you could sauté it in a small amount of canola oil instead. Rather than basting a turkey with fatty drippings or butter, use broth.

Few ingredients or foods need to be completely avoided. However, some ingredients should be used sparingly or less often. Saturated fat, sugar, and salt are three ingredients that should be reduced or replaced when cooking healthy meals. Gradually decrease the use of salt and sugar. Fill the flavor void with herbs, spices, lemon juice, or flavored vinegars. Marinades and rubs can be used on meats before cooking to enhance flavor.

Healthy Cooking Methods

The cooking methods you use affect the flavor and nutrient content of your food. Healthy cooking methods enable you to prepare flavorful foods while retaining nutrients and avoiding the use of too much fat or salt.

To prepare healthier foods, use cooking methods such as roasting, baking, grilling, broiling, poaching, sautéing, braising, steaming, and stir-frying. Rather than panfrying fish, try poaching it in flavorful liquid. Instead of deep-fat frying, try marinating chicken and then grilling it. To remove fat remaining in cooking liquid after braising or stewing food, place the liquid in the refrigerator. As the food cools, the fat will rise to the surface and harden. This can be skimmed off before reheating.

FOOD AND THE ENVIRONMENT

Composting

Schools generate an enormous amount of food waste by throwing away uneaten, and often untouched, fruits and vegetables. Uneaten produce and waste could be composted instead. Composting benefits the environment in a number of ways including:

- helps soil hold moisture,
- reduces the need for chemical fertilizers,
- recycles organic resources; and
- reduces the need for landfill space.

Compost adds nutrients and improves plant growth in a sustainable manner. Some of the many uses of compost include mulch, fertilizer, and soil amendment. It can be used for houseplants, in potted gardens, around trees, and on lawns.

Composting methods vary widely depending on the time, energy, and space available. For example, countertop bins enable apartment dwellers to compost. Compare this with commercial composting operations that handle large volumes of organic waste generated by entire communities.

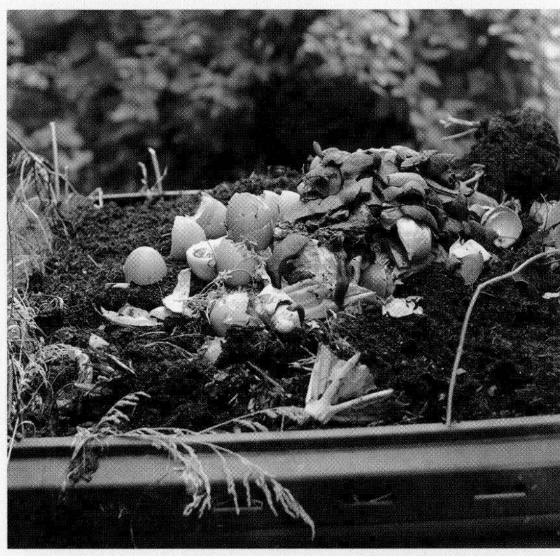

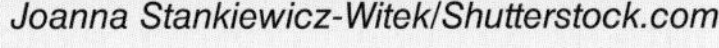

Joanna Stankiewicz-Witek/Shutterstock.com

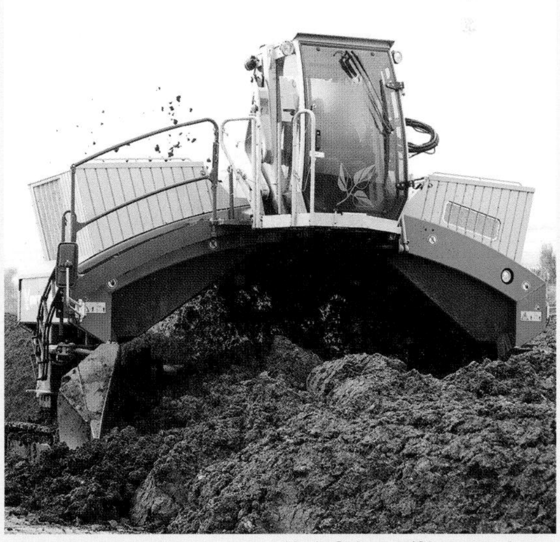

Yaniv Schwartz/Shutterstock.com

Do you know what happens with the food waste at your school? How might a compost program benefit your school and community?

Think Critically

1. Outline a plan to start a composting program at your school. Begin by interviewing the cafeteria manager and school administrators to determine how much waste is produced. Find out what policies are currently in place for food waste and recycling and where a composting pile could be placed.
2. Interview the biology teachers at your school to find out if they are interested in using a composting program in their curriculum.

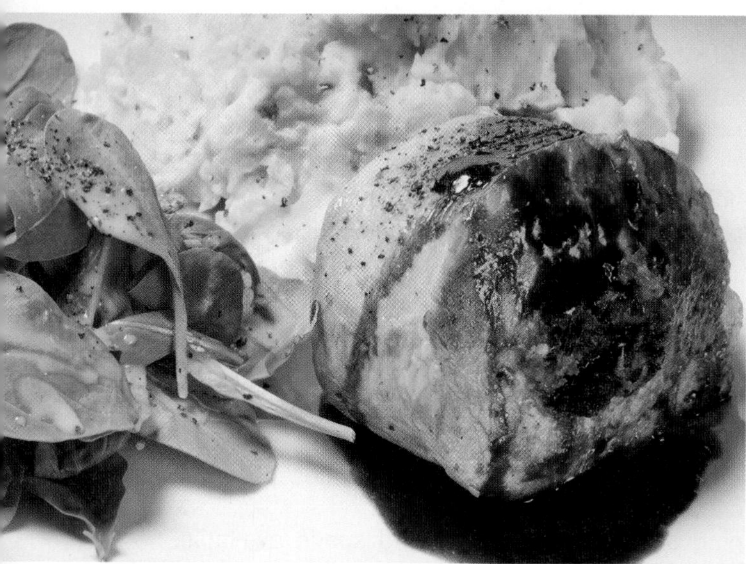

BGSmith/Shutterstock.com

Figure 19.43 Sauces like the balsamic vinegar and berry reduction in this photo can be healthier than starch-based sauces.

Make healthier sauces using reduction. *Reduction* is the process of cooking a liquid with the intent of losing volume through evaporation. This technique concentrates the flavors and thickens the liquid without the use of fat or starches (**Figure 19.43**).

When cooking washed fruits and vegetables, keep them in larger pieces and avoid peeling, if possible. This reduces the amount of exposed surface area and helps to reduce the amount of nutrients that leach into the cooking liquid. Use the smallest amount of cooking liquid possible to help preserve water-soluble nutrients. Protect heat-sensitive nutrients, such as folate and vitamin C, by cooking foods for the shortest time possible. Roasting does not significantly change nutrient content of vegetables. Roasting vegetables brings out their sweetness, which may make them more palatable to someone who dislikes vegetables. To retain as many nutrients as possible, leave vegetables in larger, uniform pieces and only roast until crisp-tender. Sautéing also minimizes nutrient loss because vegetables cook for a short time. In addition, the small amount of oil used in sautéing helps your body absorb more nutrients.

High heat and long cooking periods can result in vitamin losses. Microwave ovens cook quickly, minimizing such losses. Microwave cooking also requires less water than conventional cooking methods. Therefore, fewer nutrients leach into the cooking liquid.

Slow cookers use low heat for long periods; therefore, nutrients destroyed by high temperatures are preserved. The cooking liquid is often eaten with one-dish meals prepared in slow cookers. This means you still benefit from any nutrients that have escaped into the cooking liquid.

Do It Yourself

When you do the cooking yourself, you can control exactly what ingredients go into the food you are eating. You can decide how much salt to add or what type of fat to use. Cooking for yourself has the added benefit of injecting activity into your day. The various chores required to make a meal or snack—shopping, preparing, cleaning up—all require the expenditure of energy. In addition, time spent preparing a meal is less time spent in sedentary screen time or mindless snacking on processed foods.

Make cooking an adventure. Explore new recipes, techniques, or foods. Cooking should not be stressful. When cooking for yourself, most recipes do not have to be followed precisely. In fact, it can be fun to substitute or add ingredients that you prefer or just want to try. Most dishes (with the exception of baked products) will still turn out well. **Figure 19.44** offers some quick and healthy snack ideas to jumpstart your creativity.

Quick and Healthy Snack Ideas

Fruit Trifle: Layer nonfat yogurt, fruit, and granola in a cup.

Bean Roll-Up: Spread refried beans on a whole-grain tortilla. Sprinkle with grated, low-fat cheddar cheese and roll up. Bake at 400°F for 10 minutes. Top with salsa.

Apple and Cheese Quesadilla: Place a whole-grain tortilla in a skillet that has been sprayed with nonstick cooking spray. Cover half of tortilla with grated, low-fat cheddar cheese and thinly sliced apples. Fold tortilla over. Cook on both sides until cheese is melted and lightly browned.

Pita Pizza: Split a whole-grain pita pocket into two rounds. Brush each round with a small amount of olive oil. Spread tomato sauce or pesto on each round. Sprinkle chopped vegetables, such as mushrooms, olives, onion, and bell pepper, on each half. Top with grated, part-skim mozzarella cheese. Bake at 350°F for about 15 to 20 minutes.

Seasoned Potato Chips: Toss a thinly sliced potato with a small amount of olive oil. Place in a single layer on baking sheet. Sprinkle lightly with curry powder, Parmesan cheese, or garlic powder. Bake at 425°F for 10 minutes, or until crisp.

Thanksgiving Pinwheels: Spread a whole-grain tortilla with low-fat Neufchatel cheese, sprinkle with dried cranberries, and top with sliced, cooked turkey. Roll into a log and slice into one-inch pinwheels.

Figure 19.44 Try one or more of these snack ideas at home or school. If you do not like a particular ingredient, replace it with one you do like.

RECIPE FILE

Baked Tilapia

6 SERVINGS

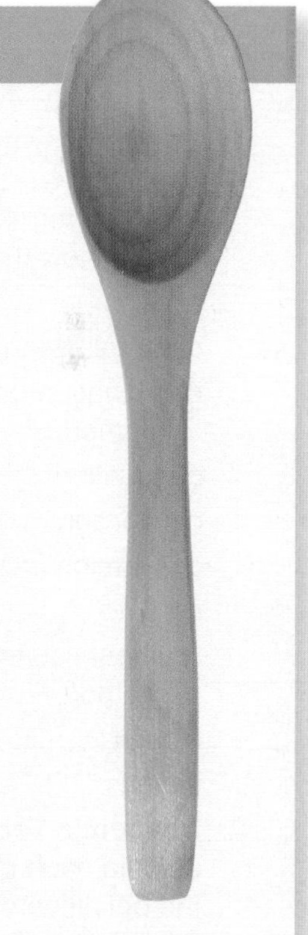

Ingredients

- 4 each (6 oz.) tilapia fillets
- cooking spray
- ¼ t. Old Bay Seasoning
- 1 clove garlic, minced
- 2 t. butter
- pepper
- 1 lemon, thinly sliced

Directions

1. Preheat oven to 350°F (177°C).
2. Rinse tilapia and pat dry with paper towels.
3. Spray a 9-inch by 13-inch pan with cooking spray.
4. Place tilapia fillets on baking sheet.
5. Sprinkle fish with seasoning and garlic.
6. Dot fish with butter.
7. Sprinkle pepper, then layer lemon slices over top.
8. Cover pan with foil.
9. Bake for 25–30 minutes, or until fish is opaque and flaky.

PER SERVING: 125 CALORIES, 23 G PROTEIN, 2 G CARBOHYDRATE, 4 G FAT, 1 G FIBER, 69 MG SODIUM.

Chapter 19 Review and Expand

Reading Summary

Successful food preparation requires organization, and organization begins with a recipe. Reading recipes requires an understanding of commonly used terms, abbreviations, and measurements.

Measurement techniques vary depending on the ingredient being measured. Learning proper knife skills saves time and avoids injuries in the kitchen. Understanding various preparation techniques and terms is necessary to read recipes and produce pleasing dishes that are consistent every time.

Heat is transferred from the heat source to food in a number of ways and using a variety of cooking methods. Different cooking methods produce different effects in foods.

Learning about foods in the various food groups and how different cooking methods affect them will help you select the best cooking method for your dish. This knowledge can help you make adjustments or substitutions to create healthier recipes.

Chapter Vocabulary

1. **Content Terms** On a separate sheet of paper, list words that relate to each of the following terms. Then, work with a partner to explain how these words are related.

al dente	homogenization
caramelization	Maillard reaction
combination cooking method	mise en place
conduction	moist-heat cooking method
convection	pasteurization
conversion factor	radiation
curdle	recipe
dry-heat cooking method	scorch
elastin	sear
gluten	tempering

2. **Academic Terms** Read the text passages that contain each of the following terms. Then write the definition of each term in your own words. Double-check your definitions by rereading the text and using the text glossary.

medium	reconstitute
opaque	residual
palatability	translucent
proximate	

Review Learning

3. List three examples of mise en place.
4. How are ingredients listed on a recipe?
5. What is the difference between an ounce and a fluid ounce?
6. Determine the conversion factor needed to change an original yield of 12 servings to a desired yield of 4 servings.
7. What steps do you need to follow when measuring liquids?
8. *True or false?* The fingertips of your guiding hand should be curled under as you grasp the food.
9. Which cutting technique would you use to produce matchstick-size pieces of carrots?
10. *True or false?* Conduction produces a circular flow that transfers heat throughout the food product.
11. Why are some moist-heat cooking methods suitable for inexpensive meat cuts?
12. *True or false?* Dry-heat cooking methods produce the Maillard reaction.
13. What is the common ratio of liquid to grains when simmering a grain product such as rice?
14. Sour cream is an example of a _____ milk product.
15. Describe the proper way to use a thermometer to check poultry for doneness.
16. Explain why ground beef must be cooked until it is no longer pink, but a beefsteak can be served rare (pink inside).
17. List five ways to help preserve nutrients in fruits and vegetables during cooking.

Self-Assessment Quiz

Complete the self-assessment quiz online to help you practice and expand your knowledge and skills.

Critical Thinking

18. **Analyze** Select a recipe from this textbook or a different source of your choosing. Analyze the recipe to determine the mise en place. Write a step-by-step description of the mise en place and submit it with a copy of the recipe.

19. **Create** Working with your lab group, choose a simple main dish recipe to prepare and perform the mise en place. Assign responsibilities to each group member and estimate how long the dish will take to prepare and create a work schedule. Create a grocery list and shop for the items you will need. In class, plan and perform a cooking show that demonstrates the proper preparation of the recipe. During the show, discuss the ingredients and skills you are using and the importance of mis en place. Be sure to follow appropriate safety and sanitation practices. After the show, write a short evaluation reflecting on the preparation process, recipe outcome, and team effectiveness. Was your recipe a success? If not, what could you have done differently? Did you learn any new skills during the preparation of this recipe? Was the work schedule accurate? Did the team work cooperatively? How did this affect the success of your recipe? Would you prepare this recipe again? Why, or why not?
20. **Evaluate** Imagine you are in college. After a long day of studying and soccer practice, you stumble into your apartment—tired and very hungry. You wander into the kitchen to prepare something quick to eat before you do some last minute studying for tomorrow's midterm. You decide you will prepare a vegetable quesadilla. You begin to gather your ingredients, but you find you do not have any tortillas. Then you remember that you ate the last one two days ago. You see you have the cheese and the vegetables, so you decide to make an omelet. You look in your refrigerator and see that you do not have any eggs! Therefore, you decide to have cereal for dinner. You pour the cereal into a bowl and grab the milk from the refrigerator. You open the milk and a noxious odor fills the kitchen. The milk is spoiled—no cereal tonight! You finally decide to have fast-food delivered. Unfortunately, your fast-food dinner cost you half your week's food budget and supplied two days' worth of sodium and fat. Evaluate your situation and decide what you can do differently in the future to avoid this problem.
21. **Analyze** Pour hot coffee into a ceramic mug. Add approximately one tablespoon of cream into the coffee. Wrap your hands around the mug as you observe the coffee and cream. How many heat transfer methods can you identify?

Core Skills

22. **Math** Change the yield for the Marinated Chicken Breasts recipe in Figure 19.1 to yield 12 servings.
23. **Technology Literacy and Writing** Plan a blog about selecting and preparing legumes. First, consider who will be reading your blog and how to make the topic appealing to them. Next, identify three main points that you want to cover. Then, be sure to give your blog a clever title. After you finish writing, be sure to edit and revise your content before posting.
24. **Science and Writing** Create a lab procedure to compare the effects of different cooking methods on chicken breasts. Use two similar-size chicken breasts. Prepare one of the breasts using a dry-heat cooking method, and prepare the other breast using a moist-heat cooking method. Record your observations. Prepare a lab report describing your experiment and analyzing your results.
25. **Writing and Speaking** Write an in-service that demonstrates basic knife safety and skills. Assume the intended audience is a class of middle school students. Use speech that is suitable for the age of the audience. Prepare questions to stimulate participation and gauge understanding. As you present your in-service, speak clearly and at a volume that can be heard by all attending.
26. **Technology Literacy** Select a recipe to make over. Create a digital poster featuring the "before and after" recipes. Identify the changes you are making to create a healthier recipe. Consider readability and appeal as you choose fonts, colors, and layout of your poster.
27. **Career Readiness Practice** In the workplace, it is important to consider the impact of your decisions on the environment. Presume you work for a restaurant that wants to offer more fish and seafood on the menu. The company has asked you to research and recommend fish to feature on the menu. You recognize the importance of promoting sustainable seafood and determine that your menu suggestions will keep the long-term health of the various fish, as well as the waters they are fished from, in mind. You will need to locate reliable sources about sustainable seafood options. Read and interpret the information and then recommend three fish dishes to offer on the menu. Write a report to support your recommendations.

Staying Physically Active

Learning Outcomes

After studying this chapter, you will be able to

- **differentiate** between physical activity and exercise;
- **recognize** common goals for physical activity;
- **summarize** the benefits of physical activity;
- **analyze** various components of physical fitness;
- **summarize** the effects of physical activity on overall heart function;
- **identify** four keys to a successful exercise program; and
- **implement** a personal exercise program.

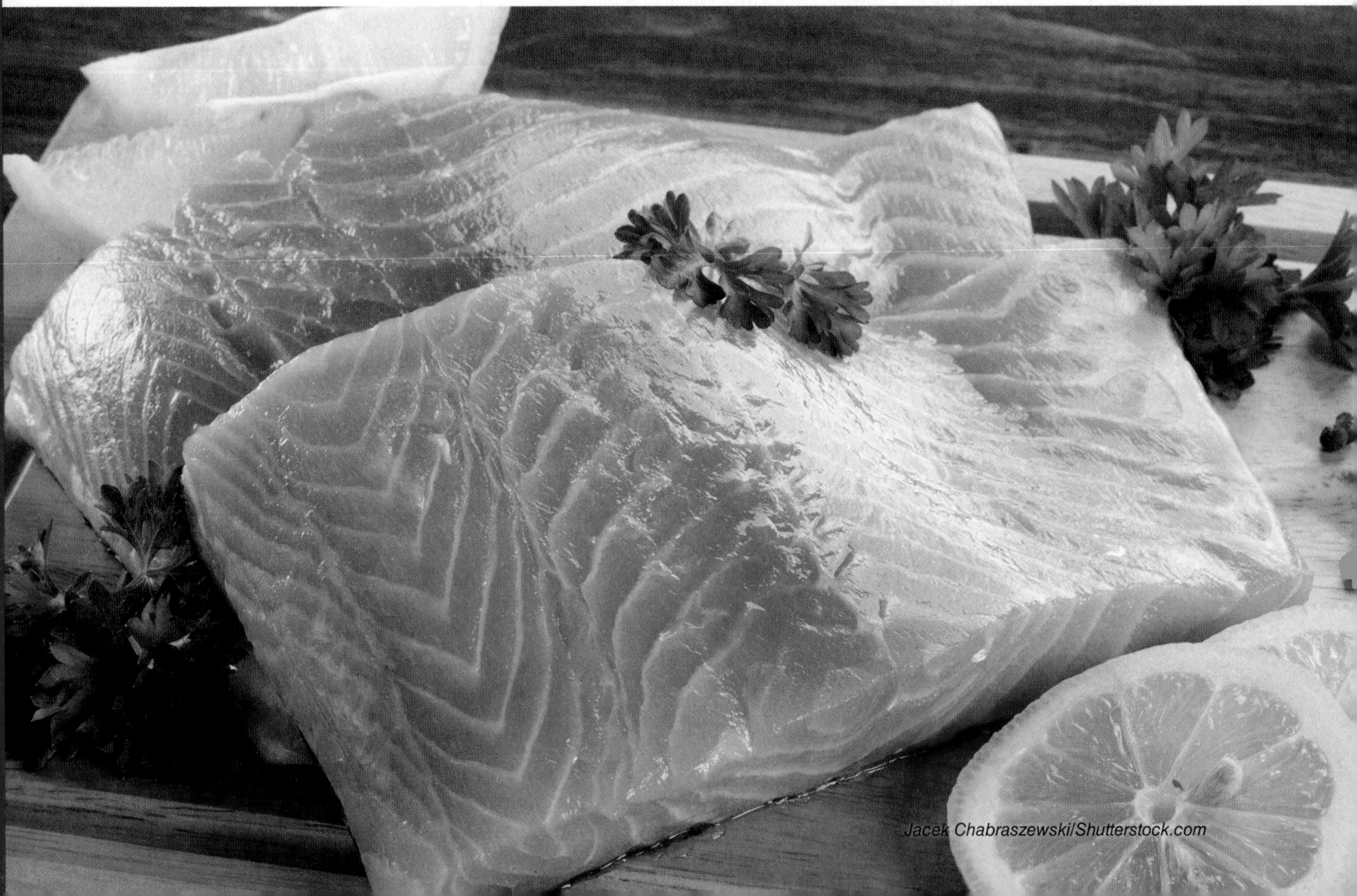

Jacek Chabraszewski/Shutterstock.com

Content Terms 

aerobic activity
agility
anaerobic activity
balance
cardiorespiratory fitness
coordination
dementia
exercise
flexibility
heart rate
maximum heart rate
muscular endurance
physical activity
physical fitness
posture
power
reaction time
resting heart rate (RHR)
speed
strength
target heart rate zone

Academic Terms 

acute
cumulative
skeptical
stamina
strenuous

What's Your Nutrition and Wellness IQ?

Take this quiz to examine how much you already know about staying physically active. If you cannot answer a question, pay extra attention to that topic as you study this chapter.

- Identify each statement as *True*, *False*, or *It Depends*. *It Depends* means in some cases the statement is true; in some cases it could be false.
- Revise false statements to make them true.
- Explain the circumstances in which each *It Depends* statement is true and when it is false.

Nutrition and Wellness IQ 

	Statement			
1.	Physical activity must be regular, structured, and performed with a purpose like at a spinning class.	True	False	It Depends
2.	The most important goal of physical activity is improved athletic performance.	True	False	It Depends
3.	A long-distance runner is an example of overall physical fitness.	True	False	It Depends
4.	A high resting heart rate (RHR) is an indication of peak physical fitness.	True	False	It Depends
5.	For the most benefit, your heart rate should be at maximum heart rate during exercise.	True	False	It Depends
6.	"I will do more exercise tomorrow than I did today" is an example of a good fitness goal.	True	False	It Depends
7.	Choosing an activity you enjoy is key to a successful exercise program.	True	False	It Depends
8.	A warm-up period prior to exercise reduces the risk of an injury.	True	False	It Depends

While studying this chapter, look for the activity icon  **to**

- **build** vocabulary with e-flash cards and interactive games;
- **assess** what you learn by completing self-assessment quizzes and completing review questions; and
- **expand** knowledge with interactive activities and activities that extend learning.

www.g-wlearning.com/foodsandnutrition/

What is your daily routine? Do you ride in a bus or car to get to and from school? After school, do you spend time studying and on social media? Is your idea of relaxation reading a book? Physical inactivity is a national health concern in the United States. This chapter will help you learn why staying physically active is important and how to incorporate it into your daily life.

Physical Activity Versus Exercise

The terms *physical activity* and *exercise* are often used interchangeably, but they have different meanings. ***Physical activity*** is any body movement that causes your muscles to work more than they would at rest. In contrast, ***exercise*** is regular, structured physical activity performed with a purpose. Regular physical activity and exercise are necessary to achieve physical fitness. ***Physical fitness*** is a condition in which all the body systems function together well. This enables you to perform daily activities with little effort or fatigue and still have the **stamina** (strength, energy) to participate in leisure activities or sports (**Figure 20.1**).

Goals for Physical Activity

Most people who are active or who want to become active have one of three main goals for becoming more physically active. They want to achieve good health, overall physical fitness, or peak athletic performance.

Good Health

Most experts agree exercise plays a key role in achieving and maintaining good physical, mental, and social health. Nearly everyone can be at least moderately active, regardless of age or physical limitations. The health benefits of physical activity outweigh the risks. Many activities that promote good health are free and require no special equipment.

To achieve the goal of good health, most of your daily activity should be aerobic. ***Aerobic activities*** use large muscles and are performed at a moderate, steady pace for long periods. *Aerobic* means "with oxygen." Aerobic activities improve heart and lung health. Certain types of exercise improve bone health.

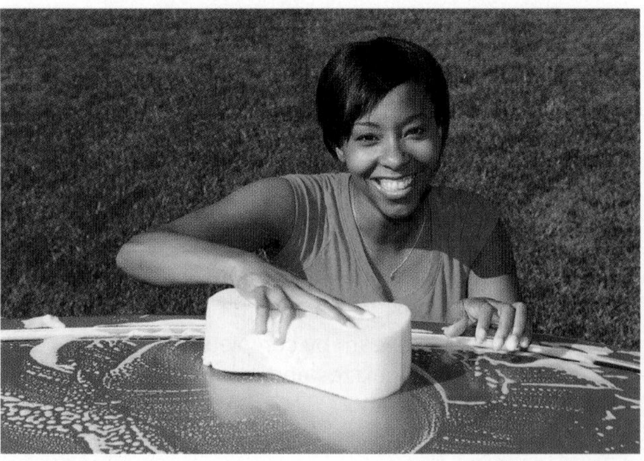

A sirtravelalot/Shutterstock.com

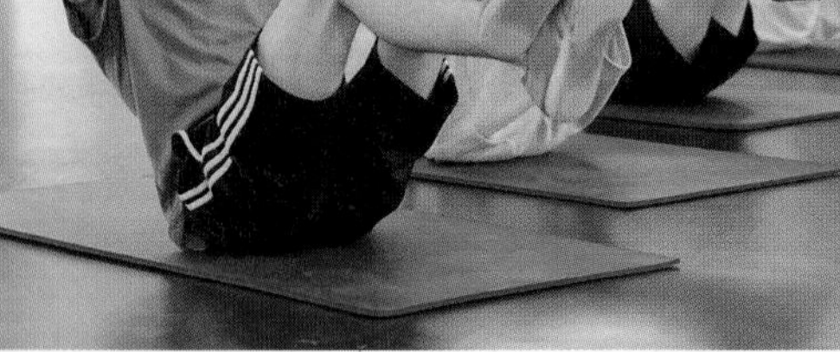

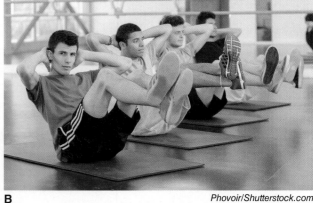

B Phovoir/Shutterstock.com

Figure 20.1 Exercise is structured physical activity performed with a purpose. *Which of these images is an example of exercise?*

Physical activities involving impact with a hard surface—such as running or jumping—stimulate bone growth and strength. Muscle strengthening exercises also increase bone strength. If you have been relatively inactive, a moderate level of activity would be a good place for you to start.

The US Department of Health and Human Services develops and publishes the *Physical Activity Guidelines for Americans*. The *Physical Activity Guidelines for Americans* is a resource that specifies amounts and types of exercise that individuals at different stages of the life cycle should perform to achieve health benefits (**Figure 20.2**). Follow these guidelines to meet your goal for good health.

You may be surprised how easy it is to include more activity in your lifestyle. Although physical activity does not need to occur in a single episode, it does need to be in addition to the light-intensity activities of daily life. Light-intensity activities include standing, walking slowly, and lifting light objects. You can meet your goal with health-enhancing physical activities that fit into your daily routine. For instance, you could spend 15 minutes riding your bicycle to school and another 15 minutes riding home. Then take your dog for a brisk 15-minute walk and spend 15 minutes shooting baskets in the driveway with friends. By the end of the day, you have accumulated a total of 60 minutes of activity.

Physical Activity Guidelines for Americans
Children and Adolescents (6–17 years)
• Perform 1 hour or more of physical activity every day.
• Most of the 1 hour or more of physical activity should be either moderate- or vigorous-intensity aerobic activity, and should include vigorous-intensity physical activity at least 3 days per week.
• Part of the daily physical activity should include muscle-strengthening activity on at least 3 days per week.
• Part of the daily physical activity should include bone-strengthening activity on at least 3 days per week.
Adults (18–64 years)
• Should do 2 hours and 30 minutes a week of moderate-intensity, or 1 hour and 15 minutes a week of vigorous-intensity aerobic physical activity, or an equivalent combination of moderate- and vigorous-intensity aerobic physical activity. Aerobic activity should be performed in episodes of at least 10 minutes, preferably spread throughout the week.
• Additional health benefits are provided by increasing to 5 hours a week of moderate-intensity aerobic physical activity, or 2 hours and 30 minutes a week of vigorous-intensity physical activity, or an equivalent combination of both.
• Should also do muscle-strengthening activities that involve all major muscle groups performed on 2 or more days per week.
Older Adults (65+ years)
• Older adults should follow the adult guidelines. If this is not possible due to limiting chronic conditions, older adults should be as physically active as their abilities allow. They should avoid inactivity.
• Older adults should do exercises that maintain or improve balance if they are at risk of falling.

Figure 20.2 Physical activity is important to the health of Americans at all ages. *How often should a 15-year-old participate in muscle-strengthening activity each week?*

Many household tasks can count as part of your daily physical activity. Pushing the lawn mower, shoveling snow, and raking leaves all require a moderate amount of physical effort. You can judge the intensity of your physical activity by using a scale of 0 to 10 based on your personal capacity for activity, or fitness level. For instance, an activity you rate 5 or 6 on your scale is considered moderate intensity. An activity you rate at 7 or 8 is considered vigorous intensity (**Figure 20.3**). As your fitness level improves, your scale will change. For example, a level of activity you once considered vigorous intensity, you may now experience as moderate intensity.

Overall Physical Fitness

Once you start feeling the benefits of being more active, you may feel like a ball picking up speed as it rolls downhill. In other words, the better you feel the more active you will want to be. You may choose to change your goal to one of achieving overall physical fitness. You may also become more interested in other aspects of your health. Many people who start exercise programs develop an interest in nutritious eating and other healthful lifestyle behaviors. Most of this chapter focuses on the goal of achieving overall physical fitness. You will learn about the different components of physical fitness and how to implement a successful exercise program.

Examples of Aerobic Activity Intensity Levels

Type of Physical Activity	Age Group	
	Children/Teens	**Adults**
Moderate-intensity aerobic	• Hiking	• Brisk walking (>3 mph, but not racewalking)
	• Skateboarding	• Water aerobics
	• Bike riding (<10 mph)	• Doubles tennis
	• Brisk walking	• Bike riding (<10 mph)
	• Pushing lawn mower	• Ballroom dancing
	• Raking leaves	• General gardening
Vigorous-intensity aerobic	• Bike riding (>10 mph)	• Singles tennis
	• Martial arts	• Swimming laps
	• Sports such as soccer, basketball, or swimming	• Racewalking, jogging, running
	• Cross-country skiing	• Heavy gardening

Photos top to bottom: JNP/Shutterstock.com; Flashon Studio/Shutterstock.com

Figure 20.3 The intensity of an activity is dependent on the amount of effort you put into it.

COMMUNITY CONNECTIONS

Advocate for a Fitness-Focused Community

What would make your community more conducive to physical activity and fitness? Fitness-focused communities have safe, well-lit places to hold biking events and run-walk challenges. These communities provide parks with paths and playground equipment that are safe and well designed. Easy access to public transportation and low-traffic areas encourage commuting and shopping by foot or bike in these communities.

You can have a voice and become an advocate for a fitness-focused community. Write letters to your school board and community council members advocating for safe and secure recreational opportunities at your school or in your community. Attend town hall meetings to voice ideas such as the following:

- Soliciting businesses or social agencies to sponsor programs that support a healthy lifestyle. For example, a local business may sponsor a fitness trail at the park, or the hospital may offer exercise classes.
- Using social media campaigns to encourage people to use areas that are safe for year-round recreation and sports activities.
- Offering incentives for wellness or walking programs in school, eldercare centers, or worksites.
- Communicating how to report safety concerns such as areas with inadequate sidewalks; unsafe intersections, recreation areas, parks, playgrounds and sports' playing fields; and poorly lit streets, bike paths, and benches.

Think Critically

1. Assess the safety and convenience issues related to walking or bicycling to your school and make a list of possible solutions. Present your list to the student council for consideration.
2. Perform an assessment to determine how fitness focused your community is. Identify an opportunity that you feel strongly about and create an action plan. Write a letter to the appropriate community leader to obtain his or her support for your plan.

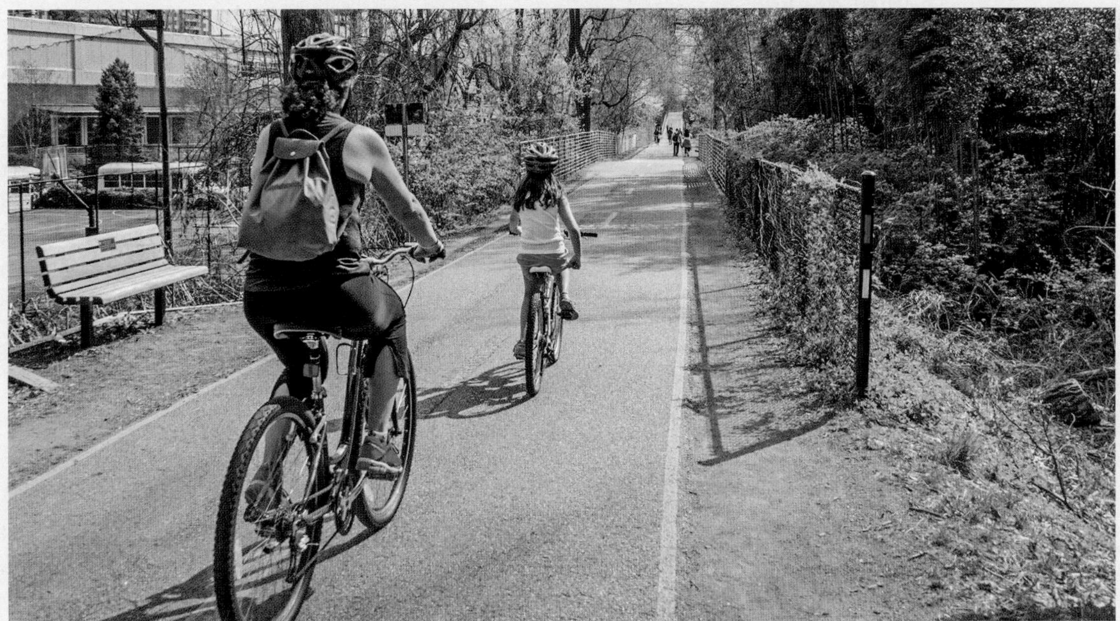

Leigh Trail/Shutterstock.com

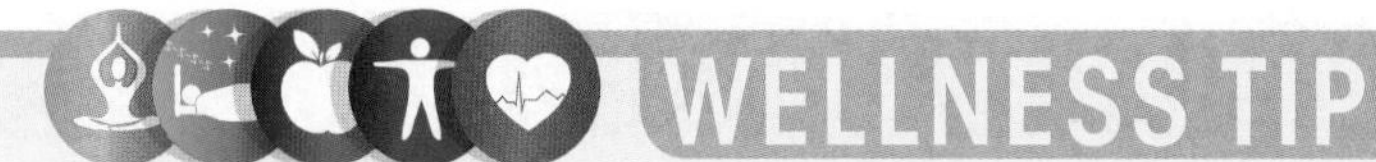

Sanitizing Sports Equipment

If you work out at the school gym or a fitness center, be sure to sanitize your sports equipment before and after use. To prevent disease transmittal, use sanitizing wipes or solution and wipe down such surfaces as handles for treadmills, stationary bikes, stair-climbers, and rowing machines; floor and wall exercise mats; free weights; weights and lifting bar; and lifting benches.

Peak Athletic Performance

A third goal for some physically active people is to reach their highest potential in sports performance. Achieving this goal requires a superior level of overall fitness. It also requires intense training designed to develop specific sports skills. For instance, the football team does drills to build speed. A gymnast does exercises intended to develop balance. A tennis player's workouts are designed to strengthen coordination.

Athletes who truly want to be the best in their sport spend many hours each week in training. They know there is always room for improvement. They also know they will not continue to improve if they do not practice nearly every day.

Benefits of Physical Activity

Any increase in physical activity can have a positive effect on your overall health. In addition to feeling the physical benefits, your mental health will improve as well. These benefits can have positive short-term and long-term effects (**Figure 20.4**).

Improved Posture

Exercise positively affects your posture. ***Posture*** is the position of the body when standing or sitting. Good posture is important to balance and movement.

Exercise develops strong back and abdominal muscles, which are necessary for maintaining good posture. Good posture reduces the chance for back problems.

Erect posture helps your clothes hang properly so you look your best and feel confident. Erect posture when sitting helps you look and feel more alert.

Many teens go through a stage when they feel clumsy and awkward. Exercise can help you move more gracefully. Agility, balance, and coordination developed through exercise are reflected in all your movements.

Weight Management

Physical activity burns calories. Thirty minutes of moderately intense activities burns about 200 calories. This may not seem like much, but the **cumulative** (increasing over time) effect is significant. For instance, engaging in 30 minutes of moderate exercise five days a week burns about 52,000 calories per year. That is nearly 15 pounds of body fat. Those who combine their exercise program with a healthy diet that is moderate in calories can lose even more weight.

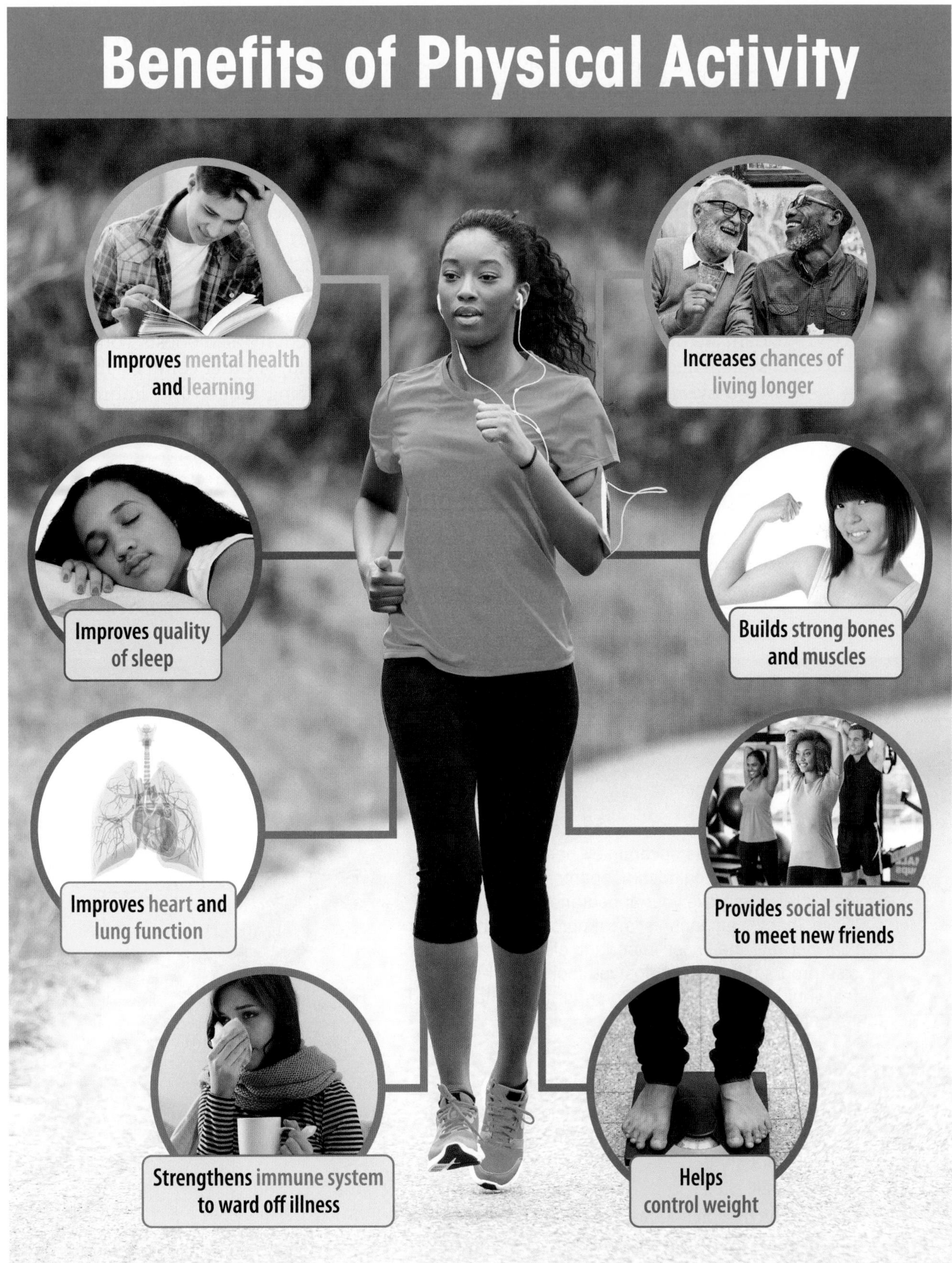
Benefits of Physical Activity
Improves mental health and learning
Increases chances of living longer
Improves quality of sleep
Builds strong bones and muscles
Improves heart and lung function
Provides social situations to meet new friends
Strengthens immune system to ward off illness
Helps control weight

Background: Samuel Borges Photography/Shutterstock.com; top row: Africa Studio/Shutterstock.com; Rawpixel.com/Shutterstock.com; 2nd row: Rob Marmion/Shutterstock.com; Arman Zhenikeyev/Shutterstock.com; 3rd row: Sebastian Kaulitzki/Shutterstock.com; Lee Torrens/Shutterstock.com; bottom row: sheff/Shutterstock.com; Chadsikan Tawanthaisong/Shutterstock.com

Figure 20.4 The benefits of physical activity apply to individuals regardless of age, race, gender, and physical ability.

People who do not have weight problems also benefit from exercise. Over a lifetime, many people experience a slow weight gain by eating an extra 75 to 150 calories per day. An exercise program could easily burn up these excess calories and help maintain weight at a healthy level throughout life.

Disease Prevention

Exercise can help reduce the risk of developing several diseases. These include osteoporosis, coronary heart disease (CHD), diabetes mellitus, high blood pressure, and some cancers. Reducing the risk of heart disease also helps reduce the risk of dementia. ***Dementia*** is the loss of brain functions such as thinking, remembering, and reasoning, and eventually the loss of ability to perform everday tasks.

Regular physical activity helps your body balance hormones to protect cells from damage that may lead to some cancers. Physical activity also boosts your immune system and reduces the chance of catching a cold, flu, or other common illnesses.

Physical activity increases your chances of living longer and improves your quality of life. You have more energy to perform your daily work and enjoy leisure activities.

Improved Mental Outlook and Performance

For many people, exercise creates a feeling of well-being. Adolescents who exercise regularly state they have improved self-control, self-esteem, and body image. They also report greater alertness and better academic performance.

THE MOVEMENT CONNECTION

Arm Circles

Why

Physical activity has several key benefits. In addition to improving the five health components, regular physical activity can also improve your appearance.

While many components are improved with regular physical activity, the most important effect of a regular exercise program is that it helps you feel your best. When you feel your best, you are able to perform daily tasks and requirements at your best.

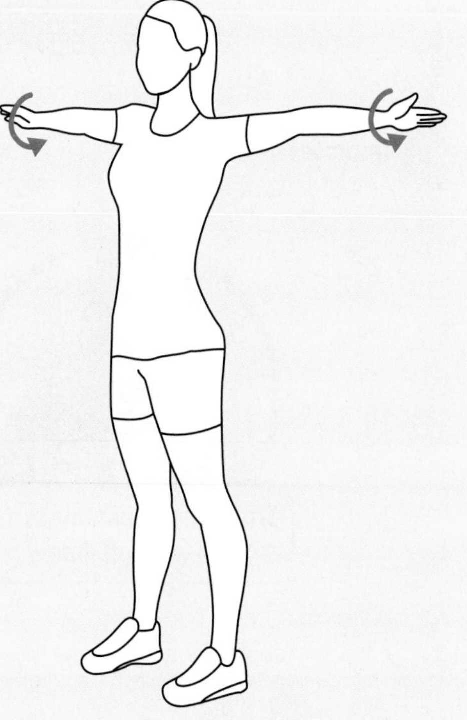

Apply

- Stand with good posture while you engage your core muscles and raise your arms to form a "T" with arms parallel to the floor.
- Make 5 small circles forward.
- Reverse the motion and make 5 circles backward.
- Try different size circles to sense how your shoulders stretch.

Although exercise does not solve problems, it helps relieve anxiety and tension. When exercising, your thoughts focus on the physical activity rather than school or family pressures. Following a workout, you are likely to feel mentally refreshed and better prepared to cope with day-to-day problems. For adults, exercise can reduce feelings of depression and strengthen social skills.

For older adults, the benefits of daily exercise include improved cognitive functioning. Regular physical activity can help to maintain or enhance various aspects of perception, thinking, and reasoning in older adults (**Figure 20.5**).

In addition, being physically active 150 minutes or more per week can improve sleep quality and duration. Adequate sleep contributes to greater alertness during the day.

Overall Physical Fitness

Is a weight lifter who has difficulty running a mile physically fit? How would you rate the fitness of a distance runner who can only manage two push-ups? Physical fitness involves more than being strong or fast. There are many components to physical fitness. Someone who has athletic skill may not be fit in all aspects. However, striving for at least a moderate level of fitness in each component promotes good health and athletic skill.

Health Components of Physical Fitness

Five major components are used to measure the impact of physical fitness on your health—cardiorespiratory fitness, muscular endurance, strength, flexibility, and body composition. Being fit in each of these areas reduces your risk for certain health problems, including heart disease and certain cancers. It also improves your body's ability to perform its various functions.

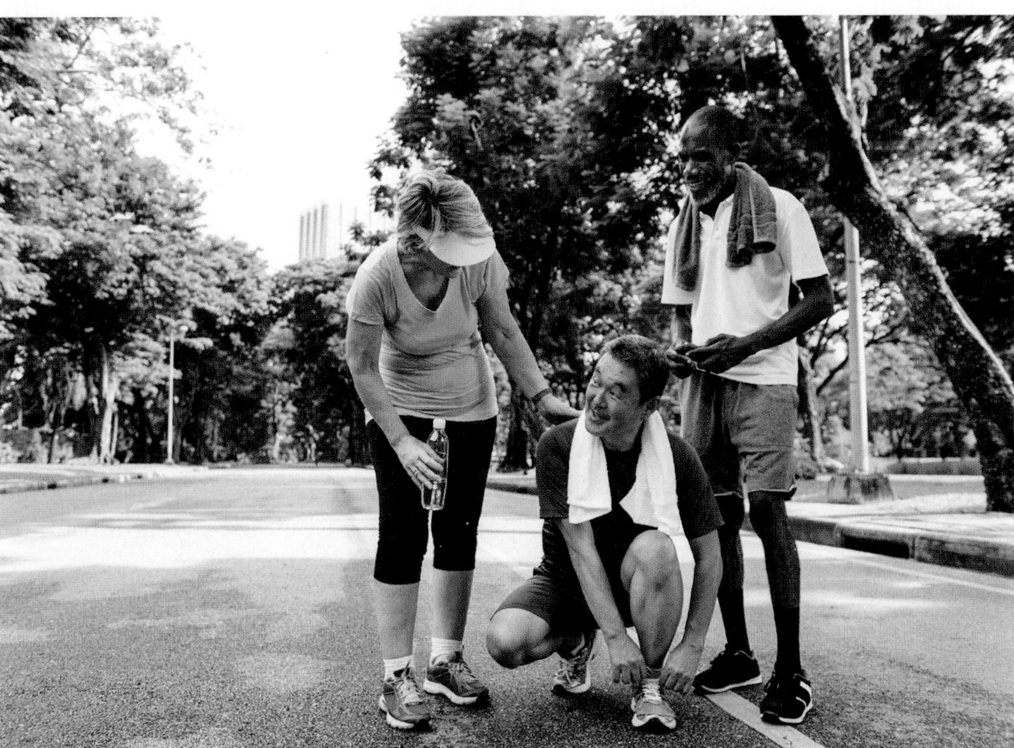

Rawpixel.com/Shutterstock.com

Figure 20.5 Regular physical activity helps maintain mental sharpness as you age.

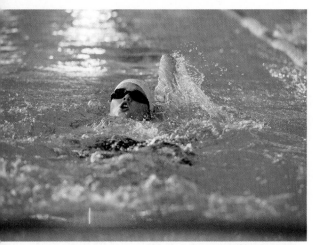

Jose Luis Carrascosa/Shutterstock.com

Figure 20.6 Swimming is an aerobic activity that works the core, arms, legs, back, and even the buttocks without stressing bones and joints.

Cardiorespiratory Fitness

The greatest sign of good health is cardiorespiratory fitness. ***Cardiorespiratory fitness*** is measured by the body's ability to take in adequate amounts of oxygen and carry oxygen efficiently through the blood to body cells. It is an indication of the efficiency of your lungs, heart, and blood vessels.

Aerobic activities build cardiorespiratory fitness. Throughout an aerobic activity, your heart and lungs should be able to supply all the oxygen your muscles need. Health benefits increase as the exercise intensity increases. The goal of aerobic exercise is to increase your heart and breathing rates to safe levels for an extended time. Most fitness experts recommend sustaining these elevated levels for 20 to 60 minutes to get the most cardiorespiratory benefits. Walking, jogging, in-line skating, bicycling, and swimming laps are examples of aerobic activities (**Figure 20.6**).

During ***anaerobic activity***, your muscles are using oxygen faster than your heart and lungs can deliver it. Anaerobic fitness means you are able to lift or move objects forcefully as required in everyday activities. Anaerobic activities use short, intense bursts of energy that induce shortness of breath. Muscles rely on a limited supply of glucose and energy is released quickly. For example, sprint events and sports such as football, baseball, tennis, or a 100-meter race are anaerobic activities. They cannot be sustained long enough to help you increase cardiorespiratory fitness. This is because you must stop often during anaerobic activities to catch your breath. Anaerobic activities can help you build strength, power, and speed.

Muscular Endurance

Muscular endurance refers to your ability to use a group of muscles repeatedly without becoming tired. For instance, muscular endurance allows you to use your leg muscles to pedal a bicycle throughout an hour-long ride. Muscular endurance helps you perform physical activities comfortably. It also enables you to remain active for extended periods.

Some people have more endurance in one muscle group than in another. For instance, people trained as runners have developed endurance in their leg muscles. Nonetheless, they may find it hard to swim several laps without their arms tiring. This is why it is important to work on developing all your muscle groups. Hiking, rowing, skating, and gymnastics can help you develop muscular endurance.

Muscular Strength

Strength is the ability of the muscles to move objects. It is usually measured in terms of how much weight you can lift. You move your body by contracting your muscles. Strong muscles enable your body to move more efficiently. Developing strength can also help you avoid some sports injuries. Obviously, weight training is an excellent activity for developing strength and lean muscle mass.

Flexibility

Flexibility is the ability to move your joints through a full range of motion. Joints are the places in your body where two bones meet. Elbows, knees, shoulders, hips, and ankles are all examples of joints. A high degree of flexibility helps prevent injury to muscles that control movement of the joints.

Females generally have the potential for greater flexibility than males. Stretching exercises can help increase flexibility.

Body Composition

Body composition is the percentage of different types of tissues in the body. High body fat percentage is a risk factor for a number of diseases. Therefore, body composition is a component of physical fitness.

If you are at or below a healthy weight, you may ask, "Do I really need to be physically active?" The answer is "yes." Everyone at all ages needs to be physically active. As described earlier, physical activity has many benefits besides helping people maintain a healthy weight. It is an essential component in maintaining overall good health and fitness.

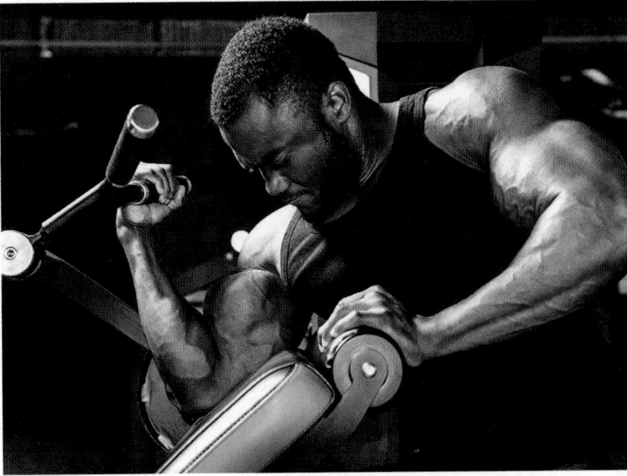

ThomsonD/Shutterstock.com

Figure 20.7 This bodybuilder's weight (245 pounds) and height (6 feet 2 inches) yields a BMI value (31.5) that classifies him as obese. *How do you explain this BMI value?*

Remember, weight is not a reliable indicator of body composition. Someone who has a large percentage of lean body tissue may be overweight according to his or her body mass index (BMI); however, he or she is not overfat (**Figure. 20.7**).

Exercise helps the body burn fat and build muscle. Glucose is the body's chief source of energy. After about 20 minutes of aerobic activity, however, the body begins to use fat for energy. Activities that increase muscular endurance and strength help build muscle tissue. Increasing the proportion of muscle mass in the body raises the basal metabolic rate (BMR), thus helping to burn even more calories. Along with a healthy diet, exercise is a key factor in achieving and maintaining a healthy body composition.

You will not see changes in body composition after a single workout. Over time, you will notice a gradual increase in lean body tissue and a decrease in body fat. Cross-country skiing, racquetball, soccer, and other aerobic exercises are among the sports that are especially good for controlling body fatness.

EXTEND YOUR KNOWLEDGE

Boost Workouts with Interval Training

Interval training is a method of fitness training that uses alternating bursts of intense activity with intervals of lighter activity or recovery. Any exercise should begin with a warm-up period. Then the interval training might begin with a two-minute walk at an intensity roughly 40 to 50 percent of your maximum heart rate. This is followed by a two-minute sprint at or above 80 percent of your maximum heart rate. This pattern is repeated.

Interval training should not be attempted by individuals who have been physically inactive or sedentary. Individuals who are being treated for a heart condition, experience chest pain during activity, or have bone or joint problems should consult their physician before trying interval training. A basic level of fitness should be achieved before starting this program.

Interval training can be used with other sports, such as swimming, crewing, stair climbing, cycling, and even walking. This form of training is more efficient and can be modified for use at all fitness levels.

Skill Components of Physical Fitness

There are six skill components of physical fitness—power, agility, balance, coordination, speed, and reaction time. For some people, strength in these components seems to come naturally; however, most people must work to improve their ability in these areas.

Having a high level of the various skill components can improve your performance in certain sports. You are more likely to take part in activities when you are confident in your performance. Therefore, developing your skill components can motivate you to be active. This, in turn, can bring you the benefits that come from an active lifestyle.

Skill-related fitness can benefit you in everyday activities as well as sports. For instance, having good balance, agility, and coordination can help you avoid accidents. Older people who possess these skills are less likely to fall and experience the problems associated with injuries.

You are likely to find you are strong in some components but weak in others. For overall fitness, you should be moderately strong in all the health components. If necessary, set goals to improve your areas of weakness. Building strength in the health components of physical fitness helps you develop your skill components.

Power

Power is your ability to do maximum work in a short time. It requires a combination of strength and speed. People need power to excel in some sports activities, such as football and many track and field events. Lifting or stacking boxes and pushing a child on a swing are everyday activities that require power.

FEATURED CAREER

Personal Trainer

Personal trainers work one-on-one or with two or three clients, either in a gym or in the clients' homes. They help clients assess their level of physical fitness. Personal trainers also help clients set and reach fitness goals. They demonstrate various exercises and help clients improve their exercise techniques. Trainers may also advise clients on lifestyle modifications outside of the gym to improve their fitness.

Education

Although the education and training required depends on the specific type of personal training, employers increasingly require fitness workers to have a bachelor's degree. This degree is generally in a field related to health and fitness, such as exercise science or physical education. Some personal trainers often start out by taking classes to become certified. Then they may begin by working alongside an experienced trainer before being allowed to train clients alone.

Job Outlook

Jobs for fitness workers are expected to increase about as fast as the average for all occupations. Aging baby boomers, one group that wants to stay healthy and fit, will be the main driver of employment growth for personal trainers. With fewer physical education programs in schools and parents' growing concern about childhood obesity, parents are often hiring personal trainers for their children.

As muscles get stronger, they also become more powerful. Joining a softball league or shooting baskets in the gym can help you develop power.

Coordination

Coordination is your ability to integrate the use of two or more parts of your body. Many sports require coordination of the eyes and hands or the eyes and feet. Many daily tasks also require these types of coordination. A football player needs good coordination to catch a pass. A soccer player needs coordination to maintain possession of the ball when dribbling down the field. You need coordination to avoid tripping over unexpected obstacles. Bowling, golf, volleyball, and tennis are all activities that help develop coordination (**Figure 20.8**).

Agility

Agility is your ability to change the position of your body with speed and control. Agility is an advantage in many sports. It is also important to everyday living. An agile player can easily move down a sports field in and around other players. Agility can also help you react quickly to move out of the path of a bike or car. Downhill skiing, soccer, and modern dance can help develop agility.

Balance

Balance is your ability to keep your body in an upright position while standing still or moving. Balance requires concentration on the task, coordination, and muscle control. Practice is needed to improve balance skills. Some sports, such as gymnastics and dancing, require **acute** (extremely great) balance to excel. A good sense of balance can also help anyone avoid falls and feel more graceful. Ice skating and bicycling can help you develop balance.

Speed

Speed is the quickness with which you are able to complete a motion. Obviously, athletes who compete in sprint events need speed. You use speed when you run to catch a bus. Martial arts classes may help you develop speed. Handball, table tennis, and roller skating are also activities that build speed.

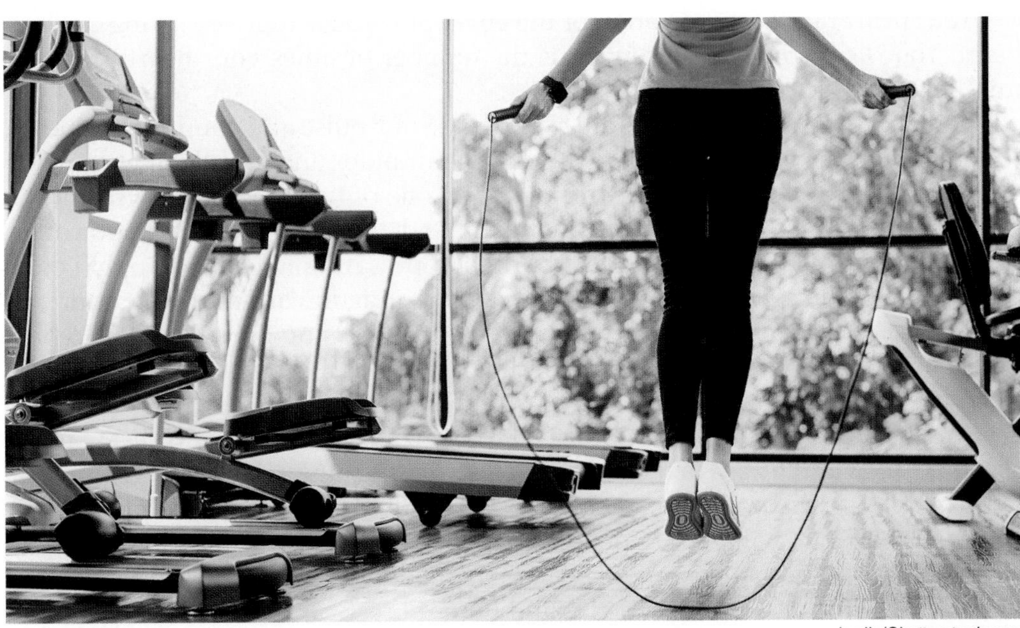
kudla/Shutterstock.com

Figure 20.8
Jumping rope develops coordination between your eyes, feet, and hands.

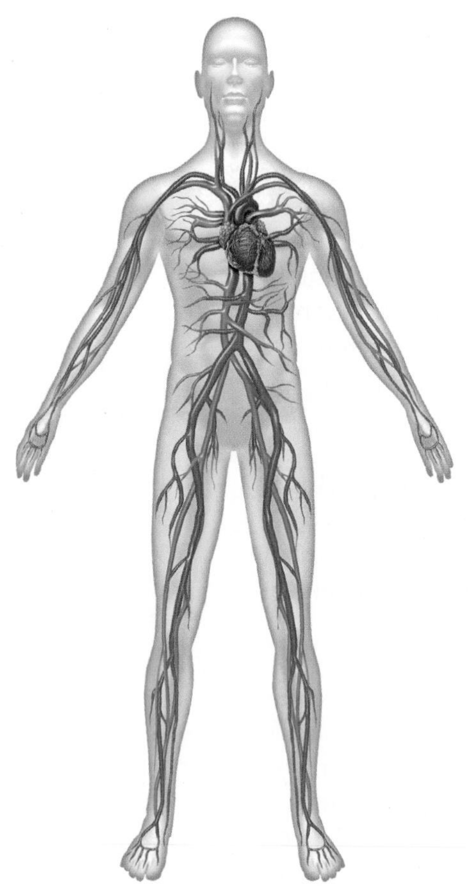

Lightspring/Shutterstock.com

Figure 20.9 A strong heart muscle is better able to pump blood to the body's extremities and back. *How might a weak heart muscle affect blood circulation?*

Reaction Time

Reaction time is the amount of time it takes you to respond to a signal once you receive the signal. In most physical activities, your response will be some type of movement. A soccer goalie needs good reaction time to block a ball headed for the net. A driver needs to be able to react to sudden changes in traffic. Playing baseball, basketball, football, or softball can help you improve your reaction time.

Physical Activity and Your Heart

Exercise affects the cardiovascular system (the heart and blood vessels) in several ways to improve overall heart function.

Remember that certain types of physical activity develop cardiorespiratory fitness. A by-product of cardiorespiratory fitness is a slower heartbeat. The heart beats slower because it is able to work more efficiently. It pumps more blood with each beat. This improved efficiency puts less strain on the heart muscle to circulate blood (**Figure 20.9**).

Another way exercise affects heart function is through its impact on blood lipids. Regular exercise—especially when combined with a healthy eating pattern—reduces levels of certain types of blood lipids that form plaque in the arteries. Plaque-clogged arteries force the heart to work harder to circulate blood through the body.

Exercise also encourages the formation of additional branches in the arteries of the heart. This increases blood flow and allows the heart to work more efficiently.

Measuring Your Heart Rate

Your heart rate is an indication of the effect physical activity is having on your heart. Your ***heart rate***, or pulse rate, is the number of times your heart beats per minute.

You can measure your heart rate by finding your pulse and counting the beats. When measuring your heart rate, always use your index and middle fingers, never your thumb. Heart rate is usually measured in one of two places: the wrist or the neck. At your wrist, slide the fingers of one hand along the thumb of your other hand to your wrist. You should feel your blood pulsating when you apply gentle pressure. You should be able to feel a similar pulsating in your neck. Put your two fingers just to the left or right of your Adam's apple. Using the second hand on a watch or clock, count the beats for 15 seconds. Then multiply the number of beats by four to find the number of beats per minute.

Another way to count your heart rate is to count the number of beats in six seconds. Then add a zero to the number to figure the number of beats per minute. For example, seven beats in six seconds equals a heart rate of 70 beats per minute.

Your heart rate will vary depending on your level of activity. The harder you work out, the faster your heart will beat. Many people are choosing fitness trackers to measure heart rate during exercise and times of rest.

Resting Heart Rate

Resting heart rate (RHR) is the baseline speed at which your heart muscle contracts when you are sitting quietly. As mentioned earlier, improved cardiorespiratory fitness results in a slower heart rate because the heart muscles work more efficiently. Someone who has been training for several months may have a resting heart rate of about 50 to 60 beats per minute (**Figure 20.10**). For children 10 years and older, and adults, normal resting heart rate can range between 60 and 100 beats per minute. Factors such as fitness level, air temperature and quality, body position, emotions, stress levels, body size, illness, and medications affect resting heart rate. A consistently high resting heart rate above 100 beats per minute or an unexplained very low heart rate may signal a health problem.

Maximum Heart Rate

Maximum heart rate is the highest speed at which your heart muscle is able to contract. Your age dictates your maximum heart rate. It is higher for a younger person than for an older person. You can calculate your maximum heart rate using the following formula:

Maximum heart rate = 220 – age in years

A 16-year-old using this formula would calculate his or her maximum heart rate as follows:

Maximum heart rate = 220 – 16 years = 204 beats per minute

A 50-year-old would calculate his or her maximum heart rate as follows:

Maximum heart rate = 220 – 50 years = 170 beats per minute

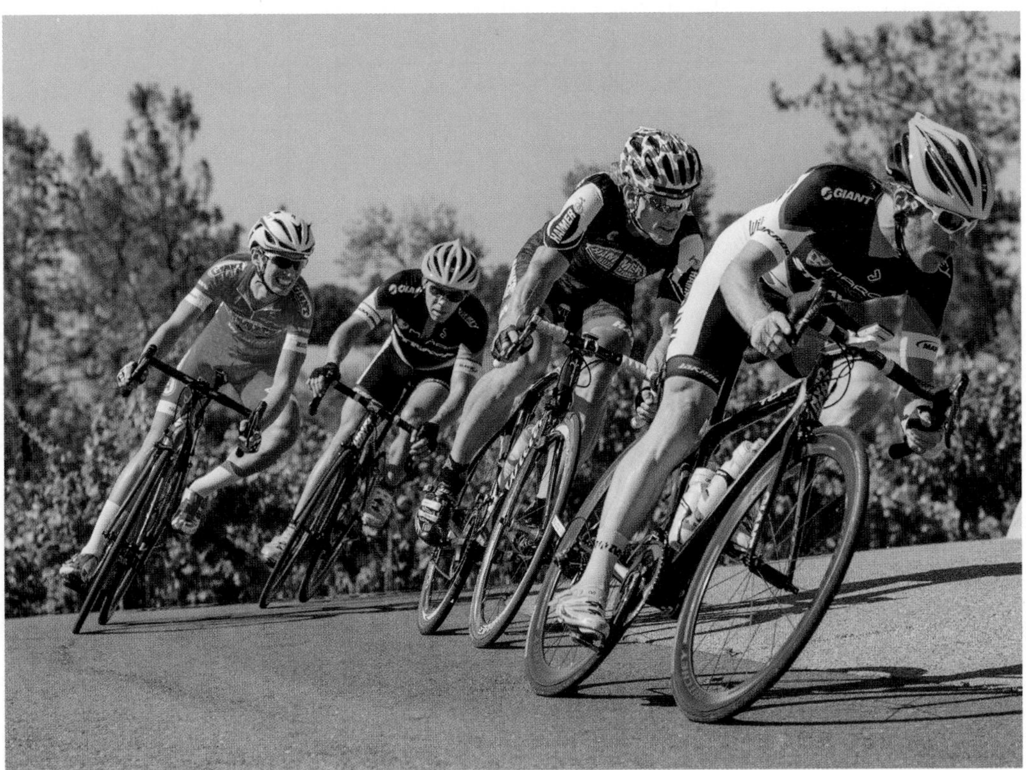

Paul Higley/Shutterstock.com

Figure 20.10 Well-trained endurance athletes such as bicyclists can have resting heart rates as low as 40 beats per minute.

Exercising Your Heart

The heart is a muscle. Like other muscles, the heart needs exercise. Measuring your heart rate can help you see if you are giving your heart enough exercise.

For effective exercise, your heart needs to beat faster than its resting rate. However, it should not beat so fast that it is unsafe. Your heart rate should not reach your maximum heart rate during exercise. Instead, exercise should be performed at an intensity that is both safe and beneficial to your heart, or the *target heart rate zone*. The ***target heart rate zone*** is the range of heartbeats per minute at which the heart muscle receives the best workout. Your target heart rate zone is 60 to 90 percent of your maximum heart rate. A 16-year-old would calculate target heart rate zone as follows:

Maximum heart rate = 220 – 16 years = 204 beats per minute

Minimum target heart rate = 204 × 0.6 = 122 beats per minute

Maximum target heart rate = 204 × 0.9 = 184 beats per minute

Target heart rate zone = 122 to 184 beats per minute

When you begin an exercise program, count your heart rate frequently during your workouts. This will help you decide whether you are pushing yourself too little or too much. Your initial goal should be to keep your heart rate at the low end of your target zone. As your fitness improves, you should be keeping your heart rate closer to the high end of your target zone (**Figure 20.11**).

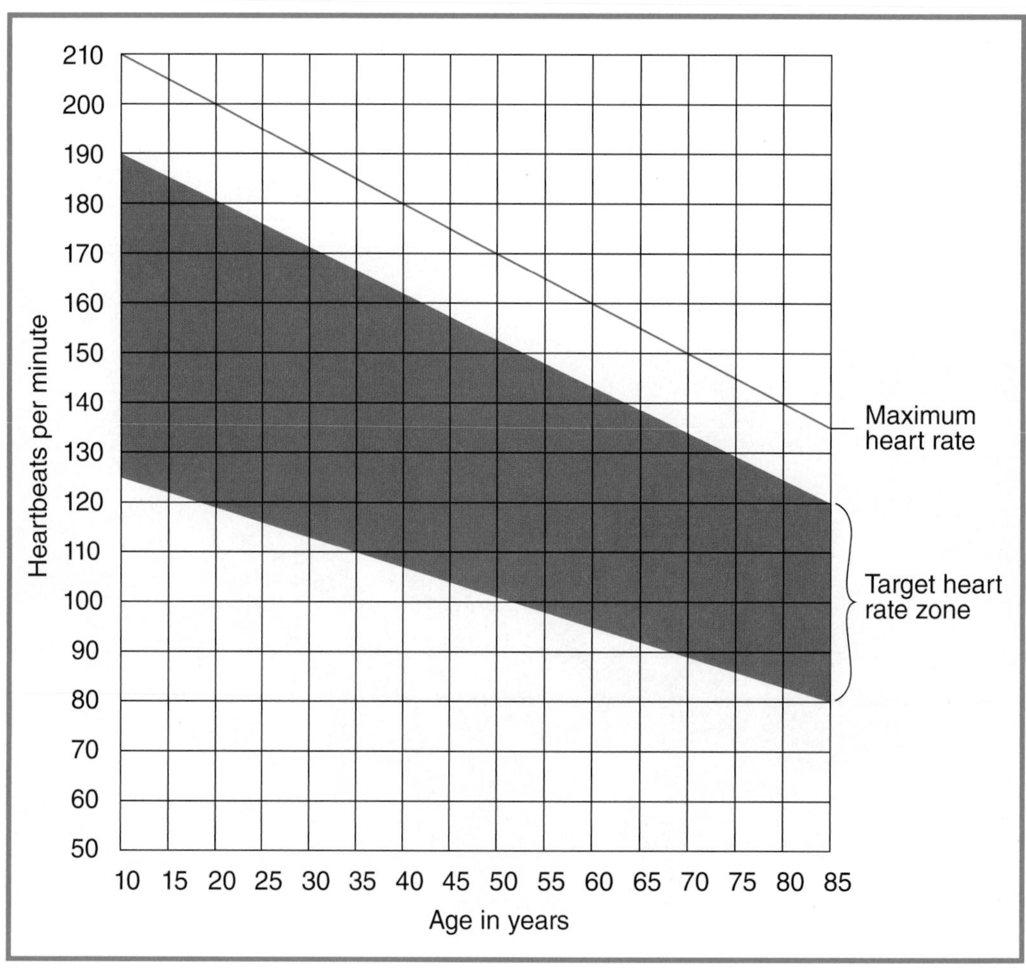

Figure 20.11
Maintain your heart rate in your target zone when exercising for a good cardiorespiratory workout.

Keys to a Successful Exercise Program

Beginning an exercise program can be hard. You may be **skeptical** (doubtful) that the rewards are worth the effort. Talk with people who exercise regularly and ask them about the benefits of being physically active. Their answers may inspire you to begin an exercise program that includes more than just daily lifestyle activities.

Researchers have identified some factors that help people stick with their exercise programs. These factors include written goals, enjoyable activities, a convenient exercise schedule, knowledge of personal fitness level, and safety. Consider these factors as you plan a program for yourself.

Put Fitness Goals in Writing

Your physical fitness efforts are most likely to be effective if you set some specific goals for them. Your long-term goal may be to achieve and maintain physical fitness. For most people, however, trying to fulfill such a big goal would be overwhelming. You need to break this goal down into smaller, more manageable goals.

Begin by identifying which component of fitness you want to improve first. Then think about activities that can help you improve in that area. Select activities that are of interest to you. Make a specific plan to include those activities in your weekly routine.

CASE STUDY

Jake's Fitness Goals

Jake stopped playing soccer two years ago. He hasn't been active in any sports since then. He spends much of his free time studying and playing video games. Lately, he has noticed that his muscle tone is gone and he can't run up the stairs as easily as he once could. Yesterday in gym class, he was winded just a few minutes into a game of basketball! Jake decides he needs to take action before his fitness level gets any worse.

That night, Jake sets the alarm on his clock for one hour earlier in the morning. Even though he hates exercising in the morning, he is determined to start his new fitness plan first thing the next day. His fitness plan is to run three miles and lift weights before school every morning.

When the alarm goes off the next morning, Jake hits the snooze button four times before he finally drags himself out of bed. He throws on some clothes and sets off for a run. Jake is out of breath and begins to walk after running just two blocks. He is so discouraged that he turns around and goes home. By the time Jake showers and has breakfast, he is running late and misses the bus for school. As his mom is driving him to school, Jake decides being fit just isn't worth the trouble.

Case Review

1. How do you think Jake felt after deciding to give up on his fitness plan?
2. Why do you think Jake's new fitness plan failed?
3. What suggestions would you give to Jake about improving his fitness plan?

One way to stay focused in your exercise program is to write down your fitness goals. Start with one specific and attainable goal. Your goal might read, "I will improve my cardiovascular fitness until my pulse drops to 100 beats per minute following a three-minute step test." Then list specific steps for achieving your goal. You might write, "I will bicycle for 30 minutes after school on Monday and Thursday. I will skate for 30 minutes after school on Tuesday and Friday." You might want to write your goal and the steps for achieving it as a personal exercise contract. Post a copy of the contract in a spot where you will see it several times a day.

Your chances for success are much better if you write down what you accomplish. Keep a record of when you are physically active and for how long. You will be less likely to skip an exercise session if you know it will show up on your record (**Figure 20.12**). You will feel good about yourself when you see how faithfully you are following your exercise contract. Be sure to praise yourself for your success.

Personal Exercise Contract

Goal
I will improve my cardiovascular fitness until my pulse drops to 100 beats per minute following a three-minute step test.

Action Plan
I will do one of the following activities at least five days a week.

Progress—Week 1

Activity	Sunday	Monday	Tuesday	Wednesday	Thursday	Friday	Saturday
Bicycle 30 minutes	✔						
Skate 30 minutes							✔
Swim 20 laps			✔		✔		
Walk 30 minutes				✔			

Progress—Week 2

Activity	Sunday	Monday	Tuesday	Wednesday	Thursday	Friday	Saturday
Bicycle 30 minutes							✔
Skate 30 minutes		✔				✔	
Swim 20 laps			✔		✔		
Walk 30 minutes	✔						

Figure 20.12 A personal exercise contract can help you adhere to an exercise program and meet your fitness goals.

Fitness goals take time to achieve. However, you should see some signs of improvement within a few weeks. If you have been following your contract and do not see improvement, evaluate your exercise plan carefully. You may need to revise the steps you are using to reach your goal. You may also want to consider seeing a fitness counselor. When you achieve your goal, congratulate yourself for a job well done. Then set a new goal and begin working toward it.

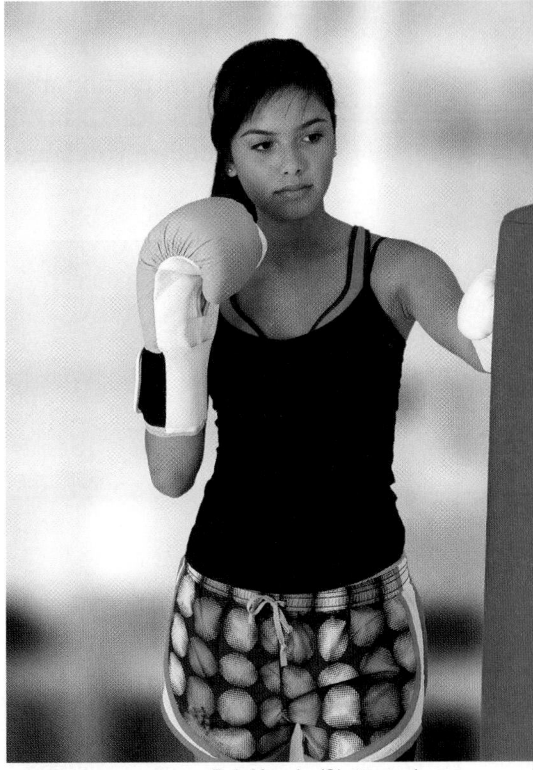

Rob Marmion/Shutterstock.com

Figure 20.13 In addition to boosting strength and cardiorespiratory fitness, boxing improves balance, coordination, and agility. Boxing is also great for releasing stress.

Choose Activities You Enjoy

Physical activity should be fun, not a chore. If you choose activities you enjoy, you are more likely to persist with your exercise program. You may enjoy outdoor activities such as hiking and canoeing. Perhaps you like the competition of team sports. Maybe you prefer such partner sports as tennis or handball that you can play with a friend. No matter what activity you choose, the important point is to be active.

Variety can help keep an exercise program enjoyable. You may become bored following the same exercise routine day after day. Varying the activities can prevent boredom and develop different components of fitness (**Figure 20.13**). This will help you reach your long-term goal of achieving an overall level of physical fitness. If you enjoy anaerobic activities, try to include some aerobic activities in your exercise program also. Choose activities that focus on different large muscle groups. For instance, you might try rowing to develop upper body strength and jogging to build leg muscles.

Although your exercise program should meet your personal fitness needs, you do not need to exercise alone. Working out with friends or family members can make a fitness program more fun. Doing activities with other people can also help you stay motivated. On a day when you are tempted to cancel your workout, a friend can encourage you to get going.

Choose a Convenient Time

Scheduling physical activity at a convenient time will increase your likelihood of following through with your exercise program. You may want to work out first thing in the morning to get your day off to a good start. You might have some free time after school when you can enjoy activities with friends. Perhaps you would rather exercise at night before going to bed. It does not matter when you exercise.

Once you find an exercise time that is convenient for you, make it a set part of your daily schedule. This will help you form a habit that is easy to follow.

Know Your Fitness Level

For your exercise program to be successful, you need to know your fitness level. In striving to meet your goal for overall physical fitness, resist the temptation to begin **strenuous** (demanding) workouts too quickly. This increases your risk of fatigue and injury, and increases the likelihood of discontinuing your fitness program.

Before you begin an exercise program, measure your level of fitness in each of the health components. Ask a health or physical education instructor for information about self-assessment tools or perform your own simple evaluation (**Figure 20.14**). If you have any health concerns, be sure to consult a physician before you begin an exercise program.

Assess Your Fitness

Fitness Component	Test
Cardiorespiratory	1. Walk for 10 minutes at a brisk pace. 2. Check and record your heart rate. (See The Movement Connection in Chapter 7.) 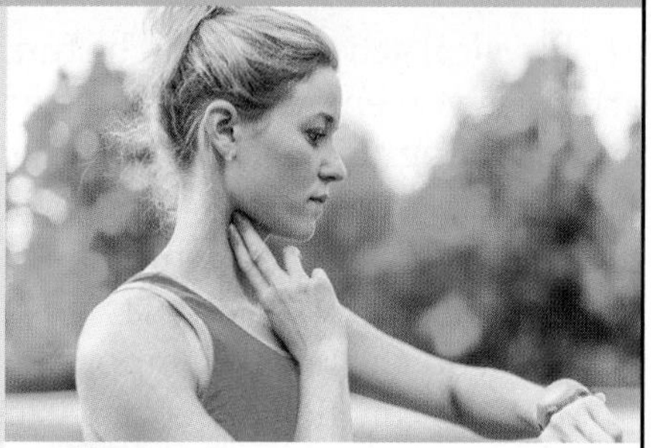
Muscular strength and endurance	1. Perform as many push-ups as you are able. If you are unable to do a classic push-up, do a modified push-up on your knees. 2. Record the number of push-ups. 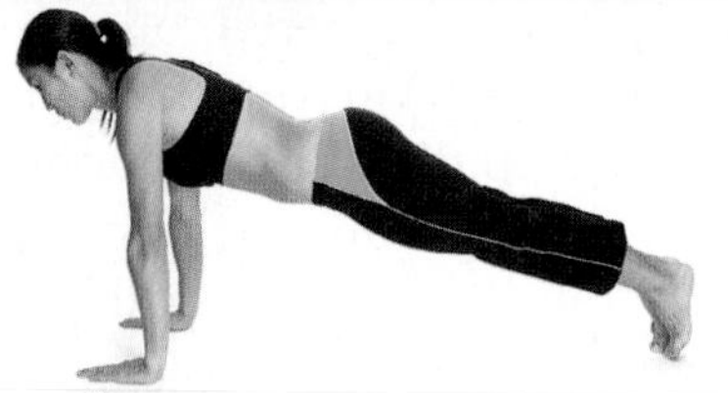 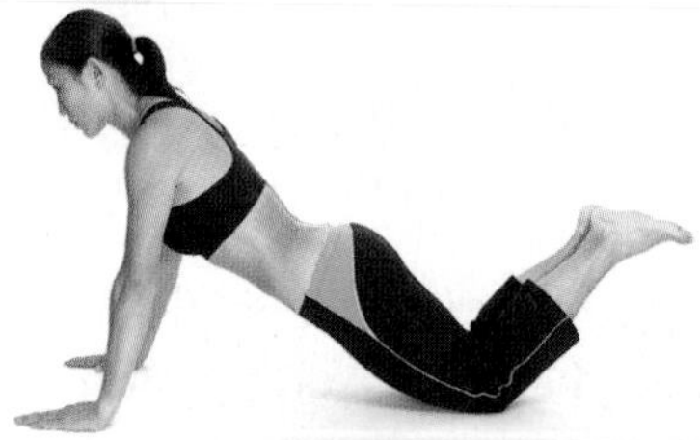
Body composition	1. Use a measuring tape to measure around your waist just above the navel. 2. Record this measurement. 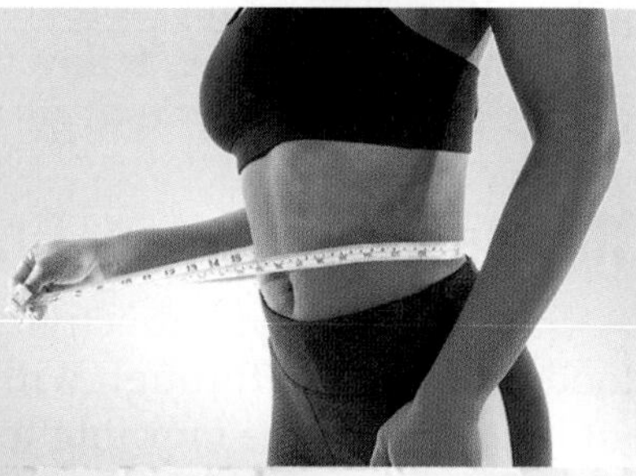
Flexibility	1. Sit tall with legs straight in front of you and your back against the wall. 2. Hold a piece of masking tape and reach your arms out in front of you. 3. Lead with your arms and chest as you stretch forward and place the tape on the floor between your legs at the furthest point of your reach. 4. Use a measuring tape to record the distance from the wall to the piece of tape. 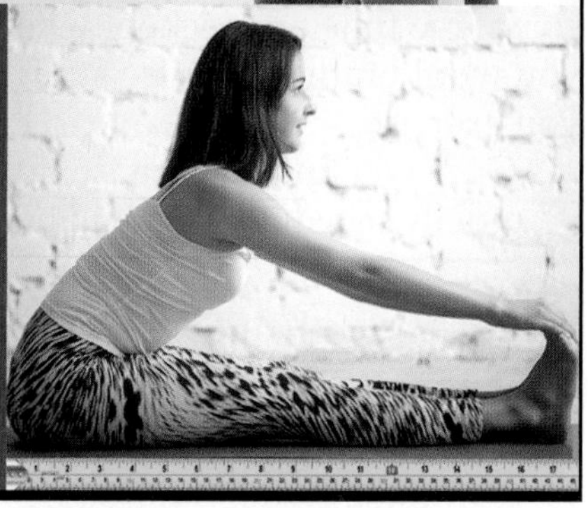

Photos top to bottom: ESB Basic/Shutterstock.com; Philip Date/Shutterstock.com; Philip Date/Shutterstock.com; Horst Petzold/Shutterstock.com; fizkes/Shutterstock.com; Jason Winter/Shutterstock.com

Figure 20.14 Establish your fitness level at the start of your exercise program so you can measure your progress.

Gaining physical fitness is a building process. It involves three key factors—frequency, intensity, and duration.

- *Frequency* is how often you exercise.
- *Intensity* is how hard you exercise.
- *Duration* refers to how long an exercise session lasts.

Begin your exercise program with moderate frequency, low intensity, and short duration. You might start by exercising three times a week. Keep your pulse at about 60 percent of your maximum heart rate for 20 minutes. As you notice improvements in your state of fitness, gradually increase the frequency, intensity, and duration of your exercise. Compete with yourself to achieve new, higher-level goals. Try increasing your frequency to five to seven days per week. Build your intensity up to 70 or 80 percent of your maximum heart rate. Extend the duration of your workouts up to 60 minutes.

Practice Safety

Being aware of your fitness level protects you from injuries caused by too much stress on your body. Exercise should not be painful. Be aware of signals your body is sending. Burning muscles and feeling as if you cannot catch your breath are signs you are working too hard. These symptoms may occur more rapidly as you increase your speed, exercise in heat or high humidity, or grow tired. If you experience these symptoms, you need to slow down your exercise pace.

Following basic safety precautions can help you avoid other types of injuries when exercising. Know how to use equipment and use it correctly. Wear protective gear, such as helmets and body pads, when appropriate. If you will be exercising outdoors, be prepared for the environmental conditions (**Figure 20.15**). If you are injured, follow first-aid practices or seek prompt medical attention if necessary.

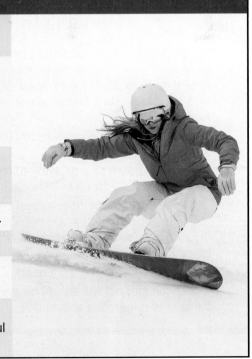

Practice Safety
• Use proper safety equipment, such as helmets, goggles, wrist guards, reflective gear, and pads.
• Use caution when exercising in hot, humid weather. High temperatures combined with high humidity increase the risk of heat exhaustion and heatstroke. Wait until temperatures have cooled or choose to exercise in an air-conditioned facility. Be sure to drink plenty of water before, during, and after exercise.
• Use caution when exercising in extremely cold weather. Cold temperatures can cause frostbite and a drop in body temperature. If you feel cold, stop the activity and get to a warmer place.
• Use caution when exercising on wet, icy, and snow-covered surfaces.
• Move indoors at the first sight of lightning.
• Allow the body time to adjust to the lower air pressure before exercising vigorously in high altitudes (over 5,000 feet).
• Avoid exercising in areas that have high levels of fume exhaust from cars and industry. Polluted air can cause headaches, painful breathing, and watery eyes.

Photo: Vadim Zakharishchev/Shutterstock.com

Figure 20.15 Take the necessary precautions when participating in physical activities to avoid illness or injury.

Planning an Exercise Program

Your exercise program should include three phases for each workout session. You need a warm-up period, workout period, and cooldown period.

Warm-Up Period

On a cold morning, a car engine needs to warm up before you start driving. In a similar way, your muscles need to warm up before you start exercising. Warming up prepares your heart and other muscles for work. Many people ignore this important phase of an exercise program. If you do not warm up, you may be more likely to end up with sore muscles or an injury.

The warm-up period should last about 5 to 10 minutes. Begin by gradually increasing your heart rate to minimize stress on the heart. Some people choose a slow jog for this purpose. If you will be swimming or bicycling, you can simply start the activity at a slow pace. Gradually increase to a moderate pace to bring your heart rate near your target zone.

Following your heart warm-up, warm up the muscles you will be using in your workout. To reduce the risks of injury, do a series of gentle stretches. Avoid bouncing motions. Your movements should resemble those you will use in your exercise activity. If you will be playing tennis, slowly move your arms as though you are making broad forehand and backhand strokes. Make these motions several times with empty hands. Then pick up a tennis racquet and repeat them several more times. After a brief warm-up session such as this, you will be ready for a more vigorous workout.

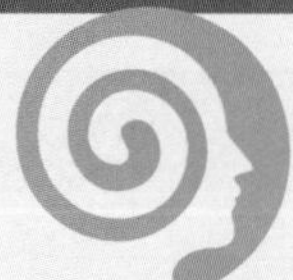

EXTEND YOUR KNOWLEDGE

Treating Injuries with R.I.C.E.

Regardless how safe and physically fit you are, it is likely that you will experience a minor (or major) injury sometime in your life. A minor injury, such as a sprain, may be difficult to differentiate from major injury, such as a break. Unless the injury is mild, a doctor should evaluate and treat the injury. Nonetheless, you can initiate care for a sprain by following the R.I.C.E. treatment plan.

- **Rest:** Move the injured body part as little as possible.
- **Ice:** Apply a cold pack for 20 minutes periodically for 48 to 72 hours.
- **Compression:** Wrap injured body part with an elastic bandage. Do not wrap so tightly that blood flow is restricted.
- **Elevate:** Raise injured body part so it is above the level of your heart.

These four actions should be performed at the same time rather than sequentially.

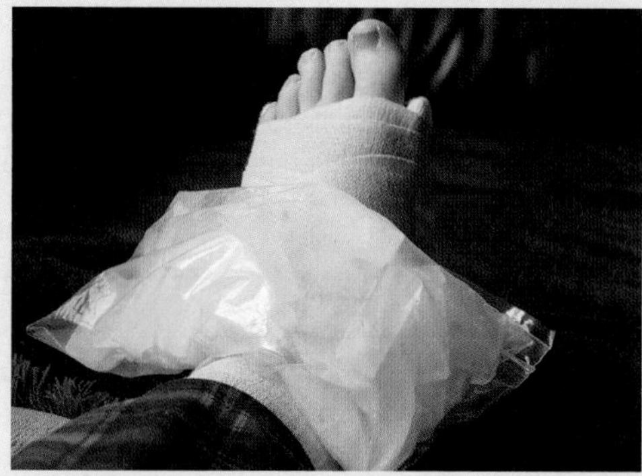

SEASTOCK/Shutterstock.com

Workout Period

The workout period is the main part of your exercise program. It should last at least 20 minutes. These activities develop the health components of fitness. When choosing activities for your workout period, remember the keys for success you read about earlier in the chapter.

Cooldown Period

Never sit down or enter a hot shower immediately after exercise without a cooldown period. The body needs to return to its pre-exercise state slowly.

During exercise, your heart pumps extra blood to your muscles to meet their increased demand for oxygen and energy. The action of your muscles keeps blood circulating back to the heart. If you stop muscle action too quickly, the extra blood temporarily collects in your muscles. This reduces the amount of oxygen-rich blood available for the heart to pump to the brain and dizziness results.

The cooldown period should last about 10 minutes. You can use the same activities for your cooldown as you used for your warm-up. A slow jog will help reduce your heart rate and allow the muscles to push more blood toward the heart. Some stretching exercises will help prevent muscle cramps and soreness by loosening muscles that have become tight from exercise.

RECIPE FILE

Baked Sweet Potato Fries

6 SERVINGS

Ingredients

- 1 lb. sweet potatoes
- ¾ t. smoked paprika
- ½ t. garlic powder
- ¼ t. salt
- 1 T. olive oil

Directions

1. Preheat oven to 450°F (232°C).
2. Wash and peel sweet potatoes. Slice into ½-inch wedges and place in a large bowl.
3. Sprinkle with paprika, garlic, and salt.
4. Drizzle with olive oil.
5. Toss until all wedges are coated with seasonings and olive oil.
6. Place in one layer on a foil-lined baking sheet that has been sprayed with cooking spray.
7. Roast for 15 minutes. Turn and roast until wedges are crispy on the outside and tender on the inside, about 10 minutes more.
8. Serve immediately.

PER SERVING: 85 CALORIES, 3 G PROTEIN, 18 G CARBOHYDRATE, 2 G FAT, 2 G FIBER, 180 MG SODIUM.

Chapter 20 Review and Expand

Reading Summary

There is a difference between physical activity and exercise, but both are necessary for physical fitness. Physical activity can help you achieve the goals of good health, overall physical fitness, or peak athletic performance.

Increased physical activity has a positive effect on your overall heath. There are long-term and short-term benefits from increased physical activity. Overall, physical fitness includes both health components and skill components. Physical activity improves heart function. You can measure your heart rate to determine how physical activity is affecting your heart and to maintain a level of intensity that is safe.

There are several keys to a successful exercise program. Put your fitness goals in writing. Choose activities you enjoy and do them at a convenient time. Also, be sure to keep your workouts in line with your fitness level.

Each exercise session should have a warm-up, workout, and cooldown period. The workout period should last at least 20 minutes. You will find physical activity is a lifestyle choice with lifetime benefits.

Chapter Vocabulary

1. **Content Terms** With a partner, choose two words from the following list to compare. Create a Venn diagram to compare your words and identify differences. Write one term under the left circle and the other term under the right. Where the circles overlap, write two characteristics the terms have in common. For each term, write a difference of the term for each characteristic in its respective outer circle.

aerobic activity	muscular endurance
agility	physical activity
anaerobic activity	physical fitness
balance	posture
cardiorespiratory fitness	power
coordination	reaction time
dementia	resting heart rate
exercise	speed
flexibility	strength
heart rate	target heart rate zone
maximum heart rate	

2. **Academic Terms** Individually or with a partner, create a T-chart on a sheet of paper and list each of the following terms in the left column. In the right column, list an *antonym* (a word of opposite meaning) for each term in the left column.

acute	stamina
cumulative	strenuous
skeptical	

Review Learning

3. Compare physical activity and exercise.
4. List three main goals for becoming physically active.
5. *True or false?* Anaerobic activities are performed using large muscles at a moderate, steady pace for long periods.
6. What physical activity guidelines should teens follow for achieving good health?
7. List four benefits of physical activity.
8. _____ activities build cardiorespiratory fitness.
9. The ability to use muscles repeatedly without tiring demonstrates muscular _____.
10. List six skill components of physical fitness and give an example of an activity that would help develop each component.
11. Explain how physical activity improves heart function.
12. *True or false?* Maximum heart rate is higher for a younger person than for an older person.
13. List five keys to a successful exercise program.
14. What is the purpose of the warm-up period before exercise?
15. Explain why dizziness may occur if you forego a cooldown period at the end of an exercise session.

Self-Assessment Quiz

Complete the self-assessment quiz online to help you practice and expand your knowledge and skills.

Critical Thinking

16. **Evaluate** Identify factors that affect your motivation to develop and maintain a personal exercise program. Make a T-chart listing the obstacles on the left side and ways to overcome the obstacles on the right side of the chart.

17. **Apply** Measure your resting heart rate after sitting for 30 minutes or more. Record your resting heart rate. Were the results what you expected? (If your results are consistently high, you should consult your healthcare provider.)
18. **Assess** Create an exercise program and write a personal exercise contract. Identify a specific, attainable fitness goal(s) and list the steps you intend to follow to achieve it. Before you begin your exercise plan, assess your current fitness level by measuring your aerobic fitness, muscle strength and endurance, flexibility, and body composition using the methods discussed in Figure 20.14. Record and save your results. Test your fitness levels at two-week intervals throughout this course and compare to previous measures to determine your progress. Write a summary of your experience.
19. **Evaluate** List 10 sports on a sheet of paper. Rank the importance of each skill component for each sport. Compare your list with the rest of the class.

Core Skills

20. **Technology Literacy** Challenge an adult friend, parent, or grandparent to join you in adopting a more physically active lifestyle and healthier eating habits. Locate the *SuperTracker Groups and Challenges User Guide* online to learn how to create a group and record data. Then, use the *SuperTracker's Quick Tracker* on your group page to record foods and physical activities for each of the participants in the challenge. Work with your family or friends to select the activities best suited to their lifestyles.
21. **Math** Identify the calorie content for your favorite fast-food item. Then select five physical activities of varying intensity. Use Internet resources to learn how many calories per hour each activity burns. Use spreadsheet or graphing software to prepare a bar graph comparing how much time each activity must be performed in order to expend the calories supplied by the fast-food item.
22. **Writing** Prepare an appealing flyer on the importance of physical activity. Address your flyer to the needs for physical activity for a particular life-cycle stage. Share your flyer with a community group where people of that age group gather.
23. **Speech** Research the causes and prevention of common sports injuries using reliable sources. Create a public service announcement (PSA) to help athletes at your school avoid injury. Be sure to address warm-up and cooldown sessions as part of your presentation. Present your PSA in class.
24. **Technology Literacy and Speaking** Working with a partner, prepare a video demonstration about physical activity targeted at a specific age group. Possible presentation ideas might include parents building more exercise into their children's daily activities, teens helping teens stay fit, or fitness activities for older adults. Use at least three reliable sources for your planning and cite them at the end of the video. When planning your presentation, adjust your rate of speech, word choice, and approach to fit the intended audience. Be sure to make the video fun to encourage participation.
25. **Science and Speaking** Select one muscle or group of muscles and research how it works in physically fit people. Prepare a speech to present your findings to the class. Use a diagram of the muscular system to show the location of the particular muscle(s) in the human body. As part of your presentation, demonstrate one stretch or physical activity that benefits this muscle.
26. **Reading** Locate and read the CDC's position statement on youth's need for physical activity. Write a summary including five key points that you identify as important to future health of adolescents in the United States.
27. **Technology Literacy and Writing** Write a tweet to motivate people to be physically active. Be sure your message is fun, interesting, accurate, and grabs the reader's attention. Remember, the tweet can be no longer than 280 characters. Use a discovery tool to help you identify popular hashtags and spread your message.
28. **Career Readiness Practice** As part of an ongoing health and wellness program at your workplace, you have been asked to organize a voluntary lunchtime exercise program for employees. With an hour for lunch, 30 minutes can be devoted to daily exercise. Using the information from the *Physical Activity Guidelines for Americans* website, organize exercise activities centered on cardiorespiratory, endurance, strength, and flexibility. Be sure to allow time for adequate warm-up, workout, and cooldown periods. Note that employees can perform some of the activities before or after work. Include ideas for keeping employees motivated to participate. Share your plan.

CHAPTER 21 Mental and Social Wellness

Learning Outcomes

After studying this chapter, you will be able to

- **analyze** the effect of physical, social, and mental health on overall wellness;
- **summarize** the aspects that are indicators of mental health;
- **identify** strategies for promoting positive mental health;
- **understand** contributing factors to social health;
- **explain** techniques for promoting positive social health;
- **create** a self-management plan to make a positive behavior change; and
- **recognize** barriers to and options for help with mental health issues.

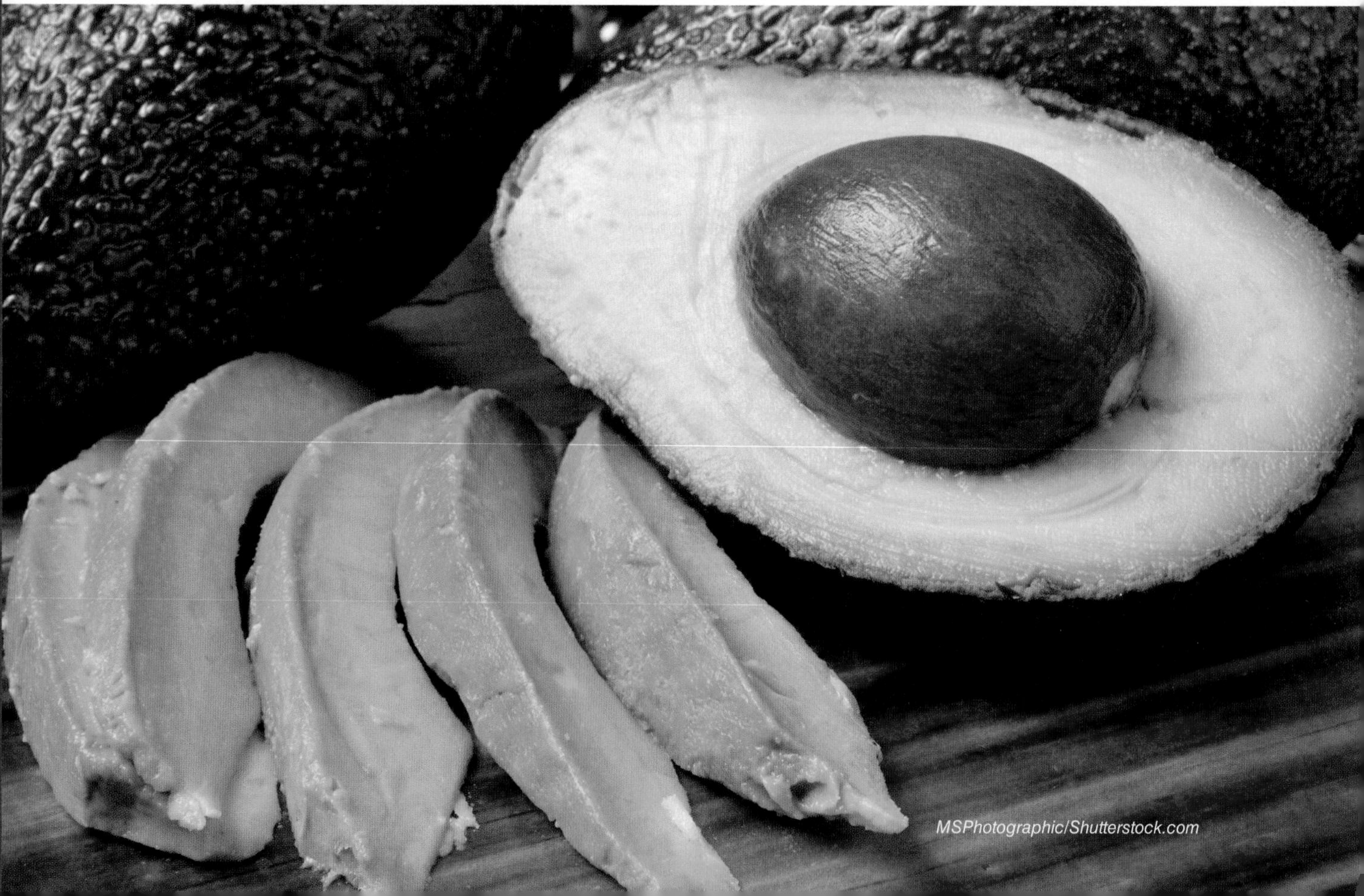

MSPhotographic/Shutterstock.com

Content Terms

assertiveness
burnout
communication
compromise
conflict
emotion
emotional intelligence (EI)
empathy
gratitude
nonverbal communication
relationship
resilience
self-actualization
self-concept
self-esteem
social development
verbal communication

Academic Terms

adversity
hierarchy
jeopardy
offensive
perspective
utmost

What's Your Nutrition and Wellness IQ?

Take this quiz to examine how much you already know about mental and social wellness. If you cannot answer a question, pay extra attention to that topic as you study this chapter.

- Identify each statement as *True*, *False*, or *It Depends*. *It Depends* means in some cases the statement is true; in some cases it could be false.
- Revise false statements to make them true.
- Explain the circumstances in which each *It Depends* statement is true and when it is false.

Nutrition and Wellness IQ 

1.	Achieving positive social and mental health is dependent on having basic human needs met.	True	False	It Depends
2.	Physical health has little to do with mental or social health.	True	False	It Depends
3.	You can learn to manage your emotions.	True	False	It Depends
4.	Nutrition has no effect on mental health.	True	False	It Depends
5.	Social skills are useful when communicating with people from different backgrounds.	True	False	It Depends
6.	Your communication skills do not affect your social health.	True	False	It Depends
7.	Making positive behavior changes requires analyzing your goals, priorities, and choices.	True	False	It Depends
8.	As with physical health conditions, mental health conditions require treatment by a physician.	True	False	It Depends

While studying this chapter, look for the activity icon  **to**

- **build** vocabulary with e-flash cards and interactive games;
- **assess** what you learn by completing self-assessment quizzes and completing review questions; and
- **expand** knowledge with interactive activities and activities that extend learning.

www.g-wlearning.com/foodsandnutrition/

Have you ever felt torn when you and your friends were on opposite sides of an issue? Has there been a time when you felt overwhelmed by more school assignments than you had time to complete? Have you skipped meals because your work and after-school practice schedule was too hectic for you to find time to eat? These situations often cause teens to lose sleep, and make poor food and exercise choices. They may even begin to feel physically ill.

In this chapter, you will learn how your mental health and social health affect your overall wellness. You will also learn actions you can take to promote your mental and social health.

Human Needs and Wellness

As a human being, you have basic needs. The degree to which these needs are met affects your physical, social, and mental health. In addition, your physical, social, and mental health affect your overall wellness (**Figure 21.1**). The potential for achieving a high level of wellness improves when human needs are met.

Psychologist Abraham Maslow proposed a theory that human needs form a **hierarchy** (ranking). He grouped needs into five basic levels. He believed people must meet their needs at the lowest level first, at least in part. Until these needs are addressed, people cannot focus on needs at the next level. Maslow's theory is represented as a triangle, which has a base broader than the peak. This suggests needs shown at the base of the triangle provide a foundation for healthy growth and development (**Figure 21.2**).

Figure 21.1
Mental, physical, and social health are equally important to your overall wellness. *Why is a triangle used to illustrate this concept?*

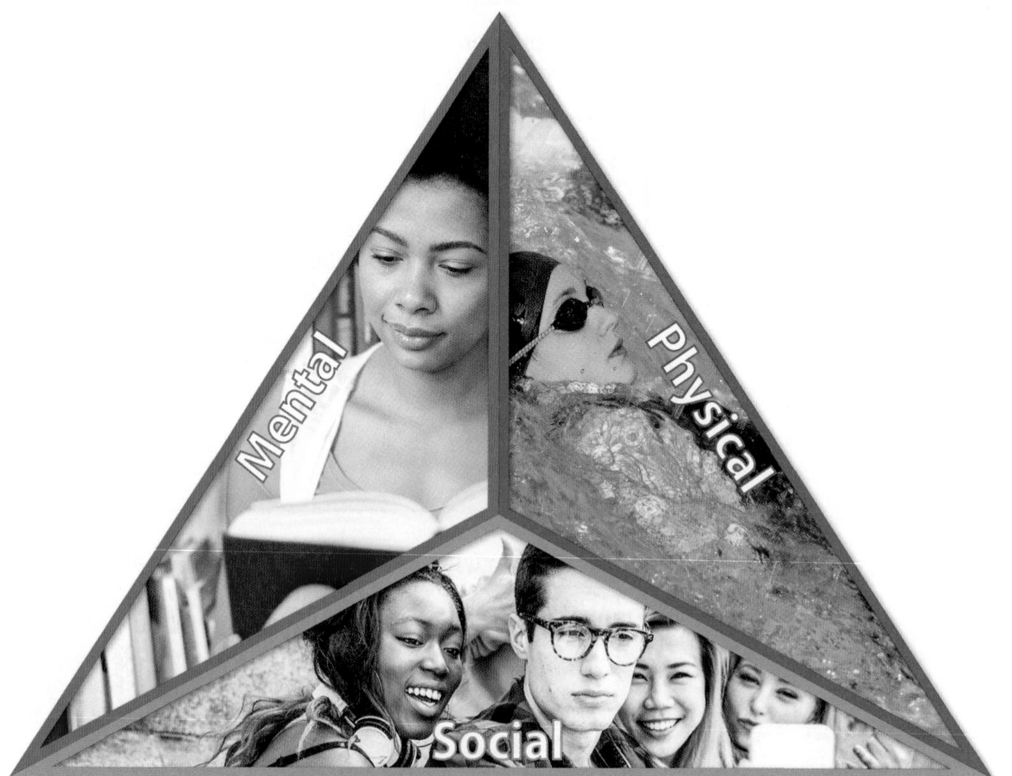

(mental) Syda/Shutterstock.com; (physical) Nate Allred/Shutterstock.com; (social) oneinchpunch/Shutterstock.com

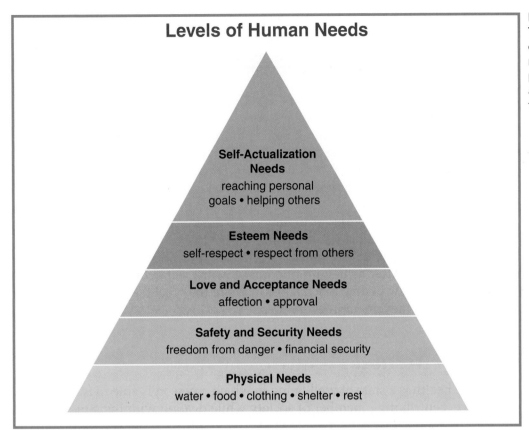

Figure 21.2
The needs at the base of Maslow's hierarchy must be at least partially met before addressing needs at the next level.

Physical Needs

The first level of needs in Maslow's hierarchy is physical needs that are basic to survival. These include needs for oxygen, water, nourishing food, shelter, clothing, and sleep. You are likely to have trouble thinking about much else until these needs are met to some degree. For instance, imagine you are sitting in a football stadium when a terrible storm suddenly begins. Watching the game is likely to become less important than finding some way to meet your basic need for shelter.

Safety and security needs—the second level in the hierarchy—also affect physical health. You need to feel protected from physical harm. You also need to feel financially secure. When these needs are threatened or not met, your state of overall health is in **jeopardy** (danger). For instance, safety needs are not being met if someone who has been drinking alcohol is driving you. Until you remove yourself from this situation, your life is at risk.

Social Needs

If basic physical and security needs are met adequately, it is possible to fulfill needs for love and acceptance. This third level of the hierarchy affects social health. These needs stem from a human desire to experience positive connections with people. All people need to know others care about them. Everyone needs to feel wanted as a member of a group. You may feel loved when a parent expresses concern about you. Perhaps you feel acceptance when a friend invites you to join in an activity. The third level also includes your need to express love and acceptance for others. Loving others helps you feel good about yourself.

Another set of social needs falls at Maslow's fourth level in the hierarchy. This level includes needs for esteem. You need to feel others value you as a person. You must also value yourself. When others recognize your achievements or ask for your opinion, they are helping to address this need.

Mental Needs

The peak of Maslow's hierarchy relates to mental needs. These are needs for people to believe they are doing their **utmost** (maximum) to reach their full human potential. Maslow referred to this as ***self-actualization***. Meeting needs at this level involves more than facing and managing daily tasks. It requires you to work at the peak of your abilities.

People who volunteer are addressing their need for self-actualization. They find the experience rewarding and feel they are helping others.

The need for self-actualization expands as you pursue it. Meeting this need is a lifelong process. After achieving one goal toward self-actualization, you need to set new goals. Few people reach a point where they feel they have reached the highest level of achievement in every area.

What Is Mental Health?

Mental health is a state of well-being in which a person is able to function as a productive, contributing member of society while dealing with the stress of daily life. Positive mental health enables a person to pursue his or her capabilities to the fullest. People with positive mental health feel comfortable with their work and family lives. They can usually adapt to the demands and challenges they must face each day. The three aspects that are indicators of mental health include emotional, psychological, and social.

Emotional

Emotion is a natural state of mind in response to the environment. Although there are many emotions, the six basic emotions include happiness, surprise, fear, sadness, disgust, and anger. These emotions influence your behavior or response to situations and events. That response is most often a lifestyle decision. For example, taking public transportation to work because traffic congestion makes you angry is a lifestyle choice (**Figure 21.3**). However, an emotion can be lifesaving if fear steers you away from an unsafe situation. For instance, fear of attack may prevent you from walking home alone at night.

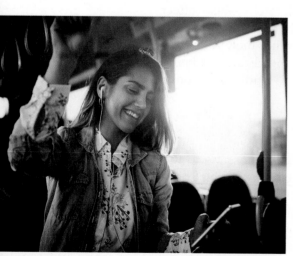

Uber Images/Shutterstock.com

Figure 21.3 Choosing environmentally friendly transportation because it makes you happy is an example of a lifestyle choice influenced by an emotion.

The ability to recognize and manage your emotions as well as the emotions of others is ***emotional intelligence (EI)***. People with a high level of emotional intelligence are able to regulate their emotions. In addition, they are able to recognize and affect the emotions of others in positive ways by encouraging them or calming them down. People with high emotional intelligence are able to identify with the wants, needs, and viewpoints of the other person. They recognize all the good that life offers and are able to recover from **adversity** (difficulty).

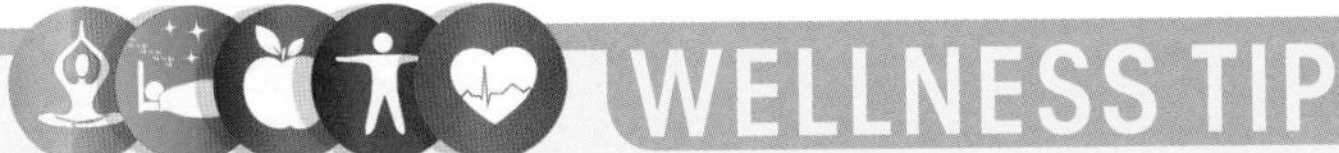
WELLNESS TIP

Exercise to Boost Mental Health

Exercise appears to decrease the symptoms of anxiety and depression in a number of ways. Participating in regular structured exercise is shown to provide the following mental health benefits:

- releases chemicals (endorphins and other neurotransmitters) in the body that help to ease anxiety and depression;
- reduces the negative effects of other chemicals (norepinephrine and other neurotransmitter faults) in the body associated with depression;
- warms the body, producing a calming effect;
- detracts from negative thinking and improves problem solving;
- reduces the long-term risk of cognitive impairment or mental decline; and
- limits time spent in negative behaviors that increase risk of depression.

Controlling Emotions

Recognizing and controlling your emotions begins with identifying your feelings. This may require spending time to evaluate how and why you are responding to a situation. The next step is accepting your feelings rather than ignoring them. Ignoring or suppressing feelings is not healthy. Talking to a friend or writing in your journal can help you accept what you are feeling and prepare you for the next step. The last step is to express your feelings. To express your feelings in a productive way, you must be calm and clear in your communication. Using angry, harsh language to express your feelings is not helpful and can damage your relationship with the other person (**Figure 21.4**).

People with high emotional intelligence are able to not only control their emotions, but also edit them. In other words, they change their outlook from a negative one to a positive one—they think positive!

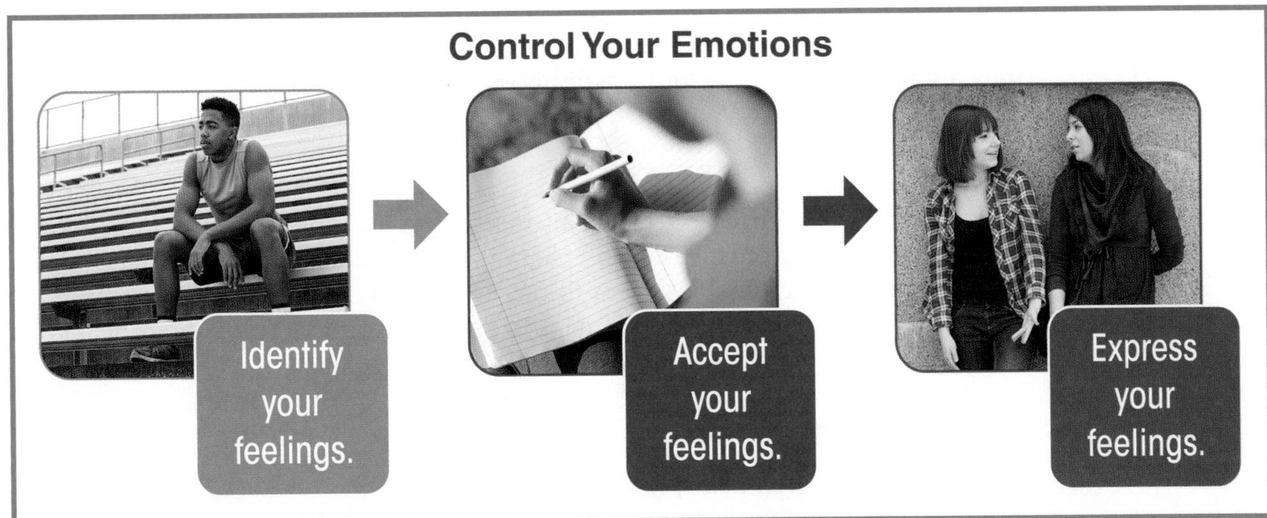
Control Your Emotions
Identify your feelings.
Accept your feelings.
Express your feelings.

L to r: digitalskillet/Shutterstock.com; Christopher Edwin Nuzzaco/Shutterstock.com; Elena Rostunova/Shutterstock.com

Figure 21.4 The ability to control your emotions demonstrates emotional intelligence (EI). *Why is controlling your emotions important?*

FEATURED CAREER

School Counselor

School counselors provide students with career, personal, social, and educational counseling. They help students evaluate their abilities, interests, talents, and personalities to develop realistic academic and career goals. Counselors often work with students who have academic and social development problems or other special needs.

Education

A master's degree usually is required to become a licensed or certified counselor, although requirements for counselors are often very detailed and vary by state.

Job Outlook

Employment for educational, vocational, and school counselors is expected to grow about as fast as the average for all occupations. Expansion of the responsibilities of school counselors also is likely to lead to increases in their employment. For example, counselors are becoming more involved in crisis and preventive counseling—helping students deal with issues ranging from drug and alcohol abuse to death and suicide.

Empathy

Recognizing the emotions of others can be equally challenging. Although emotions are often easy to see on a person's face, recognizing the underlying reasons for the response can be more difficult. The ability to understand other people's emotions develops with experience and effort. It requires empathy. ***Empathy*** is the ability to recognize the feelings, thoughts, or experiences of another person. Developing empathy requires keeping an open mind and listening carefully.

Gratitude

People with emotional intelligence recognize the goodness in life, or gratitude. ***Gratitude*** is thankful appreciation for what is valuable and meaningful in your life. Gratitude helps people form and maintain social relationships. As a result, they are happier and more optimistic about life.

Resilience

Positive mental health does not mean you are always smiling and happy. It is normal to experience bouts of fear, insecurity, and loss of control. These are normal emotional events. However, people with good mental health demonstrate resilience. ***Resilience*** enables them to deal effectively with stressful or traumatic events. This flexibility and willingness to adapt and grow helps them deal with life's challenges and move forward.

Psychological

Psychological well-being contributes to overall mental health. Positive psychological health includes positive emotions, behaviors, and attitudes. Mentally healthy people react positively to major life events. An emotional crisis, such as losing a job or ending a relationship, may cause distress. A lifestyle change, such as a move to a new community, may create discomfort. Nonetheless, they find ways to control and reshape the effects of these emotional upheavals. They focus on improving the conditions they can change.

Mentally healthy people are likely to view life's challenges as opportunities for growth. When an event occurs, they identify the issues involved. They consider their goals as they search for solutions to the problem. If a situation becomes too overwhelming, mentally healthy people are not afraid to ask others for help.

Social

Early social interactions with family and friends develop your self-concept. ***Self-concept***, also called *self-image*, is how you perceive your abilities, appearance, and personality. It is how you view your behavior in relation to other people and tasks.

A positive self-concept is a sign of good mental health. You have a realistic view of yourself and the events in your life. You realize there are positives and negatives to most situations.

Your self-concept is often a reflection of the way you believe other people see you. If other people focus only on your strengths, you may form a negative self-concept. This means you have an inaccurate picture of yourself. You fail to realize you have faults as well as gifts. You are also likely to form a negative self-concept if other people dwell on your failures. You may not recognize you have both positive and negative qualities. If other people acknowledge both your strengths and weaknesses, you are likely to form a positive self-concept. This means you have an accurate picture of yourself. You understand you have abilities as well as shortcomings.

As you grow and change, your self-concept can change. Feedback from family members, friends, teachers, and community leaders may reinforce your self-concept (**Figure 21.5**). It may also cause you to reevaluate and redefine your self-concept. This is part of human growth over the life cycle.

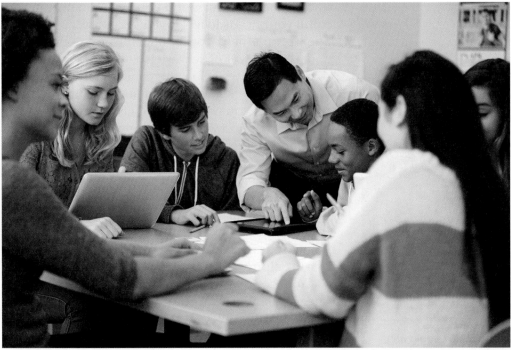

Monkey Business Images/Shutterstock.com

Figure 21.5
Feedback from people in your life helps you develop an accurate self-concept.

A high level of self-esteem is also an indication of good mental health. ***Self-esteem*** is how you value yourself and your perception of your value to others. Like your self-concept, the people around you affect your self-esteem. When people give you the impression you do not matter, it may damage your self-esteem. For instance, picture your teachers refusing to call on you when you raise your hand. Imagine your family members ignoring your opinions. Think about your friends always interrupting you. Over time, these actions may cause you to feel worthless.

A person who has low self-esteem may feel helpless to make decisions. He or she may not feel deserving of good fortune. This person may be easily influenced by peer pressure.

When people express the opinion that you are worthwhile and important, they help build your self-esteem. For example, a teacher may say you did a good job on your science report. Your parents may show pride when you make a mature decision. Your friend may thank you for your loyalty. These types of positive feedback help you feel good about yourself.

With high self-esteem, you feel like a capable, secure, and creative person most of the time. You care about how situations affect you. This empowers you to recognize negative peer pressure and to resist taking part in activities that could be harmful to you. A high level of self-esteem enables you to set goals and take actions to achieve them. Your self-esteem grows as you accomplish tasks that are important to you.

Promoting Mental Health

You can take steps to promote good mental health. Having positive mental health can help you meet your mental needs. A realistic self-assessment can help move you toward self-actualization.

Surround Yourself with Supportive People

Your mental health is enhanced when you surround yourself with people who fulfill your needs to feel loved, accepted, and valued. Such people help you build a positive self-concept and a high level of self-esteem. Their love and support help you develop the confidence you need to succeed. They show support for the nutrition and fitness goals you choose.

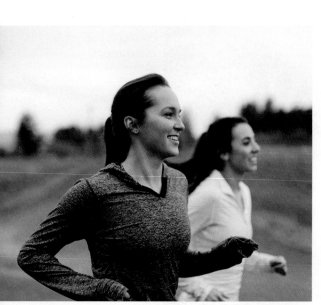

Twin Sails/Shutterstock.com

Figure 21.6 Surround yourself with people who support your nutrition and fitness goals.

Try to connect with encouraging friends and adult role models (**Figure 21.6**). These supportive people can help you build on your strengths and learn from your mistakes. Avoid people who are negative.

Keep in mind that healthy relationships involve giving as well as receiving. Just as you need support from others, others need support from you. When you encourage others, you are playing an important role in helping to fulfill their social and mental needs.

You also need to be supportive of yourself. Encouragement from others will not go very far if you have a poor opinion of yourself. Try to avoid negative thoughts about yourself. Concentrate on using your strengths and improving your weaknesses.

EXTEND YOUR KNOWLEDGE

Feed Your MIND

Is it possible that eating certain foods could improve your brain health as you age? Studies have shown improved cognitive function in people who follow the MIND diet. *MIND* stands for *Mediterranean-DASH Intervention for Neurodegenerative Delay*. The diet combines many of the recommendations of the Mediterranean and DASH diets.

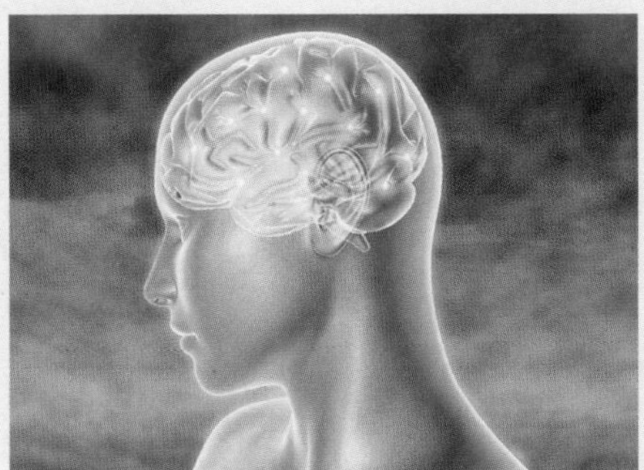

Illustration Forest/Shutterstock.com

The MIND diet does not identify one particular superfood that makes you happier or improves cognitive abilities. Rather, the diet recommends adding or increasing specific foods that have been shown to provide benefits to the brain.

The MIND diet recommends including the following foods in your meals:

- Green, leafy vegetables—six or more servings per week
- All other vegetables—minimum of one serving a day
- Berries—at least two servings per week
- Nuts—five servings or more per week
- Olive oil—use as your primary cooking oil
- Whole grains—at least three servings per day
- Fish—at least one serving per week; select fatty fish that are high in omega-3 fatty acids more often
- Beans—at least four servings per week; includes lentils, dried beans, and soybeans
- Poultry—at least two servings per week; avoid fried poultry
- Wine—adults should limit to one glass per day

The diet also suggests limiting five foods:

- Butter and margarine—less than one tablespoon per day
- Cheese—less than one serving per week
- Red meat—no more than three servings per week
- Fried food—less than one serving per week; best to avoid altogether
- Pastries and sweets—less than four servings per week

Although more research is necessary to prove a definitive link between the MIND diet and improved cognitive function, the early studies showed promising results.

The connection between mental health and social health goes both ways. When you have good mental health, you will find it easier to attract people who meet your social needs. Other people will be drawn to your positive outlook. They will appreciate your realistic view of yourself.

Adopt a Healthy Lifestyle

A healthy lifestyle includes regular physical activity and good nutrition. A healthy lifestyle supplies the energy and strength necessary to face your problems.

Regular physical activity improves mental health. It reduces anxiety, depression, and negative moods while improving self-esteem and mental function. On a basic level, performing regular physical activity provides a sense of accomplishment.

THE MOVEMENT CONNECTION

Mindful Breathing with a Twist

Why

Positive mental health benefits your physical health. Promote positive mental health by focusing on something other than negative thoughts. Mindful breathing focuses your attention on the act of breathing and away from stressors. This can help to relax your central nervous system, slow your heart rate, and alleviate stress.

Apply

Practice mindful breathing as you perform the following stretch:

- Sit up straight and place feet flat on the floor.
- Extend arms out to the sides at shoulder height with palms facing down.
- Inhale for 5 seconds.
- Slowly—to the count of 6 seconds—rotate your arms and torso to the left while exhaling. Your hips should remain stationary during this move. Imagine your slow, deliberate exhalation pushing stressful thoughts out of your body as you twist.
- Return to center, inhaling for 5 seconds.
- Repeat this move to the right.
- Alternate stretching sides for one minute.

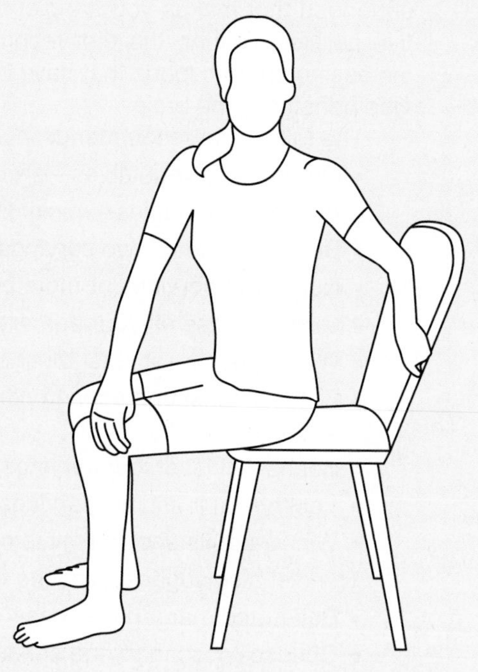

Notice how you feel twisting from side to side. Does one side feel more restricted than the other or do you feel balance on both sides? If you notice significant limitations on one side, ask your health or physical education instructor how you could alleviate this.

The connection between nutrition and physical health is clear. Understanding of the link between diet and mental health is growing. The research that specifically looks at nutrition and mental health as it affects mood, depression, and dementia continues to grow. Consider the following ways to improve your mental health with nutrition:

- *Eat breakfast to benefit mental health.* Performance and learning behaviors noticeably improve when individuals begin the day with breakfast.
- *Drink adequate fluids to protect against dehydration.* Dehydration affects your ability to think clearly and concentrate.
- *Eat meals on a regular basis to promote calmness and satisfaction.* A hungry person can feel irritable and restless.
- *Choose foods that are digested slowly and are a good source of fiber to moderate swings in blood sugar levels.* Mood and energy swings can be associated with big fluctuations in blood sugar levels that result from eating foods high in sugar and other simple carbohydrates. Include more fruits, vegetables, and whole grains in your diet.

- *Include high-quality proteins every day to supply all the amino acids needed for brain function.* Protein intake can affect brain function and mental health. Many of the neurotransmitters in the brain are made from amino acids. When these essential amino acids are missing from the diet, there is evidence of mood-lowering effects, increased anxiety, loss of concentration, and fatigue.
- *Select foods and beverages rich in vitamins, minerals, and omega-3 fatty acids to support healthy brain function and a positive mental outlook.* Researchers have observed the prevalence of mental health disorders increases as the nutritious quality of food and beverage choices deteriorates. Deficiencies of certain vitamins or minerals can result in damaged brain cells and reduced memory, problem-solving abilities, and brain function.
- *Consume sufficient calories to support the energy needs of a developing body and brain.* Developing fetuses and young children are susceptible to brain damage from malnutrition. Decrease in brain size, poor growth, and weak, brittle bones are some of the risks of eating disorders during a growth phase. Balanced nutrition is vital for reaching full brain development.

Maintain Balance in Your Life

Have you ever been so busy going out with your friends that you barely have time to see your family? Have you ever been so involved with a school project that you forgot to eat a meal? From time to time, people focus too much energy on one area of their lives. As a result, they lose touch with other areas and their lives lack balance.

You must distribute time and energy among your many roles and responsibilities in a balanced way. A lack of balance can have a negative effect on mental health. People whose lives are out of balance become exhausted emotionally. They are likely to experience ***burnout*** or a lack of energy and motivation to work toward goals. Burnout causes a reduced sense of personal accomplishment.

Look at your life from an outsider's point of view to assess the balance in your life. This provides a better **perspective** (mental view) of how your daily actions affect the quality of your life. You may discover you need to reconsider your allocation of time and energy.

Balance comes from devoting an appropriate amount of time and energy to each of your roles. These roles may include family, school or job, and community roles (**Figure 21.7**).

While dividing your time among your roles, remember to save some time for yourself. You need to take care of your physical, social, and mental needs. You need to allow yourself the time to select nutritious foods and get adequate amounts of rest and exercise. You also need to take the time to relax and enjoy hobbies and friends. Taking time for yourself makes you better prepared to face your roles and responsibilities.

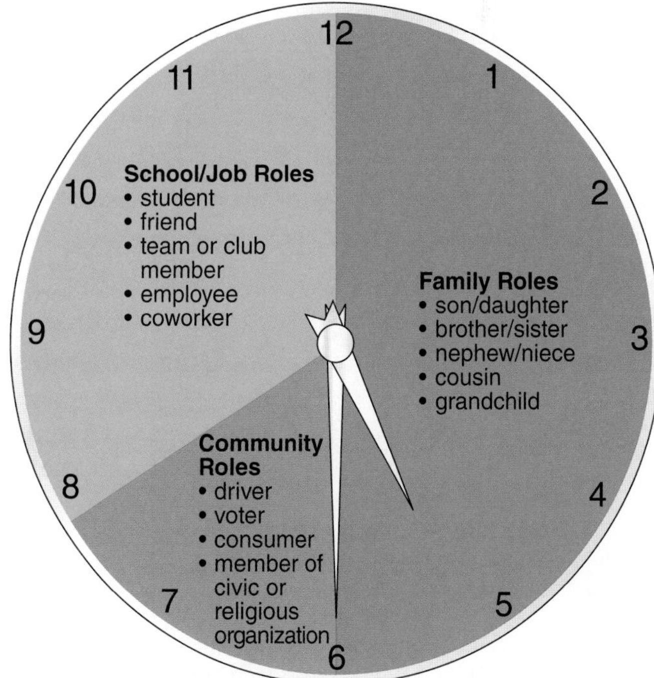

Figure 21.7 Promoting positive mental health involves allotting time to each of your roles. ***How do you allocate your time?***

What Is Social Health?

The degree to which your social needs for love, acceptance, and esteem are met affects your social health. Social health is reflected in your ability to get along with the people around you. It is measured by the quality of your relationships. ***Relationships*** are the connections you form with family members, friends, and other people.

Building relationships with others enriches your life and helps you understand what types of interactions meet your social needs. You learn how to interact with people from other cultures who may have values different from your own. As you understand what is important to you, you are able to form stronger relationships. You will enjoy making new friends while keeping old ones.

Certain traits are common in people with good social health. These traits help them relate to others. Such traits include patience, courtesy, respect, selflessness, and empathy. Socially healthy people exhibit these traits through their daily words and actions. They share thoughts and ideas while showing respect for the needs of others.

Social Development

One sign of social health is positive social development during childhood and adolescence. ***Social development*** is learning how to get along well with others. In addition to being able to form close personal relationships, it involves the ability to act appropriately in different social situations. For example, not talking in a movie theater, thanking a clerk for help, and raising your hand in class are social skills. Social skills are used to communicate effectively with people from different backgrounds. These skills may not be enough to help you form close friendships, but help you feel more at ease in social settings.

Food encounters are often used as a way to build social connections. At social gatherings, food is a symbol of welcoming hospitality. Teen parties usually include favorite foods and beverages. The mere presence of food often suggests fun, relaxation, and a time to get to know each other. You learn how to interact with friends informally.

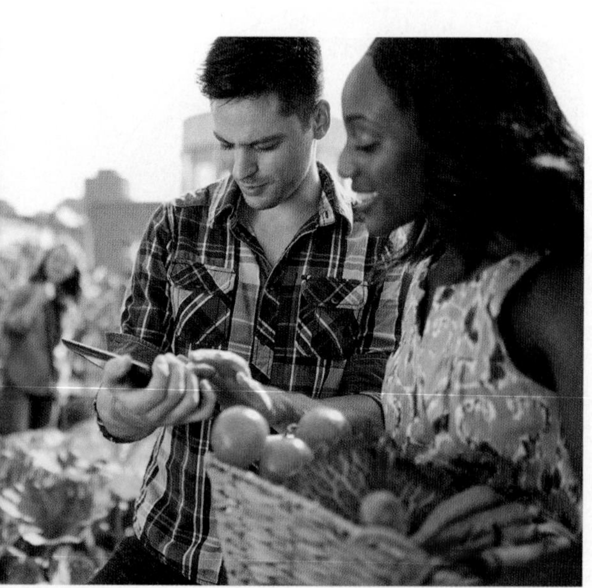

AYA images/Shutterstock.com

Figure 21.8 Community garden projects offer an opportunity to demonstrate cooperation and responsibility.

Another example of how food can become a focus for social development is with school or community garden projects (**Figure 21.8**). Even young children can learn the importance of group cooperation and social responsibilities while planting and growing food in a common area. "Many hands make light work" is a quote that expresses the benefit of working together. Children learn from each other and from adults who model cooperative behaviors.

Like children, teens tend to model the conduct of their peers. Peers who model inappropriate social actions can have a negative effect on social development. Teens who learn to recognize and reject inappropriate behavior can protect their social health status.

Adult relationships involve getting along with coworkers as well as friends and family members. Job success depends on achieving social competence. Aging family members need positive social contacts to thrive. Positive social skills learned early in life will carry you through healthy teen years, to your career successes and advancements, and through the healthy aging process.

Your Social Circle

For most people, the closest and most continuous relationships occur within families. These relationships begin at birth as family members respond to a baby's needs. A family that demonstrates care and respect for each of its members displays signs of positive social health (**Figure 21.9**).

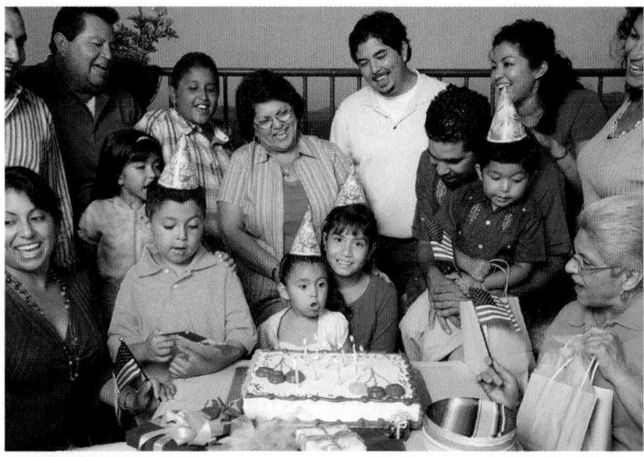

Blend Images/Shutterstock.com

Figure 21.9 Much early social development occurs within the family unit.

Sharing friendship is an important way to achieve social health. Friends provide people with a source of fun and companionship. You feel free to exchange joys and sorrows with a friend. Most importantly, friends help you work through problems and supply feedback. As your friends provide this type of support for you, you provide it for them. This two-way exchange can be a valuable source of self-discovery.

Beyond family members and friends, your social connections can expand through Internet communications, travel, media, and group activities. For example, it is more fun to exercise with friends and even challenge each other to reach higher levels of skill through friendly competition. You face new social challenges as you include people from other cultures in your social network. As you interact with others, they influence your thoughts and feelings and you influence theirs. Sharing friendships is an important way to achieve social health.

EXTEND YOUR KNOWLEDGE

Safe Use of Social Media

Using social media is a common part of a teen's life. Social media refers to the many ways to communicate by sharing ideas and information online. Through social media, individuals can make social and professional contacts. However, caution is advised because many people read information shared on social media.

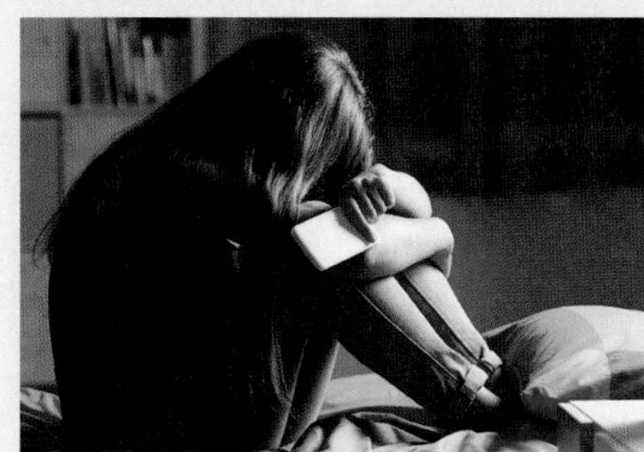

Antonio Guillem/Shutterstock.com

To be safe and to protect yourself, follow these guidelines:

- Check or update your privacy settings.
- Avoid posting sensitive data, personal phone numbers, or your location.
- Keep social profiles private so only friends or selected contacts can see your posts.
- Be suspicious of strangers who want information or wish to be friends. Flirting with strangers on social media can have serious consequences.
- Follow school policies regarding smartphone use and sharing photos.
- Never use social media to send mean or hurtful content. Online bullying and de-friending may lead others to symptoms of depression. Resolve conflicts in person.

Consider your experiences using social media. Can you cite examples of both positive and negative effects on mental health?

Be proactive when choosing a circle of friends. Being *proactive* is taking steps to deal with anticipated situations. Select friends who support your choice to live a healthy lifestyle. Avoid friends who encourage you to participate in destructive behaviors. If your friends support your interests in good health and fitness, you will find extra motivation to make health-promoting choices.

Promoting Social Health

Take steps to build positive relationships that meet your social needs. Many experts agree that an ability to share ideas with others is the most important social skill. With this skill, you can solve problems with others and make your needs known to them. You can also express care for others and work with them to achieve goals.

Develop Communication Skills

Communication is the sending of a message from one source to another. Two basic types of communication are used to convey messages. ***Verbal communication*** uses words. It may be spoken or unspoken. Speaking to someone and writing a letter are both examples of verbal communication. ***Nonverbal communication*** transmits messages without the use of words. Posture, facial expressions, tone of voice, and symbols are nonverbal ways of communicating. When verbal and nonverbal communication both send the same message, communication is clear.

You need effective communication skills to exchange ideas with others. These skills can greatly affect your relationships and, thus, your social health (**Figure 21.10**).

The increasing use of e-mail, text messaging, and other electronic communication makes clear communication skills more important than ever. A message containing errors or inaccurate information could spread a bad impression around the world in a matter of seconds.

Learn how to write effectively and take time to select the right words and construct clear sentences. Use a writing style that conveys your intended tone. Be sure the message you send cannot be interpreted as **offensive** (rude, insulting) to another person or group of people. For informative writing, keep sentences short. Sentences that are long and use technical terms are harder for people to read and understand. Following these suggestions will help you represent yourself well as you use written communication to build personal relationships.

Resolve Conflicts

A ***conflict*** is a disagreement. Conflicts tend to arise between people in social situations. Perhaps someone has blamed you for something you did not do. You may have gotten into an argument with a good friend. These are examples of conflict.

If you do not handle conflicts carefully, they can grow. A conflict that gets out of hand can eventually destroy a relationship. This is why an ability to resolve, or settle, conflicts is important for maintaining good social health. You can use your communication skills to help you resolve conflicts.

Handling conflicts promptly helps keep them under control. However, you should wait until you have a chance to talk about the problem privately. Airing your disagreement publicly is likely to make the other person uncomfortable and defensive.

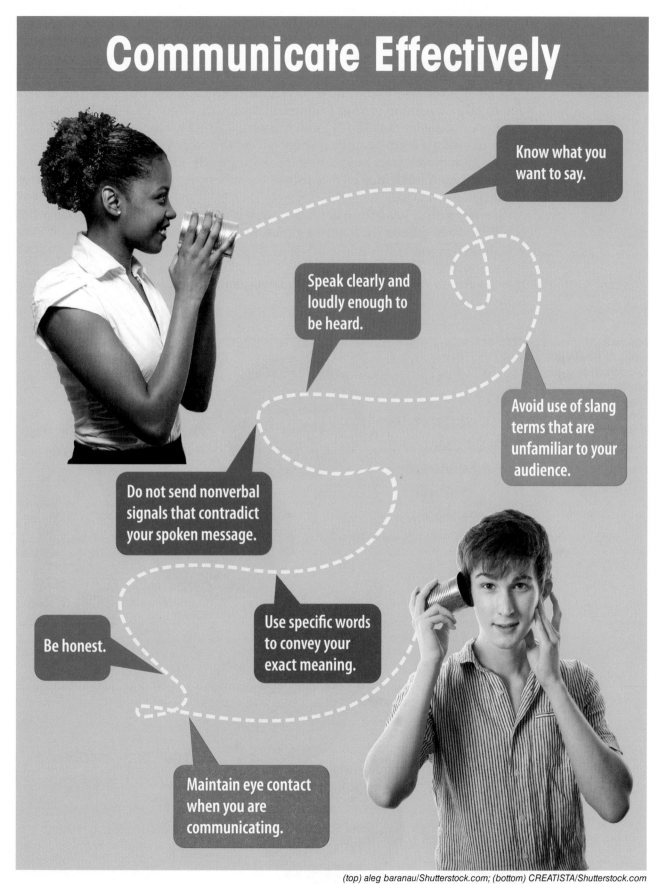

(top) aleg baranau/Shutterstock.com; (bottom) CREATISTA/Shutterstock.com

Figure 21.10 Effective communication skills facilitate the exchange of ideas in an accurate and clear manner. *Can you remember a time when your message was misunderstood? How did that make you feel?*

Stay focused on the facts related to the problem. Try not to bring emotions into your discussion. Also, avoid being distracted by other issues. Explain why you are unhappy with the person's *actions*, rather than why you are unhappy with the *person*.

Use "I" messages to state how you feel and why you feel that way. This allows you to take ownership of your feelings. In contrast, a "you" message blames your feelings on someone else. The "I" statements in the first example in **Figure 21.11** are likely to evoke a more positive response from the other person.

Try to monitor your voice. Tone of voice greatly influences the quality of a conversation. A loud, angry voice causes the other person to feel as though he or she is being attacked.

Do not simply criticize what is wrong with a situation; rather, explain what could be done differently. Suggest a plan that might work better. Describe why you think this solution would work. Stay flexible as you discuss various solutions to the problem. The other person may also have some good ideas. Together you may be able to reach a compromise. A ***compromise*** is a solution that blends ideas from differing parties.

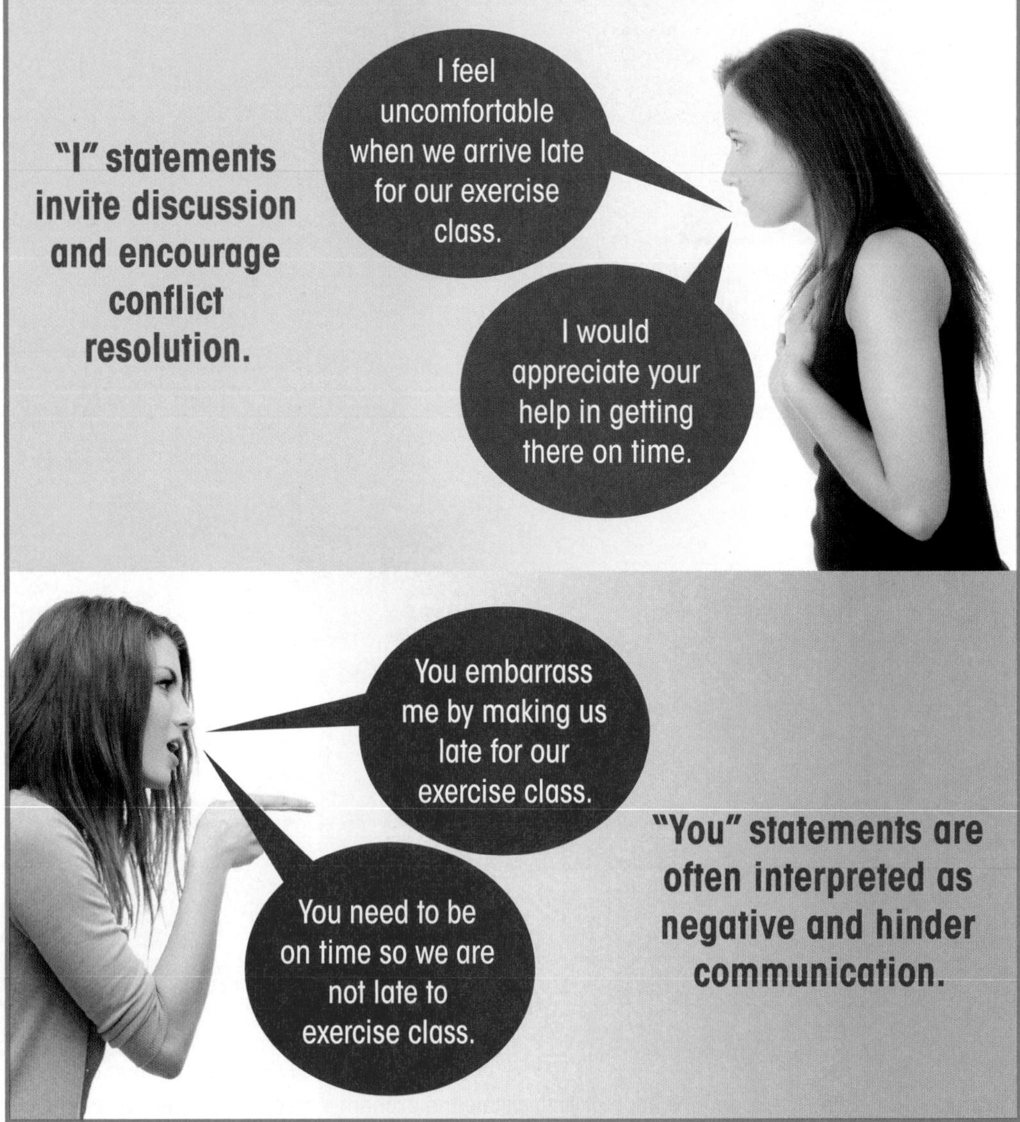

Figure 21.11
Using "I" statements to communicate a problem is more likely to promote a cooperative interaction and possible solution.

(top) PhotoMediaGroup/Shutterstock.com; (bottom) Syda Productions/Shutterstock.com

Practice Assertiveness

Learning to be assertive helps you develop positive social health. ***Assertiveness*** is a personality trait. It is the boldness to express what you think and feel in a way that does not offend others. It is different from aggressiveness and goes beyond passiveness. To be *aggressive* is to express your feelings in a way that is pushy and offensive. To be *passive* may mean failing to express your feelings at all.

Assertiveness allows you to take steps to reach desired outcomes. You feel actively involved in the decisions. Assertiveness is demonstrated when you ask important questions and locate necessary resources to achieve your needs and interests.

Assertiveness can help you feel more confident in socially challenging situations. You are able to say "no" when an activity does not agree with your personal values and beliefs. You are able to turn down offers to join in activities that do not fit into your schedule. You are able to pursue opportunities that are important to you.

You can practice assertiveness if it does not come naturally to you. Make a point of expressing your opinions to others. Be firm when asking for what you want. However, if the answer is "no," let go of the issue. Avoid becoming angry, demanding, and argumentative. (This would be aggressive behavior.) Do not be afraid of your position or feel you must defend it. (This would be passive behavior.) Just state your feelings calmly and openly. In most cases, people will respect your honesty.

When you encounter someone who is aggressive, your most assertive response is to leave. You will not be able to reason with someone who is out of control. To protect yourself from potential violence, you need to remove yourself from the situation.

Be a Good Listener

Communication involves listening as well as speaking. You need to listen carefully to be sure you understand the message someone else is sending. Try restating information that has been shared. Ask questions about any points that are not clear. These steps allow you to confirm that you have correctly understood what the other person said.

CASE STUDY

Social Health on the Menu

Mia and her friends decide to go out to eat after play practice. The group goes to a nearby fast-food restaurant. They each stand in line to place their orders. Mia is the last person to arrive at the table with her food. The rest of her group has ordered fries, sodas, milkshakes, and cheeseburgers. When they see Mia has a grilled chicken sandwich (no mayonnaise), nonfat milk, and a small salad on her tray, they begin teasing her. They tell her she eats like an old person and ask if her mom ordered her meal for her. They laugh and wonder if she is trying to get extra credit with the health teacher.

Case Review

1. Why do you think Mia's friends are reacting to her food choices in this manner?
2. How could Mia respond in an assertive manner without endangering the friendship of the group?

Good friends are good listeners. You know you can rely on them and they can rely on you. Friends need to be understanding and sensitive about how you feel at any given time. Friends also show they care. Communicating a sense of caring and understanding is a way to empathize with another. A good listener demonstrates she values your feelings and words as much as her own. At the same time, you need to offer others the same qualities you desire in a friend. Friends listen carefully to what each other is saying.

Be a Team Member

A socially healthy person functions effectively as a member of a group and is willing to participate in teamwork. *Teamwork* is the effort of two or more people toward a common goal. Teamwork is often required to solve complex problems or complete involved tasks. For instance, making a parade float for a school club would require teamwork among club members. Each person contributes unique talents, giving the project balance and completeness. A club member with artistic skill could design the float. Someone with consumer skills could buy the supplies. A member who has construction skills could help build the float.

Completing the project successfully would be much more difficult without the addition of each person's unique abilities. By helping and encouraging one another, team members can accomplish more as a group than they can individually (**Figure 21.12**).

Making Positive Behavior Changes

Perhaps you have a desire to improve your overall mental health. You have read several suggestions for helping you reach this goal; however, it may require the adoption of new behaviors. Making such changes in your life can be difficult. It involves conscious and responsible efforts.

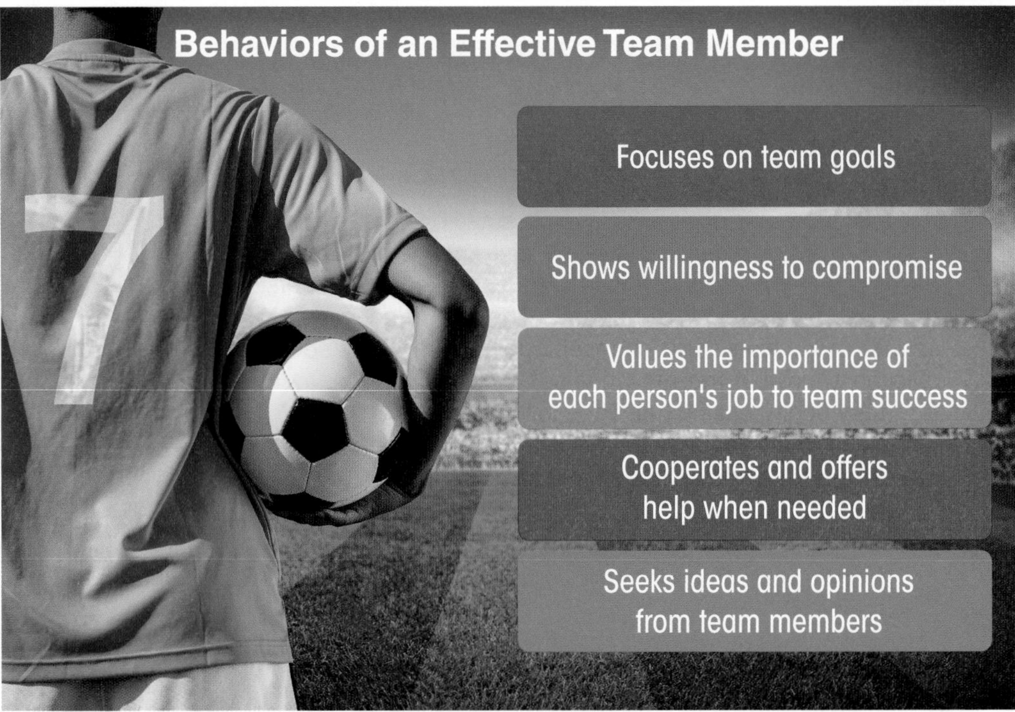
Behaviors of an Effective Team Member
Focuses on team goals
Shows willingness to compromise
Values the importance of each person's job to team success
Cooperates and offers help when needed
Seeks ideas and opinions from team members
7

pixfly/Shutterstock.com

Figure 21.12 Participating as a member of a team teaches conflict-resolution skills and builds self-esteem.

Using a self-management plan can make this change process easier. A self-management plan is an action-oriented tool for making a positive behavior change. It involves carefully analyzing goals, priorities, and choices. It requires you to identify options before making and acting on decisions. As you read about each step in the self-management plan, prepare a plan of your own (**Figure 21.13**).

List Your Strengths

Most people have experienced many successes in life. No one has a life full of failures. Begin your self-management plan by examining your strengths in the health area you want to improve. For example, suppose you want to improve your social health. Your current social strengths may include your honesty as a friend and your cooperative attitude when working on a team.

List Your "Needs Improvement" Behaviors

Identify health-related behaviors you feel you need to improve. You might believe being assertive is one of your weaker social skills. Maybe you feel you often hesitate to express your needs to others. As a result, your wishes go unnoticed. You might also feel you have trouble resolving conflicts. Perhaps you do not tell other people when you disagree with them. Instead, you allow negative feelings to build up until you have an outburst of temper.

Prioritize Your "Needs Improvement" Behaviors

After you have identified the "needs improvement" behaviors, you must narrow your focus. You are less likely to be successful if you scatter your attention in too many directions. Look at the list of behaviors you identified in the second step.

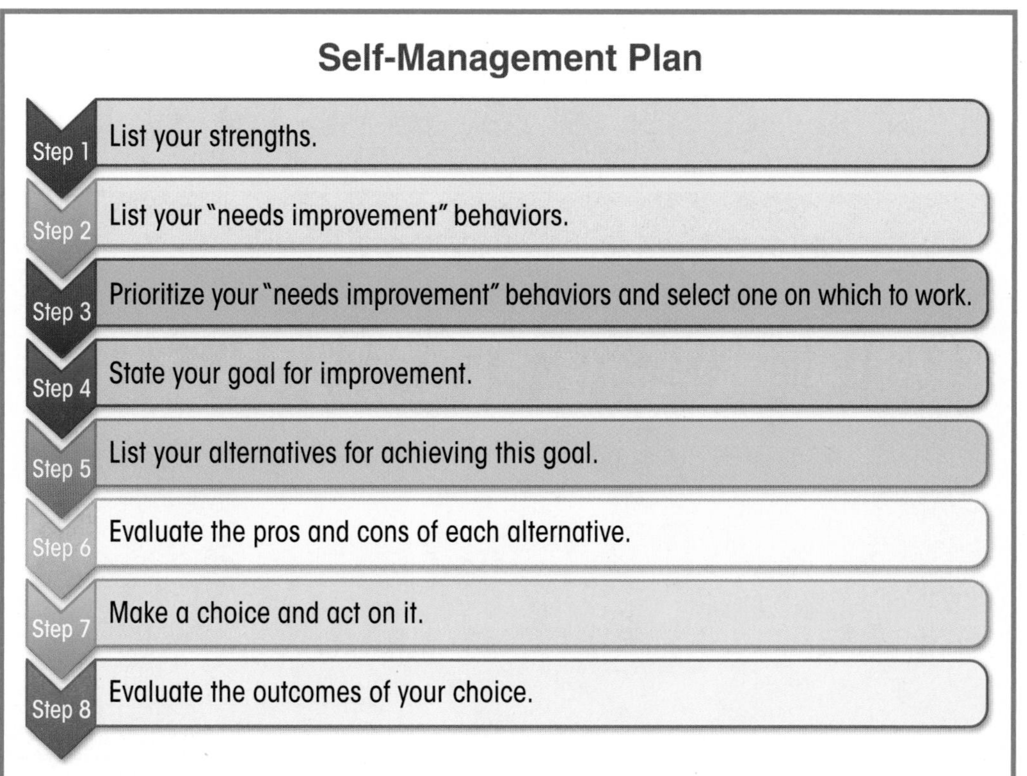

Self-Management Plan
Step 1
List your strengths.
Step 2
List your "needs improvement" behaviors.
Step 3
Prioritize your "needs improvement" behaviors and select one on which to work.
Step 4
State your goal for improvement.
Step 5
List your alternatives for achieving this goal.
Step 6
Evaluate the pros and cons of each alternative.
Step 7
Make a choice and act on it.
Step 8
Evaluate the outcomes of your choice.

Figure 21.13 Self-management plans promote self-reliance and develop useful life skills.

Rank your list, placing the behavior that concerns you most at the top. You may believe assertiveness will help you resolve conflicts. Therefore, you decide to put "being more assertive" at the top of your "needs improvement" list.

State Your Goal

Now that you have identified your main area for self-improvement, shape it into a specific goal. This will give you a sense of direction. State your goal in writing, using concrete, measurable terms. (Use the guidelines for SMART goals discussed in Chapter 1 of this text.) Be realistic about what you can achieve.

Divide your goal into manageable subgoals. For example, your main goal is "I want to be more assertive." This is a broad goal. A measurable subgoal might be "I will ask one question or state one opinion every day." Another subgoal might be "I will not apologize when I have to say 'no' to participating in an activity." You can easily see how well you are achieving these specific subgoals. This will give you motivation to continue working toward your main goal.

As you are clarifying your goal, decide how important it is to you. Consider if you are willing to do what is required to create a change. Also, consider how the achievement of your goal will affect others (**Figure 21.14**).

List Your Alternatives

For each subgoal you have identified, list all the ways you can think of to achieve it. Usually there will be more than one choice available. For example, to learn how to ask questions and state opinions boldly, you could attend an assertiveness workshop. You might read a book about expressing yourself with confidence. You could ask advice from someone who has an ability to speak out. You could also ask a trusted friend to help you practice asking questions and stating opinions. All these choices have the possibility of helping you develop assertiveness skills.

You may want to research alternatives for reaching your goal. The more options you know about, the more likely you are to find one that works for you. Use the Internet or your community library to gather information. Seek the advice of a school counselor or someone else who may be knowledgeable on the subject.

Figure 21.14
A goal to spend more time with a younger sibling will have a positive effect on his self-esteem as well as your own.

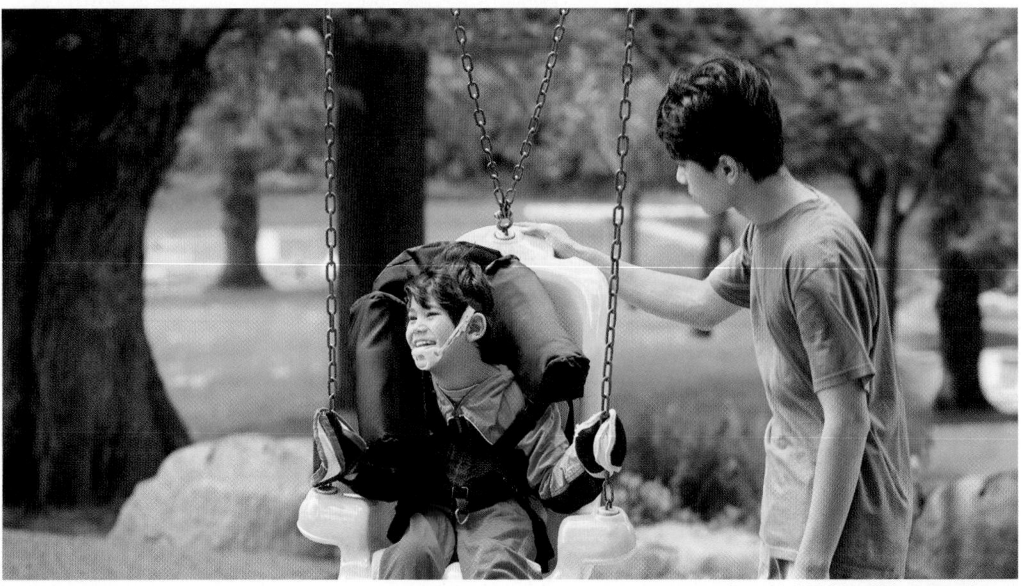

Jaren Jai Wicklund/Shutterstock.com

Evaluate the Pros and Cons

Identify as many advantages and disadvantages as you can for each alternative on your list. For example, an assertiveness workshop has the advantage of acquiring new skills quickly. On the other hand, it may have the disadvantage of being costly. Weigh the pros against the cons for each alternative. Delete any options on your list that have more drawbacks than benefits.

Think about how each alternative affects your resources, including time, money, and physical energy. Also, consider the results of choosing one alternative over another. Choosing one option can often remove other options. If you spend your money to attend a workshop, you can no longer use that money to buy a book.

COMMUNITY CONNECTIONS

Fund-Raising to Help Others

Resources for community welfare programs are often scarce. Fund-raising is one way to help. *Fund-raising* means collecting contributions, in the form of money or other needed resources. It may require requesting donations from individuals, clubs, businesses, and even government agencies. The funds or items collected are given to the agency, organization, or persons in need.

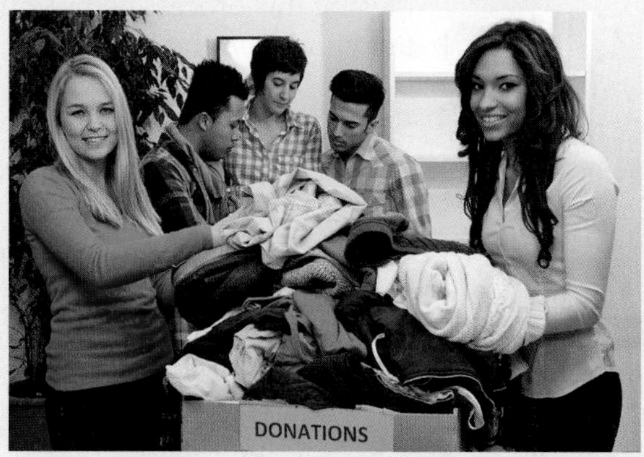

mangostock/Shutterstock.com

If you want to help solve social issues, consider fund-raising. First, you must identify a project that is important to you. Be sure to choose a charitable organization with a history of using most, if not all, of donations for the work of helping those in need. A number of free sites are available online that evaluate how efficiently charities use donations. Then, learn what the organization's needs are. Seek approval to organize a collection center in your school. Use social media and school bulletins to communicate the collection location, date, and purpose.

If the fund-raiser is an event, such as a food sale, informal dinner, dance, or party, then detailed planning is required. Form a committee to identify goals, detail arrangements, and assign roles. Be sure that money is spent judiciously (carefully) so that most funds collected go to the charity.

After the event, "thank-you" notes should be mailed to donors. In addition, proceeds must be calculated and reported. This information is shared with the donors. Most importantly, donations must be distributed to the charity. A fund-raiser can be a fun way to show support for helping your community.

Think Critically

1. Research three charitable organizations that interest you. Learn about their needs for volunteers and donations. Compare each for how efficiently donations are used.
2. Identify ways that volunteering makes your community a better place to live. What motivates people to volunteer?

Make a Choice and Act on It

After comparing your various alternatives, choose the one that best suits you and act on your choice. Suppose you decide to read a book on expressing yourself with confidence. Go to a bookstore or library. Find a book on this topic that seems engaging. Buy or check out the book and read it. Begin to employ advice from the book in your daily interactions with others.

Evaluate Outcomes

As a final step, you need to evaluate the effectiveness of your plan. Spend time reflecting on your outcomes: Did your chosen action help you meet your goal? Are modifications needed? (**Figure 21.15**).

After time spent in reflection, write your evaluation. This will help you to focus and clarify your results. Evaluation is a valuable step in making permanent and meaningful change.

If your evaluation reveals your chosen action failed to produce the desired change, do not view it as a failure. Instead, consider this as information that brings you one step closer to genuine, lasting change. Use this information to modify your original goal and try again.

Using this process helps you learn more about yourself and will help you make better choices in the future.

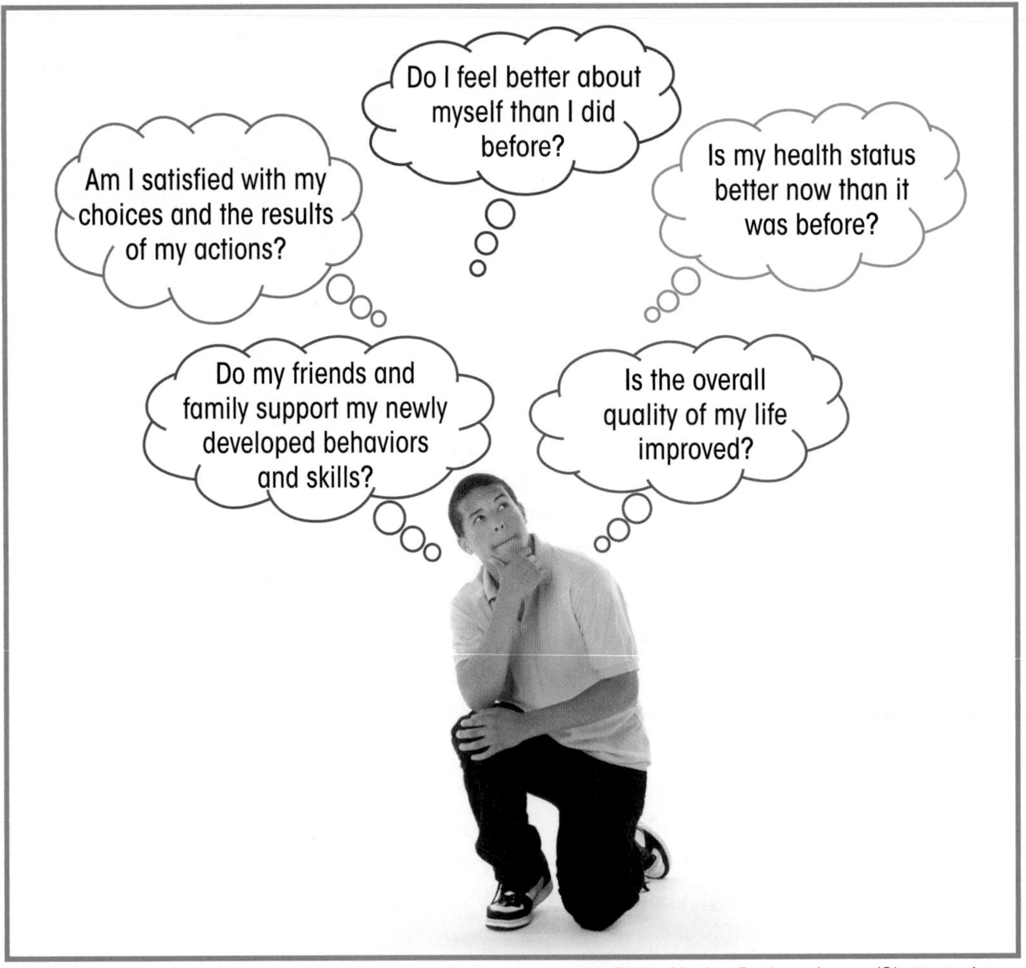
Do I feel better about myself than I did before?
Am I satisfied with my choices and the results of my actions?
Is my health status better now than it was before?
Do my friends and family support my newly developed behaviors and skills?
Is the overall quality of my life improved?

Photo: Monkey Business Images/Shutterstock.com

Figure 21.15 Evaluation is a critical step in creating meaningful change that is often overlooked. *Why do you think people choose to skip this step?*

Seeking Help for Mental Health Problems

Positive mental and social health are key elements of overall wellness. Many people find the methods described earlier helpful for improving mental and social health. However, some people have mental and social health problems that cannot be solved with self-help techniques. Such problems require the help of healthcare professionals.

Mental and social health problems can occur for many reasons. Some are the result of specific crisis events, such as divorce, death of a person close to you, or school relocation. Other problems arise out of long-term situations, such as emotional neglect or substance abuse. No matter what is causing the problem, the important point is to find needed help.

A physician can recommend professionals who can help people with social or mental problems. A professional will begin by helping a client define the problem. Treatment may involve individual, family, or group therapy. Therapy often focuses on helping clients develop the tools they need to help themselves. Treatment for some clients also involves medication.

Helpful therapists convey interest, understanding, and respect to clients. They offer advice and support to help clients improve their mental and social health. However, the clients are responsible for making needed behavior changes.

Often people fail to seek help for mental health issues. The cost of treatment may present a barrier to pursuing needed help. Many health insurance policies cover some portion of the cost. Free clinics, community health centers, and hotlines are low-cost or free options. In addition to cost, the social stigma associated with a mental health issue is a barrier for many people. However, mental health issues are common to many people and should not be a reason for embarrassment. As with physical health conditions, mental health conditions require treatment by a physician.

RECIPE FILE

Strawberry Compote

6 SERVINGS

Ingredients

- 1½ c. fresh strawberries, stems removed
- 1 T. orange juice
- 1 t. clover honey
- ½ t. chia seeds

Directions

1. Cut strawberries in half and place in small saucepan over medium heat.
2. When fruit begins to simmer, reduce heat and smash the fruit in the pan.
3. Add orange juice and honey.
4. Simmer for about 10–15 minutes.
5. Remove from heat, add chia seeds, and stir well.
6. Refrigerate in a covered container.

PER SERVING: 19 CALORIES, 0.5 G PROTEIN, 4 G CARBOHYDRATE, 0 G FAT, 1 G FIBER, 1 MG SODIUM.

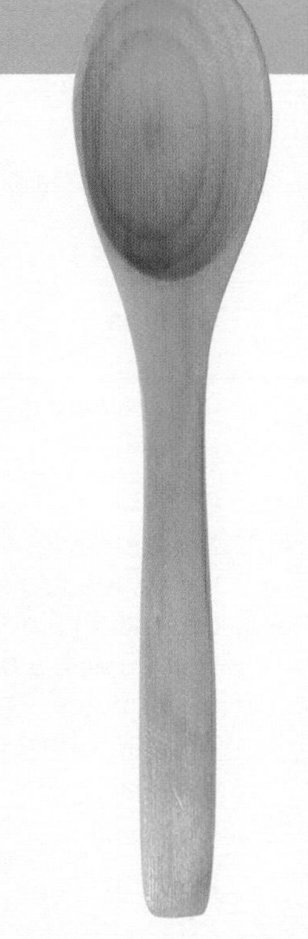

Chapter 21 Review and Expand

Reading Summary

Mental, social, and physical health areas are interrelated and affect overall wellness. These three health areas are affected by the degree to which human needs are met.

People with positive mental health are able to function as productive, contributing members of society while dealing with the stresses of daily life. Positive mental health is promoted by surrounding yourself with supportive people, adopting a healthy lifestyle, and maintaining balance in your life.

Social health is the ability to form quality relationships with others. Acquisition of social skills and a positive, caring social circle contribute to positive social health. Positive social health is promoted by developing effective communication skills, learning to resolve conflicts, practicing assertiveness, listening well, and functioning as an effective team member.

A self-management plan is helpful for making positive behavior changes that promote overall wellness. However, some problems require treatment from health-care professionals.

Chapter Vocabulary

1. **Content Terms** In teams, create categories for the following terms and classify as many of the terms as possible. Then, share your ideas with the remainder of the class.

assertiveness	nonverbal communication
burnout	relationship
communication	resilience
compromise	self-actualization
conflict	self-concept
emotion	self-esteem
emotional intelligence (EI)	social development
empathy	verbal communication
gratitude	

2. **Academic Terms** For each of the following terms, identify a word or group of words describing a quality of the term—an *attribute*. Pair up with a classmate and discuss your list of attributes. Then, discuss your list of attributes with the whole class to increase understanding.

adversity	offensive
hierarchy	perspective
jeopardy	utmost

Review Learning

3. Why are physical needs the first (bottom) level of Maslow's hierarchy of human needs?
4. *True or false?* The need to express love and acceptance for others is a component of self-actualization.
5. Explain why meeting the need for self-actualization is a lifelong process.
6. What are three aspects that are indicators of mental health?
7. Why is learning to control your emotions important?
8. *True or false?* You are likely to form a positive self-concept when others acknowledge only your strengths.
9. Social health is measured by the _____ of your relationships.
10. What are four traits that help people with good social health relate to others?
11. Explain why developing effective communication skills is important to your social health.
12. List five tips for resolving conflict.
13. "Anyone who likes that rock band is an idiot. That music stinks!" is an example of a(n) _____ statement.
14. Why should a person prioritize "needs improvement" behaviors when preparing a self-management plan?
15. What could you tell a friend who refuses to seek treatment because he is embarrassed to admit he has a mental health issue?

Self-Assessment Quiz

Complete the self-assessment quiz online to help you practice and expand your knowledge and skills.

Critical Thinking

16. **Analyze** How you choose to balance your roles and responsibilities is a product of your values and your actions. Reflect on the amount of time you dedicate to your various roles and responsibilities. Prepare a pie chart to illustrate how you allocate your time. Analyze how you allocate your time and determine if this accurately reflects your values.

17. **Draw Conclusions** Why do you think there is a stigma associated with mental health problems? How might that stigma affect the course of the individual's mental health problem? What conclusion can you draw about the importance of erasing the stigma?
18. **Role-Play** Write a brief description of a situation that would benefit from assertiveness skills. In a small group, role-play the situation to practice using assertiveness skills. Video your role-play and invite your classmates to critique your use of the skills.
19. **Apply** Start a gratitude journal. A gratitude journal is a record of the good things that occur in your life. Maintaining a gratitude journal can decrease stress, provide perspective, supply clarity, and help you understand yourself. To start, you simply record the good things in your life on a daily basis. It can be a simple listing of events or a more detailed description. For example, perhaps you made the debate club, received a college acceptance letter, or spent time cooking with your grandmother. When you are feeling down, you can read your gratitude journal to help you focus on what is important in your life.

Core Skills

20. **Write** Research and write an informative paper about Abraham Maslow. Discuss what led him to the development of his hierarchy of human needs theory. Cite your sources.
21. **Technology Literacy** Plan and write three entries for a blog that promotes self-esteem. The blog should highlight the importance of self-esteem and discuss how it relates to human needs in Maslow's hierarchy. The blog should include ideas for building self-esteem. First, consider the audience who will be reading your blog. What does your audience want and need to know about this topic? Then, determine the content and its organization. Select three main points that you want to address each day. Next, create an appealing title to capture your reader's attention. Write each blog entry, providing supporting facts for each main point. Consider providing an action item for each entry.
22. **Write** Develop a questionnaire to measure how working families balance their daily lives. Learn how much time each member of the family allots to family, work, community, and other roles. Ask respondents to rate their satisfaction with the balance in their lives. Ask them to provide helpful tips they use to maintain balance. Compile the results of your questionnaire and write an analysis of your findings.
23. **Speaking** Research the effects of nutrition on brain development, function, and health. Prepare and give a presentation to share what you learned with the class. Adjust the style and content of your presentation to your audience. Use digital media to add visual interest and improve understanding.
24. **Writing** Community or school-based support programs that provide counseling can help teens resolve personal conflicts and deal with trauma. Write a proposal recommending the creation of a local program to promote social and mental health for students. State the purpose of your proposal in a clear, concise manner. Explain why the program is needed to ensure the reader understands the problem. Outline how the program will resolve the problem. Provide a brief description of how the program would operate, who would oversee it, and the population served by it. Estimate the cost to start and maintain the program for one year. Find two references from literature or mental health professionals to verify the need for the program.
25. **Research and Speaking** Research issues regarding mental health services in the United States. Make a list of talking points in preparation for a discussion of the topic with another classmate. During the discussion, the two of you will sit in the center of the room surrounded by the rest of the class. To promote communication, use skills such as asking follow-up questions and restating or expanding on the other person's point. Students who are not in the center will observe and critique the exchange.
26. **Career Readiness Practice** Presume you have just started a new job. In your previous job, you were overworked and life was out of balance. You developed many habits that were not good for your physical, social, and mental health. You know you need to make some changes. Use the steps in the self-management plan to create a step-by-step plan for making positive behavior changes to improve your social and mental health.

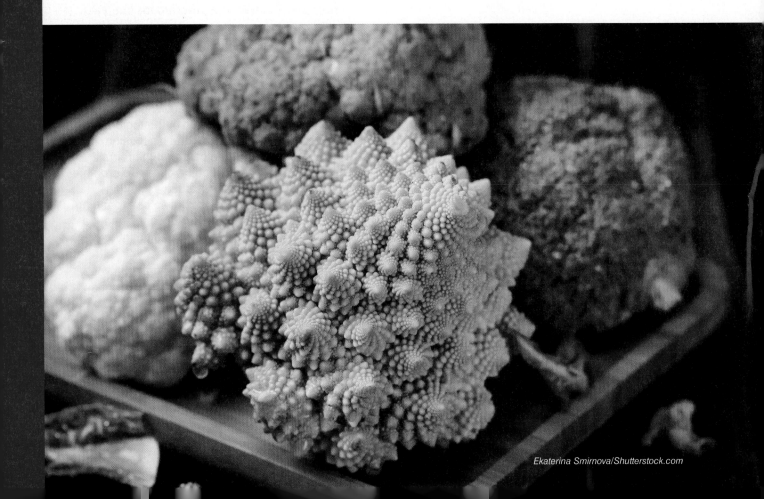

Stress and Wellness

Learning Outcomes

After studying this chapter, you will be able to

- **differentiate** between types of stressors;
- **understand** the body's response to stress;
- **summarize** the effects of stress on your health; and
- **implement** strategies to prevent stress.

Ekaterina Smirnova/Shutterstock.com

Content Terms

distress
eustress
fight-or-flight response
progressive muscle relaxation
self-talk
stress
stressor
support system
visualization

Academic Terms

acuity
alleviate
insurmountable
prohibit
ubiquitous

What's Your Nutrition and Wellness IQ?

Take this quiz to examine how much you already know about stress and wellness. If you cannot answer a question, pay extra attention to that topic as you study this chapter.

- Identify each statement as *True*, *False*, or *It Depends*. *It Depends* means in some cases the statement is true; in some cases it could be false.
- Revise false statements to make them true.
- Explain the circumstances in which each *It Depends* statement is true and when it is false.

Nutrition and Wellness IQ

	Statement			
1.	All stress is negative and unhealthy.	True	False	It Depends
2.	The body's normal response to a physical threat is to "freeze."	True	False	It Depends
3.	After experiencing a high level of stress, a person may be more susceptible to a cold.	True	False	It Depends
4.	Stress management strategies can be applied to stress situations throughout life.	True	False	It Depends
5.	A person's attitude about a stressful event does not affect the stressor's impact.	True	False	It Depends
6.	It is impossible to manage stress caused by stressors you cannot control.	True	False	It Depends
7.	Negative self-talk tends to increase stress.	True	False	It Depends
8.	The best way to avoid stress caused by conflict is to refrain from sharing your feelings and opinions.	True	False	It Depends

While studying this chapter, look for the activity icon to

- **build** vocabulary with e-flash cards and interactive games;
- **assess** what you learn by completing self-assessment quizzes and completing review questions; and
- **expand** knowledge with interactive activities and activities that extend learning.

www.g-wlearning.com/foodsandnutrition/

How would the following events affect you physically and emotionally?

- Your teacher announces there will be a unit test in two days, and you have not yet read the chapters.
- You and your dating partner had a major disagreement last night and now you have no date for the prom.
- Varsity basketball tryouts are tomorrow afternoon, and making the team has been your goal for years.
- You were invited to be a bridesmaid in a cousin's wedding. She has not offered to pay for the dress, and you cannot afford it.
- High school graduation is in four months. You are excited, but undecided about your plans for the fall.

Each situation described above can produce stress. You experience stress throughout your life. Some stress is good for you and some is bad. To understand how stress can affect your life, you need to examine what causes stress and how your body reacts to it. In this chapter, you will learn to recognize and manage the stress in your life.

What Is Stress?

Stress is the physical, mental, and emotional reactions you experience in response to challenges you face. Those challenges, or sources of stress, are called ***stressors***. Stressors produce the inner agitation you feel when you are exposed to change, difficulty, or danger.

Types of Stressors

Typically, stressors are categorized as either chronic or acute. Chronic stressors include circumstances that endure for an extended period. For example, living in an unsafe community or caring for a family member with an ongoing illness are chronic stressors. On the other hand, acute stressors are usually short-lived episodes, such as giving a presentation in class or going on a first date.

Stressors range in severity from routine to traumatic. Routine, minor stressors that produce tension are often known as *daily hassles*. Long lines at the supermarket, heavy traffic, and misplaced belongings are common daily hassles. These types of persistent annoyances can place strain on a person's body, mind, or relationships.

Life event stressors are situations that greatly alter a person's life. Death of a loved one, divorce, remarriage, legal problems, and sudden unemployment are examples of life event stressors. Life events cause significant changes in an individual's life and adjusting to the changes requires time (**Figure 22.1**).

Life Event Stressors for Teens
Death of a family member
Parents' divorce or separation
Personal injury
Change in health of family member
Loss of a job or financial resources
Death of a close friend
Pregnancy
New baby in the household
Relocation due to parent's job
Being bullied
Breakup with dating partner
Transfer to new school

Figure 22.1 Teens may react to stressors differently, but all teens experience some level of stress. *What other stressors could you add to this list?*

Traumatic stressors are life-threatening or abusive experiences. These types of stressors are experienced by survivors of physical or sexual abuse; survivors of hurricanes, earthquakes, or floods; troops serving in wars; and witnesses of traumatic events. These experiences can have long-lasting effects and recovery may take years.

Teens have many stressors in their lives. They face the physical changes associated with body growth and hormonal influences. Teens may also encounter emotional and social changes in relationships with family members and friends. Taking classes that are more challenging and making decisions that affect their future are also sources of stress for teens.

Positive Versus Negative Stress

Some types of stress provide motivation to achieve and perform well. Other types of stress can produce negative results.

Positive stress, or ***eustress***, motivates individuals to be productive and accomplish challenging goals. For example, athletes often feel positive stress when they are competing. The atmosphere during practice may not always prompt athletes to excel. At times, practice can feel like drudgery, and some athletes must push themselves to keep working. However, the atmosphere changes when opponents, fans, and officials are present. How athletes respond to this change in atmosphere is a form of positive stress (**Figure 22.2**). The stress of competition is the force that spurs athletes to give their best performance. They are inspired to achieve the goal of winning.

When you see an event or situation as a threat to your well-being, you are likely to feel negative stress. Negative stress, or ***distress***, is harmful stress. Negative stress can reduce your effectiveness by causing you to be fearful and perform poorly. If a classmate threatens to tell a teacher you cheated on a test, you will probably feel negative stress. Fear over whether the teacher will confront you about cheating may prevent you from focusing on class material. This, in turn, may hinder your performance in the class.

Distress also results when you experience a number of minor changes within a short period. For instance, suppose you have a job and are regularly scheduled to work from six to nine on Thursday evenings. On Wednesday, your manager calls and asks you to work on Friday evening instead of Thursday. This change in your schedule might not seem like a problem. However, imagine it occurred on the same weekend your best friend from out of town was planning to visit you. Suppose you have no car available to get to work. Now your work schedule, your visiting plans, and your travel arrangements are changed simultaneously. This many changes can cause distress.

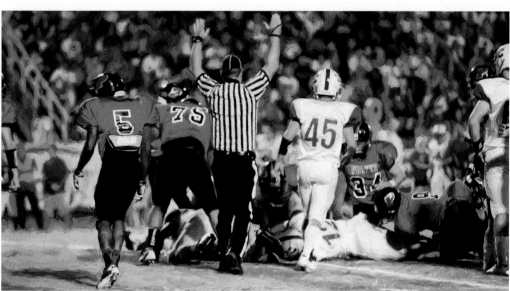

B. Franklin/Shutterstock.com

Figure 22.2
The positive stress of competition helps athletes work toward the reward of winning.

CASE STUDY

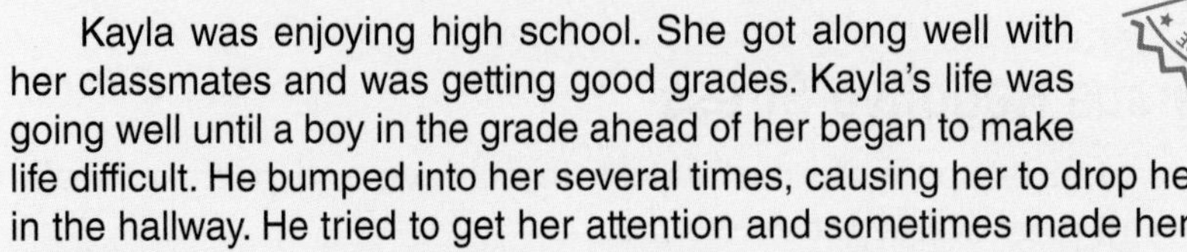

Daily Hassles or Major Stressors?

Kayla was enjoying high school. She got along well with her classmates and was getting good grades. Kayla's life was going well until a boy in the grade ahead of her began to make life difficult. He bumped into her several times, causing her to drop her books in the hallway. He tried to get her attention and sometimes made her late for classes. He even text messaged her asking when they could meet.

People began to tease her about her new "boyfriend." Kayla did not want the boy's attention, much less to be his girlfriend! He constantly behaved rudely around her friends. One day, the boy wrote a nasty message about her in the boys' restroom. When Kayla learned about it, she didn't know what to do. Now Kayla was so worried that she felt sick. She was stressed out!

Case Review

1. Do you believe Kayla is experiencing a major stressor?
2. How do you think Kayla should handle this situation?

Reactions to Stressors Vary

Many factors, such as heredity, experiences, and outlook, determine how you react to the stressors in your life. A source of negative stress for you may not be a source of negative stress for your friend. The same stressors affect each of you differently because perception of a situation influences the level of stress that is experienced. For example, one student may agonize over getting a *C* on a test. Another student might be pleased to do that well. A third student may see it as an opportunity to do better next time.

In addition, events that cause stress may vary from one time in your life to another. A mosquito bite can seem stressful to young children, but many adults would scarcely notice a mosquito bite.

Your reactions to stress depend partly on your personality and your outlook on life. People display different behaviors as they work toward their goals. Some people are relaxed and easygoing; others may be tense and hostile. A person with a tense personality tends to display impatient, angry, and pushy behaviors. They easily become irritated over stressful events. People in this group can be at greatest risk for stress-related health problems.

A person with an easygoing personality is less likely to become upset over stressful events. The ability to turn a negative stress into positive stress is a valuable wellness behavior that can be learned.

The Body's Response to Stress

Your body goes through three stages when responding to a stressful event—alarm, resistance, and exhaustion. To understand these three stages, imagine you just started a job in a fast-food restaurant. It is dinnertime and a long line of people is forming at your counter. Customers are reeling off orders, coworkers are bustling around, and children are crying in the background. You are trying to listen to orders, make change, package food, and keep the line moving. Suddenly one of your coworkers bumps into you. Your initial *alarm* response may include fear of spilling the food you are carrying. You may also feel mad at the coworker and discouraged about the delay in filling the customer's order.

These emotional responses during the alarm stage couple with physical responses. Inside your body, hormones release into your bloodstream. These hormones cause your heart rate, blood pressure, and breathing rate to increase. Brain function increases and you become more alert. You start breathing faster. Your face flushes, and you begin to perspire. The muscles in your arms, legs, and stomach become tense. Your hearing sharpens and your pupils widen. All these reactions indicate your body is gathering its resources to conquer danger or escape to safety. This reaction to stress is often called the ***fight-or-flight response***. You can choose to strike out (*fight*) or flee the situation (*flight*). This response is automatic, fast, and more common when physical threat is perceived (**Figure 22.3**).

The next stage of the body's response to stress is *resistance*. During resistance, your body devotes efforts to coping with the situation. Your entire body is engaged in responding to the event.

As the line of customers at your counter becomes shorter, your stress level subsides. Your body systems return to their prestress state. You stop perspiring and your arms, legs, and stomach begin to relax. However, if the rush of customers continues for several hours, your body may never have a chance to recover. In this case, you progress to the third response stage of *exhaustion*. Physical and mental fatigue are a part of this stage. You feel tired and have a hard time thinking clearly. Your inner resources to resist and adapt to stress are gone.

Suppose you experience this kind of stress every evening at work. Soon your body automatically becomes tense each day as you begin your shift. After months of working under these stressful conditions, tension spills over into other areas of your life. You are less able to handle minor daily stressors. Over time, your body begins to show signs of weakness. If lifestyle changes and stress reduction methods do not occur, physical illness may follow.

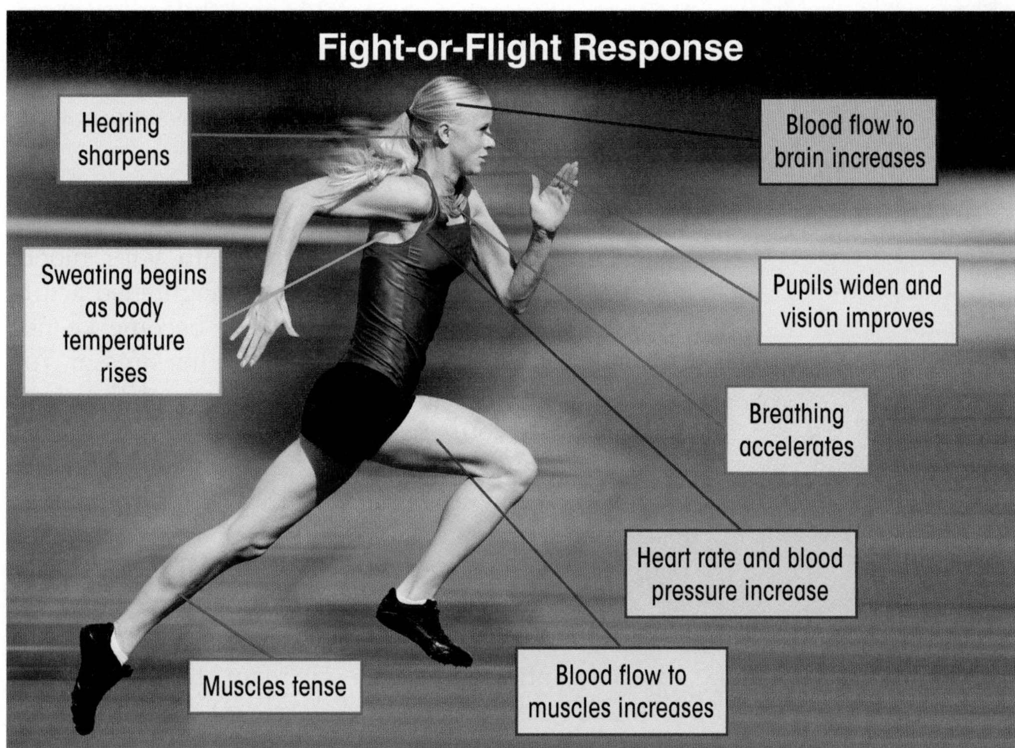

Stephen Mcsweeny/Shutterstock.com

Figure 22.3
A teen's body responds more quickly to challenges than an adult's body. *What are the potential consequences of a quicker response?*

Effects of Stress on Health

Stress affects your health. A continuous high level of negative stress weakens body systems and increases your risk for certain diseases. Stress also taxes your emotional well-being.

Effects on Physical Health

Over time and without your awareness, too much stress damages your physical health. Some researchers believe stress may be one of the greatest contributors to illness in the modern industrialized world.

You read earlier about physical reactions triggered by the release of stress hormones into your bloodstream. You breathe harder and faster to bring more oxygen into your body. Your heart beats more rapidly to pump oxygen out to the muscles. Your liver releases glucose and fat cells release fat into the bloodstream. Your blood pressure increases to speed the glucose and fat to the muscles for use as energy. All these reactions prepare your body to take action. Your muscles are getting ready to either defend you against the source of stress or run from it.

Many sources of stress in today's society do not require a physical battle or escape to safety. For instance, you may feel stress about auditioning for a part in the school play; however, dealing with this stress will not involve fighting or running from the director of the play. Therefore, the increase in your heart rate and blood pressure serve only to strain your heart and blood vessels. The extra fat released into your bloodstream may accumulate in your arteries. The overall effect is an increased risk for coronary heart disease, hypertension, and stroke.

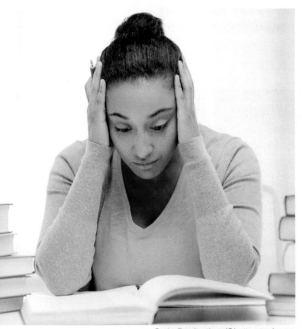

Syda Productions/Shutterstock.com

Figure 22.4 The pressure you exert on yourself to perform well academically can cause stress.

Effects on the Immune System

Your body's immune system helps protect you from disease. During periods of stress, your immune system defenses may be diminished. As a result, your resistance to infection, such as colds and flu, is decreased. For example, during midterms or finals, you may be very worried about passing the tests (**Figure 22.4**). When the tests are over, your immune system may be so depressed that you develop a cold.

Effects on Sleep Patterns

When stress hormones release into your bloodstream, you are likely to experience heightened **acuity** (awareness). Your sight and hearing become keener. Your mind races as it tries to deal with the stressor. You may have reached the exhaustion stage of the stress response, but your increased level of mental activity **prohibits** (prevents) you from falling asleep. Once you are able to sleep, it is a poor quality sleep that fails to restore and refresh you. This lack of rest can add to your stress and further depress your immune system.

Effects on Eating Habits

When stress hormones are circulating in the bloodstream, the body treats digesting food as a low priority. The body focuses its resources on the needs of the muscles and nerves rather than the digestive system.

FOOD AND THE ENVIRONMENT

Fast Food and the Environment

How many fast-food restaurants are within one-half mile of your school or home? Fast-food restaurants are **ubiquitous** (everywhere). This ready availability coupled with a stressful, hectic lifestyle makes fast food a popular choice for meals. For time-crunched families, ready-made meals are considered a necessity. The portability of fast foods makes them easy to eat while working or driving.

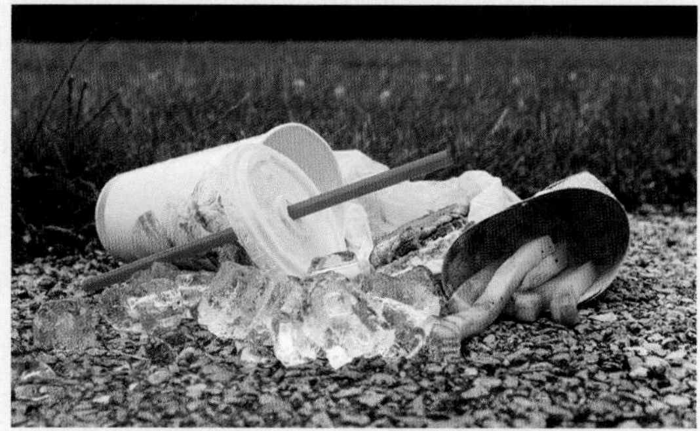

Burlingham/Shutterstock.com

It is reported that 25 percent of Americans eat fast food every day. The waste that results affects the environment. Consider the following effects on the environment:

- Litter is frequently made up of the discards from fast-food sales, such as wrappers, straws, cups, napkins, bags, boxes, and plastic packaging. The Environmental Protection Agency (EPA) reports that 65 percent of fast-food waste ends up in the landfill. Only 35 percent is recycled or otherwise diverted from the landfill. The Clean Water Action (CWA) group found that nearly half of the trash in one of the waterways they studied was from fast-food packaging.
- Many containers are made of polystyrene foam (Styrofoam™), which is hard to recycle and does not easily biodegrade.
- Fast-food trash discarded on the roadside can clog drainage gutters and contribute to flooding.
- As with most retail food establishments, fast-food products are often transported long distances, which impacts air quality.
- Many fast-food restaurants specialize in serving beef and/or chicken. For example, one international fast-food giant purchases approximately 2½ billion pounds of beef, poultry, and pork each year. The production and distribution of meat and chicken products contribute to climate change.

Think Critically

1. What is a possible solution to fast food and its negative effect on the environment?
2. How are fast food's effects on the environment analogous to its effects on your health?

Stress often affects people's eating habits and emotional responses to food. This is why stress is sometimes a factor in body weight problems. During emotional stress, some people nibble foods nervously or binge. Eating may seem to relieve their feelings of frustration. In contrast, some people cannot eat when under stress. They do not feel hunger because they are focused on the source of stress. Others may experience an upset stomach. Stress can also contribute to the development of anorexia nervosa and bulimia nervosa.

Eating habits affected by stress may change your nutritional status. Eating out of boredom or tension may cause you to eat excess calories. An extra trip to a fast-food restaurant may give temporary comfort. Weight gains can lead to overweight. Not eating because you are too excited, nervous, or constantly worried may cause you to lose weight and feel tired and cranky. Eating disorders can compound the effects of stress.

Effects on Emotional Health

Too much stress can make you irritable, tense, and anxious. You may reach a point where you are unable to keep preventable sources of stress out of your life. When this happens, worry can overtake productive thinking.

Many social and emotional problems for teens are the result of undue amounts of stress in their lives and their inability to manage it. Reports of substance abuse and suicide are often tied to an inability to cope with high stress levels. For adults, stress at work as well as in the family can take a toll on emotional health.

Stress Management

You cannot avoid all stress; however, you can learn to manage it. Viewing stress as positive promotes creativity and personal growth. Learning to minimize or adapt to negative stress makes you resilient and better able to deal with the changes that occur throughout life (**Figure 22.5**).

You can use a number of strategies to manage your stress. The key is to choose the strategies that work for you. Try to combine a variety of strategies to achieve the greatest effects on overall health.

Use Support Systems

Identify your support system and seek them out in times of crisis or need. A ***support system*** is a person or group of people who can provide help and emotional comfort. Family members and friends can listen and offer insights to problems. School counselors, social workers, and psychologists can give their professional opinions about how to deal with stressful situations. Turn to these people when you are feeling overwhelmed.

It is likely that you are part of someone else's support system. In this role, you can lend support by listening. You may need to encourage the other person to talk about concerns and worries. If she wants to talk, listen attentively and avoid offering advice unless it is requested. Many times, the person is not seeking advice, but simply wants someone to listen.

Someone who mentions suicide is at great risk. Someone who talks about drinking or getting high to handle stress may also need professional help. You may need to seek the help of an adult on your friend's behalf. Parents, teachers, guidance counselors, and members of the clergy can provide assistance when a friend is in potential danger.

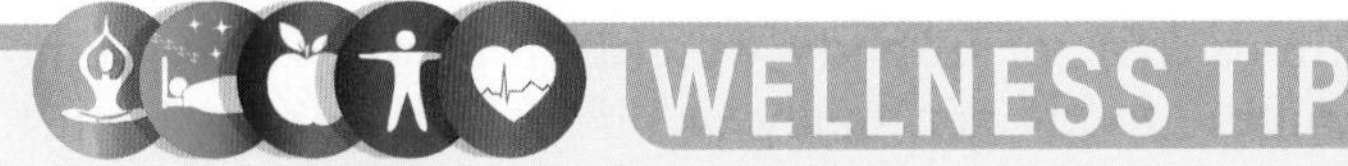

Laughter—Medicine for Stress

Have you ever noticed how well you feel after a good, hearty laugh? Research shows that laughter is an excellent source of stress relief. Not only does a hearty laugh reduce levels of stress hormones like *adrenaline*, it also increases beneficial hormones like *endorphins*. The next time you feel stressed or frustrated, laugh about the situation instead of worrying over it, watch a funny movie or your favorite cartoon, read a joke book, or join some friends for an evening of fun and laughter.

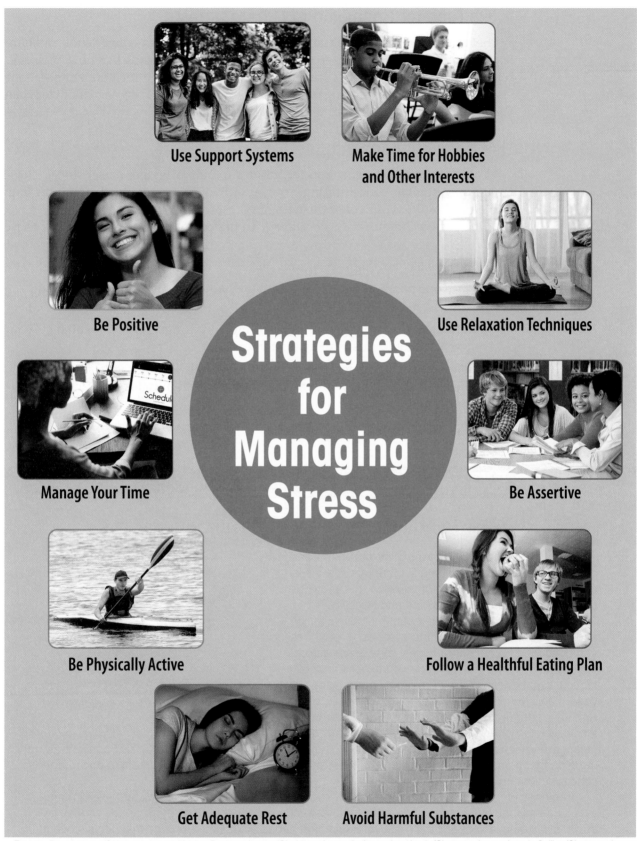

Top row: Rawpixel.com/Shutterstock.com; Monkey Business Images/Shutterstock.com; 2nd row: cheapbooks/Shutterstock.com; Antonio Guillem/Shutterstock.com; 3rd row: Rawpixel.com/Shutterstock.com; Monkey Business Images/Shutterstock.com; 4th row: Jelena Aloskina/Shutterstock.com; Pressmaster/Shutterstock.com; bottom row: Africa Studio/Shutterstock.com; threerocksimages/Shutterstock.com

Figure 22.5 You may not be able to avoid all stress, but you can control how you react to it. *How do you manage stress in your life?*

Make Time for Hobbies and Other Interests

Set aside time to enjoy hobbies and leisure activities with your friends and family. Different people find different activities relaxing. Perhaps listening to music, reading a book, or enjoying your favorite hobby is relaxing for you. For someone else, playing sports or working out may be more relaxing. Learn to recognize when you need to take a break from work or other demands.

Use Relaxation Techniques

Learn and employ relaxation techniques to help **alleviate** (ease) stress. These techniques involve concentrating your attention on something that is calming, while heightening your consciousness of your physical self.

One such technique is *deep breathing*. To perform deep breathing, follow these steps:

- Assume a comfortable position.
- Place one hand on your stomach below your ribs and the other hand on your chest.
- Inhale slowly through your nose, filling your lungs. As you breathe in, your stomach should push out against your hand.
- Release each breath in a long, controlled exhale through your mouth. The hand should move inward as your stomach muscles contract to empty your lungs.
- Repeat this process 5–10 times, focusing on each breath.

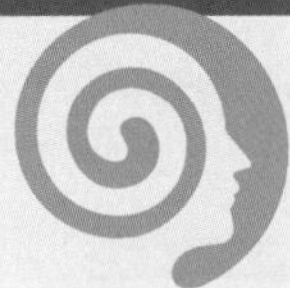

EXTEND YOUR KNOWLEDGE

How to Manage Stress with Yoga

Yoga is a mind and body practice that has been performed for thousands of years. More recently, it has gained popularity as a form of exercise that provides stress relief and improves balance and flexibility.

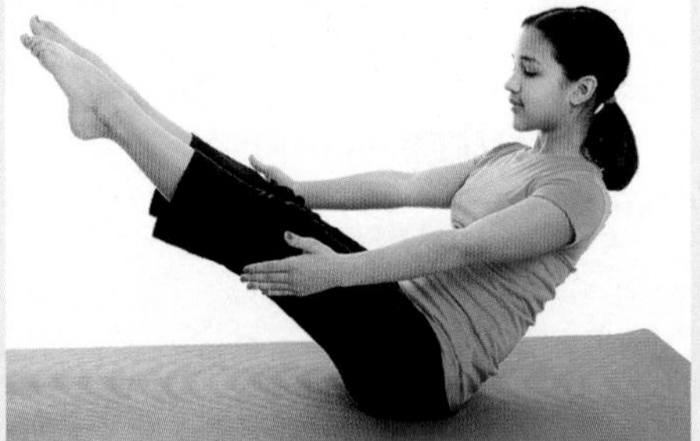

Rob Marmion/Shutterstock.com

The form of yoga that is popular in fitness classes and centers involves performing a series of postures and controlled breathing exercises. Yoga is not a competitive activity. The level of effort you expend is solely for your own benefit. While there are many variations of yoga, basic yoga helps develop a more flexible body. Stretch postures that use your body weight as resistance develop strength. The various postures require balance and concentration. The result is that you focus less on your stressors, and concentrate more on the moments of relaxation and calmness. Breathing is performed with intent to encourage concentration and relaxation.

Beginner yoga is suitable for all ages; however, the type of yoga should match the joint and muscle conditions of the person. A well-trained instructor is necessary and medical advice may be advised if you have specific health issues. Equipment needs are minimal. A yoga mat helps prevent sliding and provides comfort for sitting or prone positions. Sometimes a ball is used for balance, a block can be used for some stretch positions, and a strap can be used to reach your feet or link your hands behind your head.

Deep breathing forces you to slow down and focus on something other than stressors. You can use this breathing technique almost anywhere. You might be waiting in a traffic jam, standing in a long line, or sitting in class before a test. A few minutes of deep breathing in any of these situations can help you feel more relaxed.

Another technique for reducing stress is ***progressive muscle relaxation***. This method involves slowly tensing and then relaxing different groups of muscles. Begin with your feet. Then gradually work your way up the body to your legs, midsection, hands, arms, shoulders, neck, and face. Tense each muscle group, hold for five seconds, then release. Try to clear your mind of all thoughts, focusing only on your muscle groups. As you release the tension in your muscles, you are also releasing stress. This technique works best in a setting where you can be alone for a few minutes. You may find listening to quiet music while you perform this technique improves your results.

Visualization is a relaxation technique during which you form mental images of peaceful, tranquil settings. Try to involve as many senses as possible during your imaginary journey. For example, if you are visualizing hiking in the mountains, try to imagine the smell of the pine needles or the sound of wind blowing through the trees.

There are many other relaxation techniques. For instance, yoga, meditation, or art therapy are useful for stress management.

FEATURED CAREER

Group Exercise Instructor

Group exercise instructors conduct group exercise sessions. They lead, instruct, and motivate people in a variety of aerobic, stretching, and muscle-conditioning exercises. Many instructors choose music and choreograph a sequence of exercise routines to the music that many participants find fun and relaxing. This conditioning of the body helps reduce the effects caused by stress and other health conditions. They demonstrate different positions and moves and carefully observe students to make sure they are doing the exercises correctly to avoid injury. Group exercise instructors are responsible for making classes motivating and safe while ensuring the exercises are not too hard for participants.

Education

Entry-level group fitness instructors may not be required to have certification; however, most organizations generally require group instructors to become certified. Achieving certification from a top organization is important. The National Commission for Certifying Agencies accredits reputable certification organizations (see their website). Once certified, continuing education is a requirement to keep certification. Some certifying organizations require an associate's or bachelor's degree in an exercise-related field.

Job Outlook

Demand for group exercise instructors is expected to remain strong at health clubs and fitness centers. Instructors with a degree in a fitness-related subject will likely have better opportunities because people will view them as having higher qualifications.

Be Positive

You can reduce stress by adopting a positive attitude. Learn to regard problems as opportunities rather than threats. Try to view new ideas and problems as exciting and challenging. This approach helps you adapt to stressful events and reduces anxiety and fear. Learn to recognize the joys of living to help change your attitude.

Use positive self-talk to reduce stress. ***Self-talk*** is the internal conversations that take place in your mind (**Figure 22.6**). Self-talk can be positive or negative. Unfortunately, self-talk often consists of negative statements such as "I'm stupid. I'll never be able to figure out how to solve this problem." This negative self-talk is harmful. It drains your emotional energy and produces stress.

Positive self-talk, on the other hand, is beneficial and helps reduce stress. This type of self-talk uses statements such as "I'm as smart as the next person. If I take my time, I'm sure I'll be able to figure out how to solve this problem." As you substitute positive statements for negative ones in your self-talk, you build your confidence. When you feel positive about your abilities, you can deal with life's stressors more effectively.

Be Assertive

Express your feelings, opinions, or beliefs instead of being aggressive or passive. Aggressive behavior can cause others to resent or mistrust you. People may begin to avoid you or offer resistance. On the other hand, when you routinely go along with the decisions of others, you may think you are "keeping the peace." However, this passive behavior gives others the permission to ignore your needs. This can create internal conflict, resentment, and stress in your life.

Learn how to become more assertive if it does not come naturally to you. This may require learning to say "no" on occasion. Learn to speak up for yourself in a respectful, thoughtful manner. Take charge of your life and make decisions that help you achieve your goals.

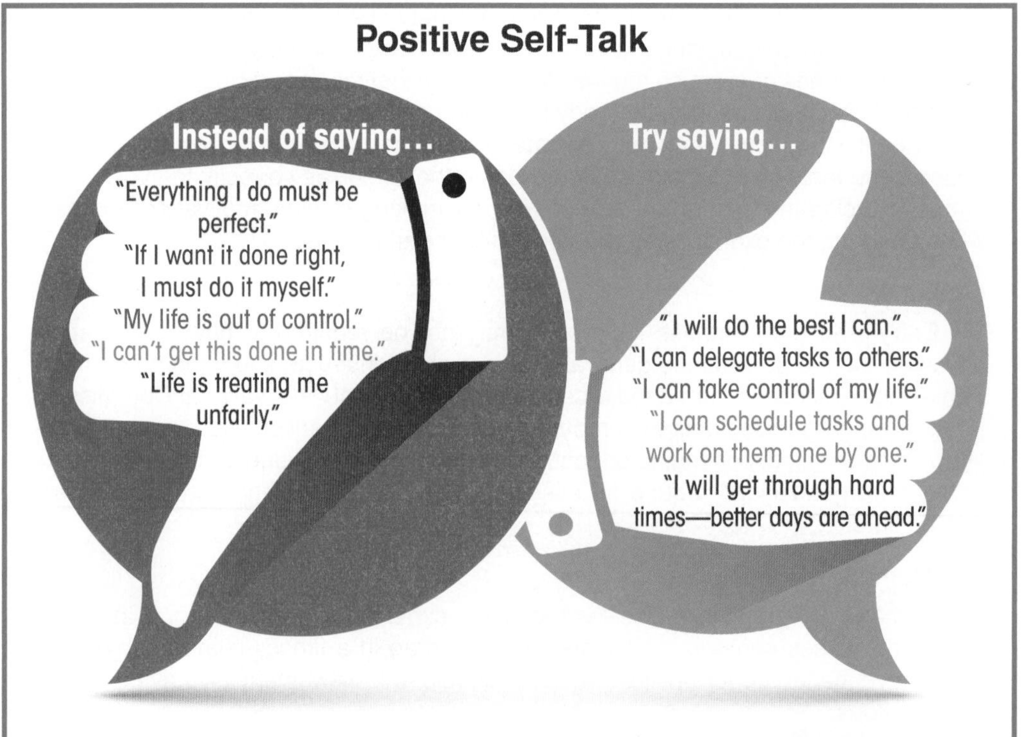
Positive Self-Talk
Instead of saying...
"Everything I do must be perfect."
"If I want it done right, I must do it myself."
"My life is out of control."
"I can't get this done in time."
"Life is treating me unfairly."
Try saying...
"I will do the best I can."
"I can delegate tasks to others."
"I can take control of my life."
"I can schedule tasks and work on them one by one."
"I will get through hard times—better days are ahead."

Figure 22.6 Revising the negative dialogue in your mind can help reduce stress and improve your outlook on life.

Hollygraphic/Shutterstock.com

Manage Your Time

One cause of stress for many people is poor time management. Imagine you have three tests tomorrow, a paper to write, and an after-school job. Having insufficient time for all you need to accomplish can produce stress. The number or size of the tasks can be paralyzing. Perhaps you are uncertain how to begin or believe your workload is **insurmountable** (impossible). Overcoming your fear and creating a time-management plan is the only way to eliminate this source of stress (**Figure 22.7**).

Begin by tracking how you currently use your time with an activity log. Record how you spend the minutes of your day. Evaluate your results. Identify time wasters that you need to address. Next, list all of the tasks you need to accomplish. If a task seems too large to accomplish, break it into smaller tasks. Assign a priority to each task and estimate the time needed to complete each. Create a schedule showing when you plan to do each task. Schedule the tasks with the highest priority first. Be realistic about what you can accomplish in one day. Consider delegating tasks to others. You may not be able to do everything, but using a schedule will help you optimize your time. Most importantly, stop procrastinating.

Review your progress periodically and cross items off your schedule as you complete them. Your confidence will increase and your stress will decrease with each task you complete.

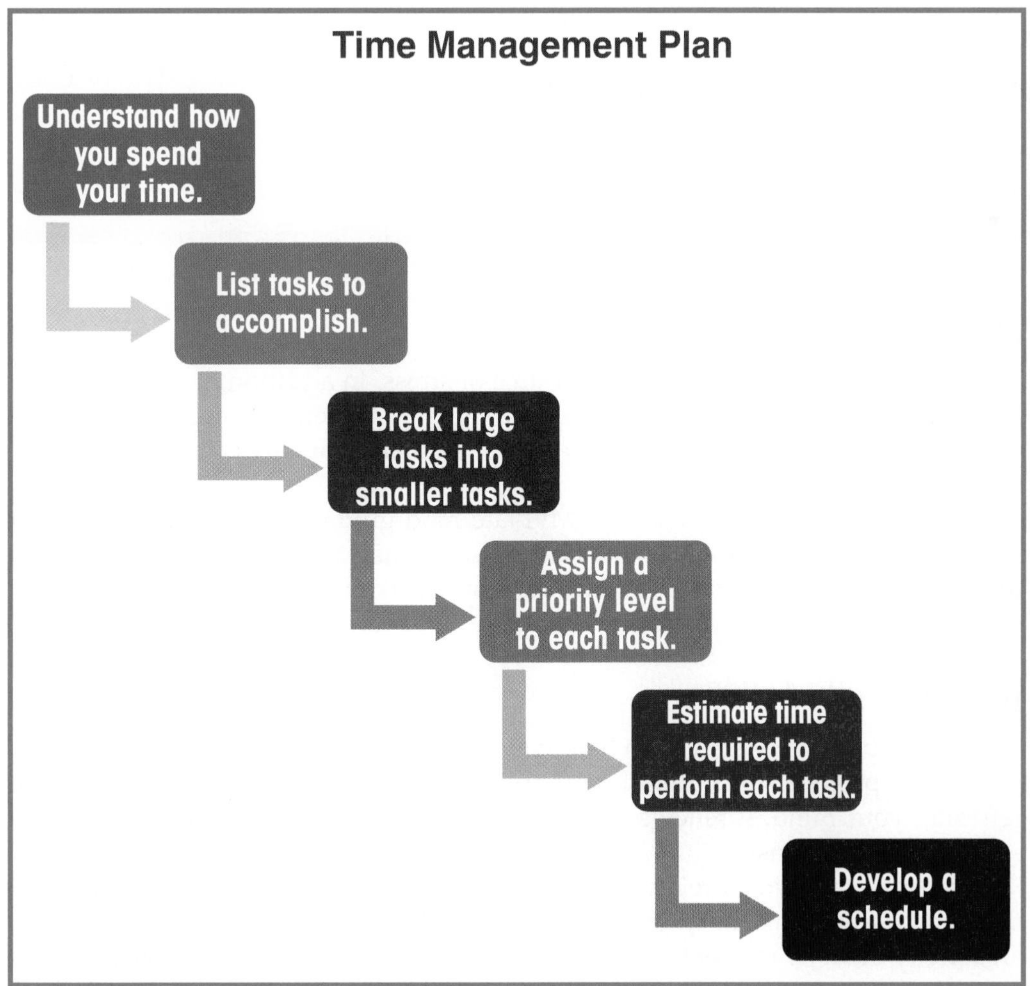

Figure 22.7 Managing your time well is guaranteed to make you more productive and reduce your stress levels.

THE MOVEMENT CONNECTION

Destressing Stretch

Why

Stress causes the muscles in your body to tense. Often, you may be unaware how tight your muscles are. Stretching helps reduce stress and fatigue while calming the mind and soothing the nerves.

The following stretch targets the hamstrings and knees while helping to keep your spine strong and flexible.

Apply

- Stand with feet hip-distance apart and good posture.
- Bend over until your stomach touches the tops of your legs. If your hamstrings are tight, bend your knees to your level of comfort.
- Hold this position for five relaxed breaths.
- Grab opposite elbows and let your head hang down, allowing the weight of your head to aid in the stretch.
- Return to standing and reach overhead with both arms as you inhale to fill your lungs.
- Exhale and repeat the move five times.

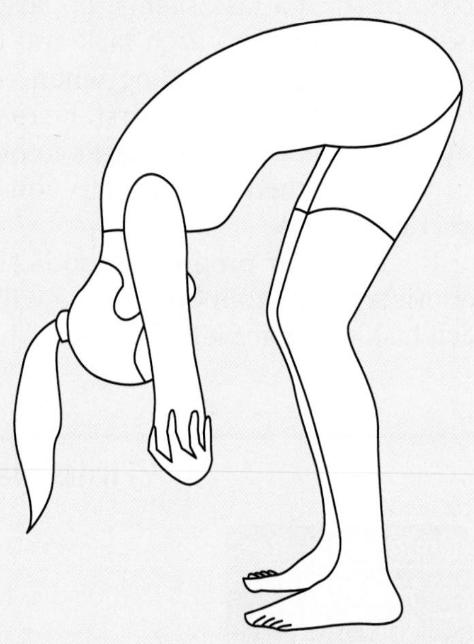

Modification

For an additional stretch on your neck, perform the destressing stretch above and try gently shaking your head "no" and nodding your head "yes" before returning to a standing position.

Follow a Healthful Eating Plan

Health problems can be a major source of stress. In addition, you learned earlier in this chapter that stress contributes to health problems. Therefore, steps you take to maintain good health are also steps for managing stress. Eating nutrient-dense foods daily is one such step.

Follow the guidelines from the MyPlate food guidance system to meet your nutrient needs and maintain your health. Limit snacks that are high in calories, unhealthy fats, sugar, and sodium. In addition, drink plenty of liquids—preferably water—to replenish body fluids and keep kidneys functioning properly.

Be Physically Active

Staying physically active can help you manage stress. Regular, vigorous physical activity promotes health and your ability to fight stress. Physical activity also refreshes your mind. It renews your energy so you can think more clearly about solutions to problems.

Physical activity can relieve stress when it occurs. You can work out frustrations and release tensions through movement. When you are feeling stressed, plan an activity break. Participate in a favorite sport or other physical activity such as walking, swimming, jogging, skating, or biking. While your body is moving, your mind is less likely to focus on your problems. After your activity, you may find you are able to face troubles with a clear mind and new insights.

Get Adequate Rest

Like staying fit and eating well, getting enough rest safeguards your health and helps you recover from stressful events. Most people need at least seven to eight hours of sleep each night; however, teens require about nine hours of sleep. Getting enough sleep can make you more alert, less irritable, and better able to manage stressful situations. When you have adequate sleep, you awaken feeling refreshed and ready to start your daily tasks.

Avoid Harmful Substances

Harmful substances such as alcohol, tobacco, and drugs do not reduce stress. In fact, they can lead to problems that are more serious. These substances temporarily mask the symptoms of stress.

The use of alcohol and drugs can cause stress by creating physical and mental health problems. Substance abuse can be a tremendous source of tension in relationships. Academic performance is likely to suffer. In addition, it adds to stress by increasing the risk of violence, accidents, and arrests. Harmful substances should be avoided.

Seek Professional Help

Despite your best efforts, you may be unable to recover from a major stress event such as the death of someone close to you. Stress can be difficult to manage on your own. If you feel overwhelmed by life or are unable to perform daily tasks, it may be time to seek professional help.

RECIPE FILE

Mock Cheesecake

1 SERVING

Ingredients

- 1 c. low-fat vanilla yogurt
- ½ c. fruit (strawberries, blueberries, mangoes, peaches, or your favorite fruit)

Directions

1. Line a sieve with two paper towels.
2. Place sieve over a bowl.
3. Smooth paper towels so there are no wrinkles or folds.
4. Stir yogurt and pour on top of paper towels.
5. Cover with plastic wrap and refrigerate for 24 hours. Yogurt should be very thick.
6. When ready to serve, invert yogurt onto a plate.
7. Top with the fruit of your choice.

PER SERVING: 258 CALORIES, 13 G PROTEIN, 46 G CARBOHYDRATE, 3 G FAT, 0 G FIBER, 164 MG SODIUM.

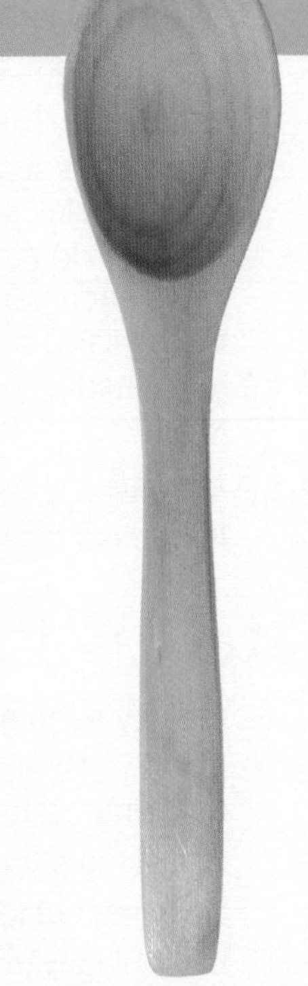

Chapter 22 Review and Expand

Reading Summary

Stress is the physical, mental, and emotional reactions you experience in response to challenges you face. The sources of stress can be acute or chronic. Stress can provide motivation to achieve and perform well or be harmful and cause you to perform poorly.

Your body progresses through three stages—alarm, resistance, and exhaustion—in response to stress. Stress can affect health in a variety of ways. Physical health outcomes include effects on the immune system as well as effects on sleep patterns and eating habits.

You cannot avoid all stress, but you can learn to manage it. Learning to minimize or adapt to negative stress makes your resilient and better able deal with the changes that occur throughout life.

Chapter Vocabulary

1. **Content Terms** Work with a partner to write the definitions of the following terms based on your current understanding before reading the chapter. Then join another pair of students to discuss your definitions and any discrepancies. Finally, discuss the definitions with the class and ask your instructor for necessary correction or clarification.

distress	self-talk
eustress	stress
fight-or-flight response	stressor
progressive muscle relaxation	support system
	visualization

2. **Academic Terms** Write each of the following terms on a separate sheet of paper. For each term, quickly write a word you think relates to the term. In small groups, exchange papers. Have each person in the group explain a term on the list. Take turns until all terms have been explained.

acuity	prohibit
alleviate	ubiquitous
insurmountable	

Review Learning

3. Identify each of the following stressors as either acute or chronic:
   A. being bullied at school
   B. asking someone for a date
   C. trying out for the school play
   D. coping with your parents' divorce
4. A hurricane destroying your home is an example of a _____ stressor.
5. *True or false?* A source of negative stress for you may be a source of positive stress for your friend.
6. What are the three stages of the body's response to stress?
7. What are three physical responses that occur when the body releases stress hormones?
8. How does stress affect the body's immune system?
9. How does stress affect your sleep pattern?
10. List three people who may be part of a person's support system.
11. Describe three relaxation techniques to help alleviate stress.
12. *True or false?* Aggressive behavior causes stress.
13. What is a time-management strategy for dealing with a task that seems too large?
14. How does the use of harmful substances affect stress?

Self-Assessment Quiz

Complete the self-assessment quiz online to help you practice and expand your knowledge and skills.

Critical Thinking

15. **Cause and Effect** Work with a partner to create a list of positive and negative stresses that teens face today. Identify the stressors that cause each stress on the list. Next, explain the effect(s) on the individual due to each stressful event. Share your answers with the class.
16. **Evaluate** Perform two of the relaxation techniques described in the chapter. Write a brief evaluation stating which technique you found more effective. What were the benefits of using this technique? Explain.
17. **Analyze** Keep a stress diary for one day. Every time you feel stress, record the source of the stress. At the end of the day, organize your list into two groups—stressors you can and cannot change. For each stressor you can change, propose steps you can take to reduce the source of stress. Implement the steps and reevaluate in two weeks to determine if they worked.

18. **Apply** Practice changing negative self-talk into positive self-talk. Working in pairs, list 10 negative self-talk statements that you or friends often make. Take turns suggesting how to turn each statement into positive self-talk.
19. **Analyze** Use spreadsheet software to create an activity log. Make columns labeled *Time of Day*, *Activity*, and *Emotional State* (for example, alert, flat, tired, energetic, etc.). Select a typical day and record how you spend your time. Then use your log to reflect on how you spend your time and what you value as important. Flag those activities that are time wasters. Use this information to analyze your time management and make changes if needed.
20. **Create** Research to learn what types of music have a calming effect. Then create a playlist of relaxing music. The playlist should be about three to four minutes long. Analyze your choices to identify the characteristics that make a piece of music relaxing. Write a paragraph or two sharing the characteristics that make music relaxing for you.

Core Skills

21. **Writing** Research to learn what drugs are commonly prescribed to treat stress- or anxiety-related disorders. Select one of the drugs and write an informative paper describing how it works, its effectiveness, and possible side effects. Identify and discuss any contraindications for its use. Cite your sources.
22. **Technology Literacy** Prepare a digital bulletin board sharing ways to manage stress. Create a digital collage of images, text, and video to convey stress-management concepts.
23. **Speaking** Find reliable print or online sources to learn more about strategies for relaxing before giving a public or group speech. Prepare and give a demonstration to teach your classmates two methods to reduce stress when giving a presentation.
24. **Math** Prepare a pie chart of the activity log you created for Activity 19. Then prepare a second version that reflects changes you would like to make by either adding more hours to a particular activity or subtracting hours.
25. **Writing** Keep a personal journal of your worries and concerns. Be sure to journal at least three days a week. Include the sources and reasons for the worry. After you make an entry, reflect on your level of stress. Do you find that writing down your concerns is helpful for reducing your stress and anxiety? After a few weeks of journaling, review your entries. Can you detect any patterns or gain insights about your sources of stress? Write a few paragraphs describing how keeping the journal affected you.
26. **Listening** Interview your parents, guardians, or grandparents to learn more about stressors in their lives. Discover what techniques they use to manage stress. List commonly mentioned adult stressors. As a class, generate a list of stress-management strategies adults and older adults use. Evaluate each strategy to determine if it is healthy.
27. **Math** Measure and record your heart rate every hour for eight hours. Next to each heart rate measurement, record your perceived stress level at the time. Compute your average heart rate for the eight hours. Create a graph of your results and include a line indicating your average heart rate. Do you see any correlation between your heart rate and stress level?
28. **Technology Literacy** Plan and write three entries about stress management techniques for the class blog. First, consider the audience who will be reading your blog. What does your audience want and need to know about this topic? Then, determine the content and its organization. Select three main points that you want to address each day. Next, create an appealing title to capture your reader's attention. Write each blog entry, providing supporting facts for each main point. Consider providing a tip or action item for each entry.
29. **Career Readiness Practice** Imagine it is five years in the future and you are starting your first full-time job. Your new employer is a digital media developer, and you know the work is fast-paced and demanding. You have watched some family members and friends suffer the effects of workplace stress on their health and wellness over the years. Your goal is to maintain your health and wellness by developing a plan for handling workplace stress. Investigate and evaluate the resources on the National Institute for Occupational Safety and Health link on the Centers for Disease Control and Prevention website. Then write your plan for preventing job stress.

CHAPTER 23 Drug and Supplement Use and Your Health

Learning Outcomes

After studying this chapter, you will be able to

- **compare and contrast** medications, drugs, and dietary supplements;
- **recognize** various types of medications;
- **summarize** how your body processes drugs;
- **classify** an undesired health event resulting from medication use;
- **distinguish between** medication misuse and medication or drug abuse;
- **identify** health risks associated with the abuse of stimulants, depressants, narcotics, marijuana, and hallucinogens;
- **summarize** the possible consequences of the use of drugs and dietary supplements to enhance physical performance; and
- **describe** treatment options for help with substance abuse disorders.

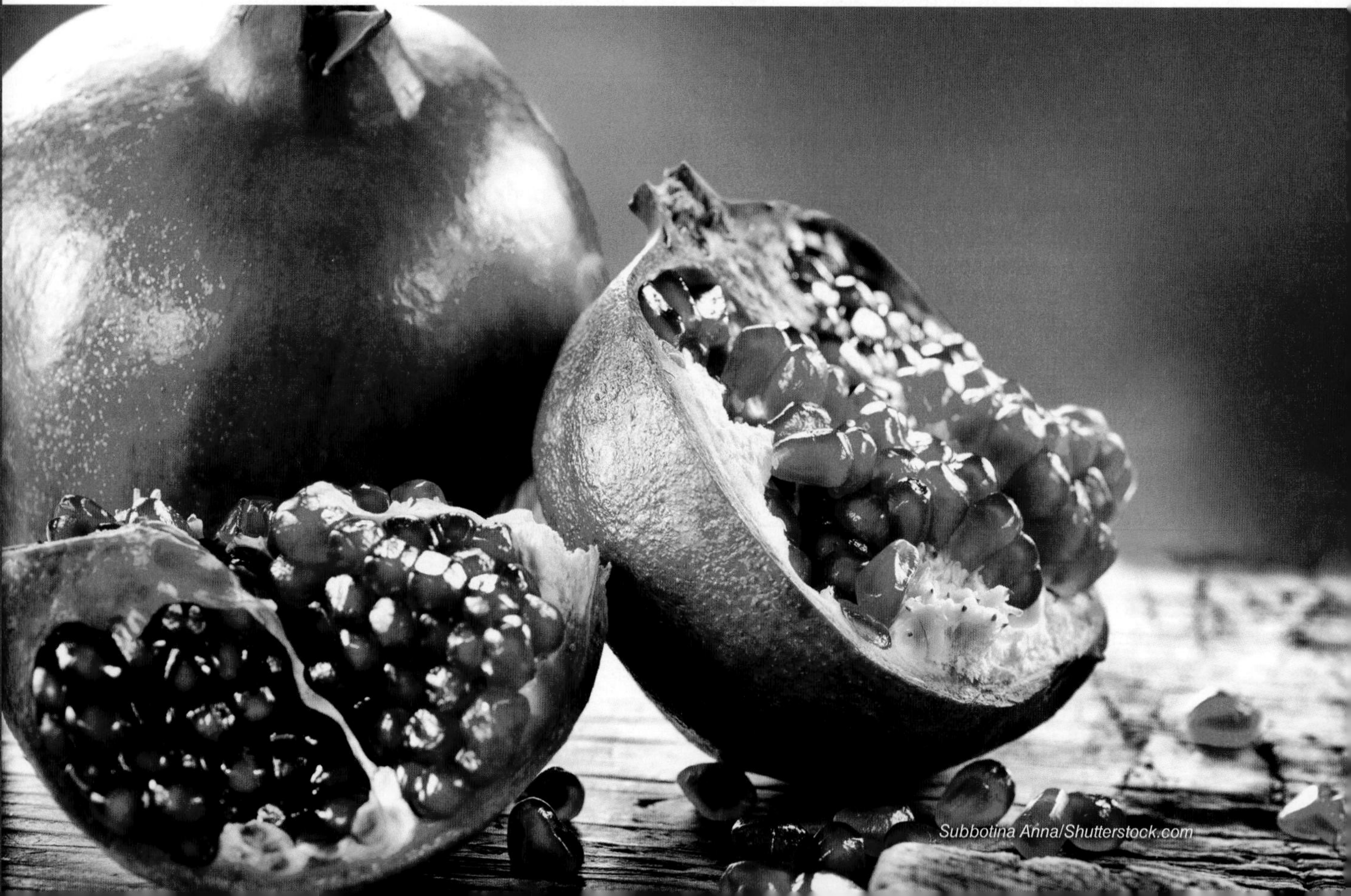

Subbotina Anna/Shutterstock.com

Content Terms

addiction
alcohol use disorder (AUD)
amphetamine
anabolic steroid
blood alcohol concentration (BAC)
cirrhosis
designer drug
dietary supplement
drug
drug-drug interaction
drug overdose
ergogenic aids
food-drug interaction
generic medication
hallucinogen
heroin
illegal drug
inhalant
medication
medication abuse
medication misuse
methamphetamine
narcotic
opioids
over-the-counter (OTC) medication
prescription medication
psychoactive drug
relapse
secondhand smoke
side effect
smokeless tobacco
stimulant
tolerance
withdrawal

Academic Terms

adverse
counterpart
euphoria
partake

What's Your Nutrition and Wellness IQ?

Take this quiz to examine how much you already know about drug and supplement use. If you cannot answer a question, pay extra attention to that topic as you study this chapter.

- Identify each statement as *True*, *False*, or *It Depends*. *It Depends* means in some cases the statement is true; in some cases it could be false.
- Revise false statements to make them true.
- Explain the circumstances in which each *It Depends* statement is true and when it is false.

Nutrition and Wellness IQ

	Statement			
1.	Over-the-counter medications can be harmful when used incorrectly.	True	False	It Depends
2.	A drug has the same effect on everyone who takes it.	True	False	It Depends
3.	Drugs and foods you consume can interact and change how they affect your body.	True	False	It Depends
4.	It is safe to take a friend's prescription medication because a doctor prescribed it.	True	False	It Depends
5.	Crystal meth is a dangerous, highly addictive drug that ages the user very quickly.	True	False	It Depends
6.	There are no health risks from using e-cigarettes because no tobacco is used and no smoke is produced.	True	False	It Depends
7.	Abuse of prescription painkillers often leads to heroin use.	True	False	It Depends
8.	Substance use disorder (SUD) is a curable disease.	True	False	It Depends

While studying this chapter, look for the activity icon  **to**

- **build** vocabulary with e-flash cards and interactive games;
- **assess** what you learn by completing self-assessment quizzes and completing review questions; and
- **expand** knowledge with interactive activities and activities that extend learning.

www.g-wlearning.com/foodsandnutrition/

This chapter will describe how various types of drugs and supplements can affect your health and physical performance. It will also discuss the physical, emotional, and social effects of the misuse and abuse of drugs.

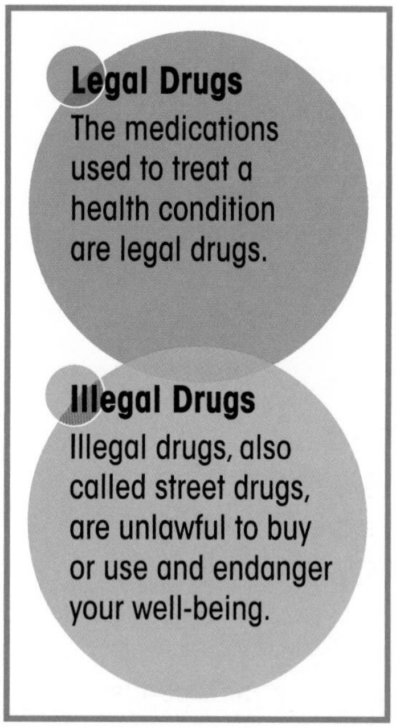

Legal Drugs
The medications used to treat a health condition are legal drugs.

Illegal Drugs
Illegal drugs, also called street drugs, are unlawful to buy or use and endanger your well-being.

Figure 23.1 Illegal drugs are dangerous because there is no way to know how strong they are, what else has been added to them, or how your body will react to them.

Medications Versus Drugs

According to the Centers for Disease Control and Prevention (CDC), nearly half of all US citizens used a prescription medication in the past 30 days. A ***medication*** is a drug used to treat an ailment or improve a disabling condition. A ***drug*** is any chemical substance that changes the way the body or mind operates. In other words, all medications are drugs, but not all drugs are medications. The medications used to treat an illness are *legal drugs*. ***Illegal drugs***, also called *street drugs*, are unlawful to buy or use and endanger your well-being (**Figure 23.1**).

Many people purchase dietary supplements in an attempt to improve their health or performance. An estimated 68 percent of Americans use dietary supplements in an attempt to improve their overall health. According to the Food and Drug Administration (FDA), a ***dietary supplement*** is a product that is ingested to add nutritional value to the diet and includes one or more of the following: vitamins, minerals, amino acids, botanicals, enzymes, metabolites, concentrates, or extracts. The FDA does not review and approve dietary supplements for safety or efficacy, however.

Taking unnecessary drugs and high doses of dietary supplements or other performance aids often adds health risks, not health benefits. Misuse of any of these substances can have serious health consequences and cause harm, rather than benefit you.

Types of Medications

The FDA regulates and oversees the safety of medications. A drug manufacturer must provide conclusive evidence to the FDA that a medication is safe and effective for the intended use. Only then is it approved for sale. Some of these medications require a physician's prescription and other medications are available in an over-the-counter form.

WELLNESS TIP

Ask a Pharmacist

Before taking any prescription drugs, ask your pharmacist about potential food-drug interactions. Ask whether you can take the medication with other drugs or whether you should avoid certain foods or beverages when taking the medicine. Read the literature that comes with the medicine for knowing about the precautions and potential side effects.

Prescription Medications

A ***prescription medication*** is a drug that can only be obtained from a pharmacy with an order from a doctor. A physician has the training to decide which prescription medication best suits the needs of a patient.

When a doctor prescribes medication for you, you need to be sure you know how to use it safely and effectively. A ***side effect*** is a reaction that differs from the drug's desired effect. Side effects may occur simultaneously with the desired effect. For instance, many medications that relieve the sneezing and runny nose associated with colds and allergies cause drowsiness. Most drugs produce some side effects in some people. For most people, however, the side effects are not even noticeable.

With each prescription, pharmacists often provide an information sheet explaining what the medication is and how it should be used (**Figure 23.2**).

Over-the-Counter Medications

Over-the-counter (OTC) medications are the drugs sold legally that do not require a physician's prescription. OTC medications are often called *nonprescription medications*. They are generally purchased off the shelves of supermarkets, drugstores, and convenience stores. When used as directed, OTC medications are not as strong as prescription medications. They also pose less potential risk than prescription medications, even when self-administered.

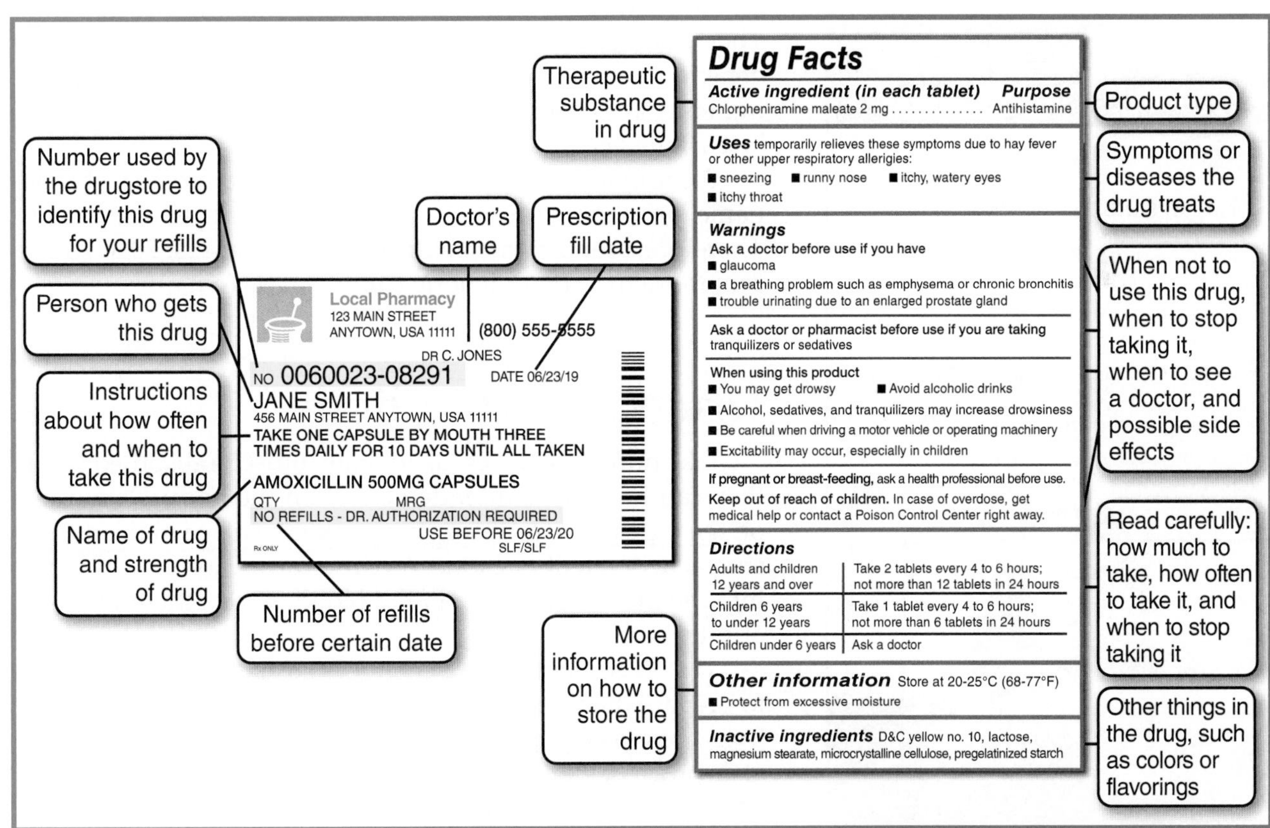

Courtesy of the US Department of Health and Human Services

Figure 23.2 All prescription medication labels must include at least the information shown. *How often and when should this medication be taken?*

As a consumer, you decide which OTC medication to buy to treat a health problem or ailment. Read package labels carefully when choosing these products. Avoid buying OTC products designed to relieve symptoms you do not have.

When you have questions, ask your doctor or pharmacist. After choosing a product, be sure to read all information that comes with the medication. Heed all cautions and do not take more than the recommended dosage. Using the medication incorrectly could be dangerous and may damage your health.

Generic Versus Brand-Name Medications

Most medications have both a generic and a brand name. The generic name is the chemical name of the medication. A brand or trade name is the name a manufacturer uses to promote a product.

When the FDA approves a new medication for sale, the manufacturer has exclusive marketing rights to it for approximately 17 years. During this period, the drug is available only under the company's brand name. After this time, other manufacturers can sell the product under their own brand names and/or under the generic name. This is true for both prescription and OTC medications.

A ***generic medication*** is a drug sold under its generic name. For example, *acetaminophen* is the generic name for a common OTC medication. People who are sensitive to aspirin use it to relieve headache and pain. You can buy this medication in one of its brand-name forms such as *Tylenol* or *Datril*, or you can purchase the generic product labeled *acetaminophen*.

Many manufacturers produce a drug product in various forms, such as powder, liquid, tablets, caplets, and capsules. They often sell a product under a brand name as well as a generic name. Generic medications contain the same active ingredients as comparable brand-name medication. They are just as safe and effective as the brand-name products.

A company usually spends money to advertise its brand-name products. These costs are passed on to consumers. Therefore, brand-name medications usually cost 20 to 70 percent more than their generic **counterparts** (equal).

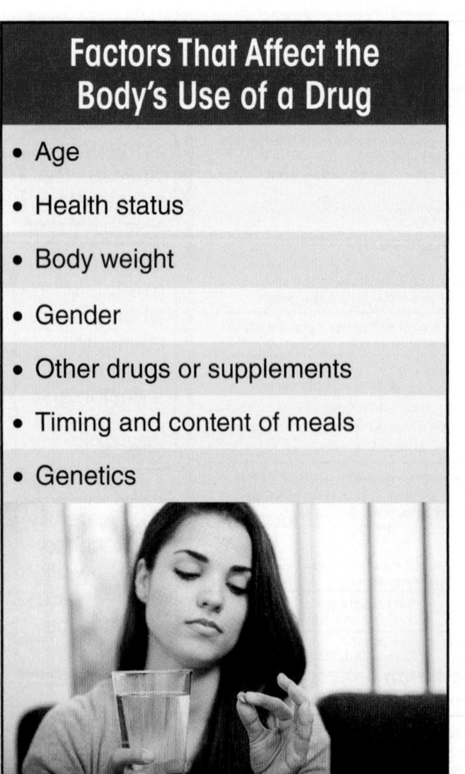

Factors That Affect the Body's Use of a Drug
• Age
• Health status
• Body weight
• Gender
• Other drugs or supplements
• Timing and content of meals
• Genetics

Photo: antoniodiaz/Shutterstock.com

Figure 23.3 Different people may be affected by the same drug in different ways.

Drugs and Your Body

Like nutrients, drugs taken orally must be absorbed before they can have their intended effect on the body. Depending on the type of drug, absorption may take place in the mouth, stomach, or small intestine. As drugs are absorbed, they pass into the bloodstream. Then the blood carries them throughout the body.

The liver changes the chemical structure of some drugs to prepare them for use in the body. If the drugs are toxic, the liver tries to convert them to less toxic substances. The liver also processes some drugs for elimination, which usually occurs via the kidneys through the urine.

A variety of factors affects how the body responds to and utilizes a drug (**Figure 23.3**). Some drugs may not be absorbed at all. Others may be absorbed, but not reduced to usable forms.

The way the body uses the drugs depends on many factors. These include the person's age, health status, body weight, use of other drugs or dietary supplements, and diet. The timing and content of meals also affect the body's use of a drug. In addition, genetics play a role in drug utilization. This means the same drug can affect two individuals differently due to their genetic differences.

Undesired Health Events from Medication Use

Undesired health events can result from the use of both over-the-counter and prescription medications as well as dietary supplements. It is important to inform your doctor about all the substances you are taking and to read the instructions that accompany the medications. The labels and information sheets that come with the medicine provide warnings of side effects and potential interactions with foods or other drugs. You should consult your physician or pharmacist with any specific concerns you may have. Provide a list of all the drugs and supplements you are currently taking to let the physician decide which ones may interact negatively with each other (**Figure 23.4**). In addition, some medications may have a negative impact on your nutritional status. The instructions also describe potential allergic reactions that may occur.

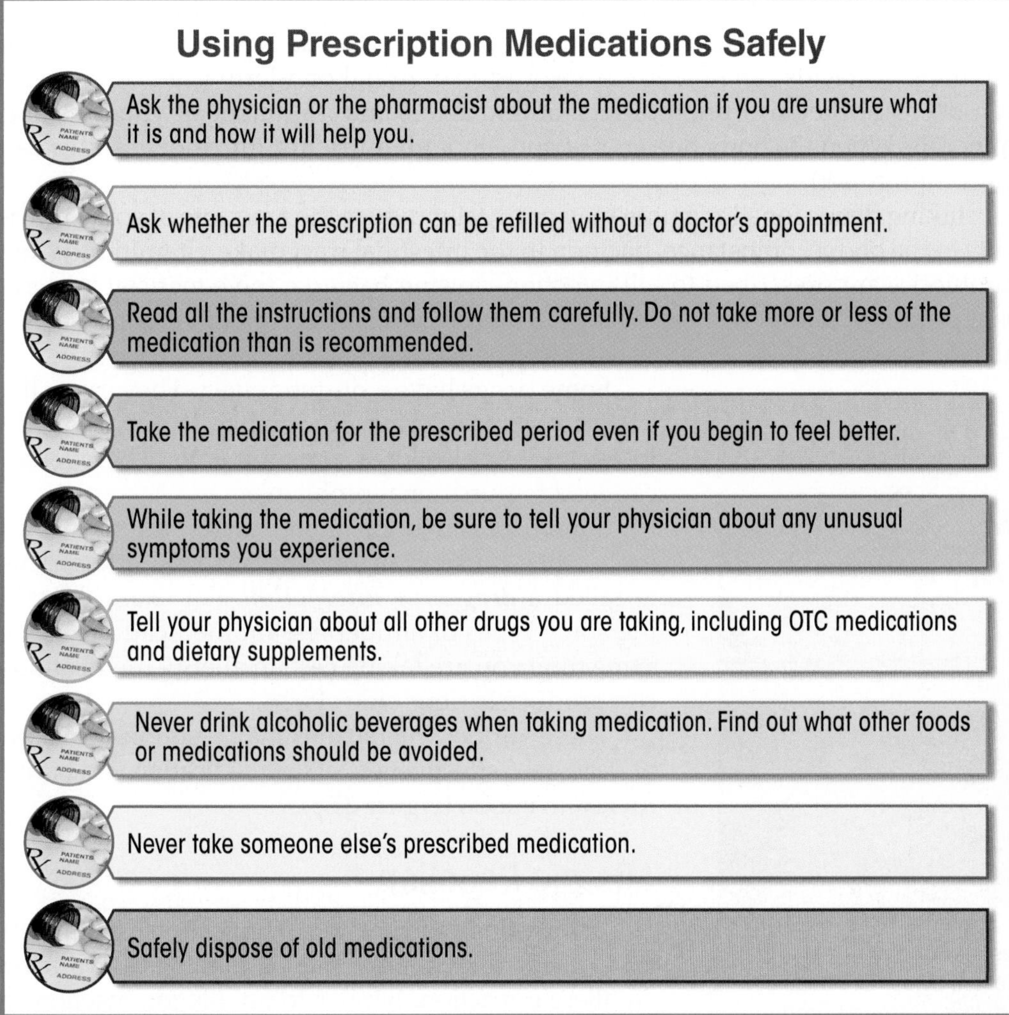
Using Prescription Medications Safely
Ask the physician or the pharmacist about the medication if you are unsure what it is and how it will help you.
Ask whether the prescription can be refilled without a doctor's appointment.
Read all the instructions and follow them carefully. Do not take more or less of the medication than is recommended.
Take the medication for the prescribed period even if you begin to feel better.
While taking the medication, be sure to tell your physician about any unusual symptoms you experience.
Tell your physician about all other drugs you are taking, including OTC medications and dietary supplements.
Never drink alcoholic beverages when taking medication. Find out what other foods or medications should be avoided.
Never take someone else's prescribed medication.
Safely dispose of old medications.

Photo: Soru Epotok/Shutterstock.com

Figure 23.4
To ensure that a prescription medication is safe and effective, you must be an active participant in your health and follow these guidelines. *Is it okay to take your friend's prescription medication if he has the same health issue as you?*

Side Effects

Medications approved by the FDA must be safe and effective; however, *safe* means the benefits of the medication are greater than the risks. In other words, side effects can still occur. Both prescription and OTC medications can produce side effects. Those side effects may range from minor events such as an upset stomach to serious events such as internal bleeding.

To reduce the chance of experiencing side effects, take the medication as described on the packaging. You can also ask the pharmacist or your doctor about ways to help avoid side effects. If you experience a side effect, consult with your doctor to learn if a different dose or a different medication is a solution.

Interactions with Foods or Other Drugs

Some drugs, dietary supplements, and foods can interact with each other in unintended ways. This can influence their effect on the body. A food and a drug may affect the body differently when consumed together than when consumed separately. This effect is called a ***food-drug interaction***. For instance, grapefruit increases absorption of some medications. Supplements may also interact with drugs. For example, calcium supplements interfere with thyroid medication when consumed at the same time.

Just as food can interfere with drug absorption, drugs can interfere with nutrient absorption. For instance, laxatives can reduce the absorption of fat-soluble vitamins. Antacids can hinder the absorption of iron. Long-term use of antibiotics can decrease the absorption of fats, amino acids, and a number of vitamins and minerals. When the body does not absorb enough nutrients, nutritional status can be compromised.

Taking drugs for a long time may gradually reduce the amounts of some nutrients in the body. For instance, bacteria in the intestinal tract make vitamin K. When antibiotics are prescribed to kill infection-causing bacteria, the beneficial bacteria that produce vitamin K are also killed. This reduces the amount of vitamin K available in the body.

Some drugs have a diuretic effect. They cause the body to increase urine production. When the body loses fluids, it also loses some minerals. These losses can lead to nutritional problems.

Sometimes two or more drugs interact with each other causing an unexpected side effect. This is called a ***drug-drug interaction***. For example, taking some types of antidepressant medications at the same time you are taking certain allergy medications can produce serious side effects.

These various interactions may result in increased or decreased effectiveness of the medication and harmful health effects **(Figure 23.5)**.

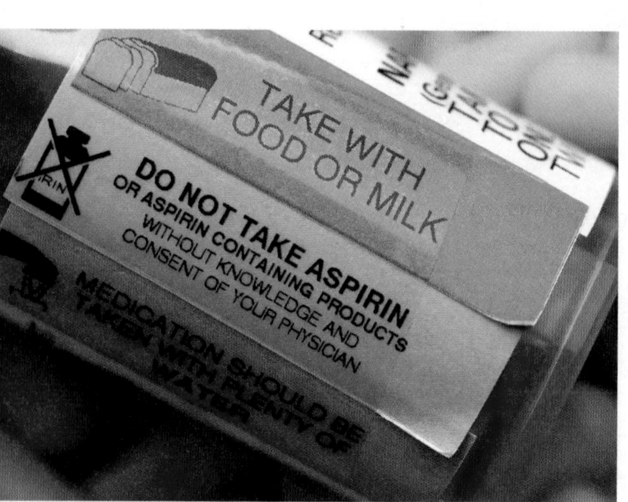
TAKE WITH
FOOD OR MILK
DO NOT TAKE ASPIRIN
OR ASPIRIN CONTAINING PRODUCTS
WITHOUT KNOWLEDGE AND
CONSENT OF YOUR PHYSICIAN
MEDICATION SHOULD BE
TAKEN WITH PLENTY OF
WATER

Steve Cukrov/Shutterstock.com

Figure 23.5 The effectiveness and safety of some medications are affected by certain foods or other drugs you are taking. *What drug should be avoided when taking the medication shown in this figure?*

Allergic Reaction

An allergic reaction to a medication is different from a side effect. Any drug is capable of inducing an allergic reaction. Similar to an allergic reaction to food, an allergic reaction to a medication is the result of your immune system responding to a perceived threat.

The reaction may occur within hours of taking the medication or may not become apparent for weeks. Allergic reactions may include itching, rash, swelling of the face or throat, wheezing, vomiting, light-headedness, and shock.

A number of factors including your genetic makeup, your body chemistry, number of prior exposures to the drug, and the existence of other diseases influence the likelihood of experiencing an allergic reaction to a medication. A doctor should be seen as soon as possible if you believe you are having an allergic reaction to a medication.

Medication Misuse

Medication misuse occurs when medicines are unintentionally used in a manner that could cause harm to the individual. Medication misuse occurs among people, especially older adults, who take several medicines daily. Sometimes they confuse *what* to take *when*. Common examples of medication misuse include the following:

- taking more or less medicine than the recommended dose
- taking medicine more or less frequently per day or for longer or shorter periods than the directions state
- leaving medicine within children's reach (**Figure 23.6**)

Misusing medication presents a serious health risk because it may result in **adverse** (unfavorable) reactions. Dangerous interactions can occur when various drugs are combined. One medication may increase or decrease the effectiveness of other medications. Therefore, medications should not be taken in combination unless directed by a doctor.

Medications should never be taken with alcohol. Depending on the quantity consumed and the frequency of use, alcohol can dull or magnify a medication's effects. In addition, too much alcohol can damage the liver, making it less able to process certain medications.

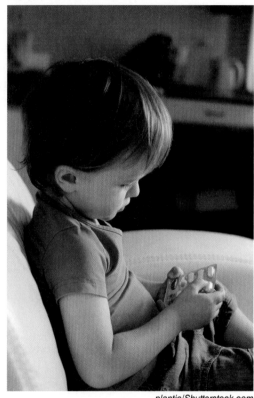

plantic/Shutterstock.com

Figure 23.6 Special care must be taken to keep medications away from children.

Medication and Drug Abuse

Medication abuse is the deliberate use of a prescription or OTC drug in a manner or dosage other than prescribed. Medication abuse also includes taking someone else's prescription medication even if the reason is for a medical issue. These drugs are legal when prescribed by a physician for treating patients; however, obtaining legal drugs through illegal means is against the law. These medications are only safe when taken for their intended purpose, in the prescribed dose, and by the patient for whom it was prescribed. Most often, medication abuse involves opioids, depressants, and stimulants.

Much drug abuse occurs with the use of illegal drugs. Many drugs that fall in this category include hallucinogens such as LSD and ecstasy as well as marijuana.

People who misuse or abuse drugs are likely to form addictions. An ***addiction*** is a psychological and/or physical dependence on a drug. When people stop taking an addictive drug, they are likely to go through ***withdrawal***. Withdrawal symptoms vary from person to person. Symptoms also depend on how long and how much of the drug has been consumed. Withdrawal usually includes one or more symptoms such as irritability, nervousness, sleeplessness, nausea, vomiting, trembling, and cramps. To avoid forming dependencies, patients must carefully follow their doctors' directions when taking drugs that can be addictive.

The most commonly misused and abused type of drugs is psychoactive drugs. A ***psychoactive drug*** is a chemical that affects the central nervous system. It interferes with normal brain activity and can affect moods and feelings. Psychoactive drugs can serve beneficial purposes when administered according to accepted medical use; however, a few psychoactive drugs have no known medical benefits or are too unsafe to use. Psychoactive drugs include stimulants, depressants, narcotics, marijuana, and hallucinogens. When an overdose occurs through misuse, the chemical reactions affect the central nervous system and consequently, respiratory depression may result causing death.

Stimulants

Stimulants are a kind of psychoactive drug that speeds up the nervous system. They produce feelings of keen alertness and boundless energy. Stimulants have a number of effects on the body. They increase heart rate, blood pressure, and breathing rate. They can also affect appetite and cause headaches, dizziness, and insomnia. Many coffees, colas, and teas contain caffeine, a mild stimulant. Other well-known stimulants include amphetamines, cocaine, and nicotine.

FEATURED CAREER

Substance Abuse Counselor

Substance abuse counselors help people who have problems with alcohol, drugs, gambling, and eating disorders. They counsel individuals to help them to identify behaviors and problems related to their addictions. Counselors are trained to assist in developing personalized recovery programs that help to establish healthy behaviors and provide coping strategies. Some counselors conduct programs and community outreach aimed at preventing addiction and educating the public.

Education

A master's degree usually is required to be licensed or certified as a counselor. Depending on the specialty, state licensure and certification requirements will vary. Fields of study for counselors may include substance abuse or addictions, rehabilitation, agency or community counseling, clinical mental health counseling, and related fields.

Job Outlook

Employment of substance abuse and behavioral disorder counselors is expected to grow much faster than the average for all occupations. As society becomes more knowledgeable about addiction, more people are seeking treatment. States are also tending toward treatment and counseling services for drug offenders rather than or in conjunction with jail time.

Caffeine

Caffeine is a mild stimulant drug that occurs naturally in the leaves, seeds, or fruits of more than 60 plants. It is found in coffee, tea, cola drinks, and cocoa products. Caffeine is often used in OTC and prescription drugs. Be sure to check medication labels for caffeine in the list of active ingredients.

Many people in the United States consume caffeine on a daily basis. A morning mug of coffee may have 100 to 200 milligrams of caffeine. An after-school cola may contain approximately 50 milligrams. A cup of tea at bedtime contributes about 40 milligrams, whereas cocoa provides fewer than 20. Some popular energy drinks can contain as much as 160 milligrams or more of caffeine.

Some individuals believe caffeine improves their performance; however, the effect of caffeine can vary greatly from person to person. Consuming too much caffeine is ill-advised and may result in dizziness, headaches, and gastrointestinal distress.

Caffeine affects the body in a number of ways. As with all stimulants, it increases breathing rate, heart rate, blood pressure, and the secretion of stress hormones. Too much caffeine may lead to irritability, lack of sleep, and an upset stomach (**Figure 23.7**). Caffeine causes diarrhea in some people. Caffeine has been the subject of much research, but the *2015–2020 Dietary Guidelines* states, "Moderate coffee consumption (three to five 8-ounce cups/day or up to 400 mg/day of caffeine) can be incorporated into healthy eating patterns." However, individuals who do not currently consume caffeine are not encouraged to start.

To avoid the physical effects of caffeine, many people prefer to use caffeine-free products. Today, many choices of decaffeinated soft drinks, coffees, and teas are available. These products contain very little or no caffeine.

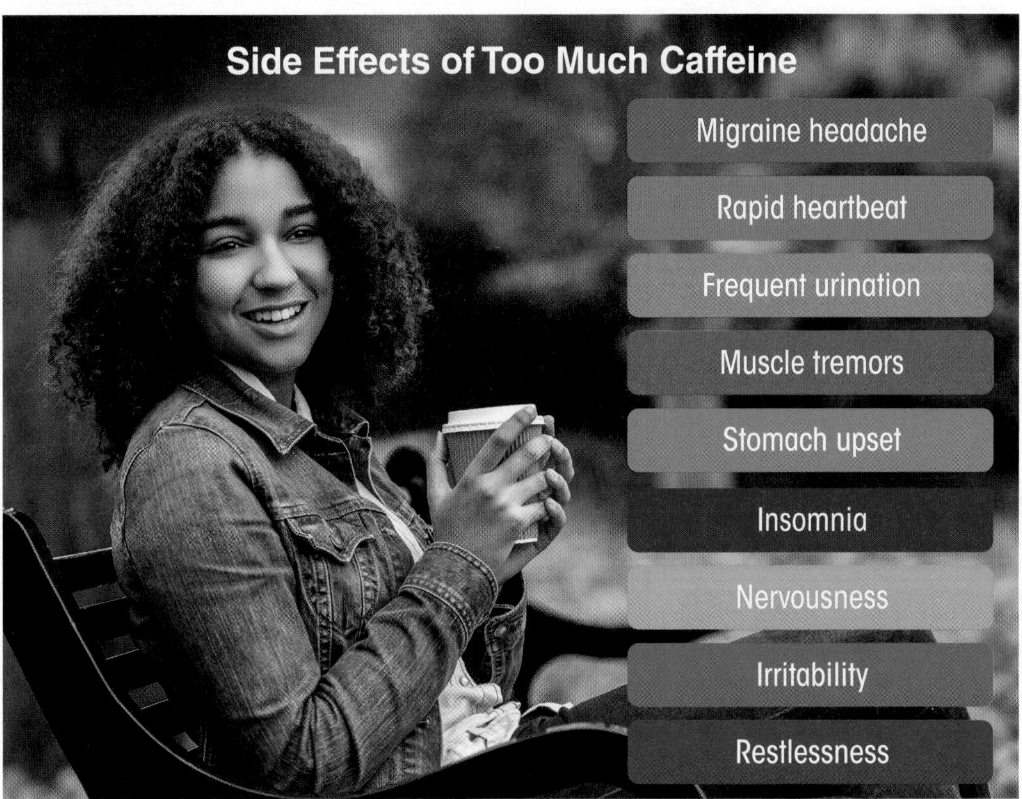
Side Effects of Too Much Caffeine
Migraine headache
Rapid heartbeat
Frequent urination
Muscle tremors
Stomach upset
Insomnia
Nervousness
Irritability
Restlessness

Darren Baker/Shutterstock.com

Figure 23.7 Coffee contains caffeine, a stimulant drug, and too much caffeine can cause side effects. ***Have you experienced any of these side effects?***

Caffeine is not an addictive drug, but it can be habit forming. People who suddenly stop drinking three or four cups of cola or coffee a day may experience withdrawal-like symptoms. These symptoms may include headaches, nausea, drowsiness, and irritability. A gradual withdrawal of caffeine will reduce these symptoms. To avoid feelings of fatigue from caffeine withdrawal, add daily exercise to your lifestyle.

Amphetamines

Amphetamines are commonly abused stimulant drugs. They are found in medicines used to treat certain sleep and attention disorders. They are also in some prescription medicines used to curb appetite for weight control. National and international sports associations ban the use of stimulants, such as amphetamines.

Use of amphetamines to control weight is usually unsuccessful. The drugs only reduce appetite. They do not help the individual learn new eating behaviors. Once the amphetamine use stops, weight is regained rapidly.

Amphetamines cause the same physical effects as other stimulants. They tend to increase physical performance, competitiveness, and aggression; however, side effects include sweating, poor sleep patterns, dizziness, and irregular cardiac rates. In addition, long-term use can result in malnutrition and various nutrient deficiency diseases. Amphetamine abusers sometimes report having strange visions and thoughts.

Continued use of the drug can result in the development of ***tolerance***. This is the ability of the body and mind to become less responsive to a drug. When a user develops a drug tolerance, he or she must take increasingly larger doses to feel the drug's effects. The accidental or intentional ingestion of a toxic amount of a substance is a ***drug overdose***. A drug overdose can cause a slowdown in brain activity, coma, or even death.

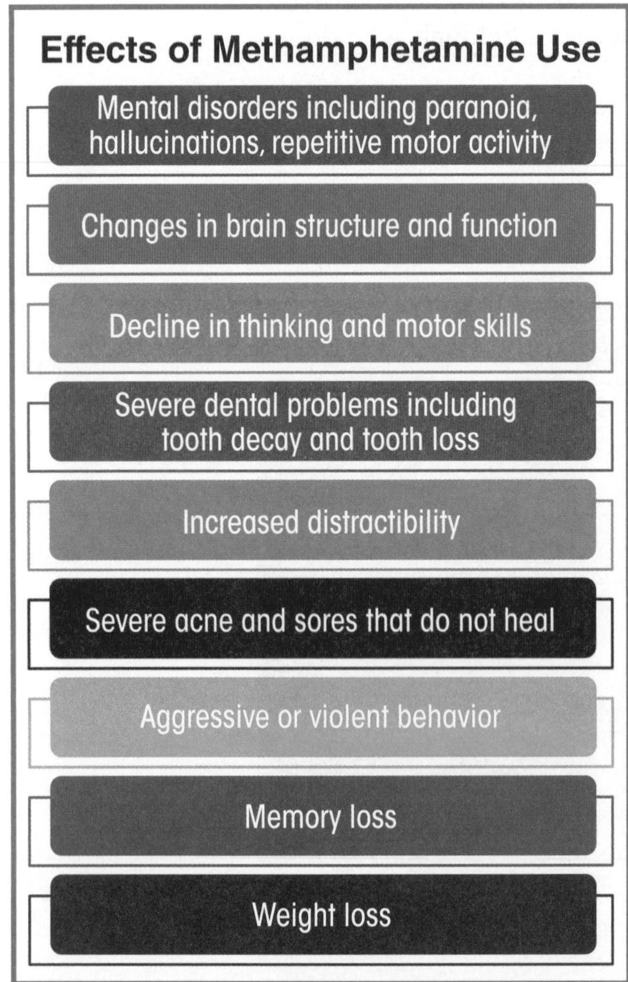

Effects of Methamphetamine Use
Mental disorders including paranoia, hallucinations, repetitive motor activity
Changes in brain structure and function
Decline in thinking and motor skills
Severe dental problems including tooth decay and tooth loss
Increased distractibility
Severe acne and sores that do not heal
Aggressive or violent behavior
Memory loss
Weight loss

Figure 23.8 Methamphetamine users often feel as though bugs are crawling on or under their skin. This results in constant scratching to get rid of the "bugs" and subsequent skin sores that never heal.

Methamphetamine

Methamphetamine, also known as *crystal meth*, is an illegal stimulant that is never prescribed for medical treatment. It is far more potent, fast acting, and addictive than amphetamines. Crystal meth is a synthetic chemical that is manufactured illegally in secretive laboratories.

This dangerous drug produces a sense of **euphoria** (extreme pleasure) in the user and a desire to continue use. Crystal meth produces increased pulse, hyperactivity, dizziness, loss of appetite, and an inability to sleep.

Crystal meth is never safe to use and ages the user very quickly. Side effects include developing sores and pimples that do not heal. Teeth become stained, break, and rot in the mouth. The user becomes paranoid, violent, and experiences hallucinations. A crystal meth overdose can be life-threatening (**Figure 23.8**).

Cocaine

Cocaine is a white powder made from the coca plant. The powder, often called *coke*, is usually inhaled through the nose. When consumed, cocaine causes impulses that flood the brain within seconds. These chemical reactions affect appetite, sleep, and emotions. A feeling of high energy is often followed by an emotional letdown, anger, and irritability. Cocaine is illegal and highly addictive.

Crack cocaine is a newer, less expensive form of cocaine. Because crack cocaine is smoked, its effects are felt quickly, usually within seconds.

Cocaine can cause a number of nutritional and health problems related to weight loss and poor sleep patterns. Just one use can cause a heart attack or lung failure, resulting in death. Use of this stimulant is illegal.

Nicotine

Nicotine is a drug that occurs naturally in tobacco leaves. When you use tobacco products, the nicotine is absorbed into the bloodstream and reaches your brain within 10 seconds. This highly addictive drug is inhaled when smoking tobacco products or using *electronic nicotine delivery systems (ENDS)*. Electronic nicotine delivery systems produce a vapor by heating nicotine-containing liquid. The user inhales the vapor, which contains nicotine. ENDS include e-cigarettes, personal vaporizers, vape pens, and e-hookahs. These systems deliver nicotine without the smoke and tar produced when smoking cigarettes. Smokeless tobacco products, such as chew and snuff, also deliver nicotine to the user. Some people mistakenly believe that these methods are healthier and safer than smoking tobacco; however, both of these smokeless options can result in addiction and health concerns.

Health Risks of Nicotine and Tobacco

Smoking leads to 480,000 deaths per year and kills more people per year than all other drugs. According to estimates, each cigarette a person smokes shortens his or her life by about 11 minutes. Longtime smokers can expect to lose 10 or more years of life expectancy. The main reasons for a smoker's reduced life expectancy are the effects of tobacco on the heart and lungs and the increased risk of cancer.

Smoking is a major contributor to heart disease. Carbon monoxide, a poisonous gas in cigarette smoke, decreases the amount of oxygen available in the blood. The carbon monoxide stresses the heart by making it work harder. Smoking also causes blood clots to form more easily. This increases the risk of heart attack and stroke.

Tobacco smoke is the major cause of lung diseases, including lung cancer and chronic obstructive pulmonary disease (COPD). When someone inhales smoke, irritating gases and particles slow the functioning of the lung's defense systems. Cigarette smoke can cause air passages to close up and make breathing more difficult. Cigarette smoke causes a sticky substance called *tar* to collect in the lungs. It can cause chronic swelling in the lungs, leading to coughs and bronchial infections. Lung tissue can be destroyed.

Smoking seems to increase the rate at which the body breaks down vitamin C. Nutrition researchers have found cigarette smokers need 35 milligrams more vitamin C each day than nonsmokers. Smokers must include extra sources of vitamin C in their diets to prevent deficiency.

Health Risks of Smokeless Options

You may think that smokeless options such as ENDS are healthier, but some studies show that nicotine bores holes in the smooth muscle of heart tissue and can lead to plaque buildup in arteries. Nicotine initiates the release of the hormone *adrenaline*.

Adrenaline acts to increase the heart rate, breathing rate, and blood pressure. The combination of the effects from the adrenaline coupled with plaque buildup in the arteries produce more strain on the heart.

Tobacco products that are not intended to be smoked, such as chewing tobacco or snuff, are called ***smokeless tobacco***. These products also contain nicotine, making them addictive and harmful to health. Chewing tobacco is associated with cancer of the cheeks, gums, and throat. Some people's mouths are affected within a few weeks after starting to use smokeless tobacco. Gums and lips can sting, crack, bleed, wrinkle, and develop sores and white patches.

Health Risks to Others

A smoker is not the only one affected by his or her smoke. In fact, secondhand smoke causes more than 41,000 deaths each year. ***Secondhand smoke*** is the tobacco smoke released into the air by smokers, which other people inhale involuntarily. According to the American Lung Association, secondhand smoke can contain more cancer-causing compounds than the smoke inhaled by the smoker. The presence of smoke is especially harmful to infants and children. According to studies, babies of parents who smoke have a higher rate of respiratory problems than babies of nonsmokers.

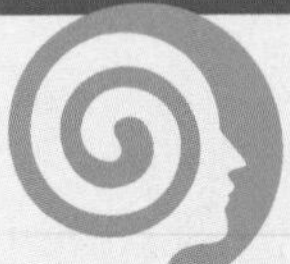

EXTEND YOUR KNOWLEDGE

What's the News on E-Cigarettes?

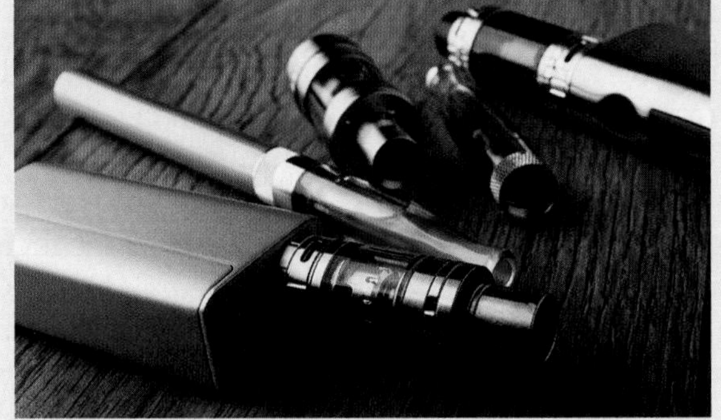

Hazem.m.kamal/Shutterstock.com

The good news is that the number of young people who smoke tobacco cigarettes has dropped to six percent. The bad news is that the use of electronic cigarettes tripled among middle school and high school students. Electronic cigarettes, also known as *e-cigs*, are battery-powered devices that simulate the experience of smoking. A cartridge of liquid containing flavoring, nicotine, and other chemicals is heated to produce a vapor. The user inhales the vapor.

Approximately 14–16 percent of high school students have used or are using e-cigarettes despite the USDA's ban on e-cigarette sales to people under 18 years of age. In fact, marketing efforts appear to be directed at youth.

Is there harm in e-cigs? Although e-cigs do not produce tar and carbon monoxide like tobacco cigarettes, there is evidence that shows teens who use e-cigs are more likely to start smoking tobacco cigarettes. In addition, the nicotine delivered in the vapor is highly addictive and particularly harmful to the teen's developing brain. Damage caused by nicotine use can result in lifelong problems, including mental health problems and changes in brain structure. Furthermore, the vapor from some e-cigarettes has been found to contain known cancer-causing substances and toxic chemicals.

The secondhand vapors from e-cigs are harmful to people nearby and young children are especially vulnerable. In addition, the residue from the vapors, referred to as *thirdhand smoke*, deposits nicotine on clothing, chairs, and other surfaces.

The safety of e-cigarettes needs further scientific study. As use of e-cigarettes continues, more evidence will be gathered for reporting long-term health outcomes.

Say "No" to Tobacco

Fortunately, information about the dangers of tobacco and nicotine has prompted many people to quit. Roughly six percent of middle school and high school students smoke cigarettes, compared with about 25 percent in 1997 (**Figure 23.9**).

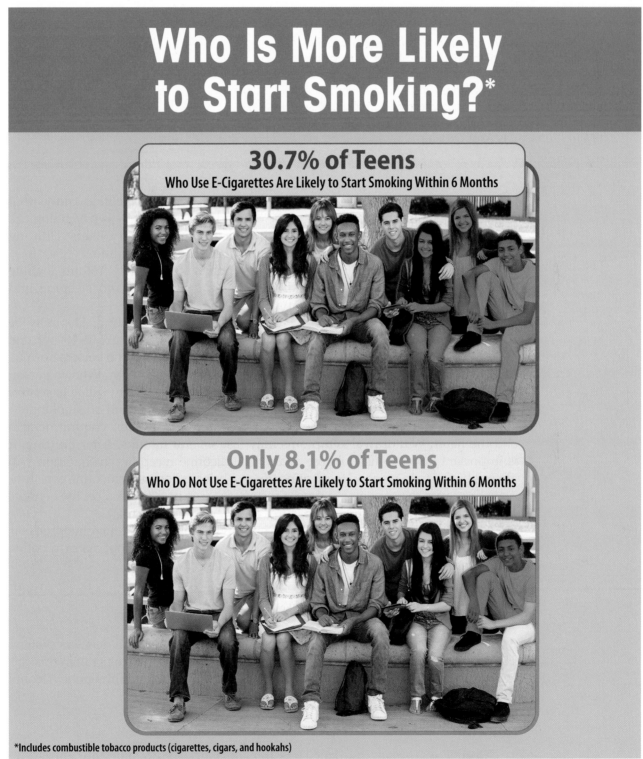

Photos: Monkey Business Images/Shutterstock.com

Figure 23.9 Many people believe e-cigarettes are a healthier option than smoking; however, many teens who use e-cigarettes switch to smoking tobacco. *Why do you think e-cigarette users are more likely to start smoking than nonusers?*

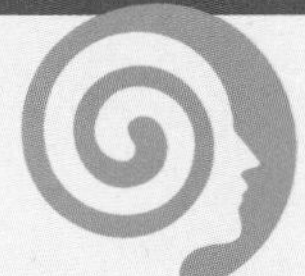

EXTEND YOUR KNOWLEDGE

Within 20 Minutes of Quitting…

Smoking causes damage to nearly every organ of the body. It causes disease and negatively affects the health of not only smokers, but also the people in their lives. Fortunately, the human body is capable of reversing some of the negative effects of smoking. Visit the Centers for Disease Control and Prevention (CDC) website for *Smoking & Tobacco Use* for more information on tobacco addiction and quitting. Discover the series of changes to your body that begin "Within 20 Minutes After Quitting…"

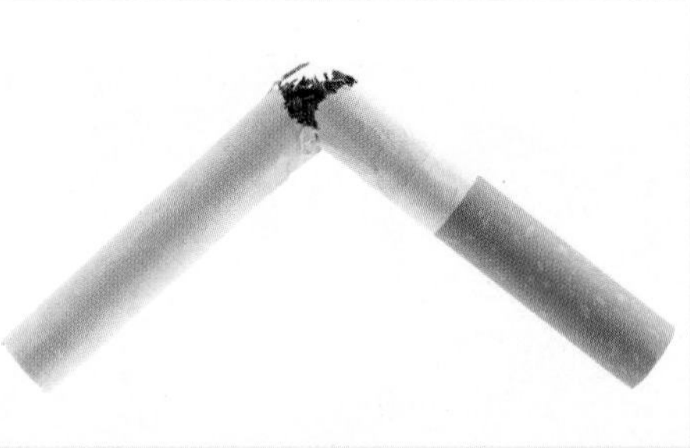

Gary Woodard/Shutterstock.com

Anyone who smokes or uses other forms of tobacco or nicotine knows that breaking the habit is not easy. Part of the dependence on nicotine is psychological. Some users associate the habit with relaxation, good food, and friends. Quitting can be especially difficult when your friends use tobacco or nicotine.

Nicotine addiction is also physical. Common withdrawal symptoms include shakiness, anxiety, and grouchiness. Dizziness, headaches, difficulty sleeping, and changes in appetite are also symptoms.

Some people claim they gain weight when they stop smoking. This may be partly because smoking elevates the body's basal metabolism about 10 percent. When a person quits smoking, his or her basal metabolism will drop back to normal. This accounts for a reduced energy need of about 100 calories a day. When a person is adjusting to not smoking, an extra walk or other physical activity will help control weight. Added activity will also help a smoker take his or her mind off smoking.

Former tobacco users must be patient and stay firm in their commitment to end the habit. Withdrawal symptoms may last several months. After quitting, it is important never to use tobacco again. The nicotine receptors in the brain will always be ready to respond to nicotine. Even a brief exposure to nicotine can stimulate the desire to use again. In time, a former tobacco user will realize the benefits of abstaining far outweigh any pleasures received from smoking.

In addition, the financial rewards of not buying tobacco and nicotine products can add up quickly. The best option is never to begin using tobacco or nicotine products at all.

Depressants

Depressants are drugs that decrease the activity of the central nervous system. They slow down certain body functions and reactions. Many drugs fall in this category. They can be grouped as barbiturates, tranquilizers, and inhalants. Alcohol is the most often abused depressant.

Alcohol

Alcohol, or *ethanol*, is a drug. It is the substance most commonly abused by teens. The consequences of drinking alcohol at this age can be serious and some are lifelong (**Figure 23.10**).

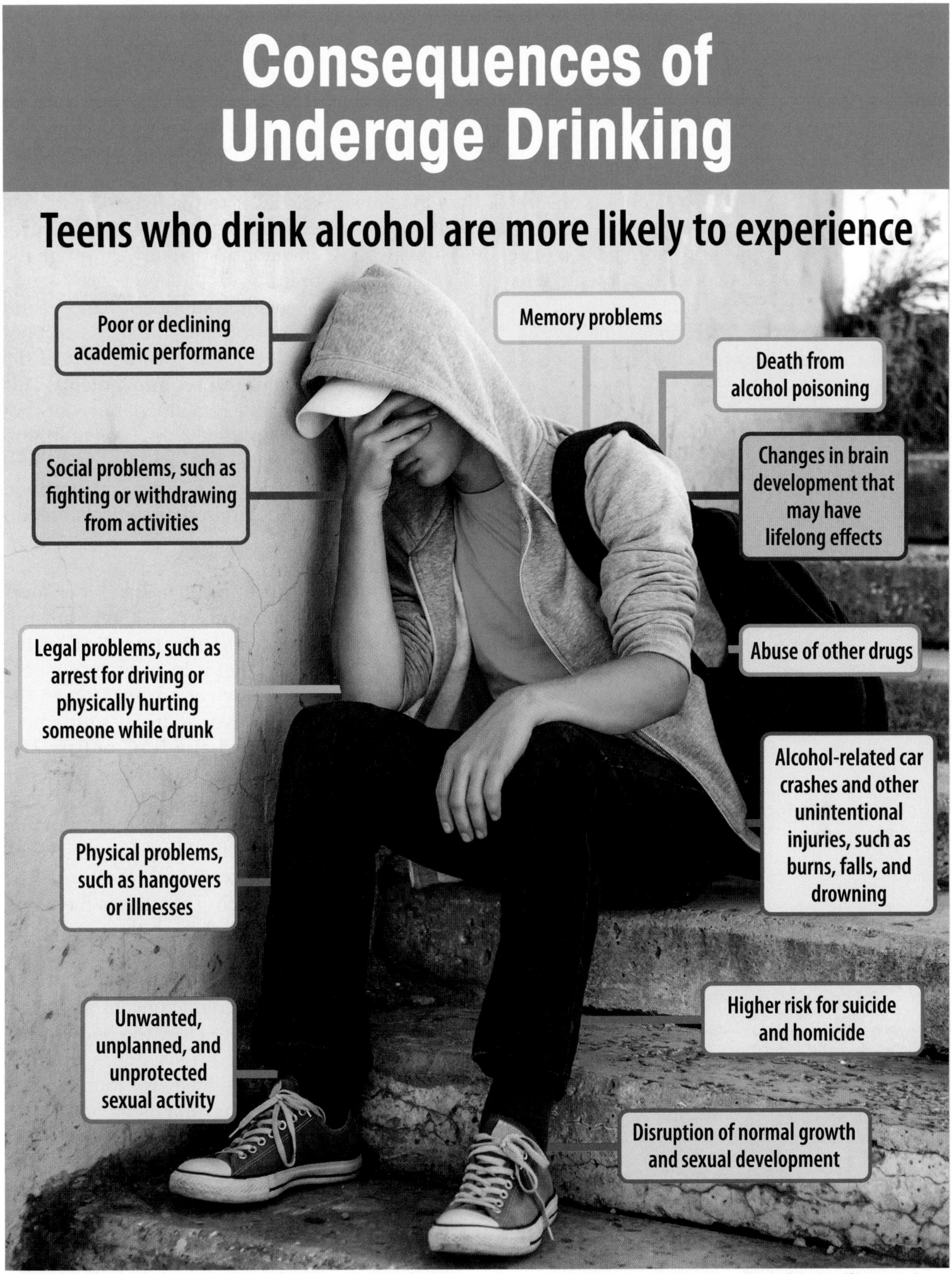

Consequences of Underage Drinking

Teens who drink alcohol are more likely to experience

Poor or declining academic performance

Memory problems

Death from alcohol poisoning

Social problems, such as fighting or withdrawing from activities

Changes in brain development that may have lifelong effects

Legal problems, such as arrest for driving or physically hurting someone while drunk

Abuse of other drugs

Alcohol-related car crashes and other unintentional injuries, such as burns, falls, and drowning

Physical problems, such as hangovers or illnesses

Higher risk for suicide and homicide

Unwanted, unplanned, and unprotected sexual activity

Disruption of normal growth and sexual development

Photo: Sabphoto/Shutterstock.com

Figure 23.10 Teens often drink as a way to cope with stress or problems in their lives, but drinking only makes these problems worse.

Physical Effects of Alcohol

Alcohol supplies seven calories of energy per gram. Carbohydrates, fats, and proteins must be digested before they are absorbed through the walls of the small intestine. Alcohol, by contrast, requires no digestion and can be absorbed through cells in the mouth and the walls of the stomach. This is what causes a person to feel the effects of alcohol so quickly. Food in the stomach helps slow the absorption of alcohol.

Once alcohol is absorbed, the bloodstream carries it to the liver. The liver is where alcohol metabolism occurs. The rate at which the liver can break down alcohol varies from person to person. Until alcohol is metabolized, it flows through the bloodstream, allowing it to reach and affect the brain.

In the brain, alcohol suppresses the action of the area that controls judgment. As alcohol consumption increases, it affects the part of the brain that controls large muscle movements. This is why people who have consumed much alcohol begin to stagger when they walk. Loss of inhibitions, confusion, drowsiness, nausea, and vomiting are other symptoms. Further consumption affects the part of the brain that controls breathing and heartbeat.

The higher the level of blood alcohol, the greater is the risk to health and life. As blood alcohol content rises, more centers of the brain shut down. ***Blood alcohol concentration (BAC)*** is the percentage of alcohol that is in a person's blood. Many states declare a driver "drunk" when the BAC reaches 0.08; however, a driver's judgment starts becoming impaired at a BAC of 0.05. Use of poor judgment may result in serious accidents even at this blood alcohol level (**Figure 23.11**).

If a person passes out, it means the entire consciousness section of the brain has closed off. Meanwhile, the body continues to absorb the alcohol still in the stomach. This causes the blood alcohol level to rise even though the person has stopped drinking.

The liver can metabolize alcohol only so fast. The higher the blood alcohol concentration, the longer it takes the liver to clear the body of the drug. The liver takes about six hours to break down the alcohol contained in four drinks. Drinking coffee, exercising, and using other techniques do not speed up this process.

A person can feel sick the day after drinking large amounts of alcohol. This condition is called a *hangover*. A person with a hangover may experience headache, nausea, vomiting, fatigue, thirst, and irritability. Alcohol consumption can also lower blood sugar levels and increase the heart rate.

Effects of Alcohol on Behavior

Percent of Blood Alcohol Concentration (BAC)	Behavioral Effect
0.00–0.05%	Slight change in feeling; decreased alertness
0.05–0.10%	Reduced social inhibitions and motor coordination; slowed reaction time; legally drunk in many states
0.10–0.15%	Unsteadiness in standing and walking; loss of peripheral (side) vision
0.15–0.30%	Staggered walk and slurred speech; impaired pain receptors
0.30% and greater	Possible shutdown of heart and lungs; complete unconsciousness; death possible

Photo: Photographee.eu/Shutterstock.com

Figure 23.11 People who drive with a blood alcohol of 0.08 or greater are breaking the law.

COMMUNITY CONNECTIONS

Teen Peer Mentoring

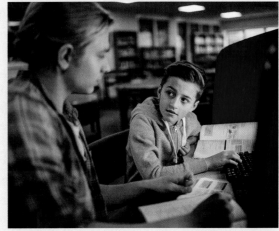
DGLimages/Shutterstock.com

A mentor is an experienced and trusted person who teaches, offers help, or gives advice to another person (mentee) in a structured program. School-based mentoring programs are becoming increasingly popular. Some of these programs match adults with students; however, mentors can be the same age as the mentee (peer-to-peer) or a slightly older student can serve as a mentor for a younger student (near peer). For example, a high school student might act as a mentor for a middle or elementary school student. The mentoring relationship tends to last for the entire school year.

Different types of mentoring programs have different goals. For example, mentor-tutoring programs are designed to help in academic areas by helping with homework or preparations for exams. Peer counseling mentor programs work on developing social and emotional skills.

Successful mentoring programs require strong support from school administrators. Careful mentor and mentee screening, selection, and training; support from parents; and safe, secure meeting spaces are also essential for favorable outcomes. As a mentor, you can expect to grow in your leadership and communication skills. If you do not have a school mentoring program, what would it take to start one in your school?

Think Critically

1. What are the risks and rewards of peer mentoring?
2. How might participating as a mentee in a peer mentoring experience during middle school have influenced your academic, social, and mental development?

Alcohol and Sports Performance

Alcohol use and athletes do not mix. It is a depressant and does not enhance performance. In fact, much evidence shows that performance is reduced when alcohol is consumed. The following reasons contribute to decreased performance.

- *Alcohol acts as a diuretic in the body.* This means the body loses more water than is consumed. During physical activity, dehydration can occur even sooner. Dehydration upsets the balance of electrolytes in the body's fluids and cells. Athletes may experience some loss of strength, energy, and performance. The imbalance must be corrected with intake of water and foods to replace lost minerals and fluids.
- *Alcohol impairs mental and physical reaction times.* The effect may even be noticed days after the consumption. Because of impaired lactic acid breakdown, the person will likely feel more soreness after exercise.
- *Alcohol can reduce balance and coordination.* As a result, rough or uneven surfaces can be the source of unexpected injuries.

- *Alcohol impairs the body's ability to regulate temperature.* During endurance training, people are more prone to overheat in hot temperatures and experience danger of harming extremities in cold weather.
- *Alcohol is not utilized efficiently by the body for energy production.* It contains seven calories per gram as compared to carbohydrates and protein that have four calories per gram. Calories from alcohol supply no nutrients.
- *Alcohol consumption can negatively affect sleep patterns and ability to concentrate during the day.* This effect can linger for days following a drinking event.

Women athletes experience adverse effects sooner and with greater intensity. One reason is due to the smaller size of the female body and lower volume of blood. The effects of alcohol also put them at greater risk for traffic accidents and date rape or other forms of interpersonal violence.

Alcohol Use Disorder (AUD)

An individual with ***alcohol use disorder (AUD)*** meets certain criteria (**Figure 23.12**). Alcohol use disorders can range from mild to severe based on the number of criteria met.

This is one of the most common substance use disorders (SUD) in the United States and is fatal if left untreated. People with AUD do not always realize they have a disease and many find it hard to seek help. Few people with this disorder seek help until they are facing a crisis.

Health Risks of Alcohol Abuse

One effect of long-term alcohol abuse is vitamin deficiencies. Many vitamins are affected, including vitamins A, C, D, K, and several B vitamins. Deficiencies may

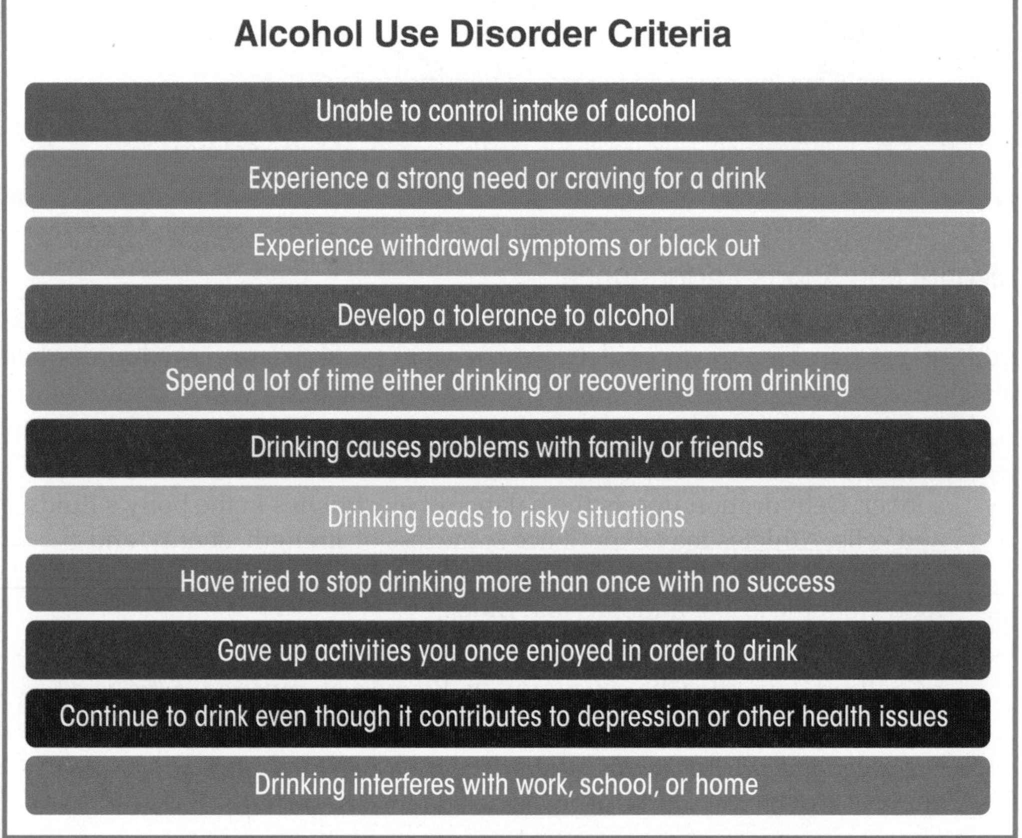

Alcohol Use Disorder Criteria
Unable to control intake of alcohol
Experience a strong need or craving for a drink
Experience withdrawal symptoms or black out
Develop a tolerance to alcohol
Spend a lot of time either drinking or recovering from drinking
Drinking causes problems with family or friends
Drinking leads to risky situations
Have tried to stop drinking more than once with no success
Gave up activities you once enjoyed in order to drink
Continue to drink even though it contributes to depression or other health issues
Drinking interferes with work, school, or home

Figure 23.12 Alcohol use disorder (AUD) ranges from mild to severe based on the number of criteria that are met.

occur due to a couple of factors. If many calories in the diet come from alcohol, the diet may be poor in nutrients. Alcohol in the system also reduces the body's ability to absorb and use nutrients.

Alcohol abuse over time causes a fat buildup in the liver. Fat accumulation in the liver eventually chokes off the supply of blood to liver cells. Scar tissue forms. Eventually, liver cells begin to die. This is characteristic of a liver disease called ***cirrhosis***. As cells die, the liver loses its ability to work. Without the function of this vital organ, a person will die. Seventy percent of deaths from cirrhosis are related to alcohol abuse.

Other health risks of alcohol abuse include stomach problems, heart disease, and brain damage. Alcohol also affects the immune system and the reproductive system. In addition, impaired judgment and slowed motor responses create health risks. These effects can lead to serious accidents.

The health risks from consuming alcohol are greatest for someone who is still growing. The body is undergoing many significant changes during the teen years, such as hormonal alterations and brain development. Researchers have found that exposing the brain to alcohol during the teen years may interrupt key processes of brain development. For some teens, this can lead to mild cognitive difficulties and can contribute to worse drinking problems.

Say "No" to Alcohol

Although drinking alcohol is illegal for teens, teens whose friends drink often feel the pressure to "fit in." Social acceptance is important; however, many studies show that most young people do not drink alcohol and wish there were less alcohol consumption in their surroundings.

The effects of alcohol can quickly interfere with the ability to make correct or safe decisions. Rates of high-risk sex, sexual assault, suicide, and other dangerous behaviors increase when alcohol is consumed.

Resisting pressure from your peers to drink alcohol is difficult, but it is easier if you are prepared. The following are strategies for refusal:

- Say "no" assertively using a firm, polite voice and while looking directly at the person.
- Use humor.
- Suggest something else to do.
- Stand up for others.
- Give a reason, fact, or excuse.
- Walk away from the situation.

Practice your refusal skills so that you are able to withstand pressure from your social circle (**Figure 23.13**). These skills are useful for refusing to **partake** (engage) in other risky behaviors as well.

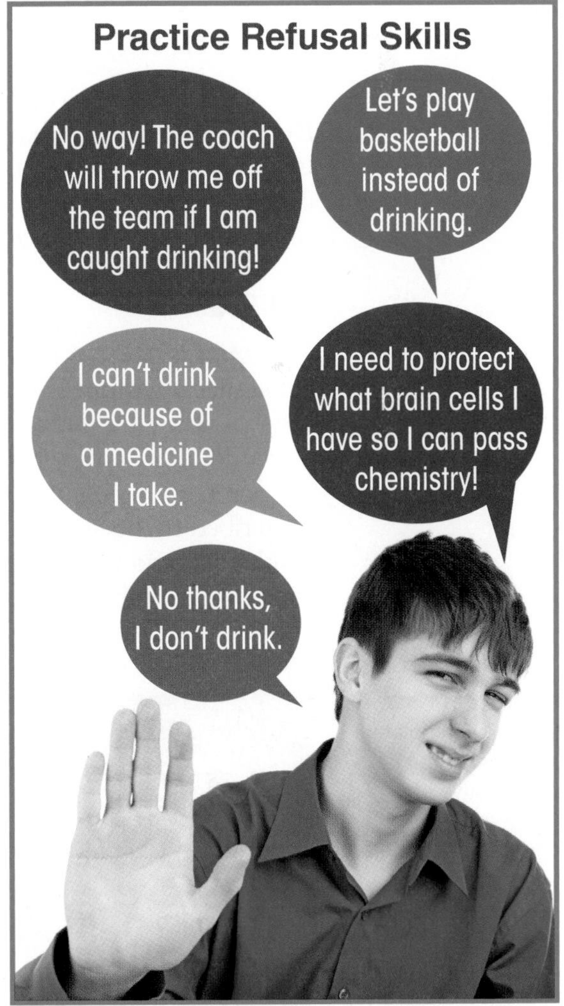
Practice Refusal Skills
No way! The coach will throw me off the team if I am caught drinking!
Let's play basketball instead of drinking.
I can't drink because of a medicine I take.
I need to protect what brain cells I have so I can pass chemistry!
No thanks, I don't drink.

Photo: Sabphoto/Shutterstock.com

Figure 23.13 Refusal skills are a powerful tool for resisting pressure in many situations. *Can you think of other strategies for withstanding peer pressure?*

Barbiturates and Tranquilizers

Two groups of depressants are barbiturates and tranquilizers. *Barbiturates* create a feeling of drowsiness.

Doctors may prescribe them for people who have trouble sleeping. *Tranquilizers* can calm emotions and relax muscles. Doctors may prescribe them for people who are feeling overly anxious or having muscle pain. Both of these groups of drugs can be addictive.

People who are taking barbiturates or tranquilizers must avoid drinking alcohol. The chemicals in the drugs and alcohol each intensify the effects of the other. The mixture can be deadly.

Inhalants

Inhalants are substances that are inhaled for their mind-numbing effects. Products used as inhalants include glue, spray paints, aerosols, and some petroleum products. People who abuse inhalants deeply breathe in their fumes. Inhalants can produce dizziness, confusion, and unconsciousness.

Abusing inhalants is very dangerous to health. Risks include a rapid increase in heart rate. Deeply breathing some substances can cause irreversible damage to lungs. Some inhalant abusers have also seen frightening visions and suffered permanent brain damage. Death from heart failure or suffocation is possible even with first-time inhalant use and addiction potential is high.

Narcotics

Narcotics are drugs that bring on sleep, relieve pain, and dull the senses. Doctors may prescribe a narcotic to help a patient relieve pain. Narcotic medications are often abused to get high or relieve anxiety. Narcotics used in excess can cause stupor, coma, and convulsions. The CDC reports that teen narcotic overdose rates have doubled since 1999.

Opioids

Opioids are a subclass of narcotics that include both natural and synthetic substances. Opium is extracted from the opium poppy plant and used to create the opioids *morphine* and *codeine*. Examples of synthetic opioids include heroin, oxycodone, fentanyl, tramadol, and methadone.

Some opioids, including codeine, morphine, oxycodone, and hydrocodone, are prescribed by doctors for pain relief. Doctors and pharmacists carefully monitor the availability and use of these drugs because *prescription painkiller use disorders (PPUD)* can develop quickly. When the prescription painkiller is no longer available, individuals with PPUD may turn to illegal and more risky substitutes like heroin (**Figure 23.14**).

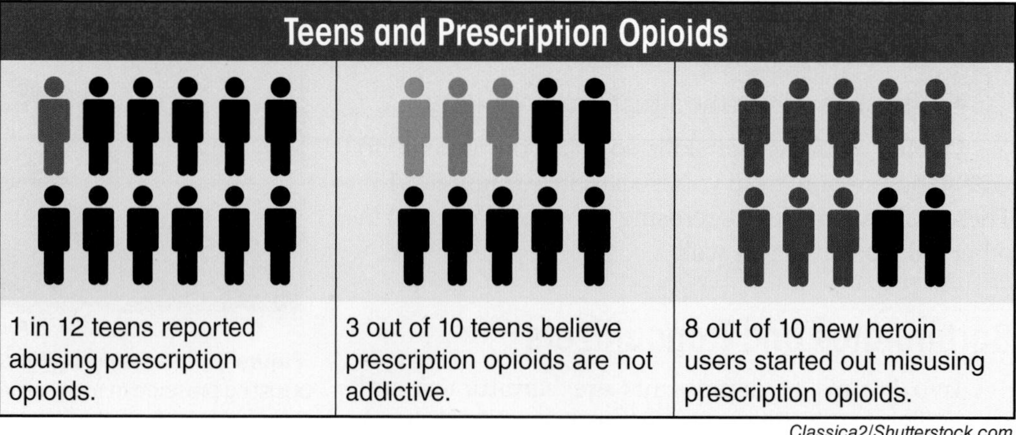

Teens and Prescription Opioids
1 in 12 teens reported abusing prescription opioids.
3 out of 10 teens believe prescription opioids are not addictive.
8 out of 10 new heroin users started out misusing prescription opioids.

Figure 23.14 Prescription opiate painkillers are just as addictive and dangerous as heroin and often lead to its use.

Classica2/Shutterstock.com

Heroin

Heroin is a highly addictive, powerful, and dangerous opioid that produces intense feelings of euphoria. It is often a white or brownish powder that may be diluted with other substances like sugar or powdered milk. This form of heroin is snorted or smoked. "Black tar" heroin is either sticky like road tar or hard like charcoal and is injected.

Repeated heroin use changes the structure of the brain and produces high levels of dependence on the drug. This dependence results in uncontrollable, risky drug seeking. A heroin overdose causes slow and shallow breathing, blue lips and fingernails, clammy skin, convulsions, coma, and possibly death.

Marijuana

Marijuana is the dry, green-brown mix of flowers, stems, seeds, and leaves from the cannabis plant. The US federal government classifies it as an illegal drug. It is usually smoked and often referred to as *pot* or *grass*. Marijuana contains over 400 chemicals. The effects of all these chemicals on the body are not fully known.

THC is the chief mood-altering ingredient in marijuana (**Figure 23.15**). It passes rapidly from the bloodstream into the brain. THC is fat-soluble and is attracted to the body's fatty tissues, where it can be stored for long periods. It takes about four weeks to rid the body of the THC from one marijuana cigarette.

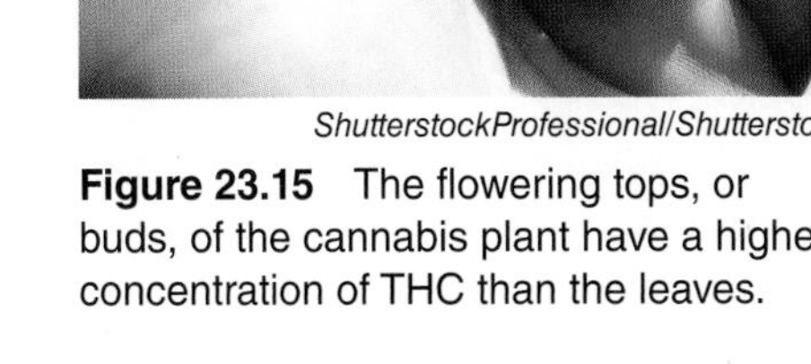

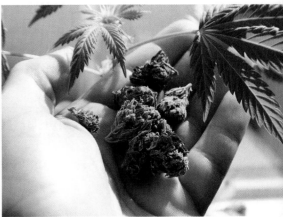

ShutterstockProfessional/Shutterstock.com

Figure 23.15 The flowering tops, or buds, of the cannabis plant have a higher concentration of THC than the leaves.

Effects of Marijuana Use

Marijuana users cannot predict what the drug's effects will be. Purity levels of the drug may vary. Other substances may also be added to marijuana. These substances can alter the drug's effects.

Short-term effects of marijuana include apathy, mood swings, and a loss of concentration. Memory, learning abilities, and coordination can also be affected. Side effects that are more serious include feelings of anxiety and even a sense of *psychosis* (a loss of contact with reality). Someone who has used marijuana may feel its effects for only an hour or two; however, his or her judgment may be impaired for four or more hours.

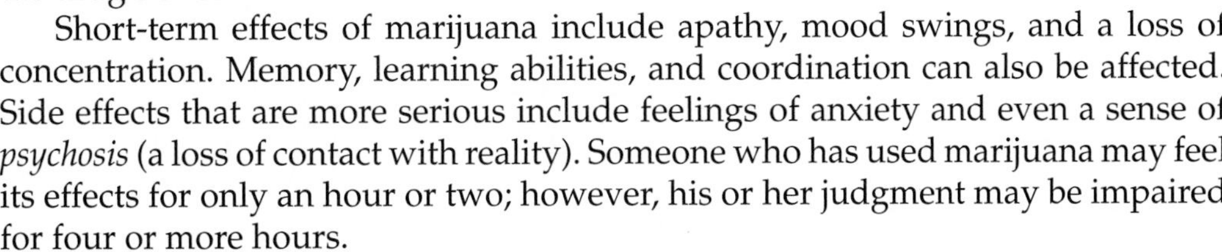

Marijuana cigarettes release five times as much carbon monoxide into the lungs as tobacco cigarettes. They also release three times as much tar. These agents can damage the heart and lungs. Marijuana also adversely affects the body's nervous and immune systems.

People who regularly use marijuana can become psychologically dependent on it. Smoking it can cause some of the same respiratory problems as smoking cigarettes. It is also common for marijuana users to experiment with drugs that are more powerful.

Legalization of Marijuana

Currently, individual states are given the right to decide the legality of growing and distributing cannabis for medical and nonmedical purposes. To grow, dispense, or possess marijuana in legally identified states, requires following specific state licensing laws.

People who are diagnosed with certain medical conditions are eligible to apply for a medical marijuana card. People must obtain written verification from their doctor that specifies their qualifying condition. Pain is the main reason people seek a prescription. It is not prescribed for people under 18 years of age. Nonmedical marijuana (or recreational marijuana) can only be purchased from approved dispensaries in very small quantities.

While some states have legalized marijuana, many others have not. The possession, use, or distribution of marijuana is still illegal in those states. Continued research is needed to help identify associated health benefits and health risks of marijuana use.

Hallucinogens

Drugs that cause the mind to create images that do not really exist are called ***hallucinogens***. The images the mind creates are called *hallucinations*. They may involve sounds and smells as well as visual images.

THE MOVEMENT CONNECTION

Strengthen Muscles and Mind

Why

Saying "no" to the offer of drugs from friends can be difficult. It is important to stay strong in these moments.

The next exercise helps develop muscular endurance. As you perform the move, imagine you are also training your mind to be strong when faced with difficult choices.

Apply

This exercise can be performed sitting or standing.

- Begin with good posture.
- Grasp a textbook with both hands and hold it above your head.
- Keep your elbows close to your ears as you slowly lower the book toward your back. Your arms should bend at the elbows while your shoulders remain stationary.
- Slowly raise the book back to the starting position.
- Repeat 10 times.

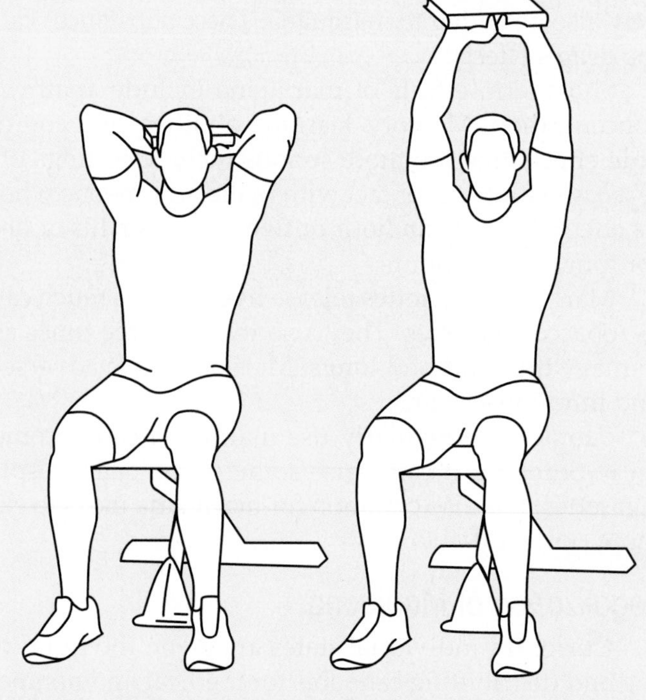

Users of hallucinogens cannot predict what effects the drugs will have from one use to the next. Some effects can be terrifying; some can be long lasting. Hallucinogens include ecstasy, LSD, PCP, and designer drugs.

Ecstasy

Ecstasy, or MDMA (methylenedioxymethamphetamine), is produced in illegal laboratories around the world. This club drug causes both hallucinogenic and stimulant effects. Ecstasy is also known by a number of street names including *disco biscuits*, *E*, *Molly*, and *clarity*.

Ecstasy is generally sold as a tablet. The tablets or capsules can be in various colors, shapes, and sizes. The drug is frequently imprinted with a design such as a butterfly, heart, star, or lightning bolt. Criminals with no education in drug manufacturing or chemistry are producing ecstasy. The amounts and types of ingredients can vary greatly from pill to pill. Ecstasy is not a safe drug for human consumption.

Ecstasy use can produce confusion, depression, sleep problems, drug craving, and severe anxiety. These problems may occur soon after taking the drug or days or weeks later. Chronic users have been identified as performing more poorly than nonusers on certain types of cognitive or memory tasks.

Using ecstasy in combination with other drugs can increase the potential for harm to the brain. When combined with methamphetamine, the health consequences increase. Major concerns include the toxic effect on the brain and interference with the body's ability to regulate temperature. When ecstasy is used with alcohol or other drugs, the chance of adverse health effects becomes even greater.

Ecstasy can be addictive for some people. Just under half of reported ecstasy users meet the criteria for dependence on the drug. Withdrawal symptoms include fatigue, loss of appetite, depressed feelings, and trouble concentrating.

LSD and PCP

LSD (lysergic acid diethylamide) and *PCP* (phencyclidine) are two very powerful, illegal, and dangerous hallucinogens. They are made in illegal laboratories. LSD can cause *flashbacks*. These are hallucinations that occur long after the drug has been used. PCP has been known to produce confusion and violent behavior.

Users of both of these drugs can quickly develop tolerance. Even a single use of either drug can cause mental illness. While under the effects of these drugs, many people engage in bizarre or dangerous behaviors. A number of users have died because of these behaviors.

Designer Drugs

Designer drugs are lab-created imitations of other street drugs. Most are much stronger than the drugs they are designed to imitate. When the drugs are being made in illegal laboratories, there is little concern for purity. They are never tested for contamination. These factors increase the already high risks of drug use.

Depending on the drug, effects may include confusion, depression, blurred vision, and nausea. Health risks include elevated blood pressure, rapid heartbeat, seizures, and permanent brain damage. Designer drugs may be hallucinogens, stimulants, or narcotics.

Drugs, Supplements, and Athletes

Drug testing of athletes is performed at all levels of competition. When tests are positive, the athlete is disqualified from the event and may be asked to leave the team. The risk of fines and even serving jail time is possible. Of course, illegal drug use is always prohibited; however, most prescription stimulants and narcotics are also banned. Diuretics and certain steroids are also banned. Most people agree athletics should be a display of natural rather than chemically altered physical ability.

Anabolic Steroids

Anabolic steroids are artificial hormones used to build a more muscular body. *Anabolic* means tissue building. These steroids are a synthetic version of the male sex hormone *testosterone*. Both males and females have been known to use anabolic steroids to help build muscles. Some people use them simply to look better. Others are motivated to use the steroids because they believe the drugs will help them excel in sports.

Some anabolic steroids are prescribed by doctors for medical reasons. However, many steroids are made and sold illegally. Like designer drugs, steroids may be produced under unsafe conditions and contamination may occur. Some products sold as muscle-building steroids are bogus. They contain no ingredients that promote muscle growth.

As long as people want to look bigger, run faster, and be stronger, the temptation to use ergogenic aids will exist. ***Ergogenic aids*** are any substances that are designed to enhance sports performance. They are promoted as providing a competitive edge. Ergogenic aids can be a drug, a dietary supplement, or other substance, and some can be harmful to your health.

Before giving in to this temptation, athletes need to know the facts about the dangers of anabolic steroid use. Even brief use of the steroids can have harmful effects on a growing body. In people of both sexes, anabolic steroids can cause problems with acne, stunted growth, digestion, sleep, urination, weight gain, hair loss, mood swings, and unusual levels of aggression. Use of these steroids has also led to coronary artery disease, liver tumors, and death. With these dangers, it is easy to understand why so many professional athletes have spoken out strongly against anabolic steroid use (**Figure 23.16**).

Possible Side Effects of Anabolic Steroid Use

For Females	For Males	For Both Males and Females
• Deepens the voice	• Increases risk of testicular or prostate cancer	• High blood pressure, heart attack, or stroke
• Increases facial and body hair	• Enlarges breasts	• Liver disease and possibly liver cancer
• Reduces breast size	• Shrinks testicles	• Acne, oily skin, and male-pattern hair loss
• Enlarges clitoris	• Decreases sperm count	• Irritability, violence, addiction, and mental disorders including mania and delusions

Marsan/Shutterstock.com

Figure 23.16 The potential health consequences of anabolic steroid use are serious.

CASE STUDY

Winning at What Cost?

Competitive sports have a long history of tragedy and even death resulting from drug or supplement use. Some athletes are driven to win at all costs and resort to drugs or supplementation to gain an advantage over their competition. These athletes often pay a dear price for their choices. Consider the following incidents in competitive sports.

In the 1960 Olympics, cyclist Knud Jensen collapsed and died during a competitive team trial. His blood contained amphetamines and nicotinyl nitrate.

In the 1976 Olympic Games, the East German women's swim team dominated the pool. The women later discovered the "vitamins" the team doctors were giving them were actually anabolic steroids. Years later, the women and their children are suffering serious health side effects as a result.

In the 1996 Olympics, Irish swimmer Michelle Smith was excited as she won her gold medals. Later, her urine sample tested positive for whiskey, which was believed to be masking the presence of other substances. This, along with other factors, cast doubt on her success.

Track star Marion Jones won five medals in the 2000 Olympic Games. She later admitted to taking steroids and the medals were taken away.

In recent years, professional baseball has had a number of high-profile players testing positive for or admitting use of steroids or other performance-enhancing substances.

Case Review

1. What are the potential consequences of performance-enhancing drug use in competitive sports?
2. Why is it important to test for drug use in athletes?

Use of Dietary Supplements

Suppose you read the following advertisement:

"Try the newly found secrets in ***Master Muscle Builder****. Two pills a day will enhance your muscle strength and endurance in just two weeks. The ingredients are all natural. Pay only $29.95 for a one-month supply! Buy it now to improve your looks and sports performance."*

Does the product in this advertisement sound too good to be true? Would you be willing to try it? Does the claim fit with what sports science professionals are saying? Perhaps if you really believed it worked, you would work out harder and then you would view the claim as true. Nonetheless, the product did not enhance your performance, your determination to achieve did.

Be aware of claims that sound too good to be true. Claims that rely on the testimonies of others to support an exaggerated expectation do not meet the rigors of scientific research.

Dietary supplements that claim to improve performance can be found in health-food stores and are frequently advertised in sports and fitness magazines as well as pop-up ads on the Internet. Some supermarkets also sell these supplements.

Dietary supplements can be very expensive. In addition, these supplements do not require approval from the Food and Drug Administration (FDA) before they are sold. This differs from drugs, which must be proven both safe and effective before they can be sold. If consumer claims are made that a supplement is "unsafe," then the FDA may choose to investigate. You cannot assume that a supplement is safe simply because it is sold at the local supermarket or health-food store.

Supplements can interact with medications. Supplement abuse may cause liver damage and even death. Most have little research to support the claims. Be sure to learn more about a dietary supplement before taking the advice of an enthusiastic coach or friend who is looking for a shortcut to "winning."

Drugs and Athletics

Drug testing in athletics usually screens for substances that either could provide an unfair advantage or could harm the athlete. Common types of drug tests used in schools include tests for marijuana, cocaine, amphetamine/methamphetamine, opiates, PCP, and alcohol.

Getting Help for a Substance Use Disorder

A substance use disorder (SUD) creates serious problems for the user as well as family, friends, and the community. Substance use disorders occur at any age and contribute to social, physical, mental, and public health problems. Someone with a substance use disorder must recognize a problem exists. Treatment is critical and the first step toward recovery is the desire to seek help. If you suspect someone you care about is abusing a substance, express your concern and offer to help (**Figure 23.17**).

Many forms of treatment are available for someone who has identified a problem with substance use. Treatments range from inpatient therapy in treatment centers, to self-help groups. No one approach is right for everyone.

Therapy programs are offered through hospitals and clinics. If needed, clients receive medical treatment for the physical effects of substance use. Trained counselors help them understand the effects at a personal level. For example, a drug problem

Figure 23.17 People who are abusing substances often try to hide the symptoms. Look for warning signs that support your suspicions.

Warning Signs of Substance Abuse
Physical Signs
• Bloodshot eyes, pupils that are larger or smaller than usual
• Changes in eating or sleeping patterns
• Decline in physical appearance and grooming
• Runny nose or persistent sniffling
• Sudden weight loss or weight gain
• Slurred speech, trembling, or impaired coordination
Behavioral Signs
• Change in relationships
• Secretive or suspicious behaviors
• Increased legal trouble from fighting or accidents
• Abrupt change in friends and activities
• Unexplained need for money

for one family member creates stress for all other members. Therapy programs help clients develop the emotional tools they need to stay drug free. Physicians and school counselors can refer people to therapy programs in their area.

Recovery from a substance use disorder is a lifelong process. Participation in self-help groups often follows other forms of treatment. These groups help people avoid *relapse* by attending regular meetings with supportive friends. ***Relapse*** is the return to use of a drug or alcohol after a period of recovery.

There are self-help groups for many substance use disorders. For example, a successful resource for help recovering from AUD is *Alcoholics Anonymous (AA).* AA is a community-based program that uses a self-help group format. Other self-help groups include *Narcotics Anonymous (NA)* and *Cocaine Anonymous (CA). Al-Anon* and *Alateen* are support groups for people who have family members with AUD. Contact information for these resources can be found on the Internet.

Health and fitness means abstaining from illegal drugs and alcohol, and taking medications only when needed, as directed by a healthcare provider, and for their intended purposes. Drug-free participation in sports protects your health and the integrity of the competition.

RECIPE FILE

Apple Crisp

8 SERVINGS

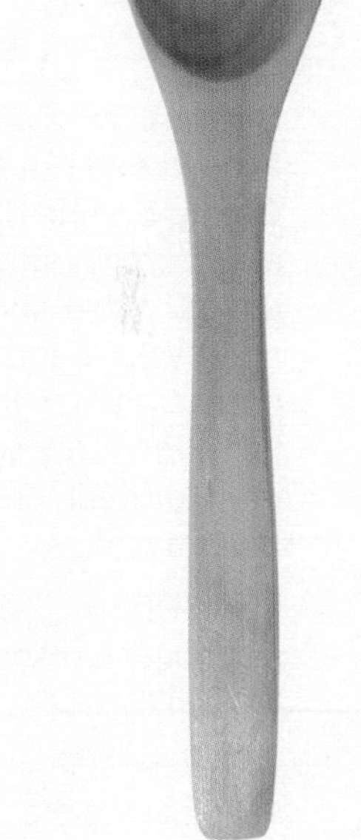

Ingredients

Topping

- ⅓ c. old-fashioned oats
- ¼ c. brown sugar
- ½ c. old-fashioned oats
- ½ t. cinnamon
- ¼ c. pecans, chopped
- 4 T. butter, cut into small pieces

Filling

- 5 medium apples, cored, peeled, and cut into ¼-inch slices
- ¼ c. maple syrup
- ½ t. cinnamon
- 1 T. pure vanilla extract

Directions

1. Preheat oven to 350°F (177°C).
2. Spray an 8-inch × 8-inch pan with cooking spray.
3. Place ⅓ cup oats in a food processor and pulse until it becomes oat flour.
4. Combine oat flour, brown sugar, old-fashioned oats, cinnamon, and pecans in a large bowl.
5. Cut butter into oat mixture using a pastry cutter. Refrigerate until ready to use.
6. Place apples, syrup, cinnamon, and vanilla in a large bowl and toss to combine.
7. Place apple mixture into pan and sprinkle evenly with topping mixture.
8. Place pan on a jelly roll pan and bake for 50 minutes, or until topping is golden brown.
9. Remove from oven and cool on wire rack.

PER SERVING: 189 CALORIES, 3 G PROTEIN, 34 G CARBOHYDRATE, 6 G FAT, 2 G FIBER, 4 MG SODIUM.

Chapter 23 Review and Expand

Reading Summary

All medications are drugs but not all drugs are medications. Illegal drugs are unlawful to buy and endanger your well-being. Dietary supplements are not reviewed and approved by the FDA for safety and effectiveness. It is important to read the information that accompanies both prescribed and over-the-counter medications to avoid undesired health events.

Drugs are absorbed and pass into the bloodstream, which carries them throughout the body. A number of factors affect how the body uses a drug.

Medication misuse is unintentional and medication abuse is intentional. Both can result in negative health effects. Psychoactive drugs are the most commonly misused or abused drugs. These include stimulants, depressants, narcotics, marijuana, and hallucinogens.

Many drugs and supplements used to enhance athletic performance can cause health problems, disqualification from competition, and worse. Many forms of treatment are available for individuals with substance use disorders.

Chapter Vocabulary

1. **Content Terms** With a partner, choose two words from the following list to compare. Create a Venn diagram to compare your words and identify differences. Write one term under the left circle and the other term under the right. Where the circles overlap, write three characteristics the terms have in common. For each term, write a difference of the term for each characteristic in its respective outer circle.

addiction
alcohol use disorder (AUD)
amphetamine
anabolic steroid
blood alcohol concentration (BAC)
cirrhosis
designer drug
dietary supplement
drug
drug-drug interaction
drug overdose
ergogenic aids
food-drug interaction
generic medication
hallucinogen
heroin
illegal drug
inhalant
medication
medication abuse
medication misuse
methamphetamine
narcotic
opioids
over-the-counter (OTC) medication
prescription medication
psychoactive drug
relapse
secondhand smoke
side effect
smokeless tobacco
stimulant
tolerance
withdrawal

2. **Academic Terms** Individually or with a partner, create a T-chart on a sheet of paper and list each of the following terms in the left column. In the right column, list an *antonym* (a word of opposite meaning) for each term in the left column.

adverse
counterpart
euphoria
partake

Review Learning

3. Explain the difference between a drug and a medication.
4. Why might a person choose a generic medication over a brand-name medication?
5. Explain the role of the liver in the body's use of drugs.
6. *True or false?* Drugs have no effect on nutrient absorption.
7. Compare medication misuse with medication abuse.
8. *True or false?* Coffee and tobacco both contain stimulants.
9. What are common health risks associated with nicotine and tobacco use?
10. What effect can drinking alcohol have on a teen's brain?
11. Why do physicians and pharmacists monitor prescribed opioids so carefully?
12. Marijuana can impair judgment for _____ or more hours.
13. List eight harmful effects anabolic steroids can have on a growing body.
14. Compare the FDA approval process for dietary supplements with drugs.

Self-Assessment Quiz

Complete the self-assessment quiz online to help you practice and expand your knowledge and skills.

Critical Thinking

15. **Apply** Predict the consequences that might result if the federal government made marijuana legal.
16. **Evaluate** What would be an appropriate warning label for electronic nicotine delivery systems (ENDS)?
17. **Create** Medication misuse is a greater problem for older adults. What is a possible solution to this problem?

Core Skills

18. **Listening** Interview a pharmacist to learn his or her opinion about the use of brand-name versus generic drugs. Prepare for the interview by developing a list of questions to help you better understand the topic. These questions will also encourage the exchange of information. If you are unclear about any answers, be sure to seek further explanation. Prepare a brief critique of the interview. Consider what aspects of the interview went well and how you could improve your interview skills for the future.
19. **Writing** Use authoritative sources to research the opioid and overdose epidemic in the United States. Write a two-page informative paper explaining what is contributing to this crisis, what conditions opioids are prescribed for, and what is being done to resolve this problem. Include a list of tips about how you and your family can protect yourselves from this danger.
20. **Science and Technology Literacy** Use presentation software to prepare an electronic presentation for middle school students to teach them how drug addiction alters the brain. Adjust the style and content of your presentation to your audience. Use digital media to add visual interest and improve understanding.
21. **Math** Search online for statistics about trends in electronic nicotine delivery system use compared with tobacco cigarettes in teens. Select data that interests you and present your findings in a bar graph.
22. **Writing** Write an opinion paper about whether the United States is a drug-dependent society compared with other developed countries in the world.
23. **Technology Literacy and Writing** Plan a blog about the dangers of anabolic steroid use. First, consider who will be reading your blog and how to make the topic appealing to them. Next, identify three main points that you want to cover. Then, be sure to give your blog a clever title. After you finish writing, be sure to edit and revise your content before posting.
24. **Math** To qualify as decaffeinated, coffee must have at least 97% of its caffeine removed. If a cup of brewed coffee contains 160 mg of caffeine, what is the maximum amount of caffeine its decaffeinated version could contain? (Round answer to nearest whole milligram.)
25. **Speaking** Prepare and give a speech discussing the benefits and drawbacks of drug testing for high school athletics. Include a discussion of current laws and school policy. Use vocabulary that is suitable for your audience. Prepare questions to stimulate participation and gauge understanding. As you present, speak clearly and at a volume that can be heard by all attending.
26. **Listening** Interview a medical professional to learn what medical conditions qualify for medical marijuana use and how it benefits those patients. Ask what form of marijuana is most effective to consume. Ask his or her opinion about why medical marijuana is only legal in some states. Discuss the implications of this.
27. **Technology Literacy** Research to learn about trends in substance abuse worldwide. Create a digital poster to share your findings. Consider readability and appeal as you choose fonts, colors, and layout of your poster.
28. **Career Readiness Practice** Suppose you work in a manufacturing facility that utilizes heavy machinery. Safe actions are important to prevent employee injuries. In an effort to promote employee safety and health, the company strictly follows a random drug testing policy. One of your coworkers often bragged to you about his off-hours alcohol and drug use—the effects of which showed in his work performance. You question whether his actions were responsible, but go about your work without saying anything. After your coworker was not at work for three days, you asked your boss about him. All that your boss said was "He won't be back." You wonder if he failed his drug test. Then you begin to ask yourself, "Did I act responsibly in this situation by not talking to my boss about my coworker's behavior? Were my coworkers in danger because of these actions?" How should you handle situations such as this in the future?

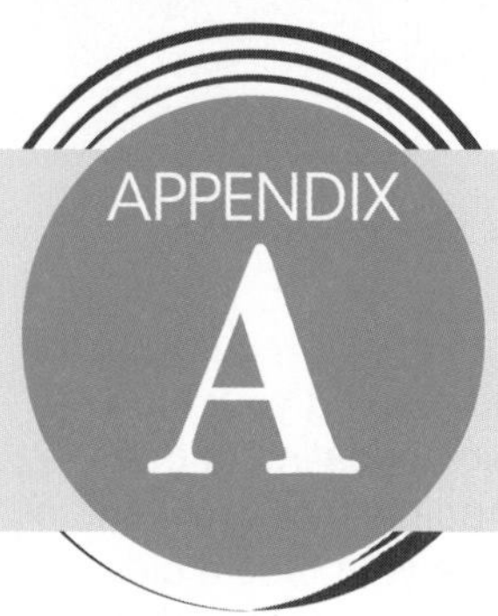

Career Planning and Preparation

Skills for the Workplace

A *job* is the work a person does regularly in order to earn money. A *career* is a series of related jobs in the same profession. A job may be a part-time position you work after school. A career is a position for which you prepare by attending school or completing specialized training. Over time, a job can turn into a career.

All employment opportunities require skills. A *skill* is something an individual does well. Skills are the foundational elements of all career fields. *Job-specific skills* are critical skills necessary to perform the required work-related tasks of a position. Job-specific skills are acquired through work experience and education or training. Without them, an individual will be unlikely to perform the job successfully.

Employability skills are applicable skills used to help an individual find a job, perform in the workplace, and gain success in a job or career. Employability skills are known as *foundation skills*. They are also known as *soft skills* or *transferrable skills*. You have already acquired many of these skills; however, some of them are gained through life experience. Others may be gained from working at a job. Some of these may be gained in social situations. These skills are not specific to one career but are transferrable to many different jobs and professional positions. Examples of employability skills are shown in **Figure A.1**.

Career Clusters

Studying the career clusters is a good way to begin analyzing the principles of career fields. The *career clusters*, shown in **Figure A.2**, are 16 groups of occupational and career specialties. Career clusters are centered on related career fields.

Employability Skills			
Basic skills	Reading Writing	Speaking Listening	Technology Mathematics
Thinking skills	Decision making Creative thinking	Problem solving Visualization	Reasoning
People skills	Social perceptiveness Leadership	Teamwork Cultural competence	
Personal qualities	Self-management Integrity	Honesty Social responsibility	

Figure A.1

The 16 Career Clusters
Agriculture, Food & Natural Resources Careers involving the production, processing, marketing, distribution, financing, and development of agricultural commodities and resources.
Architecture & Construction Careers involving the design, planning, managing, building, and maintaining of buildings and structures.
Arts, A/V Technology & Communications Careers involving the design, production, exhibition, performance, writing, and publishing of visual and performing arts.
Business Management & Administration Careers involving the planning, organizing, directing, and evaluation of functions essential to business operations.
Education & Training Careers involving the planning, management, and providing of training services.
Finance Careers involving the planning and providing of banking, insurance, and other financial-business services.
Government & Public Administration Careers involving governance, national security, foreign service, revenue and taxation, regulation, and management and administration.
Health Science Careers involving planning, managing, and providing health services, health information, and research and development.
Hospitality & Tourism Careers involving management, marketing, and operations of foodservice, lodging, and recreational businesses.
Human Services Careers involving family and human needs.
Information Technology Careers involving the design, development, support, and management of software, hardware, and other technology-related materials.
Law, Public Safety, Corrections & Security Careers involving the planning, management, and providing of legal services, public safety, protective services, and homeland security.
Manufacturing Careers involving the planning, management, and processing of materials to create completed products.
Marketing Careers involving the planning, management, and performance of marketing and sales activities.
Science, Technology, Engineering & Mathematics Careers involving the planning, management, and providing of scientific research and technical services.
Transportation, Distribution & Logistics Careers involving the planning, management, and movement of people, materials, and goods.

Figure A.2

Within each of the 16 career clusters are multiple career pathways. *Career pathways* are subgroups within the career clusters that reflect occupations requiring similar knowledge and skills. These pathways include careers that range from entry-level to those that require advanced college degrees and many years of experience. All the careers within the pathways share a foundation of common knowledge and skills.

Levels of Careers

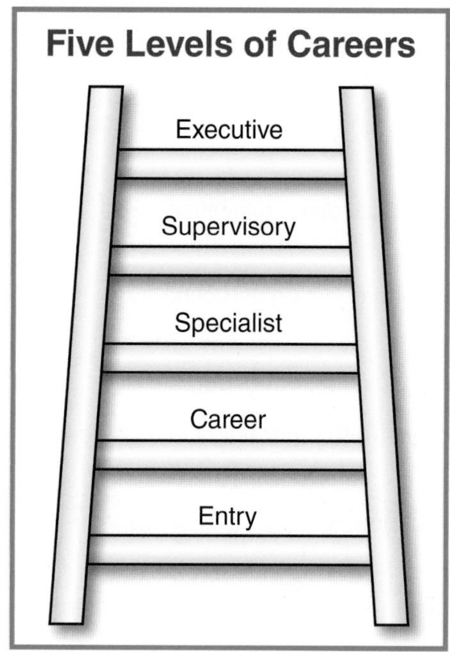

Goodheart-Willcox Publisher

In each career area, there are many opportunities for employment. Positions are generally grouped by skill level or education. A *career ladder* is an outline of jobs in a given career field that are available at different levels of education, training, and experiences. There are five levels of careers that make up a career ladder.

- An *entry-level* position is usually a person's first or beginning job. It requires very little previous training.
- A *career-level* position requires an employee to have the skills and knowledge for continued employment and advancement in the field.
- A *specialist-level* position requires specialized knowledge and skills in a specific field of study. However, someone in this position does not supervise other employees.
- A *supervisory-level* position requires specialized knowledge and skills. It also includes management responsibility over other employees.
- An *executive-level* position is the highest level. This position is responsible for the planning, organization, and management of a company.

Career Plan

A *career plan* is a list of steps on a time line an individual can follow to reach his or her career goals. It is also known as a *postsecondary plan*. A career plan should include education options. Education options include four-year colleges, two-year colleges, or technical schools. It should also address current job opportunities in your career of interest.

There is no set format for writing a career plan. Many free career plan templates can be found on the Internet. To create a plan, you should first conduct a self-assessment and then set SMART goals. You will continue revising the career plan as you achieve your goals and set new ones.

Conducting a Self-Assessment

A *self-assessment* is the first step in evaluating your aptitudes, abilities, values, and interests. By conducting a self-assessment, you can focus your energy on what is necessary for you to become successful in a career. Some self-assessment techniques are thinking or writing exercises. Others are in the form of tests, such as a personality test. Your career counselor can help you conduct a self-assessment.

Consider what you like to do and what you do well. This can give you clues to aid your self-assessment. If you always do well in math class, you may find success in a career that requires working with numbers. On the other hand, if you do not do well in English class, a career that requires writing may not be your best match. Identifying a career that you will enjoy and excel in begins with finding out what you like to do.

What is your *work style*? Some individuals prefer to work independently. Others need constant direction to accomplish a task. Mornings are more productive for some workers, while others perform better in the afternoons. Casual dress influences some people to perform well. Business dress makes others more effective on the job.

When taking a self-assessment, strive to identify your aptitudes, abilities, values, and interests. Learning this information can reveal careers for which you are well suited.

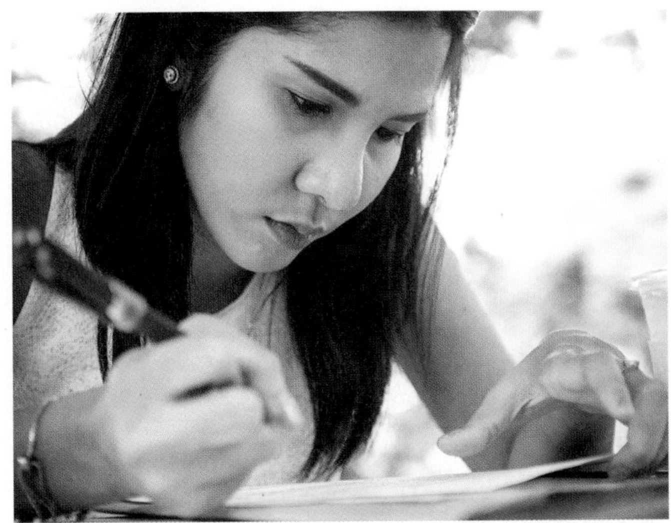
noPPonPat/Shutterstock.com

Aptitudes

An *aptitude* is a characteristic that an individual has developed naturally. Aptitudes are also called *talents*. When a person naturally excels at a task without practicing or studying, he or she has an aptitude for it. For example, a person with an aptitude for music may be very good at accurately humming a tune or keeping a beat, even if he or she has never studied music. Some examples of aptitudes include:

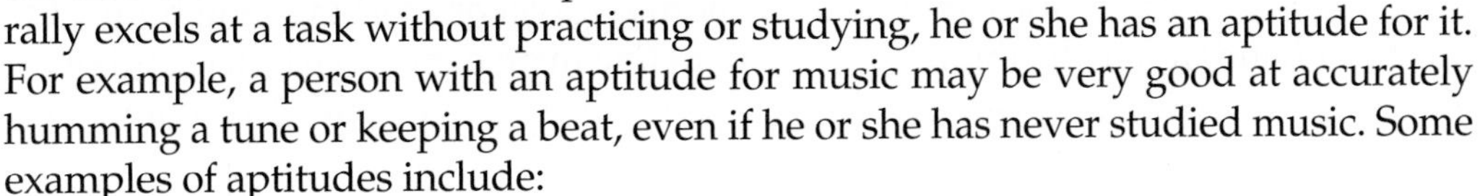

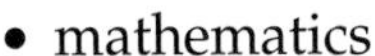

- mathematics
- drawing
- writing
- sports

Abilities

An *ability* is the mastery of a skill or the capacity to do something. Having aptitudes and skills are supported or limited by a person's abilities. For instance, a student who has musical aptitude and skill might not have the ability to perform under pressure in musical concerts. Examples of abilities are:

- teaching others
- multitasking
- thinking logically
- speaking multiple languages

While an aptitude is something a person is born with, an ability can be acquired. Often, it is easier to develop abilities that match your natural aptitudes. For example, someone with an aptitude for acquiring languages may have the ability to speak French. A person without an aptitude for acquiring language can also learn to speak French, but it may be more difficult. Aptitudes and abilities do not always match. Someone with an aptitude for repairing machines may not enjoy doing this type of work and never develop the ability.

Values

The principles and beliefs that an individual considers important are values. *Values* are beliefs about the things that matter most to an individual. They are developed as people mature and learn. Your values will affect your life in many ways.

They influence how you relate to other people and make decisions about your education and career.

Your work values can provide great insight into what kind of career will appeal to you. For some individuals, work values include job security. For others, the number of vacation days is important. Everyone has a set of work values that are taken into consideration when choosing a career path. Examples of values include:

- perfection
- equality
- harmony
- status

Closely related to values are family responsibilities and personal priorities. These can have a direct impact on career choice. For example, if you expect to have a large family, you may decide that time is a family responsibility. You may want to spend as much time as possible with your children as they grow. This may mean choosing a career that does not typically require travel or working long hours. On the other hand, it may be important to you to live in an expensive house and drive an expensive car. This personal priority will require a career with an income level that supports these choices.

Interests

An *interest* is a feeling of wanting to learn more about a topic or to be involved in an activity. Your interests might include a subject, such as history. Your interests can also include hobbies, such as biking or cooking. There is a good chance there is a career that would allow you to do what you enjoy as a profession.

Your interests may change over time. Try to determine if there is a uniting theme to your interests. When considering your interests, look at the "big picture." For example, you may enjoy being on the cross-country team right now. In a few years, a career as an arborist might suit you because you enjoy physical activity and being outdoors. Examples of interests include:

- art and creativity
- technology
- sports and adventure
- collecting

Setting Goals

Another step in the career-planning process is to set goals. A *goal* is something a person wants to achieve in a specified time period. There are two types of goals: short term and long term. A *short-term goal* is one that can be achieved in less than one year. An example of a short-term goal may be getting an after-school job for the fall semester. A *long-term goal* is one that will take a longer period of time to achieve, usually more than one year. An example of a long-term goal is to attend college to earn a four-year degree.

Goal setting is the process of deciding what a person wants to achieve. Your goals must be based on what you want for your life. Well-defined career goals follow the SMART goal model. Recall that *SMART goals* are specific, measurable, attainable, realistic, and timely, as illustrated in **Figure A.3**.

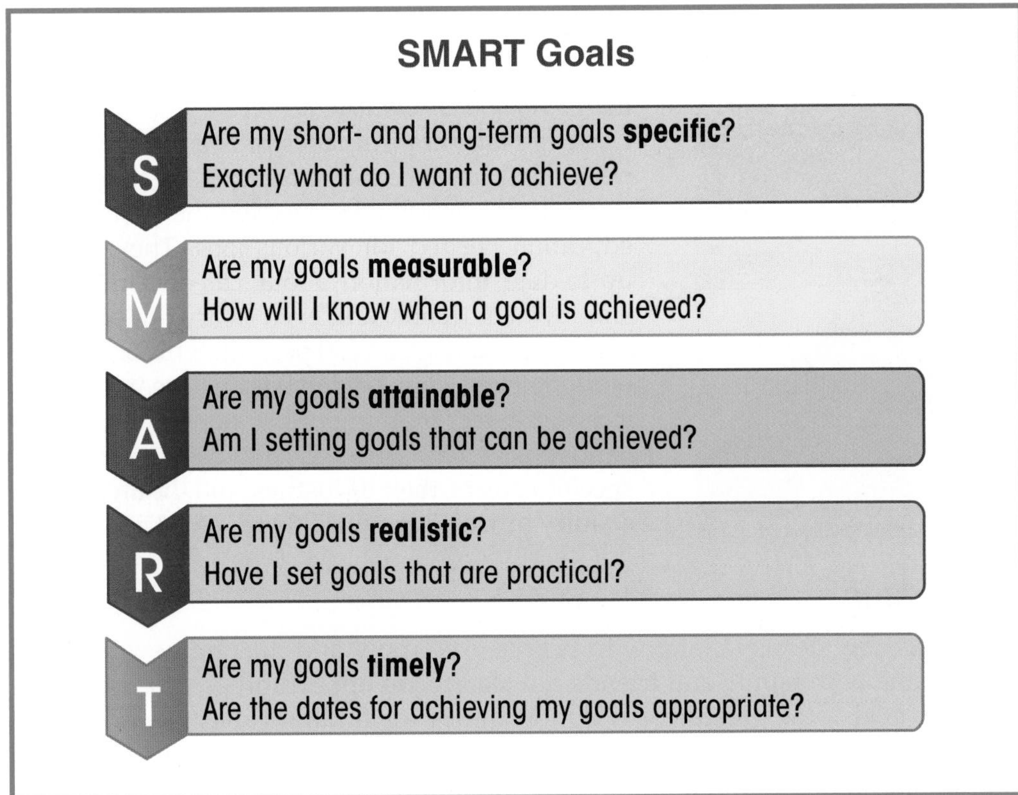
SMART Goals
S
Are my short- and long-term goals specific?
Exactly what do I want to achieve?
M
Are my goals measurable?
How will I know when a goal is achieved?
A
Are my goals attainable?
Am I setting goals that can be achieved?
R
Are my goals realistic?
Have I set goals that are practical?
T
Are my goals timely?
Are the dates for achieving my goals appropriate?

Figure A.3

Finding Career Information

There are many resources for career research. They will help you evaluate which careers and current job opportunities make the best use of your talents, skills, and interests.

Internet Research

The Internet is a good place to start when you begin researching your future career. Researching various professions, employment trends, industries, and prospective employers provides insight to careers that may interest you. It is also important to investigate current and future job opportunities for various occupations. Certain potential careers may have low demand now, but may be increasing in the future. And the opposite may be true: there are jobs that are plentiful now but will be phased out in the future.

The Occupational Information Network (O*NET) is a valuable resource for career information. The most comprehensive database of occupational information, O*NET Online, was created by the US Department of Labor and is updated regularly. This website contains data on salary, growth, openings, education requirements, skills and abilities, work tasks, and related occupations for more than 1,000 careers. The database can be searched by career cluster.

The Internet is also a great tool to use when you begin applying for jobs. You can search for available jobs in almost any career field. When you find a job that interests you, you can submit a résumé, job application, and cover letter via the Internet.

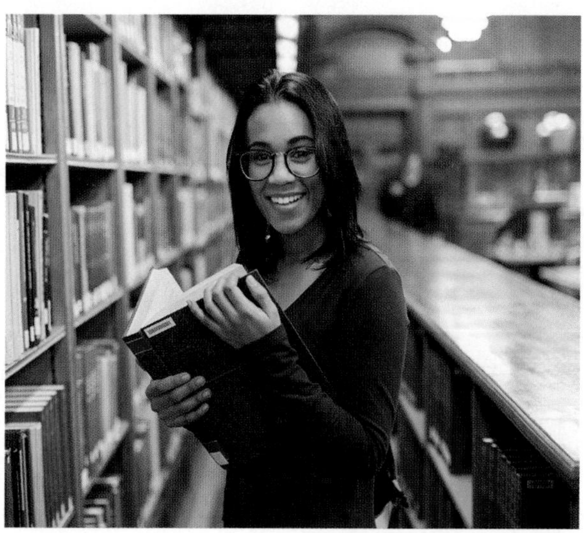

Nick Starichenko/Shutterstock.com

Career Handbooks

The US Bureau of Labor Statistics publishes the *Occupational Outlook Handbook* and the *Career Guide to Industries*. An *industry* is a group of businesses that produce the same type of goods or services. These handbooks describe the training and education needed for various jobs. They provide up-to-date information about careers, industries, employment trends, and even salary outlooks. The average person spends 30 percent of his or her time working every day. Understanding the industry of a chosen career is an important step to take. Career handbooks offer a great place to begin researching specific careers, their industries, and the areas of the country or world in which these industries thrive.

Networking

Networking means talking with people you know and making new contacts. Networking with family and friends can lead to job opportunities. The more contacts you make, the greater your opportunities for finding career ideas. Talking with people you know can help you evaluate career opportunities. It also may lead to potential jobs.

There are many professional organizations that encourage students and professionals to join and interact with other professionals. Professional organizations typically provide networking events, job opening notification, and continuing education opportunities for members. Examples of professional organizations for food and nutrition careers include:

- Academy of Nutrition and Dietetics
- American Culinary Federation
- Institute of Food Technologists

Informational Interviews

Informational interviews can give you unique insight into a career. *Informational interviewing* is a strategy used to interview a professional to ask for advice and direction, rather than for a job opportunity. This type of interview will help you get a sense of what it is like to work in that profession.

It can also be a valuable networking opportunity. By talking with someone in the field, you can learn more about what is expected. You can also learn what types of jobs are available and other information about an industry.

At informational interviews, be as professional and polite as you would in any other interview situation. Follow up with your contact after an interview. Send a thank-you message to show appreciation for his or her time.

Education, Training, and Certification

There are many steps you will take as you plan your career. Your educational needs will depend on your career interests and goals. Some careers require a high school diploma followed by technical training or a bachelor degree. Others require a master degree or doctorate, as well. Still others require professional certification. Early career planning can help you make decisions about your education. Investigating the opportunities and costs of future education, training, and certification is an investment in your future.

Education, training, and certification have a direct effect on income and career potential. Some employers pay increased salaries for those individuals who continue training in their positions and become more skilled in their areas. Certain positions may require additional training in order to advance career potential.

Education

Formal education is the education received in a school, college, or university. Most careers require a college degree. However, for an entry-level position, a high school diploma may get you in the door. Jobs higher on the career ladder often require additional formal education.

High School

During high school, a variety of subjects is covered. This gives students a well-rounded education to serve as a foundation for life-long learning. English, history, and science are some of the subjects all students study in high school. At the end of four years, students graduate and receive a *high school diploma*.

Postsecondary Education

Postsecondary education is any education achieved after high school. This includes all two- and four-year colleges and universities. Common postsecondary degrees are an associate degree and a bachelor degree. An associate degree is a two-year degree. A bachelor degree is a four-year degree.

Graduate and Postgraduate Education

Education received after an individual has earned a bachelor degree is *graduate education*. Master degrees are graduate degrees. Education beyond a master degree is called *postgraduate education*. Doctorate degrees are postgraduate degrees.

Graduate study often builds on the same subject area, or a closely related subject, in which the bachelor degree was earned. For example, a student who earned a Bachelor of Science in accounting may pursue a Master of Science degree in business.

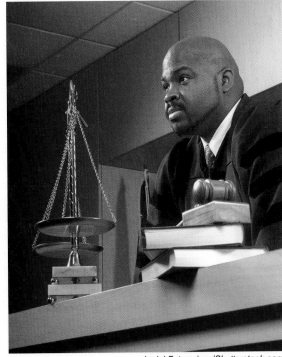

Junial Enterprises/Shutterstock.com

Continuing Education

Some careers that have professional licenses require *continuing education* classes. These classes are completed to maintain the license. Completing these classes earns the student *continuing education units (CEUs)*. If you are a teacher, for example, your school system may require that you earn a specified number of CEUs every year.

Another form of continuing education is more commonly called *adult education* or *adult ed*. These classes are for people age 18 or older and traditionally focus on basic skills. Classes are offered in a wide variety of topics ranging from learning computer skills to the English language.

Training

A college degree is not necessary for all career paths. Before taking on the expense of college classes, decide if college is right for you and your goals. There are many options for career training, including occupational training, internships, apprenticeships, and military service.

Occupational Training

Training for a specific career can be an option for many technical, trade, and technology fields. *Occupational training* is education that prepares you for a specific type of work. This type of training typically costs less than a traditional college education. It can also be completed in less time.

Internships

An *internship* is a short-term position with a sponsoring organization that gives the intern an opportunity to gain on-the-job experience in a certain field of study or occupation. Internships can be paid or unpaid. Often, high schools, colleges, and universities offer school credit for completing internships. Internships are an opportunity to gain work experience while working on an education.

Apprenticeships

An *apprenticeship* is a combination of on-the-job training, work experience, and classroom instruction. Apprenticeships are typically available to those who want to learn a trade or a technical skill. The apprentice works on mastering the skills required to work in the trade or field under the supervision of a skilled tradesperson.

Military Service

Service in the military can provide opportunities to receive skilled training, often in highly specialized technical areas. In addition to receiving this training, often it can be translated into college credit or professional credentials. After completing military service, there are many benefits available to veterans. For example, the *GI Bill* is a law that provides financial assistance for veterans pursuing education or training. Other forms of tuition assistance are also available.

Some people choose to enter the armed forces through the *Reserve Officers Training Corp (ROTC)*. Each branch of the military has an ROTC program at selected colleges and universities. Some high schools have Junior ROTC programs. The purpose of the ROTC program is to train commissioned officers for the armed forces. It can provide tuition assistance in exchange for a commitment to military service. Students enrolled in this program take classes just like other college students. The program is considered an elective; however, students also receive basic military and officer training. Information is available on the Today's Military website sponsored by the US Department of Defense. Opportunities available in the armed forces are also outlined in the *Occupational Outlook Handbook*.

Professional Certification

Some professional organizations offer certifications. *Certification* is a professional status earned by an individual after passing an exam focused on a specific body of knowledge. The individual usually prepares for the exam by taking classes and studying content that will be tested.

Some jobs require a professional certification. There are many types of certifications in most industries and trades. For example, a hospital might require a dietitian to be certified as a qualification for the job. Other employers may prefer, but not require, certification. Certification requirements should be considered when creating a career plan.

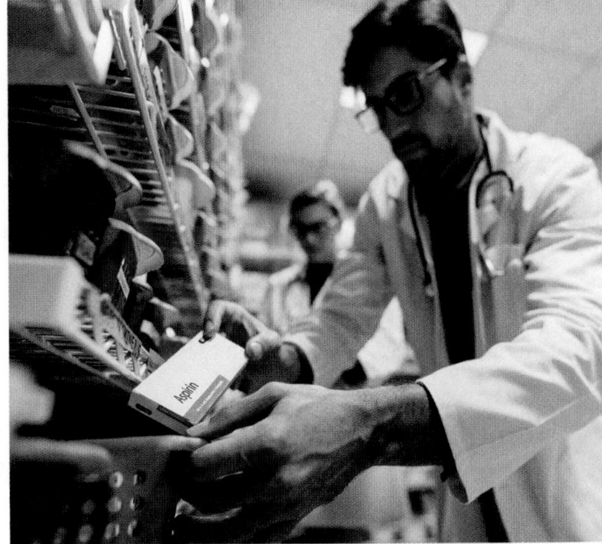

Jacob Lund/Shutterstock.com

There are certifications that must be renewed on a regular basis. For example, many certifications sponsored by Microsoft are only valid for the specific version of software. When the next version is released, another exam must be taken to be certified for the update. Other certifications require regular continuing education classes to ensure individuals are current with up-to-date information in the profession.

Some certifications are not subject-specific. Instead, they verify that an individual has employability skills. These certifications confirm that the person possesses the skills to be a contributing employee. The focus of these certifications is on workplace skills. Individuals who earn this type of certification have demonstrated they possess the qualities necessary to become effective employees.

Writing a Résumé

When looking for employment, you must sell your talents and skills to a potential employer. A job applicant must persuade the hiring manager that his or her skills and experience match the qualifications of the job being sought. A *résumé* is a document that profiles a person's career goals, education, and work history. Think of a résumé as a snapshot that shows who you are and why you would be an asset as an employee.

A résumé is the first impression that potential employers will have of you. It must be well written and free of errors. A résumé that contains typographical errors or poor language usage reflects negatively on the applicant. The *four Cs of communication* are clarity, conciseness, courtesy, and correctness. These should be applied when writing for employment. When finished, each line should be proofread and checked for correct grammar, vocabulary, and punctuation.

A general rule of thumb is that a résumé should be one page. Résumés have standard parts that employers expect to see. A typical résumé is shown in **Figure A.4**. This student is applying for a job as a dietetic technician, which is a position in the human services career cluster. Positions in the human services career cluster share many job titles with the health sciences cluster.

Jamal Barton
123 Eastwood Terrace
Saratoga Springs, NY 60123
518-555-9715
jbarton@e-mail.edu

CAREER OBJECTIVE
A mature and responsible high school senior seeks an entry-level job as a dietetic technician.

WORK EXPERIENCE
Saratoga Springs Community Hospital, Saratoga Springs, NY
September 2017 to present
Diet Office Clerk

- Maintained and updated nutrition related data in the dietary department.
- Visited patients and provided assistance with menu selection.
- Collected nutritional data for nutrition screening by the clinical dietitian.
- Reviewed patient trays for accuracy.

Saratoga Springs Assisted-Living Facility, Saratoga Springs, NY
September 2016 to September 2017
Foodservice Worker

- Set and cleared dining tables for residents.
- Served food to residents.
- Performed minor food preparation.

EDUCATION
Hunter High School, Saratoga Springs, NY
Expected graduation date: May 2020
Relevant coursework: Introduction to Foods, Nutrition for Life, Food Science

HONORS

- Hunter High School Honor Roll, 8 quarters
- Won 1st place in the National FCCLA STAR Event, 2018

ACTIVITIES

- Saratoga High School FCCLA, two years

Figure A.4

Name and Personal Information

The top of the résumé should present your name, address, telephone number, and e-mail address. Use an e-mail address that is your real name, or at least a portion of it. E-mails with nicknames or screen names do not make a professional impression. Before you begin applying for jobs via e-mail, set up an e-mail address that you will use only for professional communication.

Career Objective

A *career objective* is a summary of the type of job for which the applicant is looking. An example of an objective is, "To gain industry experience as a dietetic technician while earning my dietetics degree." The career objective should match or be related to the position for which you are applying.

Work Experience

The work experience section of a résumé includes details about the jobs you have held in the past as well as your current job. The information in this section is typically the main focus of the employer's attention.

As you begin composing this section, list your current or most recent employer first. This format is known as a chronological résumé. A *chronological résumé* lists information in reverse chronological order, with the most recent employer listed first.

For each work experience entry, include the company name, your job title, and the duration of time you worked there. List the responsibilities and details about the position you held. Do not list the addresses or telephone numbers of previous employers. This information will be provided on a job application.

Volunteer work may also be listed as work experience. Employers are especially interested in community-oriented applicants who do volunteer work. Be certain to list any volunteer activities and the length of time you have participated in the activities.

Education

The education section should list the name of your high school and where it is located. Indicate the year in which you will graduate. Briefly describe any courses you have taken that are relevant to the job for which you are applying. List any certifications you have earned, special courses or training programs completed, and any other educational achievements related to the job you are seeking.

Honors, Activities, and Publications

Employers look for well-rounded individuals. Include information on your résumé that shows your involvement in activities outside of work or school. These can be separate sections, or they can be combined into one section. List applicable honors, activities, or publications with the corresponding year in which each occurred. If you have been a leader in an organization, note that experience. If you are a

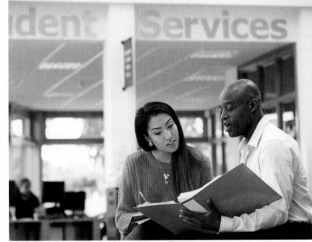

Monkey Business Images/Shutterstock.com

member of a career and technical student organization (CTSO), include the name of the organization and number of years you have been a member.

References

It is customary for references to be provided only when requested by the employer. For that reason, references should not be included on your résumé. Instead, create a separate list of references.

A *reference* is a person who can comment on the qualifications, work ethic, personal qualities, and work-related aspects of another person's character. Your list of references should include three or four people for whom you have worked and one person who knows you socially. Do not include relatives. Ask permission from the people you intend to use as references. Include each person's name, title, and contact information.

To be prepared, bring copies of your list of references to the job interview. Employers who require references in advance usually indicate this in the job advertisement. Otherwise, you will be told during the interview process when references are needed.

Portfolio

In some cases, candidates may be asked to submit a portfolio as part of the application process. A *portfolio* is a selection of related materials that an individual has created to show qualifications, skills, and talents to support a career or personal goal. For example, a dietitian may have a portfolio that includes nutrition-related blogs or articles.

Writing a Cover Message

A *cover message*, or *cover letter*, is a letter or e-mail sent with a résumé to introduce the applicant and summarize his or her reasons for applying for a job. It is a sales message written to persuade the reader to grant an interview. A cover message provides an opportunity to focus a potential employer's attention on your background, skills, and work experience that match the job you are seeking. Writing a cover message is an important part of applying for a job. It sets the tone for the résumé that follows. **Figure A.5** shows an example of a cover letter that is sent by e-mail.

Introduction

The cover message should begin with an introduction. The introduction should tell the employer who you are and why you are applying. If applying for a specific position, state the title of the position.

If responding to an advertisement, mention where you found the ad. For example, you might be responding to a posting on the company's website. Mention this in the introduction.

If sending a general letter of application, explain in specific terms how you identified the company and why you are interested in working there. If someone gave you the name of the employer to contact, mention the person and his or her connection to the company.

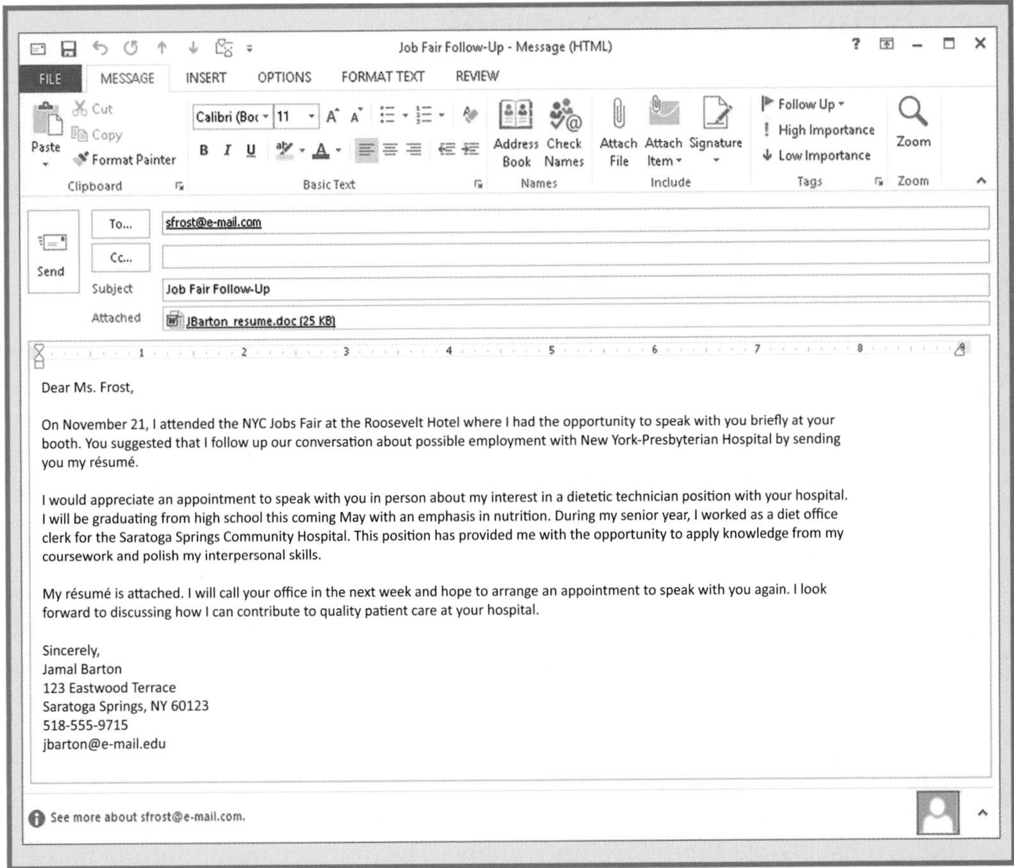

Job Fair Follow-Up - Message (HTML)

To... sfrost@e-mail.com

Cc...

Subject Job Fair Follow-Up

Attached JBarton resume.doc (25 KB)

Dear Ms. Frost,

On November 21, I attended the NYC Jobs Fair at the Roosevelt Hotel where I had the opportunity to speak with you briefly at your booth. You suggested that I follow up our conversation about possible employment with New York-Presbyterian Hospital by sending you my résumé.

I would appreciate an appointment to speak with you in person about my interest in a dietetic technician position with your hospital. I will be graduating from high school this coming May with an emphasis in nutrition. During my senior year, I worked as a diet office clerk for the Saratoga Springs Community Hospital. This position has provided me with the opportunity to apply knowledge from my coursework and polish my interpersonal skills.

My résumé is attached. I will call your office in the next week and hope to arrange an appointment to speak with you again. I look forward to discussing how I can contribute to quality patient care at your hospital.

Sincerely,
Jamal Barton
123 Eastwood Terrace
Saratoga Springs, NY 60123
518-555-9715
jbarton@e-mail.edu

See more about sfrost@e-mail.com.

Figure A.5

Body

The body of the cover message is where to demonstrate your positive work behaviors and qualities that make you employable. This may include illustrating your ambition, determination, and skills. Examine the job description for the position and identify the positive traits and skills the employer seeks. Then, focus on these traits and skills. Explain why you are qualified and how your skills and experience make you the best candidate for the job.

Conclusion

The cover message should end with a conclusion. The conclusion has two purposes:

- request an interview
- make it easy for the reader to grant an interview

Leave no doubt in the reader's mind about your desire to be contacted for an interview. Specifically request an interview. State how and when you can be reached to schedule an interview. Provide the information necessary to arrange an interview. You may also state how and when you will follow up to schedule an interview.

Applying for Employment

Applying for employment may involve completing a form, submitting a résumé, or both. This may be done in person, by mail, or online. However, before applying, it is important to do one final review of your résumé and cover message. Make sure both are accurate and free from errors. If you are submitting an application by mail, follow the rules for formatting a letter.

Applying in Person

The traditional way to apply for employment is to print your résumé, cover message, and portfolio and hand deliver them to a potential employer. All documents should be on the same high-quality white or off-white paper and printed using a laser printer. Do not fold or staple the documents. Instead, use a large envelope or paperclip the pages together. If using an envelope, print your name on the outside and list the components included.

Be prepared to complete a job application. A *job application* is a form with spaces for contact information, education, and work experience. Even though much of this information may be repeated on your résumé, many companies require a job application to be completed. Use blue or black ink and your best penmanship. Like a résumé or cover message, an employment application needs to be free of spelling, grammar, and usage errors. Carefully review the form before submitting it.

Applying Online

Today, most people submit résumés online. The first step in submitting may be to complete an online application. Next, you may be required to upload a résumé, copy and paste information into a form on the site, or send it as an e-mail attachment. Do not forego a cover message just because you are submitting online.

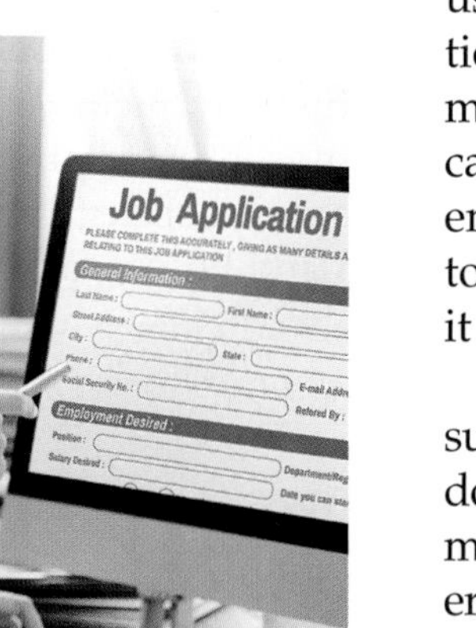

Rawpixel.com/Shutterstock.com

Be aware that copying and pasting into a form usually strips out formatting, such as tabs, indentations, and bold type. Avoid pasting text that is formatted in any way. Even if the formatting holds, it can make the information difficult to read when the employer accesses the application. You may need to adjust the layout of your résumé after uploading it or pasting it into an online application form.

Carefully review everything before clicking the submit button. Just because you are applying online does not mean you can ignore proper spelling, grammar, and usage. What you submit will be the employer's first impression of you. Submitting an application with misspellings or other errors may encourage an employer not to consider you as a serious candidate.

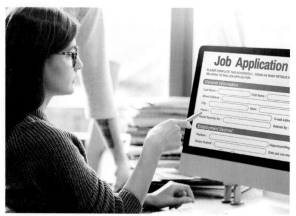

Job Interview

A *job interview* is a meeting in which an applicant and the employer discuss the job and the candidate's skills. It is the employer's opportunity to review your résumé with you and ask questions to see if you are qualified for the position. This is your opportunity to sell yourself in person and to demonstrate professionalism. Your answers to interview questions are important in the employer's decision-making process. Most job interviews are conducted face to face, but it is common to have a preliminary phone interview before the in-person meeting.

Preparing for the Interview

The first step in preparing for a job interview is to learn as much as you can about not only the position, but the company as well. There are several ways to do this. If the company has a website, thoroughly study the site. Pay special attention to the *About Us* section for an overview of the company. Look for press releases, annual reports, and information on its products or services.

While a company website can be a valuable source of information, do not limit your research to just the company site. Use your network of friends and relatives to find people who are familiar with the employer. Get as much information as you can from them.

Call the company's human resources department. The human resources department often has materials specifically for potential employees. Use your best telephone etiquette while speaking with the person who answers the phone. *Etiquette* is the art of using good manners in any situation. *Telephone etiquette* is using good manners while speaking on the telephone. Introduce yourself, state your purpose for calling, and be prepared with a list of questions to ask. Be polite and say "please" and "thank you" when speaking with each person so that you project a positive impression.

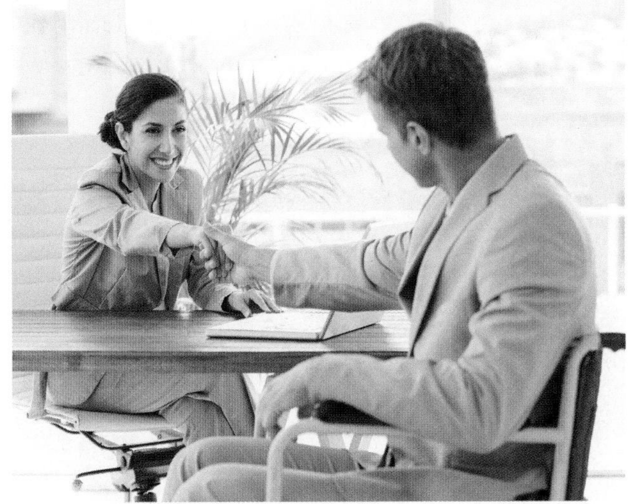

wavebreakmedia/Shutterstock.com

Depending on the position, there may be a performance test as part of the interview. For example, a cook may be asked to prepare a simple dish. Be prepared to take a performance test if needed.

Dressing for the Interview

A face-to-face interview is typically the first time you are seen by a company representative. First impressions are important, so dress appropriately. You should be well-groomed and professionally dressed. Your appearance communicates certain qualities about you to the interviewer. When dressing for an interview, consider what you wish to communicate about yourself.

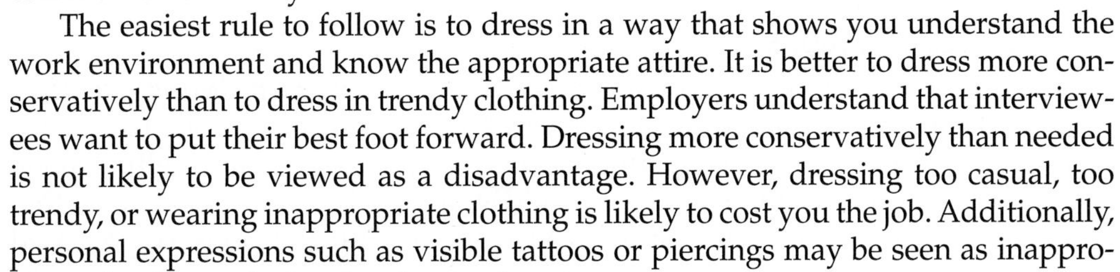

The easiest rule to follow is to dress in a way that shows you understand the work environment and know the appropriate attire. It is better to dress more conservatively than to dress in trendy clothing. Employers understand that interviewees want to put their best foot forward. Dressing more conservatively than needed is not likely to be viewed as a disadvantage. However, dressing too casual, too trendy, or wearing inappropriate clothing is likely to cost you the job. Additionally, personal expressions such as visible tattoos or piercings may be seen as inappropriate for the workplace by the employer.

Preparing for Interview Questions

Interview questions are intended to assess your skills and abilities and to explore your personality. Your answers to these questions will help determine whether you will fit in with the company team and the manager's leadership style.

Interviewers also want to assess your critical-thinking skills. They may ask you to cite specific examples of projects you have completed or problems you have solved.

Communicating effectively in an interview requires specific skills to be mastered. *Verbal communication* is speaking words to communicate. It is also known as *oral communication*. In the course of a workday, most people spend at least some portion of time talking with coworkers, supervisors, managers, or customers. This communication involves a variety of situations, such as conversations about work tasks, asking and answering questions, making requests, giving information, and participating in meetings. During the interview, your communication skills will be observed. Communicate as clearly and effectively as you can.

Common Questions

Before the interview, try to anticipate questions the interviewer is likely to ask you. The following are some common interview questions.

- What are your strengths?
- What are your weaknesses?
- What about this position interests you?
- What do you plan to be doing five years from now?
- Why do you want to work for this organization?

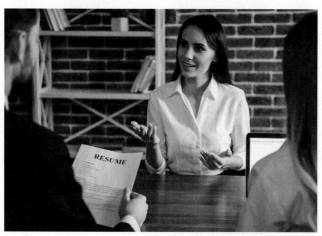

George Rudy/Shutterstock.com

Write down your answers to these questions. Practice answering the questions while in front of a mirror. An important part of the communication process is nonverbal communication. Practicing in front of a mirror will allow you to see your nonverbal communication.

Another way to prepare for an interview is to conduct a mock interview with a friend or instructor. A *mock interview* is a practice interview conducted with another person. Practice until you can give your planned responses naturally and without reading them. The more prepared you are, the more relaxed, organized, competent, and professional you will appear to the interviewer.

Hypothetical Questions

Interviewers may also ask hypothetical questions. *Hypothetical questions* require a candidate to imagine a situation and describe how he or she would act. Frequent topics of hypothetical questions relate to working with and getting along with coworkers. For example, "How would you handle a disagreement with a coworker?" You cannot prepare specific answers to these questions, so you need to rely on your ability to think on your feet.

For these types of questions, the interviewer is aware that you are being put on the spot. In addition to what you say, he or she considers other aspects of your answer as well. Body language is first and foremost. Avoid fidgeting and looking at the ceiling while thinking of your answer. Instead, look at the interviewer and calmly take a moment to compose your thoughts. Keep your answer brief. If your answer runs on too long, you risk losing your train of thought. Try to relate the question to something that is familiar to you and answer honestly.

Do not try to figure out what the interviewer wants you to say. Showing that you can remain poised and project confidence carries a lot of weight, even if your answer is not ideal. In many cases, the interviewer is not as interested in *what* your response is as much as *how* you responded. Was your response quick and thoughtful? Did you ramble? Did you stare blankly at the reviewer before responding?

Behavioral Questions

Interviewers may ask behavioral questions. *Behavioral questions* are questions that draw on an individual's previous experiences and decisions. Your answers to these types of questions indicate past behavior, which may be used to predict future behavior and success in a position. The following are some examples of behavioral questions.

- Tell me about a time when you needed to assume a leadership position in a group. What were the challenges, and how did you help the group meet its goals?
- Describe a situation where you needed to be creative in order to help a client with a problem.
- Describe a situation when you made a mistake. How did you correct the mistake and what measures did you put in place to ensure it did not happen a second time?

Again, you cannot prepare specific answers to these questions. Remain poised, answer honestly, and keep your answers focused on the question. Making direct eye contact with the interviewer can project a positive impression.

Questions an Employer Should Not Ask

State and federal laws prohibit employers from asking questions on certain topics. It is important to know these topics so you can be prepared if such a question comes up during an interview. It is illegal for employers to ask questions about a job candidate's religion, national origin, gender, or disability. Questions about age can only be asked if a minimum age is required by law for a job. The following are some examples of questions an employer is not permitted to ask a candidate.

- What is your religion?
- Are you married?
- What is your nationality?
- Are you disabled?
- Do you have children?
- How much do you weigh?

If you are presented with similar questions during the interview, remain professional. You are not obligated to provide an answer. You could respond, "Please explain how that relates to the job." Or you could completely avoid the question by saying, "I would rather not answer personal questions."

Questions to Ask the Employer

Keep in mind that the questions you ask reveal details about your personality. Asking questions can make a good impression. Questions show that you are interested and aware. Good questions cover the duties and responsibilities of the position. Be aware of how you word questions.

Some questions are not appropriate until after you have been offered the job. In the early stages of the interview process, your questions should demonstrate that you would be a valuable employee and are interested in learning about the company. The following are some questions you may want to ask.

- What are the specific duties of this position?
- What is company policy or criteria for employee promotions?
- Do you have a policy for providing on-the-job training?
- When do you expect to make your hiring decision?
- What is the anticipated start date?

Usually, questions related to pay and benefits, such as vacation time, should not be asked in the interview unless the employer brings them up. These can be asked after an offer of employment is made to you. Sometimes, however, an interviewer asks what salary you want or expect. It is also common for salary requirements to be requested in the job posting, in which case you would need to address that in your cover message. Prepare for questions about salary by researching the industry. If you are unsure, you can simply tell the interviewer that the salary is negotiable.

Evaluating the Interview

Evaluate your performance as soon as you can after the interview. Asking yourself the following questions can help in evaluating your performance.

- Was I adequately prepared with knowledge about the company and the position?
- Did I remember to bring copies of my résumé, list of references, portfolio, and any other requested documents to the interview?
- Was I on time for the interview?
- Did I talk too much or too little?
- Did I honestly and completely answer the interviewer's questions?
- Did I dress appropriately?
- Did I display nervous behavior, such as fidgeting, or forget things I wanted to say?
- Did I come across as composed and confident?
- Which questions could I have handled better?

Every job interview is an opportunity to practice. If you discover that you are not interested in the job, do not feel as though your time was wasted. Make a list of the things you feel you did right and things you would do differently next time.

Writing Follow-Up Messages

Immediately after the interview, write a *thank-you message* to each person who interviewed you. Thank the interviewer for taking the time to talk with you about the job and your career interests. A thank-you may be in the form of a printed letter sent through the mail or an e-mail. Keep the letter brief and to the point. Remind the interviewer of your name and reiterate your enthusiasm, but do not be pushy. An example of a thank-you message is shown in **Figure A.6**.

Employment decisions can take a long time. Some companies notify all applicants when a decision has been made, but some do not. If you have not heard anything after a week or two, it is appropriate to send a brief follow-up message. Simply restate your interest in the job and politely inquire whether a decision has been made.

Employment Process

The employment process can take a substantial amount of time. There are tasks that the employer completes to make sure a candidate is a fit for the position. In addition, there are forms that the employee must complete before starting a position.

Employment Verification

The employer will complete an employment verification using the information on your application or résumé. *Employment verification* is a process through which the information provided on an applicant's résumé is checked to verify that it is correct. A person's past employers typically verify only the dates of employment, position title, and other objective data. Most companies will not provide opinions about employees, such as whether or not he or she was considered a good worker.

Another important part of the employment process is a background check. A *background check* is an investigation into personal data about a job applicant. This information is available from governmental records and other sources, including public information on the Internet. The employer must inform you that a background check will be conducted, and you must grant permission before the employer can do so. Sometimes employers also run a check of your credit. Employers must have your permission to conduct this check as well.

Many employers use Internet search engines, such as Google, to search for your name. Employers may also check social networking websites, such as Facebook and Twitter. Be aware of this before posting any personal information or photos.

Dear Ms. Frost,

Thank you for the opportunity to discuss the position of dietetic technician.

I am very excited about the possibility of working for New York-Presbyterian Hospital. The job is exactly the sort of challenging opportunity I had hoped to find. I believe my educational background and experience will enable me to make a contribution, while also learning and growing on the job.

Please contact me if you need any additional information. I look forward to hearing from you.

Sincerely,
Jamal Barton

Figure A.6

These checks might work to your advantage or against you, depending on what the employer finds. It is up to you to ensure that the image you project on social networking sites, which is your *digital footprint*, is not embarrassing or, worse, prevents you from achieving your career goals.

Accepting an Offer

If an employer decides to offer you a position after the interview process and employment verification, someone will contact you with an official offer of employment. Sometimes this offer is extended via mail, e-mail, or telephone. Be sure to evaluate the offer before making a decision. If you have any questions regarding salary or benefits, this is the time to ask them. Take the time to apply critical-thinking skills to evaluate opportunities before you accept the offer.

Consider the position and whether it is right for you. Are you looking for a short-term position or one that is long term? Is the job a correct fit for you in terms of hours, location, and responsibilities? If you have taken a self-assessment, you have already identified your aptitudes, abilities, values, and interests. Does the position match these?

Compare salary and benefits before accepting the offer of employment. Evaluate what the starting salary is and what future pay increases may be expected. Ask about career rewards, such as job promotions or pay bonuses for outstanding performance. Verify whether the position is salaried or hourly. Be sure to understand what demands will be placed on you. Will you be expected to work outside of the scheduled hours? How does the employer allow employees to maintain a good work-life balance? Compare the demands with the rewards, and decide if the position is right for you. The employer should also outline the responsibilities and demands of the job. Some positions require supervising other employees. Many salaried positions require workweeks that go beyond the typical 40-hour week.

Many companies offer benefits. Health insurance is offered by most companies, but some also offer dental and vision care insurance. Other benefits that may be offered include paid time off (vacation and sick time), short-term disability insurance, tuition assistance, and flexible work hours. Opportunities for continuing education can be a big benefit, allowing you to improve your lifelong learning while enhancing chances for advancement in your career. Depending on the type of position, a company car or expense account may be offered. Evaluate the benefits offered as compared to what is standard for the type of position.

Employment Forms

The first day on the job, you will spend a considerable amount of time in the human resources department completing necessary forms for your employment. Come prepared with the personal information required for the many forms you will need to complete. You will need your social security number, contact information for emergencies, and other personal information.

Form I-9

A *Form I-9 Employment Eligibility Verification* is used to verify an employee's identity and that he or she is authorized to work in the United States. This form is from the US Citizen and Immigration Services, a governmental agency within the

US Department of Homeland Security. Both citizens and noncitizens are required to complete this form. An example of a Form I-9 is shown in **Figure A.7**.

The Form I-9 must be signed in the presence of an authorized representative of the human resources department. Documentation of identity must be presented at the time the form is signed. Acceptable documentation commonly used includes a valid driver's license, a state-issued photo ID, or a passport.

Form W-4

A *Form W-4 Employee's Withholding Allowance Certificate* is used by the employer for the information needed to withhold the appropriate amount of taxes from an employee's paycheck. Withholdings are based on marital status and the number of dependents claimed, including the employee. The amounts withheld are forwarded to the appropriate governmental agency.

At the end of the year, the employer sends the employee a *Form W-2 Wage and Tax Statement* to use when filing income tax returns. This form summarizes all wages and deductions for the year for an individual employee.

Benefits Forms

The human resources department will provide a variety of forms that are specific to the compensation package offered by the employer. Health insurance forms will need to be completed. If the position involves driving, you may need to fill out additional forms related to your driving record. Other benefits offered by the employer may also have forms that need to be completed.

Employment Eligibility Verification
Department of Homeland Security
US Citizenship and Immigration Services

USCIS
Form I-9
OMB No. 1615-0047
Expires 03/31/20XX

► START HERE. Read instructions carefully before completing this form. The instructions must be available during completion of this form.

ANTI-DISCRIMINATION NOTICE. It is illegal to discriminate against work-authorized individuals. Employers **CANNOT** specify which document(s) they will accept from an employee. The refusal to hire an individual because the documentation presented has a future expiration date may also constitute illegal discrimination.

Section 1. Employee Information and Attestation *(Employees must complete and sign Section 1 of Form I-9 no later than the **first day of employment**, but not before accepting a job offer.)*

Last Name *(Family Name)*	First Name *(Given Name)*	Middle Initial	Other Names Used *(if any)*

Address *(Street Number and Name)*	Apt. Number	City or Town	State	Zip Code

Date of Birth *(mm/dd/yyyy)*	U.S. Social Security Number	E-mail Address	Telephone Number

I am aware that federal law provides for imprisonment and/or fines for false statements or use of false documents in connection with the completion of this form.

I attest, under penalty of perjury, that I am (check one of the following):

☐ A citizen of the United States

☐ A noncitizen national of the United States *(See instructions)*

☐ A lawful permanent resident (Alien Registration Number/USCIS Number): ____________

☐ An alien authorized to work until (expiration date, if applicable, mm/dd/yy) ________. Some aliens may write "NA" in this field. *(See instructions)*

*For aliens authorized to work, provide your Alien Registration Number/USCIS Number **OR** Form 1-94 Admission Number:*

Source: US Department of Homeland Security

Figure A.7

On the Job

Landing the job you want is just a beginning. You should do all you can to succeed and advance in your chosen field. Exhibiting *professional behavior* means taking responsibility for your behavior and your work. Certain work habits and traits demonstrate professionalism in almost any job in business and industry, from stock clerk to top executive. These habits and traits include promptness, reliable attendance, dependability, a positive attitude, and eagerness to do the work as best you can. Meeting the dress standards of your work environment will help you fit in and move ahead. If there is no dress code to guide you, take your cue from reliable coworkers or ask superiors what is appropriate. This also applies to "casual Fridays."

Etiquette is the art of using good manners in any situation. *Business etiquette* is required in the workforce. You will need to master basic communication skills, such as meeting and greeting clients and customers, interacting with other employees and superiors, and handling business telephone calls and e-mails. Face-to-face communication requires eye contact, a firm handshake, and an easy conversational manner. Listening to what other people say is important as well. Concentrate on important names, dates, information, and instructions.

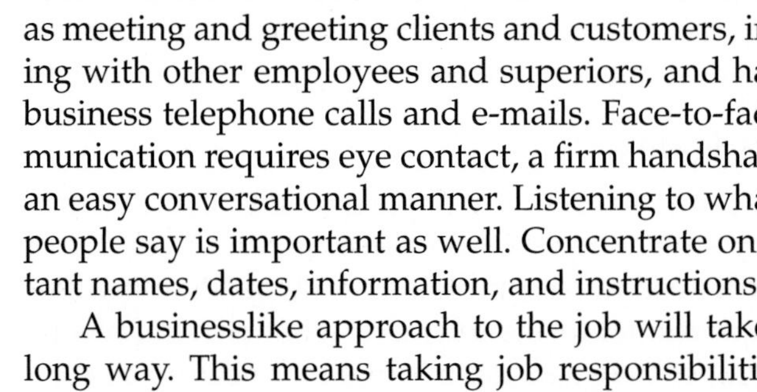

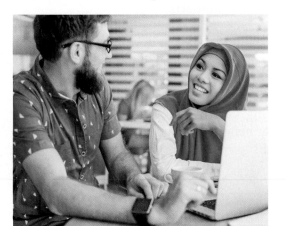

Mila Supinskaya Glashchenko/Shutterstock.com

A businesslike approach to the job will take you a long way. This means taking job responsibilities seriously. Stick to the work you have to do, and try not to be idle during working hours. If you find yourself with time on your hands, ask for more work to do. If you end up with more work than you can complete, discuss the situation with your superior before falling hopelessly behind.

There are some behaviors you should avoid on the job. Do not send and receive personal e-mail and phone calls on company time. Do not let friends drop by to see you at your workplace. Keep breaks and lunches to the amount of time allowed.

Team Member Skills

A *team* is a group of two or more people who work together to achieve a common goal. In business, the terms *team* and *group* are used interchangeably. Teams may be located under one roof, or they may have members located around the world.

Effective teams are those that accomplish the defined goals. This can happen only when the members are cooperative and focused on the assigned tasks. Effective team members are individuals who collaborate and contribute both ideas and personal effort. They are cooperative and work well with others on their team and outside of the team. Successful team members are productive and work to see the team achieve its goals.

A diverse workplace is valued in society. *Diversity* is having people from different backgrounds, cultures, or demographics come together in a group. Elements of diversity include age, race, nationality, gender, mental ability, physical ability, and other qualities that describe an individual. Diversity should never create situations of stereotyping. A *stereotype* is a belief or generalization about a group of people with a given set of characteristics. Stereotyping is not acceptable in any situation.

Interpersonal Skills

Members must interact with each other in a positive manner for the team to be successful. Acquiring positive interpersonal skills helps an employee be effective within the team and with customers of the business. A skill is something a person does well. *Interpersonal skills* are skills that help people communicate and work well with each other. These skills are important when working with team members, an employer, or customers. Some examples of important interpersonal skills necessary to be an effective employee are:

- problem-solving skills
- critical-thinking skills
- verbal skills
- nonverbal skills
- listening skills
- collaboration skills

Problem-solving skills are the ability to use the mind to solve a problem by working through specific steps. The systematic decision-making model in **Figure A.8** is a guideline that can be used when a problem needs to be solved.

Critical-thinking skills are the ability to interpret and make reasonable judgments and decisions by analyzing a situation. Then, a solution or process can be applied so that a productive action can be taken. Applying critical-thinking skills can help problem solve in a more efficient manner.

Verbal skills are the ability to communicate effectively using spoken or written words. Possessing good verbal skills helps to make communication with other team members and customers successful.

Nonverbal skills are the ability to communicate effectively using body language, eye contact, touch, personal space, behavior, and attitude. Nonverbal skills can be used to send messages.

Listening skills are the ability of an individual to not only hear what a person says, but also understand it. Listening is required for all positive communication.

Communication skills—verbal, nonverbal, and listening—may be applied in person or through digital means. Communicating digitally may take the form of e-mail, video conferencing, message boards, or forums. In many cases, nonverbal communication is difficult when communicating digitally, so the other communication skills become more important.

Collaboration skills are being able to work with others to achieve a common goal. This includes sharing ideas and compromising when the greater good of the team is at stake. To *compromise* is to give up an individual idea so that the group can come to a solution. Collaboration and compromise are two important skills to learn in the workplace.

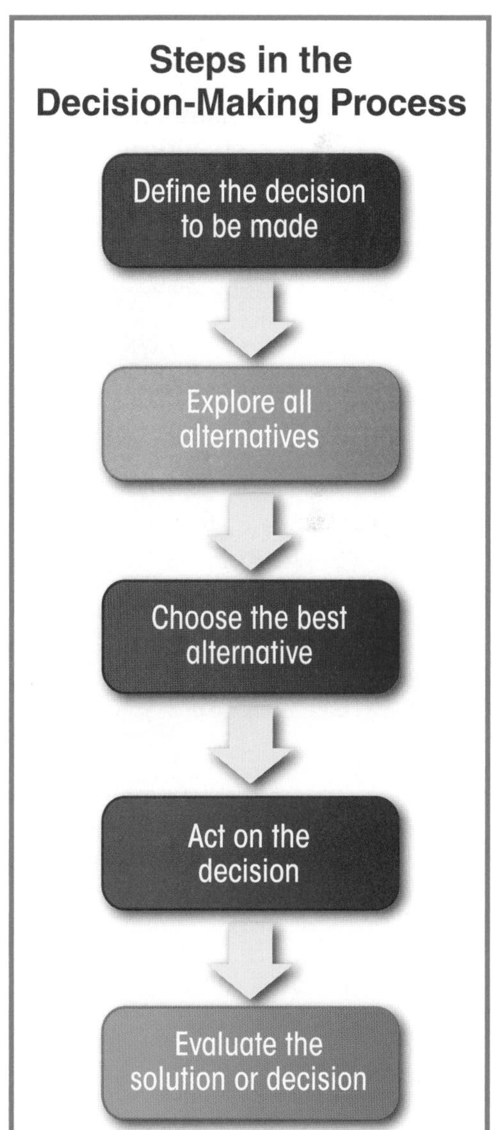

Steps in the Decision-Making Process
Define the decision to be made
Explore all alternatives
Choose the best alternative
Act on the decision
Evaluate the solution or decision

Figure A.8

Time-Management Skills

Effective teams achieve great accomplishments. In order to be productive and accomplish the goals that are set, time-management skills are needed. *Time management* is the practice of organizing time and work assignments to increase personal efficiency. Team members often work on several tasks at the same time. Tasks must be prioritized by determining which ones should be completed before others. The difference between average and excellent workers is often not how hard they work, but how well they prioritize assignments.

Customer Service Skills

All businesses require good customer service skills from their employees. *Customer service* is the ability to provide a product or service in a way it has been promised to a customer. *External customers* are the people and businesses who purchase product from an organization. *Internal customers* are the coworkers within the business with whom each employee works and collaborates. As an employee, it is necessary to apply relationship building with both types of customers.

Listening to customers, hearing their concerns, and meeting their needs are necessary for a company to exist and be profitable. Learning how to resolve complaints from outside customers can help insure that product is sold and customers return for future transactions. Understanding and collaborating with internal customers helps a business create product that meets customer needs and generates profits. Both types of customers are necessary for a successful business.

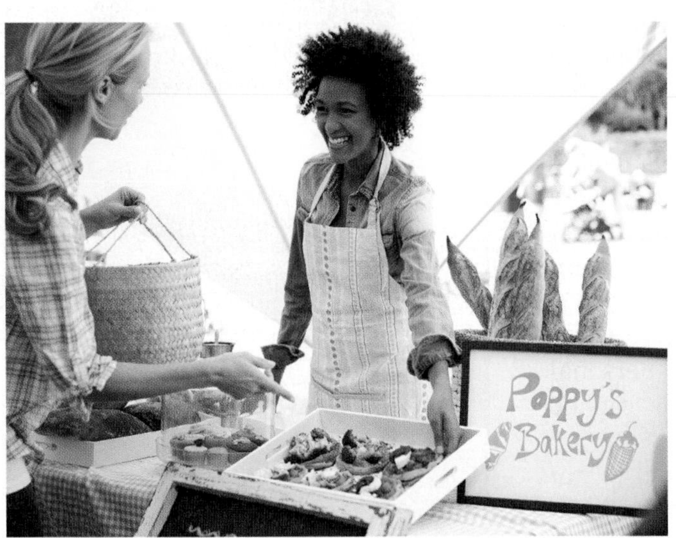

Monkey Business Images/Shutterstock.com

Workplace Ethics

Ethics are a set of moral values that guide a person's behavior. They help a person determine what is right and wrong in given situations. Ethics are based on traits such as trustworthiness, honesty, loyalty, respect, responsibility, and fairness. Ethics in the workplace is a significant issue in the business world. Over 90 percent of business schools now require ethics courses as part of their curriculum.

An employee with strong ethics will always try to do the right thing. Employees demonstrate their ethics through honesty, integrity, and loyalty. *Honesty* is the quality of being truthful and sincere. *Integrity* is strong moral character. Employees with integrity will consistently refuse to compromise their ethical principles, regardless of any outside influence, punishment, or reward. *Loyalty* is faithfulness to a commitment. In the business world, loyalty is faithfulness to an employer or a supplier.

Companies differ in their approach to workplace behavior. Some companies simply assume that employees bring their own standards to the job, and management offers very little guidance. Some companies rely on an informal corporate culture that guides job-related decisions and actions. Other businesses follow a carefully developed program. This program may include a statement of corporate values and a code of ethics to guide employees.

A company may convey its expectations for ethics on the job in different ways. These may include employee handbooks, training sessions or seminars, or printed formal statements of company values and ethics. A stated *code of ethics* generally addresses relationships of the business with employees, customers, suppliers, investors, creditors, competitors, and communities. A business code of ethics frequently relates to issues such as fair treatment of employees, teamwork, competition, and conflicts of interest. Other issues include use of business resources and assets, confidentiality, and environmental concerns.

Becoming an Entrepreneur

Would you like to start a business of your own someday? People who start, own, and operate their own businesses are called *entrepreneurs.* Many opportunities exist for entrepreneurs in the area of nutrition and fitness. For example, a dietitian may develop a program on drug-free muscle building to present to athletes at area schools. A fitness specialist may create an exercise program to help factory workers avoid repetitive-motion injuries.

Successful entrepreneurs are innovative, persistent, and risk takers.

- **Innovative.** Entrepreneurs have creativity to take old or new ideas and market them effectively to their target audience.
- **Persistent.** Willingness to repeatedly adapt a product or service until it fully meets the needs of the target market is true to the persistent nature of entrepreneurs. Most entrepreneurs are people who stick with their dreams. They know what needs to be done and they do it.
- **Risk takers.** Entrepreneurs take reasonable risks. They are willing to invest their time and resources to put their business plan into action.

Entrepreneurs get their business ideas by doing market research. Many start with observing consumer needs. Then they search for ways to meet those needs with new products or services.

Advances in technology also create new opportunities for entrepreneurs. Through technology, new research findings can be revealed and new products and services can be developed.

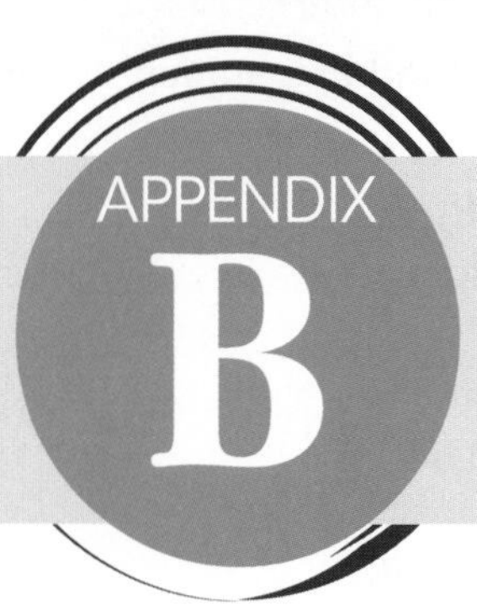

APPENDIX B

Ingredient Substitutions and Egg One-Cup Equivalents

Ingredient Substitutions		
Ingredient	**Amount**	**Substitute**
Baking powder	1 teaspoon	¼ teaspoon baking soda + ½ teaspoon cream of tartar
Baking soda	1 teaspoon	2–3 teaspoons double-acting baking powder and replace acidic ingredient with nonacidic ingredient
Bread crumbs, dry	1 cup	1 cup crushed saltine crackers, cornflakes, or matzo
Brown sugar	1 cup + 1 tablespoon	1 cup granulated sugar + 1 tablespoon molasses, pulse in food processor
Butter	1 tablespoon	1 tablespoon vegetable shortening
Buttermilk	1 cup	1 cup milk + 1 tablespoon lemon juice or vinegar 1 cup sour cream 1 cup plain yogurt
Chicken broth	1 cup	1 bouillon cube + 1 cup water
Chocolate, unsweetened	1 ounce	3 tablespoons cocoa powder + 1 tablespoon butter or margarine
Corn syrup	1 cup	1 cup granulated sugar + ¼ cup liquid 1 cup honey
Cornstarch	1 tablespoon	2 tablespoons all-purpose flour
Cottage cheese	1 cup	1 cup ricotta cheese
Cream of tartar	1 teaspoon	1 teaspoon lemon juice or white vinegar
Cream, heavy	1 cup	¾ cup whole milk + ⅓ cup butter or margarine
Egg (in baking)	1 whole	½ teaspoon baking powder + 1 tablespoon vinegar + 1 tablespoon liquid 1 mashed ripe banana
Garlic	1 clove	⅛ teaspoon garlic powder
Mayonnaise	1 cup	1 cup plain yogurt or sour cream
Milk, skim	1 cup	1 cup reconstituted nonfat dry milk ½ cup evaporated skim milk + ½ cup water

Ingredient Substitutions *(Continued)*		
Ingredient	**Amount**	**Substitute**
Milk, whole	1 cup	1 cup almond, soy, or rice milk 1 cup reconstituted nonfat dry milk + 2 tablespoons butter
Oil, in baked goods	1 cup	1 cup unsweetened applesauce
Sour cream	1 cup	1 cup plain yogurt
Tomato sauce	1 cup	½ cup tomato paste + ½ cup water
Vinegar	1 tablespoon	2 tablespoons lemon juice

Egg Size Substitutions				
Replace this number of large eggs:	**With this number of other size eggs:**			
Large	**Jumbo**	**Extra Large**	**Medium**	**Small**
1	1	1	1	1
2	2	2	2	3
3	2	3	3	4
4	3	4	5	5
5	4	4	6	7
6	5	5	7	8

Eggs: One-Cup Equivalents			
	Number of Eggs		
Egg Size	**Whole Egg**	**Whites Only**	**Yolks Only**
Jumbo	4	5	11
Extra Large	4	6	12
Large	5	7	14
Medium	5	8	16
Small	6	9	18

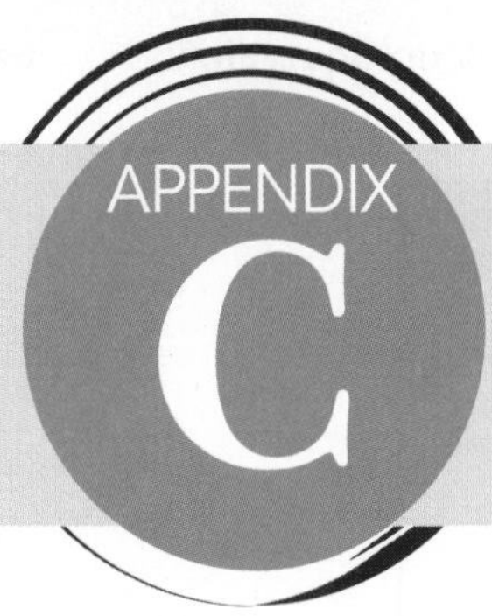

Dietary Reference Intakes

Dietary Reference Intakes (DRIs): Recommended Dietary Allowances and Adequate Intakes, Vitamins

Food and Nutrition Board, Institute of Medicine, National Academies

Life Stage Group	Vitamin A (μg/d)[a]	Vitamin C (mg/d)	Vitamin D (μg/d)[b,c]	Vitamin E (mg/d)[d]	Vitamin K (μg/d)	Thiamin (mg/d)	Riboflavin (mg/d)	Niacin (mg/d)[e]	Vitamin B_6 (mg/d)	Folate (μg/d)[f]	Vitamin B_{12} (μg/d)	Pantothenic Acid (mg/d)	Biotin (μg/d)	Choline (mg/d)[g]
Infants														
0 to 6 mo	400*	40*	10	4*	2.0*	0.2*	0.3*	2*	0.1*	65*	0.4*	1.7*	5*	125*
6 to 12 mo	500*	50*	10	5*	2.5*	0.3*	0.4*	4*	0.3*	80*	0.5*	1.8*	6*	150*
Children														
1–3 y	**300**	**15**	**15**	**6**	30*	**0.5**	**0.5**	**6**	**0.5**	**150**	**0.9**	2*	8*	200*
4–8 y	**400**	**25**	**15**	**7**	55*	**0.6**	**0.6**	**8**	**0.6**	**200**	**1.2**	3*	12*	250*
Males														
9–13 y	**600**	**45**	**15**	**11**	60*	**0.9**	**0.9**	**12**	**1.0**	**300**	**1.8**	4*	20*	375*
14–18 y	**900**	**75**	**15**	**15**	75*	**1.2**	**1.3**	**16**	**1.3**	**400**	**2.4**	5*	25*	550*
19–30 y	**900**	**90**	**15**	**15**	120*	**1.2**	**1.3**	**16**	**1.3**	**400**	**2.4**	5*	30*	550*
31–50 y	**900**	**90**	**15**	**15**	120*	**1.2**	**1.3**	**16**	**1.3**	**400**	**2.4**	5*	30*	550*
51–70 y	**900**	**90**	**15**	**15**	120*	**1.2**	**1.3**	**16**	**1.7**	**400**	**2.4**[h]	5*	30*	550*
> 70 y	**900**	**90**	**20**	**15**	120*	**1.2**	**1.3**	**16**	**1.7**	**400**	**2.4**[h]	5*	30*	550*
Females														
9–13 y	**600**	**45**	**15**	**11**	60*	**0.9**	**0.9**	**12**	**1.0**	**300**	**1.8**	4*	20*	375*
14–18 y	**700**	**65**	**15**	**15**	75*	**1.0**	**1.0**	**14**	**1.2**	**400**[i]	**2.4**	5*	25*	400*
19–30 y	**700**	**75**	**15**	**15**	90*	**1.1**	**1.1**	**14**	**1.3**	**400**[i]	**2.4**	5*	30*	425*
31–50 y	**700**	**75**	**15**	**15**	90*	**1.1**	**1.1**	**14**	**1.3**	**400**[i]	**2.4**	5*	30*	425*
51–70 y	**700**	**75**	**15**	**15**	90*	**1.1**	**1.1**	**14**	**1.5**	**400**	**2.4**[h]	5*	30*	425*
> 70 y	**700**	**75**	**20**	**15**	90*	**1.1**	**1.1**	**14**	**1.5**	**400**	**2.4**[h]	5*	30*	425*
Pregnancy														
14–18 y	**750**	**80**	**15**	**15**	75*	**1.4**	**1.4**	**18**	**1.9**	**600**[j]	**2.6**	6*	30*	450*
19–30 y	**770**	**85**	**15**	**15**	90*	**1.4**	**1.4**	**18**	**1.9**	**600**[j]	**2.6**	6*	30*	450*
31–50 y	**770**	**85**	**15**	**15**	90*	**1.4**	**1.4**	**18**	**1.9**	**600**[j]	**2.6**	6*	30*	450*
Lactation														
14–18 y	**1,200**	**115**	**15**	**19**	75*	**1.4**	**1.6**	**17**	**2.0**	**500**	**2.8**	7*	35*	550*
19–30 y	**1,300**	**120**	**15**	**19**	90*	**1.4**	**1.6**	**17**	**2.0**	**500**	**2.8**	7*	35*	550*
31–50 y	**1,300**	**120**	**15**	**19**	90*	**1.4**	**1.6**	**17**	**2.0**	**500**	**2.8**	7*	35*	550*

NOTE: This table (taken from the DRI reports, see www.nap.edu) presents Recommended Dietary Allowances (RDAs) in **bold type** and Adequate Intakes (AIs) in ordinary type followed by an asterisk (*). An RDA is the average daily dietary intake level; sufficient to meet the nutrient requirements of nearly all (97-98 percent) healthy individuals in a group. It is calculated from an Estimated Average Requirement (EAR). If sufficient scientific evidence is not available to establish an EAR, and thus calculate an RDA, an AI is usually developed. For healthy breastfed infants, an AI is the mean intake. The AI for other life stage and gender groups is believed to cover the needs of all healthy individuals in the groups, but lack of data or uncertainty in the data prevent being able to specify with confidence the percentage of individuals covered by this intake.

[a] As retinol activity equivalents (RAEs). 1 RAE = 1 μg retinol, 12 μg β-carotene, 24 μg α-carotene, or 24 μg β-cryptoxanthin. The RAE for dietary provitamin A carotenoids is two-fold greater than retinol equivalents (RE), whereas the RAE for preformed vitamin A is the same as RE.

[b] As cholecalciferol. 1 μg cholecalciferol = 40 IU vitamin D.

[c] Under the assumption of minimal sunlight.

[d] As α-tocopherol. α-Tocopherol includes *RRR*-α-tocopherol, the only form of α-tocopherol that occurs naturally in foods, and the *2R*-stereoisomeric forms of α-tocopherol (*RRR*-, *RSR*-, *RRS*-, and *RSS*-α-tocopherol) that occur in fortified foods and supplements. It does not include the *2S*-stereoisomeric forms of α-tocopherol (*SRR*-, *SSR*-, *SRS*-, and *SSS*-α-tocopherol), also found in fortified foods and supplements.

[e] As niacin equivalents (NE). 1 mg of niacin = 60 mg of tryptophan; 0–6 months = preformed niacin (not NE).

[f] As dietary folate equivalents (DFE). 1 DFE = 1 μg food folate = 0.6 μg of folic acid from fortified food or as a supplement consumed with food = 0.5 μg of a supplement taken on an empty stomach.

[g] Although AIs have been set for choline, there are few data to assess whether a dietary supply of choline is needed at all stages of the life cycle, and it may be that the choline requirement can be met by endogenous synthesis at some of these stages.

[h] Because 10 to 30 percent of older people may malabsorb food-bound B_{12}, it is advisable for those older than 50 years to meet their RDA mainly by consuming foods fortified with B_{12} or a supplement containing B_{12}.

[i] In view of evidence linking folate intake with neural tube defects in the fetus, it is recommended that all women capable of becoming pregnant consume 400 μg from supplements or fortified foods in addition to intake of food folate from a varied diet.

[j] It is assumed that women will continue consuming 400 μg from supplements or fortified food until their pregnancy is confirmed and they enter prenatal care, which ordinarily occurs after the end of the periconceptional period—the critical time for formation of the neural tube.

SOURCES: *Dietary Reference Intakes for Calcium, Phosphorous, Magnesium, Vitamin D, and Fluoride* (1997); *Dietary Reference Intakes for Thiamin, Riboflavin, Niacin, Vitamin B_6, Folate, Vitamin B_{12}, Pantothenic Acid, Biotin, and Choline* (1998); *Dietary Reference Intakes for Vitamin C, Vitamin E, Selenium, and Carotenoids* (2000); *Dietary Reference Intakes for Vitamin A, Vitamin K, Arsenic, Boron, Chromium, Copper, Iodine, Iron, Manganese, Molybdenum, Nickel, Silicon, Vanadium, and Zinc* (2001); *Dietary Reference Intakes for Water, Potassium, Sodium, Chloride, and* Sulfate (2005); and *Dietary Reference Intakes for Calcium and Vitamin D* (2011). These reports may be accessed via www.nap.edu. Reprinted with permission from the National Academies Press, National Academy of Sciences.

Dietary Reference Intakes (DRIs): Recommended Dietary Allowances and Adequate Intakes, Elements
Food and Nutrition Board, Institute of Medicine, National Academies

Life Stage Group	Calcium (mg/d)	Chromium (μg/d)	Copper (μg/d)	Fluoride (mg/d)	Iodine (μg/d)	Iron (mg/d)	Magnesium (mg/d)	Manganese (mg/d)	Molybdenum (μg/d)	Phosphorus (mg/d)	Selenium (μg/d)	Zinc (mg/d)	Potass-ium (g/d)	Sodium (g/d)	Chloride (g/d)
Infants															
0 to 6 mo	200*	0.2*	200*	0.01*	110*	0.27*	30*	0.003*	2*	100*	15*	2*	0.4*	0.12*	0.18*
6 to 12 mo	260*	5.5*	220*	0.5*	130*	**11**	75*	0.6*	3*	275*	20*	**3**	0.7*	0.37*	0.57*
Children															
1–3 y	**700**	11*	**340**	0.7*	**90**	**7**	**80**	1.2*	**17**	**460**	**20**	**3**	3.0*	1.0*	1.5*
4–8 y	**1,000**	15*	**440**	1*	**90**	**10**	**130**	1.5*	**22**	**500**	**30**	**5**	3.8*	1.2*	1.9*
Males															
9–13 y	**1,300**	25*	**700**	2*	**120**	**8**	**240**	1.9*	**34**	**1,250**	**40**	**8**	4.5*	1.5*	2.3*
14–18 y	**1,300**	35*	**890**	3*	**150**	**11**	**410**	2.2*	**43**	**1,250**	**55**	**11**	4.7*	1.5*	2.3*
19–30 y	**1,000**	35*	**900**	4*	**150**	**8**	**400**	2.3*	**45**	**700**	**55**	**11**	4.7*	1.5*	2.3*
31–50 y	**1,000**	35*	**900**	4*	**150**	**8**	**420**	2.3*	**45**	**700**	**55**	**11**	4.7*	1.5*	2.3*
51–70 y	**1,000**	30*	**900**	4*	**150**	**8**	**420**	2.3*	**45**	**700**	**55**	**11**	4.7*	1.3*	2.0*
> 70 y	**1,200**	30*	**900**	4*	**150**	**8**	**420**	2.3*	**45**	**700**	**55**	**11**	4.7*	1.2*	1.8*
Females															
9–13 y	**1,300**	21*	**700**	2*	**120**	**8**	**240**	1.6*	**34**	**1,250**	**40**	**8**	4.5*	1.5*	2.3*
14–18 y	**1,300**	24*	**890**	3*	**150**	**15**	**360**	1.6*	**43**	**1,250**	**55**	**9**	4.7*	1.5*	2.3*
19–30 y	**1,000**	25*	**900**	3*	**150**	**18**	**310**	1.8*	**45**	**700**	**55**	**8**	4.7*	1.5*	2.3*
31–50 y	**1,000**	25*	**900**	3*	**150**	**18**	**320**	1.8*	**45**	**700**	**55**	**8**	4.7*	1.5*	2.3*
51–70 y	**1,200**	20*	**900**	3*	**150**	**8**	**320**	1.8*	**45**	**700**	**55**	**8**	4.7*	1.3*	2.0*
> 70 y	**1,200**	20*	**900**	3*	**150**	**8**	**320**	1.8*	**45**	**700**	**55**	**8**	4.7*	1.2*	1.8*
Pregnancy															
14–18 y	**1,300**	29*	**1,000**	3*	**220**	**27**	**400**	2.0*	**50**	**1,250**	**60**	**12**	4.7*	1.5*	2.3*
19–30 y	**1,000**	30*	**1,000**	3*	**220**	**27**	**350**	2.0*	**50**	**700**	**60**	**11**	4.7*	1.5*	2.3*
31–50 y	**1,000**	30*	**1,000**	3*	**220**	**27**	**360**	2.0*	**50**	**700**	**60**	**11**	4.7*	1.5*	2.3*
Lactation															
14–18 y	**1,300**	44*	**1,300**	3*	**290**	**10**	**360**	2.6*	**50**	**1,250**	**70**	**13**	5.1*	1.5*	2.3*
19–30 y	**1,000**	45*	**1,300**	3*	**290**	**9**	**310**	2.6*	**50**	**700**	**70**	**12**	5.1*	1.5*	2.3*
31–50 y	**1,000**	45*	**1,300**	3*	**290**	**9**	**320**	2.6*	**50**	**700**	**70**	**12**	5.1*	1.5*	2.3*

NOTE: This table (taken from the DRI reports, see www.nap.edu) presents Recommended Dietary Allowances (RDAs) in **bold type** and Adequate Intakes (AIs) in ordinary type followed by an asterisk (*). An RDA is the average daily dietary intake level; sufficient to meet the nutrient requirements of nearly all (97-98 percent) healthy individuals in a group. It is calculated from an Estimated Average Requirement (EAR). If sufficient scientific evidence is not available to establish an EAR, and thus calculate an RDA, an AI is usually developed. For healthy breastfed infants, an AI is the mean intake. The AI for other life stage and gender groups is believed to cover the needs of all healthy individuals in the groups, but lack of data or uncertainty in the data prevent being able to specify with confidence the percentage of individuals covered by this intake.

SOURCES: *Dietary Reference Intakes for Calcium, Phosphorous, Magnesium, Vitamin D, and Fluoride* (1997); *Dietary Reference Intakes for Thiamin, Riboflavin, Niacin, Vitamin B_6, Folate, Vitamin B_{12}, Pantothenic Acid, Biotin, and Choline* (1998); *Dietary Reference Intakes for Vitamin C, Vitamin E, Selenium, and Carotenoids* (2000); and *Dietary Reference Intakes for Vitamin A, Vitamin K, Arsenic, Boron, Chromium, Copper, Iodine, Iron, Manganese, Molybdenum, Nickel, Silicon, Vanadium, and Zinc* (2001); *Dietary Reference Intakes for Water, Potassium, Sodium, Chloride, and* Sulfate (2005); and *Dietary Reference Intakes for Calcium and Vitamin D* (2011). These reports may be accessed via www.nap.edu. Reprinted with permission from the National Academies Press, National Academy of Sciences.

Dietary Reference Intakes (DRIs): Tolerable Upper Intake Levels, Vitamins
Food and Nutrition Board, Institute of Medicine, National Academies

Life Stage Group	Vitamin A (μg/d)[a]	Vitamin C (mg/d)	Vitamin D (μg/d)	Vitamin E (mg/d)[b,c]	Vitamin K	Thiamin	Riboflavin	Niacin (mg/d)[c]	Vitamin B_6 (mg/d)	Folate (μg/d)[c]	Vitamin B_{12}	Pantothenic Acid	Biotin	Choline (g/d)	Carotenoids[d]
Infants															
0 to 6 mo	600	ND[e]	25	ND	ND	ND	ND	ND	ND	ND	ND	ND	ND	ND	ND
6 to 12 mo	600	ND	38	ND	ND	ND	ND	ND	ND	ND	ND	ND	ND	ND	ND
Children															
1–3 y	600	400	63	200	ND	ND	ND	10	30	300	ND	ND	ND	1.0	ND
4–8 y	900	650	75	300	ND	ND	ND	15	40	400	ND	ND	ND	1.0	ND
Males															
9–13 y	1,700	1,200	100	600	ND	ND	ND	20	60	600	ND	ND	ND	2.0	ND
14–18 y	2,800	1,800	100	800	ND	ND	ND	30	80	800	ND	ND	ND	3.0	ND
19–30 y	3,000	2,000	100	1,000	ND	ND	ND	35	100	1,000	ND	ND	ND	3.5	ND
31–50 y	3,000	2,000	100	1,000	ND	ND	ND	35	100	1,000	ND	ND	ND	3.5	ND
51–70 y	3,000	2,000	100	1,000	ND	ND	ND	35	100	1,000	ND	ND	ND	3.5	ND
> 70 y	3,000	2,000	100	1,000	ND	ND	ND	35	100	1,000	ND	ND	ND	3.5	ND
Females															
9–13 y	1,700	1,200	100	600	ND	ND	ND	20	60	600	ND	ND	ND	2.0	ND
14–18 y	2,800	1,800	100	800	ND	ND	ND	30	80	800	ND	ND	ND	3.0	ND
19–30 y	3,000	2,000	100	1,000	ND	ND	ND	35	100	1,000	ND	ND	ND	3.5	ND
31–50 y	3,000	2,000	100	1,000	ND	ND	ND	35	100	1,000	ND	ND	ND	3.5	ND
51–70 y	3,000	2,000	100	1,000	ND	ND	ND	35	100	1,000	ND	ND	ND	3.5	ND
> 70 y	3,000	2,000	100	1,000	ND	ND	ND	35	100	1,000	ND	ND	ND	3.5	ND
Pregnancy															
14–18 y	2,800	1,800	100	800	ND	ND	ND	30	80	800	ND	ND	ND	3.0	ND
19–30 y	3,000	2,000	100	1,000	ND	ND	ND	35	100	1,000	ND	ND	ND	3.5	ND
31–50 y	3,000	2,000	100	1,000	ND	ND	ND	35	100	1,000	ND	ND	ND	3.5	ND
Lactation															
14–18 y	2,800	1,800	100	800	ND	ND	ND	30	80	800	ND	ND	ND	3.0	ND
19–30 y	3,000	2,000	100	1,000	ND	ND	ND	35	100	1,000	ND	ND	ND	3.5	ND
31–50 y	3,000	2,000	100	1,000	ND	ND	ND	35	100	1,000	ND	ND	ND	3.5	ND

NOTE: A Tolerable Upper Intake Level (UL) is the highest level of daily nutrient intake that is likely to pose no risk of adverse health effects to almost all individuals in the general population. Unless otherwise specified, the UL represents total intake from food, water, and supplements. Due to a lack of suitable data, ULs could not be established for vitamin K, thiamin, riboflavin, vitamin B_{12}, pantothenic acid, biotin, and carotenoids. In the absence of a UL, extra caution may be warranted in consuming levels above recommended intakes. Members of the general population should be advised not to routinely exceed the UL. The UL is not meant to apply to individuals who are treated with the nutrient under medical supervision or to individuals with predisposing conditions that modify their sensitivity to the nutrient.

[a] As preformed vitamin A only.

[b] As α-tocopherol; applies to any form of supplemental α-tocopherol.

[c] The ULs for vitamin E, niacin, and folate apply to synthetic forms obtained from supplements, fortified foods, or a combination of the two.

[d] β-Carotene supplements are advised only to serve as a provitamin A source for individuals at risk of vitamin A deficiency.

[e] ND = Not determinable due to lack of data of adverse effects in this age group and concern with regard to lack of ability to handle excess amounts. Source of intake should be from food only to prevent high levels of intake.

SOURCES: *Dietary Reference Intakes for Calcium, Phosphorous, Magnesium, Vitamin D, and Fluoride* (1997); *Dietary Reference Intakes for Thiamin, Riboflavin, Niacin, Vitamin B_6, Folate, Vitamin B_{12}, Pantothenic Acid, Biotin, and Choline* (1998); *Dietary Reference Intakes for Vitamin C, Vitamine E, Selenium, and Carotenoids* (2000); *Dietary Reference Intakes for Vitamin A, Vitamin K, Arsenic, Boron, Chromium, Copper, Iodine, Iron, Manganese, Molybdenum, Nickel, Silicon, Vanadium, and Zinc* (2001); and *Dietary Reference Intakes for Calcium and Vitamin D* (2011). These reports may be accessed via www.nap.edu. Reprinted with permission from the National Academies Press, National Academy of Sciences.

Dietary Reference Intakes (DRIs): Tolerable Upper Intake Levels, Elements
Food and Nutrition Board, Institute of Medicine, National Academies

Life Stage Group	Arsenic[a]	Boron (mg/d)	Calcium (mg/d)	Chromium	Copper (μg/d)	Fluoride (mg/d)	Iodine (μg/d)	Iron (mg/d)	Magnesium (mg/d)[b]	Manganese (mg/d)	Molybdenum (μg/d)	Nickel (mg/d)	Phosphorus (g/d)	Selenium (μg/d)	Silicon[c]	Vanadium (mg/d)[d]	Zinc (mg/d)	Sodium (g/d)	Chloride (g/d)
Infants																			
0 to 6 mo	ND[e]	ND	1,000	ND	ND	0.7	ND	40	ND	ND	ND	ND	ND	45	ND	ND	4	ND	ND
6 to 12 mo	ND	ND	1,500	ND	ND	0.9	ND	40	ND	ND	ND	ND	ND	60	ND	ND	5	ND	ND
Children																			
1–3 y	ND	3	2,500	ND	1,000	1.3	200	40	65	2	300	0.2	3	90	ND	ND	7	1.5	2.3
4–8 y	ND	6	2,500	ND	3,000	2.2	300	40	110	3	600	0.3	3	150	ND	ND	12	1.9	2.9
Males																			
9–13 y	ND	11	3,000	ND	5,000	10	600	40	350	6	1,100	0.6	4	280	ND	ND	23	2.2	3.4
14–18 y	ND	17	3,000	ND	8,000	10	900	45	350	9	1,700	1.0	4	400	ND	ND	34	2.3	3.6
19–30 y	ND	20	2,500	ND	10,000	10	1,100	45	350	11	2,000	1.0	4	400	ND	1.8	40	2.3	3.6
31–50 y	ND	20	2,500	ND	10,000	10	1,100	45	350	11	2,000	1.0	4	400	ND	1.8	40	2.3	3.6
51–70 y	ND	20	2,000	ND	10,000	10	1,100	45	350	11	2,000	1.0	4	400	ND	1.8	40	2.3	3.6
> 70 y	ND	20	2,000	ND	10,000	10	1,100	45	350	11	2,000	1.0	3	400	ND	1.8	40	2.3	3.6
Females																			
9–13 y	ND	11	3,000	ND	5,000	10	600	40	350	6	1,100	0.6	4	280	ND	ND	23	2.2	3.4
14–18 y	ND	17	3,000	ND	8,000	10	900	45	350	9	1,700	1.0	4	400	ND	ND	34	2.3	3.6
19–30 y	ND	20	2,500	ND	10,000	10	1,100	45	350	11	2,000	1.0	4	400	ND	1.8	40	2.3	3.6
31–50 y	ND	20	2,500	ND	10,000	10	1,100	45	350	11	2,000	1.0	4	400	ND	1.8	40	2.3	3.6
51–70 y	ND	20	2,000	ND	10,000	10	1,100	45	350	11	2,000	1.0	4	400	ND	1.8	40	2.3	3.6
> 70 y	ND	20	2,000	ND	10,000	10	1,100	45	350	11	2,000	1.0	3	400	ND	1.8	40	2.3	3.6
Pregnancy																			
14–18 y	ND	17	3,000	ND	8,000	10	900	45	350	9	1,700	1.0	3.5	400	ND	ND	34	2.3	3.6
19–30 y	ND	20	2,500	ND	10,000	10	1,100	45	350	11	2,000	1.0	3.5	400	ND	ND	40	2.3	3.6
31–50 y	ND	20	2,500	ND	10,000	10	1,100	45	350	11	2,000	1.0	3.5	400	ND	ND	40	2.3	3.6
Lactation																			
14–18 y	ND	17	3,000	ND	8,000	10	900	45	350	9	1,700	1.0	4	400	ND	ND	34	2.3	3.6
19–30 y	ND	20	2,500	ND	10,000	10	1,100	45	350	11	2,000	1.0	4	400	ND	ND	40	2.3	3.6
31–50 y	ND	20	2,500	ND	10,000	10	1,100	45	350	11	2,000	1.0	4	400	ND	ND	40	2.3	3.6

NOTE: A Tolerable Upper Intake Level (UL) is the highest level of daily nutrient intake that is likely to pose no risk of adverse health effects to almost all individuals in the general population. Unless otherwise specified, the UL represents total intake from food, water, and supplements. Due to a lack of suitable data, ULs could not be established for vitamin K, thiamin, riboflavin, vitamin B_{12}, pantothenic acid, biotin, and carotenoids. In the absence of a UL, extra caution may be warranted in consuming levels above recommended intakes. Members of the general population should be advised not to routinely exceed the UL. The UL is not meant to apply to individuals who are treated with the nutrient under medical supervision or to individuals with predisposing conditions that modify their sensitivity to the nutrient.

[a]Although the UL was not determined for arsenic, there is no justification for adding arsenic to food or supplements.

[b]The ULs for magnesium represent intake from a pharmacological agent only and do not include intake from food and water.

[c]Although silicon has not been shown to cause adverse effects in humans, there is no justification for adding silicon to supplements.

[d]Although vanadium in food has not been shown to cause adverse effects in humans, there is no justification for adding vanadium to food and vanadium supplements should be used with caution. The UL is based on adverse effects in laboratory animals and this data could be used to set a UL for adults but not children and adolescents.

[e]ND = Not determinable due to lack of data of adverse effects in this age group and concern with regard to lack of ability to handle excess amounts. Source of intake should be from food only to prevent high levels of intake.

SOURCES: *Dietary Reference Intakes for Calcium, Phosphorous, Magnesium, Vitamin D, and Fluoride* (1997); *Dietary Reference Intakes for Thiamin, Riboflavin, Niacin, Vitamin B_6, Folate, Vitamin B_{12}, Pantothenic Acid, Biotin, and Choline* (1998); *Dietary Reference Intakes for Vitamin C, Vitamin E, Selenium, and Carotenoids* (2000); *Dietary Reference Intakes for Vitamin A, Vitamin K, Arsenic, Boron, Chromium, Copper, Iodine, Iron, Manganese, Molybdenum, Nickel, Silicon, Vanadium, and Zinc* (2001); *Dietary Reference Intakes for Water, Potassium, Sodium, Chloride, and Sulfate* (2005); and *Dietary Reference Intakes for Calcium and Vitamin D* (2011). These reports may be accessed via www.nap.edu. Reprinted with permission from the National Academies Press, National Academy of Sciences.

Estimated Energy Requirements (EER)

Estimated amount of calories needed to maintain calorie balance for various gender and age groups at three different levels of physical activity. The estimates are rounded to the nearest 200 calories. An individual's calorie needs may be higher or lower than these average estimates.

Age (years)	Gender/Activity level					
	Male/ Sedentary[a]	Male/ Moderately Active[b]	Male/Active[c]	Female[d]/ Sedentary[a]	Female[d]/ Moderately Active[b]	Female[d]/ Active[c]
2	1,000	1,000	1,000	1,000	1,000	1,000
3	1,200	1,400	1,400	1,000	1,200	1,400
4	1,200	1,400	1,600	1,200	1,400	1,400
5	1,200	1,400	1,600	1,200	1,400	1,600
6	1,400	1,600	1,800	1,200	1,400	1,600
7	1,400	1,600	1,800	1,200	1,600	1,800
8	1,400	1,600	2,000	1,400	1,600	1,800
9	1,600	1,800	2,000	1,400	1,600	1,800
10	1,600	1,800	2,200	1,400	1,800	2,000
11	1,800	2,000	2,200	1,600	1,800	2,000
12	1,800	2,200	2,400	1,600	2,000	2,200
13	2,000	2,200	2,600	1,600	2,000	2,200
14	2,000	2,400	2,800	1,800	2,000	2,400
15	2,200	2,600	3,000	1,800	2,000	2,400
16	2,400	2,800	3,200	1,800	2,000	2,400
17	2,400	2,800	3,200	1,800	2,000	2,400
18	2,400	2,800	3,200	1,800	2,000	2,400
19–20	2,600	2,800	3,000	2,000	2,200	2,400
21–25	2,400	2,800	3,000	2,000	2,200	2,400
26–30	2,400	2,600	3,000	1,800	2,000	2,400
31–35	2,400	2,600	3,000	1,800	2,000	2,200
36–40	2,400	2,600	2,800	1,800	2,000	2,200
41–45	2,200	2,600	2,800	1,800	2,000	2,200
46–50	2,200	2,400	2,800	1,800	2,000	2,200
51–55	2,200	2,400	2,800	1,600	1,800	2,200
56–60	2,200	2,400	2,600	1,600	1,800	2,200
61–65	2,000	2,400	2,600	1,600	1,800	2,000
66–70	2,000	2,200	2,600	1,600	1,800	2,000
71–75	2,000	2,200	2,600	1,600	1,800	2,000
76+	2,000	2,200	2,400	1,600	1,800	2,000

[a] Sedentary means a lifestyle that includes only the physical activity of independent living.

[b] Moderately Active means a lifestyle that includes physical activity equivalent to walking about 1.5 to 3 miles per day at 3 to 4 miles per hour, in addition to the activities of independent living.

[c] Active means a lifestyle that includes physical activity equivalent to walking more than 3 miles per day at 3 to 4 miles per hour, in addition to the activities of independent living.

[d] Estimates for females do not include women who are pregnant or breastfeeding.

Source: *2015–2020 Dietary Guidelines for Americans*, 8th Edition.

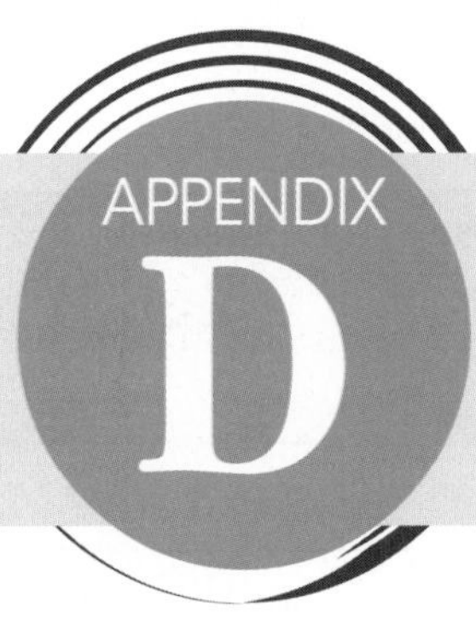

APPENDIX D Nutritive Values of Foods

(*Tr* indicates nutrient present in trace amount.)

Item	Approximate Measures (edible portion)		Food Energy	Protein	Fat	Saturated Fat	Carbo-hydrate	Dietary Fiber	Calcium	Iron	Vitamin A
			Nutrients in Indicated Quantity								
		Grams	Calories	Grams	Grams	Grams	Grams	Grams	Milligrams	Milligrams	Micrograms
BEVERAGES											
Club soda	12 fl. oz.	355	0	0	0	0.0	0	0	18	Tr	0
Cola, regular	12 fl. oz.	369	160	0	0	0.0	41	0	11	0.2	0
Coffee, brewed	6 fl. oz.	180	Tr	Tr	Tr	0.0	Tr	0	4	Tr	0
Fruit punch drink	6 fl. oz.	190	85	Tr	0	0.0	22	0	15	0.4	2
DAIRY PRODUCTS											
Cheese:											
Cheddar, cut pieces	1 oz.	28	115	7	9	0.6	Tr	0	204	0.2	86
Cottage, low-fat (2%)	1 cup	226	205	31	4	2.8	8	0	155	0.4	45
Mozzarella, whole milk	1 oz.	28	80	6	6	3.7	1	0	147	0.1	68
Mozzarella, part skim milk	1 oz.	28	80	8	5	3.1	1	0	207	0.1	54
Parmesan, grated	1 tbsp.	5	25	2	2	1.0	Tr	0	69	Tr	9
Pasteurized process cheese, American	1 oz.	28	95	6	7	4.4	2	0	163	0.2	62
Milk, fluid:											
Whole (3.3% fat)	1 cup	244	150	8	8	5.1	11	0	291	0.1	76
Low-fat (2%)	1 cup	244	120	8	5	2.9	12	0	297	0.1	139
Low-fat (1%)	1 cup	244	100	8	3	1.6	12	0	300	0.1	144
Nonfat (skim)	1 cup	245	85	8	Tr	0.3	12	0	302	0.1	149
Buttermilk	1 cup	245	100	8	2	1.3	12	0	285	0.1	20
Milk beverages:											
Chocolate milk, low-fat (2%)	1 cup	250	180	8	5	3.1	26	3	284	0.6	143
Shakes, thick, chocolate	10-oz. container	283	335	9	8	6.5	60	Tr	374	0.9	59
Milk desserts, frozen:											
Ice cream, vanilla, regular (about 11% fat)	1 cup	133	270	5	14	9.0	32	Tr	176	0.1	133
Sherbet (about 2% fat)	1 cup	193	270	2	4	2.2	59	0	103	0.3	39

Item	Approximate Measures (edible portion)		Food Energy	Protein	Fat	Saturated Fat	Carbo-hydrate	Dietary Fiber	Calcium	Iron	Vitamin A
		Grams	Calories	Grams	Grams	Grams	Grams	Grams	Milligrams	Milligrams	Micrograms
Yogurt, low-fat, fruit-flavored	8-oz. container	227	230	10	2	1.6	43	1	345	0.2	25
Yogurt, low-fat, plain	8-oz. container	227	145	12	4	2.3	16	0	415	0.2	36
EGGS											
Fried in butter	1 egg	46	95	6	7	1.9	1	0	29	1.1	94
Hard-cooked, shell removed	1 egg	50	80	6	6	1.6	1	0	28	1.0	78
Scrambled (milk added) in butter; also omelet	1 egg	64	110	7	8	2.2	2	0	54	1.0	102
FATS AND OILS											
Butter (4 sticks per lb.)	1 tbsp.	14	100	Tr	11	7.1	Tr	0	3	Tr	106
Margarine, imitation (about 40% fat), soft	1 tbsp.	14	50	Tr	5	0.9	Tr	0	2	0.0	139
Corn oil	1 cup	218	1,925	0	218	29.4	0	0	0	0.0	0
Salad dressings, commercial:											
French, low-calorie	1 tbsp.	16	25	Tr	2	0.1	2	Tr	6	Tr	Tr
Italian, regular	1 tbsp.	15	80	Tr	9	1.0	1	Tr	1	Tr	3
Thousand Island, regular	1 tbsp.	16	60	Tr	6	1.0	2	Tr	2	0.1	15
FISH AND SHELLFISH											
Fish sticks (stick, 4 × 1 × ½-in.)	1 fish stick	28	70	6	3	0.9	4	Tr	11	0.3	5
Shrimp, French fried (7 medium)	3 oz.	85	200	16	10	3.8	11	Tr	61	2.0	26
Tuna, canned, drained, water pack, solid white	3 oz.	85	135	30	1	0.2	0	0	17	0.6	32
FRUITS AND FRUIT JUICES											
Apples, raw, unpeeled, 2¾-in. diam.	1 apple	138	80	Tr	Tr	0.1	21	3	10	0.2	7
Apple juice, bottled or canned	1 cup	248	115	Tr	Tr	Tr	29	Tr	17	0.9	Tr
Applesauce, canned, unsweetened	1 cup	244	105	Tr	Tr	Tr	28	3	7	0.3	7
Avocados, raw (about 2 per lb.)	1 avocado	173	305	4	30	4.5	12	6	19	2.0	106
Bananas, raw (about 2½ per lb.)	1 banana	114	105	1	1	0.2	27	2	7	0.4	9

Item	Approximate Measures (edible portion)		Food Energy	Protein	Fat	Saturated Fat	Carbo-hydrate	Dietary Fiber	Calcium	Iron	Vitamin A
		Grams	Calories	Grams	Grams	Grams	Grams	Grams	Milligrams	Milligrams	Micrograms
Cherries, sweet, raw	10 cherries	68	50	1	1	0.1	11	Tr	10	0.3	15
Fruit cocktail, canned, juice pack	1 cup	248	115	1	Tr	Tr	29	3	20	0.5	76
Grapefruit, raw, 3¾-in. diam.	½ grapefruit	120	40	1	Tr	Tr	10	1	14	0.1	1
Grapes, raw, Thompson seedless	10 grapes	50	35	Tr	Tr	0.1	9	Tr	6	0.1	4
Grape juice, canned or bottled	1 cup	253	155	1	Tr	0.1	38	2	23	0.6	2
Melons, raw, cantaloupe, 5-in. diam.	½ melon	267	95	2	1	0.1	22	2	29	0.6	861
Nectarines, raw (about 3 per lb.)	1 nectarine	136	65	1	1	0.1	16	2	7	0.2	100
Oranges, raw, whole, 2⅝-in. diam.	1 orange	131	60	1	Tr	Tr	15	3	52	0.1	27
Orange juice, frozen concentrate, diluted per directions	1 cup	249	110	2	Tr	Tr	27	Tr	22	0.2	19
Peaches, raw, 2½-in. diam.	1 peach	87	35	1	Tr	Tr	10	2	4	0.1	47
Peaches, canned, juice pack	1 cup	248	110	2	Tr	Tr	29	4	15	0.7	94
Pears, raw with skin, Bartlett, 2½-in. diam.	1 pear	166	100	1	1	Tr	25	4	18	0.4	3
Pineapple, raw, diced	1 cup	155	75	1	1	Tr	19	2	11	0.6	4
Pineapple, canned, juice pack, chunks or tidbits	1 cup	250	150	1	Tr	Tr	39	2	35	0.7	10
Plums, raw, 2⅛-in. diam.	1 plum	66	35	1	Tr	Tr	9	1	3	0.1	21
Raisins, seedless	1 cup	145	435	5	1	0.2	115	5	71	3.0	1
Raspberries, raw	1 cup	123	60	1	1	Tr	14	5	27	0.7	16
Strawberries, raw	1 cup	149	45	1	1	Tr	10	2	21	0.6	4
Watermelon, raw, piece (4 × 8-in. wedge)	1 piece	482	155	3	2	0.6	35	1	39	0.8	176
GRAIN PRODUCTS											
Bagels, plain, enriched, 3½-in. diam.	1 bagel	68	200	7	2	0.1	38	2	29	1.8	0
Breads:											
Italian bread, enriched, slice, 4½ × 3¼ × ¾-in.	1 slice	30	85	3	Tr	0.3	17	1	5	0.8	0
Pita bread, enriched, white, 6½-in. diam.	1 pita	60	165	6	1	0.1	33	1	49	1.4	0

Item	Approximate Measures (edible portion)		Food Energy	Protein	Fat	Saturated Fat	Carbo-hydrate	Dietary Fiber	Calcium	Iron	Vitamin A
		Grams	Calories	Grams	Grams	Grams	Grams	Grams	Milligrams	Milligrams	Micrograms
Raisin bread, enriched (18 slices/loaf)	1 slice	25	65	2	1	0.3	13	1	25	0.8	Tr
White bread, enriched (18 slices/loaf)	1 slice	25	65	2	1	0.2	12	1	32	0.7	Tr
Whole-wheat bread (16 slices/loaf)	1 slice	28	70	3	1	0.3	13	2	20	1.0	Tr
Breakfast cereals:											
Corn (hominy) grits, regular and quick, enriched	1 cup	242	145	3	Tr	0.1	31	5	0	1.5	0
Oatmeal, regular, quick and instant, nonfortified	1 cup	234	145	6	2	0.4	25	4	19	1.6	4
Oatmeal, instant, fortified, plain	1 pkt.	177	105	4	2	0.3	18	3	163	6.3	453
Cap'n Crunch® (about ¾ cup)	1 oz.	28	120	1	3	2.2	23	1	5	7.5	4
Cheerios® (about 1¼ cup)	1 oz.	28	110	4	2	0.3	20	2	48	4.5	375
Froot Loops® (about 1 cup)	1 oz.	28	110	2	1	0.2	25	1	3	4.5	375
Grape-Nuts® (about ¼ cup)	1 oz.	28	100	3	Tr	Tr	23	3	11	1.2	375
Honey Nut Cheerios® (about ¾ cup)	1 oz.	28	105	3	1	0.1	23	1	20	4.5	375
Nature Valley® Granola (about ⅓ cup)	1 oz.	28	125	3	5	5.0	19	2	18	0.9	2
Rice Krispies® (about 1 cup)	1 oz.	28	110	2	Tr	Tr	25	Tr	4	1.8	375
Shredded Wheat (about ⅔ cup)	1 oz.	28	100	3	1	0.2	23	4	11	1.2	0
Frosted Flakes® (about ¾ cup)	1 oz.	28	110	1	Tr	Tr	26	1	1	1.8	375
Cakes prepared from cake mixes with enriched flour:											
Angel food, 1⁄12 of cake	1 piece	53	125	3	Tr	0.1	29	1	44	0.2	0
Coffee cake, crumb, ⅙ of cake	1 piece	72	230	5	7	1.3	38	1	44	1.2	32
Devil's food with chocolate frosting, 1⁄16 of cake	1 piece	69	235	3	8	3.2	40	2	41	1.4	31

Item	Approximate Measures (edible portion)		Food Energy	Protein	Fat	Saturated Fat	Carbo-hydrate	Dietary Fiber	Calcium	Iron	Vitamin A
		Grams	Calories	Grams	Grams	Grams	Grams	Grams	Milligrams	Milligrams	Micrograms
Devil's food with chocolate frosting, cupcake, 2½-in. diam.	1 cupcake	35	120	2	4	1.9	20	1	21	0.7	16
Carrot with cream cheese frosting, 1⁄16 of cake	1 piece	96	385	4	21	5.5	48	1	44	1.3	15
Cookies made with enriched flour:											
Brownies with nuts, commercial, with frosting, 1½ x 1¾ x ⅞-in.	1 brownie	25	100	1	4	1.1	16	1	13	0.6	18
Chocolate chip, commercial, 2¼-in. diam., ⅜-in. thick	4 cookies	42	180	2	9	3.1	28	1	13	0.8	15
Oatmeal with raisins, 2⅝-in. diam., ¼-in. thick	4 cookies	52	245	3	10	1.7	36	2	18	1.1	12
Sandwich type (chocolate or vanilla), 1¾-in. diam., ⅝-in. thick	4 cookies	40	195	2	8	1.7	29	1	12	1.4	0
Crackers:											
Cheese, plain, 1-in. square	10 crackers	10	50	1	3	0.9	6	Tr	11	0.3	5
Graham, plain, 2½-in. square	2 crackers	14	60	1	1	0.4	11	Tr	6	0.4	0
Saltines	4 crackers	12	50	1	1	0.3	9	Tr	3	0.5	0
Wheat, thin	4 crackers	8	35	1	1	0.7	5	1	3	0.3	Tr
Doughnuts made with enriched flour:											
Cake type, plain, 3¼-in. diam.	1 doughnut	50	210	3	12	1.9	24	1	22	1.0	5
Yeast-leavened, glazed, 3¾-in. diam.	1 doughnut	60	235	4	13	3.5	26	1	17	1.4	Tr
English muffins, plain, enriched	1 muffin	57	140	5	1	0.1	27	2	96	1.7	0
French toast, from home recipe	1 slice	65	155	6	7	2.0	17	Tr	72	1.3	32
Macaroni, enriched, cooked	1 cup	130	190	7	1	0.1	39	2	14	2.1	0
Muffins, 2½-in. diam., from commercial mix:											
Blueberry	1 muffin	45	140	3	5	0.7	22	1	15	0.9	11
Bran	1 muffin	45	140	3	4	1.1	24	4	27	1.7	14
Corn	1 muffin	45	145	3	6	1.3	22	2	30	1.3	16

Item	Approximate Measures (edible portion)		Food Energy	Protein	Fat	Saturated Fat	Carbo-hydrate	Dietary Fiber	Calcium	Iron	Vitamin A
		Grams	Calories	Grams	Grams	Grams	Grams	Grams	Milligrams	Milligrams	Micrograms
Noodles (egg noodles), enriched, cooked	1 cup	160	200	7	2	0.5	37	2	16	2.6	34
Pancakes, 4-in. diam., plain, from mix (egg, milk, and oil added)	1 pancake	27	60	2	2	0.1	8	Tr	36	0.7	7
Piecrust, home recipe, 9-in. diam.	1 pie shell	180	900	11	60	15.5	79	3	25	4.5	0
Pies:											
Apple, piece, ⅙ of pie	1 piece	158	405	3	18	3.3	60	3	13	1.6	5
Cream, piece, ⅙ of pie	1 piece	152	455	3	23	7.4	59	0	46	1.1	65
Pecan, piece, ⅙ of pie	1 piece	138	575	7	32	5.2	71	5	65	4.6	54
Snacks:											
Corn chips	1-oz. package	28	155	2	9	1.3	16	1	35	0.5	11
Popcorn, air-popped, unsalted	1 cup	8	30	1	Tr	Tr	6	1	1	0.2	1
Popcorn, popped in vegetable oil, salted	1 cup	11	55	1	3	0.5	6	1	3	0.3	2
Pretzels, twisted, thin, 3¼ × 2¼ × ¼-in.	10 pretzels	60	240	6	2	0.4	48	2	16	1.2	0
Rice:											
Brown, cooked	1 cup	195	230	5	1	0.4	50	4	23	1.0	0
White, enriched, cooked	1 cup	205	225	4	Tr	0.2	50	1	21	1.8	0
White, enriched, instant, ready-to-serve	1 cup	165	180	4	0	0.1	40	1	5	1.3	0
Rolls, commercial, enriched:											
Dinner, 2½-in. diam.	1 roll	28	85	2	2	0.7	14	1	33	0.8	Tr
Frankfurter and hamburger (8 per pkg.)	1 roll	40	115	3	2	0.5	20	1	54	1.2	Tr
Hard, 3¾-in. diam.	1 roll	50	155	5	2	0.3	30	1	24	1.4	0
Spaghetti, enriched, cooked	1 cup	130	190	7	1	0.1	39	2	14	2.0	0
Tortillas, corn	1 tortilla	30	65	2	1	0.1	13	2	42	0.6	8
Wheat flours:											
All-purpose or family flour, enriched, sifted	1 cup	115	420	12	1	0.2	88	3	18	5.1	0
Cake or pastry flour, enriched, sifted	1 cup	96	350	7	1	0.1	76	2	16	4.2	0
Whole-wheat, from hard wheat, stirred	1 cup	120	400	16	2	0.4	85	15	49	5.2	0

Item	Approximate Measures (edible portion)		Food Energy	Protein	Fat	Saturated Fat	Carbo-hydrate	Dietary Fiber	Calcium	Iron	Vitamin A
		Grams	Calories	Grams	Grams	Grams	Grams	Grams	Milligrams	Milligrams	Micrograms
LEGUMES, NUTS, AND SEEDS											
Almonds, shelled, slivered	1 cup	135	795	27	70	6.7	28	13	359	4.9	0
Black-eyed peas, dry, cooked	1 cup	250	190	13	1	0.2	35	12	43	3.3	3
Chickpeas, cooked, drained	1 cup	163	270	15	4	0.4	45	8	80	4.9	Tr
Lentils, dry, cooked	1 cup	200	215	16	1	0.1	38	5	50	4.2	4
Peanuts, roasted in oil, salted	1 cup	145	840	39	71	9.8	27	10	125	2.8	0
Peanut butter	1 tbsp.	16	95	5	8	1.5	3	1	5	0.3	0
Peas, split, dry, cooked	1 cup	200	230	16	1	0.2	42	6	22	3.4	8
Pistachio nuts, dried, shelled	1 oz.	28	165	6	14	1.7	7	3	38	1.9	7
Refried beans, canned	1 cup	290	295	18	3	1.0	51	14	141	5.1	0
Sesame seeds, dry, hulled	1 tbsp.	8	45	2	4	2.9	1	3	11	0.6	1
Tofu, piece, 2½ × 2¾ × 1-in.	1 piece	120	85	9	5	0.9	3	1	108	2.3	0
Sunflower seeds, dry, hulled	1 oz.	28	160	6	14	1.9	5	2	33	1.9	1
Walnuts, English or Persian, pieces or chips	1 cup	120	770	17	74	6.7	22	5	113	2.9	15
MEAT AND MEAT PRODUCTS											
Beef, cooked:											
Cuts braised, simmered, or pot roasted, such as chuck blade, 2½ × 2½ × ¾-in.	3 oz.	85	325	22	26	11.6	0	0	11	2.5	Tr
Cuts braised, simmered, or pot roasted, such as bottom round, 4⅛ × 2¼ × ½-in.	3 oz.	85	220	25	13	3.6	0	0	5	2.8	Tr
Ground beef, broiled, patty, 3 × ⅝-in., regular	3 oz.	85	245	20	18	7.9	0	0	9	2.1	Tr
Roast, such as eye of round, 2 pieces, 2½ × 2½ × ⅜-in.	3 oz.	85	205	23	12	6.2	0	0	5	1.6	Tr
Steak, sirloin, broiled, 2½ × 2½ × ¾-in.	3 oz.	85	240	23	15	8.7	0	0	9	2.6	Tr
Lamb, cooked:											
Chops	2.2 oz.	63	220	20	15	3.5	0	0	16	1.5	Tr

Item	Approximate Measures (edible portion)		Food Energy	Protein	Fat	Saturated Fat	Carbo-hydrate	Dietary Fiber	Calcium	Iron	Vitamin A
		Grams	Calories	Grams	Grams	Grams	Grams	Grams	Milligrams	Milligrams	Micrograms
Pork, cured, cooked:											
Bacon, regular	3 medium slices	19	110	6	9	3.3	Tr	0	2	0.3	0
Ham, light cure, roasted, 2 pieces, 4⅛ × 2¼ × ¼-in.	3 oz.	85	205	18	14	6.8	0	0	6	0.7	0
Luncheon meat, ham (1-oz. slice), regular	2 slices	57	105	10	6	1.9	2	0	4	0.6	0
Pork, fresh, cooked:											
Chop, loin, broiled	3.1 oz.	87	275	24	19	4.6	0	0	3	0.7	3
Rib, roasted, piece, 2½ × ¾-in.	3 oz.	85	270	21	20	6.7	0	0	9	0.8	3
Sausages:											
Bologna (1-oz. slice)	2 slices	57	180	7	16	3.2	2	0	7	0.9	0
Brown and serve	1 link	13	50	2	5	1.7	Tr	0	1	0.1	0
Frankfurter	1 frankfurter	45	145	5	13	4.9	1	0	5	0.5	0
Salami, dry type	2 slices	20	85	5	7	2.5	1	0	2	0.3	0
MIXED DISHES AND FAST FOODS											
Mixed dishes:											
Beef and vegetable stew, from home recipe	1 cup	245	220	16	11	4.9	15	2	29	2.9	568
Chicken chow mein, canned	1 cup	250	95	7	Tr	0.0	18	2	45	1.3	28
Chili con carne with beans, canned	1 cup	255	340	19	16	3.4	31	4	82	4.3	15
Macaroni (enriched) and cheese, from home recipe	1 cup	200	430	17	22	8.9	40	1	362	1.8	232
Spaghetti (enriched) with meatballs and tomato sauce, canned	1 cup	250	260	12	10	2.1	29	6	53	3.3	100
Fast-food entrees:											
Cheeseburger, 4-oz. patty	1 sandwich	194	525	30	31	10.2	40	0	236	4.5	128
Enchilada	1 enchilada	230	235	20	16	15.0	24	0	322	11.0	352
English muffin, egg, cheese, and bacon	1 sandwich	138	360	18	18	8.6	31	1	197	3.1	160
Fish sandwich, regular, with cheese	1 sandwich	140	420	16	23	6.2	39	Tr	132	1.8	25
Hamburger, 4-oz. patty	1 sandwich	174	445	25	21	9.7	38	0	75	4.8	28
Pizza, cheese, ⅛ of 15-in. diam. pizza	1 slice	120	290	15	9	2.9	39	2	220	1.6	106
Taco	1 taco	81	195	9	11	4.6	15	1	109	1.2	57

Item	Approximate Measures (edible portion)		Food Energy	Protein	Fat	Saturated Fat	Carbo-hydrate	Dietary Fiber	Calcium	Iron	Vitamin A
		Grams	Calories	Grams	Grams	Grams	Grams	Grams	Milligrams	Milligrams	Micrograms
POULTRY AND POULTRY PRODUCTS											
Chicken:											
Fried, batter-dipped breast, (5.6-oz. with bones)	4.9 oz.	140	365	35	18	4.9	13	Tr	28	1.8	28
Fried, batter-dipped drumstick	2.5 oz.	72	195	16	11	3.0	6	Tr	12	1.0	19
Roasted, flesh only, breast, (4.2-oz. with bones and skin)	3 oz.	86	140	27	3	0.9	0	0	13	0.9	5
Turkey, roasted, flesh only, dark meat, piece, 2½ × 1⅝ × ¼-in.	4 pieces	85	160	24	6	4.0	0	0	27	2.0	0
Turkey, roasted, flesh only, light meat, piece, 4 × 2 × ¼-in.	2 pieces	85	135	25	3	2.7	0	0	16	1.1	0
SOUPS, SAUCES, AND GRAVIES											
Soups, canned, condensed:											
Prepared with equal volume of milk, cream of chicken	1 cup	248	190	7	11	4.6	15	Tr	181	0.7	94
Prepared with equal volume of milk, tomato	1 cup	248	160	6	6	2.9	22	1	159	1.8	109
Prepared with equal volume of water, beef broth, bouillon, consommé	1 cup	240	15	3	1	0.3	Tr	0	14	0.4	0
Prepared with equal volume of water, chicken noodle	1 cup	241	75	4	2	0.7	9	1	17	0.8	71
Prepared with equal volume of water, green pea	1 cup	250	165	9	3	1.8	27	5	28	2.0	20
Prepared with equal volume of water, vegetable beef	1 cup	244	80	6	2	0.9	10	Tr	17	1.1	189
Sauces:											
From home recipe, white sauce, medium	1 cup	250	395	10	30	6.4	24	Tr	292	0.9	340
Ready to serve, barbecue	1 tbsp.	16	10	Tr	Tr	Tr	2	Tr	3	0.1	14
Ready to serve, soy	1 tbsp.	18	10	2	0	Tr	2	0	3	0.5	0
Gravies:											
Canned, beef	1 cup	233	125	9	5	2.7	11	1	14	1.6	0
From dry mix, chicken	1 cup	260	85	3	2	0.5	14	Tr	39	0.3	0

Item	Approximate Measures (edible portion)		Food Energy	Protein	Fat	Saturated Fat	Carbo-hydrate	Dietary Fiber	Calcium	Iron	Vitamin A
		Grams	Calories	Grams	Grams	Grams	Grams	Grams	Milligrams	Milligrams	Micrograms
SUGARS AND SWEETS											
Candy:											
Chocolate, milk, plain	1 oz.	28	145	2	9	5.2	16	1	50	0.4	10
Chocolate, milk, with peanuts	1 oz.	28	155	4	11	3.4	13	2	49	0.4	8
Fudge, chocolate, plain	1 oz.	28	115	1	3	1.5	21	Tr	22	0.3	Tr
Gumdrops	1 oz.	28	100	Tr	Tr	0.0	25	0	2	0.1	0
Jelly beans	1 oz.	28	105	Tr	Tr	0.0	26	0	1	0.3	0
Marshmallows	1 oz.	28	90	1	0	0.0	23	Tr	1	0.5	0
Gelatin dessert prepared with powder and water	½ cup	120	70	2	0	0.0	17	0	2	Tr	0
Honey	1 cup	339	1,030	1	0	0.0	279	Tr	17	1.7	0
Jams and preserves	1 tbsp.	20	55	Tr	Tr	0.0	14	Tr	4	0.2	Tr
Popsicle, 3-fl.-oz. size	1 popsicle	95	70	0	0	0.0	18	0	0	Tr	0
Pudding, canned, chocolate	5-oz. can	142	205	3	11	1.0	30	1	74	1.2	31
Sugar, brown, packed	1 cup	220	820	0	0	0.0	212	0	3	0.1	0
White, granulated	1 tbsp.	12	45	0	0	0.0	12	0	Tr	Tr	0
Syrup, chocolate-flavored syrup or topping, thin type	2 tbsp.	38	85	1	Tr	0.2	21	1	38	0.5	13
Syrup, table syrup (corn and maple)	2 tbsp.	42	122	0	0	0.0	30	0	26	0.4	0
VEGETABLES AND VEGETABLE PRODUCTS											
Asparagus, green, cooked and drained, cuts and tips	1 cup	180	45	5	1	0.2	8	4	43	1.2	149
Beans, snap, cooked, drained, from frozen (cut)	1 cup	135	35	2	Tr	Tr	8	4	61	1.1	71
Broccoli, cooked, chopped	1 cup	185	50	6	Tr	Tr	10	5	94	1.1	350
Cabbage, raw, shredded or sliced	1 cup	70	15	1	Tr	Tr	4	1	33	0.4	9
Carrots, raw, whole, 7½ × 1⅛-in.	1 carrot	72	30	1	Tr	Tr	7	2	19	0.4	2,025
Carrots, cooked, sliced	1 cup	146	55	2	Tr	Tr	12	6	41	0.7	2,585
Cauliflower, cooked	1 cup	180	35	3	Tr	Tr	7	4	31	0.7	4
Celery, pascal type, raw, stalk, large outer, 8 × 1½-in. (at root end)	1 stalk	40	5	Tr	Tr	Tr	1	1	14	0.2	5

Item	Approximate Measures (edible portion)		Food Energy	Protein	Fat	Saturated Fat	Carbo-hydrate	Dietary Fiber	Calcium	Iron	Vitamin A
		Grams	Calories	Grams	Grams	Grams	Grams	Grams	Milligrams	Milligrams	Micrograms
Collards, cooked	1 cup	170	60	5	1	0.2	12	6	357	1.9	1,017
Corn, sweet, cooked, ear, 5 × 1¾	1 ear	77	85	3	1	0.2	19	2	2	0.5	17
Corn, sweet, cooked, kernels	1 cup	165	135	5	Tr	Tr	34	4	3	0.5	41
Cucumber, with peel, slices, ⅛-in. thick	8 small slices	28	5	Tr	Tr	Tr	1	Tr	4	0.1	1
Kale, cooked, chopped	1 cup	130	40	4	1	Tr	7	2	179	1.2	826
Lettuce, raw, iceberg, wedge, ¼ of head	1 wedge	135	20	1	Tr	Tr	3	1	26	0.7	45
Mushrooms, raw, sliced or chopped	1 cup	70	20	1	Tr	Tr	3	Tr	4	0.9	0
Onions, raw, chopped	1 cup	160	55	2	Tr	Tr	12	3	40	0.6	0
Peas, green, canned, drained solids	1 cup	170	115	8	1	0.2	21	6	34	1.6	131
Peas, green, frozen, cooked, drained	1 cup	160	125	8	Tr	Tr	23	8	38	2.5	107
Peppers, hot chile, raw	1 pepper	45	20	1	Tr	Tr	4	1	8	0.5	484
Potatoes, cooked:											
Baked (about 2 per lb., raw), with skin	1 potato	202	220	5	Tr	0.1	51	5	20	2.7	0
Boiled (about 3 per lb., raw), peeled after boiling	1 potato	136	120	3	Tr	Tr	27	2	7	0.4	0
French fried, strip, 2 to 3½ in. long, frozen, oven heated	10 strips	50	110	2	4	3.8	17	1	5	0.7	0
French fried, strip, 2 to 3½ in. long, frozen, fried in vegetable oil	10 strips	50	160	2	8	2.5	20	2	10	0.4	0
Mashed, milk and margarine added	1 cup	210	225	4	9	2.2	35	4	55	0.5	42
Potato chips	10 chips	20	105	1	7	3.1	10	1	5	0.2	0
Spinach, cooked	1 cup	190	55	6	Tr	Tr	10	4	277	2.9	1,479
Sweet potatoes, (raw about 2½ per lb.), baked in skin, peeled	1 potato	114	115	2	Tr	Tr	28	4	32	0.5	2,488
Tomatoes, raw, 2⅗-in. diam.	1 tomato	123	25	1	Tr	0.1	5	1	9	0.6	139
Tomatoes, canned, solids and liquids	1 cup	240	50	2	1	0.1	10	2	62	1.5	145
Tomato products, canned, paste	1 cup	262	220	10	2	0.3	49	11	92	7.8	647
Tomato products, canned, sauce	1 cup	245	75	3	Tr	Tr	18	3	34	1.9	240
Vegetables, mixed, frozen, cooked	1 cup	182	105	5	Tr	Tr	24	5	46	1.5	778

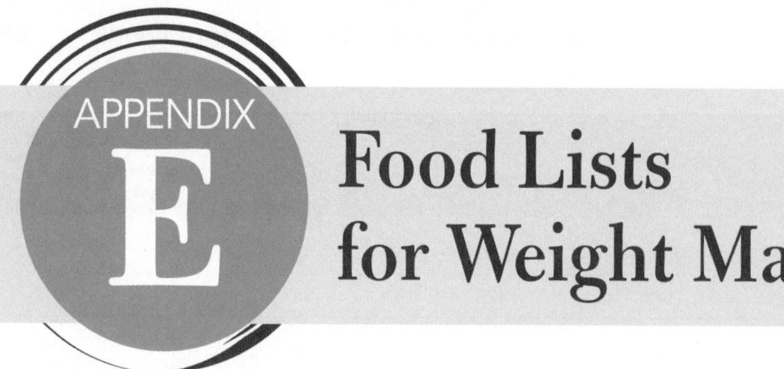

Appendix E Food Lists for Weight Management

The Food Lists

The following chart shows the amount of nutrients in one choice from each list.

Food List	Carbohydrate (grams)	Protein (grams)	Fat (grams)	Calories
Carbohydrates				
Starch: breads; cereals; grains and pasta; starchy vegetables; crackers and snacks; and beans, peas, and lentils	15	3	1	80
Fruits	15	—	—	60
Milk and Milk Substitutes				
Fat-free, low-fat, 1%	12	8	0–3	100
Reduced-fat, 2%	12	8	5	120
Whole	12	8	8	160
Nonstarchy Vegetables	5	2	—	25
Sweets, Desserts, and Other Carbohydrates	15	varies	varies	varies
Proteins				
Lean	—	7	2	45
Medium-fat	—	7	5	75
High-fat	—	7	8	100
Plant-based	varies	7	varies	varies
Fats	—	—	5	45

* = More than 3 grams of dietary fiber per serving.
♦ = A food with extra fat.
♦♦ = A food with two extra fat choices or a food prepared with added fat.
‡ = 480 milligrams or more of sodium per serving; 600 milligrams or more of sodium per serving (for combination or fast-food main dishes/meals).

Starch

Breads, cereals, grains (including pasta and rice), starchy vegetables, crackers and snacks, and cooked beans, peas, and lentils are starches. In general, **one starch choice** is

- ½ cup of cooked cereal, grain, or starchy vegetable
- ⅓ cup of cooked rice or pasta
- 1 ounce of a bread product, such as 1 slice of bread
- ¾ ounce to 1 ounce of most snack foods (some snack foods may also have extra fat)

Bread

Food	Serving Size
Bagel, large (about 4 oz.)	¼ (1 oz.)
♦ Biscuit, 2½ inches across	1
Breads, loaf-type	
white, whole-grain, French, Italian, pumpernickel, rye, sourdough, unfrosted raisin or cinnamon	1 slice (1 oz.)
* reduced-calorie	2 slices (1½ oz.)
Breads, flat-type (flatbreads)	
chapatti	1 oz.
ciabatta	1 oz.
naan, 3¼-inch square	1
pita, 6 inches across	½
roti	1 oz.
* sandwich flat buns, whole wheat	1½ oz.
♦ taco shell, 5 inches across	2
tortilla, corn, 6 inches across	1
tortilla, flour, 6 inches across	1
♦ Cornbread, 1¾-inch cube	1 (1½ oz.)
English muffin	½
Hot dog bun or hamburger bun	½ bun (¾ oz.)
Pancake, 4 inches across, ¼-inch thick	1
Roll, plain, small	1 (1 oz.)
♦ Stuffing, bread	⅓ cup
♦ Waffle, 4-inch square or 4 inches across	1

Cereals

Food	Serving Size
* Bran cereal (twigs, buds, or flakes)	½ cup
Cooked cereals (oats, oatmeal)	½ cup
Granola cereal	¼ cup
Grits, cooked	½ cup
Muesli	¼ cup
Puffed cereal	1½ cups
Shredded wheat, plain	½ cup
Sugar-coated cereal	½ cup
Unsweetened, ready-to-eat cereal	¾ cup

Grains (Including Pasta and Rice)

Unless otherwise indicated, serving sizes listed are for cooked grains.

Food	Serving Size
Barley, cooked	⅓ cup
* Bran, dry, oat	¼ cup
* Bran, dry, wheat	½ cup
* Bulgur (cooked)	½ cup
Couscous	⅓ cup
Kasha	½ cup
Millet, cooked	⅓ cup
Pasta, white or whole-wheat (all shapes and sizes)	⅓ cup
Polenta	⅓ cup
Quinoa, all colors	⅓ cup
Rice, white, brown, and other colors and types	⅓ cup
Tabbouleh (tabouli), prepared	½ cup
Wheat germ, dry	3 Tbsp.
Wild rice	½ cup

Starchy Vegetables

All of the serving sizes for starchy vegetables on this list are for cooked vegetables.

Food	Serving Size
Breadfruit	¼ cup
Cassava or dasheen	⅓ cup
Corn	½ cup
Corn on cob	4 to 4½ inch piece (½ large cob)
* Hominy, canned	¾ cup
Marinara, pasta, or spaghetti sauce	½ cup
* Mixed vegetables with corn or peas	1 cup
* Parsnips	½ cup
* Peas, green	½ cup
Plantain	⅓ cup
Potato	
baked with skin	¼ large (3 oz.)
boiled, all kinds	½ cup or ½ medium (3 oz.)
♦ mashed, with milk and fat	½ cup
French fried (oven-baked)	1 cup (2 oz.)
* Pumpkin puree, canned, no sugar added	¾ cup
* Squash, winter (acorn, butternut)	1 cup
* Succotash	½ cup
Yam or sweet potato, plain	½ cup (3½ oz.)

Note: Restaurant-style French fries are on the **Fast Foods** list.

Crackers and Snacks

Food	Serving Size
Crackers	
animal	8 crackers
* crispbread	2 to 5 pieces (¾ oz.)
graham, 2½-inch square	3 squares
nut and rice	10 crackers
oyster	20 crackers
* round, butter-type	6 crackers
saltine-type	6 crackers
* sandwich-style, cheese or peanut butter filling	3 crackers
whole-wheat, baked	5 regular 1½-inch squares or 10 thins (¾ oz.)
Granola or snack bar	1 bar (¾ oz.)
Matzoh, all shapes and sizes	¾ oz.
Melba toast, about 2-inch by 4-inch piece	4 pieces
Popcorn	
* no fat added	3 cups
♦♦ with butter added	3 cups
Pretzels	¾ oz.
Rice cakes, 4 inches across	2 cakes
Snack Chips	
baked (potato, pita)	about 8 chips (¾ oz.)
♦♦ regular (tortilla, potato)	about 13 chips (1 oz.)

Note: For other snacks, see the **Sweets, Desserts, and Other Carbohydrates** list.

Tip: An open handful is equal to about 1 cup or 1 to 2 ounces of snack food.

Beans, Peas, and Lentils

The choices on this list count as **one starch choice** and **one lean protein choice**.

Food	Serving Size
* Baked beans, canned	⅓ cup
* Beans (black, garbanzo, kidney, lima, navy, pinto, white), cooked or canned, drained and rinsed	½ cup
* Lentils (any color), cooked or canned	½ cup
* Peas (black-eyed, split), cooked	½ cup
*‡ Refried beans, canned	½ cup

Note: Beans, peas, and lentils are also found on the **Protein** list.

Fruits

Fresh, frozen, canned, and dried fruits and fruit juices are on this list. In general, **one fruit choice** is

- ½ cup of canned or fresh fruit
- 1 small fresh fruit ¾ to 1 cup)
- ½ cup unsweetened fruit juice
- 2 tablespoons of dried fruit

Fruit

The weights listed include skin, core, seeds, and rind.

Food	Serving Size
Apple, unpeeled, small	1 (4 oz.)
Apples, dried	4 rings
Applesauce, unsweetened	½ cup
Apricots	
canned	½ cup
dried	8 halves
fresh	4 whole (5½ oz.)
Banana, extra small (about 4 inches long)	1 (4 oz.)
* Blackberries	1 cup
Blueberries	¾ cup
Cantaloupe	1 cup diced
Cherries	
sweet, canned	½ cup
sweet, fresh	12 (3½ oz.)
Dates	3 small or 1 large
Dried fruits (blueberries, cherries, cranberries, mixed fruit, raisins)	2 Tbsp.
Figs	
dried	3 small figs
* fresh	1½ large or 2 medium (3½ oz. total)
Fruit cocktail	½ cup
Grapefruit	
fresh	½ large (5½ oz.)
sections, canned	¾ cup
Grapes	17 small (3 oz. total)
* Guava	2 small (2½ oz. total)
Honeydew melon	1 cup diced
Kiwi	½ cup sliced
Loquat	¾ cup cubed
Mandarin oranges, canned	¾ cup
Mango	½ small mango (5½ oz.) or ½ cup
Nectarine	1 medium (5½ oz.)
* Orange	1 medium (6½ oz.)
Papaya	½ papaya (8 oz.) or 1 cup cubed
Peaches	
canned	½ cup
fresh	1 medium (6 oz.)
Pears	
canned	½ cup
* fresh	½ large pear (4 oz.)
Pineapple	
canned	½ cup
fresh	¾ cup
Plantain, extra-ripe (black), raw	¼ plantain (2¼ oz.)
Plums	
canned	½ cup
dried (prunes)	3 prunes
fresh	2 small plums (5 oz. total)
Pomegranate seed (arils)	½ cup
* Raspberries	1 cup
* Strawberries	1¼ cup whole berries
Tangerine	1 large (6 oz.)
Watermelon	1¼ cups diced

Fruit Juice

Food	Serving Size
Apple juice/cider	½ cup
Fruit juice blends, 100% juice	⅓ cup
Grape juice	⅓ cup
Grapefruit juice	½ cup
Orange juice	½ cup
Pineapple juice	½ cup
Pomegranate juice	½ cup
Prune juice	⅓ cup

Milk

Different types of milk, milk products, and substitutes are included on this list. However, certain types of milk and milk-like products are found in other lists:

- Cheeses are on the **Protein** list (because they are rich in protein and have very little carbohydrate).
- Butter, cream, coffee creamers, and unsweetened nut milks are on the **Fats** list.
- Ice cream and frozen yogurt are on the **Sweets, Desserts, and Other Carbohydrates** list.

	Carbohydrate (grams)	Protein (grams)	Fat (grams)	Calories
Fat-free (skim)/low-fat (1%)	12	8	0–3	100
Reduced-fat (2%)	12	8	5	120
Whole	12	8	8	160

Milk and Yogurts

Food	Serving Size	Count As
Fat-free (skim) or low-fat (1%)		
milk, buttermilk, acidophilus milk, lactose-free milk	1 cup	1 fat-free milk
evaporated milk	½ cup	1 fat-free milk
yogurt, plain or Greek; may be sweetened with an artificial sweetener	⅔ cup (6 oz.)	1 fat-free milk
chocolate milk	1 cup	1 fat-free milk + 1 carbohydrate
Reduced-fat (2%)		
milk, acidophilus milk, kefir, lactose-free milk	1 cup	1 reduced-fat milk
yogurt, plain	⅔ cup (6 oz.)	1 reduced-fat milk
Whole		
milk, buttermilk, goat's milk	1 cup	1 whole milk
evaporated milk	½ cup	1 whole milk
yogurt, plain	1 cup (8 oz.)	1 whole milk
chocolate milk	1 cup	1 whole milk + 1 carbohydrate

Other Milk Foods and Milk Substitutes

Food	Serving Size	Count As
Eggnog		
fat-free	⅓ cup	1 carbohydrate
low-fat	⅓ cup	1 carbohydrate + ½ fat
whole milk	⅓ cup	1 carbohydrate + 1 fat
Rice drink		
plain, fat-free	1 cup	1 carbohydrate
flavored, low-fat	1 cup	2 carbohydrates
Soy milk		
light or low-fat, plain	1 cup	½ carbohydrate + ½ fat
regular, plain	1 cup	½ carbohydrate + 1 fat
Yogurt, with fruit, low-fat	⅔ cup (6 oz.)	1 fat-free milk + 1 carbohydrate

Note: Coconut milk is on the **Fats** list.

Nonstarchy Vegetables

Vegetables that contain a small amount of carbohydrate and few calories are on this list. (Vegetables that contain higher amounts of carbohydrate and calories can be found on the **Starch** list.) In general, one **nonstarchy vegetable choice** is

- ½ cup of cooked vegetables or juice
- 1 cup of raw vegetables

If you eat three cups or more of raw vegetables or one and one-half cups or more of cooked nonstarchy vegetables in a meal, count them as one starch choice.

Nonstarchy Vegetables

Amaranth leaves (Chinese spinach)
Artichoke
Artichoke hearts (no oil)
Asparagus
Baby corn
Bamboo shoots
Bean sprouts (alfalfa, mung, soybean)
Beans (green, wax, Italian, yard-long)
Beets
Broccoli
Broccoli slaw, packaged, no dressing
* Brussels sprouts
Cabbage (green, red, bok choy, Chinese)
* Carrots
Cauliflower
Celery
* Chayote
Coleslaw, packaged, no dressing
Cucumber
Daikon
Eggplant
Fennel
Gourds (bitter, bottle, luffa, bitter melon)
Green onions or scallions
Greens (collard, dandelion, mustard, purslane, turnip)
Hearts of palm
* Jicama
Kale
Kohlrabi
Leeks
Mixed vegetables (without starchy vegetables, legumes, or pasta)
Mung bean sprouts
Mushrooms, all kinds, fresh
Okra
Onions
Pea pods
Peppers (all varieties)
Radishes
Rutabaga
‡ Sauerkraut
Spinach
Squash, summer varieties (yellow, pattypan, crookneck, zucchini)
Sugar snap peas

- Swiss chard
- Tomato
- Tomatoes, canned
- ‡ Tomato sauce (unsweetened)
- ‡ Tomato/vegetable juice
- Turnips
- Water chestnuts

Note: Salad greens (like arugula, chicory, endive, escarole, lettuce, radicchio, romaine, and watercress) are on the **Free Foods** list.

Sweets, Desserts, and Other Carbohydrates

Foods on this list have added sugars or fat. However, you can substitute food choices from this list for other carbohydrate-containing foods. Choose foods from this list less often.

Beverages, Soda, and Energy/Sports Drinks

Food	Serving Size	Count As
Cranberry juice cocktail	½ cup	1 carbohydrate
Fruit drink or lemonade	1 cup (8 oz.)	2 carbohydrates
Hot chocolate, regular	1 envelope (2 Tbsp. or ¾ oz.) added to 8 oz. water	1 carbohydrate
Soft drink (soda), regular	1 can (12 oz.)	2½ carbohydrates
Sports drink (fluid replacement type)	1 cup (8 oz.)	1 carbohydrate

Brownies, Cake, Cookies, Gelatin, Pie, and Pudding

Food	Serving Size	Count As
Biscotti	1 oz.	1 carbohydrate + 1 fat
Brownie, small, unfrosted	1¼-inch square, ⅞-inch high (about 1 oz.)	1 carbohydrate + 1 fat
Cake		
angel food, unfrosted	1⁄12 of cake (about 2 oz.)	2 carbohydrates
frosted	2-inch square (about 2 oz.)	2 carbohydrates + 1 fat
unfrosted	2-inch square (about 1 oz.)	1 carbohydrate + 1 fat
Cookies		
100-calorie pack	1 oz.	1 carbohydrate + ½ fat
chocolate chip	2 cookies, 2¼ inches across	1 carbohydrate + 2 fats
gingersnap	3 small cookies, 1½ inches across	1 carbohydrate
large cookie	1 cookie, 6 inches across (about 3 oz.)	4 carbohydrates + 3 fats
sandwich, with crème filling	2 small cookies (about ⅔ oz.)	1 carbohydrate + 1 fat
sugar-free	3 small or 1 large (¾ to 1 oz.)	1 carbohydrate + 1 to 2 fats
vanilla wafer	5 cookies	1 carbohydrate + 1 fat
Cupcake, frosted	1 small (about 1¾ oz.)	2 carbohydrates + 1 to 1½ fats
Flan	½ cup	2½ carbohydrates + 1 fat
Fruit cobbler	½ cup (3½ oz.)	3 carbohydrates + 1 fat
Gelatin, regular	½ cup	1 carbohydrate
Pie		
commercially prepared fruit, 2 crusts	⅙ of 8-inch pie	3 carbohydrates + 2 fats
pumpkin or custard	⅛ of 8-inch pie	1½ carbohydrates + 1½ fats
Pudding		
regular (made with reduced-fat milk)	½ cup	2 carbohydrates
sugar-free or sugar- and fat-free (made with fat-free milk)	½ cup	1 carbohydrate

Candy, Spreads, Sweets, Sweeteners, Syrups, and Toppings

Food	Serving Size	Count As
Blended sweeteners (mixtures of artificial sweeteners and sugar)	1½ Tbsp.	1 carbohydrate
Candy		
chocolate, dark or milk type	1 oz.	1 carbohydrate + 2 fats
chocolate "kisses"	5 pieces	1 carbohydrate + 1 fat
hard	3 pieces	1 carbohydrate
Coffee cream, nondairy type		
powdered, flavored	4 tsp.	½ carbohydrate + ½ fat
liquid, flavored	2 Tbsp.	1 carbohydrate
Fruit snacks, chewy (pureed fruit concentrate)	1 roll (¾ oz.)	1 carbohydrate
Fruit spreads, 100% fruit	1½ Tbsp.	1 carbohydrate
Honey	1 Tbsp.	1 carbohydrate
Jam or jelly, regular	1 Tbsp.	1 carbohydrate

Food	Serving Size	Count As
Sugar	1 Tbsp.	1 carbohydrate
Syrup		
chocolate	2 Tbsp.	2 carbohydrates
light (pancake type)	2 Tbsp.	1 carbohydrate
regular (pancake type)	1 Tbsp.	1 carbohydrate

Condiments and Sauces

Food	Serving Size	Count As
Barbecue sauce	3 Tbsp.	1 carbohydrate
Cranberry sauce, jellied	¼ cup	1½ carbohydrates
‡ Curry sauce	1 oz.	1 carbohydrate + 1 fat
‡ Gravy, canned or bottled	½ cup	½ carbohydrate + ½ fat
Hoisin sauce	1 Tbsp.	½ carbohydrate
Marinade	1 Tbsp.	½ carbohydrate
Plum sauce	1 Tbsp.	½ carbohydrate
Salad dressing, fat-free, cream-based	3 Tbsp.	1 carbohydrate
Sweet and sour sauce	3 Tbsp.	1 carbohydrate

Note: You can also check the **Fats** list and **Free Foods** list for other condiments.

Doughnuts, Muffins, Pastries, and Sweet Breads

Food	Serving Size	Count As
Banana nut bread	1-inch slice (2 oz.)	2 carbohydrates + 1 fat
Doughnut		
cake, plain	1 medium (1½ oz.)	1½ carbohydrates + 2 fats
hole	2 holes (1 oz.)	1 carbohydrate + 1 fat
yeast-type, glazed	3¾ inches across (2 oz.)	2 carbohydrates + 2 fats
Muffin		
regular	1 muffin (4 oz.)	4 carbohydrates + 2½ fats
lower-fat	1 muffin (4 oz.)	4 carbohydrates + ½ fat
Scone	1 scone (4 oz.)	4 carbohydrates + 3 fats
Sweet roll or Danish	1 pastry (2½ oz.)	2½ carbohydrates + 2 fats

Frozen Bars, Frozen Desserts, Frozen Yogurt, and Ice Cream

Food	Serving Size	Count As
Frozen pops	1	½ carbohydrate
Fruit juice bars, frozen, 100% juice	1 bar (3 oz.)	1 carbohydrate
Ice cream		
fat-free	½ cup	1½ carbohydrates
light	½ cup	1 carbohydrate + 1 fat
no sugar added	½ cup	1 carbohydrate + 1 fat
regular	½ cup	1 carbohydrate + 2 fats
Sherbet, sorbet	½ cup	2 carbohydrates
Yogurt, frozen		
fat-free	⅓ cup	1 carbohydrate
regular	½ cup	1 carbohydrate + 0 to 1 fat
Greek, lower-fat or fat-free	½ cup	1½ carbohydrates

Protein

Meat, fish, poultry, cheese, eggs, and plant-based foods are all sources of protein and have varying amounts of fat. Foods from this list are divided into four groups based on the amount of fat they contain. These groups are lean protein, medium-fat protein, high-fat protein, and plant-based protein. The following chart shows you what one protein choice includes.

	Carbohydrate (grams)	Protein (grams)	Fat (grams)	Calories
Lean protein	—	7	2	45
Medium-fat protein	—	7	5	75
High-fat protein	—	7	8	100
Plant-based protein	varies	7	varies	varies

Lean Protein

One ounce is usually the serving size for meat, fish, poultry, or hard cheeses.

Food	Serving Size
Beef: ground (90% or higher lean/10% or lower fat); select or choice grades trimmed of fat: roast (chuck, round, rump, sirloin), steak (cubed, flank, porterhouse, T-bone), tenderloin	1 oz.
‡ Beef jerky	½ oz.
Cheeses with 3 grams of fat or less per ounce	1 oz.
Curd-style cheeses: cottage-type (all kinds); ricotta (fat-free or light)	¼ cup (2 oz.)
Egg substitutes, plain	¼ cup
Egg whites	2
Fish	
fresh or frozen, such as catfish, cod, flounder, haddock, halibut, orange roughy, tilapia, trout	1 oz.
salmon, fresh or canned	1 oz.
sardines, canned	2 small sardines
tuna, fresh or canned in water or oil and drained	1 oz.
‡ smoked: herring or salmon (lox)	1 oz.
Game: buffalo, ostrich, rabbit, venison	1 oz.
‡ Hot dog with 3 grams of fat or less per ounce *(Note: May contain carbohydrate.)*	1 hot dog (1¾ oz.)
Lamb: chop, leg, or roast	1 oz.
Organ meats: heart, kidney, liver *(Note: May be high in cholesterol.)*	1 oz.
Oysters, fresh or frozen	6 medium
Pork, lean	
‡ Canadian bacon	1 oz.
‡ ham	1 oz.
rib or loin chop/roast, tenderloin	1 oz.
Poultry, without skin: chicken, Cornish hen, domestic duck or goose (well-drained of fat), turkey; lean ground turkey or chicken	1 oz.
‡ Processed sandwich meats with 3 grams of fat or less per ounce: chipped beef, thin-sliced deli meats, turkey ham, turkey pastrami	1 oz.
‡ Sausage with 3 grams of fat or less per ounce	1 oz.
Shellfish: clams, crab, imitation shellfish, lobster, scallops, shrimp	1 oz.
Veal: cutlet (no breading), loin chop, roast	1 oz.

‡ **High in sodium** (based on the sodium content of a typical 3-ounce serving of meat, unless 1 ounce or 2 ounces is the normal serving size).

Medium-Fat Protein

One ounce is usually the serving size for meat, fish, poultry, or hard cheeses.

Food	Serving Size
Beef trimmed of visible fat: ground beef (85% or lower lean/15% or higher fat), corned beef, meat loaf, prime cuts of beef (rib roast), short ribs, tongue	1 oz.
Cheeses with 4 to 7 grams of fat per ounce: feta, mozzarella, pasteurized processed cheese spread, reduced-fat cheeses	1 oz.
Cheese, ricotta (regular or part-skim)	¼ cup (2 oz.)
Egg	1 egg
Fish: any fried type	1 oz.
Lamb: ground, rib roast	1 oz.
Pork: cutlet, ground, shoulder roast	1 oz.
Poultry with skin: chicken; dove, pheasant, turkey, wild duck, or goose; fried chicken	1 oz.
‡ Sausage with 4 to 7 grams of fat per ounce	1 oz.

‡ **High in sodium** (based on the sodium content of a typical 3-ounce serving of meat, unless 1 ounce or 2 ounces is the normal serving size).

High-Fat Protein

These foods are high in saturated fat, cholesterol, and calories and may raise blood cholesterol levels if eaten on a regular basis. Try to eat three or fewer choices from this group per week. One ounce is usually the serving size for meat, fish, poultry, or hard cheeses.

Food	Serving Size
Bacon, pork	2 slices (1 oz. each before cooking)
‡ Bacon, turkey	3 slices (½ oz. each before cooking)
Cheese, regular: American, blue-veined, brie, cheddar, hard goat, Monterey Jack, Parmesan, queso, and Swiss	1 oz.
♦ Hot dog: beef, pork, or combination (10 hot dogs per 1 lb.-sized package)	1 hot dog
Hot dog: turkey or chicken (10 hot dogs per 1 lb.-sized package)	1 hot dog
Pork: sausage, spareribs	1 oz.
‡ Processed sandwich meats with 8 grams of fat or more per ounce: bologna, hard salami, pastrami	1 oz.
‡ Sausage with 8 grams of fat or more per ounce: bratwurst, chorizo, Italian, knockwurst, Polish, smoked, summer	1 oz.

‡ **High in sodium** (based on the sodium content of a typical 3-ounce serving of meat, unless 1 ounce or 2 ounces is the normal serving size).

Plant-Based Protein

Because carbohydrate content varies among plant-based protein foods, you should read the food label.

Food	Serving Size	Count As
"Bacon" strips, soy-based	2 strips (½ oz.)	1 lean protein
* Baked beans, canned	⅓ cup	1 starch + 1 lean protein
* Beans (black, garbanzo, kidney, lima, navy, pinto, white), cooked or canned, drained and rinsed	½ cup	1 starch + 1 lean protein
"Beef" or "sausage" crumbles, meatless	1 oz.	1 lean protein
"Chicken" nuggets, soy-based	2 nuggets (1½ oz.)	½ carbohydrate + 1 medium-fat protein
* Edamame, shelled	½ cup	½ carbohydrate + 1 lean protein
Falafel (spiced chickpea and wheat patties)	3 patties (about 2 inches across)	1 carbohydrate + 1 high-fat protein
Hot dog, soy-based	1 (1½ oz.)	1 lean protein

* Hummus	⅓ cup	1 carbohydrate + 1 medium-fat protein
* Lentils, any color, cooked or canned, drained and rinsed	½ cup	1 carbohydrate + 1 lean protein
Meatless burger, soy-based	3 oz.	½ carbohydrate + 2 lean proteins
* Meatless burger, vegetable- and starch-based	1 patty (about 2½ oz.)	½ carbohydrate + 1 lean protein
Meatless deli slices	1 oz.	1 lean protein
Mycoprotein ("chicken" tenders or crumbles), meatless	2 oz.	½ carbohydrate + 1 lean protein
Nut spreads: almond butter, cashew butter, peanut butter, soy nut butter	1 Tbsp.	1 high-fat protein
* Peas (black-eyed and split peas), cooked or canned, drained and rinsed	½ cup	1 starch + 1 lean protein
*‡ Refried beans, canned	½ cup	1 starch + 1 lean protein
"Sausage" breakfast-type patties, meatless	1 (1½ oz.)	1 medium-fat meat
Soy nuts, unsalted	¾ oz.	½ carbohydrate + 1 medium-fat protein
Tempeh, plain, unflavored	¼ cup (1½ oz.)	1 medium-fat protein
Tofu	½ cup (4 oz.)	1 medium-fat protein
Tofu, light	½ cup (4 oz.)	1 lean protein

‡ **High in sodium** (based on the sodium content of a typical 3-ounce serving of meat, unless 1 ounce or 2 ounces is the normal serving size).

Note: Beans, peas, and lentils are also found on the **Starch** list. Nut butters in smaller amounts are found in the **Fats** list. Canned beans, lentils, and peas can be high in sodium unless they are labeled *no-salt added* or *low-sodium*. Draining and rinsing canned beans, peas, and lentils reduces sodium content by at least 40%.

Fats

The fats on this list are divided into three groups, based on the main type of fat they contain:

- **Unsaturated fats, monounsaturated** and **polyunsaturated** (including omega-3 fats), primarily come from vegetable sources and are considered healthy fats.
- **Saturated fats** primarily come from animal sources and are considered unhealthy fats.

In general, one **fat choice** equals:

- 1 teaspoon of regular margarine, vegetable oil, or butter
- 1 tablespoon of regular salad dressing

Unsaturated Fats—Monounsaturated Fats

Food	Serving Size
Almond milk (unsweetened)	1 cup
Avocado, medium	2 Tbsp. (1 oz.)
Nut butters (*trans* fat-free): almond butter, cashew butter, peanut butter (smooth or crunchy)	1½ tsp.
Nuts	
almonds	6 nuts
Brazil	2 nuts
cashews	6 nuts
filberts (hazelnuts)	5 nuts
macadamia	3 nuts
mixed (50% peanuts)	6 nuts
peanuts	10 nuts
pecans	4 halves
pistachios	16 nuts
Oil: canola, olive, peanut	1 tsp.
Olives	
black (ripe)	8
green, stuffed	10 large
Spread, plant stanol ester-type	
light	1 Tbsp.
regular	2 tsp.

Unsaturated Fats—Polyunsaturated Fats

Food	Serving Size
Margarine	
lower-fat spread (30% to 50% vegetable oil, *trans* fat-free)	1 Tbsp.
stick, tub (*trans* fat-free), or squeeze (*trans* fat-free)	1 tsp.
Mayonnaise	
reduced-fat	1 Tbsp.
regular	1 tsp.
Mayonnaise-style salad dressing	
reduced-fat	1 Tbsp.
regular	2 tsp.
Nuts	
pignolia (pine nuts)	1 Tbsp.
walnuts, English	4 halves
Oil: corn, cottonseed, flaxseed, grape-seed, safflower, soybean, sunflower	1 tsp.
Salad dressing	
reduced-fat (Note: May contain carbohydrate.)	2 Tbsp.
regular	1 Tbsp.
Seeds	
flaxseed, ground	1½ Tbsp.
pumpkin, sesame, sunflower	1 Tbsp.
Tahini or sesame paste	2 tsp.

Tip: Your thumb is about the same size and volume as one tablespoon of salad dressing, mayonnaise, margarine, or oil. It is also about the same size as one ounce of cheese. Your thumb tip is about the size of one teaspoon of margarine, mayonnaise, or other fats and oils.

Saturated Fats

Food	Serving Size
Bacon, cooked, regular or turkey	1 slice
Butter	
reduced-fat	1 Tbsp.
stick	1 tsp.
whipped	2 tsp.
Butter blends made with oil	
reduced-fat or light	1 Tbsp.
regular	1½ tsp.

Chitterlings, boiled . . . . . 2 Tbsp. (½ oz.)
Coconut, sweetened, shredded . . . . . 2 Tbsp.
Coconut milk, canned, thick
light . . . . . ⅓ cup
regular . . . . . 1½ Tbsp.
Cream
half-and-half . . . . . 2 Tbsp.
heavy . . . . . 1 Tbsp.
light . . . . . 1½ Tbsp.
whipped . . . . . 2 Tbsp.
Cream cheese
reduced-fat . . . . . 1½ Tbsp. (¾ oz.)
regular . . . . . 1 Tbsp. (½ oz.)
Lard . . . . . 1 tsp.
Oil: coconut, palm, palm kernel . . . . . 1 tsp.
Salt pork . . . . . ¼ oz.
Shortening, solid . . . . . 1 tsp.
Sour cream
reduced-fat or light . . . . . 3 Tbsp.
regular . . . . . 2 Tbsp.

Free Foods

A "free" food is any food or drink choice that has less than 20 calories and 5 grams or less of carbohydrate per serving.

- If a "free" food is listed with a serving size, that means the calories and/or carbohydrate are near the limits defined for "free." Limit yourself to three servings or fewer of that food per day, and spread the servings throughout the day.
- Food and drink choices listed here without a serving size can be eaten whenever you like.

Low-Carbohydrate Foods

Food — **Serving Size**

Candy, hard (regular or sugar-free) . . . . . 1 piece
Fruits
Cranberries or rhubarb, sweetened with sugar substitute . . . . . ½ cup
Gelatin dessert, sugar-free, any flavor
Gum, sugar-free
Jam or jelly, light or no-sugar-added . . . . . 2 tsp.
Salad greens (such as arugula, chicory, endive, escarole, leaf or iceberg lettuce, purslane, romaine, radicchio, spinach, watercress)
Sugar substitutes (artificial sweeteners)
Syrup, sugar-free . . . . . 2 Tbsp.
Vegetables: any **raw** nonstarchy vegetables (such as broccoli, cabbage, carrots, cucumber, tomato) . . . . . ½ cup
Vegetables: any **cooked** nonstarchy vegetables (such as carrots, cauliflower, green beans) . . . . . ¼ cup

Reduced-Fat or Fat-Free Foods

Food — **Serving Size**

Cream cheese, fat-free . . . . . 1 Tbsp. (½ oz.)
Coffee creamers, nondairy
liquid, flavored . . . . . 1½ tsp.
liquid, sugar-free, flavored . . . . . 4 tsp.
powdered, flavored . . . . . 1 tsp.
powdered, sugar-free, flavored . . . . . 2 tsp.
Margarine spread
fat-free . . . . . 1 Tbsp.
reduced-fat . . . . . 1 tsp.
Mayonnaise
fat-free . . . . . 1 Tbsp.
reduced-fat . . . . . 1 tsp.
Mayonnaise-style salad dressing
fat-free . . . . . 1 Tbsp.
reduced-fat . . . . . 2 tsp.
Salad dressing
fat-free . . . . . 1 Tbsp.
fat-free, Italian . . . . . 2 Tbsp.
Sour cream, fat-free or reduced fat . . . . . 1 Tbsp.
Whipped topping
light or fat-free . . . . . 2 Tbsp.
regular . . . . . 1 Tbsp.

Condiments

Food — **Serving Size**

Barbecue sauce . . . . . 2 tsp.
Catsup (ketchup) . . . . . 1 Tbsp.
Chili sauce, sweet, tomato-type . . . . . 2 tsp.
Horseradish
Hot pepper sauce
Lemon juice
Miso . . . . . 1½ tsp.
Mustard
honey . . . . . 1 Tbsp.
brown, Dijon, horseradish-flavored, wasabi-flavored
Parmesan cheese, grated . . . . . 1 Tbsp.
Pickle relish (dill or sweet) . . . . . 1 Tbsp.
Pickles
‡ dill . . . . . 1½ medium pickles
sweet, bread and butter . . . . . 2 slices
sweet, gherkin . . . . . ¾ oz.
Pimento
Salsa . . . . . ¼ cup
‡ Soy sauce, light or regular . . . . . 1 Tbsp.
Sweet and sour sauce . . . . . 2 tsp.
Taco sauce . . . . . 1 Tbsp.
Vinegar
Worcestershire sauce
Yogurt, any type . . . . . 2 Tbsp.

Drinks/Mixes

‡ Bouillon, broth, consommé
Bouillon or broth, low-sodium
Carbonated or mineral water
Club soda
Cocoa powder, unsweetened (1 Tbsp.)
Coffee, unsweetened or with sugar substitute
Diet soft drinks, sugar-free
Drink mixes, (powder or liquid drops) sugar-free
Tea, unsweetened or with sugar substitute
Tonic water, sugar-free
Water
Water, flavored, sugar-free

Seasonings

Flavoring extracts (for example, vanilla, almond, or peppermint)
Garlic, fresh or powder
Herbs, fresh or dried
Kelp
Nonstick cooking spray
Spices
Wine, used in cooking

Combination Foods

Many of the foods you eat, such as casseroles and frozen entrees, are mixed together in various combinations. These "combination" foods do not fit into any one choice list. This list of some typical "combination" food choices will help you fit these foods into your eating plan. Ask your registered dietitian nutritionist about the nutrient information for other combination foods you would like to eat, including your own recipes. One carbohydrate choice in this list has 15 grams of carbohydrate and about 70 calories.

Entrees

Food	Serving Size	Count As
‡ Casserole-type entrees (tuna noodle, lasagna, spaghetti with meatballs, chili with beans, macaroni and cheese)	1 cup (8 oz.)	2 carbohydrates + 2 medium-fat proteins
‡ Stews (beef/other meats and vegetables)	1 cup (8 oz.)	1 carbohydrate + 1 medium-fat protein + 0 to 3 fats

Frozen Meals/Entrees

Food	Serving Size	Count As
*‡ Burrito (beef and bean)	1 (5 oz.)	3 carbohydrates + 1 lean protein + 2 fats
‡ Dinner-type healthy meal (includes dessert and is usually less than 400 calories)	about 9 to 12 oz.	3 carbohydrates + 3 medium-fat meats + 3 fats
‡ "Healthy"-type entree (usually less than 300 calories)	about 7 to 10 oz.	2 carbohydrates + 2 lean proteins
Pizza		
‡ cheese/vegetarian, thin crust	¼ of a 12-inch (4½ to 5 oz.)	2 carbohydrates + 2 medium-fat proteins
‡ meat topping, thin crust	¼ of a 12-inch (5 oz.)	2 carbohydrates + 2 medium-fat proteins + 1½ fats
‡ cheese/vegetarian or meat topping, rising crust	⅙ of a 12-inch (4 oz.)	2½ carbohydrates + 2 medium-fat proteins
‡ Pocket sandwich	1 sandwich (4½ oz.)	3 carbohydrates + 1 lean protein + 1 to 2 fats
‡ Pot pie	1 pie (7 oz.)	3 carbohydrates + 1 medium-fat protein + 3 fats

Salads (Deli-Style)

Food	Serving Size	Count As
Coleslaw	½ cup	1 carbohydrate + 1½ fats
Macaroni/pasta salad	½ cup	2 carbohydrates + 3 fats
‡ Potato salad	½ cup	1½ to 2 carbohydrates + 1 to 2 fats
Tuna salad or chicken salad	½ cup (3½ oz.)	½ carbohydrate + 2 lean proteins + 1 fat

Soups

Food	Serving Size	Count As
*‡ Bean, lentil, or split pea	1 cup	1 carbohydrate + 1 lean meat
‡ Chowder (made with milk)	1 cup (8 oz.)	1 carbohydrate + 1 lean meat + 1½ fats
‡ Cream soup (made with water)	1 cup (8 oz.)	1 carbohydrate + 1 fat
‡ Miso soup	1 cup (8 oz.)	½ carbohydrate + 1 fat
‡ Ramen noodle	1 cup (8 oz.)	2 carbohydrates + 2 fats
Rice soup/porridge (congee)	1 cup (8 oz.)	1 carbohydrate
‡ Tomato soup (made with water), borscht	1 cup (8 oz.)	1 carbohydrate
‡ Vegetable beef, chicken noodle, or other broth-type soup (including "healthy"-type soups, such as those lower in sodium and/or fat)	1 cup (8 oz.)	1 carbohydrate

Fast Foods

The choices in the **Fast Foods** list are not specific fast-food meals or items, but are estimates based on popular foods. You can get specific nutrition information for almost every fast-food or restaurant chain. Ask the restaurant or check its website for nutrition information about your favorite fast foods. A carbohydrate choice has 15 grams of carbohydrate and about 70 calories.

Main Dishes/Entrees

Food	Serving Size	Count As
Chicken		
‡ breast, breaded and fried[1]	1 (about 7 oz.)	1 carbohydrate + 6 medium-fat proteins
breast, meat only[2]	1	4 lean proteins
drumstick, breaded and fried[1]	1 (about 2½ oz.)	½ carbohydrate + 2 medium-fat proteins
drumstick, meat only[2]	1	1 lean protein + ½ fat
‡ nuggets or tenders	6 (about 3½ oz.)	1 carbohydrate + 2 medium-fat proteins + 1 fat
‡ thigh, breaded and fried[1]	1 (about 5 oz.)	1 carbohydrate + 3 medium-fat proteins + 2 fats
thigh, meat only[2]	1	2 lean proteins + ½ fat
wing, breaded and fried[1]	1 wing (about 2 oz.)	½ carbohydrate + 2 medium-fat proteins
wing, meat only[2]	1 wing	1 lean protein
Pizza		
‡ cheese, pepperoni, or sausage, regular or thick crust	⅛ of a 14-inch (about 4 oz.)	2½ carbohydrates + 1 high-fat protein + 1 fat
‡ cheese, pepperoni, or sausage, thin crust	⅛ of a 14-inch (about 2¾ oz.)	1½ carbohydrates + 1 high-fat protein + 1 fat
‡ cheese, meat, and vegetable, regular crust	⅛ of a 14-inch (about 5 oz.)	2½ carbohydrates + 2 high-fat proteins

1 Definition and weight refer to food **with** bone, skin, and breading.

2 Definition refers to above food **without** bone, skin, and breading.

Asian

Food	Serving Size	Count As
‡ Beef/chicken/shrimp with vegetables in sauce	1 cup (about 6 oz.)	1 carbohydrate + 2 lean proteins + 1 fat
Egg roll, meat	1 egg roll (about 3 oz.)	1½ carbohydrates + 1 lean protein + 1½ fats
Fried rice, meatless	1 cup	2½ carbohydrates + 2 fats
Fortune cookie	1 cookie	½ carbohydrate
‡ Hot-and-sour soup	1 cup	½ carbohydrate + ½ fat
‡ Meat with sweet sauce	1 cup (about 6 oz.)	3½ carbohydrates + 3 medium-fat proteins + 3 fats
‡ Noodles and vegetables in sauce (chow mein, lo mein)	1 cup	2 carbohydrates + 2 fats

Mexican

Food	Serving Size	Count As
*‡ Burrito with beans and cheese	1 small burrito (about 6 oz.)	3½ carbohydrates + 1 medium-fat protein + 1 fat
‡ Nachos with cheese	1 small order (about 8 nachos)	2½ carbohydrates + 1 high-fat protein + 2 fats
‡ Quesadilla, cheese only	1 small order (about 5 oz.)	2½ carbohydrates + 3 high-fat proteins
Taco, crisp, with meat and cheese	1 small taco (about 3 oz.)	1 carbohydrate + 1 medium-fat protein + ½ fat
*‡ Taco salad with chicken and tortilla bowl	1 salad (1 lb. including tortilla bowl)	3½ carbohydrates + 4 medium-fat proteins + 3 fats
‡ Tostada with beans and cheese	1 small tostada (about 5 oz.)	2 carbohydrates + 1 high-fat protein

Sandwiches

Food	Serving Size	Count As
Breakfast sandwiches		
‡ breakfast burrito with sausage, egg, cheese	1 burrito	1½ carbohydrates + 2 high-fat proteins
‡ egg, cheese, meat on an English muffin	1 sandwich	2 carbohydrates + 3 medium-fat proteins + ½ fat
‡ egg, cheese, meat on a biscuit	1 sandwich	2 carbohydrates + 3 high-fat proteins + 2 fats
‡ sausage biscuit sandwich	1 sandwich	2 carbohydrates + 1 high-fat protein + 4 fats
Chicken sandwiches		
‡ grilled with bun, lettuce, tomatoes, spread	1 sandwich (about 7½ oz.)	3 carbohydrates + 4 lean proteins
‡ crispy with bun, lettuce, tomatoes, spread	1 sandwich (about 6 oz.)	3 carbohydrates + 2 lean proteins + 3½ fats
Fish sandwich with tartar sauce	1 sandwich (about 5 oz.)	2½ carbohydrates + 2 medium-fat proteins + 1½ fats
Hamburger		
regular with bun and condiments (catsup, mustard, onion, pickle)	1 burger (about 3½ oz.)	2 carbohydrates + 1 medium-fat protein + 2½ fats
‡ 4 oz. meat with cheese, bun, and condiments (catsup, mustard, onion, pickle)	1 burger (about 8½ oz.)	3 carbohydrates + 4 medium-fat proteins + 1 fat
‡ Hot dog with bun, plain	1 hot dog (about 3½ oz.)	1½ carbohydrates + 1 high-fat protein + 2 fats
Submarine sandwich (no cheese or sauce)		
‡ less than 6 grams fat	1 6-inch sub	3 carbohydrates + 2 lean proteins
‡ regular	1 6-inch sub	3 carbohydrates + 2 lean proteins + 1 fat
Wrap, grilled chicken, vegetables, cheese, and spread	1 small wrap (about 4 to 5 oz.)	2 carbohydrates + 2 lean proteins + 1½ fats

Sides/Appetizers

Food	Serving Size	Count As
‡♦ French fries	1 small order (about 3½ oz.)	2½ carbohydrates + 2 fats
‡♦ French fries	1 medium order (about 5 oz.)	3½ carbohydrates + 3 fats
‡♦ French fries	1 large order (about 6 oz.)	4½ carbohydrates + 4 fats
‡ Hashbrowns	1 cup/medium order (about 5 oz.)	3 carbohydrates + 6 fats
‡ Onion rings	1 serving (8 to 9 rings, about 4 oz.)	3½ carbohydrates + 4 fats
Salad, side (no dressing, croutons, or cheese)	1 small salad	1 nonstarchy vegetable

Beverages and Desserts

Food	Serving Size	Count As
Coffee, latte (fat-free milk)	1 small order (about 12 oz.)	1 fat-free milk
Coffee, mocha (fat-free milk, no whipped cream)	1 small order (about 12 oz.)	1 fat-free milk + 1 carbohydrate
Milkshake, any flavor	1 small shake (about 12 oz.)	5½ carbohydrates + 3 fats
Milkshake, any flavor	1 medium shake (about 16 oz.)	7 carbohydrates + 4 fats
Milkshake, any flavor	1 large shake (about 22 oz.)	10 carbohydrates + 5 fats
Soft-serve ice cream cone	1 small	2 carbohydrates + ½ fat

Note: See the **Starch** list for plain rice; see the **Starch** list and **Sweets, Desserts, and Other Carbohydrates** list for foods such as bagels and muffins; see the **Starch** list or **Protein** list for refried and other beans; see the **Sweets, Desserts, and Other Carbohydrates** list for frozen desserts such as ice cream or frozen yogurt.

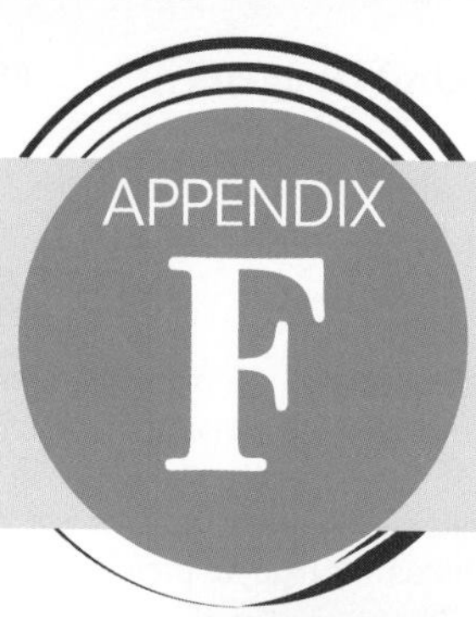

Body Mass Index-for-Age Percentiles

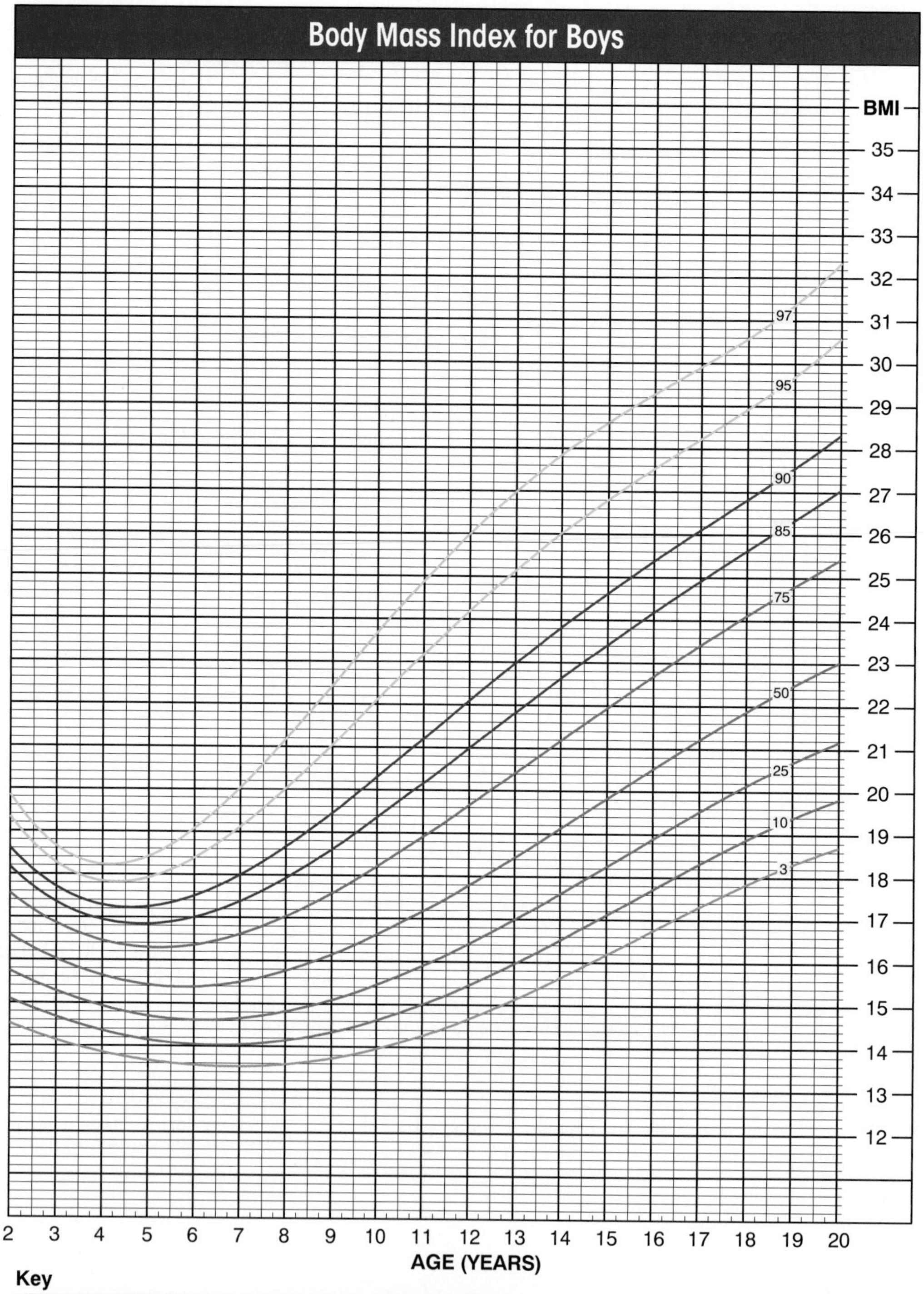

Body Mass Index for Boys

BMI

35 34 33 32 31 30 29 28 27 26 25 24 23 22 21 20 19 18 17 16 15 14 13 12

97 95 90 85 75 50 25 10 3

2 3 4 5 6 7 8 9 10 11 12 13 14 15 16 17 18 19 20

AGE (YEARS)

Key

Weight Status Category	Percentile Range
Underweight	Less than the 5th percentile
Healthy weight	5th percentile to less than the 85th percentile
Overweight	85th percentile to less than the 95th percentile
Obese	Equal to or greater than the 95th percentile

SOURCE: Developed by the National Center for Health Statistics in collaboration with the National Center for Chronic Disease Prevention and Health Promotion

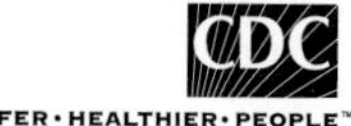

SAFER • HEALTHIER • PEOPLE™

Body Mass Index for Girls

BMI

35 34 33 32 31 30 29 28 27 26 25 24 23 22 21 20 19 18 17 16 15 14 13 12

95 90 85 75 50 25 10 5

2 3 4 5 6 7 8 9 10 11 12 13 14 15 16 17 18 19 20

AGE (YEARS)

Key

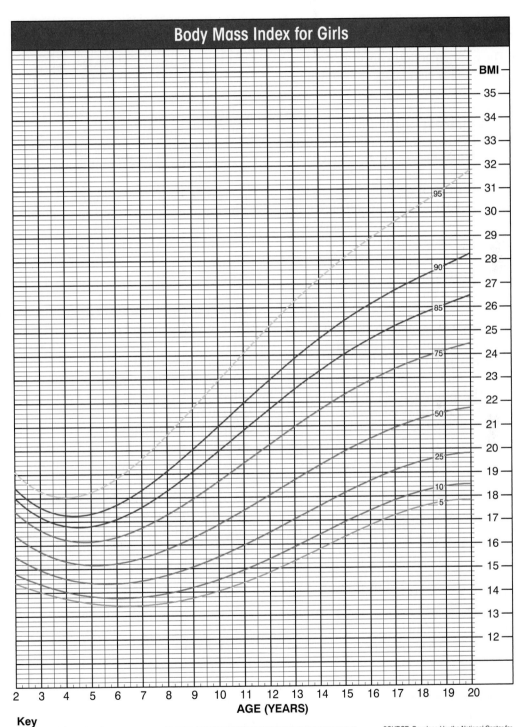

Weight Status Category	Percentile Range
Underweight	Less than the 5th percentile
Healthy weight	5th percentile to less than the 85th percentile
Overweight	85th percentile to less than the 95th percentile
Obese	Equal to or greater than the 95th percentile

SOURCE: Developed by the National Center for Health Statistics in collaboration with the National Center for Chronic Disease Prevention and Health Promotion

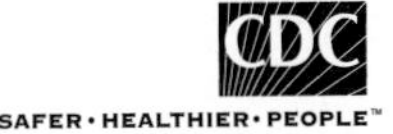

Glossary

A

absorption. The passage of nutrients from the digestive tract into the circulatory or lymphatic system. (4)

abundant. Plentiful. (7)

Acceptable Macronutrient Distribution Ranges (AMDR). Ranges of recommended dietary intake for a particular macronutrient energy source that are intended to help people achieve a balanced, healthy diet. (5)

acid. A compound that has a pH lower than 7. (10)

acid-base balance. The maintenance of stable levels of acids and bases in body fluid. (8)

acuity. Awareness. (22)

acute. Extremely great. (20)

addiction. Dependence. (6)

adept. Skilled. (5)

Adequate Intake (AI). A reference value that is used when there is insufficient scientific evidence to determine an EAR for a nutrient. (5)

adhere to. Observe. (3)

adipose tissue. The location in which the body stores a large share of excess energy for use during times when food is unavailable or insufficient. (7)

adolescence. The period of life between childhood and adulthood. (14)

adverse. Unfavorable. (23)

adversity. Difficulty. (21)

aerobic. Energy production system that requires the presence of oxygen. (15)

aerobic activity. Activity that uses large muscles and is performed at a moderate, steady pace for long periods. (20)

agility. The ability to change the position of the body with speed and control. (20)

alcohol use disorder (AUD). One of the most common substance use disorders. (23)

al dente. A term to describe pasta that has been cooked until tender but firm. (19)

alleviate. Ease. (22)

amended. Revised. (5)

amino acid. The building blocks of protein molecules. (8)

amphetamine. A commonly abused stimulant drug typically found in medicines used to treat certain sleep and attention disorders. (23)

anabolic steroid. An artificial hormone used to build a more muscular body. (23)

anerobic. Energy production system that takes place in the absence of oxygen. (15)

anaerobic activity. Activity during which the muscles use oxygen faster than the heart and lungs can deliver it. (20)

anorexia nervosa. An eating disorder characterized by self-imposed chronic and severe food restrictions, distorted body image, intense fear of weight gain, and refusal to maintain a healthy body weight. (16)

antibody. A protein that defends the body against infection and disease. (8)

antidepressant. A group of drugs that alter the nervous system and relieve depression. (16)

antioxidant. Substances that react with oxygen to protect other substances from the harmful effects of oxygen exposure. (9)

apparatus. Equipment with a purpose. (12)

apt. Fitting. (9)

ascertain. Find out. (3)

aseptic packaging. A packaging technology that preserves quality and extends the shelf life of food. (2)

assertiveness. The boldness to express thoughts and feelings in a way that does not offend others. (21)

atherosclerosis. The most common form of heart disease, caused by plaque narrowing the arteries requiring the heart to work harder to pump blood. (7)

ATP (adenosine triphosphate). The source of immediate energy found in muscle tissue. (4)

atrophy. Wasting. (12)

augment. Increase. (9)

B

bacteria. Single-celled microorganisms that live in soil, water, and the bodies of plants and animals. (3)

The numbers in parentheses following definitions represent the chapter in which the terms appear.

balance. The ability to keep your body in an upright position while standing still or moving. (20)

basal metabolic rate (BMR). The pace at which the body uses energy to support basal metabolism. (12)

basal metabolism. All of the ongoing functions in the body that sustain life. (12)

base. A compound that has a pH greater than 7 and is alkaline. (10)

beriberi. Thiamin deficiency disease. (9)

bile. A digestive juice which aids fat digestion. (4)

binge-eating disorder. An eating disorder characterized by repeatedly ingesting excessive amounts of food in a short time. (16)

bingeing. Uncontrollable eating of excessive amounts of food in a relatively short period. (16)

bioelectrical impedance. A process for measuring body fat that measures the body's resistance to a low-energy electrical current. (12)

blood alcohol concentration (BAC). The percentage of alcohol that is in a person's blood. (23)

body composition. The percentage of different tissues in the body, such as fat, muscle, and bone. (12)

body mass index (BMI). An estimate of body fatness based on an individual's height and weight. (12)

broiler. A dedicated burner found on the ceiling of the oven. (17)

budget. A spending plan. (18)

buffer. A compound that can counteract an excess of either acid or base in a fluid. (8)

built-in oven. Oven built into the cabinetry. (17)

bulimia nervosa. An eating disorder characterized by bingeing followed by partaking in one of several unhealthy practices used as attempts to prevent weight gain. (16)

buoyant. Capable of floating. (12)

burnout. A lack of energy and motivation to work toward goals. (21)

C

calorie density. The concentration of energy in a food. (12)

cancer. A general term that refers to a number of diseases in which abnormal cells grow out of control. (7)

caramelization. A browning process that occurs when heat is applied to sugars. (19)

carbohydrate loading. A technique used to trick the muscles into storing more glycogen for extra energy. (15)

carbohydrates. One of the six essential nutrients and a major source of energy for the body. (6)

cardiorespiratory fitness. A sign of health measured by the body's ability to take in adequate amounts of oxygen and carry oxygen efficiently through the blood to body cells. (20)

cardiovascular disease (CVD). Disease of the heart and blood vessels, such as narrowed or blocked blood vessels. (7)

channel. Guide. (2)

cholesterol. A white, waxy lipid that performs essential functions in the body. (7)

chronic. Recurring. (1)

chylomicron. A cluster of newly formed triglycerides that are thinly coated with cholesterol, phospholipids, and proteins. (7)

chyme. The mixture of gastric juices and chewed and swallowed food as combined in the stomach. (4)

cirrhosis. A liver disease. (23)

coagulation. Clotting. (9)

coenzyme. A nonprotein compound that combines with an inactive enzyme to form an active enzyme system. (9)

cofactor. A substance that acts with enzymes to increase enzyme activity. (10)

collagen. A protein substance in the connective tissue that holds cells together. (9)

combination cooking method. A cooking method that uses both dry- and moist-heat cooking methods. (19)

commerce. Business; trade. (2)

communication. The sending of a message from one source to another. (21)

comparison shopping. Assessing prices and quality of similar products. (18)

compel. Influence. (16)

complementary proteins. Two or more incomplete proteins that can be combined to provide all the essential amino acids. (8)

complete protein. Proteins composed of all the essential amino acids humans need. (8)

complex carbohydrate. Long chains of sugar units arranged as starch or fiber; also called polysaccharides. (6)

comprise. Make up. (5)

compromise. A solution that blends ideas from differing parties. (21)

conclusive. Convincing. (9)

conduction. The transfer of heat by direct contact. (19)

conflict. A disagreement. (21)

congenital disability. Conditions existing from birth that limit a person's ability to use his or her body or mind. (14)

congregate meal. A group meal. (18)

constipation. When chyme moves very slowly through the large intestine, causing too much water to be reabsorbed, the feces become hard, and bowel movements painful. (4)

constrict. Shrink. (11)

consumer. Someone who buys and uses products and services. (18)

contaminant. An undesirable substance that is unintentionally introduced in food. (3)

convection. The movement of molecules from a hotter area to a cooler area in a liquid or gas. (19)

convection oven. An oven with a fan that circulates hot air around the inside of the oven cavity, allowing foods to cook more evenly and quickly. (17)

conversion factor. The number used to adjust each original ingredient amount in a recipe to achieve the desired yield. (19)

convert. Change. (15)

cooktop. The top portion of a range, which consists of either gas burners or electric heating elements controlled by knobs or dials. (17)

coordination. The ability to integrate the use of two or more parts of the body. (20)

counterpart. Equal. (23)

cretinism. A developmental impairment of a fetus caused by iodine deficiency in the mother's diet during pregnancy. (10)

cross-contamination. When harmful bacteria from one food are transferred to another food. (3)

crucial. Important. (8)

cultural heritage. Learned behavior about a way of life that is passed from one generation to the next. (2)

culture. The beliefs and social customs of a group of people. (2)

cumulative. Increasing over time. (20)

curdle. Coagulate. (19)

D

Daily Values (DV). Recommended nutrient intakes developed to represent the needs of a typical individual. (5)

deficiency disease. A sickness caused by the lack of an essential nutrient. (8)

deficient. Lacking. (8)

dehydration. A condition resulting from excessive loss of body fluids. (11)

demeanor. Attitude. (16)

dementia. The loss of brain functions such as thinking, remembering, and reasoning, and eventually the loss of ability to perform everyday tasks. (20)

denaturation. The changing of the structure of a protein caused by heat, acids, bases, alcohol, agitation, and oxidation. (8)

dental caries. Tooth decay. (6)

deplete. Consume. (15)

depress. Reduce. (12)

designer drug. A lab-created imitation of other street drugs. (23)

destine. Make unavoidable. (13)

diabetes mellitus. A disease characterized by a lack of or an inability to use the hormone insulin. (6)

diagnosis. The identification of a disease. (1)

diarrhea. Frequent expulsion of watery feces. (4)

dietary fiber. The carbohydrates and lignins found in plants, which cannot be digested by human enzymes. (6)

Dietary Guidelines for Americans. Information and advice published by the United States Departments of Health and Human Services and Agriculture that promote health through improved nutrition and physical activity. (5)

Dietary Reference Intakes (DRI). Reference values for nutrients and food components that can be used to plan and assess diets for healthy people. (5)

dietary supplement. A product that is ingested to add nutritional value to the diet and includes one or more of the following: vitamins, minerals, amino acids, botanicals, enzymes, metabolites, concentrates, or extracts. (23)

digestion. The process by which the body breaks down food, and the nutrients in food, into simpler substances. (4)

dilated. Enlarged. (9)

diminished. Reduced. (1)

disaccharide. A carbohydrate made up of two sugar units. (6)

dishwasher. An appliance with spray arms that distribute detergent and rinse water over, under, and around dishes to loosen and remove soil. (17)

disordered eating. Unhealthy eating behaviors. (16)

disparity. Difference. (16)

disperse. Distribute. (4)

dissipate. Lose. (11)

distress. Negative stress. (22)

diuretic. A substance that increases urine production. (11)

diverticulosis. A disorder in which many abnormal pouches form in the intestinal wall. (4)

drug. Any chemical substance that changes the way the body or mind operates. (23)

drug-drug interaction. The creation of an unexpected side effect caused by the interaction of two or more drugs. (23)

drug overdose. The accidental or intentional ingestion of a toxic amount of a substance. (23)
dry-heat cooking method. A cooking method that uses hot air or fat to transfer heat to foods. (19)
dynamics. Patterns. (16)

E

eating disorder. A serious mental illness that is characterized by abnormal eating patterns focusing on body weight and food issues. (16)
eating pattern. All of the foods and beverages a person routinely consumes over time, or their dietary intake. (1)
elastin. A tough, elastic, yellowish tissue; cannot be softened by heat. (19)
emigrate. Leave one's country to live elsewhere. (2)
emotion. A natural state of mind in response to the environment. (21)
emotional intelligence (EI). The ability to recognize and manage one's own emotions as well as the emotions of others. (21)
empathy. The ability to recognize the feelings, thoughts, or experiences of another person. (21)
emulsifier. A substance that can mix with both water and fat. (7)
endeavor. Effort. (1)
endurance athlete. Athletes who participate in sports and activities that require them to use their muscles for long periods. (15)
energy. The ability to do work. (12)
enhanced water. Bottled sports, health, and energy drinks that contain added ingredients such as artificial flavors, sugar, sweeteners, vitamins, minerals, amino acids, caffeine, and other "enhancers." (11)
enriched food. A food to which vitamins and minerals have been added to replace those lost during processing. (9)
entice. Tempt. (18)
environmental contaminant. Substances released into the air or water by industrial plants. (3)
environmental cue. An event or situation around you that stimulates eating. (13)
environmental quality. The state of the physical world. (1)
enzyme. A type of protein produced by cells that causes specific chemical reactions. (4)
epithelial cells. The surface cells that line the outside of the body. (9)
ergogenic aids. Any substances that are designed to enhance sports performance. (23)
erode. Wear away. (6)
erratic. Irregular. (4)
erythrocyte hemolysis. A vitamin E deficiency often found in premature babies that causes red blood cells to break, which makes the babies weak and listless. (9)
essential amino acid. An amino acid the body cannot make for itself and must obtain from foods. (8)
essential fatty acid. A polyunsaturated fatty acids that the body cannot synthesize and must obtain from foods. (7)
Estimated Average Requirement (EAR). A nutrient recommendation estimated to meet the needs of 50 percent of the people in a defined group. (5)
Estimated Energy Requirement (EER). An estimate of the calories a healthy person needs based on height, weight, age, sex, and physical activity level. (5)
euphoria. Extreme pleasure. (23)
eustress. Positive stress that motivates individuals to be productive and accomplish challenging goals. (22)
exacerbate. Make worse. (14)
excreted. Eliminated. (8)
exercise. Regular, structured physical activity performed with a purpose. (20)
expend. Use up. (15)
extracellular water. The water outside the cells. (11)
extracted. Separated. (7)

F

fad diet. An eating plan that promises rapid weight loss and is popular for a short time. (13)
fallacy. Falsehood. (13)
fasting. To refrain from consuming most or all sources of calories. (13)
fat-soluble vitamin. Vitamins that dissolve in fats. (9)
fatty acid. An organic compound made up of a chain of carbon atoms to which hydrogen atoms are attached. (7)
feces. Solid wastes that result from digestion. (4)
female athlete triad. A trio of health problems—including disordered eating, amenorrhea, and osteoporosis—many females face. (16)
fetal alcohol syndrome (FAS). A set of symptoms that can occur in newborns when a mother drinks alcohol while pregnant. (14)
fetus. A developing human from nine weeks after conception until birth. (14)
fight-or-flight response. The body's natural response during the alarm stage to either conquer danger or escape to safety. (22)
flexibility. The ability to move the joints through a full range of motion. (20)
fluctuation. Change. (12)

fluorosis. A spotty discoloration of the teeth caused by a very high fluoride intake. (10)

food additive. A substance added to food products to cause desired changes in the products. (18)

food allergy. A reaction of the body's immune system to certain proteins found in foods. (4)

food biotechnology. A science that uses knowledge of plant or animal science and genetics to develop plants and animals with specific desirable traits while eliminating traits that are not wanted. (2)

foodborne illness. A disease transmitted by food. (3)

food-drug interaction. The effect a food and drug may have on the body when they are consumed together. (23)

food intolerance. An unpleasant reaction of the body to food that does not cause an immune system response. (4)

food irradiation. The treatment of approved foods with ionizing energy. (18)

food journal. A record of the kinds and amounts of foods and beverages consumed for a given time. (5)

food norm. A typical standard and pattern related to food and eating behaviors. (2)

food processing. Any procedure performed on food to prepare it for consumers. (18)

food taboo. Customs prohibiting the use of certain edible resources as food. (2)

fortified food. Foods that have one or more nutrients added during processing. (9)

free radical. A highly reactive, unstable, single oxygen molecule. (9)

frugal. Thrifty; economical. (18)

functional fiber. Isolated, nondigestible carbohydrates that have been proven to have beneficial effects on human health. (6)

functional food. Food with ingredients, such as fiber, added in order to provide health benefits beyond basic nutrition. (6)

fundamental. Important. (18)

fungi. Organisms that vary greatly in size and structure, and are classified as plants. (3)

G

gallstones. Small crystals that form from bile in the gallbladder. (4)

gastric juices. Hydrochloric acid, digestive enzymes, and mucus. (4)

gastrointestinal (GI) tract. A muscular tube leading from the mouth to the anus. (4)

generally recognized as safe (GRAS) list. A list created by the FDA containing all of the food additives that have proven to be safe. (18)

generic medication. A drug sold under its generic name. (23)

generic product. An unbranded product that has no trade name. (18)

genetically modified (GM) food. Foods derived from organisms whose genetic material (DNA) has been modified in a way that does not occur naturally. (2)

glucose. The monosaccharide that circulates in the bloodstream, supplies energy to the body's cells, and is the only fuel used by the brain. (6)

gluten. A protein found in wheat and other cereals that is formed when gliadin and glutenin combine during mixing. (19)

glycemic index (GI). A measure of the speed at which various carbohydrates are digested into glucose, absorbed, and enter the bloodstream. (6)

glycogen. The body's stored form of glucose. (6)

goiter. An enlargement of the thyroid gland caused by low iodine levels in the thyroid gland. (10)

gratitude. Thankful appreciation for what is valuable and meaningful in life. (21)

growth spurt. A period of rapid physical growth. (14)

H

habit. A routine behavior that is often difficult to break. (13)

hallucinogen. A drug that causes the mind to create images that do not really exist. (23)

hazard analysis critical control point (HACCP) system. A system that identifies the steps at which a food product is at risk of biological, chemical, or physical contamination as it moves through an operation. (3)

healthy body weight. A body weight specific to gender, height, and body frame size that is associated with health and longevity. (12)

heart attack. The destruction of heart cells due to a buildup of plaque in the arteries feeding oxygen and nutrients to the heart muscle. (7)

heartburn. A burning pain in the middle of the chest caused by stomach acid flowing back into the esophagus. (4)

heart rate. The number of times the heart beats per minute. (20)

hemoglobin. A molecule that includes a large protein called *globin* and an iron molecule called *heme* that helps red blood cells carry oxygen from the lungs to cells throughout the body and carbon dioxide from body tissues back to the lungs for excretion. (10)

heroin. A highly addictive, powerful, and dangerous opioid that produces intense feelings of euphoria. (23)
hierarchy. Ranking. (21)
high-density lipoprotein (HDL). A type of lipoprotein that picks up cholesterol from around the body and transfers it to other lipoproteins for transport back to the liver. (7)
hinder. Prevent. (10)
holistic medicine. An approach to healthcare that focuses on all aspects of patient care—physical, mental, and social. (1)
homogenization. A process to suspend butterfat in milk permanently. (19)
homogenous. Similar. (17)
hormone. Chemicals produced in the body and released into the bloodstream to regulate specific body processes. (6)
hydrogenation. The process of breaking the double carbon bonds in an unsaturated fatty acid and adding hydrogen. (7)
hygiene. Practices that promote good health. (3)
hypertension. Abnormally high blood pressure. (7)
hypoglycemia. A low blood glucose level. (6)
hypothesis. A proposed answer to a scientific question, which can be tested and verified. (1)

I

iconic. Important; recognizable. (2)
illegal drug. Drugs that are unlawful to buy or use and endanger the user's well-being. (23)
impair. Damage. (1)
impede. Slow. (8)
impulse buying. Making unplanned purchases. (18)
incomplete protein. The protein provided by plants. (8)
indigestion. Abdominal discomfort that begins soon after eating and relates to difficulty digesting food. (4)
induce. Cause. (1)
infant. A child in the first year of life. (14)
ingrained. Firmly fixed. (7)
inhalant. A substance that is inhaled for its mind-numbing effects. (23)
inherent. Belonging by nature. (7)
insulin. A chemical that helps the body lower blood glucose back to a normal level. (6)
insurmountable. Impossible. (22)
intracellular water. The water inside the cells. (11)
iron-deficiency anemia. An iron deficiency where the body makes fewer red blood cells, and which means the blood has a decreased ability to carry oxygen to body tissues. (10)

J

jeopardy. Danger. (21)
judicious. Sensible. (17)

K

ketone bodies. Compounds used by the nervous system to meet some of its energy needs. (12)
ketosis. An abnormal buildup of ketone bodies in the bloodstream. (12)
kilocalorie. The unit in which the energy value of food is measured. (4)
kosher food. Foods prepared according to the laws of Orthodox Judaism that forbid the eating of pork and shellfish and specify that meat and dairy foods may not be stored, prepared, or eaten together. (2)
kwashiorkor. A protein deficiency disease. (8)

L

lactation. The ability of a new mother's body to produce breast milk following the birth of the baby. (14)
lactic acid. A substance that builds up in muscles caused by the incomplete breakdown of glucose in the absence of oxygen. (15)
lactose intolerance. An inability to digest lactose, the main carbohydrate in milk. (6)
lecithin. A phospholipid that is made by the liver and is also found in many foods of animal origin. (7)
legume. Plants that have a special ability to capture nitrogen from the air and transfer it to their protein-rich seeds. (8)
lethargic. Lacking energy. (15)
liberate. Set free; release. (10)
life cycle. The series of growth and development stages through which people pass from before birth through death. (14)
life expectancy. The average length of life of people living in the same environment. (1)
lipid. A broader term for a group of compounds that includes fats, oils, lecithin, and cholesterol. (7)
lipoprotein. A particle consisting of fats and proteins that helps transport fats in the body. (7)
longevity. Long life. (12)
low-birthweight baby. A baby that weighs less than 5½ pounds (2,500 g) at birth. (14)
low-density lipoprotein (LDL). A type of lipoprotein that carries cholesterol through the bloodstream to body cells. (7)
lubricant. A substance that reduces friction between surfaces. (11)

M

macromineral. Minerals required in the diet in amounts of 100 or more milligrams per day. (10)

macronutrient. A nutrient needed in relatively large amounts, including carbohydrates, protein, lipids, and water. (4)

Maillard reaction. A chemical reaction between the amino acids and sugars in a protein food that occurs when dry heat is applied. (19)

mandate. Direct. (2)

manifest. Is made evident. (14)

marasmus. A wasting disease caused by a lack of calories and protein. (8)

mastication. Chewing. (4)

maximum heart rate. The highest speed at which the heart muscle is able to contract. (20)

medication. A drug used to treat an ailment or improve a disabling condition. (23)

medication abuse. The deliberate use of a prescription or OTC drug in a manner or dosage other than prescribed. (23)

medication misuse. When medicines are unintentionally used in a manner that could cause harm to the individual. (23)

medium. Substance. (19)

menopause. The time of life when menstruation ends due to a decrease in production of the hormone estrogen. (14)

mental health. The way a person feels about herself, her life, and the people around her. (1)

metabolic syndrome. A term used to describe a cluster of conditions that increase a person's risk of heart disease, stroke, and diabetes. (13)

metabolism. All the chemical changes that occur as cells produce energy and materials needed to sustain life. (4)

methamphetamine. An illegal stimulant that is never prescribed for medical treatment. It is also known as *crystal meth.* (23)

micromineral. Minerals required in amounts of less than 100 milligrams per day. (10)

micronutrient. Nutrients the body needs in smaller amounts, including vitamins and minerals. (4)

microorganism. Living beings so small they are only visible under a microscope. (3)

minerals. Inorganic elements that are nutrients needed in small amounts to perform various functions in the body. (10)

minimally processed food. A food that preserves most of its innate physical and nutritional properties. (17)

mise en place. Organization for successful food preparation. (19)

moist-heat cooking method. A cooking method that uses liquid or steam to transfer heat to food; these methods use temperatures ranging from 160°F to 212°F. (19)

monochromatic. Similar color. (17)

monosaccharide. A carbohydrate composed of single sugar units. (6)

monounsaturated fatty acid. Fatty acid molecule that has only one double bond between carbon atoms. (7)

muscular endurance. The ability to use a group of muscles repeatedly without becoming tired. (20)

myoglobin. A protein that carries oxygen and carbon dioxide in muscle tissue. (10)

MyPlate. A food guidance system that is based on the *Dietary Guidelines for Americans* and offers tools and resources that help individuals make changes to their eating habits. (5)

N

narcotic. A drug that brings on sleep, relieves pain, and dulls the senses. (23)

national brand. Products that are distributed and advertised throughout the country by major food companies. (18)

necessitate. Require. (14)

negligible. Slight. (10)

neutralize. To counterbalance. (4)

night blindness. A condition where the eyes adapt slowly to darkness and night vision becomes poor. (9)

nitrogen balance. A comparison of the nitrogen a person consumes with the nitrogen he or she excretes. (8)

nonessential amino acid. The amino acids the body can make for itself. (8)

nonverbal communication. Communication that transmits messages without the use of words. (21)

nutrient. The basic component of food that nourishes the body. (1)

nutrient dense. Foods and beverages that provide vitamins, minerals, and other substances that contribute to adequate nutrition or may have positive health effects; nutrient-dense foods contain little or no solid fats, added sugars, refined starches, and sodium. (5)

nutrition. The sum of the processes by which a person takes in and uses food substances. (1)

O

obese. A BMI of 30 or more. (12)

offensive. Rude; insulting. (21)

omega-3 fatty acids. Polyunsaturated fatty acids with the first double bond located between the third and fourth carbon atoms. (7)

opaque. Not see-through. (19)

opioids. A subclass of narcotics that include both natural and synthetic substances that are sometimes prescribed by doctors for pain relief. (23)

optimum health. A state of wellness characterized by peak physical, mental, and social well-being. (1)

organic foods. Foods produced without the use of synthetic fertilizers, pesticides, antibiotics, herbicides, or growth hormones. (18)

osmosis. The movement of water across cell membranes. (10)

osteomalacia. A vitamin D deficiency disease—similar to rickets—that afflicts adults and can cause the leg and spine bones to soften and bend. (9)

osteoporosis. A condition that results when bones become porous and fragile due to a loss of calcium. (10)

outpatient treatment. Medical care that does not require a hospital stay. (16)

oversee. Monitor. (14)

over-the-counter (OTC) medication. The drugs sold legally that do not require a physician's prescription. (23)

overweight. A BMI of 25 to 29.9. (12)

P

palatability. Agreeable taste. (19)

parasite. An organism that lives off another organism. (3)

partake. Engage. (23)

pasteurization. The process of heating every particle of the milk or milk product to a precise temperature for a specified time to destroy harmful bacteria. (19)

pathogen. A microorganism that causes foodborne illness. (3)

peer pressure. The influence people in one's age and social group have on his or her behavior. (1)

pellagra. Niacin deficiency disease. (9)

perforation. Hole. (17)

perishable. Prone to spoil and decay. (17)

peristalsis. A series of squeezing actions by the muscles in the esophagus. (4)

pernicious anemia. A deficiency disease caused by an inability to absorb vitamin B_{12}. (9)

perspective. Mental view. (21)

pesticide residue. Chemical pesticide particles that remain on or in food after it is prepared for consumption. (3)

pH. The measure of a substance's acidity or alkalinity. (10)

phospholipids. Lipids that have a phosphorus-containing compound in their chemical structure. (7)

physical activity. Any body movement that causes your muscles to work more than they would at rest. (20)

Physical Activity Guidelines for Americans. A set of recommendations that specify amounts and types of exercise that individuals at different life-cycle stages need each day. (5)

physical fitness. A condition in which all the body systems function together well and with sufficient stamina to perform daily activities as well as leisure activities or sports. (20)

physical health. The fitness of the body. (1)

phytochemicals. Health-enhancing compounds in plant-based foods that are active in the body's cells. (9)

pica. The craving for and ingestion of nonfood materials such as clay, soil, or chalk. (14)

pilot light. A small gas flame that burns continuously and lights the larger burner flame when needed. (17)

placebo effect. A change in a person's condition that is not a result of treatment given, but of the individual's belief that the treatment is working. (9)

placenta. An organ that forms inside the uterus during pregnancy, where oxygen and nutrients are carried from the mother's bloodstream to the fetus via their entwined blood vessels. (14)

plaque. A buildup formed by fatty compounds made largely of cholesterol attaching to the inside walls of arteries. (7)

polysaccharide. Carbohydrates that are made up of many sugar units. (6)

polyunsaturated fatty acid. Fatty acid molecule that has two or more double bonds. (7)

posture. The position of the body when standing or sitting. (20)

power. The ability to do maximum work in a short time. (20)

prebiotics. The nondigestible food ingredients that stimulate the growth of good microorganisms in the colon. (9)

predominant. Main. (7)

preheat. To allow an oven to reach the selected temperature before baking or roasting. (17)

premature baby. A baby born before the 37th week of pregnancy. (14)

premature death. Death that occurs earlier than expected due to lifestyle behaviors that lead to a fatal accident or the development of an avoidable disease. (1)

prescription medication. A drug that can only be obtained from a pharmacy with an order from a doctor. (23)

prevalent. Main. (2)

probiotics. The "good" microorganisms found in foods that offer health benefits when eaten in sufficient amounts. (9)

progressive muscle relaxation. A method for reducing stress that involves slowly tensing and then relaxing different groups of muscles. (22)

prohibit. Prevent. (22)

protein. An energy-yielding macronutrient composed of carbon, hydrogen, oxygen, and nitrogen. (8)

protein-energy malnutrition (PEM). A condition caused by a lack of calories and protein in a person's eating pattern. (8)

protozoa. Single-celled organisms. (3)

provitamin. A compound that is not a vitamin, but that can be converted into the active form of a vitamin by the body. (9)

provoke. Bring about. (10)

proximate. Close. (19)

psychoactive drug. A chemical that affects the central nervous system. (23)

puberty. The time during which a person develops sexual maturity. (14)

purging. Clearing the food from the digestive system by forcing oneself to vomit or by abusing laxatives, diuretics, or enemas. (16)

Q

quality of life. A person's satisfaction with his or her looks, lifestyle, and responses to daily events. (1)

R

radiation. The transfer of heat through waves of energy that penetrate food and bump into the molecules of water and fat. (19)

rancid. A term to describe a food oil in which the fatty acid molecules have combined with oxygen, causing them to break down and the oil to spoil. (7)

range. A large kitchen appliance that usually consists of an oven, cooktop, and broiler. (17)

reactant. A substance that enters into a chemical reaction and is changed by it. (11)

reaction time. The amount of time it takes to respond to a signal once it is received. (20)

recidivism. Relapse. (13)

recipe. A set of instructions for preparing a particular food item, including a list of ingredients and a preparation method. (19)

Recommended Dietary Allowance (RDA). The average daily intake of a nutrient required to meet the needs of most (97 to 98 percent) healthy individuals. (5)

reconstitute. Restore. (19)

recovery. The phase after exercise when glycogen stores are replenished to pre-exercise levels. (15)

refrigerator-freezer. The cold storage center of the kitchen. (17)

relapse. Recurrences. (16)

relationship. A connection formed with family members, friends, and other people. (21)

repel. Keep away. (3)

replenish. Restock. (6)

reputable. Trustworthy. (3)

residual. Remaining. (19)

resilience. The ability to deal effectively with stressful or traumatic events. (21)

resting heart rate (RHR). The baseline speed at which the heart muscle contracts when a person is sitting quietly. (20)

resting metabolic rate (RMR). Another method used to measure the body's resting energy expenditure, collected four hours after food has been eaten or significant physical activity. (12)

rickets. A deficiency disease in children caused by lack of vitamin D. (9)

risk factor. A characteristic or behavior that influences a person's chance of being injured or getting a disease. (1)

ruminant. An animal that chews cud. (7)

rupture. Burst. (11)

S

sanitation. The practice of clean food-handling habits to help prevent disease. (3)

sated. Fully satisfied. (13)

satiety. Feeling of fullness after eating. (6)

saturated fatty acid. Fatty acids with no double bonds in their chemical structure and a full load of hydrogen atoms. (7)

scientific method. The process researchers use to answer a question. (1)

scorch. Burn. (19)
scurvy. A disease caused by vitamin C deficiency. (9)
sear. Browning foods by cooking quickly over high heat. (19)
secondhand smoke. The tobacco smoke released into the air by smokers, which other people inhale involuntarily. (23)
secrete. To release. (4)
sedentary activity. Activities that require much sitting or little movement. (12)
self-actualization. Doing the utmost to reach one's full human potential. (21)
self-concept. How a person perceives his or her abilities, appearance, and personality. (21)
self-esteem. How a person values himself or herself and their perception of his or her value to others. (21)
self-talk. The internal conversations that take place in the mind. (22)
side effect. A reaction that differs from a drug's desired effect. (23)
simple carbohydrate. The naturally occurring sugars in fruits, vegetables, and milk, as well as added sugars such as table sugar or honey. (6)
skeptical. Doubtful. (20)
skinfold test. A test that uses a special tool called a caliper to measure the thickness of a fold of skin in order to assess body composition based on an estimate of the amount of subcutaneous fat a person has. (12)
sloughed. Shed. (4)
smokeless tobacco. Tobacco products that are not intended to be smoked, such as chewing tobacco or snuff. (23)
social development. Learning how to get along well with others. (21)
social health. The way a person gets along with other people. (1)
social media. Forms of electronic communication (such as websites) through which people create online communities to share information or ideas. (2)
solvent. Liquids in which substances can be dissolved. (11)
speed. The quickness with which one is able to complete a motion. (20)
stamina. Strength; energy. (20)
staple food. A food that is eaten routinely and supplies a large portion of the calories people need to maintain health. (2)
starch. A polysaccharide that is the stored form of energy in plants. (6)
stationary. Not movable. (11)
sterols. A class of lipids that have a molecular configuration that features complex ring structures, such as vitamin D, some hormones, and cholesterol. (7)
stigma. Shame. (13)
stimulant. A kind of psychoactive drug that speeds up the nervous system. (23)
store brand. Products that bear the name of the food store in which they are bought and are sold only in those stores. (18)
streamline. Simplify. (17)
strength. The ability of the muscles to move objects. (20)
strenuous. Demanding. (20)
stress. The physical, mental, and emotional reactions experienced in response to challenges. (22)
stressor. A source of stress. (22)
stroke. The destruction of brain cells that occurs when the blood supply is cut off to the brain due to a buildup of plaque in the arteries leading to the brain. (7)
subcutaneous fat. The fat that lies underneath the skin and accounts for about half the fat in the body. (12)
suffice. Be adequate. (18)
sugars. The collective name for all of the monosaccharides and disaccharides. (6)
supplement. A concentrated source of a nutrient, usually in pill, liquid, or powder form. (6)
support system. A person or group of people who can provide help and emotional comfort. (22)
surplus. Excess. (9)
sustain. Keep up. (15)
synthesis. Forming; building. (7)

T

target heart rate zone. The range of heartbeats per minute at which the heart muscle receives the best workout. (20)
technology. The application of scientific knowledge for useful purposes to accomplish tasks or solve problems. (2)
tempering. The gradual addition of an ingredient to milk, while stirring constantly. (19)
tepid. Lukewarm. (17)
theory. A principle that tries to explain something that happens in nature, but requires further testing. (1)
thermic effect of food (TEF). The energy required to complete the processes of digestion, absorption, and metabolism. (12)
thyroxine. A hormone created by the thyroid that helps control the body's metabolism. (10)

toddler. A child who is one to three years old. (14)
Tolerable Upper Intake Level (UL). The maximum level of ongoing daily intake for a nutrient that is unlikely to cause harm to most people in a defined group. (5)
tolerance. The ability of the body and mind to become less responsive to a drug. (23)
total fiber. The sum of dietary and functional fibers in a food. (6)
toxicity. A level or degree that is poisonous. (9)
toxin. Poisons that cause illness. (3)
***trans* fatty acid.** A fatty acid that results from hydrogenation, and is naturally found in some food sources; also known as *trans fat*. (7)
translucent. See-through. (19)
transmit. Relay. (10)
triglycerides. The major type of fat found in foods and in the body. (7)
trimester. One-third of the pregnancy period which lasts about 13 to 14 weeks. (14)

U

ubiquitous. Everywhere. (22)
ulcer. An open sore in the lining of the stomach or small intestine. (4)
undermine. Weaken. (5)
underweight. A BMI below 18.5. (12)
unit price. A product's cost per standard unit of weight or volume. (18)
unsaturated fatty acid. Fatty acid that has at least one double bond between two carbon atoms in each molecule. (7)
utmost. Maximum. (21)

V

value. A belief and attitude that is important to people. (2)
vegetarianism. The practice of making eating choices consisting entirely or largely of plant foods. (8)
verbal communication. Communication using spoken or written words. (21)
verified. Confirmed. (18)
versatile. Capable of many uses. (9)
very low-density lipoprotein (VLDL). A type of lipoprotein that carries triglycerides and cholesterol made by the liver to body cells. (7)
villi. Tiny, fingerlike projections that give the lining of the small intestine a velvetlike texture. (4)
virus. A disease-causing agent that must inhabit the living cell of another organism to grow or multiply. (3)
viscous. Thick. (11)
visualization. A relaxation technique during which one forms mental images of peaceful, tranquil settings. (22)
vital. Needed. (8)
vitamin. An organic compound that is an essential nutrient needed in very small amounts to regulate body processes. (9)

W

wane. Decrease. (14)
water intoxication. A condition caused by drinking too much water and consuming too few electrolytes. (11)
water-soluble vitamin. Vitamins that dissolve in water. (9)
weight cycling. A pattern of repeatedly losing and gaining weight over time. (13)
weight management. Attaining healthy weight and maintaining it throughout life. (13)
wellness. The state of being in good health. (1)
withdrawal. Symptoms experienced when people stop taking an addictive drug. (23)

Index

E

Q

R

S

T

U

V

W

Y

Z